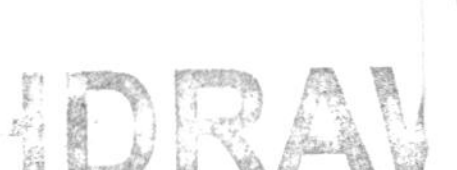

Psychiatric Nursing

Contemporary Practice

Psychiatric Nursing

Contemporary Practice

FOURTH EDITION

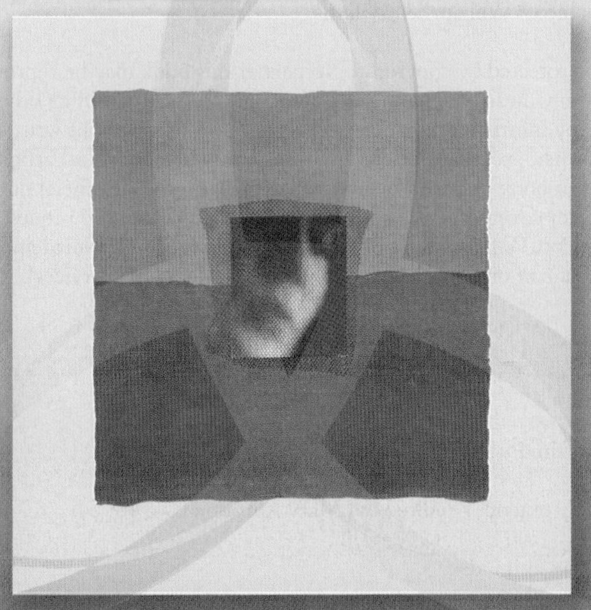

Mary Ann Boyd, PhD, DNS, RN, APRN, BC
Professor and Associate Dean of Academic Programs
Southern Illinois University Edwardsville
Edwardsville, IL

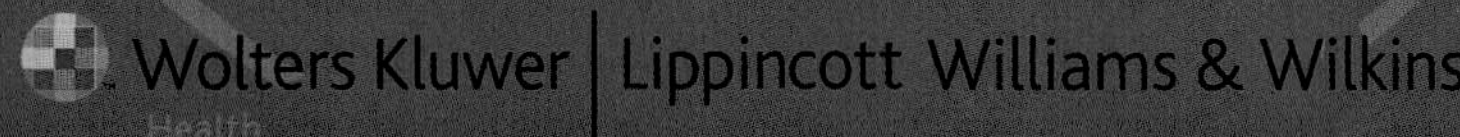

Philadelphia • Baltimore • New York • London
Buenos Aires • Hong Kong • Sydney • Tokyo

Acquisitions Editor: Pete Darcy
Managing Editor: Helen Kogut
Editorial Assistant: Season Evans
Senior Production Editor: Marian A. Bellus
Director of Nursing Production: Helen Ewan
Senior Managing Editor/Production: Erika Kors
Art Director, Design: Joan Wendt
Art Director, Illustration: Brett MacNaughton
Senior Manufacturing Manager: William Alberti
Manufacturing Coordinator: Karin Duffield
Indexer: Alexandra Nickerson
Compositor: Spearhead

4th Edition

Printed in China.

9 8 7 6 5 4 3 2 1

Library of Congress Cataloging-in-Publication Data

Psychiatric nursing : contemporary practice / [edited by] Mary Ann Boyd. — 4th ed.
p. ; cm.
Includes bibliographical references and index.
ISBN-13: 978-0-7817-9169-4
ISBN-10: 0-7817-9169-3
1. Psychiatric nursing. I. Boyd, M. (Mary Ann)
[DNLM: 1. Mental Disorders—nursing. 2. Nursing Care—methods. 3. Psychiatric Nursing—methods. WY 160 P9726 2008]
RC440.P749 2008
616.89′0231—dc22 2007008911

Care has been taken to confirm the accuracy of the information present and to describe generally accepted practices. However, the authors, editors, and publisher are not responsible for errors or omissions or for any consequences from application of the information in this book and make no warranty, expressed or implied, with respect to the currency, completeness, or accuracy of the contents of the publication. Application of this information in a particular situation remains the professional responsibility of the practitioner; the clinical treatments described and recommended may not be considered absolute and universal recommendations.

The authors, editors, and publisher have exerted every effort to ensure that drug selection and dosage set forth in this text are in accordance with the current recommendations and practice at the time of publication. However, in view of ongoing research, changes in government regulations, and the constant flow of information relating to drug therapy and drug reactions, the reader is urged to check the package insert for each drug for any change in indications and dosage and for added warnings and precautions. This is particularly important when the recommended agent is a new or infrequently employed drug.

Some drugs and medical devices presented in this publication have Food and Drug Administration (FDA) clearance for limited use in restricted research settings. It is the responsibility of the health care provider to ascertain the FDA status of each drug or device planned for use in their clinical practice.

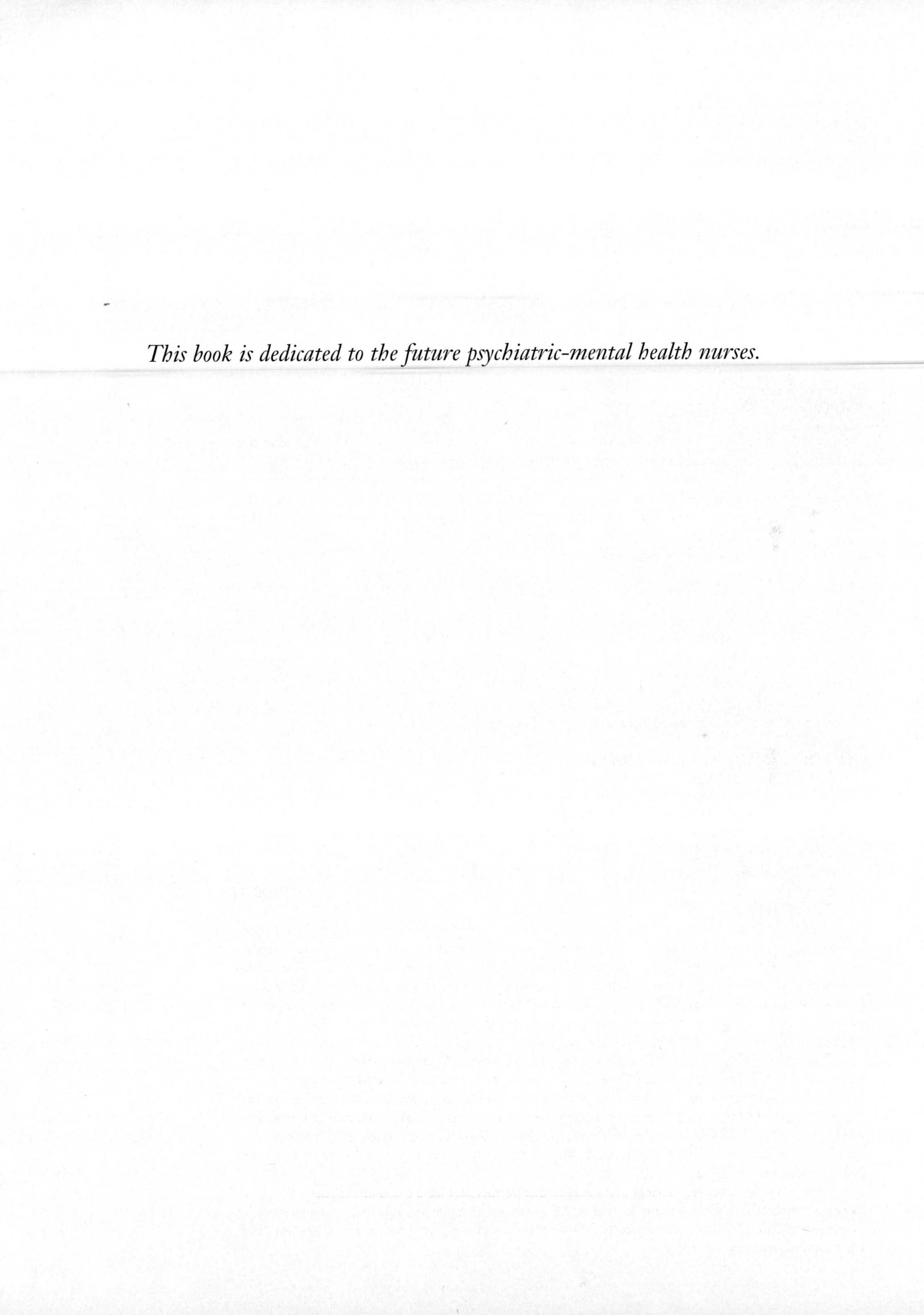

This book is dedicated to the future psychiatric-mental health nurses.

Contributors

Marjorie Baier, PhD, RN
Associate Professor
School of Nursing
Southern Illinois University Edwardsville
Edwardsville, IL

Ann R. Bland, PhD, APRN, BC
Associate Professor
Department of Baccalaureate & Graduate Nursing
Eastern Kentucky University
Richmond, KY

Andrea Bostrom, PhD, RN, APRN, BC
Associate Professor and Dean of Academic Programs
Kirkhof College of Nursing
Grand Valley State University
Allendale, MI

Mary R. Boyd, PhD, RN
Associate Professor
College of Nursing
University of South Carolina
Columbia, SC

Stephanie Burgess, PhD, APN-BC
Clinical Professor and Associate Dean for Nursing Practice
College of Nursing
University of South Carolina
Columbia, SC

Rita Canfield, RN, MSN, DNSc
School of Nursing
Southern Illinois University Edwardsville
Edwardsville, IL

Jeanne A. Clement, EdD, APRN, BC, FAAN
Associate Professor and
Director of Graduate Specialty Program in Psychiatric-Mental Health Nursing
College of Nursing
The Ohio State University
Columbus, OH

Harvey Davis, RN, PhD, CARN, PHN
School of Nursing
San Francisco State University
San Francisco, CA

Catherine Gray Deering, PhD, RN, APRN, BC
Professor
Clayton State College
Morrow, GA

Peggy El-Mallakh, PhD, RN
Post-Doctoral Scholar
College of Nursing
Chandler Medical Center
University of Kentucky
Lexington, KY

Cheryl Forchuk, RN, PhD
Professor/Scientist
Nursing, Faculty of Health Sciences
University of Western Ontario
Lawson Health Research Institute
London, Ontario
Canada

Judith E. Forker, PhD, APRN, BC
Associate Dean for Academic Affairs
School of Nursing
Aldelphi University
Garden City, NY

Vanya Hamrin, RN, MS, APRN, BC
Assistant Professor
School of Nursing
Yale University
New Haven, CT

Beverly Gilliam Hart, RN, PhD
Associate Professor of Baccalaureate and Graduate Nursing
Eastern Kentucky University
Richmond, KY

Emily J. Hauenstein, PhD, APRN, LCP, BC
Professor
School of Nursing
University of Virginia
Charlottesville, VA

Nancy Anne Hilliker, MA, RN, ANP, CS
Nurse Practitioner
Barnes-Jewish Hospital
St Louis, MO

Gail Kongable, MSN, RN, FNP
Associate Professor
Neurological Surgery
University of Virginia Health Systems
Charlottesville, VA

Ruth Beckmann Murray, MSN, EdD, N-NAP, FAAN
Professor Emerita
Doisy College of Health Sciences
School of Nursing
St. Louis University
St. Louis, MO

Maryellen C. Pachler, MSN, APRN
Child Psychiatric Nurse Practitioner
Child Study Center
School of Medicine
Yale University
New Haven, CT

Nan Roberts, MS, APRN, BC
Director of Clinical Trials
Advent Research Institute
St. Peters, MO

Lawrence Scahill, PhD, MSN, FAAN
Professor of Nursing and Child Psychiatry
Child Study Center
Yale University
New Haven, CT

Victoria Soltis-Jarrett, PhD, APRN-BC
Clinical Associate Professor and MSN Coordinator, Psychiatric Mental Health
Family Psychiatric Nurse Practitioner and Clinical Nurse Specialist
School of Nursing
University of North Carolina at Chapel Hill
Chapel Hill, NC

Mickey Stanley, PhD, RN
Associate Professor
School of Nursing
Southern Illinois University Edwardsville
Edwardsville, IL

Roberta Stock, MS, APRN, BC
Advanced Practice Nurse
Comtrea, Inc
Festus, Missouri

Sandra P. Thomas, PhD, RN, FAAN
Professor and Director, PhD Program
College of Nursing
The University of Tennessee
Knoxville, TN

Barbara Jones Warren, PhD, APRN, BC
Associate Clinical Professor
College of Nursing
The Ohio State University
Executive Nurse
Ohio Department of Mental Health
Columbus, OH

Jane White, PhD, DNSc, APRN, BC
Vera E. Bender Professor of Nursing and
Associate Dean for Research and Graduate Programs
Adelphi University
Garden City, NY

Lorraine D. Williams, RN, PhD, APRN, BC
Associate Professor
School of Nursing
Southern Illinois University Edwardsville
Edwardsville, IL

Rhonda Kay Wilson, RN, BSN, MS
Quality Manager
Chester Mental Health Center
Chester, IL

Richard Yakimo, PhD, APRN, BC
Assistant Professor
School of Nursing
Southern Illinois University Edwardsville
Edwardsville, IL

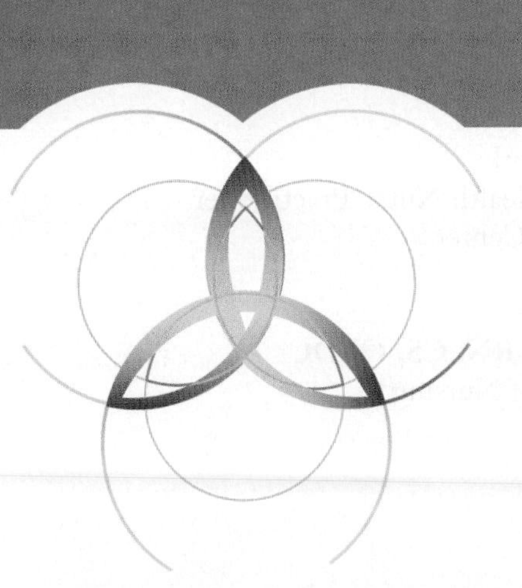

Reviewers

Elizabeth M. Andal, PhD, ARNP, FAAN
Professor of Psychiatric Mental Health Nursing
California State University
Bakersfield, California

Noreen R. Brady, PhD, APN-BC, LPCC
Assistant Professor, Director, Hirsh Institute for Best Nursing Practice Based on Evidence
Frances Payne Bolton School of Nursing
Case Western Reserve University
Cleveland, Ohio

Mary Ann Camann, PhD, APRN, BC
Associate Professor
Kennesaw State University
Kennesaw, Georgia

Kathleen Clark, RN, MSN, CNRN, APN, BC
Nursing Faculty
Thomas Jefferson University
Philadelphia, Pennsylvania

Norma Jean Eastaop, MSN, RN
Assistant Professor of Nursing
Medical University of Ohio
Toledo, Ohio

Amy H. Edgar, RN, MSN
Assistant Professor Nursing
Cedar Crest College
Allentown, Pennsylvania

Meredith Flood, PhD, APRN, BC
Assistant Professor
University of North Carolina
Charlotte, North Carolina

Vanessa Althea Johnson, PhD, MS, RN, BC
Assistant Professor
The University of Oklahoma Health Sciences Center College of Nursing
Tulsa, Oklahoma

Wendy Lewandowski, PhD, APRN, BC
Assistant Professor
Kent State University
Kent, Ohio

Dimitra Loukissa, PhD, RN
Assistant Professor
Rush University Medical Center
Chicago, Illinois

Carl H. Mangum II, RN, MSN, PhD(c), CHS
Assistant Professor
University of Mississippi School of Nursing
Jackson, Mississppi

Maryellen McHale
Associate Professor of Nursing
Bergen Community College
Paramus, New Jersey

Merryle K. Parns
Assistant Professor
Barry University
Miami Shores, Florida

Linda Anne Pfaff, MS, APRN, BC
Clinical Assistant Professor
Byrdine F. Lewis School of Nursing
Georgia State University
Atlanta, Georgia
Clinician in Private Practice
Atlanta, Georgia

Sherry L. Roper, MSN, BSN
Assistant Professor
Mountain State University
Beckley, West Virginia

Linda E. Sevidio, MSN, BC, APN, RN
Professor, Psychiatric Mental Health Nursing
Brookdale Community College
Lincroft, New Jersey

Mary-Margaret Sinclair, MSN, MEd, RN-BC
Assistant Professor
Patty Hanks Shelton School of Nursing
Abilene, Texas

Pasqua Spinelli, RN, MSN, LNC, PMHNP
Clinical Professor
Adelphi University
Garden City, New York
Psychiatric Mental Health Nurse Practitioner
Southeast Guidance Center
Seaford, New York

Carol Stewart, MS, RN, CS, CADC
Associate Professor of Nursing
College of Nursing
College of DuPage
Glen Ellyn, Illinois

Preface

The need for psychiatric nurses continues to escalate as we are constantly reminded of the importance of early recognition and treatment of mental illnesses. A new generation of young men and women are returning from military combat and are facing the challenges of living with long-term effects of trauma and violence. Suicide rates are at an all-time high for children and the older adult. Individuals with mental illnesses often are incarcerated in a correction system rather than treated in a mental health system.

Psychiatric Nursing: Contemporary Practice, Fourth Edition, was revised in response to these social changes. In this edition, there is a new unit, *Unit 4*, which addresses mental health promotion with separate chapters on stress, cultural and spiritual issues, mental health promotion of the young and middle-aged, and suicide. *New chapters*: Chapter 11, *Cognitive Interventions in Psychiatric Nursing*; Chapter 26, *Sleep Disorders*; and Chapter 35, *Care of the Mentally Ill in Forensic Settings* have been added. All other chapters have been updated to reflect the state-of-the-art care of persons with emotional problems and psychiatric disorders. For example, the relationship of drug-drug interactions and the Cytochrome P450 system is highlighted in Chapter 8 and applied throughout the text.

Today, nursing students are expected to think critically, use research evidence in their practice, and reflect upon their nursing care. This edition was written in anticipation of meeting emerging learning needs. Evidence-based studies are found throughout the book. Concept Maps of nursing diagnoses are included in Unit 5 and Reflection Boxes appear in Units 4 and 5. Students will also be challenged with the pedagogical features of previous editions, including NCLEX tips, the Nursing Care Plans, Critical Thinking Questions, Fame and Fortune highlights, and summaries of entertainment videos.

Our goal continues to be to prepare a well-rounded graduate nurse who can apply the knowledge and understanding of human behavior and psychiatric disorders to the individuals and families.

TEXT ORGANIZATION

Early chapters of *Psychiatric Nursing: Contemporary Practice, Fourth Edition*, discuss the concepts and principles underlying responsible psychiatric mental health nursing. They are the building blocks for the chapters on disorders and special populations that follow. Then, each chapter that focuses on patient care highlights a carefully selected number of the more commonly occurring disorders and patient situations that require some degree of psychiatric nursing care.

This approach permits a more in-depth exploration of current knowledge related to etiology, epidemiology, risk factors, assessment, interventions, and outcomes that are appropriate in contemporary psychiatric health care settings. The text is organized to help students assimilate the principles that are key to providing effective psychiatric nursing care within the constraints of the fast-changing health care environment. Less commonly occurring disorders are summarized in the text and tables, which provide students with the basis for developing appropriate nursing care for patients who have a variety of diagnoses and who may be encountered in any setting.

PEDAGOGICAL FEATURES

The fourth edition of *Psychiatric Nursing: Contemporary Practice* incorporates a multitude of pedagogical features to focus and direct student learning:

- Expanded Table of Contents allows readers to find and refer to concepts from one location.
- Chapter opening Learning Objectives, Key Terms, and Key Concepts cue the reader on what will be encountered and important to understand in the text.
- Summary of Key Points is at the end of each chapter and encapsulates core chapter content to focus chapter review and encourage content assimilation.

- Critical Thinking Challenges use aspects of the chapter content to stimulate analytical thinking and apply principles and concepts of psychiatric nursing to nursing practice.
- Movies and films, widely available in DVD form for rent or purchase, are exemplified as a basis for discussion in class and among students. Viewing points are provided so that students can focus on specific aspects of the film.

NEW PEDAGOGICAL FEATURES

Nursing Diagnosis Concept Maps Nurses are expected to generate a nursing diagnosis based on the synthesis of patient information. Concept maps help the student develop skills in organizing complex patient data into a meaningful nursing diagnosis. These appear in all of the chapters in Unit 5: Care of Persons with Psychiatric Disorders.

Using Reflection Boxes The use of reflection to understand the meaning of patient-nurse interaction is critical for the psychiatric nurse. The use of reflection in the interpretation of a clinical situation is highlighted in these reflection boxes appearing in Units 4 and 5.

SPECIAL FEATURES

- *NCLEX Notes:* One last hurdle the nursing student has before becoming a licensed registered nurse is successfully passing the NCLEX examination. NCLEX Notes help the student to focus on important application areas.
- *Fame and Fortune* feature highlights famous people who dealt with mental health problems. These well-known people have made important contributions to society despite their mental illnesses. In many instances, the public remained unaware of these disorders. The purposes of this feature are to emphasize that mental disorders can happen to anyone and that people with mental health problems can be productive members of society.
- *Nursing Management of Selected Disorders section* provides an in-depth study of the more commonly occurring major psychiatric disorders.
- *Case Study-based Nursing Care Plans* present actual clinical examples of patients with the highlighted diagnosis and demonstrate plans of care that follow patients through various diagnostic stages and care delivery settings. The care plans help students understand the dynamic nature of the nursing process: the ongoing need to constantly assess, develop nursing diagnoses and interventions, and identify and evaluate patient outcomes.
- *Interdisciplinary Treatment Plans (ITPs)* are linked with their respective nursing care plans in several chapters. ITPs are used extensively in the real world of practice.
- *Therapeutic Dialogue Boxes* compare and contrast therapeutic and nontherapeutic conversations to encourage by example the development of helpful and effective communication.
- *Psychoeducation Checklists* identify content areas for patient and family education related to specific disorders and their treatment. These checklists support critical thinking by encouraging students to develop patient-specific teaching plans based on chapter content.
- *Clinical Vignette Boxes* present vivid reality-based clinical portraits of patients who exhibit the symptoms described in the text. Questions are posed to help the student express his or her thoughts and solutions to issues presented in the vignettes.
- *Drug Profile Boxes* present a thorough picture of commonly prescribed medications for patients with mental health problems. Examples include lorazepam (Ativan), an anxiolytic, and mirtazapine (Remeron), an antidepressant. The profiles complement the text discussions of biologic processes known to be associated with various mental health disorders.
- *Research Boxes*: Today's focus on evidence-based practice for *best practice*, is highlighted by findings and implications of studies that ask and answer questions that are applicable to psychiatric nursing practice.
- *Key Diagnostic Characteristics* DSM IV tables and summaries describe diagnostic criteria treatment parameters, and more, for various disorders as standardized in the *Diagnostic and Statistical Manual of Mental Disorders, 4th edition, text revision*, (DSM-IV-TR) authored by the American Psychiatric Association.
- *Patient education*, *family*, and *emergency content* are highlighted to help link concepts to practice.
- *Line art, photos, scan images, and flow charts* colorfully illustrate the interrelationship of the biologic, psychological, and social domains of mental health and illness.

TEACHING–LEARNING PACKAGE

Student Resources

Free and bound in the book, this CD-ROM supplies the following learning tools:

- *Movie Viewing Guides* that highlight films depicting individuals with mental health disorders and provide students the opportunity to approach nursing care related to mental health and illness in a novel way.

- *Clinical Simulations* on Schizophrenia, Depression, and the Acutely Manic Phase that walk students through case studies and put them in real-life situations.

These and other valuable student resources are also available on thePoint, along with NCLEX-style psychiatric nursing questions that help prepare students to face exams armed with confidence and knowledge.

INSTRUCTOR RESOURCES

The Instructor's Resource CD-ROM contains additional information and activities that will help you engage your students from the semester's beginning to its end including:

- PowerPoint slides
- Image Bank
- Test Generator

Additionally, advanced technology and superior content combine at thePoint—http://thepoint.lww.com—to allow instructors easy access to an extensive selection of materials for each chapter, including

- Pre-Lecture Quizzes
- Discussion Topics
- Written, Group, Clinical, and Web Assignments
- Guided Lecture Notes
- Chapter-Specific Journal Articles

THE POINT

ThePoint thePoint (*http://thepoint.lww.com*), a trademark of Wolters Kluwer Health, is a web-based course and content management system providing every resource that instructors and students need in one easy-to-use site. Advanced technology and superior content combine at thePoint to allow instructors to design and deliver on-line and off-line courses, maintain grades and class rosters, and communicate with students. Students can visit thePoint to access supplemental multimedia resources to enhance their learning experience, check the course syllabus, download content, upload assignments, and join an on-line study group. ThePoint...where teaching, learning, and technology click!

Mary Ann Boyd, PhD, DNS, RN, APRN, BC
Professor and Associate Dean of Academic Programs

Contents

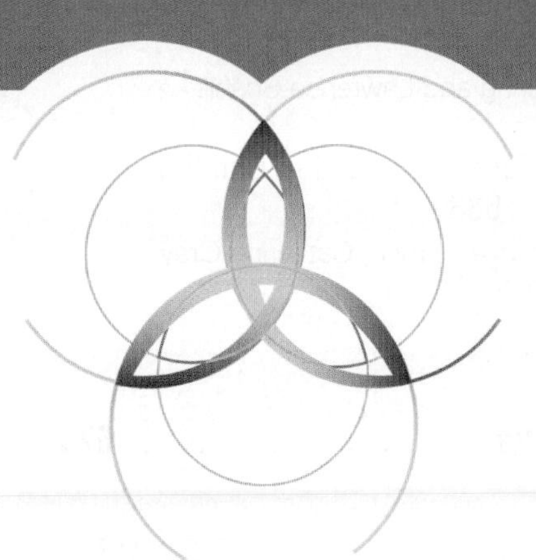

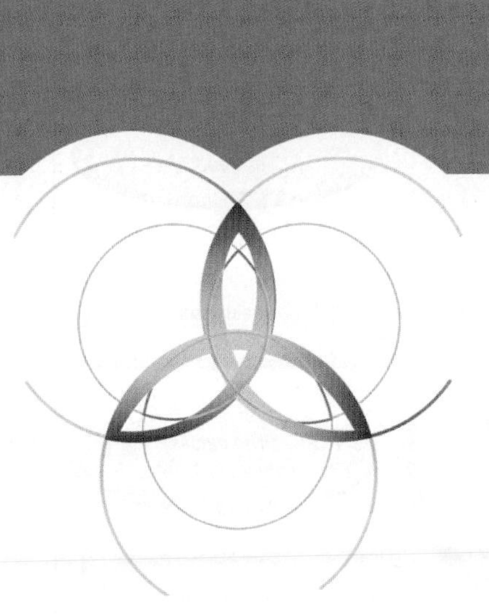

How To Use *Psychiatric Nursing: Contemporary Practice*

LEARNING OBJECTIVES let students know what they'll learn upon chapter completion.

LEARNING OBJECTIVES

After studying this chapter, you will be able to:

- Discuss the concept of stress related to mental health and mental illness.
- Discuss evidence that supports theoretical models of stress.
- Evaluate person–environment factors that contribute to the stress experience.
- Discuss the importance of cognitive appraisal in experiencing stress.
- Determine when problem-focused and emotion-focused coping should be used.
- ...ation in terms of health, psychological well-being, and ...n.

BOX 14.3

Clinical Vignette: Stress Responses to an Examination

Two students are preparing for the same examination. Susan is genuinely interested in the subject, prepares by studying throughout the semester, and reviews the content 2 days before test day. The night before the examination, she goes to bed early, gets a good night's sleep, and wakes refreshed but is slightly nervous about the test. She wants to do well and expects a difficult test but knows that she can retake it at a later date if she does poorly.

In contrast, Joanne is not interested in the subject matter and does not study throughout the semester. She "crams" 2 days before the test date and does an "all nighter" the night before. This is the last time that Joanne can take the exami... she h... tions. ... schoo... and s... at the... tion s... hyper... the te... tresse...

What...

- Ho... any...
- Are... situ...

CLINICAL VIGNETTES engage students through real-world examples.

Biologic
Health/wellness
Positive physical functioning in all systems (immune, cardiovascular, etc.)
Adequate sleep and rest
Adequate nutrition
Social
Social functioning
Positive interpersonal relationships
Positive work experience
Maintenance of social activities
Psychological
Psychological well-being
Positive self-esteem
Confidence

BIOPSYCHOSOCIAL model provides students with a strong knowledge base grounded in theory and research.

• NCLEXNOTE

Recognition of side effects, including movement disorders, tardive dyskinesia, and weight gain, should lead to interventions. Neuroleptic malignant syndrome is a medical emergency.

NCLEX NOTES highlight pertinent information to help students enhance exam performance.

KEY CONCEPT Negative symptoms reflect a lessening or loss of normal functions, such as restriction or flattening in the range and intensity of emotion (affective flattening or blunting); reduced fluency and productivity of thought and speech (alogia); withdrawal and inability to initiate and persist in goal-directed activity (avolition); and inability to experience pleasure (anhedonia).

KEY CONCEPTS boxes highlight critical terminology.

NURSING DIAGNOSIS CONCEPT MAP visually link key concepts of a disorder to in-practice examples.

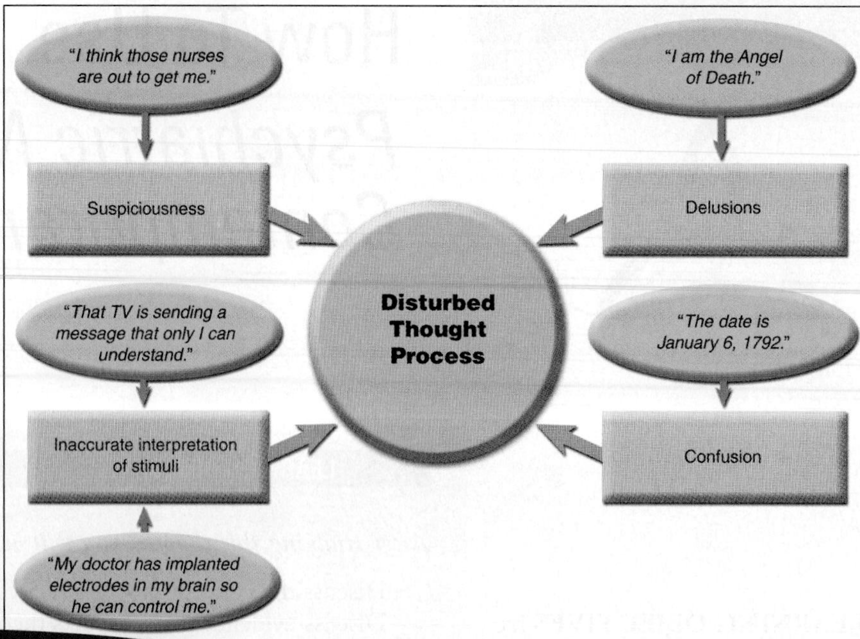
"I think those nurses are out to get me."
Suspiciousness
"That TV is sending a message that only I can understand."
Inaccurate interpretation of stimuli
"My doctor has implanted electrodes in my brain so he can control me."
Disturbed Thought Process
"I am the Angel of Death."
Delusions
"The date is January 6, 1792."
Confusion

FAME AND FORTUNE

Abraham Lincoln (1809–1865)
Civil War President

Public Persona

The 16th President of the United States led a nation through turbulent times during a civil war. Ultimately his leadership preserved the United States as the republic we know today, despite periods of "melancholy" or depression throughout his life. At times, he had strong thoughts of committing suicide. Yet he had an enormous ability to cope with depression, especially in later life. He generally coped with the depression through his work, humor, fatalistic resignation, and even religious feelings. He generally did not let his depression interfere with his work as President. In 1841, he wrote of his ongoing depression, "A tendency to melancholy .... let it be observed, is a misfortune, not a fault." (Letter to Mary Speed, September 27, 1841)

Personal Realities

Lincoln's depression began in early childhood and can be traced to multiple causes. There is evidence that there was a genetic basis because both of his parents suffered from depression. Lincoln was partially isolated from his peers because of his unique interests in politics and reading. Additionally, he suffered through the deaths of his younger brother, mother, and older sister. There is speculation that Lincoln's depression may have dated to Thomas Lincoln's cold treatment of his son. There is also evidence that Abraham Lincoln took a commonly prescribed medication called *blue mass,* which contained mercury. Consequently, some speculate that he suffered from mercury poisoning.

SOURCE: Hirschhorn, N., Feldman, R.G., & Greaves, I.A. (2001). *Abraham Lincoln's Blue Pills: Did Our 16th President Suffer from Mercury Poisoning? Perspectives in Biology and Medicine, 44* (3), 315–322.

FAME AND FORTUNE highlights nursing of famous persons who dealt with mental health issues.

NURSING MANAGEMENT: HUMAN RESPONSE TO GENERALIZED ANXIETY DISORDER

Nursing assessment and intervention for individuals with GAD include many of the same biopsychosocial considerations that apply to panic disorder. Assessment of the patient's anxiety symptoms should include the following questions; answers are used to tailor individual approaches:

- How do you experience anxiety symptoms?
- Are your symptoms primarily physical, psychological, or both?
- Are you aware when you are becoming anxious?
- Are you aware that anxiety induces the physical symptoms?
- What coping mechanisms do you routinely use to deal with anxiety?
- What life stressors add to these symptoms? What changes can you make to reduce these stressors?

NURSING MANAGEMENT sections provide in-depth information to inform the nurse about specific disorders.

NURSING CARE PLANS present case scenarios followed by appropriate diagnoses and actions.

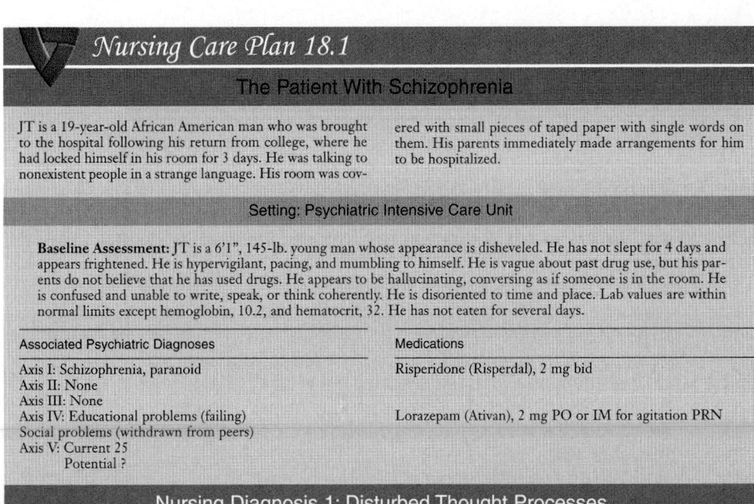

Nursing Care Plan 18.1

The Patient With Schizophrenia

JT is a 19-year-old African American man who was brought to the hospital following his return from college, where he had locked himself in his room for 3 days. He was talking to nonexistent people in a strange language. His room was covered with small pieces of taped paper with single words on them. His parents immediately made arrangements for him to be hospitalized.

Setting: Psychiatric Intensive Care Unit

Baseline Assessment: JT is a 6′1″, 145-lb. young man whose appearance is disheveled. He has not slept for 4 days and appears frightened. He is hypervigilant, pacing, and mumbling to himself. He is vague about past drug use, but his parents do not believe that he has used drugs. He appears to be hallucinating, conversing as if someone is in the room. He is confused and unable to write, speak, or think coherently. He is disoriented to time and place. Lab values are within normal limits except hemoglobin, 10.2, and hematocrit, 32. He has not eaten for several days.

Associated Psychiatric Diagnoses	Medications
Axis I: Schizophrenia, paranoid Axis II: None Axis III: None	Risperidone (Risperdal), 2 mg bid
Axis IV: Educational problems (failing) Social problems (withdrawn from peers) Axis V: Current 25 Potential ?	Lorazepam (Ativan), 2 mg PO or IM for agitation PRN

Nursing Diagnosis 1: Disturbed Thought Processes

Defining Characteristics	Rela
• Delusional thinking (people are thinking his thoughts; CIA agents are searching for him because of the plan he has developed) • Suspiciousness • Hallucinations (responding to voices that are not heard by others) • Cognitive impairment—attention, memory, and executive function impairments	• U

Outcomes

Initial	Long
• Decreased delusional thinking through accurate interpretation of environment • Conversations include fewer references to thought broadcasting and concerns about the CIA • Expresses less suspiciousness about staff and other patients • Decreased evidence of talking to people that others can't see (fewer vocalizations and observations of responding to sounds that others can't hear) • Able to participate in activities of increasing length and complexity (e.g., sitting through group and group activities, able to make projects that require increased concentration and contain more steps)	• Al sy in • Al mi tic fa • Al on • Al th an im

BOX 18.8

Drug Profile: Risperidone (Risperdal)

DRUG CLASS: Atypical antipsychotic

RECEPTOR AFFINITY: Antagonist with high affinity for D_2 and 5-HT_2, also histamine (H_1) and $_{\alpha 1-, \alpha 2}$-adrenergic receptors, weak affinity for D_1 and other serotonin receptor subtypes; no affinity for acetylcholine or β-adrenergic receptors.

INDICATIONS: Treatment of schizophrenia, short-term treatment of acute manic or mixed episodes associated with bipolar I disorder, irritability associated with autistic disorder in children and adolescents, including symptoms of aggression towards others, deliberate self-injuriousness, temper tantrums, and quickly changing moods.

ROUTES AND DOSAGE: 0.25-, 0.5-, 1-, 2-, 3-, and 4-mg tablets and liquid concentrate (1 mg/mL). Orally disintegrating tablets, 0.5-, 1-, 2-, 3-, and 4-mg.

Adult: Schizophrenia: Initial dose: typically 1 mg bid. Maximal effect at 6 mg/d. Safety not established above 16 mg/d. Use lowest possible dose to alleviate symptoms.

Bipolar mania: 2 to 3 mg per day

Geriatric: Initial dose, 0.5 mg/d, increase slowly

Children: 0.25 mg per day for patients < 20 kg day > 20 kg.

HALF-LIFE (PEAK EFFECT): mean, 20 h (1 h, metabolite = 3–17 h).

SELECT ADVERSE REACTIONS: Insomnia, ag ety, extrapyramidal symptoms, headache, rhi lence, dizziness, headache, constipation, nausea, dyspepsia, vomiting, abdominal pain, hypersalivation, tachycardia, orthostatic hypotension, fever, chest pain, coughing, photosensitivity, weight gain.

BOXED WARNING: Increased mortality in elderly patients with dementia-related psychosis

WARNING: Rare development of neuroleptic malignant syndrome. Observe frequently for early signs of tardive dyskinesia. Use caution with individuals who have cardiovascular disease; risperidone can cause ECG changes. Avoid use during pregnancy or while breastfeeding. Hepatic or renal impairments increase plasma concentration.

SPECIFIC PATIENT/FAMILY EDUCATION

- Notify prescriber if tremor, motor restlessness, abnormal movements, chest pain, or other unusual symptoms develop.
- Avoid alcohol and other CNS depressant drugs.
- Notify prescriber if pregnancy is possible or planning to become pregnant. Do not breastfeed while taking this med-

DRUG PROFILES: Psychopharmacologic content throughout, with an emphasis on patient and family education.

BOX 14.1

Research for Best Practice

Moneyham, L., Murdaugh, C., Phillips, K., Jackson, K., Tavakoli, A., Boyd, M., et al. (2005). Patterns of risk of depressive symptoms among HIV-positive women in the Southeastern United States. Journal of the Association of Nurses in Aids Care, 16(4), 25–38.

The Question: What factors contribute to depression among rural women with HIV/AIDS?

Methods: This study used the Lazarus stress theory for the framework to identify potential risk factors of depressive symptoms in women with HIV/AIDS. A sample of 278 HIV-infected women was interviewed in rural areas of South Carolina, Georgia, and Alabama. HIV symptoms, function, social support, coping, and depressive symptoms were measured.

Findings: The researchers were able to identify factors that correlated with the development of depression. The frequency of HIV symptoms, feeling sadness and hopeless in the past 12 months, and coping with HIV by isolation/withdrawal and denial/avoidance were all associated with depressive symptoms. Availability of social support and coping by living positively with HIV were both negatively associated with less depression.

Implications for Nursing: Results can guide the development of interventions in preventing depression in this population Assessing women with HIV/AIDS for depressive symptoms is important in the care of these patients. Developing interventions that increase social support and teaching patients how to live positively with HIV are useful in reducing the likelihood of developing depressive symptoms.

Schindler's List: 1993. The film presents the true story of Oskar Schindler, member of the Nazi party, womanizer, zed. Yet, fear underliple's daily lives. Crises erupt at different times during the very long period of chronic stress.

VIEWING POINTS: Differentiate the periods of chronic stress from crisis in this film. Own feelings throughout the movie. Did you experience stress?

MOVIE VIEWING POINTS highlight films that depict various mental health disorders.

RESEARCH BOXES emphasize nursing implications of recent findings.

BOX 17.6

Therapeutic Dialogue: Suicide

When Caroline sought medical care for a cold from her nurse practitioner, the nurse observed more than a cough and runny nose. Caroline appeared downcast and unusually sad. As the nurse and patient talked, the subject of family life came up, whereupon Caroline began to cry softly. As words tumbled out, she said that she had been unhappy at home for a long time. When she was very young, she recalled being happy, but things changed when her brother was born, 4 years after her. Her father began to abuse her sexually, starting when Caroline was 5 years old and continuing until he moved out of the house when she was 12 years old. Caroline suspects her mother knew of the abuse, although she did nothing about it.

Two years ago, Caroline's father committed suicide. Caroline feels relieved about his death but frustrated that she never got a chance to tell him how angry she was with him. Caroline's relationship with her mother has not improved. Caroline says that her mother favors her brother and is always telling her she won't amount to anything. Caroline begins to cry harder.

Ineffective Approach

Nurse: Clearly, many things are troubling you. Don't you think that things seem worse now because you have a cold?

Caroline: Well, that could be. What are you going to do to make me feel better?

Nurse: Give you some medicine to help you sleep and clear your nose. I think you should see a psychiatrist, too.

Caroline: I don't need a psychiatrist. I came here for my cold.

Nurse: I know you did, but you seem to be depressed.

Caroline: What are you, some kind of social worker? I am just tired.

Nurse: I am a nurse, and you seem down to me. Are you thinking about suicide?

Caroline: I don't think you know what you're talking about. I want to go now. Could you give me my medicine?

Effective Approach

Nurse: It seems as though many things have been piling up on you. Does it seem that way to you, too?

Caroline: It sure does. I've just been trying to get through one day at a time, but now with this cold and no sleep, I feel like I can't go on.

Nurse: When you say you can't go on, what does that mean to you?

Caroline: Lately, I have been thinking about running away to some place where I can't be found and maybe starting over. But then I think, where would I go? Where would I stay? Who would take care of me?

Nurse: When you think that your plan for escape won't work, what happens?

Caroline: (Starting to cry again.) Then I think that maybe it would be better if I just did what my father did. I really don't think anyone would miss me.

Nurse: So you think you might take your life, like your Dad did?

Caroline: Yeah, and what really scares me is lately I have been thinking about that a lot. I keep saying to myself, "You're just tired," but I am so exhausted now that I can't chase the thoughts away.

Nurse: So, do you think about suicide every day?

Caroline: It seems like I never stop thinking about it.

Nurse: Is there anything you can do to make the thoughts go away?

Caroline: Nothing. (Silence.)

Nurse: What would you do?

Caroline: I think I would get as many pills as I could find, drink a lot of alcohol, and maybe smoke some pot and just go to sleep.

Nurse: Do you have enough pills at home to kill yourself?

Caroline (wan smile): I was hoping that the sleeping medicine you would give me might do the job.

Nurse: It sounds like you need some help getting through this time in your life. Would you like some?

Caroline: I honestly don't know—I just want to sleep for a long time.

Critical Thinking Challenge

- In the first interaction, the nurse made two key blunders. What were they? What effect did they have on the patient? How did they interfere with the patient's care?
- What did Caroline do that might have contributed to the nurse's behavior in the first interaction?
- In the second interaction, the nurse did several things that ensu… they?… nurse…

THERAPEUTIC DIALOGUES juxtapose effective and ineffective approaches to client communication.

BOX 17.7

Psychoeducation Checklist: Suicide Prevention

When teaching the patient and family about suicide and its prevention, be sure to address the following topics:

- Importance of talking to someone
- Suicidal behavior
- Identification of stressors
- Coping mechanisms
- Positive self-talk
- Information about medications and treatments of underlying mental disorders

PSYCHOEDUCATION CHECKLISTS assist the student in developing patient-specific teaching plans based on chapter content.

BOX 15.4

Using Reflection: Facilitating Spiritual Connections

Incident: A young gay man with severe depression, psychosis, and HIV was shunned by his family and church. He is homeless and sleeps at a shelter each night, roaming the streets during the day. As a veteran, he seeks health services at a local Veterans Administration. He is reluctant to seek out mental health care. In an interview, he asks the nurse if God is punishing him for being gay.

Reflection: The nurse's immediate thought was to assure him that he was not being punished. As the nurse reflected on the situation, she realized that he might be asking for help in understanding the meaning of his situation and how he could understand his connection to his God. She initiated a therapeutic relationship with him and then conducted a spiritual assessment.

USING REFLECTION provides opportunities for students to think critically about a situation.

UNIT I

The Nature of Mental Health and Mental Illness

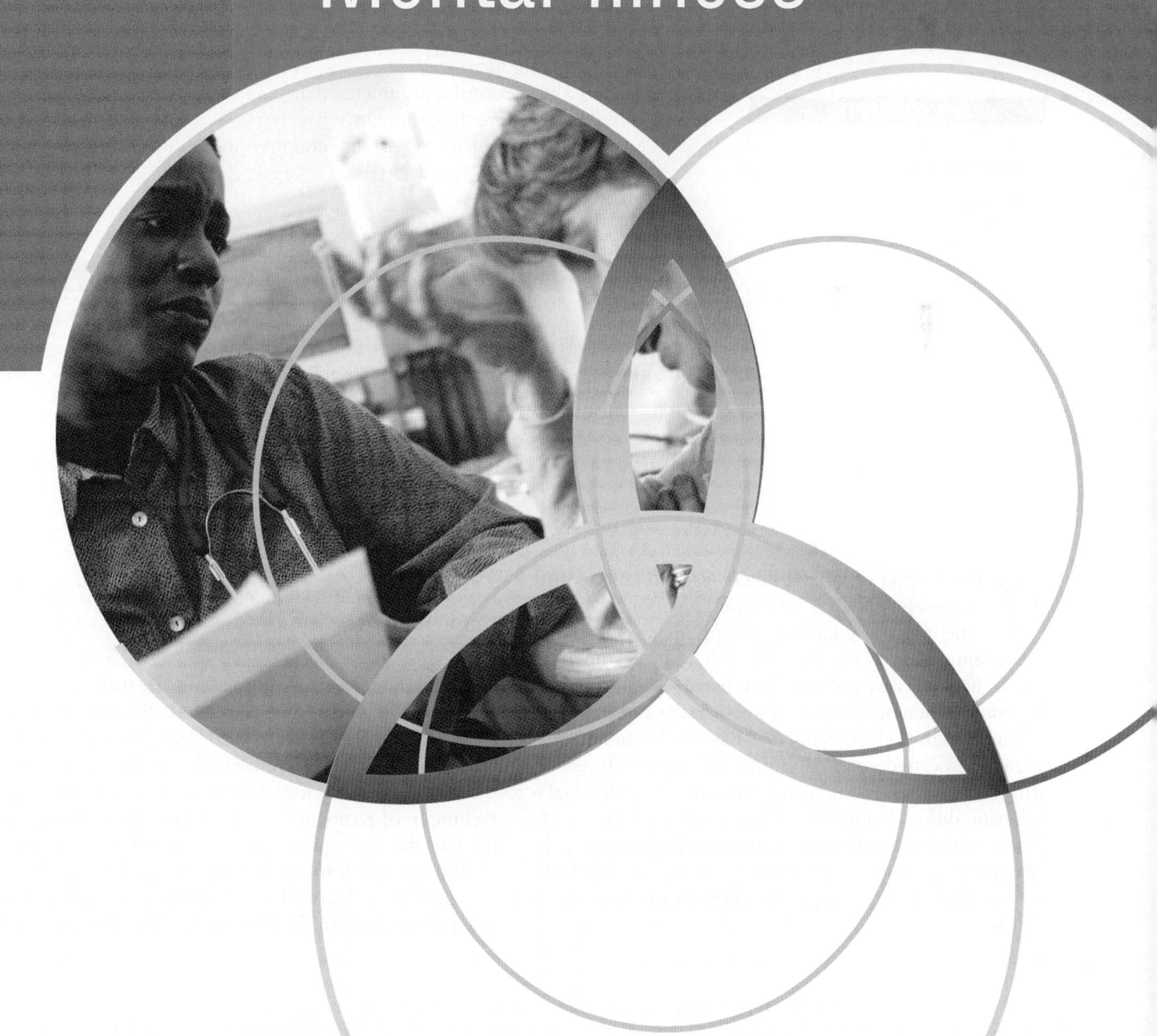

CHAPTER 1

Stigma, Social Change, and Mental Health

Mary Ann Boyd

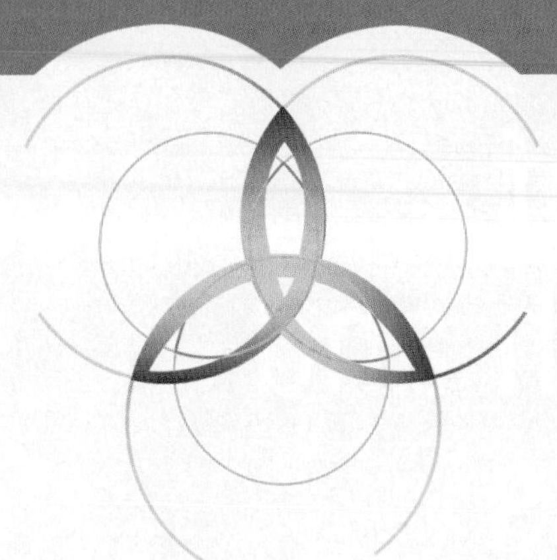

KEY CONCEPTS

- social change
- stigma

LEARNING OBJECTIVES

After studying this chapter, you will be able to:

- Discuss the impact of the stigma of mental illness.
- Identify agents of social change that affect the delivery of mental health care.
- Relate the concept of social change to the history of psychiatric–mental health care.
- Discuss the history of psychiatric–mental health nursing and its place within nursing history.
- Analyze the theoretical arguments that shaped the development of contemporary scientific thought.
- Summarize the impact of current economic and political forces on the delivery of mental health services.

KEY TERMS

• biologic view • deinstitutionalization • marginalization • moral treatment • psychiatric pluralism • psychoanalytic movement • psychosocial theory

The **stigma** of mental illness leads to community misunderstanding and discrimination. One of the most stigmatized groups includes persons with mental illness. The mentally ill have been stoned to death, hanged, and publicly humiliated. Stigmatization has robbed these individuals of work, independent living, and meaningful relationships (see Fame & Fortune). The stigma associated with all forms of mental illness is strong but generally increases the more an individual's behavior differs from the cultural norm (see Box 1-1). The result of stigmatization is the **marginalization** (relegation to a lower social standing or to the outskirts of society) of a group of people solely on the basis of an illness.

> **KEY CONCEPT Stigma** can be defined as a mark of shame, disgrace, or disapproval that results in an individual being shunned or rejected by others.

Throughout history, prevailing treatment methods reflected the underlying popular beliefs of the times. When the causes of mental disorders were believed to be biologic, individuals were treated with the latest biologic therapy. Prehistoric healers practiced an ancient surgical technique of removing a disk of bone from the skull to let out the evil spirits. In the early Christian period (1–100 AD), when sin or demonic possession was thought to cause mental disorders, clergymen treated patients, often through prescribed exorcisms. If such measures did

BOX 1.1

Hidden Burden

Because of stigma, persons suffering from a mental illness are:

- Often rejected by friends, relatives, neighbors and employers, leading to aggravated feelings of rejection, loneliness, and depression
- Often denied equal participation in family life, normal social networks, and productive employment

Stigma has a detrimental effect on a mentally ill person's recovery, ability to find access to services, the type of treatment and level of support received, and acceptance in the community.

Rejection of people with mental illness also affects the family and caretakers of the mentally ill person and leads to isolation and humiliation.

A major cause of stigma associated with mental illness are the myths, misconceptions, and negative stereotypes about mental illness held by many people in the community.

Stigma can be reduced by:

- Openly talking about mental illness in the community
- Providing accurate information on the causes, prevalence, course, and effects of mental illness
- Countering the negative stereotypes and misconceptions surrounding mental illness
- Providing support and treatment services that enable persons suffering from a mental illness to participate fully in all aspects of community life
- Ensuring the existence of legislation to reduce discrimination in the workplace, in access to health and social community services.

Adapted from World Health Organization (2001). Mental health problems: The undefined and hidden burden. Fact sheet N281. *http://www.who.int;mediacentre/factsheets/fs218/en/print.html.* Retrieved September 18, 2005.

FAME AND FORTUNE

Thomas Eagleton, LL.B (1929–2007)

U.S. Senator from Missouri (1968–1987)

Public Persona

Thomas Eagleton was born in St. Louis, Missouri. He graduated from Amherst College in 1950 and Harvard Law School in 1953. He was elected circuit attorney of St. Louis and Attorney General of Missouri in 1960. He was elected to the United States Senate in 1968 and served in the Senate for 19 years. He was instrumental in the Senate's passage of the Clean Air and Water Acts and sponsored the Eagleton Amendment, which halted the bombing in Cambodia and effectively ended American involvement in the Vietnam War. He was active in matters dealing with foreign relations, intelligence, defense, education, health care, and the environment. He served in public office for more than 30 years, wrote three books, and currently holds the title of Professor of Public Affairs at Washington University in St. Louis. The U.S. Courthouse in downtown St. Louis was named for him.

Personal Realities

Thomas Eagleton was nominated to run for Vice President at the 1972 Democratic Party convention with George McGovern as the presidential candidate. Following the convention, Mr. Eagleton's hospitalization and treatment for depression was revealed. He was replaced on the Democratic presidential ticket within a few weeks.

Source: Biographical Directory of the United States Congress, 1774–Present. Retrieved from *http://bioguide.congress.gov/scripts/biodisplay.pl?index=E000004.* Retrieved March 8, 2007.

not succeed, patients were excluded from the community and sometimes even put to death. Later in the Medieval era (1000–1300), many believed disorders were products of dysfunctional environments, and individuals were removed from their "sick" environments and placed in protected asylums.

The safety of mentally ill patients depends on the community's perceived notions and fears of those with mental disorders. People with mental illnesses or emotional problems were often stigmatized, ostracized, and isolated by the society in which they live. History reflects that generally, in periods of relative social stability, there is less fear and more tolerance for deviant behaviors, and it is easier for individuals with mental disorders to live safely within their communities.

KEY CONCEPT Social change, the structural and cultural evolution of society, is constant and at times erratic. Psychiatric mental health care has evolved within the social framework and cannot be separated from economic and political realities.

During periods of rapid **social change** and instability, there is more general anxiety and fear and subsequently more intolerance and ill treatment of people with mental disorders. See Table 1-1 for a summary of historical events and correlating perspectives on mental health during the Premoral Treatment Era (800 BC to the Colonial Period).

A REVOLUTIONARY IDEA: HUMANE TREATMENT

The emergence of enlightened political ideas and an increasing availability of economic resources in the late 18th century led to the advent of **moral treatment** in mental health care, which was characterized by kindness, compassion, and a pleasant environment for patients. Publicly and privately supported asylums for individuals with mental disorders were built during this time, and patients were routinely removed from their home environments, which were believed to be causing the illnesses. It was the first humane treatment period since the Greek and Roman eras.

Table 1.1 Social Change in the Premoral Treatment Era

Period	Socioeconomic and Political Events and People	Changing Attitudes and Practice in Mental Health Care
Ancient Times to 800 BCE	Sickness was an indication of the displeasure of deities for sins. Viewed as supernatural.	Persons with psychiatric symptoms were driven from homes and ostracized by relatives. When behavioral manifestations were viewed as supernatural powers, the persons who exhibited them were revered.
Periods of Inquiry: 800 BCE to 1 CE	Egypt and Greek periods of inquiry. Physical and mental health viewed as interrelated. Hippocrates argued abnormal behaviors were due to brain disturbances. Aristotle related mental to physical disorders.	Counseling, work, music were provided in temples by priests to relieve the distress of those with mental disorders. Observation and documentation were a part of the care. The mental disorders were treated as diseases. The aim of treatment was to correct imbalances.
Early Christian and Early Medieval: 1–1000 CE	Power of Christian church grew. St. Augustine pronounced all diseases ascribed to demons.	Persons with psychiatric symptoms were incarcerated in dungeons, beaten, and starved.
Later Medieval: 1000–1300	In Western Europe, spirit of inquiry dead. Healing by theologians and witchdoctors. Persons with psychiatric symptoms were incarcerated in dungeons, beaten, and starved. In Mideast, Avicenna said mental disorders are illnesses.	First asylums built by Muslims. Persons with psychiatric symptoms were treated as being sick.
Renaissance: 1300–1600	In England, differentiated insane from criminal. In colonies, mental illness believed caused by demonic possession. Witch hunts were common. 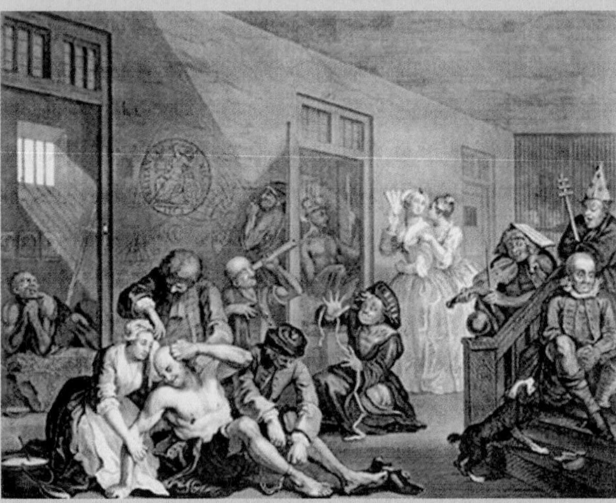 Interior of Bethlehem Asylum, London	Persons with psychiatric symptoms who presented a threat to society were apprehended and locked up. There were no public provisions for persons with mental disorders except jail. Private hospitalization for the wealthy who could pay. Bethlehem Asylum was used as a private institution.
Colonial: 1700–1790	1751: Benjamin Franklin established Pennsylvania Hospital (in Philadelphia)—the first institution in United States to receive those with mental disorders for treatment and cure.	The beginnings of mental diseases viewed as illness to be treated.

(Continued)

Table 1.1 Social Change in the Premoral Treatment Era (continued)

Period	Socioeconomic and Political Events and People	Changing Attitudes and Practice in Mental Health Care
The Tranquilizer Chair of Benjamin Rush. A patient is sitting in a chair, his body immobilized, a bucket attached beneath the seat. U.S. National Library of Medicine, *Images from the History of Medicine*, National Institutes of Health, Department of Health and Human Services.	1773: First public, free-standing asylum at Williamsburg, Virginia 1783: Benjamin Rush categorized mental illnesses and began to treat mental disorders with medical interventions, such as bloodletting, mechanical devices.	

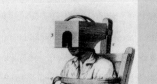

By the height of the French Revolution in 1792, moral treatment had become standard practice. It was during this time that Philippe Pinel (1745–1826) was appointed physician to Bicetre, a men's hospital that had the unfortunate distinction of being the worst asylum in the world. Pinel believed that the insane were sick patients who needed special treatment, and once installed in his position, he ordered the removal of the chains, stopped the abuses of drugging and bloodletting, and placed the patients under the care of physicians. Three years later, the same standards were extended to Salpetriere, the asylum for female patients. At about the same time in England, William Tuke (1732–1822), a member of the Society of Friends, raised funds for a retreat for members who had mental disorders. The York Retreat was opened in 1796; restraints were abandoned, and sympathetic care in quiet, pleasant surroundings with some form of industrial occupation, such as weaving or farming, was provided (Fig. 1-1).

While Tuke was influential in England, the Quakers also exercised their influence in the United States, where they were instrumental in stopping the practice of bloodletting; they also placed great emphasis on providing a proper religious atmosphere (Deutsch, 1949). The Quaker Friends Asylum was proposed in 1811 and opened 6 years later in Frankford, Pennsylvania (now Philadelphia), to become the second asylum in the United States. The humane and supportive rehabilitative attitude of the Quakers was seen as an extremely important influence in changing techniques of caring for those with mental disorders. As states were founded, new hospitals were opened that were dedicated to the care of patients with mental disorders.

Even with these hospitals, only a fraction of people with mental disorders received treatment. Those who

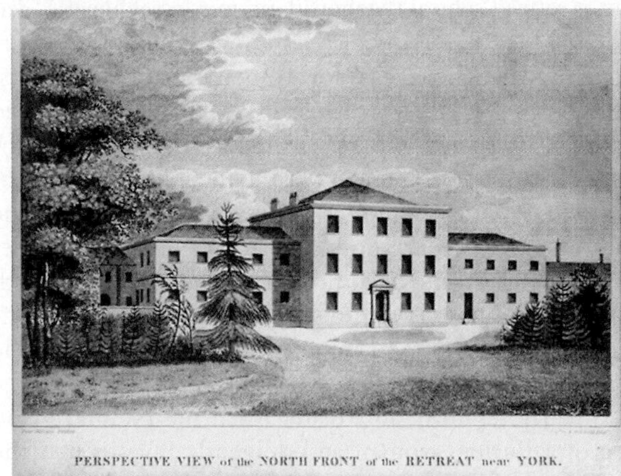
PERSPECTIVE VIEW of the NORTH FRONT of the RETREAT near YORK.

FIGURE 1.1. The perspective view of the north front of the retreat near York. U.S. National Library of Medicine, *Images from the History of Medicine*. National Institutes of Health, Department of Health and Human Services.

were judged dangerous were hospitalized; those deemed harmless or mildly insane were treated the same as other indigents and given no public support. In farm communities, as was the custom during the first half of the 19th century, the poor and indigent were often auctioned and bought by landowners to provide cheap labor. Landowners eagerly sought them for their strong backs and weak minds. The arrangement had its own economic usefulness because it provided the community with a low-cost way to care for its mentally ill. Some states used almshouses (poorhouses) for housing the mentally ill.

THE 19TH AND EARLY 20TH CENTURIES

Horace Mann and the Beginning of Public Responsibility

In 1828, Horace Mann, a representative in the Massachusetts state legislature, saw his plea that the "insane are wards of the state" become a reality. State governments were expected to assume financial responsibility for the care of people with mental illnesses. This is an important milestone because it set a precedent for tax-supported mental health funding. In Canada also, mental health care was embraced as a public responsibility, and by 1867 when the British North America Act was passed, creating the Dominion of Canada, the care of the mentally ill was the responsibility of provinces.

A Social Reformer: Dorothea Lynde Dix

Dorothea Lynde Dix (1802–1887), a militant crusader for the humane treatment of patients with mental illness, was responsible for much of the reform of the mental health care system in the 19th century. At nearly 40 years of age, Dix, a retired school teacher living in Massachusetts, was solicited by a young theology student to help in preparing a Sunday School class for women inmates at the East Cambridge jail. Dix led the class herself and was shocked by the filth and dirt in the jail. She was particularly struck by the treatment of inmates with mental disorders. It was the dead of winter, and no heat was provided. When she questioned the jailer about the lack of heat, his answer was that "the insane need no heat." The prevailing myth was that the insane were insensible to extremes of temperature. Dix's outrage initiated a long struggle in the reform of care.

An early feminist, Dix disregarded the New England role of a Puritan woman and diligently investigated the conditions of jails and the plight of the mentally ill. Her solution was state hospitals. She first influenced the Massachusetts legislature to expand the Massachusetts State Hospital. Then, through public awareness campaigns and lobbying efforts, she managed to convince state after state to build hospitals. She also turned her attention to the plight of the mentally ill in Canada, where she was instrumental in creating mental hospitals in Halifax, Nova Scotia, and St. John, Newfoundland (Fig. 1-2).

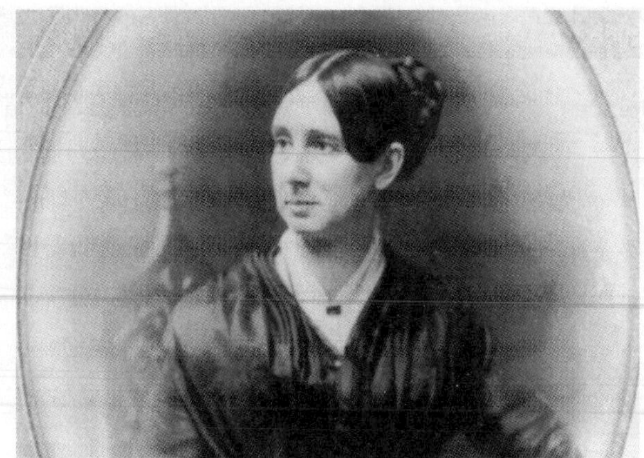

FIGURE 1.2. Dorothea Lynde Dix. U.S. National Library of Medicine, *Images from the History of Medicine.* National Institutes of Health, Department of Health and Human Services.

At the end of Dix's long career, 20 states had responded directly to her appeals by establishing or enlarging state hospitals. Dix played an important role in the establishment of the Government Hospital for the Insane in Washington, DC (which later became St. Elizabeth's Hospital). She also extended her work into Great Britain and other parts of Europe. During the Civil War, she was appointed to the post of Superintendent of Women Nurses, the highest position held by a woman during the war.

Life Within Early Institutions

The approach inside the institution was one of practical management, not treatment. The patients did not possess the interpersonal and social skills to live within a family setting, let alone in the complex group-living environment of a state hospital with others who were equally ill. The major concern was the management of a large number of people who had bizarre thoughts and behaviors and who lived in close quarters.

Women had a particularly difficult time and often were institutionalized at the convenience of their fathers or husbands. Because a woman's role in the late 1800s was to function as a domestic extension of her husband, any behaviors or beliefs that did not conform to male expectations could be used to justify the claim of insanity. These women were literally held prisoner for years. In the asylums, women were psychologically degraded, used as servants, and physically tortured by male physicians and female attendants (Lightner, 1999).

These institutions had little more to offer than food, clothing, pleasant surroundings, and perhaps some means of employment and exercise. Because the scientific hypotheses linking mental disorders to brain dysfunction were generally ignored, the emphasis in the institutions was on humane custodial care within an efficient organization. Many people believed that this custodial care was the highest possible level of treatment that could be provided.

People with mental disorders who were warehoused in state mental institutions had little hope of reentering society. In 1908, Clifford Beers (1876–1943) published an autobiography, *A Mind That Found Itself*, depicting his 3-year experience in three different types of hospitals: a private for-profit hospital, a private nonprofit hospital, and a state institution. In all of these facilities, he was beaten, choked, imprisoned for long periods in dark, dank, padded cells, and confined many days in a straightjacket. At the end of his book, he recommended that a national society be established for the purpose of reforming care and treatment, disseminating information, and encouraging and conducting research. Beers' cause was supported by a prominent neuropathologist, Adolf Meyer (1866–1950), who suggested the term "mental hygiene" to denote mental health. By 1909, Beers formed a National Committee for Mental Hygiene. Through the committee's efforts, child guidance clinics, prison clinics, and industrial mental health approaches were developed.

Early institutions eventually evolved into self-contained communities that produced their own food and made their own clothing. A medical superintendent, who was usually more adept in executive and business ability than in treatment, managed the closed mental health community. Attendants, many of whom were untrained, staffed these institutions. Nursing care was not introduced until the very late 1800s.

The Development of Psychiatric–Mental Health Nursing Thought

Early Views

The roots of contemporary psychiatric–mental health nursing thought can be traced to Florence Nightingale's seminal work *Notes on Nursing*, originally published in 1839 (Nightingale, 1859). The holistic view of the patient, with the body and soul seen as inseparable and the patient viewed as a member of a family and community, was central to Nightingale's view of nursing. Although she did not address the care of patients in asylums, Nightingale was sensitive to human emotion and recommended interactions that today would be classified as therapeutic communication (see Chapter 9). This early nursing leader advocated promotion of health and development of independence by encouraging patients to perform their own health care. She believed that this, in turn, would reduce their anxiety in the face of illness.

BOX 1.2

History of Psychiatric Mental Health Nursing

1882 First training school for psychiatric nursing at McLean Asylum by E. Cowles; first nursing program to admit men.

1913 First nurse-organized program of study for psychiatric training by Euphemia (Effie) Jane Taylor at Johns Hopkins Phipps Clinic.

1914 Mary Adelaide Nutting emphasized nursing role development.

1920 First psychiatric nursing text published, *Nursing Mental Disease*, by Harriet Bailey.

1950 Accredited schools required to offer a psychiatric nursing experience.

1952 Publication of Hildegarde E. Peplau's *Interpersonal Relations in Nursing.*

1954 First graduate program in psychiatric nursing established at Rutgers University by Hildegarde E. Peplau.

1963 *Perspectives in Psychiatric Care* and *Journal of Psychiatric Nursing* published.

1967 *Standards of Psychiatric-Mental Health Nursing Practice* published. American Nurses Association (ANA) initiated the certification of generalists in psychiatric mental health nursing.

1979 *Issues in Mental Health Nursing* published. ANA initiated the certification of specialists in psychiatric mental health nursing.

1980 *Nursing: A Social Policy Statement* published by the ANA.

1982 *Revised Standards of Psychiatric and Mental Health Nursing Practice* issued by the ANA.

1985 *Standards of Child and Adolescent Psychiatric and Mental Health Nursing Practice* published by the ANA.

1987 *Archives of Psychiatric Nursing and Journal of Child and Adolescent Psychiatric and Mental Health Nursing* published.

1994 *Statement on Psychiatric-Mental Health Clinical Nursing Practice* and *Standards of Psychiatric–Mental Health Clinical Nursing Practice.*

1996 Guidelines specifying course content and competencies published by Society for Education and Research in Psychiatric–Mental Health Nursing (SERPN).

2000 *Scope and Standards of Psychiatric–Mental Health Nursing Practice.*

The need for specialized psychiatric–mental health nursing was recognized when the humane care that characterized the Moral Treatment Era was emerging as a model for practice. Dr. Edward Cowles, director of the McLean Asylum in Massachusetts, firmly believed that patients in mental hospitals should receive nursing care. His attempts to employ nurses proved fruitless. Cowles encouraged Linda Richards, the United States' first trained nurse, to open a training school for psychiatric–mental health nurses (Cowles, 1887). The Boston City Hospital Training School for Nurses was established in 1882 at McLean Hospital (Box 1-2).

Although nurses were trained in the care of patients in psychiatric institutions, their training depended financially and academically on the institution's organizational structure and was outside mainstream nursing education. In 1913 at Johns Hopkins' Phipps Clinic, Effie Taylor initiated the first nursing program of study organized by nurses for psychiatric training. Taylor sought to integrate the concepts from general and mental health nursing into a more comprehensive knowledge base for all nursing care. She was committed to the concept of wholeness and warned that mental health nursing and general nursing could not and should not exist independently of each other. In Taylor's classes at Johns Hopkins, the psychobiologic orientation was basic to all patients, not just to those labeled mentally ill. Taylor, like Nightingale before her, encouraged nurses to avoid the dichotomy of mind and body (Church, 1987). She believed that the integrated whole was the focus of nursing.

In 1914, distinguished nursing leader and educator Mary Adelaide Nutting (1858–1948) addressed a conference at the new Psychopathic Hospital in Boston on the role of the psychopathic nurse. Her unique message was that nursing care should be based on scientific study and conceptualized in terms of diagnosis, care, and treatment.

Social Influences

The development of nursing thought has been significantly influenced by the larger social climate in which women in the profession operated. During Cowles' era, women could neither vote nor own property, and nursing training reflected the societal view of women as helpmates of men (physicians). In the early 1900s, nurses were expected to stay subservient to physicians and administrators and quietly play out the maternal role outside the home (Church, 1987). Although this may have been an acceptable social policy, it effectively barred nurses from obtaining full access to information they needed to treat their patients properly. For example, in 1920, Effie Taylor complained bitterly to Adolf Meyer that nurses were not allowed to view medical records, whereas medical students (men) were.

Despite the oppressive social climate for psychiatric nurses, nursing thought continued to develop. The first psychiatric nursing textbook, *Nursing Mental Disease*, was written by Harriet Bailey in 1920. The content of the book reflected an understanding of mental disorders of the times and set forth nursing care in terms of procedures.

MODERN THINKING

As psychiatric–mental health nursing continued to develop as a profession in the early part of the 20th century, modern perspectives on mental illness were emerging in research, and these new theories would profoundly shape the future of mental health care for all practitioners. Chapter 7 examines the underlying ideologies, but it is important to understand their development within the social and historical context to appreciate fully their impact on treatment approaches.

Evolution of Scientific Thought

In the early 1900s, two opposing views were held regarding mental illnesses: the belief that mental disorders had biologic origins and the belief that the problems were attributed to environmental and social stresses. The **psychosocial theory** proposed that mental disorders resulted from environmental and social deprivation. Moral management (nonrestraint, kindness, and hygiene) in an asylum was the answer. The **biologic view** held that mental illnesses had a biologic cause and could be treated with physical interventions. However, biologic science was not far enough advanced to offer reasonable treatment approaches, and existing primitive physical treatments, such as venesections (bloodletting) and gyrations (strapping patients to a rotating board), were either painful or considered barbaric.

Meyer and Psychiatric Pluralism

Adolf Meyer attempted to bridge the ideologic gap between the two groups by introducing the concept of **psychiatric pluralism**, an integration of human biologic functions with the environment. His approach focused on investigating how the organs related to the person and how the person, constituted of these organs, related to the environment (Neill, 1980). However, the biologic explanations were so far removed from later scientific evidence that Meyer's concept of psychiatric pluralism won little support. The times were right for another approach.

Freud and the Psychoanalytic Theory

Sigmund Freud (1856–1939) and the **psychoanalytic movement** of the early 1900s promised an even more radical approach to psychiatric–mental health care. Freud, trained as a neuropathologist, developed a personality theory based on unconscious motivations for behavior, or drives. Using a new technique, psychoanalysis, he delved into the patient's feelings and emotions regarding past experiences, particularly early childhood and adolescent memories, to explain the basis of aberrant behavior. He showed that symptoms of hysteria could be produced and made to disappear while patients were in a subconscious state of hypnosis.

As psychoanalytic theory gained in popularity, ideas of the mind–body relationship were lost. According to the

Freudian model, normal development occurred in stages, with the first three being the most important: oral, anal, and genital. The infant progressed through the oral stage, experiencing the world through symbolic oral ingestion; through the anal stage, in which the toddler developed a sense of autonomy through withholding; and on to the genital stage, in which a beginning sense of sexuality emerged within the framework of the oedipal relationship. If there was any interference in normal development, such as psychological trauma, psychosis or neurosis would develop.

Primary causes of mental illnesses were now viewed as psychological, and any physical manifestations or social influences were considered secondary (Malamud, 1944). It was generally believed within the psychiatric community that mental illnesses were a result of disturbed personality development and faulty parenting. Mental illnesses were categorized either as a psychosis (severe) or neurosis (less severe). A psychosis impaired daily functioning because of breaks in contact with reality. A neurosis was less severe, but individuals were often distressed about their problems. The terms *psychosis* and *neurosis* entered common, everyday language and added credibility to Freud's conceptualization of mental disorders. Soon, Freud's ideas represented the forefront of psychiatric thought and began to shape society's view of mental health care. Freudian ideology dominated psychiatric thought well into the 1970s.

Intensive psychoanalysis, which focused on repairing the trauma of the original psychological injury, was the treatment of choice. Psychoanalysis was costly, time-consuming, and required lengthy training. Few could perform it. Thousands of patients in state institutions with severe mental illnesses were essentially ignored.

Integration of Biologic Theories Into Psychosocial Treatment

Until the 1940s, the biologic understanding of mental illness was fairly unsophisticated and often misguided. Biologic treatments during this century often were unsuccessful because of the lack of understanding and knowledge of the biologic basis of mental disorders. For example, the use of hydrotherapy, or baths, was an established procedure in mental institutions. The use of warm baths and, in some instances, ice cold baths produced calming effects for patients with mental disorders. However, the treatment's success was ascribed to its effectiveness as a form of restraint because the physiologic responses that hydrotherapy produced were not understood.

Baths were applied indiscriminately and used as a form of restraint, rather than a therapeutic practice. Other examples of biologic procedures applied either indiscriminately or inappropriately include psychosurgery and electroconvulsive therapy (see Chapter 8). Thanks to modern technology, neurosurgical techniques and electroconvulsive therapy can be humanely applied with positive therapeutic outcomes for some psychiatric disorders.

Support for the biologic approaches increased as successful symptom management with psychopharmacologic agents was reported. When a pharmacologic agent made a difference in care, a biologic hypothesis was considered. Modern psychopharmacology began in the 1930s, when barbiturates, particularly amobarbital sodium (Amytal Sodium), were tried for treating mental diseases (Malamud, 1944). Psychopharmacology revolutionized the treatment of mental illness and led to an increased number of patients discharged into the community and the eventual focus on the brain as the key to understanding psychiatric disorders.

Increased Government Involvement in Mental Health Care

As scientific advances led to an increased intellectual understanding of the biologic foundations of mental illness, social change and historical events fostered a new level of empathy on an emotional level. During World War II, mental illness was beginning to be seen as a problem that could happen to anyone. Many "normal" people who volunteered for the armed services were disqualified on the grounds that they were psychologically unfit to serve. Others who had already served a tour of duty received diagnoses of psychiatric and emotional problems believed to be caused by the war. Consequently, in 1946, President Truman signed into law the National Mental Health Act, which supported research, training, and the establishment of clinics and treatment centers. This act created a six-member National Mental Health Advisory Council that established the National Institute of Mental Health (NIMH), which was responsible for overseeing and coordinating research and training.

The Hill-Burton Act of 1946 provided substantial federal support for hospital construction, which facilitated the expansion of psychiatric units in general hospitals. With the passage of the National Mental Health Act, the federal government became more involved in financing and controlling the deliv ery of care. Under the Act's provisions, the federal government provided grants to states to support existing outpatient facilities and programs to establish new ones. Before 1948, more than half of all states had no clinics; by 1949, all but five had one or more. Six years later, there were 1,234 outpatient clinics.

Continued Evolution of Psychiatric–Mental Health Nursing

Another outcome of the Act's passage was the provision of training grants to institutions for stipends and fellowships to prepare specialty nurses in advanced practice (Chamberlain, 1983). The first graduate nursing program, developed by Hildegarde E. Peplau in 1954 at Rutgers University, was in the specialty of psychiatric nursing. Subspecialties began to emerge focusing on children, adolescents, or elderly people. Today in the United States, many master's degree programs offer specializations in psychiatric–mental health.

In 1952, Peplau published the landmark work *Interpersonal Relations in Nursing*. It introduced psychiatric mental health nursing practice to the concepts of interpersonal relations and the importance of the therapeutic relationship. In fact, the nurse–patient relationship was defined as the very essence of psychiatric–mental health nursing (see Chapters 5 and 9). This was a significant switch in perspective from the neurobiologic approach that had characterized the discipline before that time. Peplau's perspective was also important in its conceptualization of nursing care as truly independent of physicians. The nurse's use of self as a nursing tool was outside the dominance of both hospital administrators and physicians.

Gradually, nursing education programs in specialized hospitals were phased into generalized programs in nursing (Peplau, 1989). Nursing programs offered in psychiatric hospitals closed. This mainstreaming of psychiatric–mental health nursing education into the general nursing curriculum made the need for specialized hospitals unnecessary.

THE LATE 20TH CENTURY

Community Health Movement and Deinstitutionalization

In 1955, the Joint Commission on Mental Illness and Health was formed to study the problems of mental health care delivery. During its 6-year existence, the commission sponsored several scholarly studies and created an atmosphere conducive to the discussion of new federal policy initiatives that eventually would undermine the traditional emphasis on institutional care. In 1961, the Commission transmitted its final report: "Action for Mental Health." The report called for larger investments in basic research; national personnel recruitment and training programs; one full-time clinic for every 50,000 individuals, supplemented by general hospital units and state-run regional intensive psychiatric treatment centers; and access to emergency care and treatment in general, both in mental hospitals and community clinics. The Commission recommended that planning and implementation of the system would include the consumers and that funding for the construction and operation of the community mental health system would be shared by federal, state, and local governments.

"Action for Mental Health" was presented at a time that was politically ripe for the new ideas. The 1960 presidential election of John F. Kennedy brought a new type of leadership to the United States. The ideas expressed in the report clearly shifted authority for mental health programming to the federal government. This report was the basis of the federal legislation, the Mental Retardation Facilities and Community Mental Health Centers Construction Act, which Kennedy signed into law in 1963.

In reality, this act included only some of the ideas proposed by the Commission and did not encompass state-run regional intensive psychiatric centers. Supporters of the legislation believed that the new community-oriented policy would provide better care and eliminate the need for institutions providing custodial care. The supporters of this 1963 legislation believed the exact opposite of what the supporters of Dorothea Dix believed during the previous century. That is, instead of viewing custodial care as the treatment of mental disorders, institutionalization was viewed as contributing to the illness. The predominant view was that many of the problems of mental disorders were caused by the deplorable conditions of the state mental institutions and that, if patients were moved into a "normal" community-living setting, the symptoms of mental disorders could easily be treated and eventually would disappear. Thus, **deinstitutionalization**, the discharge of the institutionalized people into the community, became a national objective. The inpatient population fell by about 15% between 1955 and 1965 and by about 59% during the succeeding decade.

The goal of the Community Mental Health Centers Construction Act was to expand community mental health services and diminish society's sole reliance on mental hospitals. Guidelines for implementing the act were somewhat vague, and administering the program became the responsibility of the federal government. Any mention of the role for or linkages to state hospitals was absent.

The Community Mental Health Construction Act, originally a construction grant, was amended in 1965 to strengthen the funding for staffing new facilities. Even so, the number of community mental health centers (CMHCs) grew slowly. There were a limited number of communities with populations large enough to support the centers and a shortage of trained personnel, even in urban areas. In smaller and rural communities, there was often no one (or no mental health provider) prepared for the new role. By the spring of 1967, only 173 funded projects existed.

There was no evidence that deinstitutionalized patients constituted a significant population of those receiving services at the new CMHCs. One problem was that the treatment of choice in most of the centers, individual psychotherapy, had not proved effective for patients with long-term mental disorders. Many urban

CMHC patients, as compared with former state hospital patients, tended to be younger and poorer and were disproportionately drawn from minority backgrounds. In addition, many centers focused on the treatment of alcoholism and drug addiction.

Sanctioning of Holistic Nursing Care

By 1963, two nursing journals focused on psychiatric nursing: the *Journal of Psychiatric Nursing* (now the *Journal of Psychosocial Nursing and Mental Health Services*) and *Perspectives in Psychiatric Care*. In 1967, the Division of Psychiatric and Mental Health Nursing Practice of the American Nurses Association (ANA) published the *Statement on Psychiatric Nursing Practice*. For the first time, there was official sanction of a holistic approach to nursing care, with psychiatric–mental health nurses practicing in a variety of settings with a variety of clientele. The emphasis was on activities ranging from health promotion to health restoration. Since 1967, there have been three more updates of the psychiatric–mental health nursing practice statement that continue to expand the role of the psychiatric nurse and delineate practice functions and roles.

Contemporary Issues

Changing Demographics

The social changes of the 1980s set the stage for the continuing evolution of mental health care. The population was rapidly aging. Family structure was diversifying through divorce, cohabitation, and a variety of family configurations. Women entered the work force in record numbers. Rapid growth of cities, or urbanization, was the single most characteristic phenomenon in the United States (Aldrich, 1986). The population in the United States was shifting toward the southwest. (In 1983, Los Angeles replaced Chicago as the second largest U.S. city.) Many of the new residents had migrated to the Southwest from Mexico and Asian countries; they had not simply relocated from other areas of the country. In North America, because of favorable immigration policies, the population was expected to grow (Deming, 1996).

By the 1990s, wrinkles in the social fabric became apparent. The deinstitutionalization movement, so long hailed as an efficient, cost-effective means of reabsorbing the mentally ill into society, was considered a failure. People with mental disorders were discharged into communities that were prepared to offer them only meager treatment, housing, or vocational opportunities. These communities were also sometimes vastly different from the ones the patients had left behind at the time of their hospitalization. In addition, fewer community-based facilities were in place to serve the growing population of people with mental disorders.

The 2,000 projected CMHCs that should have been in place by 1980 never materialized. By 1990, about 1,300 programs provided various types of psychosocial rehabilitation services, such as vocational, educational, or social-recreational services (International Association of Psychosocial Rehabilitation, 1990). The CMHCs, by and large, ignored the legions of people with serious mental illnesses. Today mental health services are inadequate and fragmented. Millions of adults and children are disabled by mental illness every year. When compared with all other diseases, mental illness ranks first in terms of causing disability in the United States, Canada, and Western Europe (World Health Organization [WHO], 2001).

The Age of Managed Care

Both public and private expenditures for health care services have increased in the United States. Financial barriers account for the different resource allocation rules for financing mental health services compared with general health care services, which leads to less overall funding for mental health. To control costs, privately "insured" mental health care has been "carved out" from the rest of health care and is managed separately. Privately owned behavioral health care firms not only manage care but also provide services through directly owned or contracted networks of providers. In theory, people with psychiatric problems have direct access to the specialists who provide the best care. In reality, services are still limited and sometimes withheld. Once care is limited or denied, individuals once again turn to public funds, which may or may not be available.

Now, large networks of public and private organizations share responsibility for mental health care, with the state remaining as the major decision maker for resource allocation. Emphasis is on reducing expensive institutional care and increasing the resources devoted to communities of individuals with mental disorders. The mental health work force is shifting from providing care in traditional health care institutions to community settings: clinics, homes, schools, and treatment centers.

National Mental Health Objectives

In 1999, *Mental Health: A Report of the Surgeon General* was the first report by the Office of the Surgeon General and supported two main findings (U.S. Department of Health and Human Services, 1999):

- The efficacy of mental health treatments is well documented.
- A range of treatments exists for most mental disorders.

The following year, another landmark report, *Report of the Surgeon General's Conference on Children's Mental Health: A National Action Agenda*, was published. This report highlights consensus recommendations for identifying, recognizing, and referring children to services, increasing access to services for families, and identifying the evidence in treatment services, systems of care, and financing (U.S. Public Health Service, 2000). In 2001, the World Health Organization focused its annual *World Health Report* on mental health, emphasizing the importance of mental health to the well-being of individuals (WHO, 2001).

In 2003, the President's New Freedom Commission on Mental Health presented its report on mental illness in the United States. It recommended the development of efficient and effective services that should be integrated into the community (New Freedom Commission on Mental Health, 2003). See Box 1-3.

One of the most important documents for the advancement of a mental health agenda is *Healthy People 2010: National Health Promotion and Disease Prevention Objectives*, which contains many health care goals that pertain specifically to mental health (Box 1-4) (U.S. Department of Health and Human Services, 2000). The challenge before nurses is to strive to meet these goals while obeying marketplace demands to provide the most cost-effective care possible. This translates into an emphasis on preventing the symptoms of mental disorders and using hospitalization as a treatment of last resort. Devising and implementing a continuum of mental health services that provides access for all is an integral part of the strategy for accomplishing these goals.

BOX 1.3

U.S. Goals in a Transformed Mental Health System

Goal 1 Americans understand that mental health is essential to overall health.
Goal 2 Mental health care is consumer and family driven.
Goal 3 Disparities in mental health services are eliminated.
Goal 4 Early mental health screening, assessment, and referral to services are common practice.
Goal 5 Excellent mental health care is delivered and research is accelerated.
Goal 6 Technology is used to access mental health care and information.

Source: New Freedom Commission on Mental Health. (2003). Achieving the promise: Transforming mental health care in America, p. 8. DHHS Publication No. SMA-03-3831. Rockville, MD.

BOX 1.4

Mental Health and Mental Disorders Objectives for the Year 2010

Mental Health Status Improvement
- Reduce the suicide rate to no more than 6.0 per 100,000 (baseline, 10.8/100,000 in 1998)
- Reduce the suicide attempts by adolescents to no more than 1% (baseline, 2.6% in 1997)
- Reduce the proportion of homeless adults who have serious mental illness (SMI)
- Increase the proportion of persons with serious mental illness who are employed

Treatment Expansion
- Reduce the relapse rates for persons with eating disorders, including anorexia nervosa and bulimia nervosa.
- Increase the number of persons seen in primary health care who receive mental health screening and assessment.
- Increase the proportion of children with mental health problems who receive treatment.
- Increase the proportion of juvenile justice facilities that screen new admissions for mental health problems.
- Increase the proportion of adults with mental disorders who receive treatment.
- Increase the proportion of persons with co-occurring substance abuse and mental disorders who receive treatment for both disorders.
- Increase the proportion of local governments with community-based jail diversion programs for adults with serious mental illness.

State Activities
- Increase the number of states and the District of Columbia that track consumers' satisfaction with the mental health services they receive.
- Increase the number of states, territories, and the District of Columbia with an operational mental health plan that addresses cultural competence.
- Increase the number of states, territories, and the District of Columbia with an operational mental health plan that addresses mental health crisis interventions, ongoing screening, and treatment services for elderly persons.

SUMMARY OF KEY POINTS

- Stigma significantly impacts the person with mental illness. Even though there is greater understanding of the basis of mental illness, the mentally ill continue to be stigmatized.
- Throughout history, attitudes and treatment toward those with mental disorders have drastically changed as a result of the changing socioeconomic backdrop of our society and the development

of new theories and study by key individuals and groups.

- During the 1800s, as mental illness began to be viewed as an illness, more humane and moral treatments began to develop.
- True social reformers, such as Dorothea Dix, Horace Mann, and Clifford Beers, dedicated their efforts to raising society's awareness and advocating public responsibility for proper treatment of patients with mental disorders.
- Theoretical arguments characterized the evolution of scientific thought and psychiatric practice. Gradually, the importance of the biologic aspect of mental disorders has been recognized.
- Although the need for psychiatric–mental health nursing was recognized near the end of the 19th century, there was much resistance to training women for the care of the insane. Linda Richards opened the Boston City Hospital Training School for Nurses in 1882.
- Gradually, all psychiatric nursing education in the United States was phased into basic nursing education, and nursing programs offered in psychiatric hospitals closed. The first graduate program in psychiatric–mental health nursing was initiated in 1954 by Hildegarde Peplau at Rutgers University.
- Through key federal and state legislative initiatives, mental health services were funded, but remain inadequate.
- The U.S. Surgeon General's reports, The President's *New Freedom Commission on Mental Health*, and the goals of *Healthy People 2010* continue to highlight the need for resources for the care of persons with mental illness.

CRITICAL THINKING CHALLENGES

1. Examine how family and friends describe people with mental illness. Do you think their description of mental illness is based on fact or myth? Explain.
2. Compare the ideas of psychiatric care during the 1800s with those of the 1990s and 2000s and identify the major political and economic forces that influenced care.
3. Analyze the social, political, and economic changes that influenced the community mental health movement.
4. Present an argument for the moral treatment of people with mental disorders.
5. Trace the history of biologic psychiatry and highlight major ideas and treatments.

One Flew Over the Cuckoo's Nest: 1975. This classic film stars Jack Nicholson as Randle P. McMurphy, who takes on the state hospital establishment. This picture won all five of the top Academy Awards: Best Picture, Best Actor, Best Actress, Best Director, and Best Adapted Screenplay. The film depicts life in an inpatient psychiatric ward of the late 1960s and increased public awareness of the potential human rights violations inherent in a large, public mental system. However, the portrayal of electroconvulsive therapy is stereotyped and inaccurate, and the suicide of Billy appears to be simplistically linked to his domineering mother. Overall, this film probably contributes to the stigma of mental illness.

VIEWING POINTS: This film should be viewed from several different perspectives: What is the basis of McMurphy's admission? How does Nurse Ratchet interact with the patients? What is missing? What is different in today's public mental health systems?

An Angel at My Table: 1989, New Zealand. This thought-provoking three-part television mini-series is based on Janet Frame's autobiography that traces her life from being a shy, socially inept little girl to New Zealand's most famous writer/poet. Produced by Jane Campion and starring Kerry Fox, the story is told in three stages of the main character's life: childhood, young adulthood, and adulthood. During the second period, Janet Frame received an inaccurate diagnosis of schizophrenia and was hospitalized for 8 years. She barely avoided a leukotomy.

VIEWING POINTS: Observe how the role of the woman in society influenced Janet Frame's admission to the hospital. Would she be considered "mentally ill and needing hospitalization" by today's standard?

Beautiful Dreamers: 1992, Canada. This film is based on a true story about poet Walt Whitman's visit to an asylum in London, Ontario, Canada. Whitman, played by Rip Torn, is shocked by what he sees and persuades the hospital director to offer humane treatment. Eventually, the patients wind up playing the townspeople in a game of cricket.

VIEWING POINTS: Observe the stigma that is associated with having a mental illness.

REFERENCES

Aldrich, R. (1986). The social context of change. *Psychiatric Annals, 16* (10), 613–618.

Bailey, H. (1920). *Nursing mental diseases.* New York: Macmillan.

Beers, C. (1908). *A mind that found itself.* New York: Longmans, Green, & Co.

Campinha, J. (1987). The training of a 'mental nurse': An historical look at McLean Training School for Nurses. *Virginia Nurse, 55* (1), 18–20.

Chamberlain, J. (1983). The role of the federal government in the development of psychiatric nursing. *Journal of Psychosocial Nursing and Mental Health Services, 21* (4), 11–18.

Church, O. (1987). From custody to community in psychiatric nursing. *Nursing Research, 36* (10), 48–55.

Cowles, E. (1887, October). Nursing reform for the insane. *American Journal of Insanity, 44*, 176, 191.

Deming, W. G. (1996). A decade of economic change and population shifts in U.S. regions. *Monthly Labor Review, 119* (11), 3–14.

Deutsch, S. (1949). *The mentally ill in America.* London: Oxford University Press.

International Association of Psychosocial Rehabilitation Services (IAPRS). (1990). *A national directory: Organizations providing psychosocial rehabilitation and related community support services in the United States.* Boston: Center for Psychiatric Rehabilitation, Boston University.

Lightner, D. L. (1999). *Asylum prison and poorhouse. The writings and reform work of Dorothea Dix in Illinois.* Carbondale and Edwardsville, IL: Southern Illinois University Press.

Malamud, W. (1944). The history of psychiatric therapies. In J. K. Hall, G. Zilboorg, & H. Bunker (Eds.), *One hundred years of American psychiatry*, 273–323. New York: Columbia University Press.

Neill, J. (1980). Adolf Meyer and American psychiatry today. *American Journal of Psychiatry, 137* (4), 460–464.

New Freedom Commission on Mental Health. (2003). *Achieving the promise: Transforming mental health care in America.* Department of Health and Human Services Publication No. SMA-03-3831. Rockville, MD.

Nightingale, F. (1859). *Notes on nursing: What it is and what it is not.* London: Harrison & Son.

Peplau, H. (1952). *Interpersonal relations in nursing.* New York: Putnam.

Peplau, H. (1989). Future directions in psychiatric nursing from the perspective of history. *Journal of Psychosocial Nursing and Mental Health Services, 27* (2), 18–21.

U.S. Department of Health and Human Services. (1999). *Mental health: A report of the Surgeon General.* Washington, DC: U.S. Department of Health and Human Services, Substance Abuse and Mental Health Services Administration, Center for Mental Health Services, National Institutes of Health, National Institute of Mental Health.

U.S. Department of Health and Human Services. (2000). *Healthy people 2010* (2nd ed.) With: Understanding and improving health and objectives for improving health. Washington, DC: U.S. Government Printing Office.

U.S. Public Health Service. (2000). *Report of the Surgeon General's Conference on Children's Mental Health: A national action agenda.* Washington, DC: Department of Health and Human Services.

World Health Organization. (2001). *The world health report: Mental health 2001: Mental health: New understanding, new hope.* Geneva: Author.

World Health Organization (2001). Mental health problems: the undefined and hidden burden. Fact sheet N281. http://www.who.int;mediacentre/factsheets/fs218/en/print.html. Retrieved September 18, 2005.

CHAPTER 2

Classification of Mental Illnesses and Evidence-Based Nursing Care

Mary Ann Boyd

LEARNING OBJECTIVES

After studying this chapter, you will be able to:

- Differentiate mental illnesses from medical diseases.
- Differentiate the five axes used in making a psychiatric diagnosis.
- Discuss the significance of epidemiology in understanding the impact of mental disorders.
- Discuss the role of evidence-based care in psychiatric nursing.

KEY CONCEPTS

- mental disorder
- epidemiology
- evidence-based practice

KEY TERMS

• axes • cultural-bound syndrome • DSM-IV-TR • epidemiology • incidence • mental disorder • mental illness • multiaxial diagnostic system • point prevalence • prevalence

Mental illness is a term used to mean a diagnosable mental disorder. A mental illness or **mental disorder** is a syndrome that has multiple causes and may represent several different disease states that have not yet been defined.

OVERVIEW OF MENTAL HEALTH CONDITIONS

Mental illness is a term used to mean a diagnosable mental disorder. A mental illness or mental disorder is a syndrome that has multiple causes and may represent several different disease states that have not yet been defined. Unlike many medical diseases, mental disorders are defined by clusters of symptoms or manifestations, not underlying pathology. A diagnosis becomes a way of labeling a particular patient problem, but there can be negative consequences of the label. Just as a person with diabetes mellitus should not be referred to as a "diabetic," but rather as a "person with diabetes," a person with a mental disorder should never be referred to as a "schizophrenic" or "bipolar," but rather as a "person with schizophrenia" or a "person with bipolar disorder."

> **KEY CONCEPT Mental disorders** are health conditions characterized by alterations in thinking, mood, or behavior. They are associated with distress or impaired functioning.

These alterations are unexpected and are outside the limits of expected psychological states, such as the normal sadness, grief, and mild depression associated with the death of a partner. Cultural definitions of "normal" are also taken into consideration. If a behavior is considered normal within a specific culture, it is not viewed as a symptom by members of that group. For example, it is common in some religious groups to "speak in tongues." To an observer, it appears that the individuals are having

FAME AND FORTUNE

Winston Churchill (1874-1965)
Great Statesman

Public Persona

Winston Churchill, former Prime Minister of England and one of the greatest statesmen of the 20th century, led the British people to victory during WWII. He ultimately had a major role in bringing peace to the world.

Personal Realities

Churchill's bouts with depression, mania, grandiose behaviors, and insomnia are well documented. "Black Dog" was the name Churchill gave to his unrelenting depressive moods that immobilized him for months, sometimes years. Several of his ancestors also suffered mood disorders. In spite of his personal problems, he instilled in the British people his own fiery resolve and will to resist the tyranny of war. When Churchill died in 1965, he received the first state funeral given to a commoner since that of the Duke of Wellington.

Churchill's childhood was privileged, but not particularly happy. He was a younger son of the Duke of Marlborough and Jennie Jerome, the daughter of an American business tycoon. Like many Victorian parents, Lord and Lady Randolph Churchill were distant figures. Letters from his schooldays reveal that Winston was often willful and rebellious. One of Winston's school reports showed him to be last in the class. He performed particularly badly in composition, writing, and spelling; yet 70 years later he would win the Nobel Prize for Literature.

Source: Storr, A (1989). *Churchill's black dog, Kafka's mice, and other phenomena of the human mind.* Grove/ Atlantic, Inc: New York.

hallucinations (see Chapter 18), a psychiatric symptom, but this behavior is normal for this group within a particular setting.

Diagnostic Classification of Mental Health Conditions

The diagnosis of mental disorders is based on the classification system of the fourth edition (text revision) of the *Diagnostic and Statistical Manual of Mental Disorders* (DSM-IV-TR) (American Psychiatric Association, 2000). The purpose of this manual is to provide a helpful guide to clinical practice that is practical for clinical, research, and educational purposes. The **DSM-IV-TR** system contains subtypes and other specifiers to describe further the characteristics of the diagnosis as exhibited in a given individual. Although the DSM-IV-TR provides criteria for diagnosing mental disorders, there are no absolute boundaries separating one disorder from another, and similar disorders may have different manifestations at different points in time.

Labeling is a negative consequence of the diagnostic process. Sometimes persons are wrongly classified as a disorder rather than having a disorder. A person with schizophrenia becomes a "schizophrenic" and is not viewed as a holistic being who has a chronic, treatable disorder. Labeling becomes especially problematic in mental health because of the universal stigma associated with mental disorders (see Chapter 1).

Some disorders are influenced by cultural factors and others are culture-bound syndromes that are present only in a particular setting (Box 2.1). Negative views of mental illness by several of the Asian cultures influence the willingness of its members to seek treatment. They may ignore symptoms or refuse to seek treatment because of the stigma associated with being mentally ill (see Chapter 15). A **culture-bound syndrome** is a recurrent, locality-specific pattern of aberrant behavior and troubling experience that is limited to specific societies or

BOX 2.1

Selected Culture-Bound Syndromes

DEFINITION: Behaviors limited to specific cultures that have meaning within that culture

ATAQUE DE NERVIOS: An idiom of distress principally reported among Latinos from the Caribbean. Symptoms include uncontrollable shouting, attacks of crying, trembling, heat in the chest rising into the head, and verbal or physical aggression. Dissociative experiences, seizurelike or fainting episodes and suicidal gestures may be present. Ataques de nervios frequently occur as a direct result of a stressful event relating to the family. Amnesia for what happened during the attack may also occur.

BRAIN FAG: Condition experienced by high school or university students in response to the challenges of schooling. Symptoms include difficulties in concentrating, remembering, and thinking. A term originally used in West Africa.

FALLING-OUT OR BLACKING OUT: An episode of sudden collapse that is sometimes preceded by feelings of dizziness. Individuals' eyes are usually open, but the person claims an inability to see. Occurs primarily in southern United States and Caribbean groups.

MAL DE OJO: Known as the "evil eye" in Mediterranean cultures and elsewhere in the world. Symptoms include fitful sleep, crying without apparent cause, diarrhea, vomiting, and fever in a child or infant.

SHENJING SHUAIRO ("neurasthenia"): In China, a condition characterized by physical and mental fatigue, dizziness, headaches, pain, concentration difficulties, sleep disturbance, and memory loss. Other symptoms include gastrointestinal problems, sexual dysfunction, irritability, excitability, and various signs suggesting disturbance of the autonomic nervous system. Symptoms may meet the criteria for Mood or Anxiety Disorders.

Adapted from American Psychiatric Association. (2000). *Diagnostic and Statistical Manual of Mental Disorders,* 4th ed, Text Revision (pp. 898–903). Washington, DC: Author.

BOX 2.2

***Research for Best Practice:* Hwa-Byung in Middle-Aged Korean Women**

Park, Y., Hesook, S.K. Schwartz-Barcott, D., Jong-Woo, K. (2002). The conceptual structure of hwa-byung in middle-aged Korean women. *Health Care for Women International, 23*, 389–397.

THE QUESTION: Hwa-byung (HB) is a Korean folk illness that is not well described, but literally means *an illness of fire.* The DSM-IV-TR translated it into meaning *anger syndrome.* It was believed to be a result of suppression of anger or projection of anger into the body. HB symptoms include characteristic physical symptoms such as insomnia; a sensation of heat in the face, eyes, mouth, or elsewhere in the body; pins and needles sensation; headache; and/or a sensation of an epigastric mass. Psychologic symptoms include anxiety, tearfulness, loss of motivation for life, fear of impending death, sense of suffocation, grief, exhaustion, depression, feelings of meaninglessness, and/or hopelessness.

METHODS: Nurse researcher Park and colleagues conducted a qualitative study that examined the experiences of six women, aged 40 to 65 years, visiting the HB clinic in Seoul, Korea. An open-ended interview was used to obtain information as to the conceptual meaning of HB.

FINDINGS: Common themes in the interview results included a strong commitment to traditional values, a quick-tempered personality, a conflicted marital relationship, a hard life, and an unhappy life. Their responses were endurance (forbearance), feeling of victimization or mortification, anger, and deep sorrow.

IMPLICATIONS FOR NURSING: This study emphasizes the importance of listening to the patient's experience and responses before using the DSM-IV-TR to diagnose a "Western" psychiatric disorder. Even though culture-bound syndromes do not meet the criteria for a DSM-IV-TR diagnosis, these syndromes are real psychiatric disorders in need of nursing assessment and interventions.

culture areas. These syndromes do not fit the DSM-IV-TR classification of mental disorders, which is dominated by Western thought. See Box 2.2.

Multiaxial Diagnostic System

The DSM-IV-TR diagnostic criteria are based on a **multiaxial diagnostic system** that includes five **axes**, or domains of information. Axis I includes most *clinical disorders* and other conditions that may be the focus of clinical attention, and Axis II contains *personality disorders* and *mental retardation*. Axis III includes the *general medical conditions* that must be considered in the diagnosis and treatment of the primary psychiatric disorders. Each axis is essential to the complete understanding and treatment of an individual with psychiatric concerns. For example, a person with a major depression (Axis I) may meet the criteria for having a dependent personality disorder (Axis II) and may also have diabetes (Axis III). See Table 2.1 for a listing of disorders and conditions that might be considered under each axis and Box 2.3 for a clinical example.

Although the first three axes appear to contain all of the diagnostic information, a truly accurate picture of the individual is incomplete without considering other factors, such as life stressors and current level of functioning. Axis IV concerns any *psychosocial or environmental problems* that may produce added stress, confound the diagnosis, or must be considered in the treatment of the primary psychiatric problem. These problems may be conceptualized in terms of life stressors, which may be negative or positive. For example, a negative life event, such as the death of a spouse, a recent divorce, or job discrimination, may exacerbate symptoms of depression. On the other hand, positive stressors, such as starting a new job, getting married, or having a baby, may also prompt the symptoms to emerge. Although the DSM-IV-TR suggests a number of problem areas to be considered, the clinician making the diagnosis should write out the individual's specific problems on this axis.

Ratings given on Axis V provide an estimate of *overall functioning* in psychological, social, and occupational spheres of life. These data are useful in planning treatment and measuring its impact. The Global Assessment Functioning (GAF) scale is used most often and is scored from low functioning of 0 to 10, to high functioning of 91 to 100 (see Table 2.1). This rating may be made at the beginning of treatment, at discharge from the hospital, or at any point thereafter. When including this rating, the point of time should also be indicated, such as "current," or "at discharge from the hospital."

BOX 2.3

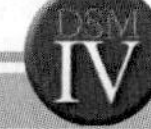

Diagnostic Axes and Their Disorders and Conditions

Clinical Example

Axis I: 300.21* Panic Disorder With Agoraphobia
Axis II: 301.4 Obsessive-Compulsive Personality Disorder
Axis III: 250.00† Diabetes Mellitus
Axis IV: Occupational Problems: Frequent Absences From Work
Axis V: Global Assessment of Function
GAF = 55 (current)
90 (potential)

*In this example, code numbers are used and can be found in the *Diagnostic and Statistical Manual of Mental Disorders,* 4th ed, text revision *(DSM-IV-TR)*. To improve readability, these code numbers are not used when discussing the various disorders. The student will see them used in the clinical setting.

†The medical conditions in Axis III are coded according to the *International Classification of Diseases (ICD).*

Table 2.1 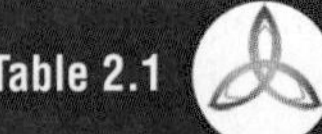 DSM-IV Multiaxial Diagnoses for Persons With Mental Disorders 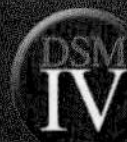

Diagnostic Axes and Their Disorders and Conditions

Axis I: Clinical Disorders and Other Conditions That May Be a Focus of Clinical Attention

Disorders Usually First Diagnosed During Infancy, Childhood, or Adolescence
Delirium, Dementia, Amnestic, and Other Cognitive Disorders
Mental Disorders Due to General Medical Conditions
Substance-Related Disorders
Schizophrenia and Other Psychotic Disorders
Mood Disorders
Anxiety Disorders
Somatoform Disorders
Factitious Disorders
Dissociative Disorders
Sexual and Gender Identity Disorders
Eating Disorders
Sleep Disorders
Impulse Control Disorders (Not Elsewhere Classified)
Adjustment Disorders
Other Conditions That May Be a Focus of Clinical Attention

Axis II: Personality Disorders and Mental Retardation

Personality Disorders:
- Paranoid Personality Disorder
- Schizoid Personality Disorder
- Schizotypal Personality Disorder
- Antisocial Personality Disorder
- Borderline Personality Disorder
- Histrionic Personality Disorder
- Narcissistic Personality Disorder
- Avoidant Personality Disorder
- Dependent Personality Disorder
- Obsessive-Compulsive Personality Disorder
- Personality Disorder Not Otherwise Specified
- Mental Retardation

Axis III: General Medical Conditions

Infectious and Parasitic Diseases
Neoplasms
Endocrine, Nutritional, and Metabolic Diseases and Immunity Disorders
Diseases of the Blood and Blood-Forming Organs
Diseases of the Nervous and Sense Organs
Diseases of the Circulatory System
Diseases of the Respiratory System
Diseases of the Digestive System
Diseases of the Genitourinary System
Complications of Pregnancy, Childbirth, and the Puerperium
Diseases of the Skin and Subcutaneous Tissue
Diseases of the Musculoskeletal System and Connective Tissue
Congenital Anomalies
Certain Conditions Originating in the Perinatal Period
Symptoms, Signs, and Ill-Defined Conditions
Injury and Poisoning

Axis IV: Psychosocial and Environmental Problems

Problems with primary support group
Problems related to the social environment
Educational problems
Occupational problems
Housing problems
Economic problems
Problems with access to health care services
Problems related to interaction with the legal system/crime
Other psychosocial and environmental problems

Axis V: Global Assessment of Functioning

Current =
Potential =
Psychologic, social, and occupational functioning on a hypothetical continuum of mental health-illness.

Scores	
91–100	Superior functioning, no symptoms
81–90	Absent or minimal symptoms, good functioning in all areas
71–80	If symptoms are present, they are transient and expectable reactions to psychosocial stressors; no more than slight impairment in social, occupational, or school functioning
61–70	Some mild symptoms or some difficulty in social, occupational, or school functioning, but generally functioning well; has some meaningful interpersonal relationships
51–60	Moderate symptoms or moderate difficulty in social, occupational, or school functioning
41–50	Serious symptoms or any serious impairment in social, occupational, or school functioning
31–40	Some impairment in reality testing or communication or major impairment in several areas, such as work or school, family relations, judgment, thinking, or mood
21–30	Behavior is considerably influenced by delusions or hallucinations or serious impairment in communication or judgment or inability to function in almost all areas
11–20	Some danger of hurting self or others or occasionally fails to maintain minimal personal hygiene or gross impairment in communication
1–10	Persistent danger of severely hurting self or others or persistent inability to maintain minimal personal hygiene or serious suicidal act with clear expectation of death

EPIDEMIOLOGY IN MENTAL HEALTH

The occurrence of mental disorders is studied through epidemiological research, just like any other disorder.

KEY CONCEPT Epidemiology is the study of patterns of disease distribution and determinants of health within populations. It focuses on the health status of population groups, or aggregates, and associated factors.

Epidemiology is not only the study of disease, particularly infectious diseases; it is also concerned with all aspects of health including acute and chronic disease, genetics, and the behavioral aspects of health such as self-care, exercise, diet, recreation, and substance abuse. Throughout this book, epidemiologic data are included in discussions of mental health problems and mental disorders. See Box 2.4 for an explanation of terms. Epidemiological studies examine associations among possible factors related to an area of investigation, not causes of a disorder. The Centers for Disease Control and Prevention (CDC) tracks and reports mental health epidemiological data.

BOX 2.4

Epidemiologic Terms

In epidemiology, certain terms have specific meanings relative to what they measure. When expressing the number of cases of a disorder, population rates, rather than raw numbers, are used.

Rate is a proportion of the cases in the population when compared with the total population. It is expressed as a fraction, in which the numerator is the number of cases and the denominator is the total number in the population, including the cases and noncases. The term *average rate* is used for measures that involve rates over specified time periods:

$$\text{Rate} = \frac{\text{Cases in the population}}{\text{Total population}}$$

(includes cases and noncases)

Prevalence refers to the total number of people who have the disorder within a given population at a specified time, regardless of how long ago the disorder started.

Point prevalence is the basic measure that refers to the proportion of individuals in the population who have the disorder at a specified point in time. This point can be a day on the calendar, such as April 1, 2010, or a point defined in relation to the study assessment, such as the day of the interview. This is also expressed as a fraction:

$$\text{Point prevalence rate} = \frac{\text{cases at } t}{\text{Population at } t}$$

Incidence refers to a rate that includes only *new* cases that have occurred within a clearly defined time period. The most common time period evaluated is 1 year. The study of incidence cases is more difficult than a study of prevalent cases because a study of incidence cases requires at least two measurements to be taken: one at the start of the prescribed time period and another at the end of it.

EVIDENCE-BASED NURSING CARE

Understanding the mental disorders, diagnostic axes, and the usefulness of epidemiological studies is only the beginning of competent nursing care. Traditionally, nursing interventions have been selected based solely on clinicians' own experiences and unsystematic trial and error. Today, the focus of care is on an evidence-based approach that involves defining clinical questions, finding and analyzing the evidence, applying the research in a practical manner, and evaluating outcomes. The state of evidence-based psychiatric nursing practice is evolving and research findings are slowly making their way into practice (Zauszniewski & Suresky, 2003).

KEY CONCEPT Evidence-based practice (EBP) is the conscientious use and integration of the best research evidence with clinical expertise and patient values in making decisions about patient care (Sackett, Straus, Richardson, & Haynes, 2000; Melnyk & Fineout-Overholt, 2005).

Evidence-based approaches rely heavily on the research literature, but this approach involves much more than using one or two studies to justify an intervention. Evidence-based practice is based on a critical analysis of all of the research studies related to a specific area. Unlike research utilization, which is the use of knowledge typically based on a single study, EBP takes into account the expertise of the clinician and the analyses of several studies. Meta-analyses are found in databases that are available through the Internet and libraries. The Cochrane Collaboration, an international nonprofit and independent organization, produces and disseminates systematic reviews of health care interventions and promotes the search for evidence in the form of clinical trials and other studies of intervention. The major product of the Collaboration is the *Cochrane Database of Systematic Reviews* (http://www.cochrane.org).

SUMMARY OF KEY POINTS

- Mental disorders are health conditions characterized by alterations in thinking, mood, or behavior and are associated with distress or impaired functioning.
- The use of diagnosis in mental health can be problematic because of the negative association of the label *mental illness*. The psychiatric diagnoses outlined in the DSM-IV-TR are the standardized, accepted language

in the mental health field. There are five diagnostic axes: psychiatric clinical disorders, personality disorders and mental retardation, general medical problems, psychosocial or environmental problems, and overall functioning.

- Culture-bound syndromes are specific disorders found within a particular locality and/or culture. They do not meet criteria for any of the DSM-IV-TR disorders, but are real psychiatric syndromes that need to be understood and treated.
- Epidemiology is important in understanding the distribution of mental illness and determinants of health within a given population. The rate of occurrence refers to the proportion of the population that has the disorder. The incidence is the rate of new cases within a specified time. The prevalence is the rate of occurrence of all cases at a particular point in time.
- Research evidence for psychiatric nursing interventions is increasing. Nurses should regularly update their knowledge through evidence-based sources.

CRITICAL THINKING CHALLENGES

1 Examine the concept "syndrome" and explain how a mental disorder syndrome differs from a medical disease.
2 Examine the description of people with mental illness in the media, including television programs, news, and newspapers. Are negative connotations evident?
3 Explain the purposes of the five axes of the DSM-IV-TR.
4 Discuss the negative impact of labeling someone with a psychiatric diagnosis.
5 Conduct a literature search on culture-bound syndromes and compare the symptom patterns and treatment.
6 Use the Global Assessment Functioning (GAF) scale to determine current level of functioning for the following patient scenarios:
   a An 83-year-old person who lives in a nursing home and who is confused and needs support from nursing staff in activities of daily living.
   b A 16-year-old male who refuses to go to school, stays in his room most of the time, and talks to people who are not apparent to anyone but him.
   c A 50-year-old person who has returned to work from a recent hospitalization. Symptoms are minimal.
7 Define the epidemiologic terms *prevalence*, *incidence*, and *rate*.
8 Access the Centers for Disease Control (CDC) website (www.cdc.gov) and identify major mental health problems in the United States.

REFERENCES

American Psychiatric Association. (2000). *Diagnostic and statistical manual of mental disorders*, 4th ed., text revision. Washington, DC: Author.

Melnyk, B.M., & Fineout-Overholt, E. (2005). *Evidence-based practice in nursing & healthcare.* Philadelphia: Lippincott Williams & Wilkins.

Sackett, D.L., Straus, S., Richardson, S.W., & Haynes, R.B. (2000). *Evidence-based medicine: how to practice and teach EBM.* (2nd ed.). London, U. K.: Churchill Livingstone.

Zauszniewski, J., & Suresky, J. (2003). Evidence for psychiatric nursing practice: An analysis of three years of published research. *Online Journal of Issues in Nursing, 9* (1), Retrieved from http://nursingworld.org/ojin/hirsh/topic4/tpc4_htm.

CHAPTER 3

Patient Rights and Legal Issues

Mary Ann Boyd

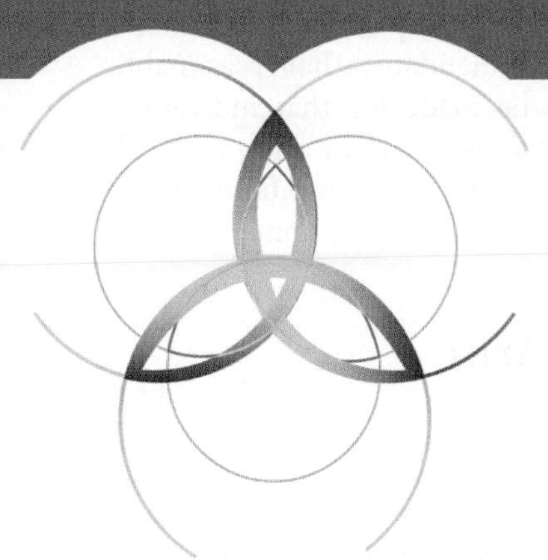

KEY CONCEPT

- self-determinism

LEARNING OBJECTIVES

After studying this chapter, you will be able to:

- Use the concepts of self-determinism and competence in discussing patient treatment choices.
- Discuss the role of informed consent in the delivery of psychiatric–mental health care.
- Delineate the differences between voluntary and involuntary treatment.
- Explain the rationale for providing the least restrictive treatment environment.
- Discuss HIPAA and mandates to inform and their implications in psychiatric–mental health care.
- Identify the importance of accurate, descriptive documentation of the biopsychosocial areas.
- Discuss the laws that protect patients' rights.

KEY TERMS

• assault • accreditation • advance care directives • breach of confidentiality • competence • confidentiality • external advocacy systems • incompetent • informed consent • internal rights protection system • involuntary commitment • least restrictive environment • medical battery • negligence • privacy • voluntary admission • voluntary commitment

In the past, people with mental disorders often received inadequate treatment and were punished because their disorder was misunderstood. It was difficult to protect human rights and maintain ethical practice standards. Today, legal rights of those with mental disorders and ethical health care practices of mental health providers are ongoing concerns for psychiatric–mental health nurses. For example, who decides the care plan for a person with a mental disorder? Can a person be forced into a hospital if his or her behavior is bizarre but harmless? What human rights can be denied to a person who has a mental disorder and under what circumstances? These questions are not easily answered. This chapter summarizes some of the key patient rights and legal issues that underlie psychiatric–mental health nursing practice across the continuum of care. The care of the mentally ill in forensic settings is found in Chapter 35.

PATIENT RIGHTS

People with psychiatric problems are vulnerable to mistreatment and abuse; consequently, laws have been passed that guarantee them legal protection. The specific laws and regulations are discussed later in the chapter.

Bill of Rights

In some instances, people with mental disorders are unable to make sound decisions regarding their treatment and care. Fortunately, certain laws protect them from their own poor decision-making abilities. The following is a discussion of certain important patient rights outlined in the Universal Bill of Rights for Mental Health Patients (Box 3.1), first established by the President's Commission on Mental Health and later made into law by the Mental Health Systems Act of 1980.

Americans With Disabilities Act and Job Discrimination

The Americans With Disabilities Act of 1990 (ADA) makes it unlawful to discriminate in employment against a qualified individual with a disability. The ADA also outlaws discrimination against individuals with disabilities in state and local government services, public accommodations, transportation, and telecommunication. The ADA defines an individual with a disability as a person who has a physical or mental impairment that substantially limits one or more major life activities, has a record of such impairment, or is regarded as having such an impairment (U.S. Equal Employment Opportunity Commission, 2002). An employer is free to select the most qualified applicant available, but if the most qualified person has a mental disorder, this law mandates that reasonable accommodations need to be made for that individual. Accommodations are any adjustments to a job or work environment, such as restructuring a job, modifying work schedules, and acquiring or modifying equipment.

ISSUES OF CONSENT

Self-Determinism

A self-determined individual chooses a course of action without being restrained by others' expectations. Personal autonomy and avoidance of dependence on others are key values.

BOX 3.1

Universal Bill of Rights for Mental Health Patients

1. The right to appropriate treatment and related services in a setting and under conditions that are the most supportive of such person's personal liberty, and restrict such liberty only to the extent necessary consistent with such person's treatment needs, applicable requirement of law, and applicable judicial orders.
2. The right to an individualized, written treatment or service plan (such plan to be developed promptly after admission of such person), the right to treatment based on such plan, the right to periodic review and reassessment of treatment and related service needs, and the right to appropriate revision of such plan, including any revision necessary to provide a description of mental health services that may be needed after such person is discharged from such program or facility.
3. The right to ongoing participation, in a manner appropriate to a person's capabilities, in the planning of mental health services to be provided (including the right to participate in the development and periodic revision of the plan).
4. The right to be provided with a reasonable explanation, in terms and language appropriate to a person's condition and ability to understand, regarding the person's general mental and physical (if appropriate) condition, the objectives of treatment, the nature and significant possible adverse effects of recommended treatment, the reasons a particular treatment is considered, the reasons access to certain visitors may not be appropriate, and any appropriate and available alternative treatments, services, and types of providers of mental health services.
5. The right not to receive a mode or course of treatment in the absence of informed, voluntary, written consent to treatment except during an emergency situation.
6. The right not to participate in experimentation in the absence of informed, voluntary, written consent (includes human subject protection).
7. The right to freedom from restraint or seclusion, other than as a mode or course of treatment or restraint or seclusion during an emergency situation with a written order by a responsible mental health professional.
8. The right to a humane treatment environment that affords reasonable protection from harm and appropriate privacy with regard to personal needs.
9. The right to access, on request, to such person's mental health care records.
10. The right, in the case of a person admitted on a residential or inpatient care basis, to converse with others privately, to have convenient and reasonable access to the telephone and mails, and to see visitors during regularly scheduled hours. (For treatment purposes, specific individuals may be excluded.)
11. The right to be informed promptly and in writing at the time of admission.
12. The right to assert grievances with respect to infringement of these rights.
13. The right to exercise these rights without reprisal.
14. The right of referral to other providers.

Title II, Public Law 99-319, *Restatement of Bill of Rights for Mental Health Patients,* Title II—Restatement of Bill of Rights for Mental Health Patients established by Mental Health Systems Act of 1980.

KEY CONCEPT Self-determinism can be defined as being empowered or having the free will to make moral judgments.

A self-determined individual has intrinsic motivation to make choices based on personal goals, not to please others or to be rewarded. That is, a person engages in activities that are interesting, challenging, pleasing, exciting, or fun, requiring no rewards other than the positive feelings that accompany them (Eisenberger & Rhoades, 2001). Researchers believe that self-determinism is a basic and fundamental psychological need.

In mental health care, self-determinism is the right to choose one's own health-related behaviors, which at times differ from those recommended by health professionals. A patient's right to refuse treatment; to choose the second or third best health care recommendation, rather than the first; and to seek a second opinion are all self-deterministic acts. In mental health care, compliance with treatment regimens may be at odds with the self-deterministic views of an individual. Supporting an individual's ability to choose treatment becomes complex because of related issues of competency, informed consent, voluntary and involuntary commitment, and public safety.

Self-Determination Act

A competent individual can make a decision about a treatment—a decision that can be honored if that person becomes incompetent. The Patient Self-Determination Act (PSDA) was implemented on December 1, 1991, as a part of the Omnibus Budget Reconciliation Act of 1990 and requires hospitals, health maintenance organizations, skilled nursing facilities, home health agencies, and hospices receiving Medicare and Medicaid reimbursement to inform patients at the time of admission of their right to be a central part of any and all health care decisions made about them or for them. These rights include that patients

- Be provided with information regarding advance care documents
- Be asked at admission or enrollment whether they have an advance care document and that this fact be recorded in the medical record
- Be provided with information on their rights to complete advance care documents and refuse medical care (Omnibus Budget Reconciliation Act, 1990).

The Act also requires health care institutions receiving Medicare and Medicaid reimbursement to educate health care personnel and the local community about advance care planning.

Advance Care Directives in Mental Health

Advance care directives include treatment directives, often referred to as living wills, and appointment directives, often referred to as power of attorney or health proxies. A living will states what treatment should be omitted or refused in the event that a person is unable to make those decisions. A durable power of attorney for health care appoints a proxy, usually a relative or trusted friend, to make health care decisions on that individual's behalf if that person is incapacitated. An advance directive does not need to be written, reviewed, or signed by an attorney. It must be witnessed by two people and notarized and applies only if the individual is unable to make his or her own decisions as a result of being incapacitated or if, in the opinion of two physicians, the person is otherwise unable to make decisions for himself or herself.

States have started to legislate separate statutes for advance care directives in mental health. This declaration must be made in advance and signed by the patient and two witnesses. Although a physician can override this declaration during times when the patient's decision-making capacity is clearly distorted because of mental illness, the patient must be informed first and the order made by the court.

Competency

In psychiatric–mental health care, individuals may make poor treatment decisions because they are experiencing symptoms of their illness. These individuals would most likely make different choices if they did not have symptoms. One of the most important concepts underlying the legal rights of individuals is competency to consent to or to refuse treatment.

Although competency is a legal determination, it is not clearly defined across the states. It is generally agreed that **competence**, or the degree to which the patient can understand and appreciate the information given during the consent process, refers to a patient's cognitive ability to process information at a specific time. A patient may be competent to make a treatment decision at one time and not be competent at another time. Competence is also decision specific, so that a patient may be competent to decide on a simple treatment with a relatively clear consequence, but may not be competent to decide about a treatment with a complex set of outcomes. A competent patient can refuse any aspect of the treatment plan, except in the case of an emergency (Masten & Curtis, 2000).

Competency is different from rationality, which is a characteristic of a patient's decision, not of the patient's ability to make a decision. An irrational decision is one that involves hurting oneself pointlessly, such as stopping recommended treatment even though symptoms return. A person who is competent may make what appears to be an irrational decision, and it cannot be overruled by health care providers; however, if a person is judged **incompetent** (i.e., unable to understand and appreciate the information given during the consent process), it is possible to force treatment on the individual. Strong arguments are made, however, against forced treatment under these circumstances. Forced treatment denigrates individuals, and according to self-determinism theory, individuals are not as likely to experience treatment success if it is externally imposed.

Informed Consent

Individuals seeking mental health care must provide **informed consent**, the right to determine what shall be done with their body and mind. To provide informed consent, the patient must be given adequate information upon which to base decisions about care and is thus an active participant who ultimately decides the course of treatment. Informed consent is not an option but is mandated by state and provincial laws. In most states or provinces, the law mandates that a mental health provider must inform a patient in such a way that an average reasonable person would be able to make an educated decision about the interventions.

Informed consent is complicated in mental health treatment. A patient must be competent to give consent, but the individual's decision-making ability often is compromised by the mental illness. This dilemma might be illustrated by a situation in which a person who is informed of medication side effects refuses treatment, not because of the potential negative impact of the medication, but because he or she denies the illness outright. The health care provider knows that once the person begins taking the medication, the symptoms of the illness will subside, and the decision-making ability will return. Thus, an adequate mental status of the patient is the basis of the informed consent dilemma.

How is it determined that a patient is competent to give informed consent? Mental health legal experts generally agree that four areas should be directly assessed (Applebaum & Grisso, 1988; Galen, 1993). The patient who is competent to give informed consent should be able to achieve the following:

- Communicate choices
- Understand relevant information
- Appreciate the situation and its consequences
- Use a logical thought process to compare the risks and benefits of treatment options.

These areas are further explained in Table 3.1. In mental health care, informed consent is important because of the potential side effects of many of the treatments, including medications and electroconvulsive therapy. Once consent is given, nursing and medical personnel are absolved from legal liability for actions they take, provided they practice according to discipline standards (see Chapter 5). Most institutions have policies that outline the nursing responsibilities within the informed consent process. The nurse has a key role in the process of informed consent, from structuring the written informed consent document to educating the patient about a particular procedure. The nurse makes sure that consent has been obtained before any treatment is given. Informed consent is especially important in research projects involving experimental drugs or therapies.

Voluntary and Involuntary Treatment

Patients seeking mental health treatment gain access to the delivery system by seeking the care of a mental health provider. The process is similar to that of seeking any other type of health care. Treatment is recommended and agreed on by both the provider and the individual, and the individual then complies with the treatment. If hospitalization is required, the person enters the treatment facility, participates in the treatment planning process, and follows through with the treatment. This individual maintains all civil rights and is free to leave at any time, even if it is against medical advice. In most set-

Table 3.1 Determination of Competency

Assessment Area	Definition	Patient Attributes
Communicate choices	Ability to express choices	Patient should be able to repeat what he or she has heard
Understand relevant information	Capacity to comprehend the meaning of the information given about treatment	Patient should be able to paraphrase understanding of treatment
Appreciate the situation and its consequence	Capacity to grasp what the information means specifically to the patient	Patient should be able to discuss the disorder, the need for treatment, the likely outcomes, and the reason the treatment is being suggested
Use a logical thought process to compare the risks and benefits of treatment options	Capacity to reach a logical conclusion consistent with the starting premise	Patient should be able to discuss logical reasons for the choice of treatment

tings, this type of admission is called a **voluntary admission**. If an individual is admitted to a public facility, the state statute may refer to the process as **voluntary commitment**, rather than admission; however, in both instances, full legal rights are retained.

Involuntary commitment is the confined hospitalization of a person without the person's consent but with a court order. There are also legal provisions for people to be involuntarily committed to outpatient mental health facilities through state civil laws. Because involuntary commitment to mental health agencies is a province of state laws, each state and the District of Columbia have separate commitment statutes; however, three common elements are found in most of these statutes. The individual must be (1) mentally disordered, (2) dangerous to self or others, or (3) unable to provide for basic needs (i.e., "gravely disabled"). Involuntary commitment is a fairly common occurrence. In one study conducted in an urban psychiatric emergency service, most (N = 347 or 55.9%) of the patients entered the psychiatric emergency service with an involuntary legal status (Segal, Laurie, & Segal, 2001).

Commitment procedures vary considerably among the states and provinces. Most have provisions for an emergency short-term hospitalization of 48 to 92 hours authorized by a certified mental health provider without court approval. At the end of that period, the individual either agrees to voluntary treatment, or extended commitment procedures are begun that can be renewed for periods of 90 days or 6 months. The judge must order the commitment, and the individual is afforded several legal rights, including notice of the proceedings, a full hearing (jury trial if requested) in which the government must prove the grounds for commitment, and the right to legal counsel at state expense.

• NCLEXNOTE

NCLEXNOTE

Which patient is most likely a candidate for involuntary commitment? A patient who refuses to take medication or one who is singing in the street in the middle of the night disturbing the neighbors?

The patient who is singing in the night disturbing the neighbors. Rationale: patients have a right to refuse medication in many states and provinces. Refusing medication does not pose an immediate danger to self or others. The patient who is singing in the street is more likely to be judged as a danger to self or to others.

RIGHT TO TREATMENT IN THE LEAST RESTRICTIVE ENVIRONMENT

Not only do people who are involuntarily committed have the right to receive treatment, but they also may have the right to refuse it. Arguments over the rights of civilly committed patients to refuse treatment first surfaced in 1975, when a federal district court judge issued a temporary restraining order prohibiting the use of psychotropic medication against the patient's will at a state hospital in Boston. Today, laws about commitment and refusal of medication vary from state to state. Many states recognize the rights of involuntary patients to refuse medication (National Mental Health Information Center, 2007). The state trend is to grant patients the right to refuse treatment.

The right to refuse treatment is related to a larger concept—the right to be treated in the **least restrictive environment**—which means that an individual cannot be restricted to an institution when he or she can be successfully treated in the community. In 1975, the courts ruled that a person committed to psychiatric treatment had a right to be treated in the least restrictive environment (Dixon *v.* Weinberger, 1975). Medication cannot be given unnecessarily. An individual cannot be restrained or locked in a room unless all other "less restrictive" interventions are tried first.

ISSUES OF CONFIDENTIALITY

Communication between patient and health care provider is protected by law. Psychiatric mental health care requires an intense level of communication in which extremely personal information is shared. Often, the information relates to other people; for example, information regarding a married woman's sexual fantasy about her coworker is confidential and cannot be shared with her husband. However, under certain circumstances, confidential information needs to be shared with others, such as when a patient relates an intention to harm someone else. Although laws have been enacted to protect patients' privacy, maintain confidentiality, and protect human rights, laws have also been enacted to protect society from actions of people with symptoms that may endanger others. The following section discusses the issues related to privacy and confidentiality.

Privacy Versus Confidentiality

Privacy refers to that part of an individual's personal life that is not governed by society's laws and government intrusion. Protecting an individual from intrusion is a responsibility of health care providers. **Confidentiality** can be defined as an ethical duty of nondisclosure. The provider who receives confidential information must protect that information from being accessed by others and resist disclosing it. Confidentiality involves two people: the individual who discloses and the person with whom the information is shared. If confidentiality is broken, a person's privacy is also violated; however, a person's privacy can be violated but confidentiality maintained. For example, if a nurse observes an adult patient reading pornography alone in his or her room, the patient's privacy has been violated. If the patient asks the nurse not to tell anyone and the request is honored, confidentiality is maintained.

Maintaining a person's privacy and protecting confidentiality involve legal and ethical considerations. A **breach of confidentiality** is the release of patient information without the patient's consent in the absence of legal compulsion or authorization to release information (Wettstein, 1994). For example, discussing a patient's problem with one of his or her relatives without the patient's consent is a **breach of confidentiality**. Even sharing patient information with another professional who is not involved in the patient's care is a breach of confidentiality because the individual has not given permission for the information to be shared. Maintaining confidentiality is not as easy as it first appears. Because of confidentiality laws, family members are legally excluded from receiving any information about an adult member without consent, even if that member is receiving care from the family. Ideally, a patient gives consent for information to be shared with the family.

Health Insurance Portability and Accountability Act

The Health Insurance Portability and Accountability Act of 1996 (HIPAA) provides legal protection in several areas of health care, including privacy and confidentiality. This act protects working Americans from losing existing health care coverage when changing jobs and increases opportunities for purchasing health care. It regulates the use and release of patient information, especially electronic transfer of health information. Effective April 2003, HIPAA regulations require patient authorization for the release of information with the exception of that required for treatment, payment, and health care administrative operations. The release of information related to psychotherapy requires patient permission. The underlying intent is to prevent the release of information to agencies not related to health care, such as employers, without the patient's consent. When this information is released, the patient must agree to the exact information that is being disclosed, the purpose of disclosure, the recipient of the information, and an expiration date for the disclosure of information (U.S. Department of Health and Human Services, 2002).

Mandates to Inform

At certain times, a professional is legally obligated to breach confidentiality. When there is a judgment that the patient has harmed any person or is about to injure someone, the professional is mandated by law to report it to authorities. The legal "duty to warn" was a result of the 1976 decision of *Tarasoff v. Regents of the University of California*. In this case, a 26-year-old graduate student told university psychologists about his obsession with another student, Tatiana Tarasoff, whom he subsequently killed. Tatiana Tarasoff's parents initiated a separate civil action and brought suit against the therapist, the university, and the campus police, claiming that Tatiana's death was a result of negligence on the part of the defendants.

The plaintiffs claimed that the therapists should have warned Ms. Tarasoff that the graduate student presented a danger to her and that he should have been confined to a hospital. Both claims were originally dismissed in the lower courts, but in 1974, the California Supreme Court reversed the lower courts' decisions and said that Ms. Tarasoff should have been warned. The high court said that psychotherapists have a duty to warn the foreseeable victims of their patients' violent actions. Because of the outcry from professional mental health organizations, the court agreed to review the case, and in 1976, the original decision was revised by the ruling that psychotherapists have a duty to exercise reasonable care in protecting the foreseeable victims of their patients' violent actions. The results of this case have had far-reaching consequences and have influenced many decisions in the United States and Canada (Borum & Reddy, 2001; Gutheil, 2001).

Although many lawsuits have been based on the Tarasoff case, most have failed. Usually, if there are clear threats of violence toward others, the therapist is mandated to warn potential victims.

• NCLEXNOTE

NCLEXNOTE

What guides the intervention for a patient who tells the nurse that he (she) wants to hurt a family member: mandate to inform or HIPAA?

Mandate to inform. Rationale: Because others are at risk for injury, the Tarasoff decision will prevail.

DOCUMENTATION AND LEGAL ISSUES

Documentation is a portrayal of the patient, nursing care, and responses to nursing care. It can be handwritten or computer generated. Patient records contain the data for evidence-based care. It is very common in psychiatric care that all disciplines record their activities on one progress note. Patients also have access to their records. Nursing documentation is based on nursing standards (see Chapter 5) and the policies of the particular facility. Of the various documentation styles that are used, many are problem focused. That is, documentation is focused on specific problems that are identified on the nursing care plan or interdisciplinary treatment plan. No matter the setting or structure of the documentation, nurses are responsible for documenting the following:

- Observations of patients' subjective and objective physical, psychological, and social responses to mental disorders and emotional problems
- Interventions implemented
- Evaluation of outcomes of interventions.

Particular attention should be paid to the reason the patient is admitted for care. Nurses are always responsible for monitoring therapeutic actions and side effects of medications that are administered. If the person's initial problem was suicide or homicidal ideation, the patient should routinely be assessed for suicidal and homicidal thoughts, even if the treatment plan does not specifically identify suicide and homicide as potential problems. Careful documentation is always needed for patients who are suicidal, homicidal, aggressive, or restrained in any way. Medications prescribed on an as-needed (PRN) basis also require a separate entry, including reason for administration, dosage, route, and response to the medication.

Patient records are legal documents. As such, they can be used in courts of law. The records often are the only written evidence of a patient's problems at the time of care and are the only documentation verifying the behavior of the patient and that care has been provided. Courts consider acts not recorded as acts not done. The entries should always be written in pen, with no erasures. If an entry is corrected, it should be initialed by the person making the correction. Any entry should be clear, well written, and void of jargon. Judgmental statements, such as "patient is manipulating staff" have no place in patients' records. Only meaningful, accurate, objective descriptions of the behavior should be used. General, stereotypic statements, such as "had a good night" or "no complaints" are meaningless and should be avoided.

Legal Processes and Psychiatric Nursing Practice

Malpractice is based on a set of **torts** (a civil wrong not based on contract committed by one person that causes injury to another). An **assault** is the threat of unlawful force to inflict bodily injury upon another. An assault must be imminent and cause reasonable apprehension in the individual. Battery is the intentional and unpermitted contact with another. **Medical battery**, intentional and unauthorized harmful or offensive contact, occurs when a patient is treated without informed consent. For example, a clinician who fails to obtain consent prior to performing a procedure is subject to medical battery. Also, failure to respect a patient's advance directives is considered medical battery. **False imprisonment** is the detention or imprisonment contrary to provision of the law. Facilities who do not discharge voluntarily committed patients upon request can be subject to this type of litigation.

Negligence is a breach of duty of reasonable care for a patient that the nurse is responsible for that results in personal injuries. A clinician who does get consent, but does not disclose the nature of the procedure and the risks involved is subject to a negligence claim. Five elements are required to prove negligence: duty (accepting assignment to care for patient), breach of duty (failure to practice according to acceptable standards of care), cause in fact (the injury would not have happened if the standards had been followed), cause in proximity (harm actually occurred within the scope of foreseeable consequence), and damages (physical or emotional injury caused by breach of standard of care). Simple mistakes are not negligent acts.

Lawsuits in Psychiatric Mental Health Care

Few lawsuits are filed against mental health clinicians and facilities when compared with other health care areas. If psychiatric nurses are included in lawsuits, they are usually included in the lawsuit filed against agency. Common areas of litigation surround the nursing care of patients who are suicidal or violent. See chapters 17 and 38. Maintaining and documenting an appropriate standard of care can protect a nurse from complicated legal proceedings. See Chapter 5. The following can help prevent negative outcomes of malpractice litigations:

- Evaluate risks, especially when privileges broaden or care is transferred
- Document decisional processes and reasons for choices among alternatives
- Involve family in important decisions
- Make decisions within team model and document this shared responsibility
- Adhere to agency's policy and procedures
- Seek consultation and record input

LAWS AND SYSTEMS THAT PROTECT HUMAN RIGHTS

The rights of people with mental disorders, emotional problems, and mental retardation are of special concern because of the vulnerability of this population to stigmatization and societal abuse. Title II of Public Law 99-319, Restatement of Bill of Rights for Mental Health Patients, reaffirms the Bill of Rights for Mental Health Patients originally recommended by the President's Commission on Mental Health and part of the Mental Health Systems Act of 1980. These rights are guaranteed by federal law to each person admitted to a program or facility for the purpose of receiving mental health services.

Internal Rights Protection System

To help combat any violation of rights, mental health care systems in the United States have developed protective mechanisms that exist within their organizations and make up the **internal rights protection system**. This system was set up by Public Law 99-319, the Protection and Advocacy for Mentally Ill Individuals Act of 1986, which requires each state mental health provider to establish and operate a system that protects and advocates the rights of individuals with mental illnesses and investigates any incidents of abuse and neglect. As states authorized the formation of their respective advocacy and protection systems, they developed their own Bill of Rights based on the federal Bill of Rights. Although there may be variation among states, all states incorporate the rights listed in Box 3.1.

FAME AND FORTUNE

Elizabeth Parsons Ware Packard (1816–1895)

Author and Social Reformer

Public Persona

Elizabeth Packard, social reformer in the latter half of the 19th century, lived in Chicago and, later, in Springfield, Illinois. She supported herself and her six children through her writings and books that exposed the abuse of patients committed to insane asylums of the day. After her children were grown, Elizabeth Packard lobbied legislators in the Illinois state capital on behalf of her reforms.

Personal Realities

In 1864, Elizabeth Packard was committed to the Illinois State Hospital for the Insane based solely on her husband's assertion that her religious views were different from his. In reality, she was not sufficiently subordinate to her husband. Illinois law at the time permitted any married man to consign his wife to the asylum with no requirement other than consent of the asylum superintendent. Elizabeth Packard was incarcerated in the hospital for 3 years, during which she rejected any treatment offered.

Source: Lightner, D.L. (1999). *Asylum, prison, and poorhouse: The writings and reform work of Dorothea Dix in Illinois.* Carbondale and Edwardsville: Southern Illinois University Press.

External Advocacy Systems

Organizations that operate outside these mental health agencies and serve as advocates for the rights and treatment of mental health patients are part of an **external advocacy system**. Some of these organizations include the American Hospital Association, American Healthcare Association, the American Public Health Association, and the United Nations. They are financially and administratively independent from the state agencies. These groups advocate through negotiation and recommendations but have no legal authority. In instances in which agencies believe their advocacy attempts are unsuccessful, they can resort to litigation that leads to lawsuits and consent decrees (legal mandates that are monitored by the U.S. Department of Justice) or, in some instances, a denial of **accreditation** to the health care institution by their certifying body.

Accreditation of Mental Health Care Delivery Systems

Mental health care is regulated by many different agencies, and nursing is integrally involved with meeting the agency accreditation standards. **Accreditation** is the process by which any mental health agency is judged by established standards to be providing acceptable quality of care. Accreditation is important to the consumer because it not only ensures that the institution meets the acceptable standards of quality of care but also is necessary for third-party payers (managed care companies, Medicare) to reimburse facilities.

Mental health agencies are accredited by a variety of organizations. One of the most influential organizations in the United States health care system is the Joint Commission on Accreditation of Healthcare Organizations (JCAHO), the body that accredits hospitals in the United States. One of JCAHO's survey areas is patient rights. Thus, all institutions seeking accreditation from this organization must also meet its patients' rights standards. The Centers for Medicare and Medicaid Services (CMS) sets accreditation standards for institutions seeking Medicare and Medicaid funding. Community mental health centers are not accredited by either JCAHO or CMS, but by another accrediting agency, the Commission on Accreditation of Rehabilitation Facilities.

SUMMARY OF KEY POINTS

- The right of self-determination entitles all patients to refuse treatment, to obtain other opinions, and to choose other forms of treatment. It is one of the basic patients' rights established by Title II, Public Law 99-139, outlining the Universal Bill of Rights for Mental Health Patients.

- Informed consent is another protective right that helps patients decide what can be done to their bodies and minds. It must be obtained from a competent individual before any treatment is begun to ensure that the information is not only received but understood. A competent person can refuse any treatment. Incompetence is determined by the court when the patient cannot understand the information. Nurses play a key role in informed consent by making sure that the patient is competent and understands the risks and interventions.
- The right to the least restrictive environment entitles patients to be treated in the least restrictive setting and by the least restrictive interventions, and protects patients from unnecessary confinement and medication.
- Laws and systems are established to protect the rights of the mentally disordered. The internal rights protection system operates from within the state mental health system and consists of special departments or agencies that monitor the treatment of patients in the system according to the Universal Patient Bill of Rights and state regulations and laws.
- The external advocacy system comprises organizations working outside the state and federal systems to protect the rights of the mentally disordered or handicapped and includes the American Hospital Association, American Healthcare Association, American Public Health Association, and the United Nations, all of which are involved in setting standards and licensing procedures.

CRITICAL THINKING CHALLENGES

1. Consider the relationship of self-determinism to competence by differentiating patients who are competent to give consent and those who are incompetent. Discuss the steps in determining whether a patient is competent to provide informed consent for a treatment.
2. Define competency to consent to or refuse treatment and relate the definition to the Self-Determination Act.
3. A patient is involuntarily admitted to a psychiatric unit and refuses all medication. After being unable to persuade the patient to take prescribed medication, the nurse documents the patient's refusal and notifies the prescriber. Should the nurse attempt to give the medication without patient consent? Support your answer.
4. A person who is homeless with a mental illness refuses any treatment. While he is clearly psychotic and would benefit from treatment, he is not a danger to himself or others and seems to be able to provide basic needs. His family is desperate for him to be treated. What are the ethical issues underlying this situation?
5. Discuss the purposes of living wills and health proxies. Discuss their use in psychiatric–mental health care.
6. Identify the legal and ethical issues underlying the Tarasoff case and mandates to inform.
7. Compare the authority and responsibilities of the internal rights protection system with those of the external advocacy system.

Nuts: 1987. Starring Barbra Streisand, Richard Dreyfuss, Maureen Stapleton, Eli Wallach, Robert Webber. A strong-willed, high-priced prostitute is accused of manslaughter. Her family and attorney want her to plead guilty by reason of insanity. The movie revolves around the family's attempt to have her declared incompetent to stand trial, which would commit her to a mental health center before she can go to trial. She insists on proving her sanity, and to discover the truth, her lawyer must battle his prejudice and her inexplicable belligerence.

VIEWING POINTS: Watch how the family members attempt to use the competency hearings for maintaining family secrets.

REFERENCES

Applebaum, P., & Grisso, T. (1988). Assessing patients' capacities to consent to treatment. *New England Journal of Medicine, 319,* 1635–1638.

Borum, R., & Reddy, M. (2001). Assessing violence risk in Tarasoff situations: A fact-based model of inquiry. *Behavioral Science and the Law, 19* (3), 375–386.

Dixon v. Weinberger, 405 F. Supp. 974 (D.D.C. 1975).

Eisenberger, R., & Rhoades, L. (2001). Incremental effects of reward on creativity. *Journal of Personality Social Psychology, 81,* 728–741.

Galen, K. (1993). Assessing psychiatric patients' competency to agree to treatment plans. *Hospital and Community Psychiatry, 44,* 362–364.

Gutheil, T. G. (2001). Moral justification for Tarasoff-type warnings and breach of confidentiality: A clinician's perspective. *Behavioral Science and the Law, 19,* 345–354.

Masten, A.S., & Curtis, W. J. (2000). Integrating competence and psychopathology: Pathways toward a comprehensive science of adaptation in development. *Development and Psychopathology, 12,* 529–550.

National Mental Health Information Center (2007). Know your rights. Center for Mental Health Service. Substance Abuse and Mental Health Services Administration. http://mentalhealth.Samhoa.gov. Retrieved March 8, 2007.

Omnibus Budget Reconciliation Act of 1990. Public Law No. 101–158, Paragraph 4206, 4751.

Segal, S. P., Laurie, T. A., & Segal, M. J. (2001). Factors in the use of coercive retention in civil commitment evaluations in psychiatric emergency services. *Psychiatric Services, 52*, 514–520.

Tarasoff v. Regents of the University of California, 551P. 2d 334 (Cal. 1976).

U.S. Department of Health and Human Services. (2002). Standards for privacy of individually identifiable health information; final rule. *Federal Register, 65*, 53182–53273.

U.S. Equal Employment Opportunity Commission, Office of the Americans With Disabilities Act. (2002). The Americans With Disabilities Act: Questions and answers. Washington, DC: U.S. Government Printing Office. Available at: www.usdoj.gov/q&aeng02.htm.

Wettstein, R. (1994). Confidentiality. In J. Oldham & M. Riba (Eds.), *Review of Psychiatry* (Vol. 13, pp. 343–364). Washington, DC: American Psychiatric Press.

CHAPTER

4

Mental Health Care in the Community

Denise M. Gibson, Robert B. Noud, & Peggy El-Mallakh

KEY CONCEPT

- continuum of care

LEARNING OBJECTIVES

After studying this chapter, you will be able to:

- Identify the different treatment settings and associated programs along the continuum of care.
- Discuss the role of the nurse at different points along the continuum of care.
- Describe current health care trends in psychiatric services.
- Explain how the concept of the least restrictive environment influences the assessment of patients for placement in different treatment settings.
- Discuss the influence of managed care on services and use of services in the continuum of care.

KEY TERMS

Assertive Community Treatment • board-and-care homes • case management • clubhouse model • continuum of care • coordination of care • crisis intervention • in-home mental health care • intensive case management • intensive residential services • intensive outpatient program • least restrictive environment • managed care organizations • outpatient detoxification • partial hospitalization • psychiatric rehabilitation programs • referral • reintegration • relapse • residential services • stabilization • therapeutic foster care • transfer • 23-hour observation

The evolution of a behavioral health care system is affected by scientific advances and social factors. The long-term nature of mental illnesses requires varying levels of care at different stages of the disorders as well as family and community support. Treatment costs are shared among public and private sectors. A demand exists for a comprehensive, holistic approach to care that encompasses all levels of need. Consumers, families, providers, advocacy groups, and third-party payers of mental health care no longer accept long-term institutionalization, once the hallmark of psychiatric care. Instead, they advocate for short-term treatment in an environment that promotes dignity and well-being while meeting the patient's biologic, psychological, and social needs.

Reimbursement issues have influenced health care. In the United States, health maintenance organizations (HMOs), preferred provider organizations (PPOs), Medicaid, and Medicare have set limits on the type and length of treatment for which they provide reimbursement coverage, which in turn influences the kind of care the patient receives. In other countries, other regulatory bodies influence access and treatment options. Fragmentation of services is a constant threat. Today, psychiatric–mental health nurses face the challenge of providing mental health care within a complex system that is affected by financial constraints and narrowed treatment requirements.

DEFINING THE CONTINUUM OF CARE

An individual's needs for ongoing clinical treatment and care are matched with the intensity of professional health services. The **continuum of care** for mental health services can be viewed from various perspectives and ranges from intense treatment (hospitalization) to supportive interventions (outpatient therapy).

KEY CONCEPT A **continuum of care** consists of an integrated system of settings, services, health care clinicians, and care levels, spanning illness-to-wellness states.

In a continuum, continuity of care is provided over an extended time. The appropriate medical, nursing, psychological, or social services may be delivered within one organization or across multiple organizations. The continuum facilitates the stability, continuity, and comprehensiveness of service to an individual and maximizes the **coordination of care** and services.

Least Restrictive Environment

The primary goal of the continuum of care is to provide treatment that allows the patient to achieve the highest level of functioning in the **least restrictive environment** (see Chapter 3). In 1999, the U.S. Supreme Court reinforced the principle of least restrictive environment with the Olmstead decision, which states that the unjustified institutionalization of people with disabilities is discrimination and a violation of the Americans with Disabilities Act (Center for Mental Health Services, 2004). Therefore, treatment is usually delivered in the community (as opposed to a hospital or institution) and, ideally, in an outpatient setting (Wasylenki et al., 2000).

Coordination of Care

Coordination of care is the integration of appropriate services so that individualized care is provided. Appropriate services are those that are tailored to address a client's strengths and weaknesses, cultural context, service preferences, and recovery goals, including **referral** to community resources and liaisons with others (e.g., physician, health care organizations, community services). Several agencies could be involved, but when care is coordinated, a person's needs are met without duplication of services. Coordination of care requires collaborative and cooperative relationships among many services, including primary care, public health, mental health, social services, housing, education, and criminal justice, to name a few.

In some instances, a whole array of integrated services are needed. For example, children can benefit from treatment and specialized support at home and school. These wraparound services represent a unique set of community services and natural supports individualized for the child or adult and family to achieve a positive set of outcomes.

Case Management

Coordinated care is often accomplished through a **case management** service model, in which a case manager locates services, links the patient with these services, and then monitors the patient's receipt of these services. This type of case management is referred to as the "broker" model. Case management can be provided by an individual or a team; it may include both face-to-face and telephone contact with the patient, as well as contact with other service providers. **Intensive case management** is targeted for adults with serious mental illnesses or children with serious emotional disturbances. Managers of such cases have fewer caseloads and higher levels of professional training than do traditional case managers.

Case management is an integral part of mental health services and is organized around fundamental elements, including a comprehensive needs assessment, development of a plan of care to meet those needs, a method of ensuring the individual has access to care, and a method of monitoring the care provided. Case management services are most effective when a strong working alliance develops between the patient and the case manager (Hopkins & Ramsundar, 2006). Through case management, access to care is increased through coordinated efforts that reduce fragmentation of care and diminish health care costs (Chan, Mackenzie, Tin-Fu, & Ka-yi Leung, 2000). In addition, case managers can optimize a patient's use of resources by developing a treatment plan that closely matches the individual needs of the patient (Hopkins & Ramsundar, 2006) and by matching the most appropriate treatment to the phase of illness that the patient is in (Herrick & Bartlett, 2004).

The Nurse As Case Manager

Psychiatric nurses serve in various pivotal functions across the continuum of care. These functions can involve both direct care and coordination of the care delivered by others. The case manager role is one in which the nurse must have commanding knowledge and special training in individual and group psychotherapy, psychopharmacology, and psychosocial rehabilitation. The nurse must have expertise not only in psychopathology and up-to-date treatment modalities, but also in treating the family as a unit. Modalities include the therapeutic use of self, networking and social systems, **crisis intervention,** pharmacology, physical assessment, psychosocial and functional assessment, and psychiatric rehabilitation. The repertoire of required skills includes collaborative, teaching, management, leadership, group, and research skills. The nurse as case manager probably is the most diverse role within the psychiatric continuum.

Mental Health Services in a Continuum of Care

Crisis Intervention

An organized approach is required to treat individuals in crisis, including a mechanism for rapid access to care (within 24 hours), a referral for hospitalization, or access to outpatient services. Crisis intervention treatment is brief, usually fewer than 6 hours (see Chapter 37). This type of short-term care focuses on **stabilization,** symptom reduction, and prevention of **relapse** requiring inpatient services.

Crisis intervention units can be found in the emergency department of a general or psychiatric hospital or in crisis centers within a community mental health center. Patients in crisis demonstrate severe symptoms of acute mental illness, including labile mood swings, suicidal ideation, or self-injurious behaviors. Therefore, this treatment option commands a high degree of nursing expertise. Patients in crisis usually require medications such as anxiolytics or benzodiazepines for symptom management. Key nursing roles include assessment of short-term therapeutic interventions and medication administration. Nurses also facilitate referrals for admission to the hospital or for outpatient services.

23-Hour Observation

The use of **23-hour observation** is a short-term treatment that serves the patient in immediate but short-term crisis. This type of care admits individuals to an inpatient setting for as long as 23 hours, during which time services are provided at a less-than-acute care level. The clinical problem usually is a transient disruption of baseline function, which will resolve quickly. Usually, the individual presents a threat to self or others. The nurse's role in this treatment modality is assessment and monitoring. Medications also are usually administered. This treatment is used for acute trauma, such as rape, alcohol and narcotic detoxification, and for individuals with Axis II personality disorders who present with self-injurious behaviors.

Crisis Stabilization

When the immediate crisis does not resolve quickly, crisis stabilization is the next step. This type of care usually lasts fewer than 7 days and has a symptom-based indication for hospital admission. The primary purpose of stabilization is control of precipitating symptoms through medications, behavioral interventions, and coordination with other agencies for appropriate after-care. The major focus of nursing care in a short-term inpatient setting is symptom management. Ongoing assessment; short-term, focused interventions; and medication administration and monitoring of efficacy and side effects are major components of nursing care during stabilization. Nurses also may provide focused group psychotherapy designed to develop and strengthen the personal management strategies of patients. When treating aggressive or violent patients, the nurse monitors the appropriate use of seclusion and restraints. The 1-hour rule that requires a physician or licensed independent practitioner to evaluate a patient within 1 hour after restraint or seclusion applies (Lee & Gurney, 2002).

Acute Inpatient Care

Acute inpatient hospitalization involves the most intensive treatment and is considered the most restrictive setting in the continuum. Inpatient treatment is reserved for acutely ill patients who, because of a mental illness, meet one or more of three criteria: high risk for harming themselves, high risk for harming others, or unable to care for their basic needs. Delivery of inpatient care can occur in a psychiatric hospital, psychiatric unit within a general hospital, or a state-operated mental hospital.

Admission to inpatient environments can be voluntary or involuntary (see Chapter 3). The average length of stay for an involuntary admission ranges between 24 hours and several days, depending on the state or province laws; whereas the length of stay for a voluntary admission depends on the acuity of symptoms and the patient's ability to pay the costs of treatment. It is unconstitutional in the United States to confine a nondangerous mentally ill person who can survive independently with the help of willing and responsible family or friends (Davison, 2000). Nevertheless, the interdisciplinary treatment team determines that the patient is no longer at risk to self or others before discharge can occur.

Both the number of available beds in psychiatric hospitals in the United States and length of inpatient stay have continually decreased since the 1980s, a trend attributed to managed care and expansion of multidisciplinary, intensive community-based services, such as Assertive Community Treatment (ACT) (Center for Mental Health Services, 2004; Schreter, 2004). Additional contributors to decreased length of stay include cost-containment mechanisms, such as strict admission criteria, utilization review, case management, and contractual arrangements with third-party payers (Leslie & Rosenheck, 2000).

Partial Hospitalization

During the 1980s, the costs associated with inpatient adult psychiatric and substance abuse treatment exceeded the clinical benefits when compared with outpatient care (Wise, 2000). **Partial hospitalization** programs (PHPs) or "day hospital" care were developed. Day hospital services complement inpatient mental health care and outpatient services and provide treatment to patients with acute psychiatric symptoms who are experiencing a decline in social or occupational functioning, who cannot function autonomously on a daily basis, or who do not pose imminent danger to themselves or others. It is a time-limited, ambulatory, active treatment program that offers therapeutically intensive, coordinated, and structured clinical services within a stable milieu. The aim of PHPs is patient stabilization without hospitalization or reduced length of inpatient care. An alternative to inpatient treatment, PHP usually provides the resources to support therapeutic activities both for full-day and half-day programs. This level of care does not include overnight hospital care; however, the patient can be admitted for inpatient care within 24 hours. The now-dwindling number of PHPs peaked in 2000 (National Association of Psychiatric Health Systems, 2002). Admissions and visits to the PHPs that remain have increased.

In partial hospitalization, the interdisciplinary treatment team devises and executes a comprehensive plan of care encompassing behavioral therapy, social skills training, basic living skills training, education regarding illness and symptom identification and relapse prevention, community survival skills training, relaxation training, nutrition and exercise counseling, and other forms of expressive therapy. Compared with other outpatient programs, PHPs offer more intensive nursing care.

Residential Services

Residential services provide a place for people to reside during a 24-hour period or any portion of the day, on an ongoing basis. A residential facility can be publicly or privately owned. **Intensive residential services** are intensively staffed for patient treatment. These services may include medical, nursing, psychosocial, vocational, recreational, or other support services. Combining residential care and mental health services, this treatment form offers rehabilitation and therapy to people with serious and persistent mental illnesses, including chronic schizophrenia, bipolar disorder, and unrelenting depression. These services may provide short-term treatment for stays from 24 hours to 3 or 6 months or long-term treatment for several months to years.

As a result of deinstitutionalization, many patients who were unable to live independently were discharged from state hospitals to intermediate- or skilled-care nursing facilities. The use of nursing homes for residential care is controversial because many of these facilities lack mental health services. Residential care in nursing homes varies from state to state. If a facility serves a primarily geriatric population, placement of younger persons there can be problematic. If a facility with more than 16 beds is engaged primarily in providing diagnosis, treatment, or care of persons with mental disorders (including medical attention, nursing care, and related services), it is designated by the federal government as an institution for mental disease (IMD). A Medicare-certified facility having more than 16 beds and at least 50% of residents with a mental disorder is also considered an IMD. An IMD does not qualify for matching federal Medicaid dollars, which means that the state has principal responsibility for funding inpatient psychiatric services (Centers for Medicaid and Medicare Services, 2002).

Nursing plays an important role in the care of people who have severe and persistent mental illnesses and who

FAME AND FORTUNE

Gheel, Belgium

Community With Mission

Since the 13th century, the entire village of Gheel, Belgium has been committed to helping the mentally ill. In this small community, people with mental illness are adopted into families and truly become a part of their foster family system throughout their lives. The commitment is carried through from generation to generation. This legendary system of foster family care for the mentally ill began centuries ago. The following describes how it all began.

Dymphna was born in Northern Ireland in the 7th century to a pagan chieftain and Christian mother. Her mother died when Dymphna was young. Her father became mentally ill following her death and was unable to find a woman to replace her. When Dymphna was 14, the father wanted to marry his daughter. She refused and fled to Gheel with the assistance of others, including a Christian priest. The father hunted them down and beheaded Dymphna and the priest. The spot where they were killed became a shrine. Miraculous cures of mental illnesses and epilepsy have been reported at the shrine. In the Catholic church, Saint Dymphna is invoked as the patron of those suffering from nervous and mental illnesses.

Source: Goldstein, J. L., & Godemont, M. M. L. (2003). The legend and lessons of Gheel, Belgium: A 1500-year-old legend, a 21st century model. *Community Mental Health Journal, 39(5)*, 441–438.

require long-term stays at residential treatment facilities. Nurses provide basic psychiatric nursing care with a focus on psychoeducation, basic social skills training, aggression management, activities of daily living (ADLs) training, and group living. Education on symptom management, understanding mental illnesses, and medication is essential to recovery. The Scope and Standards of Psychiatric–Mental Health Nursing Practice guide the nurse in delivering patient care (American Nurses Association, American Psychiatric Nurses Association, 2000). See Chapter 5.

Respite Residential Care

Sometimes families of a person with mental illness who lives at home may be unable to provide care continuously. In such cases, respite residential care can provide short-term necessary housing for the patient and periodic relief for the caregivers.

In-home Mental Health Care

If at all possible, a person with a mental illness lives at home, not a residential treatment setting. Choices, not placement; physical and social integration, not segregated and congregate grouping by disability; and individualized flexible services and support, not standardized levels of service, are the goals. When a person can live at home but outpatient care does not meet the treatment needs, in-**home mental health care** may be provided. Home care emphasizes the personal autonomy of the patient and the need for a trusting, collaborative relationship between the nurse and the patient (Magnusson, Severinsson, & Lutzen, 2003). In this setting, direct patient care and case management skills are used to decrease hospital stays and increase the functionality of the patient within the home. Individuals who most benefit from in-home mental health care include patients with chronic, persistent mental illness or patients with mental illness and co-morbid medical conditions that require ongoing monitoring.

In-home mental health care services rely on the skills of the mental health nurse in providing ongoing assessment and implementing a comprehensive, individualized treatment plan of care. Components of the care plan and the ongoing assessment include data on mental health status, the environment, medication compliance, family dynamics and home safety, supportive psychotherapy, psychoeducation, coordination of services delivered by other home care staff, and communication of clinical issues to the patient's psychiatrist. In addition, the plan should address care related to collecting laboratory specimens (blood tests) and crisis intervention to reduce rehospitalization (see Box 4-1).

BOX 4.1

Research for Best Practice: Reaching Out to Elderly With Psychiatric Illness

Rabins, P. V., et al. (2000). Effectiveness of a nursing-based outreach program for identifying and treating psychiatric illness in the elderly. Journal of the American Medical Association, 283(21), 2802–2809.

The Question: This study asked whether a nurse-based mobile outreach program for seriously mentally ill elderly persons is more effective than usual care in reducing levels of depression, psychiatric symptoms, and undesirable moves (nursing home placement eviction, board and care placement).

Methods: A prospective randomized trial was conducted in six urban public housing sites for elderly persons in Baltimore, Maryland. A total of 945 (83%) of 1,195 residents underwent screening for psychiatric illness. Among those screened, 342 screened positive and 603 screened negative. Residents in three buildings were randomized to receive the PATCH model intervention, which included educating building staff to be case finders, performing assessment in resident apartments, and providing care when indicated. Residents in the other three buildings were randomized to receive usual care.

Findings: At 26 months, people with psychiatric diagnoses at the intervention sites had significantly lower depression and psychiatric symptom scores than did those at the nontreatment comparison sites.

Implications for Nursing: This research supports the effectiveness of home visits and providing education to the support network as well as to patients.

Outpatient Care

Outpatient care is a level of care that occurs outside of a hospital or institution. Outpatient services usually are less intensive and are provided to patients who do not require inpatient, residential, or home care environments. Many patients enroll in outpatient services immediately upon discharge from an inpatient setting. Outpatient treatment can include ongoing medication management, skills training, supportive group therapy, substance abuse counseling, social support services, and case management (Timko, Dixon, & Moos, 2005). Many outpatient mental health clinics have developed integrated mental health–primary care treatment models to address the physical health needs of those with mental illnesses (Druss, Rohrbaugh, Levinson, & Rosenheck, 2002). These varying services promote community reintegration, symptom management, and optimal patient functioning. Outpatient services are provided by private practices, clinics, and community mental health centers.

Intensive Outpatient Programs

The primary focus of **intensive outpatient programs** is on stabilization and relapse prevention for highly vulnerable individuals who function autonomously on a daily basis. People who meet these criteria have returned to their previous lifestyle, e.g., interacting with family, resuming work, or returning to school. Attendance in this type of program benefits individuals who still require frequent monitoring and support within a therapeutic milieu that enables them to remain connected to the community. The duration of treatment and level of services rendered are based on the patient's immediate needs. Treatment duration usually is time limited, with sessions offered 3 to 4 hours per day and 2 to 3 days per week. The treatment activities of the intensive outpatient program are similar to those offered in PHPs, but PHPs emphasize social skills training, whereas intensive outpatient programs teach patients about stress management, illness, medication, and relapse prevention.

Supportive Employment

Supportive employment services assist individuals to find work; assess individuals' skills, attitudes, behaviors, and interest relevant to work; offer vocational rehabilitation or other training; and provide work opportunities. Supportive employment programs are new, highly individualized, and competitive. They provide on-site support and job-coaching services on a one-to-one basis. They occur in real work settings and are used for patients with severe mental illnesses. The primary focus is to maintain attachment between the mentally ill person and the work force. Transitional employment programs offer the same support as supported employment programs, but the employment is temporary. This type of work has a time frame agreed on by the employer and the participant. The person works at the temporary position until he or she can find permanent, competitive employment (Bustillo, Laurillo, Horan, & Keith, 2001).

Other Services Integrated into a Continuum of Care

Within the continuum of care, other outpatient services may be received separately or simultaneously within various settings. They involve discrete services and patient variables. Table 4-1 defines the six levels of service variables along the continuum. Table 4-2 outlines the patient variables.

Outpatient Detoxification

Except for situations involving severe or complicated withdrawal, alcohol and drug rehabilitation is now almost exclusively outpatient based. Patients with alcohol dependence who show signs of tolerance and withdrawal can undergo detoxification in an ambulatory care setting. However, patients who undergo ambulatory detoxification must have reliable family members who are available to provide monitoring. In addition, those who have a history of a seizure disorder, pregnancy, or current severe alcohol withdrawal, especially with delirium, cannot be treated for alcohol withdrawal in an ambulatory care setting (Blondell, 2005). **Outpatient detoxification** is a specialized form of partial hospitalization for patients requiring medical supervision. During the initial withdrawal phase, use of a 23-hour bed may be a treatment option, depending on the stage of withdrawal and the type of addictive substance used. Or the patient may be required to attend a detoxification program 4 to 5 days per week until symptoms resolve. The length of participation depends on the severity of addiction.

Outpatient detoxification includes the 12-step recovery model, such as Alcoholics Anonymous (AA) and Narcotics Anonymous (NA), which provides outpatient involvement with professionals experienced in addiction counseling. It encourages abstinence and provides training in stress management and relapse prevention. Ala-Non and Ala-Teen rely on 12-step support for families, who are usually included in the treatment program.

In-home Detoxification

There is an increasing shift toward outpatient detoxification of patients with alcohol addiction. Although a reported 64,000–140,000 Americans die from an alcohol related factor, few with alcohol problems receive formal treatment (USDHH, 2007). Except for situations involving severe or complicated withdrawal or for adolescents, alcohol detoxification may be implemented on an outpatient basis. In such cases, the nurse is required to visit the patient daily for medication monitoring during the patient's first week of sobriety. Daily visits are necessary until the patient is in medically stable condition. Referrals may come from primary care physicians, court mandates, or employee assistance programs.

Assertive Community Treatment

The **Assertive Community Treatment** (ACT) model is a multidisciplinary clinical team approach providing 24-hour, intensive community services in the individual's natural setting that helps individuals with serious mental illness live in the community. The ACT approach provides a comprehensive range of treatment, rehabilitation, and supportive services to help patients meet the requirements of community living. Concentration of services for high-risk patients within a single multiservice team enhances continuity and coordination of care, improving both the quality of care and its cost-effectiveness (Bustillo et al., 2001). Initially, patients receive frequent direct

Table 4.1 The Continuum of Behavioral Health Care: Service Variables

Primary Care	Outpatient	Multimodal Outpatient	Intermediate Ambulatory	Acute Ambulatory	Inpatient Residential
Service Function					
Provision of screening, early identification, and education; medication management	Decrease symptoms related to mild to moderate disorders; maintenance of stability (patient with severe disorders)	Coordinated treatment to prevent decline in functioning when outpatient service cannot meet patient need	Stabilization, symptom reduction, and prevention of relapse	Crisis stabilization and acute symptom reduction; alternative to and prevention of hospitalization	Provision of 24-hour monitoring, supervision, and intensive intervention
Scheduled Programming					
Incorporated with visits for general medical care	Sessions as needed with maximum of 3 hours per week	A minimum of 4 hours per week	Minimum of 3–4 hours per day, at least 2–3 days per week	Minimum of 4 hours per day scheduled 4–7 days	24 hours per day
Crisis Backup Availability					
Decision-assistance programs; established liaison with behavioral health specialty care	On-call coverage	A 24-hour crisis and consultation service	A 24-hour crisis and consultation service	An organized, integrated 24-hour crisis backup system with immediate access to current clinical and treatment information	24-hour-per-day staffing with personnel skilled in crisis intervention
Medical Involvement					
Not applicable	Medical consultation PRN	Medical consultation PRN	Medical consultation	Medical supervision	Medical management
Accessibility					
Regular appointments scheduled within 3–5 days	Regular appointments scheduled within 3–5 days	Capable of admitting within 72 hours	Capable of admitting within 48 hours	Capable of admitting within 24 hours	Capable of admitting within 1 hour
Milieu					
Relationship between provider and patient	Within the session and relationship between provider and patient	Active therapeutic; primarily within home and community	Active therapeutic within treatment setting and home and community	Preplanned, consistent, and therapeutic; primarily within treatment setting	Preplanned, consistent, and therapeutic within treatment setting
Structure					
Minimal structure via scheduled appointments	Minimal structure via scheduled appointments	Individualized and coordinated	Regularly scheduled, individualized	High degree of structure and scheduling	High degree of structure, security, and supervision
Responsibility and Control					
Patient functions independently with support from family and community	Patient functions independently with support from family and community	Monitoring and support mostly by patient, family, and support system	Monitoring and support shared with patient, family, and support system	Staff aggressively monitors and supports patients and family	Staff assumes responsibility for safety and security of patient
Service Examples					
Regular medical check-up	Outpatient office visit; speciality group; psychotherapy	After-care; clubhouse programs	Psychosocial rehabilitation; day-treatment programs; intensive outpatient; 23-hour respite beds	Day hospital; intensive in-home crisis intervention; outpatient detoxification; 23-hour observation beds	Acute inpatient unit; crisis stabilization bed

From http://www.aabh.org/public.

Table 4.2 The Continuum of Behavioral Health Care: Patient Variables

Primary Care	Outpatient	Multimodal Outpatient	Intermediate Ambulatory	Acute Ambulatory	Inpatient Residential
Level of Functioning					
At-risk, subclinical, or mild impairment	Mild to moderate impairment in at least one area of daily life	Moderate impairment in at least one area of daily life	Marked impairment in at least one area of daily life	Severe impairment in multiple areas of daily life	Significant impairment with inability to maintain activities of daily living without 24-hour assistance
Psychiatric Signs and Symptoms					
At-risk, subclinical presentation, or mild symptoms related to behavioral health disorder	Mild to moderate symptoms related to acute condition or exacerbation of severe or persistent disorder	Moderate symptoms related to acute condition or exacerbation of severe or persistent disorder	Moderate to severe symptoms related to acute condition or exacerbation of severe or persistent disorder	Severe to disabling symptoms related to acute condition or exacerbation of severe or persistent disorder	Disabling symptoms related to acute condition or exacerbation of severe or persistent disorder
Risk, Dangerousness					
At-risk or limited with minimal need for confinement	Limited, transient dangerousness and minimal risk for confinement	Mild instability with limited dangerousness and low risk for confinement	Moderate instability and/or dangerousness with some risk for confinement	Marked instability and/or dangerousness with high risk for confinement	Significant danger to self or others
Commitment to Treatment Follow-through					
Ability to form and maintain treatment contract	Ability to form and sustain treatment contract	Ability to sustain treatment contract with intermittent monitoring and support	Limited ability to form extended treatment contract; requires frequent monitoring and support	Inability to form more than initial treatment contract; requires close monitoring and support	Inability to form treatment contract; requires constant monitoring and supervision
Social Support System					
Ability to form and maintain relationships outside of treatment	Ability to form and maintain relationships outside of treatment	Ability to form and maintain relationships outside of treatment	Limited ability to form relationships or seek support	Impaired ability to access or use caregiver, family, or community support	Insufficient resources and/or inability to access or use caregiver, family, or community support

From http://www.aabh.org/public.

assistance while reintegrating into the community. Emergency telephone numbers, or crisis numbers, are shared with patients and their families in the event that immediate assistance is needed. The ACT program is staffed 24 hours a day for emergency referral. Mobile treatment teams often are a part of the ACT model and provide assertive outreach, crisis intervention, and independent-living assistance with linkage to necessary support services. ACT services have been effective in reducing hospitalizations and use of costly emergency room services (Kane & Blank, 2004).

Psychiatric Rehabilitation and the Nurse's Role

Psychiatric rehabilitation programs, also termed psychosocial rehabilitation, focus on the reintegration of people with psychiatric disabilities into the community through work, education, and social avenues while addressing their medical and residential needs. The goal is to empower patients to achieve the highest level of functioning possible. Therapeutic activities or interventions are provided individually or in groups. They may include development and maintenance of daily and community-living skills, such as communication (basic language), vocational, self-care (grooming, bodily care, feeding), and social skills that help patients function in the community. These programs promote increased functioning with the least necessary ongoing professional intervention. Psychiatric rehabilitation provides a highly structured environment, similar to a PHP, in a variety of settings, such as office buildings, hospital outpatient units, and freestanding structures.

The mental health nurse's role continues to adapt to the changing needs of persons with mental illness. As behavioral health care delivery occurs more in outpatient settings, so does the work of the nurse. Most rehabilitation programs have a full-time nurse who functions as part of the multidisciplinary team.

The psychiatric-rehabilitation nurse is concerned with the holistic evaluation of the person and with assessing and educating the patient on compliance issues, necessary laboratory work, and environmental and lifestyle issues. This evaluation assesses the five dimensions of a person—physical, emotional, intellectual, social, and spiritual—and emphasizes psychiatric rehabilitation. Issues of psychotropic medication—evaluation of response, monitoring of side effects, and connection with pharmacy services—also fall to the nurse.

Clubhouse Model

The **clubhouse model** is a form of psychosocial rehabilitation that aims to reintegrate a person with mental illness into the community. Fountain House in New York City developed the clubhouse model in the 1940s. Its belief system involves membership and belonging—being wanted, needed, and expected. Additional fundamental beliefs include: all members of society can be productive; every human aspires to achieve gainful employment; humans require social contacts, and programs are incomplete if they offer recreational, social, and vocational opportunities but neglect housing needs (Bustillo et al., 2001).

Fountain House seeks to improve its members' quality of life by organizing daytime support, providing meaningful daytime activities, and offering opportunities for paid labor. Clubhouses are a unique treatment form because they are entirely run by patients with psychiatric illnesses with minimal assistance from mental health professionals. Patients who join a clubhouse are voluntary members, and they are expected to help operate the house. Membership is not time limited. Generally, members do not live in the clubhouse; however, the clubhouse may have formed relationships with providers of low-cost housing. Open 365 days a year, services are available any time an individual needs them. Fountain House remains the model for other clubhouses. Today, about 200 clubhouses are active across the United States.

Members of the clubhouse are expected to assist with household chores, follow instructions of others, volunteer for tasks, and be punctual. Most new members begin vocational training by participating in work units at the clubhouse, such as janitorial services, meal preparation, clerical services, public relations, and maintenance services. As members improve, they may move on to transitional employment, which is part-time paid work outside the clubhouse setting. When vocational skills have been acquired, members move into competitive employment.

The role of the staff person in this unique setting is different than in other inpatient and outpatient settings. Because a clubhouse is operated by its members, staff roles are limited. The focus of the staff member is to accentuate the skills and performance of the members. The employee works with, rather than for, the member. The clubhouse model requires the employee nurse to function as a member of the clubhouse and be active in all components of the program. Although the nurse has expertise in pathology of mental illness, the focus is strictly on the individual's recovery. Case management in the clubhouse setting requires staff to participate in work units or transitional employment settings with members. More commonly, a nurse plays a pivotal role in urging a patient's participation in a clubhouse program and may actually refer patients to the program.

Relapse Prevention After-Care Programs

Relapse of mental illness symptoms and substance abuse is the major reason for rehospitalization in the United States. Relapse is the recurrence or marked increase in severity of the symptoms of a disease, especially after a period of apparent improvement or stability. Many issues affect a person's well-being. First and foremost, patients must feel that their lives are meaningful and worthwhile. Homelessness and unemployment create tremendous threats to a person's identity and feelings of wellness.

Much work has gone into relapse-prevention programs for the major mental illnesses and addiction disorders. Relapse prevention programs involve both patients and families and seek to (1) educate them about the illness, (2) enable them to cope with the chronic nature of the illness, (3) teach them to recognize early warning signs of relapse, (4) educate them about prescribed medications and the need for compliance, and (5) inform them about other disease management strategies (i.e., stress management, exercise) in preventing relapse.

Nurses become involved in relapse prevention programs in several different ways. They can act as a referral source for the programs, trainer or leader of the programs, or an after-care source for patients when the program is completed. In addition, mental health nurses can help the patient and family by promoting optimism, sticking to goals and aspirations, and focusing on individual strengths.

Technology-Based Care

Access to mental health services is frequently inadequate in rural communities due to clinician shortages, lack of public transportation, and poverty. Rural communities are addressing barriers to care by creating alternative, technology-based ways to connect nurses with their patients. Telephone contact with patients after discharge from the hospital allows nurses to assess psychiatric symptoms, check on medication adherence, discuss approaches to solving problems associated with community living, and provide emotional support (Beebe & Tian, 2004). Patients who receive telephone contacts from nurses after discharge are more comfortable talking on the phone if the nurse meets with the patient before discharge to establish rapport. Telemedicine uses video teleconferencing equipment to link health care professionals with patients in remote rural areas. Providers of specialty psychiatric services in university settings can use telemedicine to conduct psychiatric assessments, diagnose, provide education, and consult with local providers in the care of community-based patients who need special individualized care (Tschirch, Walker, & Calvacca, 2006).

Alternative Housing Arrangements

Housing is an important factor in successful community transition. Patients with psychiatric disabilities who are homeless are a vulnerable population. Over 40% of homeless people have a serious mental illness, which increases their risk for substance abuse, inability to access health care, assaults, incarceration, and physical health problems (Folsom et al., 2005). Therefore, one of the largest hurdles to overcome in treating the severely mentally ill patient is finding appropriate housing that will meet the patient's immediate social, financial, and safety needs. The course of chronic mental illness, as symptoms wax and wane, preys on the stamina of families and caregivers. Most individuals live in some form of supervised or supported community living situation, which ranges from highly supervised congregate settings to independent apartments. The following discussion focuses on four models of alternative housing and the role of the nurse. These include personal care homes, **board-and-care homes,** supervised apartments, and **therapeutic foster care.**

Personal Care Homes

Personal care homes operate within houses in the community. Usually, 6 to 10 people live in one house, with a health care attendant providing 24-hour supervision to assist with medication monitoring or other minor activities, including transportation to appointments, meals, and self-care skills. The clientele generally are heterogenous and include elderly, mildly mentally retarded, and mentally ill patients whose severity of illness is chronic and subacute. Most states require these homes to be licensed.

Board-and-Care Homes

Board-and-care homes provide 24-hour supervision and assistance with medication, meals, and some self-care skills. Individualized attention to self-care skills and other ADLs generally is not available. These homes are licensed to house 50 to 150 people in one location. Rooms are shared, with two to four occupants per bedroom.

Therapeutic Foster Care

Therapeutic foster care is indicated for patients in need of a family-like environment and a high level of support. Therapeutic foster care is available for child, adolescent, and adult populations. This level of care actually places patients in residences of families specially trained to handle individuals with mental illnesses. The training usually consists of crisis management, medication education, and illness education. The family provides supervision, structure, and support for the individual living with them. The person who receives these services shares the responsibility of completing household chores and may be required to attend an outpatient program during the day.

Supervised Apartments

In a supervised apartment setting, individuals live in their own apartments, usually alone or with one roommate, and are responsible for all household chores and self-care. A staff member or "supervisor" stops by each apartment routinely to evaluate how well the patients are doing, make sure they are taking their medications, and ensure that the household is being maintained. The supervisor may also be required to mediate disagreements between roommates.

Role of the Nurse in Alternative Housing

The professional registered nurse typically is not employed in alternative housing settings. However, nurses play a pivotal role in the successful reintegration of patients from more restrictive inpatient settings into society. Nurses are employed in partial hospitalization programs, inpatient units, and as case managers. Therefore, nurses act as liaisons for the residential placement of patients. Nurses are employed directly as consultants or provide consultation to treatment teams during discharge planning in determining appropriate outpatient settings, evaluating medication follow-up needs, and making recommendations for necessary medical care for existing physical conditions. Feedback from the residential care providers and follow-up by the treatment team regarding the patient's response to treatment interventions are essential. Rehospitalization can be curtailed if the residential care operators identify and for-

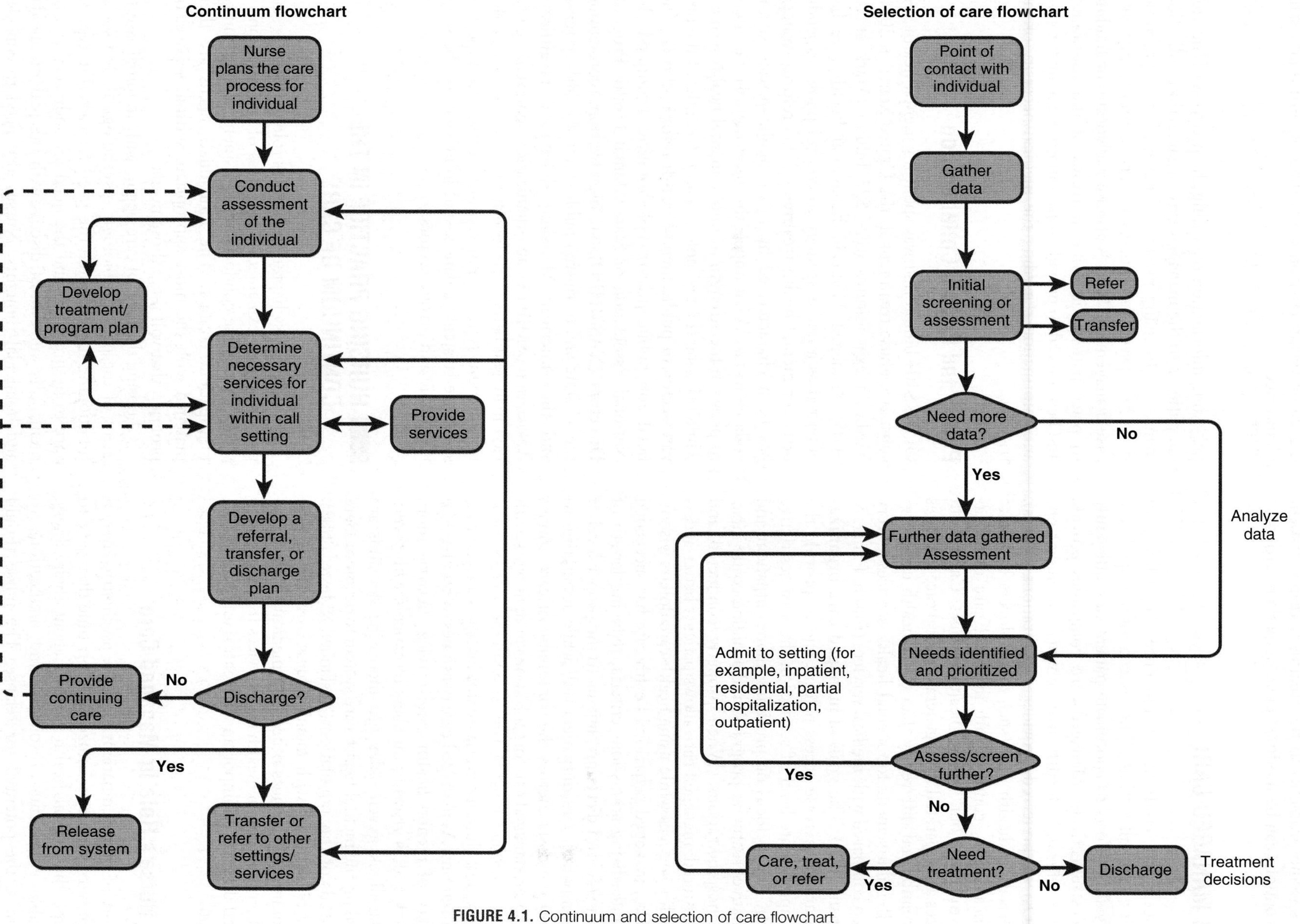

FIGURE 4.1. Continuum and selection of care flowchart

ward specific problems to the treatment teams. Patient interventions can be modified in an outpatient setting.

MANAGED CARE

Managed care continues to influence the delivery of health care in all settings. The concept of managed care emerged in efforts to coordinate patient care efficiently and cost-effectively. Managed care companies provide services through health maintenance organizations (HMOs) or preferred provider organizations (PPOs). Purchasers of health care, such as employers and state health agencies, contract with managed care organizations to "carve out" mental health services. Carved out services are separated from general medical care packages and reimbursed differently than other health care services. Reimbursement for mental health services is very limited compared with medical services (Busch, Frank, & Lehman, 2004). The goals of **managed care organizations** are to increase access to care and to provide the most appropriate level of services in the least restrictive setting. Efforts focus on providing more outpatient and alternative treatment programs and avoiding costly inpatient hospitalizations. When properly conducted and administered, managed care allows patients better access to quality services while using health care dollars wisely.

Today, managed behavioral health care has succeeded in standardizing admissions criteria, reducing length of patient stay, and directing patients to the proper level of care—inpatient and outpatient—all while attempting to control the costs. Across the continuum of care, nurses encounter managed care organizations in their work with patients, and they must be familiar with the policies, procedures, and clinical criteria established by managed care organizations. As managed care continues to regulate the delivery of mental health care, services become more limited, and as growing numbers of patients with severe mental illness reach older age, increasing demands are placed on the mental health care system to accommodate the needs of this population (Auslander & Jeste, 2002). Many older adults with mental illness currently receive no community services other than medication monitoring. Increasing home health care services for people with mental illness is an important alternative to institutionalization.

The Nurse's Role in Managed Care

Because of shorter inpatient stays, the psychiatric–mental health nurses must maximize the short time they have to educate the mental health patients about their illness, available community resources, and medications to minimize the potential for relapse. The nurse should focus on teaching social skills and self-reliance and creating empowering environments that, in turn, build self-confidence.

The interface of psychiatric–mental health nurses with managed care organizations is primarily in the form of providing information regarding the progress of individual patients to the managed care organization utilization managers. In many instances, managed care organizations hire psychiatric nurses for crisis intervention and case management. Nurses also may advocate for funding to place patients in other portions of the continuum and be required to provide substantiating documentation and information regarding the medical necessity of the transfer.

Public and Private Collaboration

Of the $104 billion that was spent for mental health and substance abuse treatment in the United States in 2001, Medicaid expenditures were $27 billion (Mark et al., 2005). Managed Medicaid behavioral health care has emerged as a major strategy to control public expenditures for mental health treatment. This reform strategy has been characterized by many public–private sector collaborations. What impels this movement is the intent to preserve the strength of public mental health systems while bringing the technologies and strengths of the private sector to public mental health reform efforts. The need for public–private collaboration prompted the National Association of State Mental Health Program Directors (NASMHPD), an organization representing the 55 state and territorial public mental health systems, and the American Managed Behavioral Healthcare Association (AMBHA), an organization representing private managed behavioral health care firms, to set guidelines for this type of joint venture. Nurses can expect to see more strategic alliances and joint ventures between the public and private sectors.

NURSING PRACTICE IN THE CONTINUUM OF CARE

Throughout this chapter, the nurse's role in different settings has been explained. Regardless of the situation or setting, the nurse conducts an assessment at the point of first patient contact. The individual's needs are then matched with the most appropriate setting, service, or program that will meet those needs.

Choosing the level of care begins with an initial assessment of the patient's biologic, psychological, and social functioning to determine the need for care, the type of care to be provided, and the need for additional assessment. The nurse must discuss with the patient suicidal and homicidal thoughts. Nurses also need to consider financial issues because funding considerations may play a part in placement options. Other factors affecting the selection of care include the type of treatment the individual seeks, his or her current physical condition and ability to consent to treatment, and the organization's ability to provide direct care or to deflect care to another service provider.

Based on the results of the initial assessment, the nurse may admit the patient into services provided at that agency or initiate a referral or transfer to provide the intensity and scope of treatment required by the individual at that point in time (Fig. 4-1). Referral involves sending an individual from one clinician to another or from one service setting to another for care or consultation. Transfer involves formally shifting responsibility for the care of an individual from one clinician to another or from one care unit to another. The processes of referral and transfer to other levels of care are integral for effective use of services along the continuum. These processes are based on the individual's assessed needs and the organization's capability to provide the care. Figure 4-1 depicts the process of assessment, treatment, transfer, and referral when considering appropriate levels of care.

Discharge Planning

Discharge planning begins upon admission of the individual at any level of health care. Most facilities have a written procedure for the discharge planning. This procedure often provides for a transfer of clinical care information when a person is referred, transferred, or discharged to another facility or level of care. All discharge planning activities should be documented in the clinical record, including the patient's response to proposed after-care treatment, follow-up for psychiatric and physical health problems, and discharge instructions. Medication education, food-drug interactions, drug-drug interactions, and special diet instructions (if applicable) are extremely important in ensuring patient safety. Discharge planning is an integral part of psychiatric nursing care and should be considered a part of the psychiatric rehabilitation process. In addressing an individual's biopsychosocial needs, one can coordinate after-care and discharge interventions for optimal outcomes. The overall goal of discharge planning is to provide the patient with all the resources he or she needs to function as independently as possible in the least restrictive environment and to avoid rehospitalization.

The nurse can optimize discharge plan compliance by involving the patient at various levels in the psychiatric milieu. Because patients with mental illnesses may have limited cognitive abilities and residual motivational and anxiety problems, nurses should explain in detail all after-care plans and instructions to the patient. It is helpful also to schedule all after-care appointments before the patient leaves the facility. The nurse should then give the patient written instructions about where and when to go for the appointment and a contact person's name and telephone number at the after-care placement. Finally, the nurse should review emergency telephone numbers and contacts and medication instructions with the patient.

Recent research has focused on the unique needs of patients who have been hospitalized for several years in state psychiatric hospitals and are ambivalent about leaving the hospital to live in the community. Supportive group therapy has been used to help patients explore conflicting thoughts and feelings about leaving a hospital setting, examine discharge goals, determine their own readiness to change living situations, and take responsibility for behaviors that promote a successful move toward discharge (Patrick, Smith, Schleifer, Morris, & McLennon, 2006). Nursing research has also involved transitional discharge nurses who work with peer support volunteers to promote successful discharge from the hospital (Reynolds et al., 2004). The transitional discharge nurse creates a working therapeutic relationship with the hospitalized patient, and continues this relationship with the patient after discharge until community-based staff members develop a working therapeutic relationship with the patient. Peer support volunteers, who are recovered mental health service users, visit the patient before discharge to offer support and encouragement and discuss issues related to re-entry into the community. They also work with the patient to develop community skills, including shopping and cooking, money management, and planning recreational activities (Reynolds et al., 2004).

SUMMARY OF KEY POINTS

- The continuum of care is a comprehensive system of services and programs designed to match the needs of the individual with the appropriate treatment in settings that vary according to levels of service, structure, and intensity of care.
- The psychiatric-mental health nurse's specific responsibilities vary according to the setting. In most settings, nurses function as members of a multidisciplinary team and assume responsibility for assessment and selection of level of care, education, evaluation of response to treatment, referral or transfer to a more appropriate level of care, and discharge planning. Discharge planning provides patients with all the resources they need to function effectively in the community and avoid rehospitalization.
- Managed care influences the continuum of care by standardizing admissions criteria and clinical guidelines for practitioners, encouraging alternative treatment

programs that avoid costly inpatient hospitalizations, and providing consumers with an integrated network of credentialed specialty behavioral health providers to help meet their needs within the community.

CRITICAL THINKING CHALLENGES

1. Define the continuum of care and discuss the importance of the least restrictive environment.
2. Differentiate the role of the nurse in each of the following continuum settings:
   a. Crisis stabilization
   b. In-home detoxification
   c. Partial hospitalization
   d. Assertive community treatment
3. Compare alternative housing arrangements, including personal care homes, board-and-care homes, therapeutic foster care, and supervised apartments.
4. Envision using more than one service at a time. What combinations of services could benefit patients and families?

REFERENCES

American Nurses Association, American Psychiatric Nurses Association. (2000). International Society for Psychiatric-Mental Health Nursing Practice. *The scope and standards of psychiatric-mental health nursing practice*. Washington, DC: American Nurses Publishing.

Auslander, L., & Jeste, D. (2002). Perceptions of problems and needs for service among middle-aged and elderly outpatients with schizophrenia and related psychotic disorders. *Community Mental Health Journal, 38* (5), 391–402.

Beebe, L. H, & Tian, L. (2004). TIPS: Telephone intervention-problem solving for persons with schizophrenia. *Issues in Mental Health Nursing, 25*, 317–329.

Blondell, R. D. (2005). Ambulatory detoxification of patients with alcohol dependence. *American Family Physician, 71* (3), 495–502, 509–510.

Busch, A. B., Frank, R. G., & Lehman, A. F. (2004). The effect of a managed behavioral health carve-out on quality of care for Medicaid patients diagnosed as having schizophrenia. *Archives of General Psychiatry, 61*, 442–448.

Bustillo, J. R., Laurillo, J., Horan, W. P., & Keith, S. J. (2001). The psychosocial treatment of schizophrenia. *American Journal of Psychiatry, 158* (2), 163–175.

Centers for Medicaid and Medicare Services. (May 15, 2002). *Institutions for mental disease*. Author: Baltimore, MD. Retrieved June 29, 2003, from www.cms.hhs.gov/medicaid/services/imd.asp.

Center for Mental Health Services. (2004). *Mental Health, United States, 2002*. Manderscheid, R. W., & Henderson, M. J. (eds.), DHHS Pub No. (SMA) 3938. Rockville, MD: Substance Abuse and Mental Health Services Administration.

Chan, S., Mackenzie, A., Tin-Fu, N. G. D., & Ka-yi Leung, J. (2000). An evaluation of the implementation of case management in the community of psychiatric nursing service. *Journal of Advanced Nursing, 31* (1), 144–156.

Davison, G. (2000). Stepped care: Doing more with less? *Journal of Consulting and Clinical Psychology, 68* (4), 580–585.

Druss, B. G., Rohrbaugh, R. M., Levinson, C. M., & Rosenheck, R. A. (2001). Integrated medical care for patients with serious psychiatric illness: A randomized trial. *Archives of General Psychiatry, 58* (9), 891–898.

Folsom, D. P., Hawthorne, W., Lindamer, L., Gilmer, T., Bailey, A., Golshan, S., et al. (2005). Prevalence and risk factors for homelessness and utilization of mental health services among 10,340 patients with serious mental illness in a large public mental health system. *American Journal of Psychiatry, 162*, 370–376.

Gold, M., & Mittler, J. (2000). Medicaid-complex goals: Challenges for managed care and behavioral health. *Health Care Financing Review, 22* (2), 85–101.

Herrick , C. A., & Bartlett, R. (2004). Psychiatric nursing case management: Past, present, and future. *Issues in Mental Health Nursing, 25*, 589–602.

Hopkins, M., & Ramsundar, N. (2006). Which factors predict case management services and how do these services relate to client outcomes? *Psychiatric Rehabilitation Services, 29* (3), 219–222.

Kane, C. F., & Blank, M. B. (2004). NPACT: Enhancing programs of assertive community treatment for the seriously mentally ill. *Community Mental Health Journal, 40* (6), 549–559.

Lee, G., & Gurney, D. (2002). The legal use of restraints. *Journal of Emergency Nursing, 28* (4), 335–337.

Leslie, D., & Rosenheck, R. (2000). Comparing quality of mental health care for public-sector and privately insured populations. *Psychiatric Services, 51* (5), 650–655.

Magnusson, A., Severinsson, E., & Lutzen, K. (2003). Reconstructing mental health nursing in home care. *Journal of Advanced Nursing, 43* (4), 351–359.

Mark, T. L., Coffey, R. M., Vandivort-Warren, R., Harwood, H. J., King, E.C., et al. (2005). US spending for mental health and substance abuse treatment, 1991–2001. *Health Affairs*, Jan-June, Supplemental Web Exclusives, W5-133 – W5-142. Retrieved August 8, 2006, from http://content.healthaffairs.org

National Association of Psychiatric Health Systems. (2003). *The annual survey report: Trends in behavioral healthcare systems*. Washington, DC: Author.

Patrick, V., Smith, R. C., Schleifer, S. J., Morris, M. E., & McLennon, K. (2006). Facilitating discharge in state psychiatric institutions: A group intervention strategy. *Psychiatric Rehabilitation Journal, 29* (3), 183–188.

Rabins, P. V., Black, B. S., Roca, R., German, P., McGuire, M., Robbins, B., et al. (2000). Effectiveness of a nurse-based outreach program for identifying and treating psychiatric illness in the elderly. *Journal of the American Medical Association, 283* (21), 2802–2809.

Reynolds, W., Lauder, W., Sharkey, S., Maciver, S., Veitch, T., & Cameron, D. (2004). The effects of a transitional discharge model for psychiatric nurses. *Journal of Psychiatric and Mental Health Nursing, 11*, 82–88.

Schreter, R. (2004). Making do with less: The latest challenge for psychiatry. *Psychiatric Services, 55* (7), 761–763.

Timko, C., Dixon, K., & Moos, R. H. (2005). Treatment for dual diagnosis patients in the psychiatric and substance abuse systems. *Mental Health Services Research, 7* (4), 229–242.

Tschirch, P., Walker, G., & Calvacca, L. T. (2006). Nursing in tele-mental health. *Journal of Psychosocial Nursing, 44* (5), 20–27.

U.S. Department of Health and Human Services. The Surgeon General's call to action to prevent and reduce underage drinking. U.S. Department of Health and Human Services. Office of the Surgeon General, 2007.

Wasylenki, D., Goering, P., Cochrane, J., Durbin, J., Rogus, J., & Prendergast, P. (2000). Tertiary mental health services. I. Key concepts. *Canadian Journal of Psychiatry, 45* (2), 179–184.

Wise, D. (2000). Mental health intensive outpatient programming: An outcome and satisfaction evaluation of a private practice model. *Professional Psychology: Research and Practice, 31* (4), 412–417.

UNIT II

Principles of Psychiatric Nursing

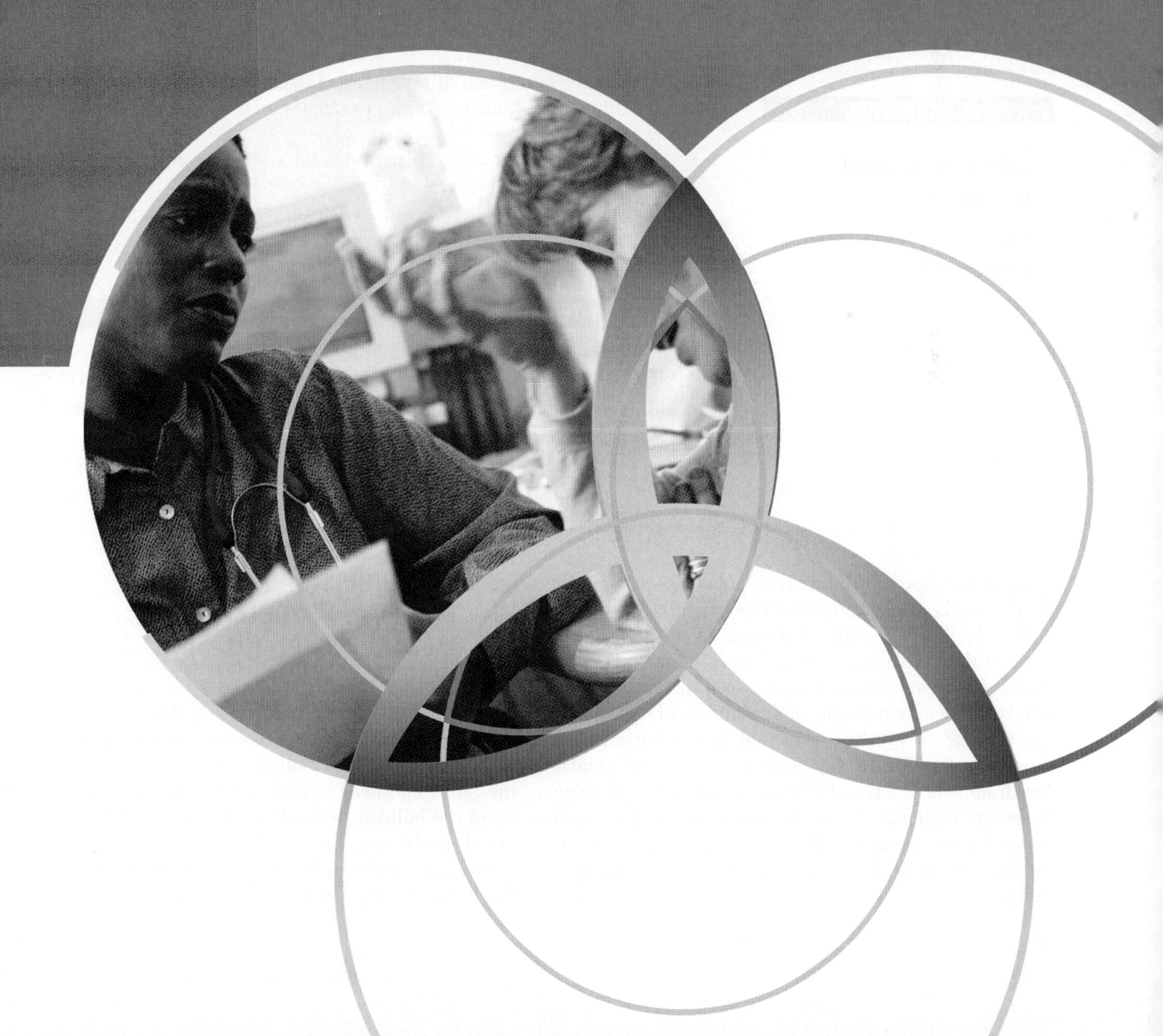

CHAPTER 5

Frameworks, Ethics, and Standards of Psychiatric Nursing

Mary Ann Boyd

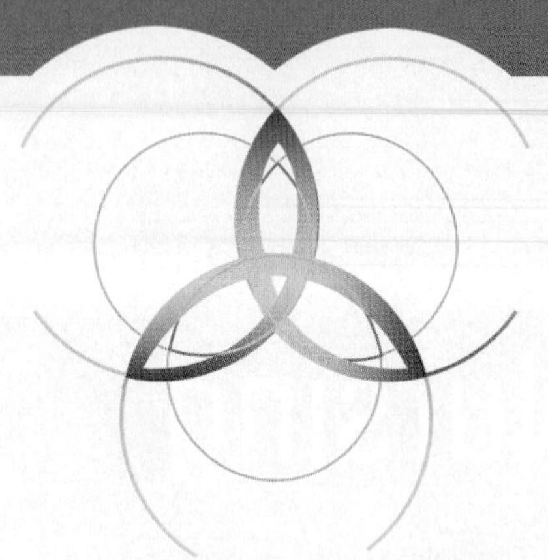

KEY CONCEPTS

- biopsychosocial model
- beneficence
- autonomy
- nursing process

LEARNING OBJECTIVES

After studying this chapter, you will be able to:

- Explain the biopsychosocial model as a psychiatric mental health nursing conceptual framework.
- Delineate the scope and standards of psychiatric–mental health nursing practice.
- Discuss the basic tools of psychiatric nursing.
- Identify ethical frameworks and principles used in the practice of psychiatric nursing.
- Discuss the impact of psychiatric–mental health nursing professional organizations on practice.
- Discuss selected challenges of psychiatric–mental health nursing.

KEY TERMS

• advanced practice psychiatric–mental health nurse • psychiatric–mental health registered nurse • clinical reasoning • fidelity • interdisciplinary approach • interdisciplinary treatment plan • justice • paternalism • nonmaleficence • reflection • standards of care • veracity

This chapter introduces the biopsychosocial model as the organizational thread for the rest of the book. The scope of practice of the psychiatric nurse is then explained, followed by a discussion of the standards of care that serve as a basis of practice. These standards are integral to the understanding of the day-to-day practice of psychiatric–mental health nursing and should be familiar to any student involved in mental health nursing practice. Ethical principles of psychiatric nurses are highlighted. The discussion of the challenges of psychiatric nursing sets the stage for the rest of the text through an overview of the dynamic nature of this specialty.

THE BIOPSYCHOSOCIAL MODEL IN PSYCHIATRIC–MENTAL HEALTH NURSING

Contemporary psychiatric nursing bases practice on many theories from the biologic, psychological, and social sciences. This holistic approach, referred to as the biopsychosocial model, is necessary to truly understand the individual who has a mental disorder or emotional problems. The model is ideal for organizing nursing care and is used throughout this text for organizing theoretic knowledge and the nursing process (see

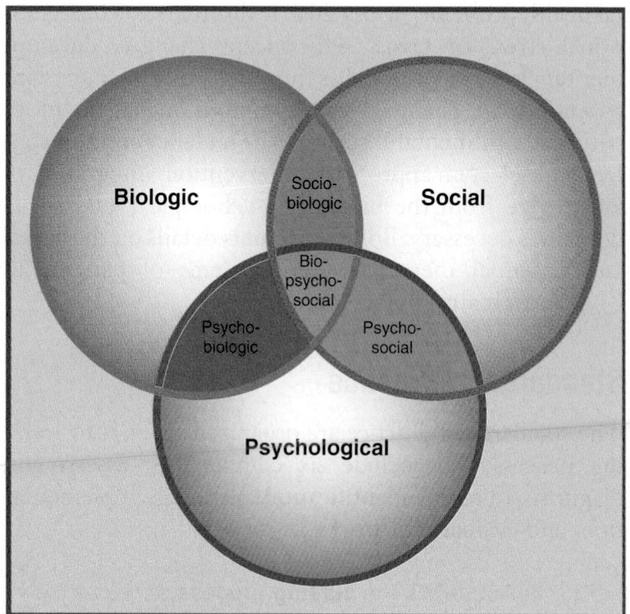

FIGURE 5.1. Continuum and selection of care flowchart.

Figure 5.1). This model is well supported in the evidence-based literature as a model of care (Currid, 2004; Borrell-Carrio, Suchman, & Epstein, 2004; Boydell, Gladstone, & Volpe, 2003). See Box 5.1 for evidence-based review.

KEY CONCEPT The **biopsychosocial model** consists of three separate but interdependent domains: biologic, psychological, and social. Each domain has an independent knowledge and treatment focus but can interact and be mutually interdependent with the other domains.

Biologic Domain

The *biologic* domain consists of the biologic theories related to mental disorders and problems as well as *all* of the biologic activity related to other health problems. Today, there is evidence of neurobiologic changes in most psychiatric disorders. Within this domain, there are also theories and concepts used as a basis of interventions focusing on the patient's physical functioning, such as exercise, sleep, and adequate nutrition. In addition, the neurobiologic theories also serve as a basis for understanding and administering pharmacologic agents (see Chapters 7 and 8).

Psychological Domain

The *psychological* domain contains the theoretical basis of the psychological processes—thoughts, feelings, and behavior (intrapersonal dynamics) that influence one's emotion, cognition, and behavior. The psychological and nursing sciences generate theories and research that are critical in understanding patient's symptoms and responses to mental disorders. Although mental disorders have a biological component, they are often manifested in psychological symptoms and physical changes. The person with a thought disorder may have bizarre behavior that needs to be interpreted within the context of the neurobiologic dysfunction of the mental disorder.

Many psychiatric nursing interventions are based on knowledge generated within this domain. Cognitive approaches, behavior therapy, and patient education are all based on the use of theories from the psychological domain. Psychiatric–mental health interventions are also based on the use of interpersonal communication techniques, which require nurses to develop awareness of their own, as well as their patient's, internal feelings and behavior. For mental health nurses, understanding their own and their patient's intrapersonal dynamics and motivation is critical in developing a therapeutic relationship and motivating patients to learn and understand their disorders and participate in their management. Motivating patients to engage in learning activities best occurs within the context of a therapeutic relationship (see Chapter 9).

Social Domain

The *social* domain includes theories that account for the influence of social forces encompassing the patient, family, and community within cultural settings. This knowledge base is generated from social and nursing sciences and explains the connections within the family and com-

BOX 5.1

Evidence-Based Review:* *Cognitive Behavior Therapy and Chronic Fatigue Syndrome

Evidence for the effectiveness of cognitive behavior therapy (CBT) in the treatment of chronic fatigue syndrome (CFS) was the focus of evidenced review. All randomized controlled trials were included in which CBT was compared with orthodox medical management. Three relevant studies met the selection criteria. These trials demonstrated that CBT significantly benefits patients with CFS when compared with orthodox medical management or relaxation.

Conclusions: Cognitive behavior therapy appears to be an effective and acceptable treatment for adult outpatients with chronic fatigue syndrome.

Price, J.R., & Couper, J. (2005) Cognitive behaviour therapy for chronic fatigue syndrome in adults (review). *Cochrane Database of Systematic Reviews*. www.cochrane.org. Retrieved May 4, 2006.

munities that affect the mental health and treatment of people with mental disorders. Psychiatric disorders are not caused by social factors, but their manifestations and treatment can be significantly affected by the society in which the patient lives. Family support can actually improve treatment outcomes. Moreover, family factors, including origin, extended family, and other significant relationships, contribute to the total understanding and treatment of patients. Community forces, including cultural and ethnic groups within larger communities, shape the patient's manifestation of disorders, response to treatment, and overall view of mental illness.

SCOPE AND STANDARDS OF PRACTICE

The practice of psychiatric nursing is regulated by law but guided by **standards of care.** The legal authority to practice nursing is granted by the states and provinces, but professional standards of care or professional nursing activities are set by professional nursing organizations. The American Nurses Association (ANA) and the psychiatric nursing organizations (discussed later in this chapter) collaborate in specifying the health problems that match the skills of psychiatric nurses and set standards of care and professional practice.

Scope of Psychiatric–Mental Health Nursing Areas of Concern

The areas of concern for the psychiatric–mental health nurse include a wide range of actual or potential mental health problems or psychiatric disorders, such as emotional stress or crisis, self-concept changes, developmental issues, physical symptoms that occur with psychological changes, and symptom management of patients with mental disorders. To understand the problem and select an appropriate intervention, integration of knowledge from the biologic, psychological, and social domain is necessary. Box 5.2 presents details on the actual and potential mental health problems of patients to whom psychiatric nurses attend.

Standards of Practice

The standards of practice are organized around the nursing process and include six components: assessment, diagnosis, outcome identification, planning, implementation, and evaluation (Box 5.3).

KEY CONCEPT The **nursing process** serves as the foundation for clinical decision-making and is used to provide an evidence base for practice (ANA, APNA, & ISPN, 2007, p. 16.).

Each standard has a measurement criteria for Psychiatric–Mental Health Registered Nurses (CRN-PMH) and Advanced Practice Registered Nurses (APRN-PMH). The fifth standard, implementation, has several subcategories that specify standards for each intervention. These standards of care represent the nursing profession's commitment to the general public. It is important that nurses know their practice standards and are able to practice at this level. Nurses ultimately are held accountable for practicing according to their standards.

BOX 5.2

Psychiatric Mental Health Nursing's Phenomena of Concern

- Promotion of optimal mental and physical health and well-being and prevention of mental illness.
- Impaired ability to function related to psychiatric, emotional, and physiological distress.
- Alterations in thinking, perceiving, and communicating due to psychiatric disorders or mental health problems.
- Behaviors and mental states that indicate potential danger to self or others.
- Emotional stress related to illness, pain, disability, and loss.
- Symptom management, side effects or toxicities associated with self-administered drugs, psychopharmacological intervention, and other treatment modalities.
- The barriers to treatment efficacy and recovery posed by alcohol and substance abuse and dependence.
- Self-concept and body image changes, developmental issues, life process changes, and end-of-life issues.
- Physical symptoms that occur along with altered psychological status.
- Psychological symptoms that occur along with altered physiological status.
- Interpersonal, organizational, sociocultural, spiritual, or environmental circumstances or events which have an effect on the mental and emotional well-being of the individual and family or community.
- Elements of recovery, including the ability to maintain housing, employment, and social support, that help individuals re-engage in seeking meaningful lives.
- Societal factors such as violence, poverty, and substance abuse.

From American Nurses Association, American Psychiatric–Mental Health Nurses Association, International Society of Psychiatric–Mental Health Nurses. (2007). Psychiatric–Mental Health Nursing: *Scope and Standards of Practice* (pp. 15–16). Silver Spring, MD: Nursebooks.org.

Standards of Professional Performance

Developing and maintaining competency is the responsibility of a professional psychiatric–mental health nurse. All nurses are expected to achieve competency in psychiatric nursing practice as specified by the standards of professional performance within the *Psychiatric–Mental Health Nursing: Scope and Standards of Practice* in the areas of quality of practice, education, professional practice evaluation, collegiality, collaboration, ethics, research, resources utilization and leadership (ANA et al., 2007) (Table 5.1).

Levels of Practice

The two levels of practice in psychiatric–mental health nursing are basic and advanced. These levels are differentiated by educational preparation, complexity of practice, and performance of nursing function (Box 5.4).

Psychiatric–Mental Health Nursing Practice

According to the *Psychiatric–Mental Health Nursing: Scope and Standards of Practice*, the RN-PMH is a registered nurse who demonstrates specialized competence and knowledge, skills, and abilities in caring for persons with mental health issues and problems and psychiatric disorders. Competency is obtained through both education and experience. The preferred educational preparation is at the baccalaureate level with credentialing by the American Nurses Credentialing Center (ANA, et al., 2007)

Nursing practice at this level is "characterized by the use of the nursing process to treat people with actual or potential mental health problems or psychiatric disorders to: promote and foster health and safety; assess dysfunction; assist persons to regain or improve their coping abilities; maximize strengths; and prevent further disability" (ANA, et al., 2007, pp. 16–17.). The nurse performs a wide range of interventions, including health promotion and health maintenance strategies, intake

BOX 5.3

Standards of Care

Standard 1. Assessment
The Psychiatric–Mental Health Registered Nurse collects comprehensive health data that is pertinent to the patient's health or situation.

Standard 2. Diagnosis
The Psychiatric–Mental Health Registered Nurse analyzes the assessment data to determine diagnoses or problems, including level of risk.

Standard 3. Outcomes Identification
The Psychiatric–Mental Health Registered Nurse identifies expected outcomes for a plan individualized to the patient or to the situation.

Standard 4. Planning
The Psychiatric–Mental Health Registered Nurse develops a plan that prescribes strategies and alternatives to attain expected outcomes.

Standard 5. Implementation
The Psychiatric–Mental Health Registered Nurse implements the identified plan.

Standard 5A Coordination of Care
The Psychiatric–Mental Health Registered Nurse coordinates care delivery.

Standard 5B Health Teaching and Health Promotion
The Psychiatric–Mental Health Registered Nurse employs strategies to promote health and a safe environment.

Standard 5C Milieu Therapy
The Psychiatric–Mental Health Registered Nurse provides structures and maintains a safe and therapeutic environment in collaboration with patients, families, and other healthcare clinicians.

Standard 5D Pharmacological, Biological, and Integrative Therapies
The Psychiatric–Mental Health Registered Nurse incorporates knowledge of pharmacological, biological, and complementary interventions with applied clinical skills to restore the patient's health and prevent further disability.

Standard 5E Prescriptive Authority and Treatment
The Psychiatric–Mental Health Advanced Practice Registered Nurse uses prescriptive authority, procedures, referrals, treatments, and therapies in accordance with state and federal laws and regulations.

Standard 5F Psychotherapy
The Psychiatric–Mental Health Advanced Practice Registered Nurse conducts individual, couples, group, and family psychotherapy using evidence-based psychotherapeutic frameworks and nurse-patient therapeutic relationships.

Standard 5G Consultation
The Psychiatric–Mental Health Advanced Practice Registered Nurse provides consultation to influence the identified plan, enhance the abilities of other clinicains to provide services for patients, and effect change.

Standard 6. Evaluation
The Psychiatric–Mental Health Registered Nurse evaluates progress toward attainment of expected outcomes.

Table 5.1 Standards of Professional Performance

Standard 7	Quality of Practice	Systematically enhances the quality and effectiveness of nursing practice
Standard 8	Education	Attains knowledge and competency that reflect current nursing practice
Standard 9	Professional Practice Evaluation	Evaluates one's own practice in relation to the professional practice standards and guidelines, relevant statures, rules, and regulations.
Standard 10	Collegiality	Interacts with and contributes to the professional development of peers and colleagues
Standard 11	Collaboration	Collaborates with patients, family and others in the conduct of nursing practice
Standard 12	Ethics	Integrates ethical provisions in all areas of practice
Standard 13	Research	Integrate research findings into practice
Standard 14	Resource Utilization	Considers factors related to safety, effectiveness, cost, and impact on practice in the planning and delivery of nursing services.
Standard 15	Leadership	Provides leadership in the professional practice setting and the profession.

From American Nurses Association, American Psychiatric–Mental Health Nurses Association, International Society of Psychiatric–Mental Health Nurses. (2007). *Psychiatric–Mental Health Nursing: Scope and Standards of Practice.* Silver Spring, MD: Nursebooks.org.

screening and evaluation and triage, case management, milieu therapy, promotion of self-care activities, psychobiologic interventions, complementary interventions, health teaching, counseling, crisis care, and psychiatric rehabilitation. An overview of psychiatric nursing interventions is presented in the chapters in Unit 3.

Advanced Practice

The **advanced practice psychiatric–mental health nurse** (APRN-PMH) is also a licensed registered nurse but is educationally prepared at the master's level and is nationally certified as a specialist by the American Nurses Credentialing Center (ANCC). The APRN-PMH is either a clinical nurse specialist (APRN-BC) or a nurse practitioner in psychiatric nursing (PMH-NP). The advanced level also includes nurses with doctoral preparation who have earned a doctorate in nursing science (DNS, DNSc) or a doctor of philosophy (PhD) degree. The emerging role of the doctorate of nursing practice (DNP) in psychiatric nursing is being developed.

The APRN-PMH's responsibilities include the complete delivery of direct primary mental health services, including, but not limited to, formulating differential diagnoses; ordering, conducting, and interpreting pertinent laboratory and diagnostic studies and procedures; conducting individual, family group, and network psychotherapy; and prescribing, monitoring, managing, and evaluating psychopharmacologic and related medication.

BOX 5.4

Clinical Activities of Psychiatric–Mental Health Nurses

Psychiatric–Mental Health Registered Nurse
Health promotion and health maintenance
Intake screening, evaluation, and triage
Case management
Provision of therapeutic and safe environments
Milieu therapy
Promotion of self-care activities
Administration of psychobiologic treatment and monitoring responses
Complementary interventions
Crisis intervention and stabilization
Psychiatric rehabilitation

Advanced Practice Registered Nurse
Psychopharmacological interventions
Psychotherapy
Community interventions
Case management
Program development and management
Clinical supervision
Consultation and liaison

TOOLS OF PSYCHIATRIC NURSING PRACTICE

Self

The most important tool of psychiatric nursing is the self. Through relationship building, patients learn to trust the nurse who then guides, teaches, and advocates for quality care and treatment. Throughout this book, the patient–nurse relationship will be emphasized.

Clinical Reasoning and Reflection

Clinical reasoning is strengthened when nurses are self-regulated learners (Kuiper & Pesut, 2004). Sound **clinical reasoning** depends on the critical thinking skills and reflection. During critical thinking activities, such as problem solving and decision making, nurses analyze evaluate, explain, infer, and interpret the biopsychosocial data. Some critical thinking activities, such as nursing assessments, take time; but many decisions are moment-to-moment, such as deciding whether a patient can leave a unit or whether a patient should receive a medication. **Reflection** involves continual self-evaluation through observing, monitoring, and judging nursing behaviors with the goal of providing ideal interventions.

Nursing Care Plans

Just like patients in medical–surgical settings, patients receiving psychiatric mental health services have a written plan of care. If only nursing care is being provided, such as in-home care, a nursing care plan may be used. If other disciplines are providing services to the same patient, which often occurs in a hospital, an individual treatment plan may be used with or instead of a traditional nursing care plan. When an interdisciplinary plan is used, components of the nursing care plan should always be easily identified. The nurse provides the care that is judged to be within the scope of practice of the psychiatric–mental health nurse. Thus, the traditional nursing care plan may or may not be used, depending on institutional policies.

Whether a nursing care plan or an individual treatment plan is used, these plans are important because they are individualized to a patient's needs. They are sometimes approved by third party payers who reimburse the cost of the service. In this text, the emphasis will be on developing nursing care plans because they serve as a basis of practice even if the interventions are included in a multidisciplinary or interdisciplinary individual treatment plan.

ETHICS OF PSYCHIATRIC NURSING

Ethical issues are clearly inherent in mental health care. The interests of the patients, nurses, health care team, and society may be in conflict and may manifest in any number of psychiatric–mental health care delivery settings. Ethical conflicts can occur when the patient is being guided by the principle of autonomy and the nurse by the principle of beneficence. The fundamental ethical principles of autonomy and beneficence are in conflict in many clinical situations.

KEY CONCEPT According to the principle of **autonomy,** each person has the fundamental right of self-determination. According to the principle of **beneficence,** the health care provider uses knowledge of science and incorporates the art of caring to develop an environment in which individuals achieve their maximal health care potential.

• NCLEXNOTE

NCLEXNOTE *Be prepared to think in terms of patient scenarios that depict the principles of beneficence versus autonomy and identify differences between views of the patient and nurse.*

Other ethical principles that guide mental health care include justice, nonmaleficence, paternalism, veracity, and fidelity. **Justice** is the duty to treat all fairly, distributing the risks and benefits equally. Justice becomes an issue when some portion of a population do not have access to health care. Basic goods should be distributed so that the least advantaged members of society are benefited. **Nonmaleficence** is the duty to cause no harm, both individual and for all. **Paternalism** is the belief that knowledge and education authorizes professionals to make decisions for the good of the patient. Mandatory use of seat belts and motorcycle helmets is an example of paternalism. This principle can be in direct conflict with the principle of autonomy. **Veracity** is the duty to tell the truth. This may seem easier than it is. Patients may ask questions where the truth is unknown. For example, if I take my medication, will the voices go away? **Fidelity** is faithfulness to obligations and duties. It is keeping promises. Fidelity is important in establishing trusting relationships.

For nurses to provide patient care within ethical frameworks, they need knowledge of basic rights and ethical principles, conceptual models as ways of thinking about ethical dilemmas, and opportunities to explore and resolve clinical dilemmas. Knowledge of the legal issues and patients' rights that have been discussed in this chapter should be used in making clinical decisions. Nursing actions in the United States are guided by the *Code for Nurses With Interpretive Statements,* adopted by the American Nurses Association (ANA) in 2001. The Code serves to inform both the nurse and society of the profession's expectations and requirements in ethical matters (Box 5.5) and provides a framework within which nurses can make ethical decisions. This document is currently being revised as a "code of ethics" for nurses.

• NCLEXNOTE

Tracking ethical decisions that the psychiatric nurse encounters in the inpatient versus outpatient setting may be a topic for examination.

Psychiatric–Mental Health Nursing Organizations

Whereas the establishment and reinforcement of standards go a long way toward legitimizing psychiatric–mental health nursing, it is professional organizations that provide leadership in shaping mental health care. They do so by providing a strong voice for meaningful legislation that promotes quality patient care and advocates for maximal use of nursing skills.

The ANA is one such organization. Although its focus is on addressing the emergent needs of nursing in general, the ANA supports psychiatric–mental health nursing practice through liaison activities, such as advocating for psychiatric–mental health nursing at the national and state levels and working closely with psychiatric–mental health nursing organizations.

The American Psychiatric Nurses Association (APNA) and the International Society of Psychiatric-Mental Health Nurses (ISPN) are two organizations for psychiatric nurses that focus on mental health care. The APNA is the largest psychiatric–mental health nursing organization, with the primary mission of advancing psychiatric–mental health nursing practice; improving mental health care for culturally diverse individuals, families, groups, and communities; and shaping health policy for the delivery of mental health services. The ISPN consists of four specialist divisions: the Association of Child and Adolescent Psychiatric Nurses, the International Society of Psychiatric Consultation Liaison Nurses, the Society for Education and Research in Psychiatric–Mental Health Nursing, and the Adult and Geropsychiatric-Mental Health Nurses. The purpose of ISPN is to unite and strengthen the presence and the voice of psychiatric–mental health nurses and to promote quality care for individuals and families with mental health problems. Both organizations have annual meetings at which new research is presented. Student memberships are available.

INTERDISCIPLINARY APPROACH AND THE NURSE'S ROLE

Psychiatric–mental health care has a long tradition of collaborating with several disciplines that are providing service to a patient at one time. An **interdisciplinary approach,** in which interventions from the different disciplines are integrated into delivery of patient care, is ideal. In the hospital, a patient may be seeing a psychiatrist for management of the disorder symptoms and for prescribed medications; a psychiatric social worker for individual psychotherapy; a psychiatric nurse for management of responses related to the mental disorder, administration of medication, and monitoring side effects; and an occupational therapist for transition into the workplace. In the community clinic, a patient may meet weekly with a therapist, monthly with a mental health provider who prescribes medication, and twice a week with a group leader in a day treatment program. All of these professionals bring a specialized skill to the patient's care.

Interdisciplinary Treatment Plans

When an **interdisciplinary treatment plan** is used, components of the nursing care plan should always be easily identified. Whether a nursing care plan or an individual treatment plan is used, these plans are important because they are individualized to a patient's needs. The psychiatric–mental health nurse can expect to collaborate with other professionals in all settings, including hospital and community. Usually, it is the nurse who coordinates the delivery of the care of these different disciplines.

CHALLENGES OF PSYCHIATRIC NURSING

The challenges of psychiatric nursing are increasing. New knowledge is being generated, technology is shaping health care into new dimensions, and nursing practice is becoming more specialized and autonomous. This section discusses a few of the challenges.

Knowledge Development, Dissemination, and Application

Knowledge is rapidly expanding in the psychiatric–mental health field. Genetic research has opened a new area of investigation into the etiology of several disorders such as schizophrenia, bipolar disorders, dementia, and autism. Neuroimmunology is investigating the role of the immune system in the development of mental disorders. The presence of comorbid medical disorders gains increasing importance in the treatment of mental disorders. For example, hypertension, hypothyroidism, hyperthyroidism, and diabetes mellitus all affect the treatment of psychiatric disorders. The challenge for psychiatric nurses today is to stay abreast

BOX 5.5

Code for Registered Nurses

1. The nurse, in all professional relationships, practices with compassion and respect for the inherent dignity, worth, and uniqueness of every individual, unrestricted by considerations of social or economic status, personal attributes, or the nature of health problems.
2. The nurse's primary commitment is to the patient, whether an individual, family, group, or community.
3. The nurse promotes, advocates for, and strives to protect the health, safety, and rights of the patients.
4. The nurse is responsible and accountable for individual nursing practice and determines the appropriate delegation of tasks consistent with the nurse's obligation to provide optimum patient care.
5. The nurse owes the same duties to self as to others, including the responsibility to preserve integrity and safety, to maintain competence, and to continue personal and professional growth.
6. The nurse participates in establishing, maintaining, and improving health care environments and conditions of employment conducive to the provision of quality health care and consistent with the values of the profession through individual and collective action.
7. The nurse participates in the advancement of the profession through contributions to practice, education, administration, and knowledge development.
8. The nurse collaborates with other health professionals and the public in promoting community, national, and international efforts to meet health needs.
9. The profession of nursing, as represented by associations and their members, is responsible for articulation of nursing values, for maintaining the integrity of the profession and its practice, and for shaping social policy.

American Nurses Association. (2001). *Code for nurses with interpretive statements.* Washington, DC: Author.

of the advances in total health care in order to provide safe, competent care to individuals with mental disorders.

Additional challenges for psychiatric nurses include updating their knowledge so that significant results of studies can be applied to the care of patients. Accessing new information through journals, electronic databases, and continuing education programs takes time and vigilance but provides a sound basis for application of new knowledge.

Overcoming Stigma

Nurses can play an important role in dispelling myths of mental illnesses. Stigma often prevents individuals from seeking help for mental health problems (see Chapter 1). The issue of stigma, identified as a major problem in *Mental Health: A Report of the Surgeon General* (U.S. Department of Health and Human Services, 1999), should be addressed by every nurse, whether or not the nurse practices psychiatric nursing. To reduce the burden of mental illness and improve access to care, nurses can educate all of their patients about the etiology, symptoms, and treatment of mental illnesses.

Health Care Delivery System Challenges

Additional continuing challenges for psychiatric nurses include providing nursing care within integrated community-based services where culturally competent, high-quality nursing care is needed to meet the emerging mental health care needs of patients. In caring for patients who require support from the social welfare system in the form of housing, job opportunities, welfare, and transportation (U.S. Department of Health and Human Services, 1999), nurses need to be knowledgeable about these systems. Moreover, in some settings, the nurse may be the only one who has a background in medical disorders, such as human immunodeficiency virus, acquired immunodeficiency syndrome, and other somatic health problems. Assertive community treatment reduces inpatient service use, promotes continuity of outpatient care, and increases the stability of people with serious mental illnesses (see Chapter 4). The nurse is involved in moving the currently fragmented health care system toward one focusing on consumer needs.

Impact of Technology

The impact of technologic advances on the delivery of psychiatric nursing care is unprecedented. Nurses are challenged to continue to develop their technical and computer skills and to use this technology in improving care. For example, telemedicine is a reality and takes many forms, from communicating with remote sites to completing educational programs. It is important that patients have the opportunity to use technology to learn about their disorders and treatment. Because many of the disorders can affect cognitive functioning, it is also important that software programs be developed that can be used by these individuals to facilitate cognitive functioning.

Another challenge related to new technology is that associated with maintaining patient confidentiality. Patient records, once stored in remote areas and rarely viewed, are now readily available and easily accessed. Nurses need to be vigilant in maintaining privacy and confidentiality. Moreover, documentation skills need to be updated continually to reflect quality patient care within the changing health care environment.

SUMMARY OF KEY POINTS

- The biopsychosocial model focuses on the three separate but interdependent dimensions of biologic, psychological, and social factors in the assessment and treatment of mental disorders. This comprehensive and holistic approach to mental disorders is the foundation for effective psychiatric–mental health nursing practice and is used as the basic organizational framework for this book.
- *Psychiatric–Mental Health Nursing, published in 2000,* established the areas of concern, standards of practice according to the nursing process, and standards of professional performance and differentiates between the functions of the RN-PMH and APRN-PMH.
- There are several ethical principles to consider when providing psychiatric nursing care, including autonomy, beneficence, justice, nonmaleficence, paternalism, veracity, and fidelity.
- Standards for ethical behaviors for professional nurses are set by national professional organizations such as the American Nurses Association.
- Nursing care plans and interdisciplinary treatment plans are written plans of care that are developed for each patient. Clinical reasoning skills are needed for developing and revising these tools.
- Several professional nursing organizations provide leadership in shaping mental health care, including the American Nurses Association, the American Psychiatric Nurses Association, and the International Society of Psychiatric–Mental Health Nurses.
- The psychiatric–mental health nurse interacts with other disciplines and many times acts as a coordinator in the delivery of care. There is always a plan of care for a patient, but it may be a nursing care plan or an individualized treatment plan that includes other disciplines.
- New challenges facing psychiatric nurses are emerging. Interpretation of research findings will assume new importance in the care of individuals with psychiatric disorders. The roles of nurses are expanding as nursing care becomes an established part of the community-based health care delivery system.

CRITICAL THINKING CHALLENGES

1 Explain the biopsychosocial model and apply it to the following three clinical examples:
   a A first-time father is extremely depressed after the birth of his child, who is perfectly healthy.
   b A child is unable to sleep at night because of terrifying nightmares.
   c An older woman is resentful of moving into a senior citizens residence even though the decision was hers.
2 Identify a clinical problem and discuss how it could have been handled better. Discuss the resources that you would need.
3 Compare the ethical concepts of *autonomy* and *beneficence.* Focus on the difference between legal consequences and ethical dilemmas.
4 Compare the variety of patients for whom psychiatric–mental health nurses care. Factors to be considered are age, health problems, and social aspects.
5 Visit the ANA website (www.nursingworld.org) for a description of the psychiatric–mental health nurse's certification credentials. Compare the basic level functions of a psychiatric nurse to those of the advanced practice psychiatric nurse.
6 Discuss the purposes of the following organizations in promoting quality mental health care and supporting nursing practice.
   a American Nurses Association (www.nursingworld.org)
   b American Psychiatric Nurses Association (www.apna.org)
   c International Society of Psychiatric–Mental Health Nurses (www.ispn-psych.org)
7 A 19-year-old patient with schizophrenia announces that he and a 47-year-old patient with bipolar disorder will be married the following week. They ask the nurse to witness the wedding. Discuss the ethical principles that may be in conflict with each other.

REFERENCES

Abraham, I., Fox, J., & Cohen, B. (1992). Integrating the bio into the biopsychosocial: Understanding and treating biological phenomena in psychiatric–mental health nursing. *Archives of Psychiatric Nursing,* 6 (5), 296–305.

American Nurses Association. (2001). *Code for nurses with interpretive statements.* Washington, DC: Author.

American Nurses Association, American Psychiatric Nurses Association, & International Society of Psychiatric-Mental Health Nurses. (2000). *Psychiatric–mental health nursing: Scope and Standards of Practice.* Silver Spring, MD.

Borrell-Carrio, F., Suchman, A. L., & Epstein, R. M. (2004). The biopsychosocial model 25 years later: Principles, practice, and scientific inquiry. *Annals of Family Medicine,* 2 (6), 576–582.

Boydell, K. M., Gladstone, B. M., & Volpe, T. (2003). Interpreting narratives of motivation and schizophrenia: a biopychosocial understanding. *Psychiatric Rehabilitation Journal, 26*(4), 422–426.

Currid, T. J., (2004). Improving perinatal mental health care. *Nursing Standards, 19* (3), 40–43.

Kuiper, R. A. O. & Pesut, D. J. (2004). Promoting cognitive and metacognitive reflective reasoning skills in nursing practice: self-regulated learning theory. *Journal of Advanced Nursing, 45* (4), 381–391.

U.S. Department of Health and Human Services. (1999). *Mental health: A report of the Surgeon General.* Rockville, MD: Author.

CHAPTER 6

Psychosocial Theoretic Basis of Psychiatric Nursing

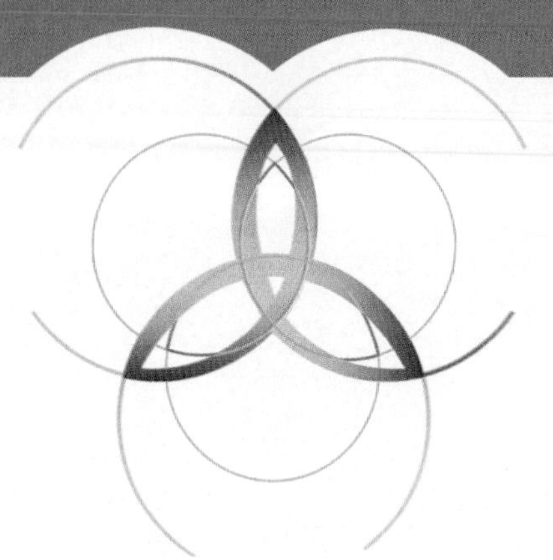

Mary Ann Boyd

KEY CONCEPT

- anxiety

LEARNING OBJECTIVES

After studying this chapter, you will be able to:

- Discuss psychosocial theories that support psychiatric nursing practice.
- Identify the underlying theories that contribute to the understanding of human beings and behavior.
- Compare the key elements of each theory that provides a basis for psychiatric–mental health nursing practice.
- Identify common nursing theoretic models used in psychiatric–mental health nursing.

KEY TERMS

• behaviorism • classical conditioning • cognition • connections • countertransference • defense levels • disconnections • disinhibition • empathy • empathic linkage • elicitation • expressed emotion • family dynamics • formal support systems • informal support systems • interpersonal relations • modeling • object relations • operant behavior • role • self-efficacy • self-system • shaping • social distance • transaction • transference

This chapter presents an overview of the psychological and social theories that serve as the knowledge base for psychiatric–mental health nursing practice. The biologic theories are discussed in Chapters 7, 8, and 14. Many of the theories underlying psychiatric nursing practice are evolving and have limited research support. Lack of research does not necessarily mean that theories are useless, but the clinician should consider the limitation when applying the theory.

PSYCHOLOGICAL THEORIES

Psychodynamic Theories

Psychodynamic theories explain the mental or emotional forces or developing processes, especially in early childhood, and their effects on behavior and mental states. The study of the unconscious is part of psychodynamic theory, and many of the models that are important in psychiatric nursing began with the Austrian physician

Sigmund Freud (1856–1939). Since his time, Freud's theories have been enhanced by so-called interpersonal and humanist models. Psychodynamic theories initially attempted to explain the cause of mental disorders, but etiologic explanations were not supported by controlled research. However, these theories proved to be especially important in the development of therapeutic relationships, techniques, and interventions (Table 6.1).

Psychoanalytic Theory

In Freud's psychoanalytic model, the human mind was conceptualized in terms of conscious mental processes (an awareness of events, thoughts, and feelings with the ability to recall them) and unconscious mental processes (thoughts and feelings that are outside awareness and are not remembered).

Study of the Unconscious

Freud believed that the unconscious part of the human mind is only rarely recognized by the conscious, as in remembered dreams (see Movies at the end of this chapter). The term "preconscious" was used to describe unconscious material that is capable of entering consciousness.

Personality and Its Development

Freud's personality structure consisted of three parts: the id, ego, and superego (Freud, 1927). The id was formed by unconscious desires, primitive instincts, and unstructured drives, including sexual and aggressive tendencies that arose from the body. The ego consisted of the sum of certain mental mechanisms, such as perception, memory, and motor control, as well as specific defense mechanisms. The ego controlled movement, perception, and contact with reality. The capacity to form mutually satisfying relationships was a fundamental function of the ego, which is not present at birth but is formed throughout the child's development. The superego was that part of the personality structure associated with ethics, standards, and self-criticism. A child's identification with important and esteemed people in early life, particularly parents, helped form the superego.

Object Relations and Identification

Freud introduced the concept of **object relations**, the psychological attachment to another person or object. He believed that the choice of a love object in adulthood and the nature of the relationship would depend on the nature and quality of the child's object relationships during the early formative years. The child's first love object was the mother, who is the source of nourishment and the provider of pleasure. Gradually, as the child separated from the mother, the nature of this initial attachment influenced any future relationships. The development of the child's capacity for relationships with others progressed from a state of narcissism to social relationships, first within the family and then within the larger community. Although the concept of object relations is fairly abstract, it can be understood in terms of a child who imitates her mother and then becomes like her mother in adulthood. This child has incorporated her mother as a love object, identifies with her, and becomes like her as an adult. This process becomes especially important in understanding an abused child who, under certain circumstances, becomes the adult abuser.

Anxiety and Defense Mechanisms

For Freud, anxiety was a specific state of unpleasantness accompanied by motor discharge along definite pathways, the reaction to danger of object loss. Defense mechanisms protected a person from unwanted anxiety. Although they are defined differently than in Freud's day, defense mechanisms still play an explanatory role in contemporary psychiatric–mental health practice. Defense mechanisms are discussed in the chapter on Communication and the Therapeutic Relationship (Chapter 9).

Sexuality

The energy or psychic drive associated with the sexual instinct, called the *libido*, literally translated from Latin to mean "pleasure" or "lust," resided in the id. When sexual desire was controlled and not expressed, tension resulted and was transformed into anxiety (Freud, 1905). Freud believed that adult sexuality was an end product of a complex process of development that began in early childhood and involved a variety of body functions or areas (oral, anal, and genital zones) that corresponded to stages of relationships, especially with parents.

Psychoanalysis

Freud developed *psychoanalysis*, a therapeutic process of accessing the unconscious and resolving the conflicts that originated in childhood with a mature adult mind. As a system of psychotherapy, psychoanalysis attempted to reconstruct the personality by examining free associations (spontaneous, uncensored verbalizations of whatever comes to mind) and the interpretation of dreams. Therapeutic relationships had their beginnings within the psychoanalytic framework.

Transference and Countertransference

Transference is the displacement of thoughts, feelings, and behaviors originally associated with significant others

Table 6.1 Psychodynamic Models

Theorist	Overview	Major Concepts	Applicability
Psychoanalytic Models			
Sigmund Freud (1856–1939)	Founder of psychoanalysis. Believed that the unconscious could be accessed through dreams and free association. Developed a personality theory and theory of infantile sexuality.	Id, ego, superego Consciousness Unconscious mental processes Libido Object relations Anxiety and defense mechanisms Free associations, transference, and countertransference	Individual therapy approach used for enhancement of personal maturity and personal growth
Anna Freud (1895–1982)	Application of ego psychology to psychoanalytic treatment and child analysis with emphasis on the adaptive function of defense mechanisms.	Refinement of concepts of anxiety, defense mechanisms	Individual therapy, childhood psychoanalysis
Neo-Freudian Models			
Alfred Adler (1870–1937)	First defected from Freud. Founded the school of individual psychology.	Inferiority	Added to the understanding of human motivation
Carl Gustav Jung (1875–1961)	After separating from Freud, founded the school of psychoanalytic psychology. Developed new therapeutic approaches.	Redefined libido Introversion Extroversion Persona	Personalities are often assessed on the introversion and extroversion dimensions
Otto Rank (1884–1939)	Introduced idea of primary trauma of birth. Active technique of therapy including more nurturing than Freud. Emphasized feeling aspect of analytic process.	Birth trauma Will	Recognized the importance of feelings within psychoanalysis
Erich Fromm (1900–1980)	Emphasized the relationship of the individual to society.	Society and individual are not separate	Individual desires are formed by society
Melanie Klein (1882–1960)	Devised play therapy techniques. Believed that complex unconscious fantasies existed in children younger than 6 months of age. Principal source of anxiety arose from the threat to existence posed by the death instinct.	Pioneer in object relations Identification	Developed different ways of applying psychoanalysis to children; influenced present-day English and American schools of child psychiatry
Karen Horney (1885–1952)	Opposed Freud's theory of castration complex in women and his emphasis on the oedipal complex. Argued that neurosis was influenced by the society in which one lived.	Situational neurosis Character	Beginning of feminist analysis of psychoanalytic thought
Interpersonal Relations			
Harry Stack Sullivan (1892–1949)	Impulses and striving need to be understood in terms of interpersonal situations.	Participant observer Parataxic distortion Consensual validation	Provided the framework for the introduction of the interpersonal theories in nursing
Humanist Theories			
Abraham Maslow (1921–1970)	Concerned himself with healthy rather than sick people. Approached individuals from a holistic-dynamic viewpoint.	Needs Motivation	Used as a model to understand how people are motivated and needs that should be met
Frederick S. Perls (1893–1970)	Awareness of emotion, physical state, and repressed needs would enhance the ability to deal with emotional problems.	Reality Here-and-now	Used as a therapeutic approach to resolve current life problems that are influenced by old, unresolved emotional problems
Carl Rogers (1902–1987)	Based theory on the view of human potential for goodness. Used the term *client* rather than *patient*. Stressed the relationship between therapist and client.	Empathy Positive regard	Individual therapy approach that involves never giving advice and always clarifying client's feelings

from childhood onto a person in a current therapeutic relationship (Moore & Fine, 1990). For example, a woman's feelings toward her parents as a child may be directed toward the therapist. If a woman were unconsciously angry with her parents, she may feel unexplainable anger and hostility toward her therapist. In psychoanalysis, the therapist uses transference as a therapeutic tool to help the patient understand emotional problems and their origin. **Countertransference**, on the other hand, is defined as the direction of all of the therapist's feelings and attitudes toward the patient. Feelings and perceptions caused by countertransference may interfere with the therapist's ability to understand the patient.

Neo-Freudian Models

Many of Freud's followers ultimately broke away, establishing their own form of psychoanalysis. Freud did not receive criticism well. The rejection of some of his basic tenets often cost his friendship as well. Various psychoanalytic schools have adopted other names because their doctrines deviated from Freudian theory.

Adler's Foundation for Individual Psychology

Alfred Adler (1870–1937), a Viennese psychiatrist and founder of the school of individual psychology, was a student of Freud who believed that the motivating force in human life is a sense of inferiority. Avoiding feelings of inferiority leads the individual to adopt a life goal that is often unrealistic and frequently expressed as an unreasoning desire for power and dominance. Because inferiority is intolerable, the compensatory mechanisms set up by the mind may get out of hand, resulting in self-centered neurotic attitudes, overcompensation, and a retreat from the real world and its problems.

Today, Adler's theories and principles have been adapted and applied to both psychotherapy and education. Adlerian theory is based on principles of mutual respect, choice, responsibility, consequences, and belonging.

Jung's Analytical Psychology

One of Freud's earliest students, Carl Gustav Jung (1875–1961), a Swiss psychoanalyst, created a model called *analytical psychology*. Jung believed in the existence of two basically different types of personalities: extroverted and introverted. Extroverted people tend to be generally interested in other people and objects of the external world, whereas introverted people tend to be interested in themselves and their internal environment. Although he argued that both tendencies exist in the normal individual, the libido usually channels itself mainly in one direction or the other. Jung rejected Freud's distinction between the ego and superego. Instead, he developed the concept of *persona* (what a person appears to be to others, in contrast with what he or she actually is) that was similar to the superego (Jung, 1966).

Horney's Feminine Psychology

Karen Horney (1885–1952), a German American psychiatrist, challenged many of Freud's basic concepts and introduced principles of feminine psychology. Recognizing a male bias in psychoanalysis, Horney was the first to challenge the traditional psychoanalytic belief that women felt disadvantaged because of their genital organs. Freud believed that women felt inferior to men because their bodies were less completely equipped, a theory he described as "penis envy." Horney rejected this concept, as well as the oedipal complex, arguing that there are significant cultural reasons why women may strive to obtain qualities or privileges that are defined by a society as being masculine. For example, university education, the right to vote, and economic independence have been available to women only recently. She argued that women truly were at a disadvantage because of the authoritarian culture in which they lived (Horney, 1939).

Other Neo-Freudian Theories

Otto Rank: Birth Trauma

Otto Rank (1884–1939), an Austrian psychologist and psychotherapist, was also a student of Freud. Introducing a theory of neurosis that attributed all neurotic disturbances to the primary trauma of birth, he described individual development as a progression from complete dependence on the mother and family to physical independence coupled with intellectual dependence on society, and finally to complete intellectual and psychological emancipation. Rank believed in the importance of will, a positive guiding organization in the integration of self.

Erich Fromm and Melanie Klein: Play Therapy

Other psychoanalytic theorists include Erich Fromm and Melanie Klein. Erich Fromm (1900–1980), an American psychoanalyst, focused on the relationship of society and the individual. He argued that individual and societal needs are not separate and opposing forces; their relationship with each other is determined by the historic background of the culture. Fromm also believed that the needs and desires of individuals are largely formed by their society. For Fromm, the fundamental problem of psychoanalysis and psychology was to bring about harmony and understanding of the relationship between the individual and society (Fromm-Reichmann, 1950).

Melanie Klein (1882–1960), an Austrian psychoanalyst, devised play therapy techniques to demonstrate how a child's interaction with toys revealed earlier infantile fantasies and anxieties. She believed that complex unconscious fantasies existed in children younger than 6 months of age. She is generally acknowledged as a pioneer in presenting an object relations viewpoint to the psychodynamic field, introducing the idea of early identification, a defense mechanism by which one patterns oneself after another person, such as a parent. Her theoretic inferences were based on her clinical observations (Klein, 1963).

Harry Stack Sullivan: Interpersonal Forces

Interpersonal theories were developed as an alternative explanation for human development and behavior. Although there are similarities between psychoanalytic and interpersonal theories, the major difference is that interpersonal theories acknowledge the importance of individual relationships in personality development. Instincts and drives are less important. Childhood relationships with parenting figures are especially significant and are believed to influence important adult relationships, such as the choice of a mate.

Harry Stack Sullivan (1892–1949), an American psychiatrist, extended the concept of **interpersonal relations** to include characteristic interaction patterns. Sullivan studied personality characteristics that could be directly observed, heard, and felt. He believed that the health or sickness of one's personality was determined by the characteristic ways in which one dealt with other people. Health also depended on the constantly changing physical, social, and interpersonal environment as well as past and current life experiences (Sullivan, 1953).

Humanistic Theories

Humanistic theories were generated as a reaction against psychoanalytic premises of instinctual drives. Humanistic therapies are based on the views of human potential for goodness. Instead of focusing on instinctual drives, humanist therapists focus on one's ability to learn about oneself, acceptance of self, and exploration of personal capabilities. Within the therapeutic relationship, the patient begins to view himself or herself as a person of worth. A positive attitude is developed. The focus is not on investigation of repressed memories, but on learning to experience the world in a different way.

Rogers' Client-Centered Therapy

Carl Rogers (1902–1987), an American psychologist, developed new methods of client-centered therapy. Rogers defined empathy as the capacity to assume the internal reference of the client in order to perceive the world in the same way as the client (Rogers, 1980). To use empathy in the therapeutic process, the counselor must be nondirect, but not passive. Thus, the counselor's attitude and nonverbal communication are crucial. He also advocated that the therapist develop unconditional positive regard, a nonjudgmental caring for the client (Rogers, 1980). Genuineness is also important in a therapist, in contrast with the passivity of the psychoanalytic therapist. Rogers believed that the therapist's emotional investment (i.e., true caring) in the client is essential in the therapeutic process.

Gestalt Therapy

Another humanistic approach created as a response to the psychoanalytic model was Gestalt therapy, developed by Frederick S. (Fritz) Perls (1893–1970), a German-born former psychoanalyst who emigrated to the United States. Perls believed that modern civilization inevitably produces neurosis because it forces people to repress natural desires and frustrates an inherent human tendency to adjust biologically and psychologically to the environment, with anxiety as the result. For a person to be cured, unmet needs must be brought back to awareness. He did not believe that the intellectual insight gained through psychoanalysis enabled people to change. Instead, he devised individual and group exercises that enhanced the person's awareness of emotions, physical state, and repressed needs as well as physical and psychological stimuli in the environment (Perls, 1969).

Abraham Maslow's Hierarchy of Needs

Abraham Maslow (1921–1970) developed a humanistic theory that is used in psychiatric–mental health nursing today. His major contributions were to the area of needs and motivation (Maslow, 1970). Maslow advocated viewing human behavior from a perspective of needs. Human beings have a hierarchy of needs that range from basic food, shelter, and warmth to a high-level requirement for self-actualization (Fig. 6.1). This model is used in understanding individual needs. For example, the need for food and shelter must be met before caring for the symptoms of a mental illness.

Applicability of Psychodynamic Theories to Psychiatric-Mental Health Nursing

Several concepts that are traced to the psychodynamic theories are important in the practice of psychiatric–mental health nursing, such as interpersonal relationships, defense mechanisms, transference, countertrans-

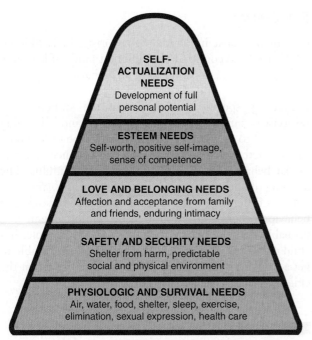

FIGURE 6.1. Maslow's hierarchy of needs.

ference, and internal objects. In particular, a therapeutic interpersonal relationship is a core of psychiatric–mental health nursing intervention. Through the strength and support of the therapeutic relationship, patients can examine and solve mental health problems (see Chapter 10 for nursing interventions).

BEHAVIORAL THEORIES

One important group of theories that serves as a knowledge base for psychiatric–mental health nursing practice is the behavioral theories, which have their roots in the discipline of psychology. Behavioral theories attempt to explain how people learn and act. Behavioral theories never attempt to explain the cause of mental disorders; instead, they focus on normal human behavior. Research results are then applied to the clinical situation (see Table 6.2).

Early Stimulus-Response Theories

Pavlovian Theory

One of the earliest behavioral theorists was Ivan P. Pavlov (1849–1936), who noticed that stomach secretions of dogs were stimulated by triggers other than food reaching the stomach. He found that the sight and smell of food triggered stomach secretions, and he became interested in this anticipatory secretion. Through his experiments, he was able to stimulate secretions with a variety of other laboratory nonphysiologic stimuli. Thus, a clear connection was made between thought processes and physiologic responses.

In Pavlov's model, there is an unconditioned stimulus (not dependent on previous training) that elicits an unconditioned (i.e., specific) response. In his experiments, meat was the unconditioned stimulus, and salivation was

Table 6.2 Behavioral Theorists

Theorist	Overview	Major Concepts	Applicability
Stimulus-Response			
Edwin R. Guthrie (1886–1959)	Continued with understanding conditioning as being important in learning	Recurrence of responses tends to follow a specific stimulus	Important in analyzing habitual behavior
Ivan P. Pavlov (1849–1936)	Classical conditioning	Unconditioned stimuli Unconditioned response Conditioned stimuli	Important in understanding learning of automatic responses such as habitual behaviors
John B. Watson (1878–1958)	Introduced behaviorism, believed that learning was classical conditioning called *reflexes*; rejected distinction between mind and body	Principle of frequency Principle of recency	Focuses on the relationship between the mind and body
Reinforcement Theories			
B. F. Skinner (1904–1990)	Developed an understanding of the importance of reinforcement and differentiated types and schedules	Operant behavior Respondent behavior Continuous reinforcement Intermittent reinforcement	Important in behavior modification
Edward L. Thorndike (1874–1949)	Believed in the importance of effects that followed behavior	Reinforcement	Important in behavior modification programs

the unconditioned response. Pavlov would then select other stimuli, such as a bell, a ticking metronome, and a triangle drawn on a large cue card, presenting this conditioned stimulus just before the meat, the unconditioned response. If the conditioned stimulus was repeatedly presented before the meat, eventually salivation was elicited only by the conditioned stimulus. This phenomenon was called **classical** (pavlovian) **conditioning** (Pavlov, 1927/1960).

John B. Watson and the Behaviorist Revolution

At about the same time Pavlov was working in Russia, John B. Watson (1878–1958) initiated the psychological revolution known as **behaviorism** in the United States. He developed two principles: frequency and recency. The principle of frequency states that the more often a given response is made to a given stimulus, the more likely the response to that stimulus will be repeated. The principle of recency states that the more recently a given response to a particular stimulus is made, the more likely it will be repeated. Watson's major contribution was the rejection of the distinction between body and mind and his emphasis on the study of objective behavior (Watson & Rayner, 1920).

Reinforecement Theories

Edward L. Thorndike

A pioneer in experimental animal psychology, Edwin L. Thorndike (1874–1949) studied the problem-solving behavior of cats to determine whether animals solved problems by reasoning or instinct. He found that neither choice was completely correct; animals gradually learn the correct response by "stamping in" the stimulus-response connection. The major difference between Thorndike and behaviorists such as Watson was that Thorndike believed in the importance of the effects that followed the response or the reinforcement of the behavior. He was the first reinforcement theorist, and his view of learning became the dominant view in American learning theory (Thorndike, 1916).

B. F. Skinner

One of the most influential behaviorists, B. F. Skinner (1904–1990), recognized two different kinds of learning, each involving a separate kind of behavior. *Respondent behavior*, or the end result of classical conditioning, is elicited by specific stimuli. Given the stimulus, the response occurs automatically. The other kind of learning is referred to as *operant behavior*. In this type of learning, the distinctive characteristic is the consequence of a particular behavioral response, not a specific stimulus. The learning of operant behavior is also known as *conditioning*, but it is different from the conditioning of reflexes. If a behavior occurs and is followed by reinforcement, it is probable that the behavior will recur. For example, if a child climbs on a chair, reaches the faucet, and is able to get a drink of water successfully, it is more likely that the child will repeat the behavior (Skinner, 1935).

COGNITIVE THEORIES

The initial behavioral studies focused attention on human actions without much attention to the internal thinking process. As complex behavior was examined and could not be accounted for by strictly behavioral explanations, thought processes became new subjects for study. Cognitive theory, an outgrowth of different theoretic perspectives, including the behavioral and the psychodynamic, attempted to link internal thought processes with human behavior (see Table 6.3).

Albert Bandura's Social Cognitive Theory

Acquiring behaviors by learning from other people is the basis of social cognitive theory, developed by Albert Bandura (b. 1925). Bandura developed his ideas after being concerned about violence on television contributing to aggression in children. He believes that important behaviors are learned by internalizing behaviors of others. His initial contribution was identifying the process of **modeling:** pervasive imitation, or one person trying to be like another. According to Bandura, the model may

Table 6.3 Cognitive Theorists

Theorist	Overview	Major Concepts	Applicability
Aaron Beck (b. 1921)	Conceptualized distorted cognitions as a basis for depression	Cognitions Beliefs	Important in cognitive therapy
Kurt Lewin (1890–1947)	Developed field theory, a system for understanding learning, motivation, personality and social behavior	Life space Positive valences	Important in understanding motivation for changing behavior
Edward Chace Tolman (1886–1959)	Introduced the concept of cognitions: believed that human beings act on beliefs and attitudes and strive toward goals	Negative valences Cognition	Important in identifying person's beliefs

not need to be a real person, but could be a character in history or generalized to an ideal person (Bandura, 1977).

The concept of **disinhibition** is important to Bandura's model and refers to the situation in which someone has learned not to make a response; then, in a given situation, when another is making the inhibited response, the individual becomes disinhibited and also makes the response. Thus, the response that was "inhibited" now becomes disinhibited through a process of imitation. For example, during severe dieting, an individual may have learned to resist eating large amounts of food. However, when at a party with a friend who eagerly fills a plate at a buffet, the person also eats large amounts of food.

In the instance of disinhibition, the desire to eat is already there, and the individual indulges that desire. However, in another instance, called **elicitation**, there is no desire present, but when one person starts an activity, others want to do the same. An example of this occurs when a child is playing with a toy, and the children also want to play with the same toy even though they showed no interest in it before that time.

An important concept of Bandura's is **self-efficacy,** a person's sense of his or her ability to deal effectively with the environment (Bandura, 1993). Efficacy beliefs influence how people feel, think, motivate themselves, and behave. The stronger the self-efficacy, the higher the goals people set for themselves and the firmer their commitment to them. The importance of self-efficacy is demonstrated by the increased research support it receives (McIntosh, 2003; Shin, Yun, Pender, and Jang, 2005).

Aaron Beck: Thinking and Feeling

American psychiatrist Aaron T. Beck (b. 1921) of the University of Pennsylvania devoted his career to understanding the relationship between cognition and mental health. For Beck, cognitions are verbal or pictorial events in the stream of consciousness. He realized the importance of cognitions when treating people with depression, finding that the depression improved when patients began viewing themselves and situations in a positive light.

He believed that people with depression had faulty information-processing systems that led to biased cognitions. These faulty beliefs cause errors in judgment that become habitual errors in thinking. These individuals incorrectly interpret life situations, judge themselves too harshly, and jump to inaccurate negative conclusions. A person may truly believe that he or she has no friends and therefore no one cares. On examination, the evidence for the beliefs is based on the fact that there has been no contact with anyone because of moving from one city to another. Thus, a distorted belief is the basis of the cognition. Beck and his colleagues developed cognitive therapy, a successful approach for the treatment of depression (see Chapters 11 and 20) (Beck, 2005). Recent research, however, suggests that the relationship between negative views of self and depression may not be present in all cultures (Box 6.1).

BOX 6.1

Research for Best Practice: Negative Cognitions and Cultural Differences

Arnault, D.S., Sakamoto, S., and Moriwaki, A. (2005). The association between negative self-descriptions and depressive symptomology: Does culture make a difference? Archives of Psychiatric Nursing, 19(2), 93–100.

The Question: What are the relationships between negative self-descriptors and depressive symptoms in Japanese and American women?

Methods: This study examined the relationships among culture, the self, and psychological distress. The samples included 79 female college students from Japan and 50 female college students from the United States. All were under the age of 25. The variables that were measured include depression (Beck Depression Inventory [BDI]), a self-description task, and a self-structure measure that had been used in people with borderline personality and other mental disorders.

Findings: Americans had more positive self-descriptors than the Japanese women. There were no cultural group differences in the negative self-descriptors. In the group from the United States, there was a significant correlation between negative core self-descriptors and the BDI.

Implication for Nursing: There is variation in the beliefs associated with the state of depression. In other cultures, negative views of self may not be associated with depression.

Applicability of Behavioral Theories to Psychiatric–Mental Health Nursing

Basing interventions on behavioral theories is widespread in psychiatric nursing. For example, patient education interventions are usually based on learning principles derived from any number of the behavioral theories. Teaching patients new coping skills for their symptoms of mental illnesses is usually based on behavioral theories. Changing an entrenched habit involves helping patients identify what motivates them and how these new lifestyle habits can become permanent. In psychiatric units, behavioral interventions include the privilege systems and token economies.

DEVELOPMENTAL THEORIES

The developmental theories explain normal human growth and development and focus on change over time. Many developmental theories are presented in terms of stages based on the assumption that normal development proceeds longitudinally from the beginning to the ending stage. Although this approach is useful, unless a stage model is truly supported by evidence, the model does not represent reality.

Erik Erikson: Psychosocial Development

Freud and Sullivan both published treatises on stages of human development, but Erik Erikson (1902–1994) outlined the psychosocial developmental model that is most often used in nursing. Erikson's model was an expansion of Freud's psychosexual development theory. Whereas Freud emphasized intrapsychic experiences, Erikson recognized the importance of culture. He believed that similar events may be experienced differently depending on a person's reaction, family background, and cultural situation.

Each of Erikson's eight stages is associated with a specific task that can be successfully or unsuccessfully resolved. The model is organized according to developmental conflicts by age: basic trust versus mistrust, autonomy versus shame and doubt, initiative versus guilt, industry versus inferiority, identity versus role diffusion, intimacy versus isolation, generativity versus stagnation, and ego integrity versus despair. Successful resolution of a crisis leads to essential strength and virtues (see Table 6.4). For example, a positive outcome of the trust versus mistrust crisis is the development of a basic sense of trust. If the crisis is unsuccessfully resolved, the infant moves into the next stage without a sense of trust. According to this model, a child who is mistrustful will have difficulty completing the next crisis successfully and, instead of developing a sense of autonomy, will more likely be full of shame and doubt (Erikson, 1963).

Identity and Adolescence

One of Erikson's major contributions was the recognition of the turbulence of adolescent development. Erikson wrote extensively about adolescence, youth, and identity formation. When adolescence begins, childhood ways must be given up, and body changes must be reconciled with the individual's social position, previous history, and identifications. An identity is formed. This task of reconciling how young people see themselves and how society perceives them can become overwhelming and lead to role confusion and alienation (Erikson, 1968).

Research Evidence for Erikson's Models

A recent longitudinal study of 86 men beginning at age 21 and reassessment 32 years later at age 53 support Erikson's psychosocial 8 stage model (Westermeyer, 2004). In this study, 48 men (56%) achieved generativity, at follow-up. Results show that generativity was significantly associated with successful marriage, work achievements, close friendships, altruistic behaviors, and overall mental health. Successful young adult predictors of Erikson's model at midlife included a warm family environment, an absence of troubled parental discipline, a mentor relationship, and, most importantly, favorable peer group relationships. In an early study, male college students who measured low on identity also scored low on intimacy ratings (Orlofsky, Marcia, & Lesser, 1973). These results lend support to the idea that identity precedes intimacy. In another study, intimacy was found to begin developing early in adolescence, before the development of identity (Ochse & Plug, 1986). Studying fathers with young children, Christiansen and Palkovitz (1998) found that generativity was associated with a paternal identity, psychosocial identity, and psychosocial intimacy. In addition, fathers who had a religious identification also had higher generativity scores than did others.

Evidence also suggests that girls' development is different than boys. One study shows that *generativity* (defined as the need or drive to produce, create, or effect a change) is associated with well-being in both males and females, but in males, generativity is related to the urge

Table 6.4 Erikson's Eight Ages of Man

Approximate Chronologic Age	Developmental Conflict*	Long-Term Outcome of Successful Resolution
Infant	Basic trust vs. mistrust	Drive and hope
Toddler	Autonomy vs. shame and doubt	Self-control and willpower
Preschool-aged child	Initiative vs. guilt	Direction and purpose
School-aged child	Industry vs. inferiority	Method and competence
Adolescence	Identity vs. role diffusion	Devotion and fidelity
Young adult	Intimacy vs. isolation	Affiliation and love
Adulthood	Generativity vs. stagnation	Production and care
Maturity	Ego integrity vs. despair	Renunciation and wisdom

*Successful outcome is evidenced by the development of the characteristic listed first.
Adapted from Erikson, E. (1963). *Childhood and society* (pp. 273–274). New York: Norton.

Table 6.5 Piaget's Periods of Intellectual Development

Age (years)	Period	Cognitive Developmental Characteristics	Description
Birth to 2	Sensorimotor	Divided into six stages, characterized by (1) inborn motor and sensory reflexes, (2) primary circular reaction and first habit, (3) secondary circular reaction, (4) use of familiar means to obtain ends, (5) tertiary circular reaction and discovery through active experimentation, and (6) insight and object permanence	The infant understands the world in terms of overt, physical action on that world. The infant moves from simple reflexes through several steps to an organized set of schemes. Significant concepts are developed, including space, time, and causality. Above all, during this period, the child develops the scheme of the permanent object.
2–7	Preoperational	Deferred imitation; symbolic play, graphic imagery (drawing); mental imagery; and language Egocentrism, rigidity of thought, semilogical reasoning, and limited social cognition	Child no longer only makes perceptual and motor adjustment to objects and events. Child can now use symbols (mental images, words, gestures) to represent these objects and events; uses these symbols in an increasingly organized and logical fashion.
7–11	Concrete operations	Conservation of quantity, weight, volume, length, and time based on reversibility by inversion or reciprocity; operations: class inclusion and seriation	Conservation is the understanding of what values remain the same. For example, if liquid is poured from a short, wide glass into a tall, narrow one, the preoperational child thinks that the quantity has changed. For the concrete operation child, the amount stays the same.
11 through end of adolescence	Formal operations	Combination system, whereby variables are isolated and all possible combinations are examined; hypothetical-deductive thinking	Mental operations are applied to objects and events.The child classifies, orders, and reverses them. Hypotheses can be generated from these concrete operations.

for self-protection, self-assertion, self-expansion, and mastery. In women, the antecedents may be the desire for contact, connection, and union (Ackerman, Zuroff, & Moskowitz, 2000).

Jean Piaget: Learning in Children

One of the most influential people in child psychology was Jean Piaget (1896–1980), who contributed more than 40 books and 100 articles on child psychology alone. Piaget viewed intelligence as an adaptation to the environment. He proposed that cognitive growth is like embryologic growth: an organized structure becomes more and more differentiated over time. Piaget developed a system that explains how knowledge develops and changes (see Table 6.5).

Each stage of cognitive development represents a particular structure with major characteristics. Piaget's theory was developed through observation of his own children and therefore never received formal testing.

The major strength of his model was its recognition of the central role of cognition in development and the discovery of surprising features of young children's thinking. For example, children in middle childhood become capable of considering more than one aspect of an object or situation at a time. Their thinking becomes more complex. They can understand that the area of a rectangle is determined by the length AND width. For psychiatric–mental health nursing, the nurse can use Piaget's model to provide a framework on which to define different levels of thinking and use the data in the assessment and intervention processes. For example, the assessment of concrete thinking would be typical of people with schizophrenia who are unable to perform abstract thinking.

Carol Gilligan: Gender Differentiation

Carol Gilligan (b. 1936) argues that most development models are male centered and therefore inappropriate for girls and women. For Gilligan, attachment within relationships is the important factor for successful female development. After comparing male and female personality development, she highlighted the differences (Gilligan, 2004). Although the first primary relationship of both boys and girls is with the mother, in developing identity, boys separate from their mother and girls attach. Thus, girls probably learn to value relationships and become interdependent at an earlier age. They learn to value the ideal of care, begin to respond to human need, and want to take care of the world by sustaining attachments so no one is left alone. According to Gilligan, female development does not follow a progression of stages but is based on experiences within relationships.

However, some researchers suggest that relationships may also be equally important for boys in their development of a strong sense of self (Nelson, 1996).

Gilligan's conclusion that female development depends on relationships has implications for everyone who provides care to women. Traditional models that advocate separation as the primary goal of human development immediately place women at a disadvantage. By negating the value and importance of attachments within relationships, the natural development of women is impaired. If Erikson's model is applied to women, their failure to separate then becomes defined as a developmental failure (Gilligan, 1982). Currently, there is considerable debate whether or not Erikson's developmental model is applicable to women.

Jean Baker Miller: A Sense of Connection

Jean Baker Miller (b. 1927) conceptualizes female development within the context of experiences and relationships. Consistent with the thinking of Carol Gilligan, the Miller relational model views the central organizing feature of women's development as a sense of connection to others. The goal of development is to increase a woman's ability to build and enlarge mutually enhancing relationships (Miller, 1994, p. 83). **Connections** (mutually responsive and enhancing relationships) lead to mutual engagement (attention), empathy, and empowerment. In those relationships in which everyone interacts beneficially, mutual psychological development can occur. **Disconnections** (lack of mutually responsive and enhancing relationships) occur when a child or adult expresses a feeling or explains an experience and does not receive any response from others. The most serious types of disconnection arise from the lack of response that occurs after abuse or attacks. The theory is currently evolving and serves as a model for psychotherapy and nursing practice on a psychiatric unit (Walker & Rosen, 2004; Riggs & Bright, 1997).

Applicability of Developmental Theories to Psychiatric–Mental Health Nursing

Developmental theories are used in understanding childhood and adolescent experiences and their manifestations as adult problems. When working with children, nurses can use developmental models to help gauge development and mood. However, because most of the models are based on the assumptions of the linear progression of stages and have not been adequately tested, applicability has limitations. In addition, these models were based on a relatively small number of children who typically were raised in a Western middle-class environment. Most do not account for gender differences and diversity in lifestyles and cultures.

SOCIAL THEORIES

Numerous social theories underlie psychiatric–mental health nursing practice. Chapter 15 presents some of the sociocultural issues and discusses various social groups. This section represents a sampling of important social theories that nurses may use. This discussion is not exhaustive and should be viewed by the student as including some of the theoretic perspectives that may be applicable.

Family Dynamics

Family dynamics are the patterned interpersonal and social interactions that occur within the family structure over the life of a family. Family dynamics models are based on systems theory describing a phenomenon in terms of a set of interrelated parts, in which the change of one part affects the total functioning of the system. A system can be "open" (interacting in the environment) or "closed" (completely self-contained and not influenced by the environment). The family is viewed organizationally as an open system in which one member's actions influence the functioning of the total system. Family theories that are important in psychiatric–mental health nursing are based on systems models but have rarely been tested for wide-range validity. Most of the theoretic explanations have emerged from case studies involved in treatment, rather than from systematic development of theory based on large samplings. Consequently, the limitation of available research should be considered when these models are used to understand family interactions and plan patient care.

Applicability of Family Theories to Psychiatric–Mental Health Nursing

Family theories are especially useful to nurses who are assessing family dynamics and planning interventions. Family systems models are used to help nurses form collaborative relationships with patients and families dealing with health problems. Generalist psychiatric–mental health nurses will not be engaged in family therapy. However, they will be caring for individuals and families. Understanding family dynamics is important in every nurse's practice. Many family interventions are consistent with these theories (see Chapter 13). Many of the symptoms of mental disorders, such as hallucinations or delusions, have implications for the total family and affect interactions.

Balance Theory and Social Distance

A useful theory for understanding caregiving activities within a community is balance theory, proposed in 1966 by sociologist Eugene Litwak (b. 1925). This theory explains the importance of informal and formal support systems in the delivery of health care.

Formal support systems are large organizations, such as hospitals and nursing homes that provide care to individuals. **Informal support systems** are family, friends, and neighbors. Litwak found that individuals with strong informal support networks actually live longer than those without this type of support. In addition, those without informal support have significantly higher mortality rates when the causes of death are accidents (e.g., smoking in bed) or suicides (Litwak, 1985).

A key concept in balance theory is **social distance,** the degree to which the values of the formal organization and primary group members differ. The formal and informal groups are considered to be balanced when they are at a midpoint of social distance, that is, close enough to communicate, but not so close to destroy each other; neither enmeshment nor isolation (Litwak, Messeri, & Silverstein, 1990; Messeri, Silverstein, & Litwak, 1993). If the primary groups and the formal care system begin performing similar caregiving services, the formal system increases the social distance by developing linkages with the primary group. Thus, a balance is maintained between the two systems. For example, if a patient relies only on the health care provider for care and support (e.g., calls the nurse every day, visits the physician weekly, refuses any help from family), the individual will be linked with an informal support system for help with some of the caregiving tasks. If the individual refuses any health promotion interventions from providers, the patient will be directly approached by the health care team.

Applicability of Balance Theory to Psychiatric–Mental Health Nursing

Balance theory is a practical model for conceptualizing delivery of mental health care in the community, particularly in rural areas where resources are limited. By using the framework of formal and informal support systems and social distance, mental health services can be developed and evaluated from this perspective. This model has been used to examine the impact of caregivers (Aberg, Sidenvall, Hepworth, O'Reilly, & Lithell, 2004) (Box 6.2). Nurse researchers at the Southeastern Rural Mental Health Research Center at the University of Virginia, Charlottesville, used this theory to develop a model for establishing linkages of formal and informal caregivers for those with serious mental illnesses (Fox, Blank, Kane, Hargrove, & David, 1994). In this model, case managers adjust the social distance between the formal and informal systems by identifying communication barriers and helping the two groups work together. For example, a patient misses an appointment because of a lack of transportation. The case manager helps the patient communicate the problem to the system to obtain another appointment. Informal caregivers are valued by the case manager, who recognizes the important services performed by family and friends. Thus, linkages between mental health providers (formal support) and the consumer network (informal support) are reinforced.

BOX 6.2

Research for Best Practice: Perceptions of informal Caregivers

Aberg, A.C., Sidenvall, B., Hepworth, M., O'Reilly, K., Lithell, H. Continuity of the self in later life. (2004). Qualitative Health Research, 14(6), 792-815.

The Question: The authors explored perceptions of informal caregivers of extremely elderly relatives or friends regarding the purpose of caregiving, including factors they considered important for the life satisfaction of the care recipients.

Methods: Qualitative interviewing of caregivers with symbolic interaction methods were used.

Findings: The purpose of the caregiving was protection of the recipient's self-care. The categories of caregiving included social, emotional, proxy, and instrumental care. Some informal caregivers encouraged the recipients to accept formal care and move to a residential facility.

Implications for Nursing: Informal caregivers are very important in the well-being of patients.

ROLE THEORIES

Perspectives

A role describes an individual's social position and function within an environment. Anthropologic theories explain members' roles that relate to a specific society. For example, the universal roles of healer may be assumed by a nurse in one culture and a spiritual leader in another. Societal expectations, social status, and rights are attached to these roles. Psychological theories, which are concerned about roles from a different perspective, focus on the relationship of an individual's role: the self. The responsibilities of a parent are often in conflict with the personal needs for time alone. All of the Neo-Freudian and humanist models that have been discussed focus on reciprocal social relationships or interactions that determine how the mind develops.

Applicability of Role Theories to Psychiatric–Mental Health Nursing

Role theories emphasize the importance of social interaction in either the individual's choice of a particular role or society's recognition of it. Psychiatric–mental health nursing uses role concepts in understanding group interaction and the role of the patient in the family and community (see Chapters 12 and 13). In addition, milieu therapy approaches discussed in later chapters are based on the patient's assumption of a role within the psychiatric environment.

SOCIOCULTURAL PERSPECTIVES

Margaret Mead: Culture and Gender

American anthropologist Margaret Mead (1901–1978) is widely known for her studies of primitive societies and her contributions to social anthropology. She conducted studies in New Guinea, Samoa, and Bali, and devoted much of her studies to the patterns of child rearing in various cultures. She was particularly interested in the cultural influences determining male and female behavior (Mead, 1970). Although her research was often criticized as not having scientific rigor and being filled with misinterpretations, it became accepted as a classic in the field of anthropology (Torrey, 1992). The importance of culture in determining human behavior was acknowledged.

Madeleine Leininger: Transcultural Health Care

Concern about the impact of culture on the treatment of children with psychiatric and emotional problems led Madeleine Leininger (b. 1924) to develop a new field, transcultural nursing, directed toward holistic, congruent, and beneficent care. Leininger developed the theory of culture care diversity and universality, which focused on diverse and universal dimensions of human caring. Thus, nursing care in one culture is different from that in another because definitions are different. Because caring is an integral part of being human, as well as a learned behavior, caring is culturally based (Leininger, 2006). Leininger developed a model to depict her theory symbolically (Fig 6.2).

Applicability of Sociocultural Theories to Psychiatric–Mental Health Nursing

The use of sociocultural theories is especially important for psychiatric–mental health nurses. In any individual or family assessment, the sociocultural aspect is integral to mental health. It would be impossible to complete an adequate assessment without considering the role of the individual within the family and society. Interventions are based on the understanding and significance of family and cultural norms. It would be impossible to interact with the family in a meaningful way without an understanding of the family's cultural values. In the inpatient setting, the nurse is responsible for designing the social environment of the unit as well as ensuring that the patient is safe from harm. To accomplish this complex task, an understanding of the unit as a small social community helps the nurse use the environment in patient treatment (see Chapter 10). In addition, many group interventions are based on sociocultural theories (see Chapter 15).

NURSING THEORIES

A number of nursing theories are applicable to psychiatric–mental health nursing. Nursing theories are useful in conceptualizing the individual, family, or community and in planning nursing interventions. Chapter 10 explains the actual implementation of the interventions. The use of a specific theory depends on the patient. For example, in people with schizophrenia who have problems related to maintaining self-care, Dorothea Orem's theory of self-care may be useful. By contrast, Hildegarde Peplau's theories may be appropriate when the nurse is developing a relationship with the patient. Because of the wide range of possible problems requiring different approaches, familiarity with a variety of nursing theories is essential. The following discussion includes nursing models typically used in psychiatric–mental health nursing.

Interpersonal Relations Models

Hildegarde Peplau: The Power of Empathy

Hildegarde Peplau's (1909–1999) theoretic perspectives continue to be an important base for the practice of psychiatric–mental health nursing. Influenced by Harry Stack Sullivan, Peplau introduced the first systematic theoretic framework for psychiatric nursing and focused on the nurse–patient relationship in her book *Interpersonal Relations in Nursing* in 1952 (Peplau, 1952). Although her work continues to stimulate debate, she led psychiatric–mental health nursing out of the confinement of custodial care into a theory-driven professional practice. One of her major contributions was the introduction of the nurse–patient relationship (see Chapter 9).

Peplau believed in the importance of the environment, defined as those external factors considered essential to human development (Peplau, 1992): cultural forces, presence of adults, secure economic status of the family, and a healthy prenatal environment. She believed in the importance of the "interpersonal environment," which included interactions between person and family, parent and child, or patient and nurse.

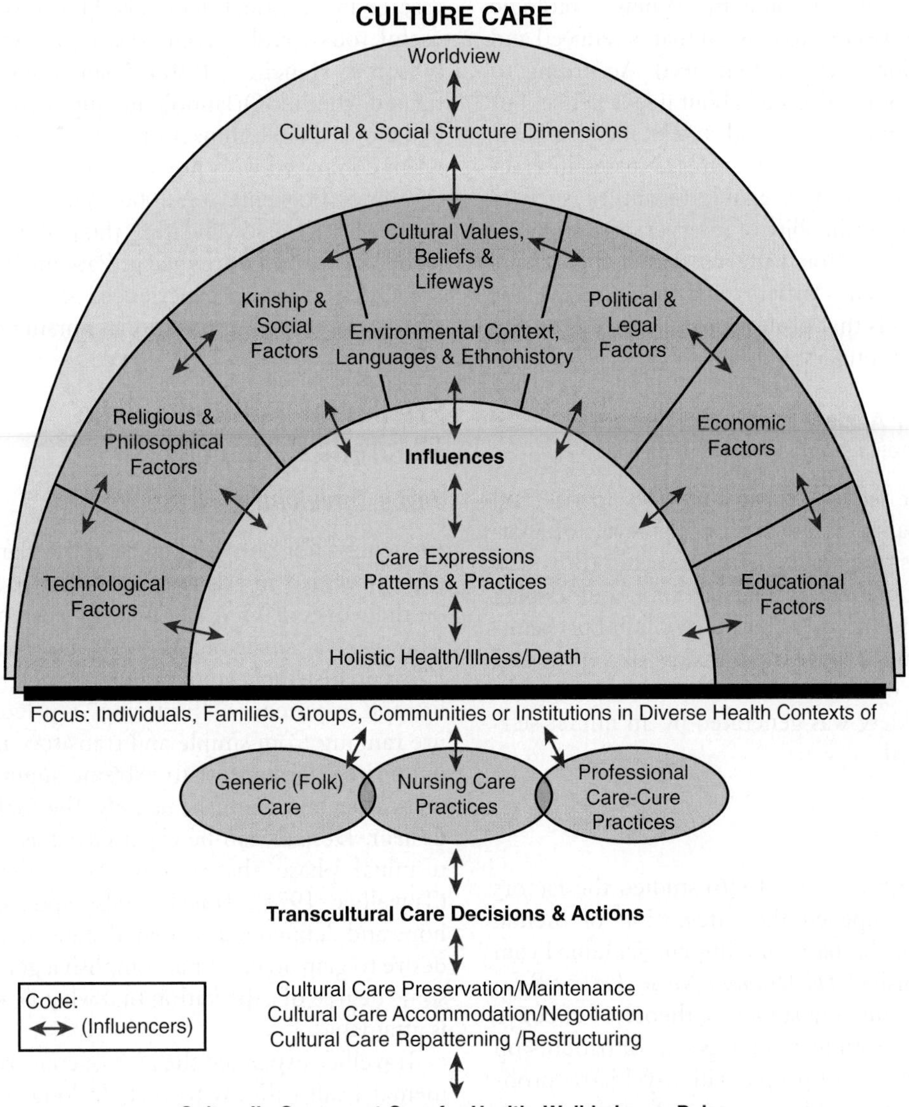

FIGURE 6.2. Leininger's Sunrise Model to depict theory of cultural care diversity and universality.

Peplau also emphasized the importance of **empathic linkage**, the ability to feel in oneself the feelings experienced by another person or people. The interpersonal transmission of anxiety or panic is the most common empathic linkage. According to Peplau, other feelings, such as anger, disgust, and envy, can also be communicated nonverbally by way of empathic transmission to others. Although the process is not yet understood, she explains that empathic communication occurs. She believes that if nurses pay attention to what they feel during a relationship with a patient, they can gain invaluable observations of feelings a patient is experiencing and has not yet noticed or talked about.

The **self-system** is an important concept in Peplau's model. Drawing from Sullivan, Peplau defined the self as an "anti-anxiety system" and a product of socialization.

• NCLEXNOTE

NCLEXNOTE Peplau's model of anxiety continues to be an important concept in psychiatric nursing. Severe anxiety interferes with learning. Mild anxiety is useful for learning.

The self proceeds through personal development that is always open to revision but tends toward a certain stability. For example, in parent–child relationships, patterns of approval, disapproval, and indifference are used by children to define themselves. If the verbal and nonverbal messages have been derogatory, children incorporate these messages and also view themselves negatively. The concept of need is important to Peplau's model. Needs are primarily of biologic origin but need to be met within a sociocultural environment. When a biologic need is present, it gives rise to tension that is reduced and relieved by behaviors meeting that need. According to Peplau, nurses are not concerned about needs per se, but recognize the patients' patterns and style of meeting their needs in relation to their health status. Nurses interact with the patient to identify available resources, such as the quantity of food, availability of interpersonal support, and support for interaction patterns that help patients obtain what is needed. Anxiety is a key concept for Peplau, who contends that professional practice is unsafe if this concept is not understood.

KEY CONCEPT Anxiety is an energy that arises when expectations that are present are not met.

If anxiety is not recognized, it continues to rise and escalates toward panic. There are various levels of anxiety, each having its observable behavioral cues (Box 6.3). These cues are sometimes called *defensive*, but Peplau argues that they are often "relief behaviors." For example, some people may relieve their anxiety by yelling and swearing, whereas others seek relief by withdrawing. In both instances, anxiety was generated by an unmet self-system security need.

Ida Jean Orlando

In 1954, Ida Jean Orlando (b. 1926) studied the factors that enhanced or impeded the integration of mental health principles in the basic nursing curriculum. From this study, she published *The Dynamic Nurse–Patient Relationship* to offer the nursing student a theory of effective nursing practice. She studied nursing care of patients on medical–surgical units, not people with psychiatric problems in mental hospitals. Orlando identified three areas of nursing concern: the nurse–patient relationship, the nurse's professional role, and the identity and development of knowledge that is distinctly nursing (Orlando, 1961). A nursing situation involves the behavior of the patient, the reaction of the nurse, and anything that does not relieve the distress of the patient. Patient distress is related to the inability of the individual to meet or communicate his or her own needs (Orlando, 1961; 1972).

Orlando's contribution to nursing practice helped nurses focus on the whole patient, rather than on the disease or institutional demands. Her ideas continue to be useful today, and current research supports her model (Olson & Hanchett, 1997). A small nursing study investigated whether Orlando's nursing theory–based practice had a measurable impact on patients' immediate distress when compared with nonspecified nursing interventions (Potter & Bockenhauer, 2000). Orlando's approach consisted of the nurse validating the patient's distress before taking any action to reduce it. Patients being cared for by the Orlando group experienced significantly less stress than those receiving traditional nursing care.

BOX 6.3

Levels of Anxiety

MILD: Awareness heightens
MODERATE: Awareness narrows
SEVERE: Focused narrow awareness
PANIC: Unable to function

Existential and Humanistic Theoretic Perspectives

Joyce Travelbee

Influenced not only by Peplau and Orlando, Joyce Travelbee provided an existential perspective to nursing based on the works of Victor Frankl, an existential philosopher who was a survivor of Nazi concentration camps. Existentialists believe that humans seek meaning in their life and experiences. "Suffering" is a feeling of displeasure ranging from simple and transitory mental, physical, or spiritual discomfort to extreme anguish, and to those phases beyond anguish, namely, the malignant phase of despair. Despair can be experienced as "not caring;" the terminal phase that follows is apathetic indifference (Travelbee, 1971). Travelbee also applied the concept of hope and defined it as a mental state characterized by the desire to gain an end or accomplish a goal combined with some degree of expectation that what is desired or sought is attainable.

Travelbee expanded the area of concern of psychiatric–mental health illness to include long-term physical illnesses. Focusing her attention on individuals who must learn to live with chronic illness, she believed that the nurse's spiritual values and philosophical beliefs about suffering would determine the extent to which the nurse could help ill people find meaning in these situations.

Travelbee's model was never subjected to empiric testing, and because of the philosophical underpinnings, it is unlikely that scientific research will be useful. However, her use of the interpersonal process as a nursing intervention and her focus on suffering and illness helped to define areas of concern for psychiatric nursing practice.

Jean Watson

The theory of transpersonal caring was initiated by Jean Watson (b. 1940). Watson believes that caring is the foundation of nursing and recommends that specific theories of caring be developed in relation to specific human conditions and health and illness experiences (Watson, 2005). There are three foundational concepts of her theory:

BOX 6.4

Nursing: Human Science and Human Care Assumptions, and Factors in Care

Assumptions

1. Caring can be effectively demonstrated and practiced only interpersonally.
2. Caring consists of factors that result in the satisfaction of certain human needs.
3. Effective caring promotes health and individual or family growth.
4. Caring responses accept a person not only as he or she is now but also as what he or she may become.
5. A caring environment offers the development of potential while allowing the person to choose the best action for him or herself at a given point in time.
6. Caring is more "healthogenic" than is curing. It integrates biophysical knowledge with knowledge of human behavior to generate or promote health and provide ministrations to those who are ill. A science of caring is complementary to the science of curing.
7. The practice of caring is central to nursing.

Clinical Caritas Processes

1. The practice of loving-kindness and equanimity within context of caring consciousness
2. Being authentically present, and enabling and sustaining the deep belief system and subjective life world of self and of one-being-cared-for
3. Cultivation of one's own spiritual practices and transpersonal self, going beyond ego self
4. Developing and sustaining a helping-trusting, authentic caring relationship
5. Being present to and supportive of the expression of positive and negative feelings as a connection with deeper spirit of self and the one-being-cared-for
6. Creative use of self and all ways of knowing as part of the caring process—to engage in the artistry of caring-healing practices
7. Engaging in genuine teaching-learning experience that attends to unity of being and meaning attempting to stay within other's frame of reference
8. Creating a healing environment at all levels (physical as well as non-physical)—a subtle environment of energy and consciousness, whereby wholeness, beauty, comfort, dignity, and peace are potentiated
9. Assisting with basic needs, with an intentional caring consciousness, administering "human care essentials," which potentiate alignment of mind-body-spirit, wholeness, and unity of being in all aspects of care—tending to both embodied spirit and evolving spiritual emergence
10. Opening and attending to spiritual-mysterious, and existential dimensions of one's own life-death—soul care for self and the one-being-cared-for

www2.uchsc.edu/sonnn/caring/content/evolution.asp

- Transpersonal Caring–Healing Relations: a relational process related to philosophic, moral, and spiritual foundation
- Clinical Caritas Process: The original 10 Carative Factors have evolved into the Clinical Caritas Processes (see Box 6.4).
- Caritas Field: A field of consciousness created when the nurse focuses on love and caring as his or her way of being, and consciously manifests a healing presence with others.

Watson's theory is especially applicable to the care of those who seek help for mental illness. This model emphasizes the importance of sensitivity to self and others, the development of helping and trusting relations, the promotion of interpersonal teaching and learning, and provision for a supportive, protective, and corrective mental, physical, sociocultural, and spiritual environment. Research studies supporting the model use qualitative approaches (Baldursdottir & Jonsdottir, 2002).

Systems Models

Imogene M. King

The theory of goal attainment developed by Imogene King (b. 1923) is based on a systems model that includes three interacting systems: personal, interpersonal, and social. She believes that human beings interact with the environment and that the individual's perceptions influence reactions and interactions (Fig. 6.3). For King, nursing involves caring for the human being, with the goal of health defined as adjusting to the stressors in both internal and external environments. She defines nursing as a "process of human interactions between nurse and patient whereby each perceives the other and the situation; and through communication, they set goals, explore means, and agree on means to achieve goals" (King, 1981, p. 144). This model focuses on the process that occurs between a nurse and a patient. The process is initiated to help the patient cope with a health problem that compromises his or her ability to maintain social roles, functions, and activities of daily living (King, 1992).

In this model, the person is goal oriented and purposeful, reacting to stressors and is viewed as an open system interacting with the environment. The variables in nursing situations are as follows:

- Geographic place of the transacting system, such as the hospital
- Perceptions of nurse and patient
- Communications of nurse and patient
- Expectations of nurse and patient
- Mutual goals of nurse and patient

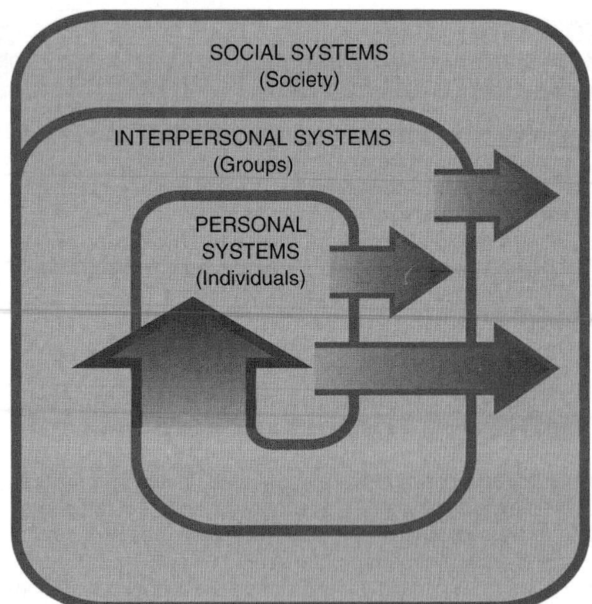

FIGURE 6.3. Imogene King's conceptual framework for nursing: dynamic interacting systems.

- Nurse and patient as a system of interdependent roles in a nursing situation (King, 1981, p. 88)

The quality of nurse–patient interactions may have positive or negative influences on the promotion of health in any nursing situation. It is within this interpersonal system of nurse and patient that the healing process is performed. Interaction is depicted in which the outcome is a **transaction,** defined as the transfer of value between two or more people. This behavior is unique, based on experience, and is goal directed (Fig. 6.3).

King's work reflects her understanding of the systematic process of theory development. She is a contemporary nursing theorist, and her model continues to be developed and applied in different settings, including psychiatric–mental health care (Goodwin, Kiehl, & Peterson, 2002). The King model was applied in group therapy for inpatient juvenile offenders, maximum security state offenders, and community parolees (Laben, Dodd, & Snead, 1991). This model has also been used as a nursing framework for individual psychotherapy (DeHowitt, 1992).

Betty Neuman

Betty Neuman (b. 1924) also used a systems approach as a model of nursing care. Neuman wanted to extend care beyond an illness model, incorporating concepts of problem finding and prevention and the newer behavioral science concepts and environmental approaches to wellness. Neuman developed her framework in the late 1960s as chairwoman of the University of California at Los Angeles graduate nursing program. The purpose of the model is to guide the actions of the professional caregiver through the assessment and intervention processes by focusing on two major components: the nature of the relationship between the nurse and patient, and the patient's response to stressors. The patient may be an individual, group (e.g., a family), or a community. The nurse is an "intervener" who attempts to reduce an individual's encounter with stress and to strengthen the person's ability to deal with stressors. The patient is viewed as a collaborator in setting health care goals and determining interventions. Neuman was one of the first psychiatric nurses to include the concept of stressors in understanding nursing care. Her work continues to be developed and applied. For example, the latest edition of the Neuman systems model is applied to a diversity of settings, including community health, family therapy, renal nursing, perinatal nursing, and mental health nursing of older adults (Neuman & Fawcett, 2001).

Dorothea Orem

Self-care is the focus of the general theory of nursing initiated by Dorothea Orem in the early 1960s. The theory consists of three separate parts: a theory of self-care, theory of self-care deficit, and theory of nursing systems (Orem, 1991). The theory of self-care defines the term as those activities performed independently by an individual to promote and maintain personal well-being throughout life. The central focus of Orem's theory is the self-care deficit theory, which describes how people can be helped by nursing. Nurses can help meet self-care requisites through five approaches: acting or doing for; guiding; teaching; supporting; and providing an environment to promote the patient's ability to meet current or future demands. The nursing systems theory refers to a series of actions a nurse takes to meet the patient's self-care requisites. This system varies from the patient being totally dependent on the nurse for care, to needing only some education and support.

Orem's model is used extensively in psychiatric–mental health nursing because of its emphasis on promoting independence of the individual and on self-care activities (Rujkorakarn & Sukmak, 2002; Campbell & Soeken, 1999). Although many psychiatric disorders have an underlying problem, such as motivation, these problems are generally manifested as difficulties conducting ordinary self-care activities (e.g., personal hygiene) or developing independent thinking skills.

Other Nursing Theories

Other nursing models are applied in psychiatric settings. Martha Rogers' model of unitary human beings and Calista Roy's adaptation model have been the basis of many psychiatric nursing approaches.

SUMMARY OF KEY POINTS

- The traditional psychodynamic framework helped form the basis of early nursing interpersonal interventions, including the development of therapeutic relationships and the use of such concepts as transference, countertransference, empathy, and object relations.
- The behavioral theories are often used in strategies that help patients change behavior and thinking.
- Sociocultural theories remain important in understanding and interacting with patients as members of families and cultures.
- Nursing theories form the conceptual basis for nursing practice and are useful in a variety of psychiatric–mental health settings.

CRITICAL THINKING CHALLENGES

1 Discuss the similarities and differences between Freud's ideas and the Neo-Freudians, including Jung, Adler, Horney, and Sullivan.
2 Compare and contrast the basic ideas of psychodynamic and behavioral theories.
3 Compare and differentiate *classic conditioning* from *operant conditioning*.
4 Define the following terms and discuss their applicability to psychiatric–mental health nursing: classical conditioning, operant conditioning, positive reinforcement, and negative reinforcement.
5 List the major developmental theorists and their main ideas.
6 Discuss the cognitive therapy approaches to mental disorders and how they can be used in psychiatric–mental health nursing practice.
7 Define formal and informal support systems. How does the concept of social distance relate to these two systems?
8 Compare and contrast the basic ideas of the nursing theorists.

Freud: 1962. This film depicts Sigmund Freud as a young physician, focusing on his early psychiatric theories and treatments. His struggles for acceptance of his ideas among the Viennese medical community are depicted. This fascinating film is well done and gives an interesting overview of the impact of psychoanalysis.

VIEWING POINTS: Watch for the impact on political thinking during the gradual acceptance of Freud's ideas. Discuss the "dream sequence" and its impact on the development of psychoanalysis as a therapeutic technique.

An Angel at My Table: 1989. New Zealand. This three-part television miniseries tells the story of Janet Frame, New Zealand's premiere novelist and poet. Based on her autobiography, the film portrays Frame as a shy, awkward child who experiences a family tragedy that alienates her socially. She studies in England to be a teacher, but her shyness and social ineptness cause extreme anxiety. Seeking mental health care, she receives a misdiagnosis of schizophrenia and spends 8 years in a mental institution. She barely escapes a lobotomy when she is notified of a literary award. She then begins to develop friendships and a new life.

VIEWING POINTS: Observe Janet Frame's childhood development. Does she "fit" any of the models that are discussed in this chapter? Consider her life in light of Gilligan and Miller's theories that it is important for women to have a sense of connection.

REFERENCES

Aberg, A. C., Sidenvall, B., Hepworth, M., O'Reilly, K., & Lithell, H. (2004). Continuity of the self in later life: perceptions of informal caregivers. *Qualitative Health Research, 14*(6), 792–815.

Ackerman, S., Zuroff, D. C., & Moskowitz, D. S. (2000). Generativity in midlife and young adults: Links to agency, communion, and subjective well-being. *International Journal of Aging and Human Development, 5*(1), 17–41.

American Psychiatric Association. (2000). *Diagnostic and statistical manual of mental disorders* (4th ed. text revision). Washington, DC: Author.

Baldursdottir, G., and Jonsdottir, H. (2002). The importance of nurse caring behaviors as perceived by patients receiving care at an emergency department *Heart & Lung, 31*(1), 67–75.

Bandura, A. (1977). *Social learning theory.* Englewood Cliffs, NJ: Prentice-Hall.

Bandura, A. (1993). Perceived self-efficacy in cognitive development and function. American Educational Research Association Annual Meeting. *Educational Psychologist, 28*(2), 117–148.

Beck, A. T. (2005). The current state of cognitive therapy: a 40-year retrospective. *Archives of General Psychiatry, 62*(9), 953–959.

Campbell, J. C., & Soeken, K. L. (1999). Women's responses to battering: A test of the model. *Research in Nursing and Health, 22*(1), 49–58.

Christiansen, S. L., & Palkovitz, R. (1998). Exploring Erikson's psychosocial theory and development: Generativity and its relationship to paternal identity, intimacy, and involvement in childcare. *The Journal of Men's Studies, 7*(1), 133–156.

DeHowitt, M. (1992). King's conceptual model and individual psychotherapy. *Perspectives in Psychiatric Care, 28(4)*, 11–14.

Erikson, E. (1963). *Childhood and society* (2nd ed.). New York: Norton.

Erikson, E. (1968). *Identity: Youth and crisis.* New York: Norton.

Freud, S. (1905). Three essays on the theory of sexuality. In J. Strachey, A. Freud, A. Strachey, & A. Tyson (Eds.). (1953). *The standard edition of the complete psychological works of Sigmund Freud* (pp. 135–248). London: Hogarth Press.

Freud, S. (1927). The ego and the id. In E. Jones (Ed.). (1957). *The international psychoanalytical library* (No. 12). London: Hogarth Press.

Fromm-Rieichmann, F. (1950). *Principles of intensive psychotherapy.* Chicago: University of Chicago Press.

Fox, J., Blank, M., Kane, C., Hargrove, C. F., & David, S. (1994). Balance theory as a model for coordinating delivery of rural mental health services. *Applied and Preventive Psychology, 3*(2), 121–129.

Gilligan, C. (2004). Recovering psyche: Reflections on life-history and history. *Annual of Psychoanalysis, 32*, 131–147.

Gilligan, C. (1982). *In a different voice.* Cambridge, MA: Harvard University Press.

Goodwin, Z., Kiehl, E. M., & Peterson, J. Z. (2002). King's theory as a foundation for an advanced directive decision-making model. *Nursing Science Quarterly, 15*(3), 237–241.

Horney, K. (1939). *New ways in psychoanalysis*. New York: Norton.

Jung, C. (1966). On the psychology of the unconscious. V. The personal and the collective unconscious. In C. Jung (Ed.), *Collected works of C. G. Jung* (2nd ed., Vol. 7, pp. 64–79). Princeton, NJ: Princeton University Press.

King, I. (1981). *A theory for nursing: Systems, concepts, process*. New York: Wiley.

King, I. (1992). King's theory of goal attainment. *Nursing Science Quarterly, 5*(1), 19–26.

Klein, M. (1963). *Our Adult World and Other Essays*. London: Heinemann Medical Books.

Laben, J., Dodd, D., & Snead, L. (1991). King's theory of goal attainment applied in group therapy for inpatient juvenile sexual offenders, maximum security state offenders, and community parolees, using visual aids. *Issues in Mental Health Nursing, 12*(1), 51–64.

Leininger, M. (2006). *Cultural care diversity and universality theory. A theory of nursing*. 2nd ed. Seaburg, MA: Jones & Bartlett Publishers.

Litwak, E. (1985). Complementary roles for formal and informal support groups: A study of nursing homes and mortality rates. *Journal of Applied Behavioral Science, 21*(4), 407–425.

Litwak, E., Messeri, P., & Silverstein, M. (1990). The role of formal and informal groups in providing help to older people. *Marriage and Family Review, 15*(1–2), 171–193.

Maslow, A. (1970). *Motivation and personality* (rev. ed.). New York: Harper & Brothers.

McIntosh, D. (2003). Testing an intervention to increase self-efficacy of staff in managing clients perceived as violent. University of Cincinnati, PhD Dissertation. www.ohiolink.edu Retrieved March 7, 2007.

Mead, M. (1970). *Culture and commitment: A study of the generation gap*. Garden City, NY: Natural History Press/Doubleday & Co.

Messeri, P., Silverstein, M., & Litwak, E. (1993). Choosing optimal support groups: A review and reformulation. *Journal of Health and Social Behavior, 34*(6), 122–137.

Miller, J. (1994). Women's psychological development. Connections, disconnections, and violations. In M. Berger (Ed.). *Women beyond Freud: New concepts of feminine psychology* (pp. 79–97). New York: Brunner Mazel.

Moore, B., & Fine, B. (Eds.). (1990). *Psychoanalytic terms and concepts*. New Haven, CT: The American Psychoanalytic Association and Yale University Press.

Nelson, M. (1996). Separation versus connection, the gender controversy: Implications for counseling women. *Journal of Counseling and Development, 74*(4), 339–344.

Neuman, B., & Fawcett, J. (2001). *The Neuman systems model* (4th ed.). Upper Saddle River, NJ: Prentice Hall.

Ochse, R., & Plug, C. (1986). Cross-cultural investigation of the validity of Erikson's theory of personality development. *Journal of Personality and Social Psychology, 50*(6), 1240–1252.

Olson, J., & Hanchett, E. (1997). Nurse-expressed empathy, patient outcomes, and the development of a middle-range theory. *Image: The Journal of Nursing Scholarship, 29*(1), 71–76.

Orem, D. (1991). *Nursing concepts of practice*. St. Louis: Mosby–Year Book.

Orlando, I. J. (1961). *The dynamic nurse–patient relationship*. New York: G. P. Putnam's Sons.

Orlando, I. J. (1972). *The discipline and teaching of nursing process*. New York: G. P. Putnam's Sons.

Orlofsky, J., Marcia, J., & Lesser, I. (1973). Ego identity status and the intimacy versus isolation crisis of young adulthood. *Journal of Personality and Social Psychology, 27*(2), 211–219.

Pavlov, I. P. (1927/1960). *Conditioned reflexes*. New York: Dover Publications.

Peplau, H. (1952). Interpersonal relations in nursing. New York: G. Putnam & Sons.

Peplau, H. (1992). Interpersonal relations: A theoretical framework for application in nursing practice. *Nursing Science Quarterly, 5*(1), 13–18.

Perls, F. (1969). *In and out of the garbage pail*. Lafayette, CA: Real People Press.

Potter, M. L., & Bockenhauer, B. J. (2000). Implementing Orlando's nursing theory. *Journal of Psychosocial Nursing and Mental Health Services, 38* (13), 14–21.

Riggs, S. R., & Bright, M. S. (1997). Dissociative identity disorder: A feminist approach to inpatient treatment using Jean Baker Miller's relational model. *Archives of Psychiatric Nursing, 11*(4), 218–224.

Rogers, C. (1980). *A way of being*. Boston: Houghton Mifflin.

Rujkorakarn, D., & Sukmak, V. (2002). Meaning of health and self-care in married men and women. *Thai Journal of Nursing Research. 6*(2): 69–75.

Shin, Y., Yun, S., Pender, N. J., & Jang, H. (2005). Test of the health promotion model as a causal model of commitment to a plan for exercise among Korean adults with chronic disease. *Research in Nursing & Health, 28*(2), 117–125.

Skinner, B. F. (1935). The generic nature of the concepts of stimulus and response. *Journal of General Psychology, 12*, 40–65.

Sullivan, H. (1953). *The interpersonal theory of psychiatry*. New York: Norton.

Thorndike, E. L. (1916, c1906). *The principles of teaching, based on psychology*. New York: A.G. Seiler.

Torrey, E. (1992). *Freudian fraud*. New York: Harper Collins.

Travelbee, J. (1971). *Interpersonal aspects of nursing* (2nd ed.). Philadelphia: F. A. Davis.

Walker, M., & Rosen, W. B. (2004). *How connections heal: Stories from relational-cultural therapy*. New York: Guilford Press.

Watson, J. (2005). *Caring science as sacred science*. Philadelphia: F. A. Davis.

Watson, J. B., & Rayner, R. (1920). Conditioned emotional reactions. *Journal of Experimental Psychology, 3*, 1–14.

Westermeyer, J. F. (2004). Predictors and characteristics of Erikson's life cycle model among men: A 32-year longitudinal study. *International Journal of Aging & Human Development, 58*(1), 29–48.

CHAPTER 7

The Biologic Foundations of Psychiatric Nursing

Susan McCabe and Mary Ann Boyd

KEY CONCEPTS

- neurotransmitters
- plasticity

LEARNING OBJECTIVES

After studying this chapter, you will be able to:

- Describe the association between biologic functioning and symptoms of psychiatric disorders.
- Locate brain structures primarily involved in psychiatric disorders; describe the primary functions of these structures.
- Describe basic mechanisms of neuronal transmission.
- Identify the location and function of neurotransmitters significant to hypotheses regarding major mental disorders.
- Discuss the basic utilization of new knowledge gained from fields of study, including psychoneuroimmunology, and chronobiology.
- Discuss the role of genetics in the development of psychiatric disorders.

KEY TERMS

• acetylcholine • amino acids • autonomic nervous system • basal ganglia • biogenic amines • biologic markers • brain stem • cerebellum • circadian cycle • chronobiology • cortex • dopamine • extrapyramidal motor system • frontal, parietal, temporal, and occipital lobes • GABA • genotype • genome • glutamate • hippocampus • histamine • limbic system • locus ceruleus • neurohormones • neuron • neuromodulators • norepinephrine • neuropeptides • phenotype • pineal body • psychoneuroimmunology • population genetics • receptors • serotonin • synaptic cleft • zeitgebers

All behavior recognized as human results from actions that originate in the brain and its amazing interconnection of neural networks. Modern research has increased understanding of how the complex circuitry of the brain interacts with external environment, memories, and experiences. Through the spinal column and peripheral nerves, along with other systems, such as the endocrine and immune systems, the brain constantly receives and processes information. As the brain shifts and sorts through the amazing amount of information it processes every hour, it decides on actions and initiates behaviors that allow each person to act in entirely unique and very human ways.

This chapter reviews the basic information necessary for understanding neuroscience as it relates to the role of the psychiatric–mental health nurse. It will review basic central nervous system (CNS) structures and functions; the peripheral nervous system (PNS); general functions of the major neurotransmitters and receptors; basic principles of neurotransmission; genetic models; circadian rhythms; and biologic tests. The chapter assumes that the reader has a basic knowledge of human biology, anatomy, and pathophysiology. It is not intended as a full presentation of neuroanatomy and physiology, but rather as an overview of the structures and functions most critical to understanding the role of the psychiatric–mental health nurse. As you read this chapter, think about what you know about the symptoms of mental illness. Psychiatric-mental health nurses must be able to make the connection between (1) patients' psychiatric symptoms, (2) the probable alterations in brain functioning linked to those symptoms, and (3) the rationale for treatment and care practices.

FAME AND FORTUNE

King George III (1739–1830)
Bipolar Illness Misdiagnosed

Public Persona

Crowned King of England at age 22, George III headed the most influential colonial power in the world at that time. England thrived in the peacetime after the Seven Years' War with France, but simultaneously taxed its American colonies so heavily and resolutely that the colonies rebelled. Could the American Revolution be blamed on King George III's state of mind?

Personal Realities

At age 50, the king first experienced abdominal pain and constipation, followed by weak limbs, fever, tachycardia, hoarseness, and dark red urine. Later, he experienced confusion, racing thoughts, visual problems, restlessness, delirium, convulsions, and stupor. His strange behavior included ripping off his wig and running about naked. Although he recovered and did not have a relapse for 13 years, he was considered to be mad. Relapses after the first relapse became more frequent and the king was eventually dethroned by the Prince of Wales.

Was George's madness in reality a genetically transmitted blood disease that caused thought disturbances, delirium, and stupor? The genetic disease porphyria is caused by defects in the body's ability to make haem. The diseases are generally inherited in an autosomal dominant fashion. The retrospective diagnosis was not made until 1966 (Macalpine & Hunter, 1966). Before that, it was believed that he suffered from bipolar disorder.

Other members of the royal family who had this hereditary disease were Queen Anne of Great Britain, Frederic the Great of Germany, George IV of Great Britain (son of George III), and George IV's daughter, Princess Charlotte, who died during childbirth from complications of the disease.

Source: Macalpine, I., & Hunter, R. (1966). The insanity of King George 3d: a classic case of porphyria. British Medical Journal, 5479 (1), 65–71.

THE BIOLOGIC BASIS OF MENTAL DISORDERS

Most human behaviors have a biologic component, but the exact neurological mechanisms are usually unknown. Mental disorders are complex syndromes consisting of biopsychosocial symptoms that more or less cluster together. These syndromes are not specific physiological disorders. Because they are not discrete physiological diseases that are easily identified by a laboratory test or x-ray, research has yet to piece together the puzzle. Many of the current theories on the pathophysiology of psychiatric disorders are inferred from the therapeutic effects of drugs (Joober, Sengupta, & Boksa, 2005). However, the effects of the drugs are often limited and affect only certain symptoms of a disorder. It is well established that genetic factors play an important role in the development of mental disorders. Genetics research is a promising area of investigation.

GENETICS AND MENTAL ILLNESS

Identifying the **genotype** or genetic make-up of the individual with reference to a specific trait or traits of mental disorders is not yet possible. There are many connections between the genetic contributions to a specific trait and the **phenotype** or observable characteristics or expressions of a specific trait. The Human Genome Project, which began in the 1990s, completed the mapping of the human **genome** in 2003. A genome is a complete set of DNA (deoxyribonucleic acid) that contains genetic instructions needed to develop and direct physiological activities. The human DNA molecules consist of two twisted, paired strands. Each strand is made of four chemical units or nucleotide bases: adenine (A), thymine (T), guanine (G), and cytosine (C). These units are paired specifically on opposite strands. A is always paired with T and C is always paired with G. This project determined the exact order or sequence of these pairs (National Human Genome Research Institute, 2005).

The sequence of the human genome is the beginning of our understanding of complex genetic connections and provides researchers with a road map of the exact sequence of the three billion nucleotide bases that make up human organisms. If printed out, the entire human genome sequence would fill a thousand 1,000-page telephone books. Many thought that once the human genome was mapped, it would be easy to determine the genes responsible for mental disorders. Unfortunately, it is not that simple. Knowing the location of the gene and its sequence are just pieces of the complex puzzle. The location of the genes does not tell us which genes are responsible for a mental illness or how mutations occur (Hough & Ursano, 2006).

Population Genetics

Population genetics is the study of inheritance. The goal of these epidemiologic studies is to show the inheritance of illnesses or traits from generation to generation. Risks and patterns of transmission are identified. These studies rely on the initial identification of an individual, a proband, who has the disorder and include the following principal methods:

- Family studies—analyze the occurrence of a disorder in first-degree relatives (biologic parents, siblings, and children), second-degree relatives (grandparents, uncles, aunts, nieces, nephews, and grandchildren), and so on.
- Twin studies—analyze the presence or absence of the disorder in pairs of twins. The *concordance rate* is the measure of similarity of occurrence in individuals with similar genetic makeup.
- Adoption studies—compare the risk for the illness developing in offspring raised in different environments. The strongest inferences may be drawn from studies that involve children separated from their parents at birth.

If mental disorders or their symptoms were an expression of a single gene, their disorder patterns would follow classic mendelian genetics. That is, a dominant allele (variant) on only one chromosome would be responsible for manifestation of a disorder. For recessive alleles, variants on both chromosomes would be required. Monozygotic (identical) twins would manifest the same disorder with 100% concordance rate. If a disorder were completely unrelated to genetics, then monozygotic twins would have the same concordance rates as dizygotic (fraternal) twins, who share roughly the same proportion of genes that ordinary siblings do (50%). If there is a genetic contribution with environmental influence, the concordance rates would be less than 100% for monozygotic twins but significantly greater than for dizygotic twins. Such is the case with several psychiatric disorders. Although no conclusive evidence exists for a complete genetic cause of most psychiatric disorders, significant evidence suggests that strong genetic contributions exist for most (Harrison & Owen, 2003; Green et al., 2003; Lea, 2000; McGuffin et al., 2003). Genetic epidemiologic studies indicate that there is usually 40% to 90% heritability for disorders such as schizophrenia, autism, and attention-deficit hyperactivity disorder (ADHD) (Sullivan, Kendler, & Neale, 2003; Bailey et al., 1995; Levy, Hay, McStephen, Wood, & Waldman, 1997).

Molecular Genetics

A gene comprises short segments of DNA and is packed with the instructions for making proteins that have a specific function. When genes are absent or malfunction, protein production is altered, and bodily functions are disrupted. In this fashion, genes play a role in cancer, heart disease, diabetes, and many psychiatric disorders.

Genes direct protein production. Gene expression is the result of the genes' direction, or the production of these proteins. It is not a static condition fixed at some point in neuronal development. Individual nerve cells may respond to neurochemical changes outside of the cell, producing different proteins for adaptation to the new environment. This dynamic nature of gene function highlights the manner in which the body and the environment interact and in how environmental factors influence gene expression.

The study of molecular genetics in psychiatric disorders is in its infancy. It is likely that psychiatric disorders are polygenic. This means that more than one gene is involved in producing a psychiatric disorder and that the disorder develops from genes interacting, which produces a risk factor, and environmental influences that lead to the expression of the illness. The environmental factors may include stress, infections, poor nutrition, catastrophic loss, complications during pregnancy, and exposure to toxins. Thus, genetic compositions convey vulnerability, or a risk for the illness, but the right set of environmental factors must be present for the disease to develop in the at-risk individual.

Genetic Susceptibility

The concept of genetic susceptibility suggests that an individual may be at increased risk for a psychiatric disorder. Research into risk factors is an important avenue of study. Just as knowledge of risk factors for diabetes and heart disease led to development of preventive interventions, learning more about risk factors for psychiatric disorders will lead to preventive care practices. Specific risk factors for psychiatric disorders are just beginning to be understood, and environmental influences are examples of risk factors (see Chapter 16). In the absence of one specific gene for the major psychiatric disorders, risk factor assessment may be a logical alternative for predicting who is more likely to experience psychiatric disorders or certain conditions, such as aggression or suicidality.

When considering information regarding risks for genetic transmission of psychiatric disorders, it is important to remember several key points:

- Psychiatric disorders have been described and labeled quite differently across generations, and errors in diagnosis may occur.
- Similar psychiatric symptoms may have considerably different causes, just as symptoms such as chest pain may occur in relation to many different causes.
- Genes that are present may not always cause the appearance of the trait.

- Several genes work together in an individual to produce a given trait or disorder.
- A biologic cause is not necessarily solely genetic in origin. Environmental influences alter the body's functioning and often mediate or worsen genetic risk factors.

NEUROANATOMY OF THE CENTRAL NERVOUS SYSTEM

Although this section discusses each functioning area of the brain separately, each area is intricately connected with the others and each functions interactively. The CNS contains the brain, brain stem, and spinal cord, whereas the total human nervous system includes the peripheral nervous system (PNS) as well. The PNS consists of the neurons that connect the CNS to the muscles, organs, and other systems in the periphery of the body. Whatever affects the CNS may also affect the PNS, and vice versa.

Cerebrum

The largest part of the human brain, the cerebrum fills the entire upper portion of the cranium. The **cortex**, or outermost surface of the cerebrum, makes up about 80% of the human brain. The cortex is four to six cellular layers thick, and each layer is composed of cell bodies mixed with capillary blood vessels. This mixture makes the cortex gray brown (thus the term *gray matter*). The cortex contains a number of bumps and grooves in a fully developed adult brain, as shown in Figure 7.1. This "wrinkling" allows for a large amount of surface area to be confined in the limited space of the skull. The increased surface area allows for more potential connections between cells within the cortex. The grooves are called *fissures* if they extend deep into the brain and *sulci* if they are shallower. The bumps or convolutions are called *gyri*. Together, they provide many of the landmarks for the subdivisions of the cortex. The longest and deepest groove, the longitudinal fissure, separates the cerebrum into left and right hemispheres. Although these two divisions are nearly symmetric, there is some variation in the location and size of the sulci and gyri in each hemisphere. Substantial variation in these convolutions is found in the cortex of different individuals.

Left And Right Hemispheres

The cerebrum can be roughly divided into two halves, or hemispheres. For most people, one hemisphere is dominant, whereas about 5% of individuals have mixed dominance. Each hemisphere controls functioning mainly on the opposite side of the body. The left hemisphere, dominant in about 95% of people, controls functions mainly on the right side of the body. The right hemisphere provides input into receptive nonverbal communication, spatial orientation and recognition; intonation of speech and aspects of music; facial recognition and facial expression of emotion; and nonverbal learning and memory. In general, the left hemisphere is more involved with verbal language function, including areas for both receptive and expressive speech control. In addition, the left hemisphere provides strong contributions to temporal order and sequencing, numeric symbols, and verbal learning and memory.

The two hemispheres are connected by the corpus callosum, a bundle of neuronal tissue that allows information to be exchanged quickly between the right and left hemispheres. An intact corpus callosum is required for the hemispheres to function in a smooth and coordinated manner.

Lobes of the Brain

The lateral surface of each hemisphere is further divided into four lobes: the **frontal, parietal, temporal, and occipital lobes** (Fig. 7.1). The lobes work in coordinated ways, but each is responsible for specific functions. An understanding of these unique functions is helpful in understanding how damage to these areas produces the symptoms of mental illness and how medications that affect the functioning of these lobes can produce certain effects.

Frontal Lobes

The right and left frontal lobes make up about one fourth of the entire cerebral cortex and are proportionately larger in humans than in any other mammal. The precentral gyrus, the gyrus immediately anterior to the central sulcus, contains the primary motor area, or homunculi. Damage to this gyrus, or to the anterior neighboring gyri, causes spastic paralysis in the opposite side of the body. The frontal lobe also contains Broca's area, which controls the motor function of speech. Damage to Broca's area produces expressive aphasia, or difficulty with the motor movements of speech. The frontal lobes are also thought to contain the highest or most complex aspects of cortical functioning, which collectively make up a large part of what we call personality. Working memory is an important aspect of frontal lobe function, including the ability to plan and initiate activity with future goals in mind. Insight, judgment, reasoning, concept formation, problem-solving skills, abstraction, and self-evaluation are all abilities that are modulated and affected by the action of the frontal lobes. These skills are often referred to as *executive functions* because they modulate more primitive impulses through numerous connections to other areas of the cerebrum.

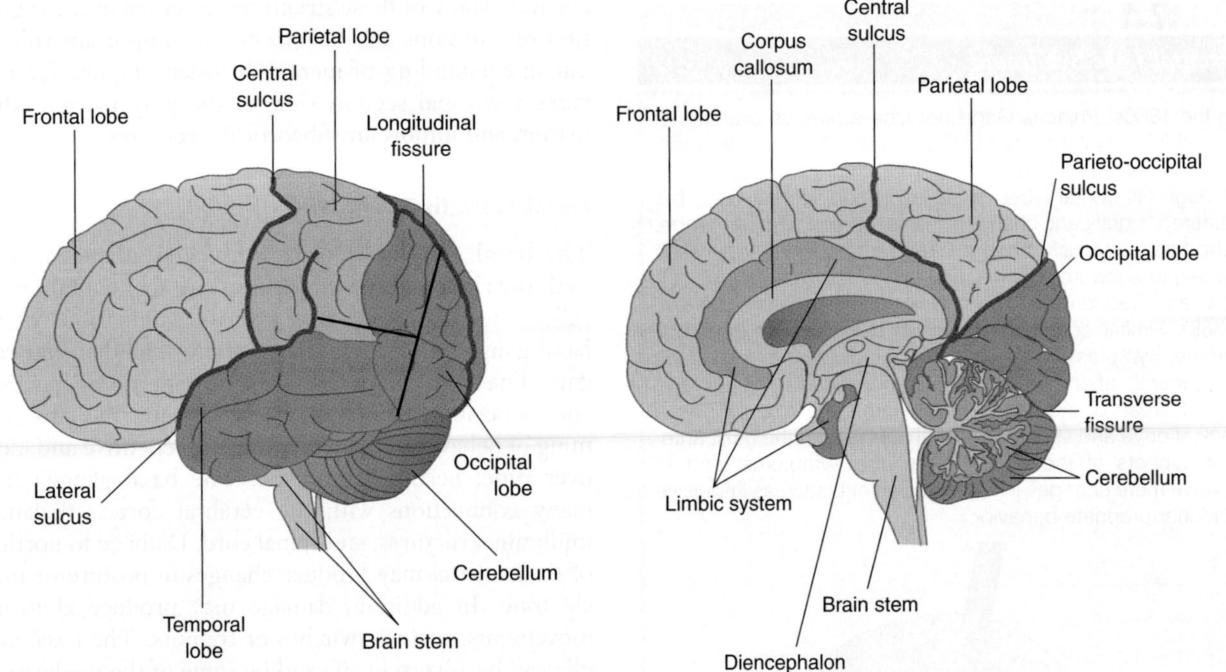

FIGURE 7.1. Lateral and medial surfaces of the brain. *Left*, the left lateral surface of the brain. *Right*, the medial surface of the right half of a sagittally hemisected brain.

When normal frontal lobe functioning is altered, executive functioning is decreased, and modulation of impulses can be lost, leading to changes in mood and personality. The importance of the frontal lobe and its role in the development of symptoms common to psychiatric disorders are emphasized in later chapters that discuss disorders such as schizophrenia, ADHD, and dementia. Box 7.1 describes how altered frontal lobe function can affect mood and personality.

PARIETAL LOBES

The postcentral gyrus, immediately behind the central sulcus, contains the primary somatosensory area. Damage to this area and neighboring gyri results in deficits in discriminative sensory function, but not in the ability to perceive sensory input. The posterior areas of the parietal lobe appear to coordinate visual and somatosensory information. Damage to this area produces complex sensory deficits, including neglect of contralateral sensory stimuli and spatial relationships. The parietal lobes contribute to the ability to recognize objects by touch, calculate, write, recognize fingers of the opposite hands, draw, and organize spatial directions, such as how to travel to familiar places.

Temporal Lobes

The temporal lobes contain the primary auditory and olfactory areas. Wernicke's area, located at the posterior aspect of the superior temporal gyrus, is primarily responsible for receptive speech. The temporal lobes also integrate sensory and visual information involved in control of written and verbal language skills as well as visual recognition. The hippocampus, an important structure discussed later, lies in the internal aspects of each temporal lobe and contributes to memory. Other internal structures of this lobe are involved in the modulation of mood and emotion.

Occipital Lobes

The primary visual area is located in the most posterior aspect of the occipital lobes. Damage to this area results in a condition called *cortical blindness*. In other words, the retina and optic nerve remain intact, but the individual cannot see. The occipital lobes are involved in many aspects of visual integration of information, including color vision, object and facial recognition, and the ability to perceive objects in motion.

Association Cortex

Although not a lobe, the association cortex is an important area that allows the lobes to work in an integrated manner. Areas of one lobe of the cortex often share functions with an area of the adjacent lobe. When these neighboring nerve fibers are related to the same sensory modality, they are often referred to as *association areas*. For example, an area in the inferior parietal, posterior temporal, and anterior occipital lobes integrates visual,

BOX 7.1

Frontal Lobe Syndrome

In the 1860s, Phineas Gage became a famous example of frontal lobe dysfunction. Mr. Gage was a New England railroad worker who had a thick iron-tamping rod propelled through his frontal lobes by an explosion. He survived, but suffered significant changes in his personality. Mr. Gage, who had previously been a capable and calm supervisor, began to show impatience, liable mood, disrespect for others, and frequent use of profanity after his injury (Harlow, 1868). Similar conditions are often called *frontal lobe syndrome*. Symptoms vary widely from individual to individual. In general, after damage to the dorsolateral (upper and outer) areas of the frontal lobes, the symptoms include a lack of drive and spontaneity. With damage to the most anterior aspects of the frontal lobes, the symptoms tend to involve more changes in mood and affect, such as impulsive and inappropriate behavior.

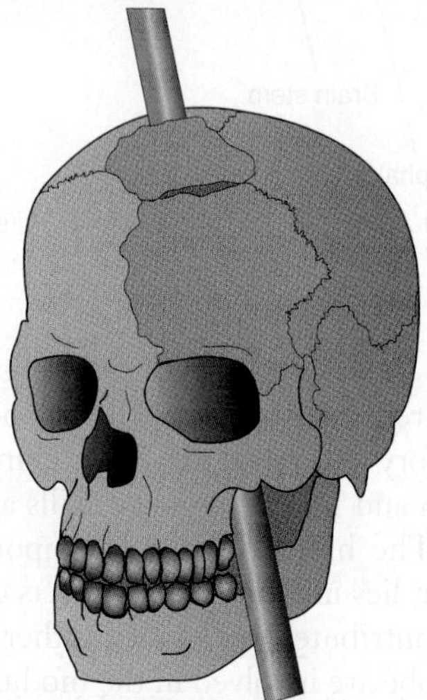

The skull of Phineas Gage, showing the route the tamping rod took through his skull. The angle of entry of the rod shot it behind the left eye and through the front part of the brain, sparing regions that are directly concerned with vital functions like breathing and heartbeat.

somatosensory, and auditory information to provide the abilities required for basic academic skills. These areas, along with numerous connections beneath the cortex, are part of the mechanisms that allow the human brain to work as an integrated whole.

Subcortical Structures

Beneath the cortex are layers of tissue composed of the axons of cell bodies. The axonal tissue forms pathways that are surrounded by glia, a fatty or lipid substance, which have a white appearance and give these layers of neuron axons their name—*white matter*. Structures inside the hemispheres, beneath the cortex, are considered subcortical. Many of these structures, essential in the regulation of emotions and behaviors, play important roles in our understanding of mental disorders. Figure 7.2 provides a coronal section view of the gray matter, white matter, and important subcortical structures.

Basal Ganglia

The **basal ganglia** are subcortical gray matter areas in both the right and the left hemisphere that contain many cell bodies or nuclei. The primary subdivisions of the basal ganglia are the putamen, globus pallidus, and caudate. The basal ganglia are involved with motor functions and association in both the learning and the programming of behavior or activities that are repetitive and, done over time, become automatic. The basal ganglia have many connections with the cerebral cortex, thalamus, midbrain structures, and spinal cord. Damage to portions of these nuclei may produce changes in posture or muscle tone. In addition, damage may produce abnormal movements, such as twitches or tremors. The basal ganglia can be adversely affected by some of the medications used to treat psychiatric disorders, leading to side effects and other motor-related problems.

Limbic System

The **limbic system** is essential to understanding the many hypotheses related to psychiatric disorders and emotional behavior in general. The limbic system is called a "system" because it comprises several small structures that work in a highly organized way. These structures include the hippocampus, thalamus, hypothalamus, amygdala, and limbic midbrain nuclei. See Figure 7.3 for identification and location of the structures within the limbic system and their relationship to other common CNS structures.

Basic emotions, needs, drives, and instinct begin and are modulated in the limbic system. Hate, love, anger, aggression, and caring are basic emotions that originate within the limbic system. Not only does the limbic system function as the seat of emotions, but, because emotions are often generated based on our personal experiences, the limbic system also is involved with aspects of memory. Hypothesized changes in the limbic system play a significant role in many theories of major mental disorders, including schizophrenia, depression, and anxiety disorders (discussed in later chapters).

Hippocampus

The **hippocampus** is involved in storing information, especially the emotions attached to a memory. Our emotional response to memories and our association with other related memories are functions of how information is stored within the hippocampus. Although memory storage is not limited to one area of the brain, destruction

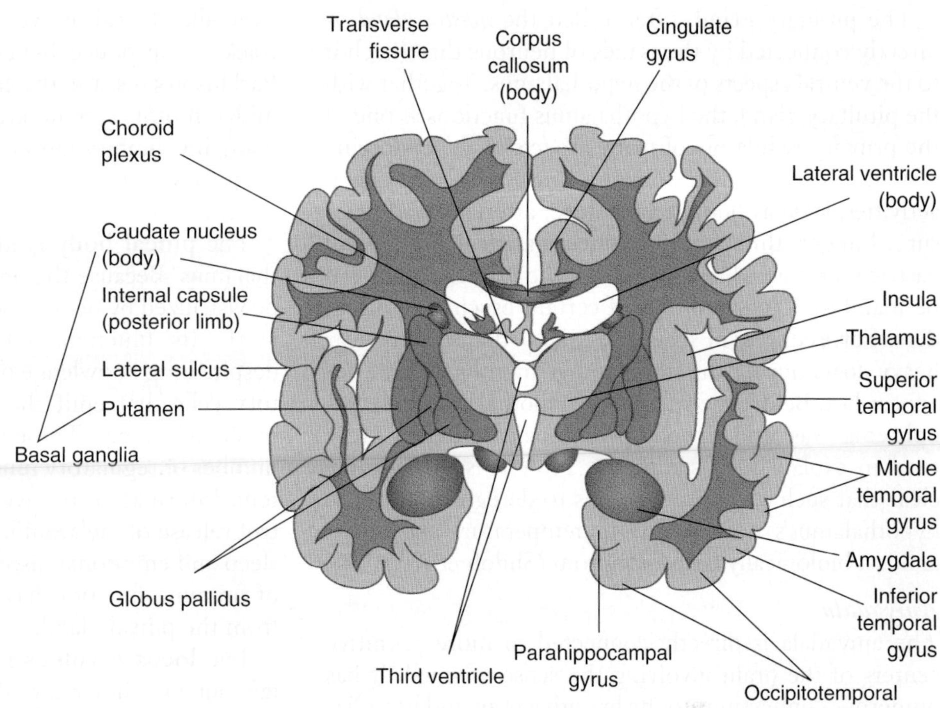

FIGURE 7.2. Coronal section of the brain, illustrating the corpus callosum, basal ganglia, and lateral ventricles.

of the left hippocampus impairs verbal memory, and damage to the right hippocampus results in difficulty with recognition and recall of complex visual and auditory patterns. Deterioration of the nerves of the hippocampus and other related temporal lobe structures found in Alzheimer's disease produces the disorder's hallmark symptoms of memory dysfunction.

Thalamus

Sometimes called the "relay-switching center of the brain," the thalamus functions as a regulatory structure to relay all sensory information, except smell, sent to the CNS from the PNS. From the thalamus, the sensory information is relayed mostly to the cerebral cortex. The thalamus relays and regulates by filtering incoming information and determining what to pass on or not pass on to the cortex. In this fashion, the thalamus prevents the cortex from becoming overloaded with sensory stimulus. The thalamus is thought to play a part in controlling electrical activity in the cortex. Because of its primary relay function, damage to a very small area of the thalamus may produce deficits in many cortical functions, thus causing behavioral abnormalities.

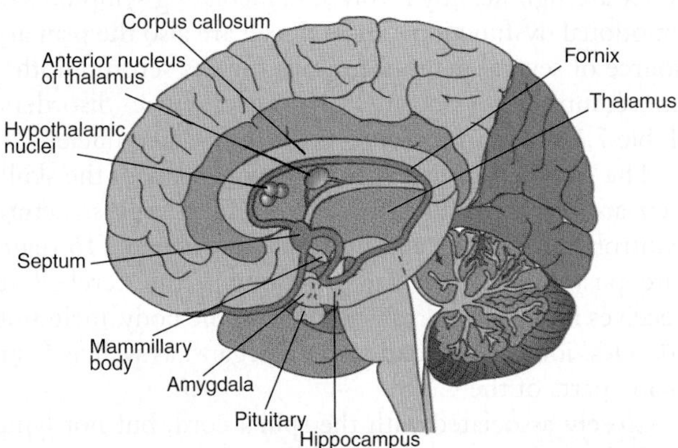

FIGURE 7.3. The structures of the limbic system are integrally involved in memory and emotional behavior. Theories link changes in the limbic system to many major mental disorders, including schizophrenia, depression, and anxiety disorders.

Hypothalamus

Basic human activities, such as sleep–rest patterns, body temperature, and physical drives such as hunger and sex, are regulated by another part of the limbic system that rests deep within the brain and is called the hypothalamus. Dysfunction of this structure, whether from disorders or as a consequence of the adverse effect of drugs used to treat mental illness, produces common psychiatric symptoms, such as appetite and sleep problems.

Nerve cells within the hypothalamus secrete hormones: for example, antidiuretic hormone, which when sent to the kidneys, accelerates the reabsorption of water; and oxytocin, which acts on smooth muscles to promote contractions, particularly within the walls of the uterus. Because cells within the nervous system produce these hormones, they are often referred to as neurohormones and form a communication mechanism through the bloodstream to control organs that are not directly connected to nervous system structures.

The pituitary gland, often called the *master gland*, is directly connected by thousands of neurons that attach it to the ventral aspects of the hypothalamus. Together with the pituitary gland, the hypothalamus functions as one of the primary regulators of many aspects of the endocrine system. Its functions are involved in control of visceral activities, such as body temperature, arterial blood pressure, hunger, thirst, fluid balance, gastric motility, and gastric secretions. Deregulation of the hypothalamus can be manifested in symptoms of certain psychiatric disorders. For example, in schizophrenia, patients often wear heavy coats during the hot summer months and do not appear hot. Before the role of the hypothalamus in schizophrenia was understood, psychological reasons were used to explain such symptoms. Now it is increasingly clear that such a symptom relates to deregulation of the hypothalamus's normal role in temperature regulation and is a biologically based symptom (Shiloh et al., 2001).

Amygdala

The amygdala is directly connected to more primitive centers of the brain involving the sense of smell. It has numerous connections to the hypothalamus and lies adjacent to the hippocampus. The amygdala provides an emotional component to memory and is involved in modulating aggression and sexuality. Impulsive acts of aggression and violence have been linked to dysregulation of the amygdala, and erratic firing of the nerve cells in the amygdala is a focus of investigation in bipolar mood disorders (see Chapter 20).

Limbic Midbrain Nuclei

The limbic midbrain nuclei are a collection of neurons (including the ventral tegmental area and the locus ceruleus) that appear to play a role in the biologic basis of addiction. Sometimes referred to as the pleasure center or reward center of the brain, the limbic midbrain nuclei function to reinforce chemically certain behaviors, ensuring their repetition. Emotions such as feeling satisfied with good food, the pleasure of nurturing young, and the enjoyment of sexual activity originate in the limbic midbrain nuclei. The reinforcement of activities such as nutrition, procreation, and nurturing young are all primitive aspects of ensuring the survival of a species. When functioning in abnormal ways, the limbic midbrain nuclei can begin to reinforce unhealthy or risky behaviors, such as drug abuse. Exploration of this area of the brain is in its infancy but offers potential insight into addictions and their treatment.

Other Central Nervous System Structures

The **extrapyramidal motor system** is a bundle of nerve fibers connecting the thalamus to the basal ganglia and cerebral cortex. Muscle tone, common reflexes, and automatic voluntary motor functioning, such as walking, are controlled by this nerve track. Dysfunction of this motor track can produce hypertonicity in muscle groups. In Parkinson's disease, the cells that compose the extrapyramidal motor system are severely affected, producing many involuntary motor movements. A number of medications, which are discussed in Chapter 8, also affect this system.

The **pineal body** is located above and medial to the thalamus. Because the pineal gland easily calcifies, it can be visualized by neuroimaging and often is a medial landmark. Its functions remain somewhat of a mystery, despite long knowledge of its existence. It contains secretory cells that emit the neurohormone melatonin and other substances. These hormones are thought to have a number of regulatory functions within the endocrine system. Information received from light–dark sources control release of melatonin, which has been associated with sleep and emotional disorders. In addition, a modulation of immune function has been postulated for melatonin from the pineal gland.

The **locus ceruleus** is a tiny cluster of neurons that fan out and innervate almost every part of the brain, including most of the cortex, the thalamus and hypothalamus, cerebellum, and the spinal cord. Just one neuron from the ceruleus can connect to more than 250,000 other neurons. Although it is very small, because of its wide-ranging neuronal connections, this tiny structure has influence in the regulation of attention, time perception, sleep–rest cycles, arousal, learning, pain, and mood and seems most involved with information processing of new, unexpected, and novel experiences. Some think its function or dysfunction may explain why individuals become addicted to substances and seek out risky behaviors, despite awareness of negative consequences.

The **brain stem,** located beneath the thalamus and composed of the midbrain, pons, and medulla, has important life-sustaining functions. Nuclei of numerous neural pathways to the cerebrum are located in the brain stem. They are significantly involved in mediating symptoms of emotional dysfunction. These nuclei are also the primary source of several neurochemicals, such as serotonin, that are commonly associated with psychiatric disorders. Table 7.1 summarizes some of the key related nuclei.

The **cerebellum** is in the posterior aspect of the skull, beneath the cerebral hemispheres. This large structure controls movements and postural adjustments. To regulate postural balance and positioning, the cerebellum receives information from all parts of the body, including muscles, joints, skin, and visceral organs, as well as from many parts of the CNS.

Closely associated with the spinal cord, but not lying entirely within its column, is the **autonomic nervous system,** a subdivision of the PNS. It was originally given this name for being independent of conscious thought, that is, automatic. However, it does not necessarily func-

Table 7.1 Classic and Putative Neurotransmitters: Their Distribution and Proposed Functions

Neurotransmitter	Cell Bodies	Projections	Proposed Function
Acetylcholine			
Dietary precursor: choline	Basal forebrain Pons Other areas	Diffuse throughout the cortex, hippocampus Peripheral nervous system	Important role in learning and memory Some role in wakefulness, and basic attention Peripherally activates muscles and is the major neurochemical in the autonomic system
Monoamines			
Dopamine (Dietary precursor: tyrosine)	Substantia nigra Ventral tegmental area Arcuate nucleus Retina olfactory bulb	Striatum (basal ganglia) Limbic system and cerebral cortex Pituitary	Involved in involuntary motor movements Some role in mood states, pleasure components in reward systems, and complex behavior such as judgment, reasoning, and insight
Norepinephrine (Dietary precursor: tyrosine)	Locus ceruleus Lateral tegmental area and others throughout the pons and medulla	Very widespread throughout the cortex, thalamus, cerebellum, brain stem, and spinal cord Basal forebrain, thalamus, hypothalamus, brain stem, and spinal cord	Proposed role in learning and memory, attributing value in reward systems, fluctuates in sleep and wakefulness Major component of the sympathetic nervous system responses, including "fight or flight"
Serotonin (Dietary precursor: tryptophan)	Raphe nuclei Others in the pons and medulla	Very widespread throughout the cortex, thalamus, cerebellum, brain stem, and spinal cord	Proposed role in the control of appetite, sleep, mood states, hallucinations, pain perception, and vomiting
Histamine (Precursor histidine)	Hypothalamus	Cerebral cortex Limbic system Hypothalamus Found in all mast cells	Control of gastric secretions, smooth muscle control, cardiac stimulation, stimulation of sensory nerve endings, and alertness
Amino Acids			
Gamma-aminobutyric acid (GABA)	Derived from glutamate without localized cell bodies	Found in cells and projections throughout the central nervous system (CNS), especially in intrinsic feedback loops and interneurons of the cerebrum Also in the extrapyramidal motor system and cerebellum	Fast inhibitory response postsynaptically, inhibits the excitability of the neurons and therefore contributes to seizure, agitation, and anxiety control
Glycine	Primarily the spinal cord and brain stem	Limited projection, but especially in the auditory system and olfactory bulb Also found in the spinal cord, medulla, midbrain, cerebellum, and cortex	Inhibitory Decreases the excitability of spinal motor neurons but not cortical
Glutamate	Diffuse	Diffuse, but especially in the sensory organs	Excitatory Responsible for the bulk of information flow
Neuropeptides			
Endogenous opioids, (i.e., endorphins, enkephalins)	A large family of neuropeptides, which has three distinct subgroups, all of which are manufactured widely throughout the CNS	Widely distributed within and outside of the CNS	Suppresses pain, modulates mood and stress Likely involvement in reward systems and addiction Also may regulate pituitary hormone release Implicated in the pathophysiology of diseases of the basal ganglia

(Continued on following page)

Table 7.1 Classic and Putative Neurotransmitters: Their Distribution and Proposed Functions (Continued)

Neurotransmitter	Cell Bodies	Projections	Proposed Function
Melatonin (One of its precursors serotonin)	Pineal body	Widely distributed within and outside of the CNS	Secreted in dark and suppressed in light, helps regulate the sleep–wake cycle as well as other biologic rhythms
Substance P	Widespread, significant in the raphe system and spinal cord	Spinal cord, cortex, brain stem and especially sensory neurons associated with pain perception	Involved in pain transmission, movement, and mood regulation
Cholecystokinin	Predominates in the ventral tegmental area of the midbrain	Frontal cortex where it is often colocalized with dopamine Widely distributed within and outside of the CNS	Primary intestinal hormone involved in satiety, also has some involvement in the control of anxiety and panic

tion as autonomously as the name indicates. This system contains efferent (nerves moving away from the CNS), or motor system neurons, which affect target tissues such as cardiac muscle, smooth muscle, and the glands. It also contains afferent nerves, which are sensory and conduct information from these organs back to the CNS.

The autonomic nervous system is further divided into the sympathetic and parasympathetic nervous systems. These systems, although peripheral, are included here because they are involved in the emergency, or "fight-or-flight," response as well as the peripheral actions of many medications (see Chapter 8). Figure 7.4 illustrates the innervations of various target organs by the autonomic nervous system. Table 7.2 identifies the actions of the sympathetic and parasympathetic nervous systems on various target organs.

Table 7.2 Peripheral Organ Response in the Autonomic Nervous System

Effector Organ	Sympathetic Response (Mostly Norepinephrine)	Parasympathetic Response (Acetylcholine)
Eye		
• Iris sphincter muscle	Dilation	Constriction
• Ciliary muscle	Relaxation	Accommodation for near vision
Heart		
• Sinoatrial node	Increased rate	Decrease is rare
• Atria	Increased contractility	Decrease in contractility
• Atrioventricular node	Increased contractility	Decrease in conduction velocity
Blood vessels	Constriction	Dilation
Lungs		
• Bronchial muscles	Relaxation	Bronchoconstriction
• Bronchial glands		Secretion
Gastrointestinal Tract		
• Motility and tone	Relaxation	Increased
• Sphincters	Contraction	Relaxation
• Secretion		Stimulation
Urinary Bladder		
• Detrusor muscle	Relaxation	Contraction
• Trigone and sphincter	Contraction	Relaxation
Uterus	Contraction (pregnant) Relaxation (nonpregnant)	Variable
Skin		
• Pilomotor muscles	Contraction	No effect
• Sweat glands	Increased secretion	No effect
Glands		
• Salivary, lachrymal		Increased secretion
• Sweat		Increased secretion

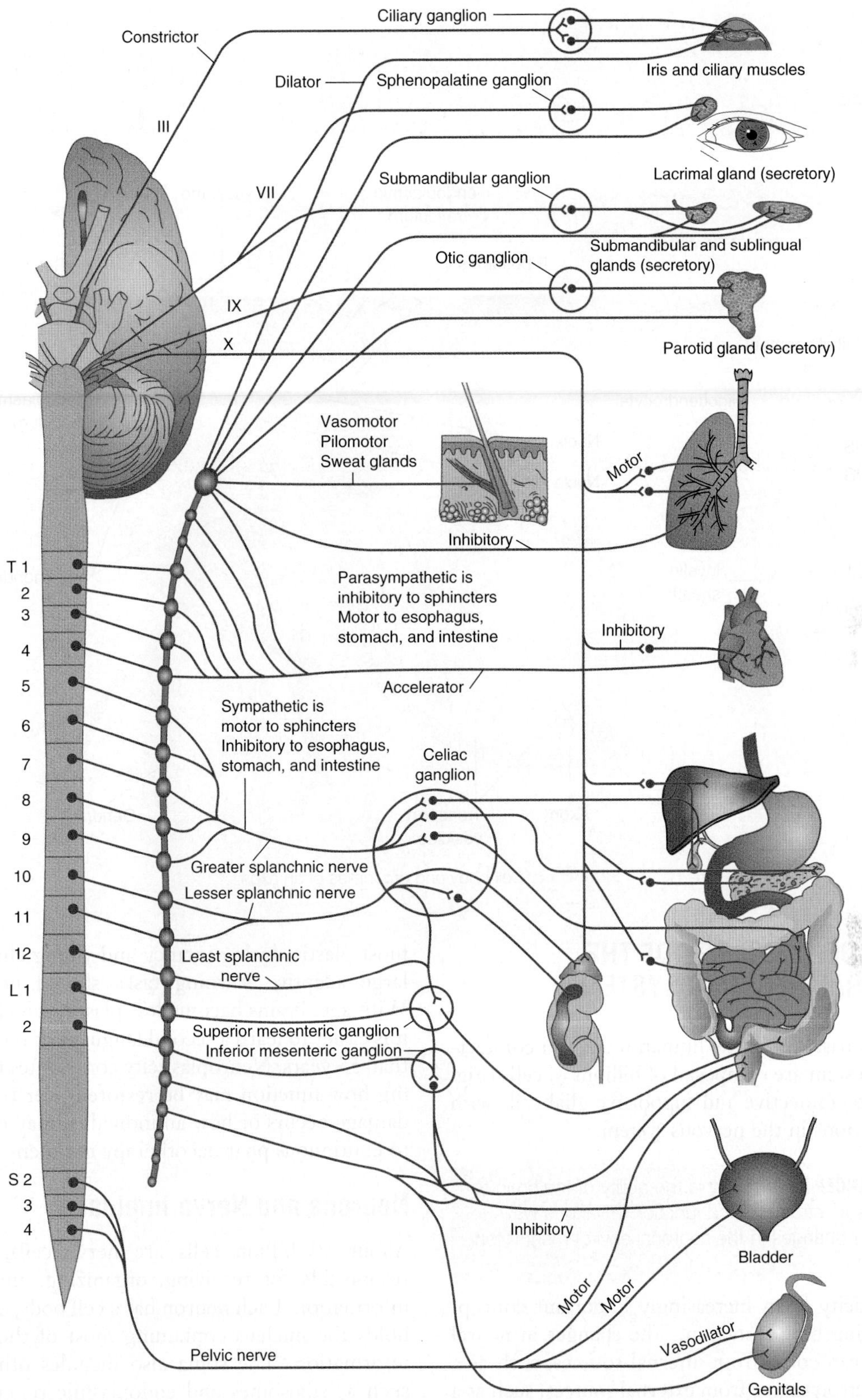

FIGURE 7.4. Diagram of the autonomic nervous system. Note that many organs are innervated by both sympathetic and parasympathetic nerves. (Adapted from Schaffe, E. E., & Lytle, I. M. [1980]. *Basic physiology and anatomy*. Philadelphia: J. B. Lippincott.)

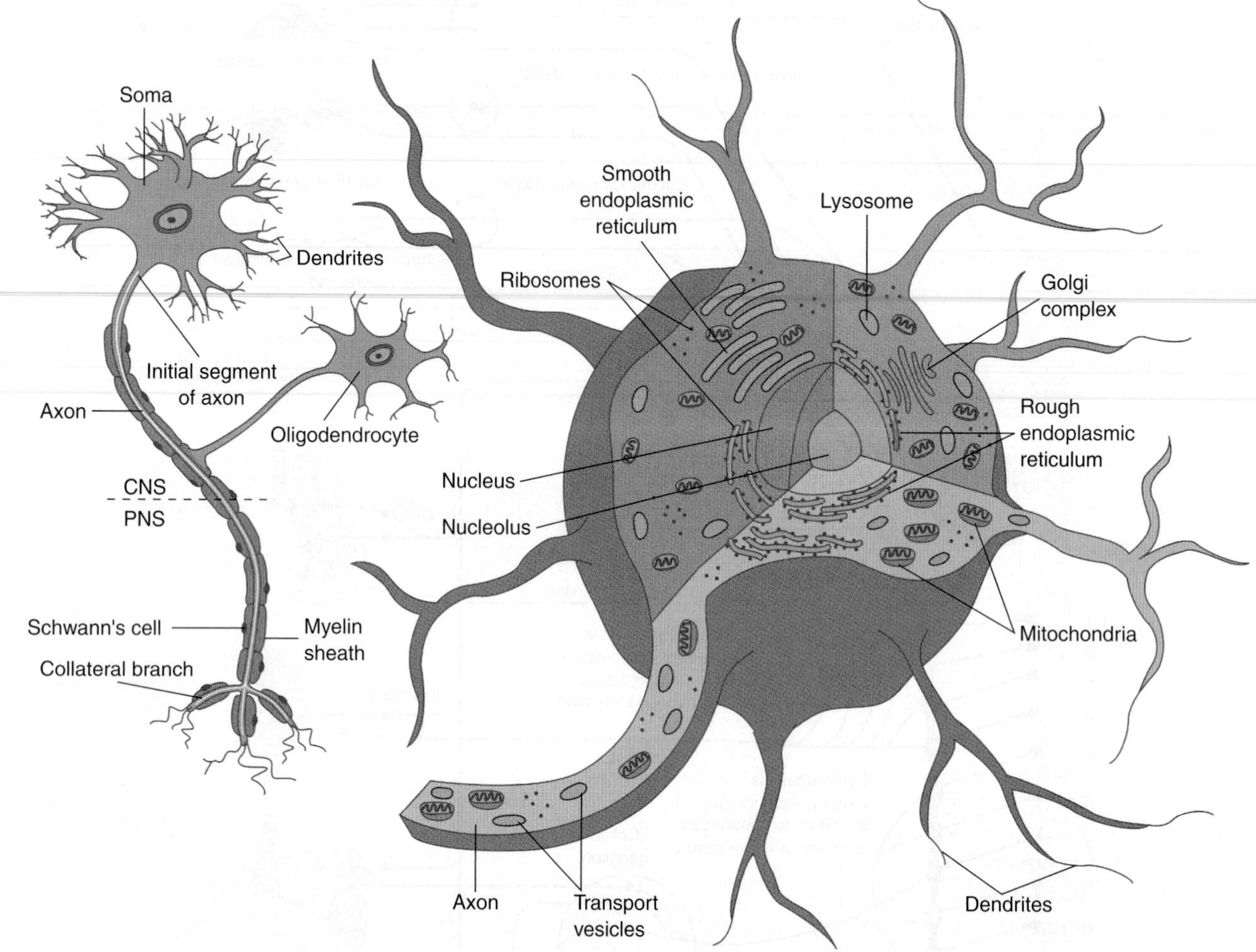

FIGURE 7.5. Cell body and organelles of an axon.

NEUROPHYSIOLOGY OF THE CENTRAL NERVOUS SYSTEM

At their most basic level, the human brain and connecting nervous system are composed of billions of cells (Fig. 7.5). Most are connective and supportive glial cells with ancillary functions in the nervous system.

> **KEY CONCEPT Plasticity** is the ability of the brain to change its structure and function in various ways to compensate for changes in the neuronal environment (Mohr & Mohr, 2001).

Neuroplasticity is an increasingly important concept when describing brain function. The changes in neural environment can come from internal sources, such as a change in electrolytes, or from external sources, such as a virus or toxin. With neuroplasticity, nerve signals may be rerouted, cells may learn new functions, sensitivity or number of cells may increase or decrease, or some nerve tissue may be regenerated in a limited way. Brains are most plastic during infancy and young childhood, when large adaptive learning tasks should normally occur. With age, brains become less plastic, which explains why it is easier to learn a second language at the age of 5 years than 55 years. Neuroplasticity contributes to understanding how function may be restored over time after brain damage occurs or how an individual may react over time to continuous pharmacotherapy regimens.

Neurons and Nerve Impulses

About 10 billion cells are nerve cells, or **neurons**, responsible for receiving, organizing, and transmitting information. Each neuron has a cell body, or soma, which holds the nucleus containing most of the cell's genetic information. The soma also includes other organelles, such as ribosomes and endoplasmic reticulum, both of which carry out protein synthesis; the Golgi apparatus, which contains enzymes to modify the proteins for specific functions; vesicles, which transport and store proteins; and lysosomes, responsible for degradation of these proteins. Located throughout the neuron, mitochondria, containing enzymes and often called the "cell's engine," are the site of many energy-producing chemical reactions. These cell structures provide the basis for secreting numerous chemicals by which neurons communicate.

It is not just the vast number of neurons that accounts for the complexities of the brain but the enormous number of neurochemical interconnections and interactions between neurons. A single motor neuron in the spinal cord may receive signals from more than 10,000 sources of interconnections with other nerves. Although most neurons have only one axon, which varies in length and conducts impulses away from the soma, each has numerous dendrites, receiving signals from other neurons. Because axons may branch as they terminate, they also have multiple contacts with other neurons.

Nerve signals are prompted to fire by a variety of chemical or physical stimuli. This firing produces an electrical impulse. The cell's membrane is a double layer of phospholipid molecules with embedded proteins. Some of these proteins provide water-filled channels through which inorganic ions may pass (Fig. 7.6). Each of the common ions—sodium, potassium, calcium, and chloride—has its own specific molecular channel. These channels are voltage gated and thus open or close in response to changes in the electrical potential across the membrane. At rest, the cell membrane is polarized with a positive charge on the outside and about a 270-millivolt charge on the inside, owing to the resting distribution of sodium and potassium ions. As potassium passively diffuses across the membrane, the sodium pump uses energy to move sodium from the inside of the cell against a concentration gradient to maintain this distribution. An action potential, or nerve impulse, is generated as the membrane is depolarized and a threshold value is reached, which triggers the opening of the voltage-gated sodium channels, allowing sodium to surge into the cell. The inside of the cell briefly becomes positively charged and the outside negatively charged. Once initiated, the action potential becomes self-propagating, opening nearby sodium channels. This electrical communication moves into the soma from the dendrites or down the axon by this mechanism.

Synaptic Transmission

For one neuron to communicate with another, the electrical process described must change to a chemical communication. The **synaptic cleft**, a junction between one nerve and another, is the space where the electrical intracellular signal becomes a chemical extracellular signal. Various substances are recognized as the chemical messengers between neurons.

As the electrical action potential reaches the ends of the axon, called *terminals*, calcium ion channels are opened, causing an influx of Ca^{++} ions into the **neuron**. This increase in calcium stimulates the release of neurotransmitters into the synapse. Rapid signaling between neurons requires a ready supply of neurotransmitter. These neurotransmitters are stored in small vesicles grouped near the cell membrane at the end of the axon. When stimulated, the vesicles containing the neurotransmitter fuse with the cell membrane, and the neurotransmitter is released into the synapse (Fig. 7.7). The neurotransmitter then crosses the synaptic cleft to a receptor site on the postsynaptic neuron and stimulates adjacent neurons. This is the process of neuronal communication.

When the neurotransmitter has completed its interaction with the postsynaptic receptor and stimulated that cell, its work is done, and it needs to be removed. It can be removed by natural diffusion away from the area of high neurotransmitter concentration at the receptors by being broken down by enzymes in the synaptic cleft, or through reuptake through highly specific mechanisms into the presynaptic terminal. The primary steps in synaptic transmission are summarized in Figure 7.7.

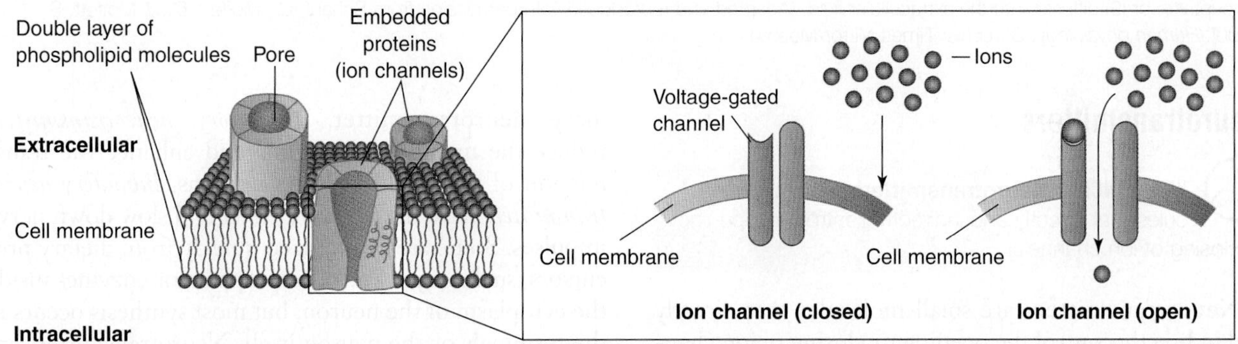

FIGURE 7.6. Initiation of a nerve impulse. The initiation of an action potential, or nerve impulse, involves the opening and closing of the voltage-gated channels on the cell membrane and the passage of ions into the cell. The resulting electrical activity sends communication impulses from the dendrites or axon into the body.

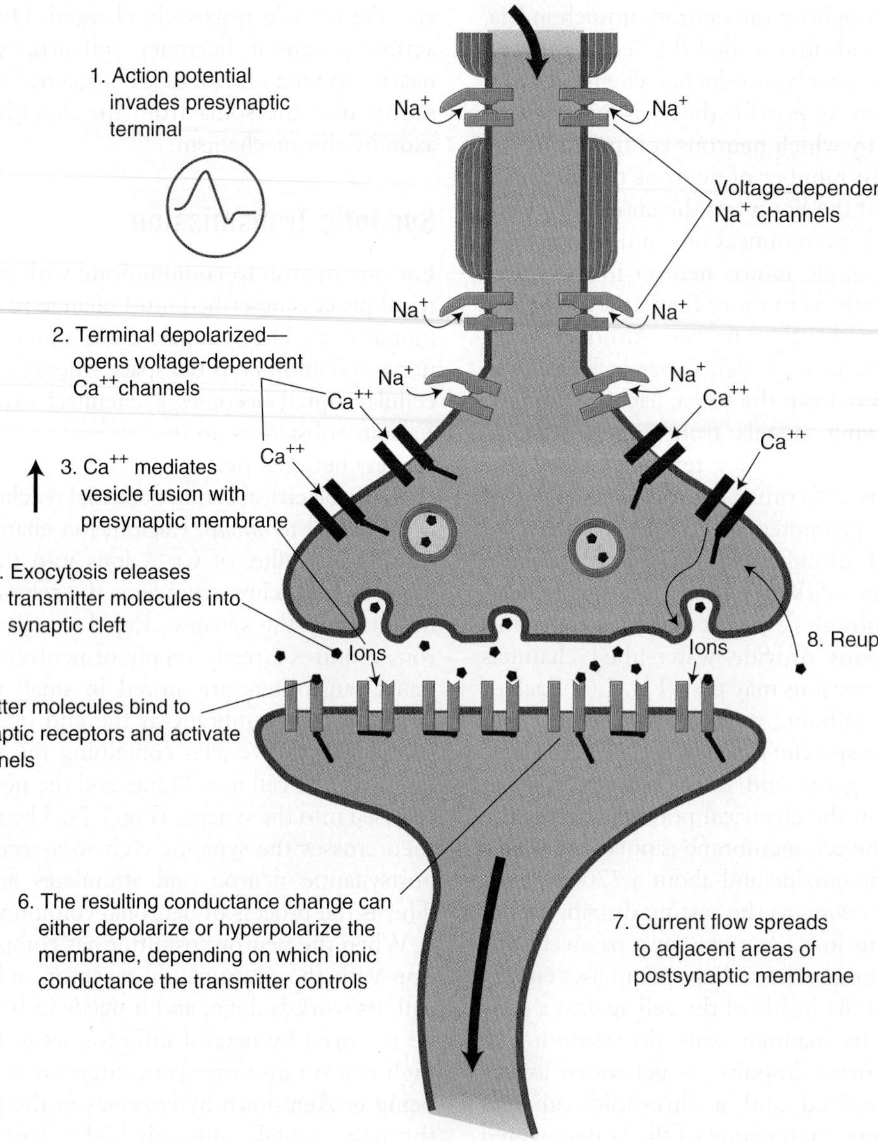

FIGURE 7.7. Synaptic transmission. The most significant events that occur during synaptic transmission: (1) the action potential reaches the presynaptic terminal; (2) membrane depolarization causes Ca^{++} terminals to open; (3) Ca^{++} mediates fusion of the vesicles with the presynaptic membrane; (4) transmitter molecules are released into the synaptic cleft, by exocytosis; (5) transmitter molecules bind to postsynaptic receptors and activate ion channels; (6) conductance changes cause an excitatory or inhibitory postsynaptic potential, depending on the specific transmitter; (7) current flow spreads along the postsynaptic membrane; (8) transmitter remaining in the synaptic cleft returns to the presynaptic terminal by reuptake; or (9) diffuses into the extracellular fluid. (Adapted and reproduced with permission from Schauf, C., Moffett, D., & Moffett, S. [1990]. *Human physiology*. St. Louis: Times Mirror/Mosby.)

Neurotransmitters

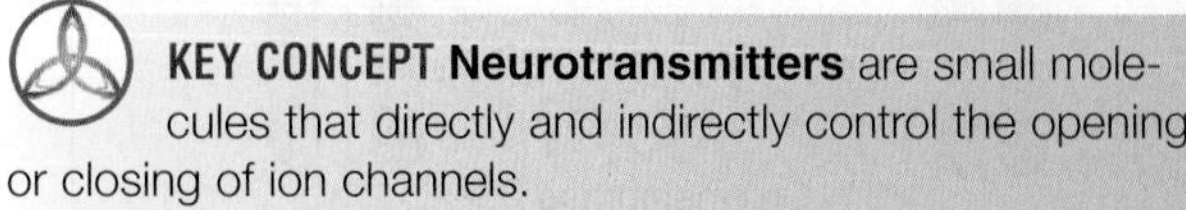

KEY CONCEPT Neurotransmitters are small molecules that directly and indirectly control the opening or closing of ion channels.

Neurotransmitters are small molecules that directly and indirectly control the opening or closing of ion channels. **Neuromodulators** are chemical messengers that make the target cell membrane or postsynaptic membrane more or less susceptible to the effects of the primary neurotransmitter. *Excitatory neurotransmitters* reduce the membrane potential and enhance the transmission of the signal between neurons. *Inhibitory neurotransmitters* have the opposite effect and slow down nerve impulses. Some are synthesized quickly from dietary precursors, such as tyrosine or tryptophan, or enzymes inside the cytoplasm of the neuron, but most synthesis occurs in the terminals or the neuron itself. Neurotransmitters are commonly classified as the following: cholinergic, biogenic amine (monoamines or bioamines), amino acid, and neuropeptides.

Acetylcholine

Acetylcholine (ACh) is the primary cholinergic neurotransmitter. Found in the greatest concentration in the PNS, ACh provides the basic synaptic communication for the parasympathetic neurons and part of the sympathetic neurons, which send information to the CNS.

ACh is an excitatory neurotransmitter and is found throughout the cerebral cortex and limbic system, arising primarily from cell bodies in the base of the frontal lobes. Pathways from this region also project throughout the hippocampus (Fig. 7.8). These connections suggest that ACh is involved in higher intellectual functioning and memory. Individuals who have Alzheimer's disease or Down syndrome often exhibit patterns of cholinergic neuron loss in regions innervated by these pathways (such as the hippocampus), which may contribute to their memory difficulties and other cognitive deficits. Some cholinergic neurons are afferent to these areas bringing information from the limbic system, highlighting the role that ACh plays in communicating emotional state to the cerebral cortex.

Biogenic Amines

The **biogenic amines** (bioamines) consist of small molecules manufactured in the neuron that contain an amine group; thus the name. These include **dopamine**, **norepinephrine**, and **epinephrine**, which are all synthesized from the amino acid tyrosine; **serotonin**, which is synthesized from tryptophan; and **histamine**, manufactured from histidine. Of all the neurotransmitters, dopamine, norepinephrine, and serotonin are most central to current hypotheses of psychiatric disorders and thus are described in more detail.

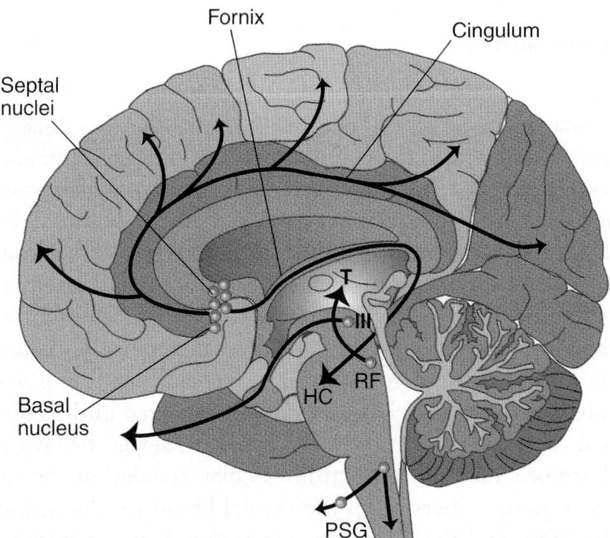

FIGURE 7.8. Cholinergic pathways. HC, hippocampal formation; PSG, parasympathetic ganglion cell; RF, reticular formation; T, thalamus. (Adapted from Nolte, J., & Angevine, J. [1995]. *The human brain: In photographs and diagrams.* St. Louis: Mosby.)

Dopamine

Dopamine is an excitatory neurotransmitter found in distinct regions of the CNS, and is involved in cognition, motor, and neuroendocrine functions. Dopamine levels are decreased in Parkinson's disease, and abnormally high production of dopamine has been associated with schizophrenia (discussed in more detail in Chapter 18). Dopamine is also the neurotransmitter that stimulates the body's natural "feel good' reward pathways, producing pleasant euphoric sensation under certain conditions. Abnormalities of dopamine use within the reward system pathways are suspected to be a critical aspect of the development of drug and other addictions. The dopamine pathways are distinct neuronal areas within the CNS in which the neurotransmitter dopamine predominates. Three major dopaminergic pathways have been identified.

The mesocortical and mesolimbic pathways originate in the ventral tegmental area and project into the medial aspects of the cortex (mesocortical) and the medial aspects of the limbic system inside the temporal lobes, including the hippocampus and amygdala (mesolimbic). Sometimes they are considered to be one pathway and at other times two separate pathways. The mesocortical pathway has major effects on cognition, including such functions as judgment, reasoning, insight, social conscience, motivation, the ability to generalize learning, and reward systems in the human brain. It contributes to some of the highest seats of cortical functioning. The mesolimbic pathway also strongly influences emotions and has projections that affect memory and auditory reception. Abnormalities in these pathways have been associated with schizophrenia.

Another major dopaminergic pathway begins in the substantia nigra and projects into the basal ganglia, parts of which are known as the *striatum*. Therefore, this pathway is called the *nigrostriatal pathway*. This influences the extrapyramidal motor system, which serves the voluntary motor system and allows involuntary motor movements. Destruction of dopaminergic neurons in this pathway has been associated with Parkinson's disease.

The next or last dopamine pathway originates from projections of the mesolimbic pathway and continues into the hypothalamus, which then projects into the pituitary gland. Therefore, this pathway, called the *tuberoinfundibular pathway*, has an impact on endocrine function and other functions, such as metabolism, hunger, thirst, sexual function, circadian rhythms, digestion, and temperature control. Figure 7.9 illustrates the dopaminergic pathways.

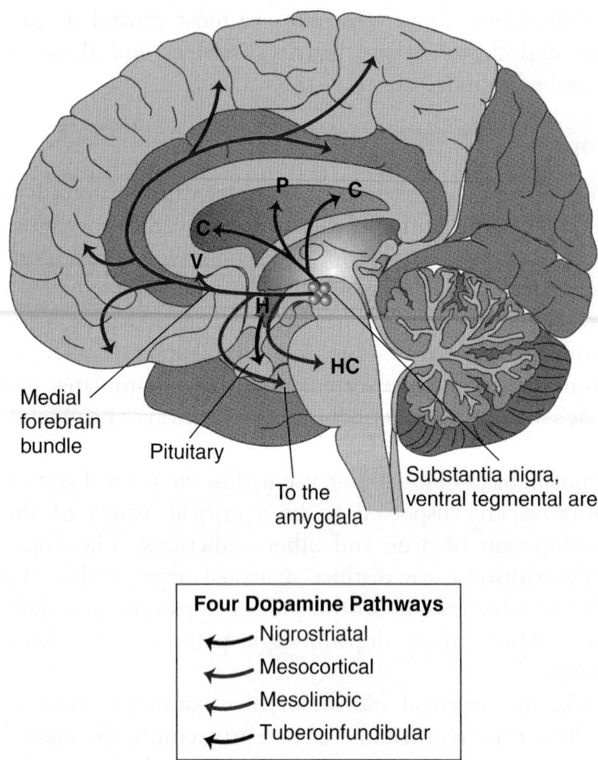

FIGURE 7.9. Dopaminergic pathways. C, caudate nucleus; H, hypothalamus; HC, hippocampal formation; P, putamen; S, striatum; V, ventral striatum. (Adapted from Nolte, J., & Angevine, J. [1995]. *The human brain: In photographs and diagrams*. St. Louis: Mosby.)

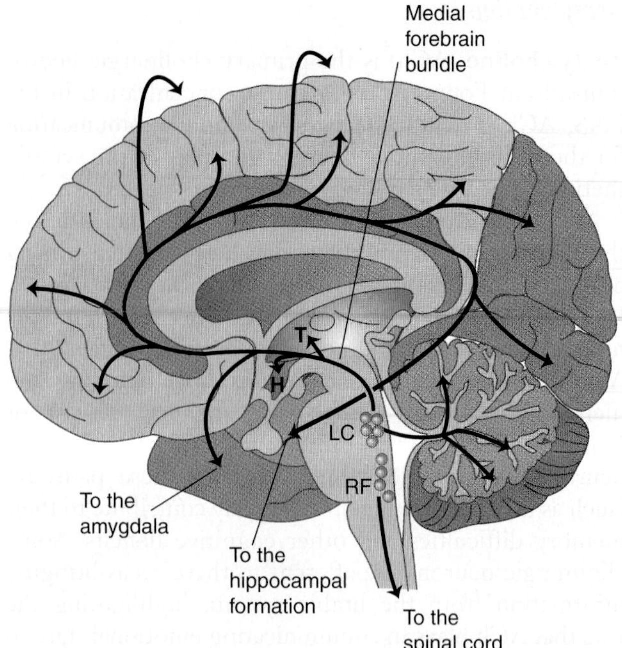

FIGURE 7.10. Noradrenergic pathways. H, hypothalamus; LC, locus ceruleus; RF, reticular formation; T, thalamus. (Adapted from Nolte, J., & Angevine, J. [1995]. *The human brain: In photographs and diagrams*. St. Louis: Mosby.)

Norepinephrine

Norepinephrine is an excitatory neurochemical that plays a major role in generating and maintaining mood states. Decreased norepinephrine has been associated with depression, and excessive norepinephrine has been associated with manic symptoms (Montgomery, 2000). Because norepinephrine is so heavily concentrated in the terminal sites of sympathetic nerves, it can be released quickly to ready the individual for a fight-or-flight response to threats in the environment. For this reason, norepinephrine is thought to play a role in the physical symptoms of anxiety.

Nerve tracts and pathways containing predominantly norepinephrine are called *noradrenergic* and are less clearly delineated than the dopamine pathways. In the CNS, noradrenergic neurons originate in the locus ceruleus, where more than half of the noradrenergic cell bodies are located. Because the locus ceruleus is one of the major timekeepers of the human body, norepinephrine is involved in sleep and wakefulness. From the locus ceruleus, noradrenergic pathways ascend into the neocortex, spread diffusely (Fig. 7.10), and enhance the ability of neurons to respond to whatever input they may be receiving. In addition, norepinephrine appears to be involved in the process of reinforcement, which facilitates learning. Noradrenergic pathways innervate the hypothalamus and thus are involved to some degree in endocrine function. Anxiety disorders and depression are examples of psychiatric illnesses in which dysfunction of the noradrenergic neurons may be involved. Table 7.2 lists the effects of ACh on various organs in the parasympathetic system.

Serotonin

Serotonin (also called 5-hydroxytryptamine or 5-HT) is primarily an excitatory neurotransmitter that is diffusely distributed within the cerebral cortex, limbic system, and basal ganglia of the CNS. Serotonergic neurons also project into the hypothalamus and cerebellum. Figure 7.11 illustrates serotonergic pathways. Serotonin plays a role in emotions, cognition, sensory perceptions, and essential biologic functions, such as sleep and appetite. During the rapid eye movement (REM) phase of sleep, or the dream state, serotonin concentrations decrease, and muscles subsequently relax. Serotonin is also involved in the control of food intake, hormone secretion, sexual behavior, thermoregulation, and cardiovascular regulation. Some serotonergic fibers reach the cranial blood vessels within the brain and the *pia mater*, where they have a vasoconstrictive effect. The potency of some new medications for migraine headaches is related to their ability to block serotonin transmission in the cranial blood vessels. Descending serotonergic pathways are important in

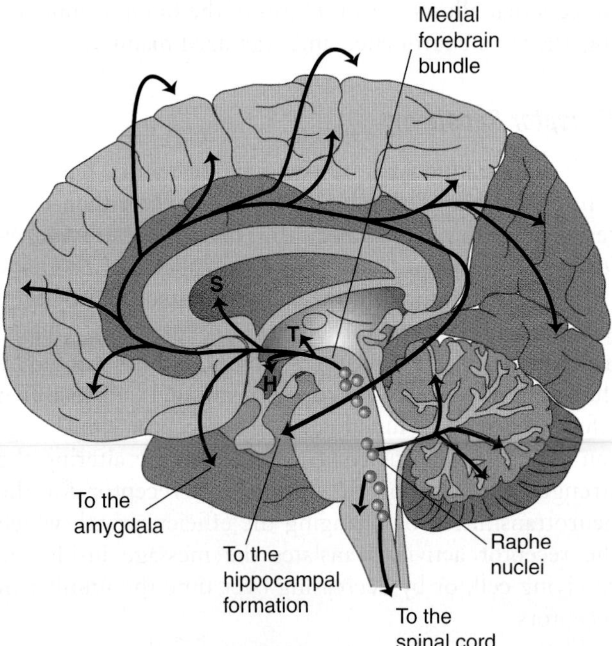

FIGURE 7.11. Serotonergic pathways. H, hypothalamus; S, septal nuclei; T, thalamus. (Adapted from Nolte, J., & Angevine, J. [1995]. *The human brain: In photographs and diagrams.* St. Louis: Mosby.)

central pain control. Depression and insomnia have been associated with decreased levels of 5-HT, whereas mania has been associated with increased 5-HT. Some of the most well-known antidepressant medications, such as Prozac and Zoloft, which are discussed in more depth in Chapter 8, function by raising serotonin levels within certain areas of the CNS (Harmer, Hill, Taylor, Cowen, & Goodwin, 2003). Obsessive-compulsive disorder, panic disorder, and other anxiety disorders are believed to be associated with dysfunction of the serotonin pathways (Kapczinski, Lima, Souza, & Schmitt, 2003).

Histamine

Histamine has only recently been identified as a neurotransmitter. Its cell bodies originate predominantly in the hypothalamus and project to all major structures in the cerebrum, brain stem, and spinal cord. Its functions are not well known, but it appears to have a role in autonomic and neuroendocrine regulation. Many psychiatric medications can block the effects of histamine postsynaptically and produce side effects such as sedation, weight gain, and hypotension.

Amino Acids

Amino acids are the building blocks of proteins and have many roles in intraneuronal metabolism. In addition, amino acids can function as neurotransmitters in as many as 60% to 70% of the synaptic sites in the brain. Amino acids are the most prevalent neurotransmitters. Virtually all of the neurons in the CNS are activated by excitatory amino acids, such as glutamate, and inhibited by inhibitory amino acids, such as GABA and glycine. Many of these amino acids coexist with other neurotransmitters.

Gamma-Aminobutyric Acid

GABA is the primary inhibitory neurotransmitter for the CNS. The pathways of GABA exist almost exclusively in the CNS, with the largest GABA concentrations in the hypothalamus, hippocampus, basal ganglia, spinal cord, and cerebellum. GABA functions in an inhibitory role in control of spinal reflexes and cerebellar reflexes. It has a major role in the control of neuronal excitability through the brain. In addition, GABA has an inhibitory influence on the activity of the dopaminergic nigrostriatal projections. GABA also has interconnections with other neurotransmitters. For example, dopamine inhibits cholinergic neurons, and GABA provides feedback and balance. Dysregulation of GABA and GABA receptors has been associated with anxiety disorders, and decreased GABA activity is involved in the development of seizure disorders.

Glutamate

Glutamate, the most widely distributed excitatory neurotransmitter, is the main transmitter in the associational areas of the cortex. Glutamate can be found in a number of pathways from the cortex to the thalamus, pons, striatum, and spinal cord. In addition, glutamate pathways have a number of connections with the hippocampus. Some glutamate receptors may play a role in the long-lasting enhancement of synaptic activity. In turn, in the hippocampus, this enhancement may have a role in learning and memory. Too much glutamate is harmful to neurons, and considerable interest has emerged regarding its neurotoxic effects.

Conditions that produce an excess of endogenous glutamate can cause neurotoxicity by overexcitation of neuronal tissue. This process, called excitotoxicity, increases the sensitivity of glutamate receptors, produces overactivation of the receptors, and is increasingly being understood as a critical piece of the cascade of events involved in physical symptoms of alcohol withdrawal in dependent individuals. Excitotoxicity is also believed to be part of the pathology of conditions such as ischemia, hypoxia, hypoglycemia, and hepatic failure. Damage to the CNS from chronic malfunctioning of the glutamate system may be involved in the psychiatric symptoms seen in neurodegenerative diseases such as Huntington's, Parkinson's, and Alzheimer's diseases; vascular dementia; amyotrophic lateral sclerosis; and acquired immune deficiency syndrome (AIDS)-related dementia (MacGregor, Avshalumov, & Rice, 2003). Degeneration of glutamate neurons has more recently been implicated in the development of schizophrenia (Kurup & Kurup, 2003).

Neuropeptides

Neuropeptides, short chains of amino acids, exist in the CNS and have a number of important roles as neurotransmitters, neuromodulators, or neurohormones. Neuropeptides were first thought to be pituitary hormones, such as adrenocorticotropin, oxytocin, and vasopressin, or hypothalamic-releasing hormones (e.g., corticotropin-releasing hormone and thyrotropin-releasing hormone [TRH]). However, when an endogenous morphine-like substance was discovered in the 1970s, the term *endorphin*, or endogenous morphine, was introduced. Although the amino acids and monoamine neurotransmitters can be produced directly from dietary precursors in any part of the neuron, neuropeptides are, almost without exception, synthesized from messenger RNA in the cell body. Currently, two types of neuropeptides have been identified. Opioid neuropeptides, such as endorphins, enkephalins, and dynorphins, function in endocrine functioning and pain suppression. The nonopioid neuropeptides, such as substance P and somatostatin, play roles in pain transmission and in endocrine functioning.

There are considerable variations in the distribution of individual neuropeptides, but some areas are especially rich in cell bodies containing neuropeptides. These areas include the amygdala, striatum, hypothalamus, raphe nuclei, brain stem, and spinal cord. Many of the interneurons of the cerebral cortex contain neuropeptides, but there are considerably fewer in the thalamus and almost none in the cerebellum.

Receptors

Embedded in the postsynaptic membrane are a number of proteins that act as receptors for the released neurotransmitters. Each neurotransmitter has a specific **receptor**, or protein, for which it and only it will fit.

Lock and Key

The "lock-and-key" analogy has often been used to describe the fit of a given neurotransmitter to its receptor site. The target cell, when stimulated by the neurotransmitter, will then respond by evoking its own action potential and either producing some action common to that cell or acting as a relay to keep the messages moving throughout the CNS. This pattern of the electrical signal from one neuron, converted to chemical signal at the synaptic cleft, picked up by an adjacent neuron, again converted to an electrical action potential, and then to a chemical signal, occurs billions of times a day in billions of different brain cells. It is this electrical-chemical communication process that allows the structures of the brain to function together in a coordinated and organized manner.

Receptor Sensitivity

Both presynaptic and postsynaptic receptors have the capacity to change, developing either a greater-than-usual response to the neurotransmitter, known as *supersensitivity*, or a less-than-usual response, called *subsensitivity*. These changes represent the concept of neuroplasticity of brain tissue discussed earlier in the chapter. The change in sensitivity of the receptor is most commonly caused by the effect of a drug on a receptor site or by disease that affects the normal functioning of a receptor site. Drugs can affect the sensitivity of the receptor by altering the strength of attraction or affinity of a receptor for the neurotransmitter, by changing the efficiency with which the receptor activity translates the message inside the receiving cell, or by decreasing over time the number of receptors.

These mechanisms may account for the long-term, sometimes severely adverse, effects of psychopharmacologic drugs, the loss of effectiveness of a given medication, or the loss of effectiveness of a medication after repeated use in treating recurring episodes of a psychiatric disorder. Disease may cause a change in the normal number or function of receptors, thereby altering their sensitivity (Garcia, Marin, & Perillo, 2002). It has been hypothesized that depression is caused by a reduction in the normal number of certain receptors, leading to an abnormality in their sensitivity to neurotransmitters such as serotonin and norepinephrine. A decreased response to continued stimulation of these receptors is usually referred to as *desensitization* or *refractoriness*. This suspected subsensitivity is referred to as *down-regulation* of the receptors.

Receptor Subtypes

The nervous system uses many different neurochemicals for communication, and each specific chemical messenger requires a specific receptor on which the chemical can act. More than 100 different chemical messengers have been identified, with new ones being uncovered. In addition to the sheer number of receptors needed to accommodate these chemicals, the neurotransmitters may produce different effects at different synaptic sites.

Each major neurotransmitter has several different subtypes of receptors, allowing the neurotransmitter to have different effects in different areas of the brain. The receptors usually have the same name as the neurotransmitter, but the classification of the subtypes varies. For example, dopamine receptors are named D1, D2, D3, and so on. Serotonin receptors are grouped in families such at 5HT 1a, 1b, etc. The receptors for acetylcholine have completely different names: muscarinic and nicotinic. Two specific subtype receptors have been identified for GABA: A, B, and C.

NEW FIELDS OF STUDY

As the complexity of the nervous system and its interrelationship with other body systems and the environment has become more fully understood, new fields of study have emerged. Although it has long been observed that individuals under stress have compromised immune systems and are more likely to acquire common diseases, only recently have changes in the immune system been noted as widespread in some psychiatric illnesses. In addition, as biologic rhythms have become more fully understood and defined, new information suggests that dysfunction of these rhythms may not only result from a psychiatric illness but also contribute to its development. Therefore, the following sections provide a brief overview of psychoneuroimmunology and chronobiology.

Psychoneuroimmunology

Psychoneuroimmunology (PNI) examines the relationships among the immune system, nervous system, and endocrine system and our behaviors, thoughts, and feelings. The immune system is comprised of the thymus, spleen, lymph nodes, lymphatic vessels, tonsils, adenoids, and bone marrow, which manufactures all the cells that eventually develop into T cells, B cells, phagocytes, macrophages, and natural killer (NK) cells (see Figure 7.12). Many contemporary stress research studies are examining the role of the NK cells in the early recognition of foreign bodies. Lower NK cell function is related to increased disease susceptibility. NK cell function is affected by stress-induced physiologic arousal in humans. NK cell activity has been shown to vary in response to many emotional, cognitive, and physiologic stressors including anxiety, depression, perceived lack of personal control, bereavement, pain, and surgery (Motzer & Hertig, 2004).

Overactivity of the immune system can occur in autoimmune diseases such as systemic lupus erythematosus (SLE), allergies, or anaphylaxis. Evidence suggests that the nervous system regulates many aspects of immune function. Specific immune system dysfunctions may result from damage to the hypothalamus, hippocampus, or pituitary and may produce symptoms of psychiatric disorders. Figure 7.13 illustrates the interaction between stress and the immune system. This figure also demonstrates the true biopsychosocial nature of the complex interrelationship of the nervous system, the endocrine system, the immune system, and environmental or emotional stress.

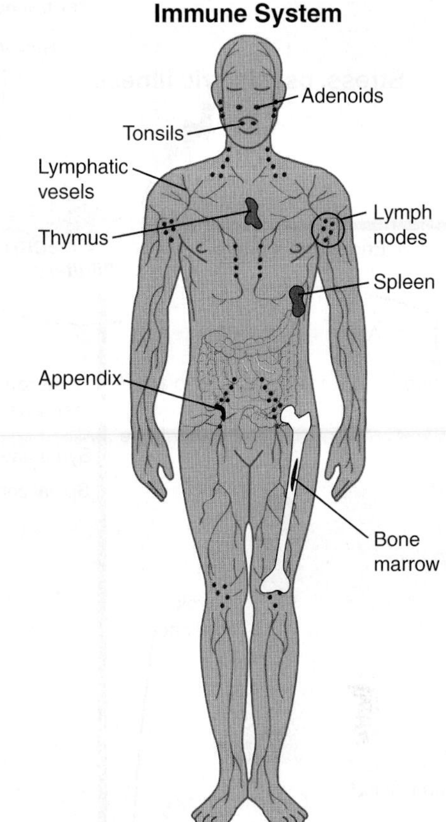

FIGURE 7.12. The immune system.

Immune dysregulation may also be involved in the development of psychiatric disorders. This can occur by allowing neurotoxins to affect the brain, damaging neuroendocrine tissue, or damaging tissues in the brain at locations such as the receptor sites. Some antidepressants have been thought to have antiviral effects. Symptoms of diseases such as depression may follow an occurrence of serious infection, and prenatal exposure to infectious organisms has been associated with the development of schizophrenia. Stress and conditioning have specific effects on the suppression of immune function (Ekman, Persson, & Nilsson, 2002; Friedman, 2000; Ishihara, Makita, Imai, Hashimoto, & Nohara, 2003).

The endocrine system also plays an important role in psychiatric disorders. Messages are conveyed within the endocrine system mainly by hormones, and neurohormones are those substances excreted by special neurons within the nervous system. **Neurohormones** are cellular substances that are secreted into the bloodstream and transported to a site where they exert their effect.

The hypothalamus sends and receives information through the pituitary, which then communicates with structures in the peripheral aspects of the body. Figure 7.14 presents an example of the communication of the anterior pituitary with a number of organs and structures. Axes, the structures within which the neurohormones are

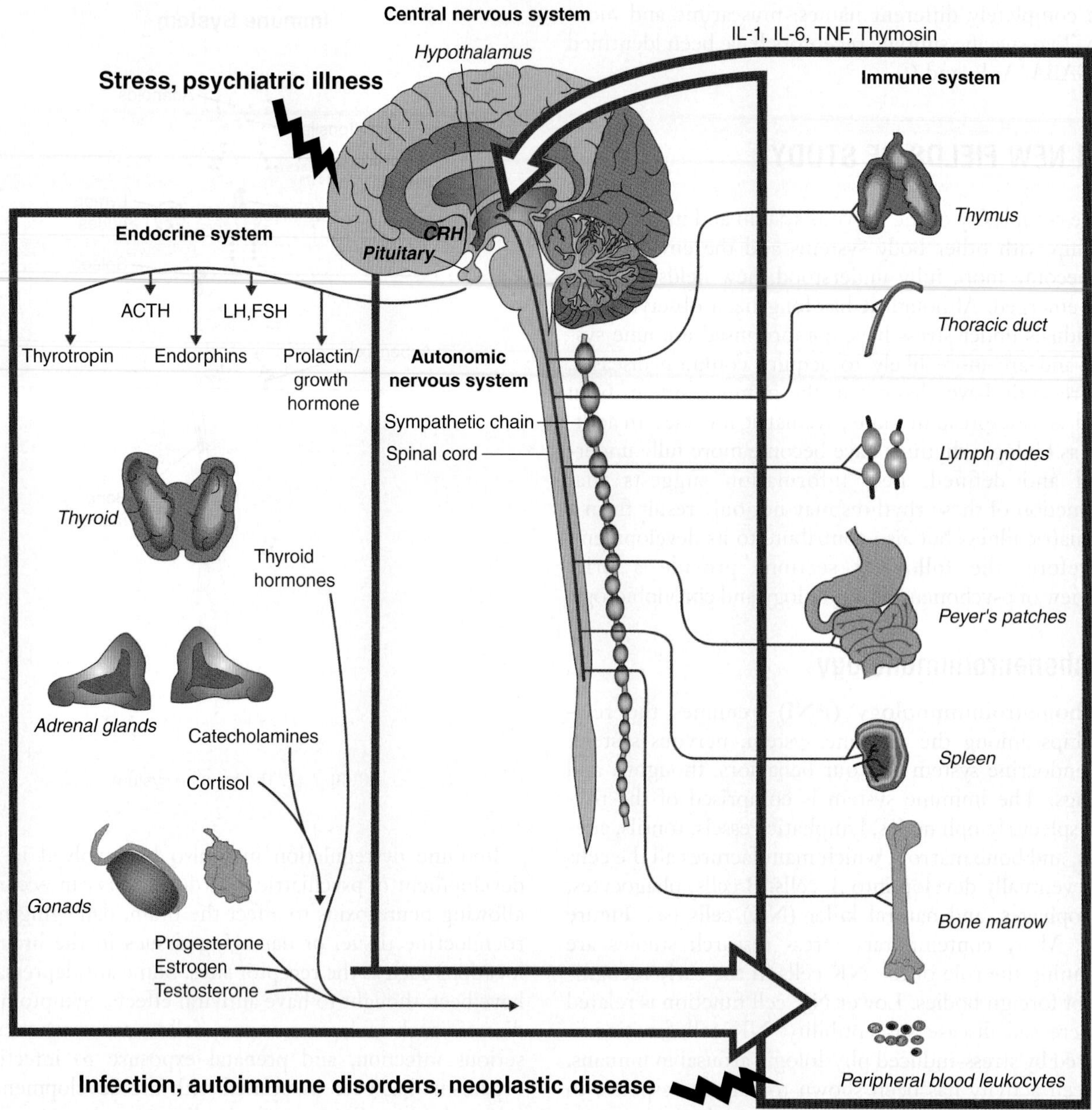

FIGURE 7.13. Examples of the interaction between stress or psychiatric illness and the immune system through the endocrine system. CRH, corticotropin-releasing hormone; IL, interleukin; TNF, tumor necrosis factor; ACTH, adrenocorticotropic hormone; LH, luteinizing hormone; FSH, follicle-stimulating hormone.

providing messages, are the most often studied aspect of the neuroendocrine system. These axes always involve a feedback mechanism. For example, the hypothalamus–pituitary–thyroid axis regulates the release of thyroid hormone by the thyroid gland using TRH hormone from the hypothalamus to the pituitary and thyroid-stimulating hormone (TSH) from the pituitary to the thyroid. Figure 7.15 illustrates the hypothalamic–pituitary–thyroid axis. The hypothalamic–pituitary–gonadal axis regulates estrogen and testosterone secretion through luteinizing hormone and follicle-stimulating hormone. Interest in the endocrine system is heightened by various endocrine disorders that produce psychiatric symptoms. Addison's disease (hypoadrenalism) produces depression, apathy, fatigue, and occasionally psychosis. Hypothyroidism produces depression and some anxiety. Administration of steroids can cause depression, hypomania, irritability, and in some cases, psychosis. Some psychiatric disorders have been associated with endocrine system dysfunction. For example, some individuals with mood disorders show evidence of dysregulation in adrenal, thyroid, and growth hormone axes (see Chapter 14).

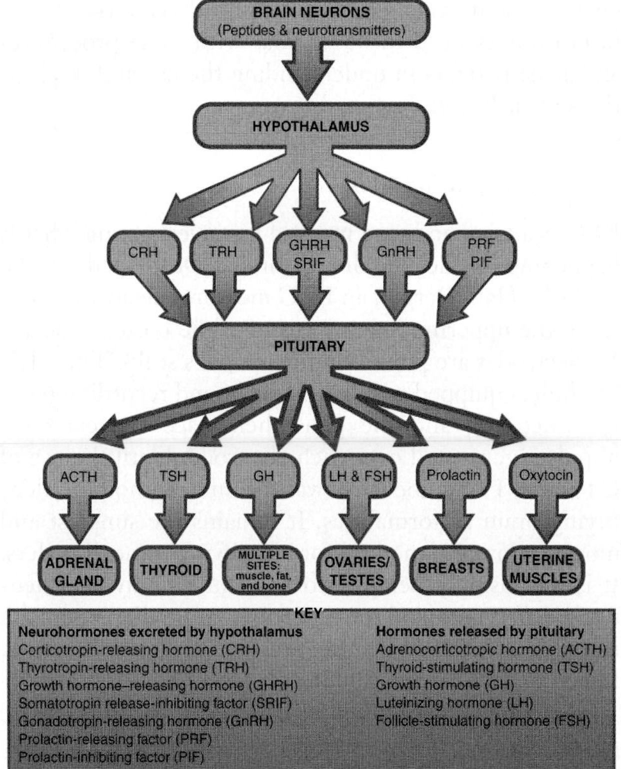

FIGURE 7.14. Hypothalamic and pituitary communication system. The neurohormonal communication system between the hypothalamus and the pituitary exerts effects on many organs and systems.

Chronobiology

Chronobiology involves the study and measure of time structures or biologic rhythms. Some rhythms have a **circadian cycle**, or 24-hour cycle, whereas others, such as the menstrual cycle, operate in different periods. Rhythms exist in the human body to control endocrine secretions, sleep–wake, body temperature, neurotransmitter synthesis, and more. These cycles may become deregulated and may begin earlier than usual, known as a phase advance, or later than usual, known as a phase delay.

Zeitgebers are specific events that function as time givers or synchronizers and that set biologic rhythms. Light is the most common example of an external zeitgeber. The suprachiasmatic nucleus of the hypothalamus is an example of an internal zeitgeber. Some theorists think that psychiatric disorders may result from one or more biologic rhythm dysfunctions. For example, depression may be, in part, a phase advance disorder, including early morning awakening and decreased time of onset of REM sleep. Seasonal affective disorder may be the result of shortened exposure to light during the winter months. Exposure to specific artificial light often relieves symptoms of fatigue, overeating, hypersomnia, and depression (see Chapters 8, 20, and 26).

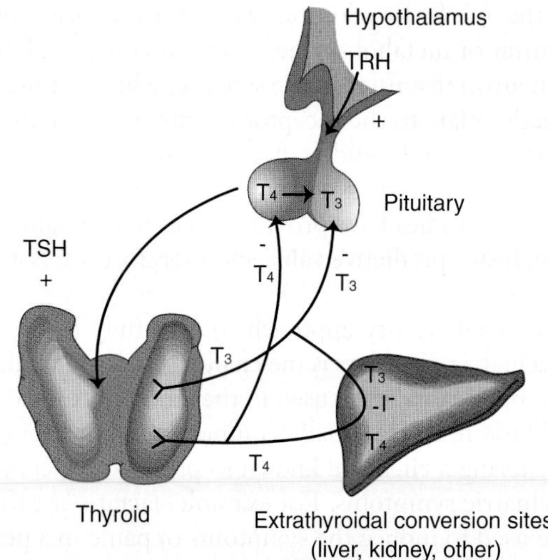

FIGURE 7.15. Hypothalamic–pituitary–thyroid axis. This figure shows the regulation of thyroid-stimulating hormone (TSH or thyrotropin) secretion by the anterior pituitary. Also depicted are the positive effects of thyrotropin-releasing hormone (TRH) from the hypothalamus and negative effects of circulating triiodothyronine (T_3) and T_3 from intrapituitary conversion of thyroxine (T_4).

DIAGNOSTIC APPROACHES

Biologic markers are diagnostic test findings that occur only in the presence of the psychiatric disorder and include such findings as laboratory and other diagnostic test results and neuropathologic changes noticeable in assessment. These markers increase diagnostic certainty, reliability, and may have predictive value, allowing for the possibility of preventive interventions to forestall or avoid the onset of illness.

In addition, biologic markers could assist in developing evidence-based care practices. If markers can be used reliably, it would be much easier to identify the most effective treatments and to determine the expected prognosis for given conditions. The psychiatric–mental health nurse should be aware of the most current information on biological markers so that information, limitations, and results can be discussed knowledgeably with the patient.

Laboratory Tests And Neurophysiologic Procedures

For many years, laboratory tests have attempted to measure levels of neurotransmitters and other CNS substances in the bloodstream. Many of the metabolites of neurotransmitters can be found in the urine and CSF as well. However, these measures have had only limited utility in elucidating what is happening in the brain. Levels of neurotransmitters and metabolites in the bloodstream or urine do not necessarily equate with levels in the CNS. In addition, availability of the neurotransmitter or metabolite does not predict the availability of the neurotransmitter in the synapse, where it must act, or directly relate to the receptor sensitivity. Nonetheless, numerous research studies have focused on changes in neurotransmitters and metabolites in blood, urine, and CSF. These studies have provided clues but remain without conclusive predictive value and therefore are not routinely used.

Another laboratory approach to the study of some of the psychiatric disorders is the challenge test. A challenge test has been most often used in the study of panic disorders. These tests are usually conducted by intravenously administering a chemical known to produce a specific set of psychiatric symptoms. For example, lactate or caffeine may be used to induce the symptoms of panic in a person who has panic disorder. The biologic response of the individual is then monitored. These tests have been developed primarily for research purposes. However, endocrine stimulation tests, such as the TRH stimulation test and the dexamethasone suppression test, have some limited clinical utility.

In the TRH stimulation test, TRH is administered and the TSH blood level is measured over time, usually at intervals during a period of 3 to 4 hours. The patient with hypothyroidism has an elevated TSH level. A blunted TRH stimulation test has been proposed as a biologic marker for major depression; however, only about 30% of individuals with major depression show the response. The dexamethasone suppression test involves administering 1 mg dexamethasone at 11 PM. Cortisol blood levels are then measured. In the healthy individual, dexamethasone suppresses cortisol levels, but results of numerous studies suggest that there is nonsuppression in certain types of depression. Typically, the cortisol levels are measured before administering the dexamethasone and then again at 7 AM, 4 PM, and 11 PM on the following day. Many medical conditions, such as diabetes mellitus, obesity, infection, pregnancy, recent surgery, and use of medications, such as carbamazepine or high doses of estrogen, may alter the test results, producing false-positive results. Overall, a positive result, or abnormal nonsuppression, appears to indicate major depression, but a negative result does not rule out depression. Considerable controversy exists regarding the clinical usefulness of this test.

Although no commonly used laboratory tests exist that directly confirm a mental disorder, laboratory tests are still an active part of care and assessment of psychiatric patients. Many physical conditions mimic the symptoms of mental illness, and many of the medications used to treat psychiatric illness can produce health problems. For these reasons, the routine care of patients with psychiatric disorders includes the use of laboratory tests such as complete blood counts, thyroid studies, electrolytes, hepatic enzymes, and other evaluative tests. Psychiatric–mental health nurses need to be familiar with these procedures and assist patients in understanding the use and implications of such tests.

Electroencephalography

EEG is a tried and true method for investigating what is happening inside the living brain. Developed in the 1920s by Hans Berger, an EEG measures electrical activity in the uppermost nerve layers of the cortex. Usually, 16 electrodes are placed on the patient's scalp. The EEG machine, equipped with graph paper and recording pens, is turned on, and the pens then trace the electrical impulses generated over each electrode. Until the use of CT in the 1970s, the EEG was the only method for identifying brain abnormalities. It remains the simplest and most noninvasive method for identifying some disorders. It is increasingly being used to identify individual neuronal differences and most recently to predict a person's response to common antidepressant medication (Cook, Leuchter, & Morgan, 2002).

An EEG may be used in psychiatry to differentiate possible causes of the patient's symptoms. For example, some types of seizure disorders, such as temporal lobe epilepsy, head injuries, or tumors, may present with predominantly psychiatric symptoms. In addition, metabolic dysfunction, delirium, dementia, altered levels of consciousness, hallucinations, and dissociative states may require EEG evaluation.

Spikes and wave-pattern changes are indications of brain abnormalities. Spikes may be the focal point from which a seizure occurs. However, abnormal activity often is not discovered on a routine EEG while the individual is awake. For this reason, additional methods are sometimes used. Nasopharyngeal leads may be used to get physically closer to the limbic regions. The patient may be exposed to a flashing strobe light while the examiner looks for activity that is not in phase with the flashing light or may be asked to hyperventilate for 3 minutes to induce abnormal activity if it exists. Sleep deprivation may also be used. This involves keeping the patient awake throughout the night before the EEG evaluation. The patient may then be drowsy and fall asleep during the procedure. Abnormalities are more likely to occur when the patient is asleep. Sleep may also be induced using medication; however, many medications change the wave patterns on an EEG. For example, the benzodiazepine class of drugs increases the rapid and fast beta activity. Many other prescribed and illicit drugs, such as lithium, which increases theta activity, can cause EEG alterations. In addition to reassuring, preparing, and educating the patient for the examination, the nurse should carefully assess the history of substance use and report this information to the examiner. If a sleep-deprivation EEG is to be done, caffeine or other stimulants that might assist the patient in staying awake should be withheld because they may change the EEG patterns.

Polysomnography

Polysomnography is a special procedure that involves recording the EEG throughout a night of sleep. This test is usually conducted in a sleep laboratory. Other tests are usually performed at the same time, including electrocardiography and electromyography. Blood oxygenation, body movement, body temperature, and other data may be collected as well, especially in research settings. This procedure is usually conducted for evaluating sleep disorders, such as sleep apnea, enuresis, or somnambulism. However, sleep pattern changes are frequently researched in mental disorders as well.

Researchers have found that normal sleep divisions and stages are affected by many factors, including drugs, alcohol, general medical conditions, and psychiatric disorders. For example, REM latency, the length of time it takes an individual to enter the first REM episode, is shortened in depression. Reduced delta sleep is also observed. These findings have been replicated so frequently that some researchers consider them biologic markers for depression.

Other Neurophysiologic Methods

Evoked potentials (EPs), also called event-related potentials, use the same basic principles as an EEG. They measure changes in electrical activity of the brain in specific regions as a response to a given stimulus. Electrodes placed on the scalp measure a large waveform that stands out after the administration of repetitive stimuli, such as a click or flash of light. There are several different types of EPs to be measured, depending on the sensory area affected by the stimulus, the cognitive task required, or the region monitored, any of which can change the length of time until the wave occurrence. EPs are used extensively in psychiatric research. In clinical practice, EPs are used primarily in the assessment of demyelinating disorders, such as multiple sclerosis.

However, brain electrical activity mapping (BEAM) studies, which involve a 20-electrode EEG that generates computerized maps of the brain's electrical activity, have found a slowing of electrical activity in the frontal lobes of individuals who have schizophrenia. These findings are consistent with other findings that suggest a "hypofrontality" in schizophrenia (see Chapter 18). Nonetheless, neurophysiologic methods provide only rough approximations compared with current structural and functional neuroimaging techniques.

SUMMARY OF KEY POINTS

- Neuroscientists now view behavior and cognitive function as a result of complex interactions within the central nervous system and its plasticity, or its ability to adapt and change in both structure and function.
- Although no one gene has been found to produce any psychiatric disorder, significant evidence indicates there is for most psychiatric disorders a genetic predisposition or susceptibility. For individuals who have such genetic susceptibility, the identification of risk factors is crucial in helping to plan interventions to prevent development of that disorder or to prevent certain behavior patterns, such as aggression or suicide.
- Each hemisphere of the brain is divided into four lobes: the frontal lobe, which controls motor speech function, personality, and working memory—often called the executive functions that govern one's ability to plan and initiate action; the parietal lobe, which controls the sensory functions; the temporal lobe, which contains the primary auditory and olfactory areas; and the occipital lobe, which controls visual integration of information.
- The structures of the limbic system are integrally involved in memory and emotional behavior. Dysfunction of the limbic system has been linked with major mental disorders, including schizophrenia, depression, and anxiety disorders.
- Neurons communicate with each other through synaptic transmission. Neurotransmitters excite or inhibit a response at the receptor sites and have been linked to certain mental disorders. These neurotransmitters include acetylcholine, dopamine, norepinephrine, serotonin, γ-aminobutyric acid, and glutamate.
- Psychoneuroimmunology examines the relationship among the immune system, the nervous system, endocrine system and thoughts, emotions, and behavior.
- Chronobiology focuses on the study and measure of time structures or biologic rhythms occurring in the body and associates dysregulation of these cycles as contributing factors to the development of psychiatric disorders.
- Biologic markers are physical indicators of disturbances within the central nervous system that differentiate one disease process from another, such as biochemical changes or neuropathologic changes. These biologic markers can be measured by several methods of testing, including challenge tests, electroencephalography, polysomnography, evoked potentials, computed tomography scanning, magnetic resonance imaging, positron emission tomography, and single-photon emission computed tomography; the psychiatric nurse must be familiar with all of these methods.

CRITICAL THINKING CHALLENGES

1. Explain the significance of mental disorders being described as polygenetic.
2. A woman who has experienced a "ministroke" continues to regain lost cognitive function months after the stroke. Her husband takes this as evidence that she never had a stroke. How would you approach patient teaching and counseling for this couple to help them understand this occurrence if the stroke did damage to her brain?
3. Your patient has "impaired executive functioning." Consider what would be a reasonable follow-up schedule for this patient for counseling sessions. Would it be reasonable to schedule visits at 1:00 PM weekly? Is the patient able to keep to this schedule? Why or why not? What would be the best schedule?
4. Mr. S. is unable to sleep after watching an upsetting documentary. Identify the neurotransmitter activity that may be interfering with sleep. (Hint: Fight or flight.)
5. Describe what behavioral symptoms or problems may be present in a patient with dysfunction of the following brain area:
   a. Basal ganglia
   b. Hippocampus
   c. Limbic system
   d. Thalamus
   e. Hypothalamus
   f. Frontal lobe
6. Compare and contrast the functions of the sympathetic and parasympathetic nervous systems.
7. Discuss the steps in synaptic transmission, beginning with the action potential and ending with how the neurotransmitter no longer communicates its message to the receiving neuron.
8. Examine how a receptor's usual response to a neurotransmitter might change.
9. Compare the role of dopamine and acetylcholine in the CNS.
10. Explain how dopamine, norepinephrine, and serotonin all contribute to endocrine system regulation. Suggest some other transmitters that may affect endocrine function.
11. Discuss how the fields of psychoneuroimmunology and chronobiology overlap.
12. Compare the methods used to find biologic markers of psychiatric disorders reviewed in this chapter. Consider the potential risks and benefits to the patient.

REFERENCES

Bailey, A., LeCouteur, A., Gottesman, I., Bolton, P., Simonoff, E., Yuzda, E., et al., (1995). Autism as a strongly genetic disorder: evidence from a British twin study. *Psychological Medicine, 25*, 63–77.

Cook, I. A., Leuchter, A. F., & Morgan, M. (2002). *Neuropsychopharmacology, 27* (1), 120–131.

Ekman, R., Persson, R., & Nilsson, C. L. (2002). Neurodevelopmental influences on the immune system reflecting brain pathology. *Neurotoxic Research, 4* (5–6), 565–572.

Friedman, M. J. (2000). What might the psychobiology of posttraumatic stress disorder teach us about the future approaches to pharmacotherapy. *Journal of Clinical Psychiatry, 61* (7), 44–51.

Garcia, D. A., Marin, R. H., & Perillo, M. A. (2002). Stress-induced decrement in the plasticity of the physical properties of chick brain membranes. *Molecular Membrane Biology, 19* (3), 221–230.

Green, R. C., Cupples, L. A., Kurz, A., Auerbach, S., Go, R., Sadovnick, D., et al. (2003). Depression as a risk factor for Alzheimer disease: The MIRAGE Study. *Archives of Neurology, 60* (5), 753–759.

Harlow, J. M. (1868). Recovery after severe injury to the head. *Publication of the Massachusetts Medical Society, 2*, 327.

Harmer, C. J., Hill, S. A., Taylor, M. J., Cowen, P. J., & Goodwin, G. M. (2003). Toward a neuropsychological theory of antidepressant drug action: Increase in positive emotional bias after potentiation of norepinephrine activity. *American Journal of Psychiatry, 160*, 990–992.

Harrison, P. J., & Owen, M. S. (2003). Genes for schizophrenia? Recent findings and their pathophysiological implications. *Lancet 361* (9355), 417–419.

Hough, D. J., & Ursano, R. J., (2006). A guide to the genetics of psychiatric disease. *Psychiatry, 69* (1), 1–19.

Ishihara, S., Makita, S., Imai, M., Hashimoto, T., & Nohara, R. (2003). Relationship between natural killer activity and anger expression in patients with coronary heart disease. *Heart Vessels, 18* (2), 85–92.

Joober, R., Sengupta, S., & Boksa, P. (2005). Genetics of developmental psychiatric disorders: pathways to discovery. *Journal of Psychiatry & Neuroscience, 30* (5), 349–353.

Kapczinski, F., Lima, M. S., Souza, J. S., & Schmitt, R. (2003). Antidepressants for generalized anxiety disorder (Cochrane Review). *Cochrane Database System Review* 2003;2:CD003592.

Kurup, R. K., & Kurup, P. A. (2003). Hypothalamic digoxin: Central role in conscious perception, neuroimmunoendocrine integration and coordination of cellular function—relation to hemispheric dominance. *Medical Hypotheses, 60* (2), 243–257.

Lea, D. H. (2000). A clinician's primer in human genetics: What nurses need to know. *Nursing Clinics of North America, 35* (3), 583–614.

Levy, R., Hay, D.A., McStephen, M., Wood, C., Waldman, I. (1997). Attention-deficit hyperactivity disorder: a category or a continuum? Genetic analysis of a large-scale twin study. *Journal of the American Academy of Child & Adolescent Psychiatry, 36*, 737–744.

MacGregor, D. G., Avshalumov, M. V., & Rice, M. E. (2003). Brain edema induced by in vitro ischemia: Causal factors and neuroprotection. *Journal of Neurochemistry, 85* (6), 1402–1411.

McGuffin, P., Rijsdijk, F., Andrew, M., Sham, P., Katz, R., & Cardno, A. (2003). The heritability of bipolar affective disorder and the genetic relationship to unipolar depression. *Archives of General Psychiatry, 60*, 497–502.

Mohr, W., & Mohr, B. (2001). Brain, behavior, connections and implications: Psychodynamics no more. *Archives of Psychiatric Nursing, 15* (4), 171–181.

Montgomery, S. A. (2000). Understanding depression and its treatment: Restoration of chemical balance or creation of conditions promoting recovery. *Journal of Clinical Psychiatry, 61* (6), 3–6.

Motzer, S. A., & Hertig, V. (2004). Stress, stress response, and health. *Nursing Clinics of North America, 39* (1), 1–17.

National Human Genome Research Institute (2005). The human genome project completion: Frequently asked questions. National Institutes of Health. Retrieved September 26, 2006 from www.genome.gov.

Nolte, J., & Angevine, J. (1995). *The human brain: In photographs and diagrams.* St. Louis: Mosby.

Shiloh, R., Weizman, A., Epstein, Y., Rosenberg, S. L., Valevski, A., Dorfman-Etrog, P., Wiezer, N., Katz., N., Munitz, H., & Hermesh, H. (2001). Abnormal thermoregulation in drug-free male schizophrenia patients. *European Neuropsychopharmacology, 11*(4), 285–288.

Sullivan, P. F., Kendler, K. S., Neale, M. C. (2003). Schizophrenia as a complex trait: evidence from a meta-analysis of twin studies. *Archives of General Psychiatry, 60*, 1187–1192.

CHAPTER 8

Psychopharmacology and Biologic Interventions

Mary Ann Boyd and Susan McCabe

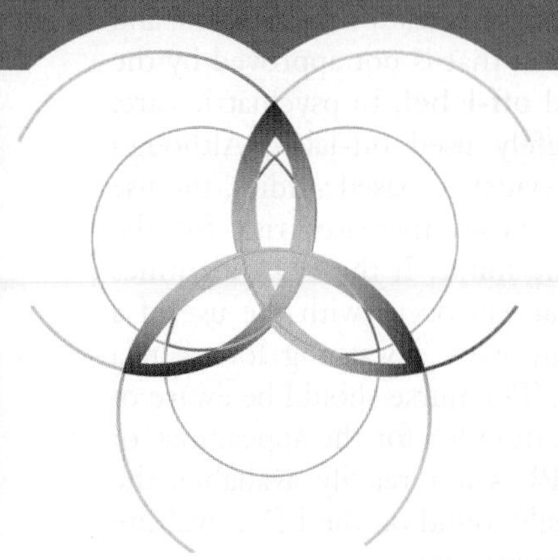

KEY CONCEPTS

- agonists
- antagonists

LEARNING OBJECTIVES

After studying this chapter, you will be able to:

- Differentiate target symptoms from side effects.
- Identify nursing interventions for common side effects of psychiatric medications.
- Explain the role of the governmental regulatory process in the approval of medication and the use of other biologic interventions.
- Discuss the pharmacodynamics related to psychiatric medications.
- Discuss the pharmacokinetics related to psychiatric medications.
- Explain the major classifications of psychiatric medications.
- Identify typical nursing interventions related to the administration of psychiatric medications.
- Analyze the potential benefits of other forms of somatic treatments, including herbal supplements, nutrition therapies, electroconvulsive therapy, light therapy, transcranial magnetic stimulation, and vagus nerve stimulation.
- Evaluate potential causes of noncompliance and implement interventions to improve compliance with treatment regimens.

KEY TERMS

• absorption • adherence • adverse reactions • affinity • agonists • akathisia • antagonists • atypical antipsychotics • augmentation • bioavailability • biotransformation • boxed warning • carrier protein • chronic syndromes • clearance • compliance • conventional antipsychotics • cytochrome P-450 (CYP450) • desensitization • distribution • dosing • drug–drug interaction • dystonia • efficacy • enzymes • ethnopsychopharmacology • excretion • extrapyramidal syndromes (EPS) • first-pass effect • half-life • inducer • inhibitor • intrinsic activity • metabolites • metabolism • pharmacogenomics • phototherapy • package insert • partial agonist • polypharmacy • potency • protein binding • off-label • pseudoparkinsonism • relapse • selectivity • serotonin syndrome • side effects • steady state • solubility • substrate • tardive dyskinesia • target symptoms • therapeutic index • tolerance • toxicity • transcranial magnetic stimulation • uptake receptors • untoward effects

Recent scientific and technologic developments opened the door for the development of new medications that produce major behavioral and psychological changes. They have become the dominant treatment of psychiatric disorders. Nurses administer these medications, monitor their effectiveness, and manage side effects. Advanced practice nurses also prescribe them. These medications are increasingly prescribed in primary care settings, and nurses practicing in nonpsychiatric settings now need an in-depth knowledge of them.

This chapter focuses on the phamacodyamics and pharmacokinetics related to psychiatric medications. Included in this chapter is an overview of the major classes of psychopharmacologic drugs used in treating mental disorders and the role of herbal supplements and nutritional therapies. In addition, other biologic treatments are discussed, including electroconvulsive therapy, light therapy, transcranial magnetic stimulation, and vagus nerve stimulation.

TARGET SYMPTOMS AND SIDE EFFECTS

Psychiatric medications and other biologic interventions are indicated for **target symptoms,** which are measurable specific symptoms expected to improve with treatment. Standards of care guide nurses in monitoring and documenting the effects of medications and other biologic treatments on target symptoms.

As yet, no drug has been developed that is so specific it affects only its target symptoms; instead, drugs act on a number of other organs and sites within the body. Even drugs with a high affinity and selectivity for a specific neurotransmitter will cause some responses in the body that are not related to the target symptoms. These unwanted effects of medications are called **side effects** or **untoward effects**. If unwanted effects have serious physiologic consequences, they are considered **adverse reactions**. Although technically different, these three terms are often used interchangeably in the literature. The nurse monitors, documents, and reports the appearance of side effects and adverse reactions and implements nursing interventions for relief of medication side effects (see Table 8.1).

REGULATORY ISSUES

The U.S. Food and Drug Administration (FDA) is responsible for assuring the safety, efficacy, and security of human and veterinary drugs, biologic products, medical devices, our nation's food supply, cosmetics, and products that emit radiation (www.FDA.gov). The FDA approves the labeling of medications and other biologic treatments after a thorough review of efficacy and safety data (see Box 8.1). Nurses administering medications are responsible for knowing the labeling content. The product labeling is found in each medication's **package insert** (PI) and includes approved indications for the medication, side effects, adverse effects, contraindications, and other important information. If a medication is ordered and administered for a condition that is not approved by the FDA, its use is considered **off-label**. In psychiatric care, many medications are safely used off-label. Although their use is supported by evidence-based studies, the use of drugs for off-label purposes increases risk for the patient and liability for the nurse. If the FDA identifies serious adverse effects that can occur with the use of a specific medication, it may issue a warning found in a **boxed warning** in the PI. The nurse should be aware of these boxed warnings and monitor for the appearance of the adverse events. If a PI is not readily available, the labeling information is easily found on the FDA's website and in most pharmacy departments.

PSYCHOPHARMACOLOGY

A comparatively small amount of medication can have a significant and large impact on cell function and resulting behavior. When tiny molecules of medication are compared with the vast amount of cell surface in the human body, the fraction seems disproportionate. Yet the drugs used to treat mental disorders often have profound effects on behavior. To understand how this occurs, one needs to understand both where and how drugs work. The following discussion highlights important concepts relevant to the psychiatric medications.

PHARMACODYNAMICS: WHERE DRUGS ACT

Psychiatric medications primarily target the central nervous system (CNS) at the cellular, synaptic level at four sites: receptors, ion channels, enzymes, and carrier proteins. Drug molecules do not act on the entire cell surface, but rather at a specific site.

Receptors

Receptors are specific proteins intended to respond to a chemical (i.e., neurotransmitter) normally present in blood or tissues (see Chapter 7). Receptors also respond to drugs with similar chemical structures. When drugs attach to a receptor, they can act as **agonists**—substances that initiate the same response as the chemical normally present in the body—or as **antagonists**—substances that

Table 8.1 Managing Common Side Effects of Psychiatric Medications

Side Effect or Discomfort	Intervention
Blurred vision	Reassurance (generally subsides in 2 to 6 wk)
Dry eyes	Warn ophthalmologist; no eye exam for new glasses for at least 3 wk after a stable dose
	Artificial tears may be required; increased use of wetting solutions for those wearing contact lens
Dry mouth and lips	Frequent rinsing of mouth, good oral hygiene, sucking sugarless candies, lozenges, lip balm, lemon juice, and glycerin mouth swabs
Constipation	High-fiber diet, encourage bran, fresh fruits and vegetables
	Metamucil (must consume at least 16 oz of fluid with dose)
	Increase hydration
	Exercise, increase fluids
	Mild laxative
Urinary hesitancy or retention	Monitor frequently for difficulty with urination, changes in starting or stopping stream
	Notify prescriber if difficulty develops
	A cholinergic agonist, such as bethanechol, may be required
Nasal congestion	Nose drops, moisturizer, *not* nasal spray
Sinus tachycardia	Assess for infections
	Monitor pulse for rate and irregularities
	Withhold medication and notify prescriber if resting rate exceeds 120 bpm
Decreased libido and ejaculatory inhibition	Reassurance (reversible). Change to another medication
Postural hypotension	Frequent monitoring of lying-to-standing blood pressure during dosage adjustment period, immediate changes and accommodation, measure pulse in both positions. Consider change to less antiadrenergic drug
	Advise patient to get up slowly, sit for at least 1 min before standing (dangling legs over side of bed), and stand for 1 min before walking or until light-headedness subsides
	Increase hydration, avoid caffeine
	Elastic stockings if necessary
	Notify prescriber if symptoms persist or significant blood pressure changes are present; medication may have to be changed if patient does not have impulse control to get up slowly
Photosensitivity	Protective clothing
	Dark glasses
	Use of sun block, remember to cover all exposed areas
Dermatitis	Stop medication usage
	Consider medication change, may require a systemic antihistamine
	Initiate comfort measures to decrease itching
Impaired psychomotor functions	Advise patient to avoid dangerous tasks, such as driving
	Avoid alcohol, which increases this impairment
Drowsiness or sedation	Encourage activity during the day to increase accommodation
	Avoid tasks that require mental alertness, such as driving
	May need to adjust dosing schedule or, if possible, give single daily dose at bedtime
	May need a cholinergic medication if sedation is the problem
	Avoid driving or operating potentially dangerous equipment
	May need change to less-sedating medication
	Provide quiet and decreased stimulation when sedation is the desired effect
Weight gain and metabolic changes	Exercise and diet teaching
	Caloric control
Edema	Check fluid retention
	Reassurance
	May need a diuretic
Irregular menstruation and/or amenorrhea	Reassurance (reversible)
	May need to change class of drug
	Reassurance and counseling (does not indicate lack of ovulation)
	Instruct patient to continue birth control measures
Vaginal dryness	Instruct in use of lubricants

block the response of a given receptor. Figure 8.1 illustrates the action of an agonist and an antagonist drug at a receptor site. A drug's ability to interact with a given receptor type may be judged by three properties: selectivity, affinity, and intrinsic activity.

Selectivity

Selectivity is the ability of the drug to be specific for a particular receptor. If a drug is highly selective, it will interact only with its specific receptors in the areas of the

BOX 8.1

Phases of New Drug Testing

- Phase I: Testing defines the range of dosages tolerated in healthy individuals
- Phase II: Effects of the drug are studied in a limited number of persons with the disorder. This phase defines the range of clinically effective dosage.
- Phase III: Extensive clinical trials are conducted at multiple sites throughout the country with larger numbers of patients. Efforts focus on corroborating the efficacy identified in phase II. Phase III concludes with a new drug application (NDA) being submitted to the FDA.
- Phase IV: Drug studies continue after FDA approval to detect new or rare adverse reactions and potentially new indications. During this period, adverse reactions from the new medication should be reported to the FDA.

Implications for Mental Health Nurses

Throughout the phases, side effects and adverse reactions are monitored closely. The studies are tightly controlled, and strict regulations are enforced at each step.

To prove drug effectiveness, diagnoses must be accurate, strict guidelines are followed, and subjects usually are not taking other medications and do not have complicating illnesses.

A newly approved drug is approved only for the indications for which it has been tested.

body where these receptors occur and, therefore, not affect tissues and organs where its receptors do not occur. Using a "lock-and-key" analogy, only a specific, highly selective key will fit a given lock. The more selective or structurally specific a drug is, the more likely it will affect only the specific receptor for which it is meant. The less selective the drug, the more receptors are affected and the more likely there will be unintended effects or side effects.

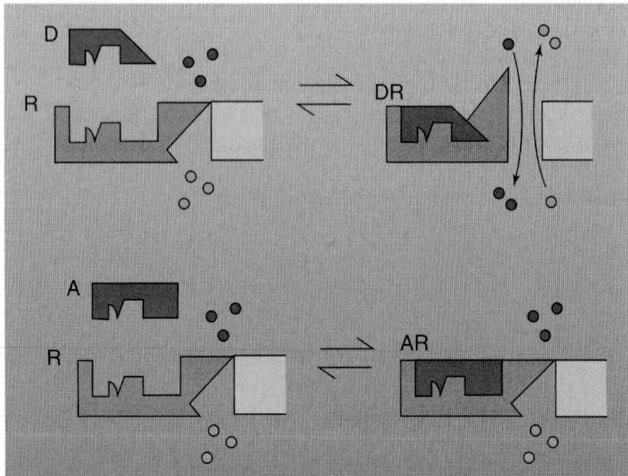

FIGURE 8.1. Agonist and antagonist drug actions at a receptor site. This schematic drawing represents drug–receptor interactions. At *top,* drug D has the correct shape to fit receptor R, forming a drug–receptor complex, which results in a conformational change in the receptor and the opening of a pore in the adjacent membrane. Drug D is an agonist. At *bottom,* drug A also has the correct shape to fit the receptor, forming a drug–receptor complex, but in this case, there is no conformational change and, therefore, no response. Drug A is, therefore, an antagonist.

Affinity

Affinity is the degree of attraction or strength of the bond between the drug and its biologic target. Affinity is strengthened when a drug has more than one type of chemical bond with its target. If a cell membrane contains several receptors to which a drug will adhere, the affinity is increased. The weaker the chemical bond, the more likely a drug's effects are reversible. Most drugs used in psychiatry adhere to receptors through weak chemical bonds, but some drugs, specifically the monoamine oxidase inhibitors (discussed later), have a different type of bond, called a *covalent bond.* A covalent bond is formed when two atoms share a pair of electrons. This type of bond is stronger and irreversible at normal temperatures. The effects of the drugs that form covalent bonds are often called "irreversible" because they are long lasting, taking several weeks to resolve. Knowledge of a medication's affinity for receptors and subtypes of receptors may give some indication of the likelihood that specific target symptoms might improve and what side effects might be predicted.

Intrinsic Activity

A drug's ability to interact with a given receptor is its **intrinsic activity,** or the ability to produce a response once it becomes attached to the receptor. Some drugs have selectivity and affinity but produce no response. An important measure of a drug is whether it produces a change in the cell containing the receptor.

KEY CONCEPTS Agonists (mimic the neurotransmitter) have all three properties: selectivity, affinity, and intrinsic activity.

Antagonists: Antagonists (block the receptor) have only selectivity and affinity because they produce no biologic response by attaching to the receptor.

Some drugs are referred to as **partial agonists** because they have some intrinsic activity (although weak). Because there are no "pure" drugs, affecting only one neurotransmitter, most drugs have multiple effects. A drug may act as an agonist for one neurotransmitter and an antagonist for another. Medications that have both agonist and antagonist effects are called *mixed agonist–antagonists.*

Ion Channels

Some drugs directly block the ion channels of the nerve cell membrane. For example the antianxiety benzodiazepine drugs, such as diazepam (Valium), bind to a region of the gamma-aminobutyric acid (GABA)-receptor chloride channel complex, which helps to open the chloride ion channel. In turn, the activity of GABA is enhanced.

Enzymes

Enzymes are usually proteins that function as catalysts for physiologic reactions and can be targets for drugs. For example, monoamine oxidase is an enzyme required to break down neurotransmitters associated with depression (norepinephrine, serotonin, and dopamine). The monoamine oxidase inhibitor (MAOI) antidepressants inhibit this enzyme, resulting in more neurotransmitter activity.

Carrier Proteins: Uptake Receptors

A **carrier protein** is a membrane protein that transports a specific molecule across the cell membrane. Carrier proteins (also referred to as **uptake receptors**) recognize sites specific for the type of molecule to be transported. When a neurotransmitter is removed from the synapse, specific carrier molecules return it to the presynaptic nerve, where most of it is stored to be used again. Medications specific for this site block or inhibit this transport and, therefore, increase the activity of the neurotransmitter in the synapse. Figure 8.2 illustrates the reuptake blockade.

CLINICAL CONCEPTS

Efficacy is the ability of a drug to produce a response and is considered when a drug is selected. The degree of receptor occupancy contributes to the drug's efficacy, but a drug may occupy a large number of receptors and not produce a response. Table 8.2 provides a brief summation of possible physiologic effects from drug actions on specific neurotransmitters. This information should serve only as a guide in predicting side effects because many

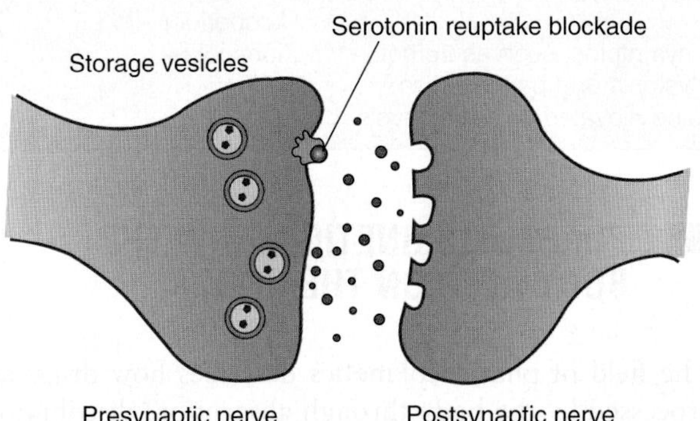

FIGURE 8.2. Reuptake blockade of a carrier molecule for serotonin by a selective serotonin reuptake inhibitor.

physical outcomes or behaviors resulting from neural transmission are controlled by multiple receptors and neurotransmitters.

Potency refers to the dose of drug required to produce a specific effect. One drug may be able to achieve the same clinical effect as another drug but at a lower dose, making it more potent. Although the drug given at the lower dose is more potent, because both drugs achieve similar effects, they may be considered to have equal efficacy.

In some instances, the effects of medications diminish with time, especially when they are given repeatedly, as in the treatment of chronic psychiatric disorders. This loss of effect is most often a form of physiologic adaptation that may develop as the cell attempts to regain homeostatic control to counteract the effects of the drug. There are many reasons for decreased drug effectiveness (Box 8.2). **Desensitization** is a rapid decrease in drug effects that may develop in a few minutes of exposure to a drug. This reaction is rare with most psychiatric medications but can occur with some medications used to treat serious side effects (e.g., physostigmine, sometimes used to relieve severe anticholinergic side effects). A rapid decrease can also occur with some drugs because of immediate transformation of the receptor when the drug molecule binds to the receptor. Other drugs cause a decrease in the number of receptors or exhaust the mediators of neurotransmission. **Tolerance** is a gradual decrease in the action of a drug at a given dose or concentration in the blood. This decrease may take days or weeks to develop and results in loss of therapeutic effect of a drug. For therapeutic drugs, this loss of effect is often called *treatment refractoriness*. In the abuse of substances such as alcohol or cocaine, tolerance is a part of the addiction (see Chapter 25).

Toxicity generally refers to the point at which concentrations of the drug in the bloodstream are high enough to become harmful or poisonous to the body. Individuals vary widely in their responses to medications. Some patients experience adverse reactions more easily than others. The **therapeutic index** is the ratio of the maximum nontoxic dose to the minimum effective dose. A high therapeutic index means that there is a large range between the dose at which the drug begins to take effect and a dose that would be toxic to the body. Drugs with a low therapeutic index have a narrow range.

This concept of toxicity has some limitations. It is only vaguely defined. The range can be affected by drug tolerance. For example, when tolerance develops, the person increases the dosage, which makes them more susceptible to an accidental suicide. The therapeutic index of a medication also may be greatly changed by the coadministration of other medications or drugs. For example, alcohol consumed with most CNS-depressant drugs will have added depressant effects, greatly increasing the likelihood of toxicity or death.

Table 8.2 Drug Affinity for Specific Neurotransmitters and Receptors and Subsequent Effects

Neurotransmitter/Receptor Action	Physiologic Effects	Example of Drugs That Exhibit High Affinity
Reuptake Inhibition		
Norepinephrine reuptake inhibition	Antidepressant action Potentiation of pressor effects of norepinephrine Interaction with guanethidine Side effects: tachycardia, tremors, insomnia, erectile and ejaculation dysfunction	Desipramine Venlafaxine
Serotonin reuptake inhibition	Antidepressant action Antiobsessional effect Increase or decrease in anxiety, dose dependent Side effects: gastrointestinal distress, nausea, headache, nervousness, motor restlessness and sexual side effects, including anorgasmia	Fluoxetine Fluvoxamine
Dopamine reuptake inhibition	Antidepressant action Antiparkinsonian effect Side effects: increase in psychomotor activity, aggravation of psychosis	Buproprion
Receptor Blockade		
Histamine receptor blockade (H_1)	Side effects: sedation, drowsiness, hypotension, and weight gain	Quetiapine Imipramine Clozapine Olanzapine
Acetylcholine receptor blockade (muscarinic)	Side effects: anticholinergic (dry mouth, blurred vision, constipation, urinary hesitancy and retention, memory dysfunction) and sinus tachycardia	Imipramine Amitriptyline Thioridazine Clozapine
Norepinephrine receptor blockade (α_1 receptor)	Potentiation of antihypertensive effect of prazosin and terazosin Side effects: postural hypotension, dizziness, reflex tachycardia, sedation	Amitriptyline Clomipramine Clozapine
Norepinephrine receptor blockade (α_2 receptor)	Increased sexual desire (yohimbine) Interactions with antihypertensive medications, blockade of the antihypertensive effects of clonidine Side effect: priapism	Amitriptyline Clomipramine Clozapine Trazodone Yohimbine
Norepinephrine receptor blockade (β_1 receptor)	Antihypertensive action (propranolol) Side effects: orthostatic hypotension, sedation, depression, sexual dysfunction (including impotence and decreased ejaculation)	Propranolol
Serotonin receptor blockade (5-HT_{1a})	Antidepressant action Antianxiety effect Possible control of aggression	Trazodone Risperidone Ziprasidone
Serotonin receptor blockade (5-HT_2)	Antipsychotic action Some antimigraine effect Decreased rhinitis Side effects: hypotension, ejaculatory problems	Risperidone Clozapine Olanzapine Ziprasidone
Dopamine receptor blockade (D_2)	Antipsychotic action Side effects: extrapyramidal symptoms, such as tremor, rigidity (especially acute dystonia and parkinsonism); endocrine changes, including elevated prolactin levels	Haloperidol Ziprasidone

BOX 8.2

Mechanisms Causing Decrease in Medication Effects

- Change in receptors
- Loss of receptors
- Exhaustion of neurotransmitter supply
- Increased metabolism of the drug
- Physiologic adaptation

PHARMACOKINETICS: HOW THE BODY ACTS ON THE DRUGS

The field of pharmacokinetics describes how drugs are processed by the body through absorption, distribution, metabolism (biotransformation), and excretion. Pharmacokinetics for specific medications are always explained in a drug's PI. Together with the principles of pharmacodynamics, this information is helpful in monitoring drug effects and predicting behavioral response.

Absorption and Routes of Administration

The first phase of **absorption** is the movement of the drug from the site of administration into the plasma. The typical routes of administration of psychiatric medications include oral (both tablet and liquid), intramuscular (short- and long-acting agents), and intravenous (rarely used for treatment of the primary psychiatric disorder, but instead for rapid treatment of adverse reactions). A transdermal patch antidepressant is also available. The advantages and disadvantages of each route and the subsequent effects on absorption are listed in Table 8.3.

Table 8.3 Selected Forms and Routes of Psychiatric Medications

Preparation and Route	Examples	Advantages	Disadvantages
Oral tablet	Basic preparation for most psychopharmacologic agents, including antidepressants, antipsychotics, mood stabilizers, anxiolytics, etc.	Usually most convenient	Variable rate and extent of absorption, depending on the drug May be affected by the contents of the intestines May show first-pass metabolism effects May not be easily swallowed by some individuals
Oral liquid	Also known as concentrates Many antipsychotics, such as haloperidol, chlorpromazine, thioridazine, risperidone The antidepressant fluoxetine Antihistamines, such as diphenhydramine Mood stabilizers, such as lithium citrate	Ease of incremental dosing Easily swallowed In some cases, more quickly absorbed	More difficult to measure accurately Depending on drug: • Possible interactions with other liquids such as juice, forming precipitants • Possible irritation to mucosal lining of mouth if not properly diluted
Rapid-dissolving tablet	Atypical antipsychotics, such as olanzapine, risperidone	Dissolves almost instantaneously in mouth Handy for people who have trouble swallowing or for patients who let medication linger in the cheek for later expectoration Can be taken when water or other liquid is unavailable	Patient needs to remember to have completely dry hands and to place tablet in mouth immediately Tablet should not linger in the hand
Intramuscular	Some antipsychotics, such as ziprasidone, haloperidol, and chlorpromazine Anxiolytics, such as lorazepam Anticholinergics, such as diphenhydramine and benztropine mesylate No antidepressants No mood stabilizers	More rapid acting than oral preparations No first-pass metabolism	Injection-site pain and irritation Some medications may have erratic absorption if heavy muscle tissue at the site of injection is not in use
Intramuscular depot (or long-acting)	Risperidone (Risperdal Consta), haloperidol decanoate, fluphenazine decanoate	May be more convenient for some individuals who have difficulty following medication regimens	Pain at injection site
Intravenous	Anticholinergics, such as diphenhydramine, benztropine mesylate Anxiolytics, such as diazepam, lorazepam, and chlordiazepoxide	Rapid and complete availability to systemic circulation	Inflammation of tissue surrounding site Often inconvenient for patient and uncomfortable Continuous dosage requires use of a constant-rate IV infusion
Transdermal patch	Antidepressant, selegiline	Avoid daily oral ingestion of medication	Skin irritation

Drugs taken orally are usually the most convenient for the patient; however, this route is also the most variable because absorption can be slowed or enhanced by a number of factors. Taking certain drugs orally with food or antacids may slow the rate of absorption or change the amount of the drug absorbed. For example, antacids containing aluminum salts decrease the absorption of most antipsychotic drugs; thus, antacids must be given at least 1 hour before administration or 2 hours after.

Oral preparations are absorbed from the gastrointestinal tract into the bloodstream through the portal vein and then to the liver. They may be metabolized within the gastrointestinal wall or liver before reaching the rest of the body. This is called the **first-pass effect**. The consequence of first-pass effect is that only a fraction of the drug reaches systemic circulation. Oral dosages are adjusted for the first-pass effect. That is, the dose of the oral form is significantly higher than the intramuscular or intravenous formulations.

Bioavailability describes the amount of the drug that actually reaches systemic circulation unchanged. The route by which a drug is administered significantly affects bioavailability. With some oral drugs, the amount of drug entering the bloodstream is decreased by first-pass metabolism and bioavailability is lower (Pandolfi et al., 2003). On the other hand, some rapid-dissolving oral medications have increased bioavailability.

Distribution

Distribution of a drug is the amount of the drug found in various tissues, particularly the target organ at the site of drug action. Factors that affect distribution include the size of the organ, amount of blood flow or perfusion within the organ, solubility of the drug, plasma **protein binding** (the degree to which the drug binds to plasma proteins), and anatomic barriers, such as the blood–brain barrier, that the drug must cross. A psychiatric drug may have rapid absorption and high bioavailability, but if it does not cross the blood–brain barrier to reach the CNS, it is of little use. Table 8.4 provides a summary of how some significant factors affect distribution. Two of these factors, **solubility** (ability of a drug to dissolve) and protein binding, warrant additional discussion with regard to how they relate to psychiatric medications.

Table 8.4 Factors Affecting Distribution of a Drug

Factor	Effect on Drug Distribution
Size of the organ	Larger organs require more drug to reach a concentration level equivalent to other organs and tissues.
Blood flow to the organ	The more blood flow to and within an organ (perfusion), the greater the drug concentration. The brain has high perfusion.
Solubility of the drug	The greater the solubility of a drug within a tissue, the greater its concentration.
Plasma protein binding	If a drug binds well to plasma proteins, particularly to albumin, it will stay in the body longer but have a slower distribution.
Anatomic barriers	Both the gastrointestinal tract and the brain are surrounded by layers of cells that control the passage or uptake of substances. Lipid-soluble substances are usually readily absorbed and pass the blood–brain barrier.

Solubility

Substances may cross a membrane in a number of ways, but passive diffusion is by far the simplest. To do this, the drug must dissolve in the structure of the cell membrane. Therefore, solubility of a drug is an important characteristic. Being soluble in lipids allows a drug to cross most of the membranes in the body and the tissues of the central nervous system (CNS) are less permeable to water-soluble drugs than are other areas of the body. Most psychopharmacologic agents are lipid soluble and easily cross the blood–brain barrier. However, this characteristic means that psychopharmacologic agents also cross the placenta; consequently most are contraindicated during pregnancy.

Protein Binding

Of considerable importance is the degree to which the drug binds to plasma proteins. Only unbound or "free" drugs act at the receptor sites. High protein binding reduces the concentration of the drug at the receptor sites. However, because the binding is reversible, as the unbound drug is metabolized, more drug is released from the protein bonds. The drugs are also released from storage in the fat depots. These processes can prolong the duration of action of the drug. When patients stop taking their medication, they often do not experience an immediate return of symptoms because they continue to receive the drug as it is released from storage sites in the body.

Metabolism

Metabolism, also called **biotransformation,** is the process by which the drug is altered and broken down into smaller substances, known as **metabolites**. Most metabolism occurs in the liver, but it can also occur in the kidneys, lungs, and intestines. Biotransformation in the liver occurs in phases. Phase I includes oxidation, hydrolysis, and reduction reactions. In most cases, metabolites are inactive, but in some psychiatric drugs, they are also active, such as norfluoxetine (metabolite of fluoxetine [Prozac]). Phase II reactions or conjugation combines a drug or metabolite with other chemicals. Through the phases of biotransformation, eventually lipid-soluble drugs become more water soluble so that they may be readily excreted.

Phase I oxidation reactions are carried out by the **cytochrome P-450 (CYP450) system**, a set of microsomal enzymes (usually hepatic) referred to as CYP1, CYP2, and CYP3. Within each CYP family, there are enzyme subgroups identified by a number-letter-sequence (i.e., 1A2 or 3A4). There are over 40 enzymes, but most of the metabolism occurs in only a few of them. A **substrate** is the drug or compound that is identified as a target of an enzyme. For example, clozapine is the substrate for the CYP1A2 enzyme.

The functioning of these enzymes is influenced by drugs and other chemical substances. An **inhibitor** of a CYP enzyme slows down metabolism, which in turn decreases the clearance of the substrate, and elevates its plasma level. An **inducer** speeds up metabolism, which in turn increases the clearance of the substrate and decreases its plasma level. For example, cigarette smoke is a potent inducer of CYP1A2, which in turn speeds up the clearance of clozapine and decreases its plasma level. A smoker will clear clozapine faster than a nonsmoker even though both take the same dose.

A **drug–drug interaction** can occur if one substance inhibits an enzyme system. For example, nortriptyline (an antidepressant with a narrow therapeutic index) is the substrate of the CYP2D6 enzyme. By adding paroxetine (a selective serotonin reuptake inhibitor [SSRI] antidepressant and an inhibitor of the CYP2D6 enzyme), the 2D6 enzyme is inhibited and nortriptyline's blood level increases. Toxicity can easily develop because of low therapeutic index (Sandson, 2003).

Each human CYP450 enzyme is an expression of a unique gene. The science of **pharmacogenomics** blends pharmacology with genetic knowledge and is concerned with understanding and determining an individual's specific CYP450 makeup, then individualizing medications to match the person's CYP450 profile. Genetically determined, some individuals are poor metabolizers and others may be rapid metabolizers. Poor metabolizers account for up to 7% of whites for CYP2D6 and up to 25% of East Asians for CYP2C19. Up to 29% in North Africa and the Middle East are ultra-rapid metabolizers for CYP2D6. There is now a test to determine an individual's metabolic capacity for certain drugs for two CYP enzymes: 2D6 and 2D19. Enzyme CYP2D6 is important in the metabolism of many antidepressants and antipsychotics, and CYP2C19 is important for some antidepressant metabolism. The practical use of this test has not yet been determined, but development of similar tests is likely in the future (Juran, Egan, & Lazaridis, 2006; de Leon, Armstrong, & Cozza, 2006).

Excretion

Excretion refers to the removal of drugs from the body either unchanged or as metabolites. **Clearance** refers to the total volume of blood, serum, or plasma from which a drug is completely removed per unit of time to account for the excretion. The half-life of a drug provides a measure of the expected rate of clearance. **Half-life** refers to the time required for plasma concentrations of the drug to be reduced by 50%. For most drugs, the rate of excretion slows while the half-life remains unchanged. It usually takes four half-lives or more of a drug in total time for more than 90% of the drug to be eliminated.

Drugs bound to plasma proteins do not cross the glomerular filter freely. These lipid-soluble drugs are passively reabsorbed by diffusion across the renal tubule and thus are not rapidly excreted in the urine. Because many psychiatric medications are protein bound and lipid soluble, most of their excretion occurs through the liver, where they are excreted in the bile and delivered into the intestine. Lithium, a mood stabilizer, is a notable example of renal excretion. Any impairment in renal function or renal disease may lead to severe toxic symptoms.

Dosing refers to the administration of medication over time, so that therapeutic levels may be achieved or maintained without reaching toxic levels. In general, it is necessary to give a drug at intervals no greater than the half-life of the medication to avoid excessive fluctuation of concentration in the plasma between doses. With repeated dosing, a certain amount of the drug is accumulated in the body.

Steady-state plasma concentration or simply **steady state** occurs when absorption equals excretion and the therapeutic level plateaus. The rate of accumulation is determined by the half-life of the drug. Drugs generally reach steady state in four to five times the elimination half-life. However, because elimination or excretion rates may vary significantly in any individual, fluctuations may still occur, and dose schedules may need to be modified.

Individual Variations in Drug Effects

Many factors affect drug absorption, distribution, metabolism, and excretion. These factors may vary among individuals, depending on their age, genetics, and ethnicity.

Age

Pharmacokinetics are significantly altered at the extremes of the life cycle. Gastric absorption changes as individuals age. Gastric pH increases and gastric emptying decreases. Gastric motility slows and splanchnic circulation is reduced. Normally, these changes do not significantly impair oral absorption of a medication, but addition of common conditions, such as diarrhea, may significantly alter and reduce absorption. Malnutrition, cancer, and liver disease decrease the production of the primary protein albumin. More free drug is acting in the system, producing higher blood levels of the medication and potentially toxic effects. The activity of hepatic enzymes also slows with age. As a result, the ability of the liver to metabolize medications may slow as much as a fourfold decrease between the ages of 20 and 70 years. Production of albumin by the liver generally declines with age. Changes in the parasympathetic nervous system produce a greater sensitivity in elderly patients to anticholinergic side effects, which are more severe with this age group.

Renal function also declines with age. Creatinine clearance in a young adult is normally 100 to 120 mL/min, but after age 40 years, this rate declines by about 10% per decade. Medical illnesses, such as diabetes and hypertension, may further the loss of renal function. When creatinine clearance falls below 30 mL/min, the excretion of drugs by the kidneys is significantly impaired, and potentially toxic levels may accumulate.

Ethnopsychopharmacology

Ethnopsychopharmacology investigates cultural variations and differences that influence the effectiveness of pharmacotherapies used in mental health. These differences include genetics and psychosocial factors. Studies of identical and nonidentical twins show that much of the individual variability in elimination half-life of a given drug is genetically determined. Some individuals of Asian descent produce higher concentrations of acetaldehyde with alcohol use than do Caucasians, resulting in a higher incidence of adverse symptoms, such as flushing and palpitations. Asian research subjects have been found to be more susceptible to the effects of drugs such as propranolol than are Caucasians, whereas those of African descent are less sensitive (Bachmann, 2002).

Regarding psychiatric medications, Asians require one half to one third the dose of antipsychotic medications that Caucasians require (Zhou, 2003). Lower doses of antidepressants are often required for those of Asian descent. Although many of these variations appear to be related to the CYP450 genetic differences discussed earlier, more research is needed to understand fully the underlying mechanisms and to identify groups that may require different approaches to medication treatment.

FAME AND FORTUNE

Abraham Lincoln (1809–1865)

Civil War President

Public Persona

The 16th President of the United States led a nation through turbulent times during a civil war. Ultimately his leadership preserved the United States as the republic we know today, despite periods of "melancholy" or depression throughout his life. At times, he had strong thoughts of committing suicide. Yet he had an enormous ability to cope with depression, especially in later life. He generally coped with the depression through his work, humor, fatalistic resignation, and even religious feelings. He generally did not let his depression interfere with his work as President. In 1841, he wrote of his ongoing depression, "A tendency to melancholy . . . . let it be observed, is a misfortune, not a fault." (Letter to Mary Speed, September 27, 1841)

Personal Realities

Lincoln's depression began in early childhood and can be traced to multiple causes. There is evidence that there was a genetic basis because both of his parents suffered from depression. Lincoln was partially isolated from his peers because of his unique interests in politics and reading. Additionally, he suffered through the deaths of his younger brother, mother, and older sister. There is speculation that Lincoln's depression may have dated to Thomas Lincoln's cold treatment of his son. There is also evidence that Abraham Lincoln took a commonly prescribed medication called *blue mass,* which contained mercury. Consequently, some speculate that he suffered from mercury poisoning.

SOURCE: Hirschhorn, N., Feldman, R.G., & Greaves, I.A. (2001). *Abraham Lincoln's Blue Pills: Did Our 16th President Suffer from Mercury Poisoning? Perspectives in Biology and Medicine, 44* (3), 315–322.

PHASES OF DRUG TREATMENT

Phases of drug treatment include initiation, stabilization, maintenance, and discontinuation of the medication. The following explains the role of the nurse in these phases.

Initiation Phase

Before the initiation of medications, patients must undergo several assessments.

- A psychiatric evaluation to determine the diagnosis and target symptoms
- A nursing assessment including cultural beliefs and practices (see Chapter 10)
- Physical examination and indicated laboratory tests, often including baseline determinations such as a complete blood count (CBC), liver and kidney function tests, electrolyte levels, and urinalysis, and possibly thyroid function tests and electrocardiogram (ECG), to determine whether a physical condition may be causing the symptoms and to establish that it is safe to initiate use of a particular medication.

During the initiation of medication, the nurse assesses, observes, and monitors the patient's response to the medication, teaches the patient about the action, dosage, frequency of administration and side effects, and develops a plan for ongoing contact with clinicians. The first medication dose should be treated as if it were a "test" dose. Patients should be monitored for adverse effects such as changes in blood pressure, pulse, or temperature; changes in mental status; allergic reactions; dizziness; ataxia; or gastric distress. If any of these symptoms develop, they should be reported to the prescriber.

Stabilization Phase

During stabilization, the medication dosage is adjusted or titrated to achieve the maximum amount of improvement with a minimum of side effects. Psychiatric–mental health nurses assess target symptoms, looking for changes or improvements and side effects. If medications are being increased rapidly, such as in a hospital setting, nurses must closely monitor temperature, blood pressure, pulse, mental status, common side effects, and unusual adverse reactions.

In the outpatient setting, nurses focus on patient education emphasizing the importance of taking the medication, expected outcomes, and potential side effects. Patients need to know how and when to take the medication, how to minimize any side effects, and which side effects require immediate attention. A plan should be developed for patients and their families to clearly identify what to do if adverse reactions develop. The plan, which should include emergency telephone numbers or available emergency treatment, should be reviewed frequently.

Therapeutic drug monitoring is most important in this phase of treatment. Many medications used in psychiatry improve target symptoms only when a therapeutic level of medication has been obtained in the individual's blood. Some medications, such as lithium, have a narrow therapeutic range and must be monitored frequently and accurately. Nurses must be aware of when and how these levels are to be determined and assist patients in learning these procedures. Because of protein binding and lipid solubility, most medications do not have obtainable plasma levels that are clinically relevant. However, plasma levels of these medications may still be requested to evaluate further such issues as absorption and adverse reactions.

Sometimes the first medication chosen does not adequately improve the patient's target symptoms. In such cases, use of the medication will be discontinued and treatment with a new medication will be started. Medications may also be changed when adverse reactions or seriously uncomfortable side effects occur or these effects substantially interfere with the individual's quality of life. Nurses should be familiar with the pharmacokinetics of both drugs to be able to monitor side effects and possible drug–drug interactions during this change.

At times, an individual may show only partial improvement from a medication, and the prescriber may try an **augmentation** strategy by adding another medication. For example, a prescriber may add a mood stabilizer, such as lithium, to an antidepressant to improve the effects of the antidepressant. **Polypharmacy**, using more than one group from a class of medications, is increasingly being used as an acceptable strategy with most psychopharmacologic agents to match the drug action to the neurochemical needs of the patient. Nurses must be familiar with the potential effects, side effects, drug interactions, and rationale for the treatment regimen.

Maintenance Phase

Once the individual's target symptoms have improved, medications are usually continued to prevent **relapse** or return of the symptoms. In some cases, this may occur despite the patient's continued use of the medication. Patients must be educated about their target symptoms and have a plan of action if the symptoms return. In other cases, the patient may experience medication side effects. The psychiatric–mental health nurse has a central role in assisting individuals to monitor their own symptoms, identify emerging side effects, manage psychosocial stressors, and avoid other factors that may cause the medications to lose effect.

Discontinuation Phase

Some psychiatric medications will be discontinued; others will not. Some require a tapered discontinuation, which involves slowly reducing dosage while monitoring closely for re-emergence of the symptoms. Some psychiatric disorders, such as mild depression, respond to treatment and do not recur. Other disorders, such as schizophrenia, usually require lifetime medication. Discontinuance of some medications, such as controlled substances, produces withdrawal symptoms; discontinuance of others does not.

ANTIPSYCHOTIC MEDICATIONS

Antipsychotic medications can be thought of as "older" and "newer" medications. Newer or **atypical antipsychotic drugs** appear to be equally or more effective, but have fewer side effects than the traditional older agents. The term *typical or conventional antipsychotic* identifies the older antipsychotic drugs. See Table 8.5 for a list of selected antipsychotics.

Indications and Mechanism of Action

Antipsychotic medications are indicated for schizophrenia, mania, and autism and to treat the symptoms of psy-

Table 8.5 Antipsychotic Medications

Generic (Trade) Drug Name	Usual Dosage Range (mg/d)	Half-Life (h)	Therapeutic Blood Level	Approximate Equivalent Dosage (mg)
Atypical Antipsychotics				
Aripiprazole (Abilify)	10–30	75–94	Not available	Not available
Clozapine (Clozaril)	300–900	4–12	141–204 ng/mL	50
Risperidone (Risperdal) Oral	2–8	20	Not available	1
Risperdal Consta	25–50 mg every 2 weeks			Not available
Olanzapine (Zyprexa)	5–15 mg	21–54	Not available	Not available
Paliperidone (Invega Extended Release)	3–12 mg once daily in AM	23 hours	Not available	Not available
Quetiapine fumarate (Seroquel)	150–750	7	Not available	Not available
Ziprasidone HCl (Geodon)	40–160	7	Not available	Not available
Conventional (Typical) Antipsychotics				
Chlorpromazine (Thorazine)	50–1200	2–30	30–100 mg/mL	100
Mesoridazine (Serentil)	50–400	24–48	Not available	50
Fluphenazine (Prolixin)	2–20	4.5–15.3	0.2–0.3 ng/mL	2
Perphenazine (Trilafon)	12–64	Unknown	0.8–12.0 ng/mL	10
Trifluoperazine (Stelazine)	5–40	47–100	1–2.3 ng/mL	5
Thiothixene (Navane)	5–60	34	2–20 ng/mL	4
Loxapine (Loxitane)	20–250	19	Not available	15
Haloperidol (Haldol)	2–60	21–24	5–15 ng/mL	2
Molindone (Moban)	50–400	1.5	Not available	10

chosis, such as hallucinations, delusions, bizarre behavior, disorganized thinking, and agitation. (These symptoms are described more fully in later chapters.) Off-label uses of these drugs are quite common. These medications also reduce agitation, aggressiveness, and inappropriate behavior associated with psychosis. Within the typical antipsychotics, haloperidol and pimozide are approved for treating Tourette's syndrome, reducing the frequency and severity of vocal tics. Some of the typical antipsychotics, particularly chlorpromazine, are used as antiemetics or for postoperative intractable hiccoughs.

The atypical antipsychotic medications differ from the typical antipsychotics in that they block serotonin receptors as well as dopamine receptors. The differences between the mechanism of action of the typical and atypical antipsychotic helps to explain their differences in terms of effect on target symptoms and in the degree of side effects they produce.

Pharmacokinetics

Antipsychotic medications administered orally have a variable rate of absorption complicated by the presence of food, antacids, smoking, and even the coadministration of anticholinergics, which slow gastric motility. Clinical effects begin to appear in about 30 to 60 minutes. Absorption after intramuscular (IM) administration is less variable because this method avoids the first-pass effects. Therefore, IM administration produces greater bioavailability. It is important to remember that IM medications are absorbed more slowly when patients are immobile because erratic absorption may occur when muscles are not in use, which is especially important to remember when administering IM antipsychotic medication to patients who are restrained. For example, the patient's arm may be more mobile than the buttocks. The deltoid has better blood perfusion, and the medication will be more readily absorbed, especially with use.

Metabolism of these drugs occurs almost entirely in the liver with the exception of paliperidone ER (Invega), which is not extensively metabolized by the liver, but is excreted largely unchanged through the kidney. These medications are subject to the effects of other drugs that induce or inhibit the CYP450 system described earlier (see Table 8.6). Careful observance of concurrent medication use, including prescribed, over-the-counter, and substances of abuse, is required to avoid drug–drug interactions. Atypical antipsychotics are unlikely to alter drugs metabolized by CYP450, but their concentrations may be affected by CYP450-inhibiting drugs such as paroxetine and fluoxetine (Kutscher & Carnahan, 2006).

Excretion of these substances tends to be slow. Most antipsychotics have a half-life of 24 hours or longer, but many also have active metabolites with longer half-lives. These two effects make it difficult to predict elimination time, and metabolites of some of these agents may be found in the urine months later. When a medication is discontinued, the adverse effects may not immediately subside. The patient may continue to experience and sometimes need treatment for the adverse effects for sev-

Table 8.6 CYP450 Metabolism of Commonly Used Antipsychotics

Drug	How Metabolized	Induces	Inhibits
Aripiprazole	2D6, 3A4	None	None
Clozapine	1A2, 2C19, 2D6, 3A4	None	None
Haloperidol	1A2, 2D6, 3A4	None	2D6
Olanzapine	1A2, 2D6	None	None
Paliperidone	Less than 10% 2D6, 3A4; primarily renal elimination	None	None
Quetiapine	3A4	None	None
Risperidone	2D6	None	Mild 2D6
Ziprasidone	1A2, 3A4	None	None

Adapted from Kutscher, E.C., & Carnahan, R. (2006). CYP450 drug interactions with psychiatric medicines: A brief review for the primary care physician. *South Dakota Journal of Medicine, 59*(1), 5–9 and from www.Janssen.com, Invega Package Insert, 12/06.

eral days. Similarly, patients who discontinue their antipsychotic drugs may still derive therapeutic benefit for several days to weeks after drug discontinuation.

High lipid solubility, accumulation in the body, and other factors have also made it difficult to correlate blood levels with therapeutic effects. Table 8.5 shows the therapeutic ranges available for some of the antipsychotic medications. Potency of the antipsychotics also varies widely and is of specific concern when considering typical antipsychotic drugs. As Table 8.5 indicates, 50 mg clozapine is roughly equivalent to 1 mg risperidone and 5 mg trifluoperazine.

Long-Acting Preparations

Currently, in the United States, atypical antipsychotic Risperdal Consta and two conventional antipsychotic drugs, haloperidol and fluphenazine, are available in long-acting forms. These antipsychotics are administered by injection once every 2 to 4 weeks. The Risperdal Consta is a water-based suspension, whereas the other two are oil-based solutions. Long-acting injectable medications maintain a fairly constant blood level between injections. Because they bypass problems with gastrointestinal absorption and first-pass metabolism, this method may enhance therapeutic outcomes for the patient.

Fluphenazine decanoate and haloperidol decanoate, referred to as depot medications, are equally effective in treating the symptoms of psychosis. Nurses should be aware that the injection site may become sore and inflamed if certain precautions are not taken. The liquids are viscous, and a large-gauge needle (at least 21 gauge) should be used. Because the medication is meant to remain in the injection site, the needle should be dry, and a deep IM injection should be given by the Z-track method. (Note: Do not massage the injection site. Rotate sites and document in the patient's record.) A change to depot preparation from oral antipsychotic is done on a gradual basis after the patient is fully informed and consents and has taken several oral doses to ensure no significant immediate adverse reactions are likely to occur.

Risperdal Consta is unique in that microspheres (encapsulated polymers containing the medication) gradually break down, releasing the active form of the medication. This medication is administered intramuscularly every 2 weeks. Initiation of this medication regimen requires that an oral antipsychotic be given during the first 3 weeks to reach a therapeutic blood level.

Side Effects, Adverse Reactions, and Toxicity

Various side effects and interactions can occur with antipsychotics, with the **conventional antipsychotics** (typical antipsychotics) producing more significant side effects than the atypical antipsychotics. The side effects vary largely based on their degree of attraction to different neurotransmitter receptors and their subtypes. See Box 8.3 for assessments that should be completed prior to starting an antipsychotic.

Cardiovascular Side Effects

Cardiovascular side effects include orthostatic hypotension and prolongation of the QTc interval. Orthostatic hypotension is very common and depends on the degree of blockade of α-adrenergic receptors. Ziprasidone (Geodon) has been associated with prolonged QTc intervals and should be used cautiously in patients who have increased Q-T intervals or are taking other medications that may prolong the Q-T interval (Taylor, 2003). Other cardiovascular side effects from typical antipsychotics have been rare, but occasionally they cause ECG changes that have a benign or undetermined clinical effect.

Anticholinergic Side Effects

Anticholinergic side effects resulting from blockade of acetylcholine are another common side effect associated

BOX 8.3

Recommended Assessments Before Starting an Antipsychotic

Weigh all patients and track BMI during treatment
- Determine if overweight (BMI 25–29.9) or obese (BMI ≥ 30)
- Monitor BMI monthly for first 3 months, then quarterly

Obtain baseline personal and family history of diabetes, obesity, dyslipidemia, hypertension, and cardiovascular disease

Get waist circumference (at umbilicus)
- Men: greater than 40 inches (102 cm)
- Women: greater than 35 inches (88)

Monitor blood pressure, fasting plasma glucose, and fasting lipid profile
- Monitor within 3 months and then annually (more frequently for patients with diabetes or have gained >5% of initial weight.
- Prediabetes (fasting plasma glucose 100–125 mg)
- Diabetes (fasting plasma glucose >126)
- Hypertension (BP > 140/90 mm Hg)
- Dyslipidemia (increased total cholesterol [>200mg], decreased HDL, and increased LDL)

Stahl, S. (2006). *Essential psychopharmacology: the prescribers guide.* Cambridge University Press: New York.

with antipsychotic drugs. Dry mouth, slowed gastric motility, constipation, urinary hesitancy or retention, vaginal dryness, blurred vision, dry eyes, nasal congestion, and confusion or decreased memory are examples of these side effects. Interventions for decreasing the impact of these side effects are outlined in Table 8.1.

This group of side effects occurs with many of the medications used for psychiatric treatment. Using more than one medication with anticholinergic effects often increases the symptoms. Elderly patients are often most susceptible to a potential toxicity that results from high blockade of acetylcholine. This toxicity is called an *anticholinergic* crisis and is described more fully, along with its treatment, in Chapter 18.

Weight Gain

Weight gain is a common side effect of the atypical antipsychotics, particularly clozapine and olanzapine (Zyprexa), which can cause a weight gain of up to 20 pounds within 1 year. Ziprasidone (Geodon) is associated with little to no weight gain during clinical trials. If a patient becomes overweight or obese, switching to another antipsychotic should be considered and weight control interventions implemented.

Diabetes

One of the more serious side effects is the risk of type II diabetes. The FDA has determined that all atypical antipsychotics increase the risk for type II diabetes. Nurses should routinely assess for emerging symptoms of diabetes and alert the prescriber of these symptoms (see Box 8.3).

Sexual Side Effects

Sexual side effects result primarily from the blockade of dopamine in the tuberoinfundibular pathways of the hypothalamus. As a result, blood levels of prolactin may increase, particularly with risperidone and the typical antipsychotics. Increased prolactin causes breast enlargement and rare but potential galactorrhea (milk production and flow), decreased sexual drive, amenorrhea, menstrual irregularities, and increased risk for growth in pre-existing breast cancers. Other sexual side effects include retrograde ejaculation (backward flow of semen) erectile dysfunction, and anorgasmia.

Blood Disorders

Blood dyscrasias are rare but have received renewed attention since the introduction of clozapine. Agranulocytosis is an acute reaction that causes the individual's white blood cell count to drop to very low levels, and concurrent neutropenia, a drop in neutrophils in the blood, develops. In the case of the antipsychotics, the medication suppresses the bone marrow precursors to blood factors. The exact mechanism by which the drugs produce this effect is unknown. The most notable symptoms of this disorder include high fever, sore throat, and mouth sores. Although benign elevations in temperature have been reported in individuals taking clozapine, no fever should go uninvestigated. Untreated agranulocytosis can be life threatening. Although agranulocytosis can occur with any of the antipsychotics, the risk with clozapine is 10 to 20 times greater than with the other antipsychotics (Bilici, Tekelioglu, Efendioglu, Ovali, & Ulgen, 2003). Therefore, prescription of clozapine requires weekly blood samples for the first 6 months of treatment, and then every 2 weeks after that for as long as the drug is taken. Drawing of these samples must continue for 4 weeks after clozapine use has been discontinued. If sore throat or fever develops, medications should be withheld until a leukocyte count can be obtained. Hospitalization, including reverse isolation to prevent infections, is usually required. Agranulocytosis is more likely to develop during the first 18 weeks of treatment. Some research indicates that it is more common in women.

Neuroleptic Malignant Syndrome

Neuroleptic malignant syndrome (NMS) is a serious complication that may result from antipsychotic medications. Characterized by rigidity and high fever, NMS is a rare condition that may occur abruptly with even one dose of medication. Temperature must always be monitored when administering antipsychotics, especially high-potency medications. This condition is discussed more fully in Chapter 18.

Other Side Effects

Photosensitivity reactions to antipsychotics, including severe sunburns or rash, most commonly develop with the use of low-potency typical medications. Sun block must be worn on all areas of exposed skin when taking these drugs. In addition, sun exposure may cause pigmentary deposits to develop, resulting in discoloration of exposed areas, especially the neck and face. This discoloration may progress from a deep orange color to a blue gray. Skin exposure should be limited and skin tone changes reported to the prescriber. Pigmentary deposits, *retinitis pigmentosa,* may also develop on the retina of the eye.

Antipsychotics may also lower the seizure threshold. Patients with an undetected seizure disorder may experience seizures early in treatment. Those who have a preexisting condition should be monitored closely.

Medication-Related Movement Disorders

Medication-related movement disorders are side effects or adverse reactions that are commonly caused by typical antipsychotic medications but less commonly with atypical antipsychotic drugs. These disorders of abnormal motor movements can be divided into two groups: **acute extrapyramidal syndromes (EPS),** which are acute abnormal movements developing early in the course of treatment (sometimes after just one dose); and **chronic syndromes**, which develop from longer exposure to antipsychotic drugs.

Acute Extrapyramidal Syndromes

Acute extrapyramidal syndromes include dystonia, pseudoparkinsonism, and akathisia. They develop early in treatment, sometimes from as little as one dose. Although the abnormal movements are treatable, they are at times dramatic and frightening, causing physical and emotional impairments that often prompt patients to stop taking their medication. EPS occurs when there is an imbalance of acetylcholine, dopamine, and GABA in the basal ganglia as a result of blocking dopamine.

Dystonia, sometimes referred to as an *acute dystonic reaction,* is impaired muscle tone that generally is the first extrapyramidal symptom to occur, usually within a few days of initiating use of an antipsychotic. Acetylcholine is overactive because one of its modulators, dopamine, is blocked. Dystonia is characterized by involuntary muscle spasms that lead to abnormal postures, especially of the head and neck muscles. Acute dystonia occurs most often in young men, adolescents, and children. Patients usually first report a thick tongue, tight jaw, or stiff neck. The syndrome can progress to a protruding tongue, oculogyric crisis (eyes rolled up in the head), torticollis (muscle stiffness in the neck, which draws the head to one side with chin pointing to the other), and laryngopharyngeal constriction. Abnormal postures of the upper limbs and torso may be held briefly or sustained. In severe cases, the spasms may progress to the intercostal muscles, producing more significant breathing difficulty for patients who already have respiratory impairment from asthma or emphysema. The treatment is the administration of a medication such as the anticholinergic agents that inhibit acetylcholine and thereby restore the balance of neurotransmitters (see Table 8.7).

Drug-induced parkinsonism is sometimes referred to as **pseudoparkinsonism** because its presentation is identical to Parkinson's disease. The difference is that the activity of dopamine is blocked in pseudoparkinsonism and in Parkinson's disease the cells of the basal ganglia are destroyed. Elderly patients are at the greatest risk for experiencing pseudoparkinsonism (O'Hara et al., 2002). Symptoms include the classic triad of rigidity, slowed movements (akinesia), and tremor. The rigid muscle stiffness is usually seen in the arms. Akinesia can be observed by the loss of spontaneous movements, such as the absence of the usual relaxed swing of the arms while walking. In addition, mask-like facies or loss of facial expression and a decrease in the ability to initiate movements also are present. Usually, tremor is more pronounced at rest, but it can also be observed with intentional movements, such as eating. If the tremor becomes severe, it may interfere with the patient's ability to eat or maintain adequate fluid intake. Hypersalivation is possible as well. Pseudoparkinsonism symptoms may occur on one or both sides of the body and develop abruptly or subtly but usually within the first 30 days of treatment. The treatment is the reduction in dosage or a change of antipsychotic that has less affinity for the dopamine receptor. Anticholinergic medication is sometimes given.

Akathisia is characterized by the inability to sit still or restlessness and is more common in the middle-aged patient. The person will pace, rock while sitting or standing, march in place, or cross and uncross the legs. All of these repetitive motions have an intensity that is frequently beyond the explanation of the individual. In addition, akathisia may be present as a primarily subjective experience without obvious motor behavior. This subjective experience includes feelings of anxiety, jitteriness, or the inability to relax, which the individual may or may not be able to communicate. It is extremely uncomfortable for a person experiencing akathisia to be forced to sit still or be confined. These symptoms are sometimes misdiagnosed as agitation or an increase in psychotic symptoms. If an antipsychotic medication is given, the symptoms will

Table 8.7 Drug Therapies for Acute Medication-Related Movement Disorders

Agents	Typical Dosage Ranges	Routes Available	Common Side Effects
Anticholinergics			
Benztropine (Cogentin)	2–6 mg/d	PO, IM, IV	Dry mouth, blurred vision, slowed gastric motility causing constipation, urinary retention, increased intraocular pressure; overdose produces toxic psychosis
Trihexyphenidyl (Artane)	4–15 mg/d	PO	Same as benztropine, plus gastrointestinal distress Elderly people are most prone to mental confusion and delirium
Biperiden (Akineton)	2–8 mg/d	PO	Fewer peripheral anticholinergic effects Euphoria and increased tremor may occur
Antihistamines			
Diphenhydramine (Benadryl)	25–50 mg qid to 400 mg daily	PO, IM, IV	Sedation and confusion, especially in elderly people
Dopamine Agonists			
Amantadine (Symmetrel)	100–400 mg daily	PO	Indigestion, decreased concentration, dizziness, anxiety, ataxia, insomnia, lethargy, tremors, and slurred speech may occur on higher doses Tolerance may develop on fixed dose
β-Blockers			
Propranolol (Inderal)	10 mg tid to 120 mg daily	PO	Hypotension and bradycardia Must monitor pulse and blood pressure Do not stop abruptly as may cause rebound tachycardia
Benzodiazepines			
Lorazepam (Ativan)	1–2 mg IM 0.5–2 mg PO	PO, IM	All may cause drowsiness, lethargy, and general sedation or paradoxical agitation Confusion and disorientation in elderly people
Diazepam (Valium)	2–5 mg tid	PO, IV	Most side effects are rare and will disappear if dose is decreased
Clonazepam (Klonopin)	1–4 mg/d	PO	Tolerance and withdrawal are potential problems

not abate and will often worsen. Differentiating akathisia from agitation may be aided by knowing the person's symptoms before the introduction of medication. Psychotic agitation does not usually begin abruptly after antipsychotic medication use has been started, whereas akathisia may occur after administration. In addition, the nurse may ask the patient if the experience is felt primarily in the muscles (akathisia) or in the mind or emotions (agitation).

Akathisia is the most difficult acute medication-related movement disorder to relieve. It does not usually respond well to anticholinergic medications. The pathology of akathisia may involve more than just the extrapyramidal motor system. It may include serotonin changes that also affect the dopamine system (Kulkarni & Naidu, 2003). The usual approach to treatment is to change or reduce the antipsychotic. A number of medications are used to reduce symptoms, including β-adrenergic blockers, anticholinergics, antihistamines, and low-dose antianxiety agents (Sajatovic, 2000). The β-adrenergic blockers, such as propranolol (Inderal), given in doses of 30 to 120 mg/d, are the most successful.

A number of nursing interventions reduce the impact of these syndromes. Individuals with acute extrapyramidal symptoms need frequent reassurance that this is not a worsening of their psychiatric condition but instead is a treatable side effect of the medication. They also need validation that what they are experiencing is real and that the nurse is concerned and will be responsive to changes in these symptoms. Physical and psychological stress appears to increase the symptoms and further frighten the patient; therefore, decreasing stressful situations becomes important. These symptoms are often physically exhausting for the patient, and nurses should ensure that the patient receives adequate rest and hydration. Because tremors, muscle rigidity, and motor restlessness may interfere with the individual's ability to eat, the nurse may need to assist the patient with eating and drinking fluids to maintain nutrition and hydration.

Risk factors for acute EPS syndromes include previous episodes of extrapyramidal symptoms. Listen closely when patients say they are "allergic" or have had "bad reactions" to antipsychotic medications. Often, they are describing one of the medication-related movement disorders, particularly dystonia, rather than a rash or other allergic symptoms. About 90% of the individuals who have experienced extrapyramidal symptoms in the past will again have these symptoms if use of an antipsychotic medication is restarted (Arana, 2000; Nasrallah, 2002).

Tardive Dyskinesia

Chronic syndromes develop from long-term use of antipsychotics. They are serious and afflict about 20% of the patients who receive typical antipsychotics for an extended period. These conditions are typically irreversible and cause significant impairment in self-image, social interactions, and occupational functioning. Early symptoms and mild forms may go unnoticed by the person experiencing them.

Tardive dyskinesia, the most well-known of the chronic syndromes, involves irregular, repetitive involuntary movements of the mouth, face, and tongue, including chewing, tongue protrusion, lip smacking, puckering of the lips, and rapid eye blinking. Abnormal finger movements are common as well. In some individuals, the trunk and extremities are also involved, and in rare cases, irregular breathing and swallowing lead to belching and grunting noises. These symptoms usually begin no earlier than after 6 months of treatment or when the medication is reduced or withdrawn. Once thought to be irreversible, considerable controversy now exists as to whether or not this is true.

Part of the difficulty in determining the irreversibility of tardive dyskinesia is that any movement disorder that persists after discontinuation of antipsychotic medication has been described as tardive dyskinesia. Atypical forms are now receiving more attention because some researchers believe they may have different underlying mechanisms of causation. Some of these forms of the disorder appear to remit spontaneously. Symptoms of what is now called *withdrawal tardive dyskinesia* appear when use of an antipsychotic medication is reduced or discontinued and remit spontaneously in 1 to 3 months. Tardive dystonia and tardive akathisia have also been described. Both appear in a manner similar to the acute syndromes but continue after the antipsychotic medication has been withdrawn. More research is needed to determine whether these syndromes are distinctly different in origin and outcome.

The risk for experiencing tardive dyskinesia increases with age. Although the prevalence of tardive dyskinesia averages 15% to 20%, the rate rises to 50% to 70% in elderly patients receiving antipsychotic medications (O'Hara et al., 2002; Yeung et al., 2000). Cumulative incidence of tardive dyskinesia appears to increase 5% per year of continued exposure to antipsychotic medications (Levy et al., 2002). Women are at higher risk than men. Anyone receiving antipsychotic medication can develop tardive dyskinesia. Risk factors are summarized in Box 8.4. The causes of tardive dyskinesia remain unclear. No one medication relieves the symptoms. Dopamine agonists, such as bromocriptine, and many other drugs have been tried with little success. Dietary precursors of acetylcholine, such as lecithin and vitamin E supplements, may prove to be beneficial.

The best approach to treatment remains avoiding the development of the chronic syndromes. Preventive measures include use of atypical antipsychotics, using the lowest possible dose of typical medication, minimizing use of as-needed (PRN) medication, and closely monitoring individuals in high-risk groups for development of the symptoms of tardive dyskinesia. All members of the mental health treatment team who have contact with individuals taking antipsychotics for longer than 3 months must be alert to the risk factors and earliest possible signs of chronic medication-related movement disorders.

Monitoring tools, such as the Abnormal Involuntary Movement Scale (AIMS), should be used routinely to standardize assessment and provide the earliest possible recognition of the symptoms. Standardized assessments should be performed at a minimum of 3- to 6-month intervals. The earlier the symptoms are recognized, the more likely they will resolve if the medication can be changed or its use discontinued. Newer, atypical antipsychotic medications have a much lower risk of causing tardive dyskinesia and are increasingly being considered first-line medications for treating schizophrenia. Other

BOX 8.4

Risk Factors for Tardive Dyskinesia

- Age more than 50 years
- Female
- Affective disorders, particularly depression
- Brain damage or dysfunction
- Increased duration of treatment
- Standard antipsychotic medication
- Possible—higher doses of antipsychotic medication

medications are under development to provide alternatives that limit the risk for tardive dyskinesia.

MOOD STABILIZERS (ANTIMANIA MEDICATIONS)

Mood stabilizers, or antimania medications, are psychopharmacologic agents used primarily for stabilizing mood swings, particularly those of mania in bipolar disorders. Lithium, the oldest, is the gold standard of treatment for acute mania and maintenance of bipolar disorders. Not all respond to lithium, and increasingly other drugs are being used as first-line agents. Anticonvulsants, calcium channel blockers, adrenergic blocking agents, and atypical antipsychotics are used for mood stabilization.

Lithium

Lithium, a naturally occurring element, is effective in only about 40% of patients with bipolar disorder. Although lithium is not a perfect drug, a great deal is known regarding its use—it is inexpensive, it has restored stability to the lives of thousands of people, and it remains the gold standard of bipolar pharmacologic treatment.

Indications and Mechanisms of Action

The target symptoms for lithium are the symptoms of mania, such as rapid speech, jumping from topic to topic (flight of ideas), irritability, grandiose thinking, impulsiveness, and agitation. Other psychiatric indications include using lithium for its mild antidepressant effects in treating depressive episodes of bipolar illness and in patients experiencing major depression that has only partially responded to antidepressants alone. Used in patients who have experienced only partial response, lithium has been used in augmentation as a potentiator (enhancing the effects) of antidepressant medications. It also has been shown to be helpful in reducing impulsivity and aggression in certain psychiatric patients.

The exact action by which lithium improves the symptoms of mania is unknown. Lithium is thought to exert multiple neurotransmitter effects, including enhancing serotonergic transmission, increasing synthesis of norepinephrine, and blocking postsynaptic dopamine (Bschor et al., 2003). Lithium is actively transported across cell membranes, altering sodium transport in both nerve and muscle cells. It replaces sodium in the sodium–potassium pump and is retained more readily than sodium inside the cell. Conditions that alter sodium content in the body, such as vomiting, diuresis, and diaphoresis, also alter lithium retention. The results of lithium influx into the nerve cell lead to increased storage of catecholamines within the cell, reduced dopamine neurotransmission, increased norepinephrine reuptake, increased GABA activity, and increased serotonin receptor sensitivity (Solomon et al., 2000). Lithium also alters the distribution of calcium and magnesium ions and inhibits second messenger systems within the neuron. Most likely, the mechanisms by which lithium improves the symptoms of mania are complex, involving the sum of all or part of these actions and more. Molecular research in the next decade may provide the answers.

Pharmacokinetics

Lithium carbonate is available orally in capsule, tablet, and liquid forms. Slow-release preparations are also available. Lithium is readily absorbed in the gastric system and may be taken with food, which does not impair absorption. Peak blood levels are reached in 1 to 4 hours, and the medication is usually completely absorbed in 8 hours. Slow-release preparations are absorbed at a slower, more variable rate.

Lithium is not protein bound, and its distribution into the CNS across the blood–brain barrier is slow. The onset of action is usually 5 to 7 days and may take as long as 2 weeks. The elimination half-life is 8 to 12 hours, and 18 to 36 hours in individuals whose blood levels have reached steady state and whose symptoms are stable. Lithium is almost entirely excreted by the kidneys but is present in all body fluids. Conditions of renal impairment or decreased renal function in elderly patients decrease lithium clearance and may lead to toxicity. Several medications affect renal function and therefore change lithium clearance. See Chapter 20 for a list of these and other medication interactions with lithium. About 80% of lithium is reabsorbed in the proximal tubule of the kidney along with water and sodium. In conditions that cause sodium depletion, such as dehydration caused by fever, strenuous exercise, hot weather, increased perspiration, and vomiting, the kidney attempts to conserve sodium. Because lithium is a salt, the kidney retains lithium as well, leading to increased blood levels and potential toxicity. Significantly increasing sodium intake causes lithium levels to fall.

Lithium is usually administered in doses of 300 mg two to three times daily. Because it is a drug with a narrow therapeutic range or index, blood levels are monitored frequently during acute mania, while the dosage is increased every 3 to 5 days. These increases may be slower in elderly patients or patients who experience uncomfortable side effects. Blood levels should be monitored 12 hours after the last dose of medication. In the hospital setting, nurses should withhold the morning dose of lithium until the serum sample is drawn to avoid falsely elevated levels. Individuals who are at home should be instructed to have their blood drawn in the morning about 12 hours after their last dose and before they take their first dose of medication. During the acute phases of mania, blood levels of 0.8 to 1.4 mEq/L are usually attained and maintained until symptoms are under control. The therapeutic range for lithium is narrow, and patients in the higher end of that range usually experience more uncomfortable side effects. During maintenance, the dosage is reduced, and dosages are adjusted to maintain blood levels of 0.4 to 1 mEq/L.

Lithium clears the body relatively quickly after discontinuation of its use. Withdrawal symptoms are rare, but occasional anxiety and emotional lability have been reported. It is important to remember that almost half of the individuals who discontinue lithium treatment abruptly experience a relapse of symptoms within a few weeks (Goodwin & Ghaemi, 2000; Kennedy et al., 2003). Some research suggests that discontinuation of the use of lithium for individuals whose symptoms have been stable may lead to lithium losing its effectiveness when use of the medication is restarted. Patients should be warned of the risks in abruptly discontinuing their medication and should be advised to consider the options carefully in consultation with their prescriber.

Side Effects, Adverse Reactions, and Toxicity

At lower therapeutic blood levels, side effects from lithium are relatively mild. These reactions correspond with peaks in plasma concentrations of the medication after administration, and most subside during the first few weeks of therapy. Frequently, individuals taking lithium complain of excessive thirst and an unpleasant metallic-like taste. Sugarless throat lozenges may be useful in minimizing this side effect. Other common side effects include increased frequency of urination, fine head tremor, drowsiness, and mild diarrhea. Weight gain occurs in about 20% of the individuals taking lithium. Nausea may be minimized by taking the medication with food or by use of a slow-release preparation. However, slow-release forms of lithium increase diarrhea. Muscle weakness, restlessness, headache, acne, rashes, and exacerbation of psoriasis have also been reported. See Chapter 20 for a summary of selected nursing interventions to minimize the impact of common side effects associated with lithium treatment. Patients most frequently discontinued their own medication use because of concerns with mental slowness, poor concentration, and memory problems.

As blood levels of lithium increase, the side effects of lithium become more numerous and severe. Early signs of lithium toxicity include severe diarrhea, vomiting, drowsiness, muscular weakness, and lack of coordination. Lithium should be withheld and the prescriber consulted if these symptoms develop. Lithium toxicity can easily be resolved in 24 to 48 hours by discontinuing the medication, but hemodialysis may be required in severe situations. See Chapter 20 for a summary of the side effects and symptoms of toxicity associated with various blood levels of lithium.

Monitoring of creatinine concentration, thyroid hormones, and CBC every 6 months during maintenance therapy helps to assess the occurrence of other potential adverse reactions. Kidney damage is considered an uncommon but potentially serious risk of long-term lithium treatment. This damage is usually reversible after discontinuation of the lithium use. A gradual rise in serum creatinine and decline in creatinine clearance indicate the development of renal dysfunction. Individuals with pre-existing kidney dysfunction are susceptible to lithium toxicity.

Lithium may alter thyroid function, usually after 6 to 18 months of treatment. About 30% of the individuals taking lithium exhibit elevations in thyroid-stimulating hormone, but most do not show suppression of circulating thyroid hormone. Thyroid dysfunction from lithium treatment is more common in women, and some individuals require the addition of thyroxine to their care. During maintenance, thyroid-stimulating hormone levels may be monitored. Nurses should observe for dry skin, constipation, bradycardia, hair loss, cold intolerance, and other symptoms of hypothyroidism. Other endocrine system effects result from hypoparathyroidism, which increases parathyroid hormone levels and calcium. Clinically, this change is not significant, but elevated calcium levels may cause mood changes, anxiety, lethargy, and sleep disturbances. These symptoms may erroneously be attributed to depression if hypercalcemia is not investigated.

Lithium use must be avoided during pregnancy because it has been associated with birth defects, especially when administered during the first trimester. If lithium is given during the third trimester, toxicity may develop in a newborn, producing signs of hypotonia, cyanosis, bradykinesia, cardiac changes, gastrointestinal bleeding, and shock. Diabetes insipidus may persist for months. Lithium is also present in breast milk, and women should not breast-feed while taking lithium. Women expecting to become pregnant should be advised to consult with their physician before discontinuing use of birth control methods.

Anticonvulsants

In the psychiatric mental health area, anticonvulsants are commonly used to treat bipolar disorder and are also considered mood stabilizers. The following discussion highlights the use of anticonvulsants as mood stabilizers in the treatment of bipolar disorder.

Indications and Mechanisms of Action

Valproate (valproic acid; Depakote), carbamazepine (Tegretol), and lamotrigine (Lamictal) have FDA approval for the treatment of bipolar disorder, mania, or mixed episodes (see Chapter 20). Other anticonvulsants, such as topiramate (Topamax), oxcarbazepine (Trileptal), and gapapentin (Neurontin) are used off-label as adjunctive treatments. In general, the anticonvulsant mood stabilizers have many actions, but it is their effects on ion channels, reducing repetitive firing of action potentials in the nerves, that most directly decreases manic symptoms. In addition, carbamazepine affects the release and reuptake of several neurotransmitters, including norepinephrine, GABA, dopamine, and glutamate. It also changes several second messenger systems. No one action has successfully accounted for the anticonvulsants' ability to stabilize mood (Loscher, 2002).

Pharmacokinetics

Valproic acid is rapidly absorbed, but the enteric coating of divalproex sodium adds a delay of as long as 1 hour. Peak serum levels occur in about 1 to 4 hours. The liquid form (sodium valproate) is absorbed more rapidly and peaks in 15 minutes to 2 hours (Loscher, 2002). Food appears to slow absorption, but does not lower bioavailability of the drug.

Carbamazepine is absorbed in a somewhat variable manner. The liquid suspension is absorbed more quickly than the tablet form, but food does not appear to interfere with absorption. Peak plasma levels occur in 2 to 6 hours. Because high doses influence peak plasma levels and increase the risk for side effects, carbamazepine should be given in divided doses two or three times a day. The suspension, which has higher peak plasma levels and lower trough levels, must be given more frequently than the tablet form.

These medications cross easily into the CNS, move into the placenta as well, and are associated with an increased risk for birth defects. Carbamazepine, valproic acid, and lamotrigine are metabolized by the CYP450 system. However, one of the metabolites of carbamazepine is potentially toxic. If other concurrent medications inhibit the enzymes that break down this toxic metabolite, severe adverse reactions are often the result. Medications that inhibit this breakdown include erythromycin, verapamil, and cimetidine (now available in nonprescription form).

Teaching Points 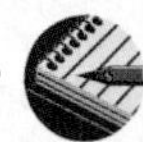

Nurses need to educate patients about potential drug interactions, especially with nonprescription medications. Nurses can also inform other health care practitioners who may be prescribing medication that these patients are taking carbamazepine. It is important to note that oral contraceptives may become ineffective, and female patients should be advised to use other methods of birth control.

Side Effects, Adverse Reactions, and Toxicity of Anticonvulsants

The most common side effects of carbamazepine are dizziness, drowsiness, tremor, visual disturbance, nausea, and vomiting. These side effects may be minimized by initiating treatment in low doses. Patients should be advised that these symptoms will diminish, but care should be taken when changing positions or performing tasks that require visual alertness. Giving the drug with food may diminish nausea. Adverse reactions include rare, aplastic anemia, agranulocytosis, severe rash, rare cardiac problems, and SIADH (syndrome of inappropriate secretion of the diuretic hormone) due to hyponatremia.

Valproic acid also causes gastrointestinal disturbances, tremor, and lethargy. In addition, it can produce weight gain and alopecia (hair loss). These symptoms are transient and should diminish with the course of treatment. Dietary supplements of zinc and selenium may be helpful to patients experiencing hair loss. Constipation and urinary retention occur in some individuals. Nurses should monitor urinary output and assist patients to increase fluid consumption to decrease constipation.

Benign skin rash, sedation, blurred or double vision, dizziness, nausea, vomiting, and other gastrointestinal symptoms are side effects of lamotrigine. In rare cases, lamotrigine (Lamictal) produces severe, life-threatening rashes that usually occur within 2 to 8 weeks of treatment. This risk is highest in children. Use of lamotrigine should be immediately discontinued if a rash is noted.

Transient elevations in liver enzymes occur with both carbamazepine and valproic acid but rarely do symptoms of hepatic injury occur. If the patient reports abnormal pain or shows signs of jaundice, the prescriber should be notified immediately. Several blood dyscrasias are associated with carbamazepine, including aplastic anemia, agranulocytosis, and leukopenia. Patients should be advised to report fever, sore throat, rash, petechiae, or bruising immediately. In addition, advise patients of the importance of completing routine blood tests throughout treatment. The increased risks for aplastic anemia and agranulocytosis with carbamazepine use still require close monitoring of CBCs during treatment. Valproate and its derivatives have had a similar course of development.

Of the off-label mood stabilizers, gabapentin (Neurontin) has relatively few side effects. Topamax (Topiramate) carries an increased risk of kidney stone formation. It can also cause a decrease in serum digoxin levels and may decrease effectiveness of oral birth control agents. In addition, ongoing ophthalmologic monitoring is required because of reports of acute myopia with secondary glaucoma. Trileptal (oxcarbazepine) has the potential for causing hyponatremia and may also decrease the effectiveness of oral birth control agents. Because of the potentially significant adverse reactions that the anticonvulsants can produce, careful patient teaching and monitoring are required.

ANTIDEPRESSANT MEDICATIONS

Medications classified as antidepressants are used not only for the treatment of depression, but in the treatment of anxiety disorders, eating disorders, and other mental health states (see Table 8.8). They are used very cautiously in persons with bipolar disorder because of the possibility of precipitating a manic episode. The exact neuromechanism for the antidepressant effect is unknown in all of them. Onset of action also varies considerably and appears to depend on factors outside of steady-state plasma levels. Initial improvement with some antidepressants, such as the SSRIs, may appear within 7 days, but complete relief of symptoms may take several weeks. Antidepressants should not be discontinued abruptly because of uncomfortable symptoms that result. Discontinuance of use of these medications requires slow tapering. Individuals taking these medications should be cautioned not to abruptly stop using them without consulting their prescriber. Antidepressant medications are well absorbed from the gastrointestinal system; however, some individual variations exist. Most of the antidepressants are metabolized by the CYP450 enzyme system so that drugs that activate this system will tend to decrease

Table 8.8 Antidepressant Medications

Generic (Trade) Drug Name	Usual Dosage Range (mg/d)	Half-Life (h)	Therapeutic Blood Level (ng/mL)
Selective Serotonin Reuptake Inhibitors (SSRIs)			
Citalopram (Celexa)	20–50	35	Not available
Escitalopram (Lexapro)	10–20	27–32	Not available
Fluoxetine (Prozac)	20–80	2–9 days	72–300
Fluvoxamine (Luvox)	50–300	17–22	Not available
Paroxetine (Paxil)	10–50	10–24	Not available
Sertraline (Zoloft)	50–200	24	Not available
Serotonin Norepinephrine Reuptake Inhibitor			
Duloxetine (Cymbalta)	40–60	8–17	Not available
Nefazodone (Serzone)	100–600	2–4	Not available
Venlafaxine (Effexor)	75–375	5–11	100–500
Norepinephrine Dopamine Reuptake Inhibitor			
Bupropion (Wellbutrin)	200–450	8–24	10–29
Alpha 2 Antagonist (NaSSA)			
Mirtazapine (Remeron)	15–45	20–40	Not available
Serotonin 2 Antagonist Reuptake Inhibitor (SARI)			
Trazodone (Desyrel)	150–600	4–9	650–1,600
Tricyclic Antidepressants			
Amitriptyline (Elavil)	50–300	31–46	110–250
Amoxapine (Asendin)	50–600	8	200–500
Clomipramine (Anafranil)	25–250	19–37	80–100
Imipramine (Tofranil)	30–300	11–25	200–350
Desipramine (Norpramin)	25–300	12–24	125–300
Doxepin (Sinequan)	25–300	8–24	100–200
Nortriptyline (Aventyl, Pamelor)	30–100	18–44	50–150
Protriptyline (Vivactil)	15–60	67–89	100–200
TETRACYCLIC			
Maprotiline (Ludiomil)	50–225	21–25	200–300
Monoamine Oxidase Inhibitors			
Phenelzine (Nardil)	15–90	24 (effect lasts 3–4 d)	Not available
Tranylcypromine (Parnate)	10–60	24 (effect lasts 3–10 d)	Not available
Selegiline (Emsam)	6–12 mg/24 hour	25%–50% delivered in 24 hours	Not available

Table 8.9 CYP450 Metabolism of Common Antidepressants

Drug	How Metabolized	Induces	Inhibits
Bupropion	2B6	None	2D6
Citalopram	2C19, 2D6, 3A4	None	Mild 2D6
Duloxetine	1A2, 2D6	None	2D6
Escitalopram	2C19, 2D6, 3A4	None	Mild 2D6
Fluoxetine	2C9, 2C19, 2D6, 3A4	None	2C19, 2D6 3A4, Norfluoxetine
Fluvoxamine	1A2, 2D6	None	1A2, 2C9, 2C19, 3A4
Mirtazepine	1A2, 2D6, 3A4	None	None
Nefazodone	2D6, 3A4	None	3A4
Paroxetine	2D6	None	2D6, 2B6
Selegiline	2A6, 2C9, 3A4/5	None	2D6, 3A4/5
Sertraline	2B6, 2C9, 2D6, 3A4	None	2B6, 2C9, 2C19, 2D6, 3A4 (dosage > 200 mg)
St. John's Wort*	3A4	3A4	None
Trazodone	2D6, 3A4	None	None
Tricyclic antidepressants	2D6, others depending on drug	None	Mild 2D6
Venlafaxine	2D6	None	Mild 2D6

*Not FDA-approved antidepressant.

Adapted from Kutscher, E. C., & Carnahan, R. (2006). CYP450 drug interactions with psychiatric medicines: A brief review for the primary care physician. *South Dakota Journal of Medicine, 59*(1), 5–9.

blood levels of the antidepressants, and inhibitors of this system will increase antidepressant blood levels (see Table 8.9). All of these medications have a "Boxed Warning" for increased risk of suicidal behavior in children and adolescents when compared to placebo.

Serotonin syndrome or serotonin intoxication syndrome can occur if there is an overactivity of serotonin or an impairment of the serotonin metabolism. Concomitant medications such as triptans used to treat migraines also can increase the serotonergic activity. With the advent of widely used antidepressants targeting the serotonergic systems, symptoms of this serious side effect should be assessed. Symptoms include mental status changes (hallucinations, agitation, and coma), autonomic instability (tachycardia, hyperthermia, changes in blood pressure), neuromuscular problems (hyperflexia, incoordination) and gastrointestinal disturbance (nausea, vomiting, diarrhea). Serotonin syndrome can be life threatening. The treatment for serotonin syndrome is discontinuation of the medication and symptom management.

Selective Serotonin Reuptake Inhibitors (SSRIs)

The serotonergic system is associated with mood, emotion, sleep, and appetite, and is implicated in the control of numerous emotional, physical, and behavioral functions (see Chapter 7). Decreased serotonergic neurotransmission has been proposed to play a key role in depression. In 1988, fluoxetine (Prozac) was the first of a class of drugs that acted "selectively" on serotonin, one group of neurotransmitters associated with depression. Other similarly selective medications, sertraline (Zoloft), paroxetine (Paxil), and fluvoxamine (Luvox), soon followed. The newest SSRI is escitalopram oxalate (Lexapro).

All of the SSRIs inhibit the reuptake of serotonin by blocking its transport into the presynaptic neuron, which in turn increases the concentration of synaptic serotonin. The concentration of synaptic serotonin is controlled directly by its reuptake; thus; drugs blocking serotonin transport have been successfully used for the treatment of depression and other conditions associated with serotonergic activity.

The SSRIs also have other properties that account for the common side effects, which include headache, anxiety, insomnia, transient nausea, vomiting, and diarrhea. Sedation may also occur, especially with paroxetine. Most often, these medications are given in the morning, but if daytime sedation occurs, they may be given in the evening. Higher doses, especially of fluoxetine, are more likely to produce sedation. Tolerance develops to the common side effects of nausea and dizziness. These symptoms, along with sexual dysfunction, sedation, diastolic hypertension, and increased perspiration, tend to be dose dependent, occurring more frequently at higher doses. Other common side effects include insomnia, constipation, dry mouth, tremors, blurred vision, and asthenia or muscle weakness.

Sexual dysfunction is a relatively common side effect with most antidepressants. Erectile and ejaculation disturbances occur in men and anorgasmia in women. This side effect is often difficult to assess if the nurse has not obtained a sexual history before initiation of use of the medication. Anorgasmia is particularly common with the SSRIs and often goes unreported, frequently because nurses and other health care providers do not ask.

Serotonin Norepinephrine Reuptake Inhibitors (SNRIs)

Decreased activity of the neurotransmitter norepinephrine (NE) is also associated with depression and anxiety disorders. Venlafaxine (Effexor), nefazodone (Serzone), and duloxetine (Cymbalta) prevent the reuptake of both serotonin and norepinephrine at the presynaptic site and are classified as SNRIs. Desipramine (Norpramine) is technically a tricyclic antidepressant, and is usually categorized as such. It works, however, on both serotonin and norepinephrine, so it can also be considered an SNRI.

Side effects are similar to the SSRIs, plus a risk for an associated increase in blood pressure. Elevations in blood pressure have been described, and nurses should monitor blood pressure, especially in patients who have a preexisting history of hypertension. Venlafaxine (Effexor) has little effect on acetylcholine and histamine; thus, it creates only mild sedation and anticholinergic symptoms. This medication is often used if the depressed patient is sleeping excessively and reports little energy. The most common side effects of nefazodone (Serzone) include dry mouth, nausea, dizziness, muscle weakness, constipation, and tremor. It is unlikely to cause sexual disturbance. Nefazodone also has a "Boxed Warning" for hepatic failure and should not be used for those with acute liver disease.

Norepinephrine Dopamine Reuptake Inhibitor (NDRI)

Bupropion (Wellbutrin, Zyban) inhibits norepinephrine, serotonin, and dopamine. Wellbutrin is indicated for depression and Zyban for nicotine addiction. The smoking cessation medication, Zyban, is given at a lower dose than Wellbutrin. Patients should not take Zyban if they are taking Wellbutrin. Bupropion has a chemical structure unlike any of the other antidepressants and somewhat resembles a few of the psychostimulants. Bupropion's activating effects may be experienced as agitation or anxiety by some patients. Others also experience insomnia and appetite suppression. For a few individuals, bupropion has produced psychosis, including hallucinations and delusions. Most likely, this is secondary to overstimulation of the dopamine system. Bupropion is contraindicated for people with seizure disorders or those at risk for seizures. It has been found that if the total daily dose of bupropion is no more than 450 mg and no individual dose is greater than 150 mg, the risk for seizures for bupropion is no greater than the risk with the other tetracyclic antidepressants (TCAs) (Ferry & Johnston, 2003). Most important, bupropion has not caused sexual dysfunction and often is used in individuals who are experiencing these side effects in other antidepressants.

Alpha-2 Antagonist (NaSSA)

Mirtazapine (Remeron) boosts norepinephrine/noradrenaline and serotonin by blocking α_2 adrenergic presynaptic receptors on a serotonin receptor ($5HT_{2A}$; $5HT_{2C}$, $5HT_3$). This is a different action than the other antidepressants. A histamine receptor is also blocked which may explain its sedative side effect. Mirtazapine is indicated for depression. Side effects include sedation (at lower doses), dizziness, weight gain, dry mouth, constipation, and change in urinary functioning.

Serotonin-2 Antagonist/ Reuptake Inhibitors (SARI)

Trazadone (Desyrel) blocks serotonin 2A receptor potently and blocks the serotonin reuptake pump less potently. It is indicated for depression, but often used off-label for insomnia and anxiety. Sedation is a very common side effect. Other side effects include weight gain, nausea, vomiting, constipation, dizziness, fatigue, incoordination, and tremor.

Tricyclic Antidepressants (TCAs)

The tricyclic antidepressants were once the primary medication used for treating depression. With the introduction of the SSRIs and other previously discussed antidepressants, the use of TCAs has significantly declined. In most cases, these medications are as effective as the other drugs, but they have more serious side effects and a higher lethal potential (see Table 8.8). The TCAs act on a variety of neurotransmitter systems including norepinephrine and serotonin reuptake systems.

Pharmacokinetics

The TCAs are highly bound to plasma proteins, which make the association between blood levels and therapeutic clinical effects difficult. However, some plasma ranges have been established (see Table 8.8). Most of the TCAs have active metabolites that act in much the same manner as the parent drug. Most of these antidepressants may be given in a once-daily single dose. If the medication causes sedation, this dose should be given at bedtime.

Side Effects, Adverse Reactions, and Toxicity

Because the TCAs act on several neurotransmitters in addition to serotonin and norepinephrine, these drugs have many unwanted effects. With the TCAs, sedation, orthostatic hypotension, and anticholinergic side effects are the most common sources of discomfort for patients receiving these medications. Other side effects of the TCAs include tremors, restlessness, insomnia, nausea and vomiting, confusion, pedal edema, headache, and seizures. Blood dyscrasias may also occur, and any fever, sore throat, malaise, or rash should be reported to the prescriber. Interventions to assist in minimizing these side effects are listed in Table 8.2.

The TCAs have the potential for cardiotoxicity. Symptoms include prolongation of cardiac conduction that may worsen pre-existing cardiac conduction problems. TCAs are contraindicated with second-degree atrioventricular block and should be used cautiously in patients who have other cardiac problems. Occasionally, they may precipitate heart failure, myocardial infarction, arrhythmias, and stroke.

Antidepressants that block the dopamine (D_2) receptor, such as amoxapine, have produced symptoms of neuroleptic malignant syndrome. Mild forms of extrapyramidal symptoms and endocrine changes, including galactorrhea and amenorrhea, may develop. Amoxapine should be avoided in elderly patients because it may be associated with the development of tardive dyskinesia with this age group (Zullino, Delacrausaz, & Baumann, 2002).

Monoamine Oxidase Inhibitor (MAOIs)

The monoamine oxidase inhibitors (MAOIs), as their name indicates, inhibit monoamine oxidase (MAO), an enzyme that breaks down the biogenic amine neurotransmitters serotonin, norepinephrine, and others. By inhibiting this enzyme, serotonin and norepinephrine activity is increased in the synapse. In the United States there are two oral formulations: phenelzine (Nardil) and tranylcypromine (Parnate). These are considered irreversible MAOIs because they form strong covalent bonds to block the enzyme monoamine oxidase. This inhibition increases with repeated administration of these medications and takes at least 2 weeks to resolve after discontinuation of use of the medication.

Selegiline (Emsam), a selective monoamine inhibitor for MOA-A and MOA-B, has recently been approved for the treatment of depressive disorder, and is available as a transdermal patch.

The major problem with the MAOIs is their interaction with tyramine-rich foods and certain medications that can result in a hypertensive crisis. All of the MAOIs have dietary modification except the 6 mg/24 hours dose of selegiline. The enzyme monoamine is important in the breakdown of dietary amines (e.g., tyramine). When the enzyme is inhibited, tyramine, a precursor for dopamine, increases in the nerve cells. Tyramine has a vasopressor action that induces hypertension. If the individual ingests food that contains high levels of tyramine while taking MAOIs, severe headaches, palpitation, neck stiffness and soreness, nausea, vomiting, sweating, and hypertension, stroke, and, in rare instances, death may result. Patients who are taking MAOIs are placed on a low-tyramine diet (see Table 8.10).

Table 8.10 Example of a Tyramine-Restricted Diet

Category of Food	Food to Avoid	Food Allowed
Cheese	All matured or aged cheeses All casseroles made with these cheeses, e.g., pizza, lasagna *Note:* All cheeses are considered matured or aged except those listed under "foods allowed"	Fresh cottage cheese, cream cheese, ricotta cheese, and processed cheese slices. All fresh milk products that have been stored properly (e.g., sour cream, yogurt, ice cream).
Meat, fish, and poultry	• Air dried, aged and fermented meats, sausages, and salamis • Pickled herring • Any spoiled or improperly stored meat • Spoiled or improperly stored animal livers	Fresh meat, poultry, and fish including fresh processed meats (such as lunch meats, hot dogs, breakfast sausage, and cooked sliced ham)
Fruits and vegetables	Broad bean pods (Fava bean pods)	All other vegetables
Alcoholic beverages	All tap beers and other beers that have not been pasteurized	Alcohol: No more than two domestic bottled or canned beers or 4-fluid-oz glasses of red or white wine per day; this applies to nonalcoholic beer also; please note that red wine may produce a headache unrelated to a rise in blood pressure
Miscellaneous foods	Marmite concentrated yeast extract Sauerkraut Soy sauce and other soybean condiments	Other yeast extracts (e.g., brewer's yeast) Soy milk Pizzas from commercial chain restaurants prepared with cheeses low in tyramine

Adapted from Gardener, D. M., Shulman, K. I., Walker, S. E., & Tailor, S. A. N. (1996). The making of a user friendly MAOI diet. *Journal of Clinical Psychiatry, 57*, 99–104.

www.fda.gov/cder/Offices/ODS/MG/selegilineMG.pdf Medication Guide, EMSAM, retrieved October 26, 2006.

In addition to food restrictions, many prescription and nonprescription medications that stimulate the sympathetic nervous system (sympathomimetic) produce the same risk for hypertensive crisis as do foods containing tyramine. The nonprescription medication interactions involve primarily diet pills and cold remedies. Patients should be advised to check the labels of any nonprescription drugs carefully for a warning against use with antidepressants, especially the MAOIs, and then consult their prescriber before consuming these medications. In addition, symptoms of other serious drug–drug interactions may develop, such as coma, hypertension, and fever, which may occur when patients receive meperidine (Demerol) while taking an MAOI. Patients should notify other health care providers, including dentists, that they are taking an MAOI before being prescribed or given any other medication.

The MAOIs frequently produce dizziness, headache, insomnia, dry mouth, blurred vision, constipation, nausea, peripheral edema, urinary hesitancy, muscle weakness, forgetfulness, and weight gain. Elderly patients are especially sensitive to the side effect of orthostatic hypotension and require frequent assessment of lying and standing blood pressures. They may be at risk for falls and subsequent bone fractures and require assistance in changing position. Sexual dysfunction, including decreased libido, impotence, and anorgasmia, also is common with MAOIs.

ANTIANXIETY AND SEDATIVE-HYPNOTIC MEDICATIONS

Sometimes called *anxiolytics*, antianxiety medications, such as buspirone (BuSpar), and sedative–hypnotic medications, such as lorazepam (Ativan) come from various pharmacologic classifications, including barbiturates, benzodiazepines, nonbenzodiazepines, and nonbarbiturate sedative–hypnotic medications, such as chloral hydrate. These drugs represent some of the most widely prescribed medications today for the short-term relief of anxiety or anxiety associated with depression.

Benzodiazepines

Commonly prescribed benzodiazepines include alprazolam (Xanax), lorazepam (Ativan), diazepam (Valium), chlordiazepoxide (Librium), flurazepam (Dalmane), and triazolam (Halcion). Although benzodiazepines are known to enhance the effects of the inhibitory neurotransmitter GABA, their exact mechanisms of action are not well understood. Of the various benzodiazepines in use to relieve anxiety (and treat insomnia), oxazepam (Serax) and lorazepam (Ativan) are often preferred for patients with liver disease and for elderly patients because of their short half-lives.

Pharmacokinetics

The variable rate of absorption of the benzodiazepines determines the speed of onset. Table 8.11 provides relative indications of the speed of onset, from very fast to slow, for some of the commonly prescribed benzodiazepines. Chlordiazepoxide (Librium) and diazepam (Valium) are slow, erratic, and sometimes incompletely absorbed when given intramuscularly, whereas lorazepam (Ativan) is rapidly and completely absorbed when given IM.

All of the benzodiazepines are highly lipid soluble and highly protein bound. They are distributed throughout the body and enter the CNS quickly. Other drugs that compete for protein-binding sites may produce drug–

Table 8.11 Antianxiety and Sedative-Hypnotic Medications

Generic (Trade) Drug Name	Usual Dosage Range (mg/d)	Half-Life (h)	Speed of Onset After Single Dose
Benzodiazepines			
Diazepam (Valium)	4–40	30–100	Very fast
Chlordiazepoxide (Librium)	15–100	50–100	Intermediate
Clorazepate (Tranxene)	15–60	30–200	Fast
Prazepam (Centrax)	20–60	30–200	Very slow
Flurazepam (Dalmane)	15–30	47–100	Fast
Lorazepam (Ativan)	2–8	10–20	Slow-intermediate
Oxazepam (Serax)	30–120	3–21	Slow-intermediate
Temazepam (Restoril)	15–30	9.5–20	Moderately fast
Triazolam (Halcion)	0.25–0.5	2–4	Fast
Alprazolam (Xanax)	0.5–10	12–15	Intermediate
Halazepam (Paxipam)	80–160	30–200	Slow-intermediate
Clonazepam (Klonopin)	1.5–20	18–50	Intermediate
Nonbenzodiazepines			
Buspirone (BuSpar)	15–30	3–11	Very slow
Zolpidem (Ambien)	5–10	2.6	Fast

drug interactions. The degree to which each of these drugs is lipid soluble affects its duration of action. Most of these drugs have active metabolites, but the degree of activity of each metabolite affects duration of action and elimination half-life. Most of these drugs vary markedly in length of half-life. Oxazepam and lorazepam have no active metabolites and thus have shorter half-lives. Elimination half-lives may also be sustained for obese patients when using diazepam, chlordiazepoxide, and halazepam (Paxipam).

Side Effects, Adverse Reactions, and Toxicity

The most commonly reported side effects result from the sedative and CNS depression effects of these medications. Drowsiness, intellectual impairment, memory impairment, ataxia, and reduced motor coordination are common adverse effects. If used for sleep, many of these medications, especially long-acting benzodiazepines, produce significant "hangover" effects experienced on awakening. Elderly patients receiving repeated doses of medications such as flurazepam (Dalmane) at bedtime may experience paradoxical confusion, agitation, and delirium, sometimes after the first dose. In addition, daytime fatigue, drowsiness, and cognitive impairments may continue while the person is awake. For most patients, the effects subside as tolerance develops; however, alcohol increases all of these symptoms and potentiates the CNS depression. Individuals using these medications should be warned to be cautious driving or performing other tasks that require mental alertness. If these tasks are part of the person's work requirements, another medication may be chosen. Administered intravenously, benzodiazepines often cause phlebitis and thrombosis at the intravenous sites, which should be monitored closely and changed if redness or swelling develops.

Because tolerance develops to most of the CNS depressant effects, individuals who wish to experience the feeling of "intoxication" from these medications may be tempted to increase their own dosage. Psychological dependence is more likely to occur when using these medications for a longer period. Abrupt discontinuation of the use of benzodiazepines may result in a recurrence of the target symptoms, such as rebound insomnia or anxiety. Other withdrawal symptoms appear rapidly, including tremors, increased perspiration, palpitations, increased sensitivity to light, abdominal discomfort or pain, and elevations in systolic blood pressure. These symptoms may be more pronounced with the short-acting benzodiazepines, such as lorazepam. Gradual tapering is recommended for discontinuing use of benzodiazepines after long-term treatment. When tapering short-acting medications, the prescriber may switch the patient to a long-acting benzodiazepine before discontinuing use of the short-acting drug.

Individual reactions to the benzodiazepines appear to be associated with sensitivity to their effects. Some patients feel apathy, fatigue, tearfulness, emotional lability, irritability, and nervousness. Symptoms of depression may worsen. The psychiatric–mental health nurse should closely monitor these symptoms when individuals are receiving benzodiazepines as adjunctive treatment for anxiety that coexists with depression. Gastrointestinal disturbances, including nausea, vomiting, anorexia, dry mouth, and constipation may develop. These medications may be taken with food to ease the gastrointestinal distress.

Elderly patients are particularly susceptible to incontinence, memory disturbances, dizziness, and increased risk for falls when using benzodiazepines. Pregnant patients should be aware that these medications cross the placenta and are associated with increased risk for birth defects, such as cleft palate, mental retardation, and pyloric stenosis. Infants born addicted to benzodiazepines often exhibit flaccid muscle tone, lethargy, and difficulties sucking. All of the benzodiazepines are excreted in breast milk, and breast-feeding women should avoid using these medications. Infants and children metabolize these medications more slowly; therefore, more drug accumulates in their bodies.

Toxicity develops in overdose or accumulation of the drug in the body from liver dysfunction or disease. Symptoms include worsening of the CNS depression, ataxia, confusion, delirium, agitation, hypotension, diminished reflexes, and lethargy. Rarely do the benzodiazepines cause respiratory depression or death. In overdose, these medications have a high therapeutic index and rarely result in death unless combined with another CNS depressant drug, such as alcohol.

Nonbenzodiazepines: Buspirone and Zolpidem

One of the nonbenzodiazepines, buspirone (BuSpar), is effective in controlling the symptoms of anxiety but has no effect on panic disorders and little effect on obsessive-compulsive disorder. Another nonbenzodiazepine, zolpidem (Ambien), is a medication for sleep that acts on the benzodiazepine–GABA receptor complex.

Indications and Mechanisms of Actions

These drugs are effective for treating anxiety disorders without the CNS depressant effects or the potential for abuse and withdrawal syndromes. Buspirone is indicated for treating generalized anxiety disorder; therefore, its target symptoms include anxiety and related symptoms, such as difficulty concentrating, tension, insomnia, restlessness, irritability, and fatigue. Because buspirone does not add to depression symptoms, it has been tried for treating anxiety that coexists with depression. In some instances, it is thought to potentiate the antidepressant actions of other medications.

Buspirone has no effect on the benzodiazepine–GABA complex, but instead appears to control anxiety by blocking the serotonin subtype of receptor, 5-HT_{1a}, at both presynaptic reuptake and postsynaptic receptor sites. It has no sedative, muscle relaxant, or anticonvulsant effects. It also lacks potential for abuse.

Zolpidem (Ambien), which is indicated for short-term insomnia treatment, appears to increase slow-wave (deep) sleep and to modulate GABA receptors and thereby suppress neurons and induce relaxation. See Chapter 26.

Pharmacokinetics

Buspirone is rapidly absorbed but undergoes extensive first-pass metabolism. Food slows absorption but appears to reduce first-pass effects, increasing the bioavailability of the medication. Buspirone is given on a continual dosing schedule of three times a day because of its short half-life of 2 to 3 hours. Clinical action depends on reaching steady-state concentrations; taking this medication with food may facilitate this process.

Buspirone is highly protein bound but does not displace most other medications. However, it does displace digoxin and may increase digoxin levels to the point of toxicity. It is metabolized in the liver and excreted predominantly by the kidneys but also via the gastrointestinal tract. Patients with liver or kidney impairment should be given this medication with caution.

Buspirone cannot be used on a PRN basis; rather, it takes 2 to 4 weeks of continual use for symptom relief to occur. It is more effective in reducing anxiety in patients who have never taken a benzodiazepine.

Buspirone does not block the withdrawal of other benzodiazepines. Therefore, a switch to buspirone must be initiated gradually to avoid withdrawal symptoms. Nurses should closely monitor patients who are undergoing this change of medication for emergence of withdrawal symptoms from the benzodiazepines and report such symptoms to the prescriber.

Zolpidem is metabolized by the liver; it crosses the placenta, and enters breast milk. It has a short half-life of 3 hours and is excreted in the urine.

Side Effects, Adverse Reactions, and Toxicity

Common side effects from buspirone include dizziness, drowsiness, nausea, excitement, and headache. Most other side effects occur at an incidence of less than 1%. There have been no reports of death from an overdose of buspirone alone. Elderly patients, pregnant women, and children have not been adequately studied. For now, buspirone can be assumed to cross the placenta and is present in breast milk; therefore, its use should be avoided in pregnant women, and women who are taking this medication should not breast-feed.

Rebound effects from zolpidem, such as insomnia and anxiety, are minimal. There are minimal effects on respiratory function and little potential for abuse, but because it acts on GABA, some of the same side effects are possible.

Sedative–Hypnotics

Zaleplon (Sonata) is in a class of drugs called sedative–hypnotics or sleep medications. Zaleplon is for short-term use, usually only a few days to 2 weeks. Longer term use must be monitored closely. The short half-life allows for sleep induction without a hangover feeling upon waking. Nurses should monitor patients taking zaleplon for side effects, including hallucinations, abnormal behavior, severe confusion, and suicidal thoughts. Other, less serious side effects that may be more likely to occur include daytime drowsiness, dizziness, ataxia, double vision or other vision problems, agitation, and vivid or abnormal dreams. Zaleplon is habit forming, and stopping use of this medication suddenly can cause withdrawal effects, including mood changes, anxiety, and restlessness. More research is needed to determine whether these and similar medications offer a substantial improvement over the benzodiazepines.

STIMULANTS

Amphetamines were first synthesized in the late 1800s but were not used for psychiatric disorders until the 1930s. Initially, amphetamines were prescribed for a variety of symptoms and disorders, but their high abuse potential soon became obvious.

Methylphenidate, Pemoline, and Modafinil

Among the medications known as stimulants are methylphenidate (Ritalin), used for attention deficit disorders; pemoline (Cylert), a central nervous system stimulant also used for hyperactivity and attention deficit disorders; and modafinil (Provigil), used for narcolepsy, a sleep disorder.

Indications and Mechanisms of Action

Medical use of these drugs is now restricted to a few disorders, including narcolepsy, attention deficit hyperactivity disorder (ADHD)—particularly in children—and obesity unresponsive to other treatments. However, stimulants are increasingly being used as an adjunctive treatment in depression and other mood disorders to address the fatigue and low energy common to these conditions.

Amphetamines indirectly stimulate the sympathetic nervous system, producing alertness, wakefulness, vasoconstriction, suppressed appetite, and hypothermia. Tolerance develops to some of these effects, such as suppression of appetite, but the CNS stimulation continues. Although the exact mechanism of action is not completely understood, stimulants cause a release of catecholamines, particularly norepinephrine and dopamine, into the synapse from the presynaptic nerve cell. They also block reuptake of these catecholamines. Methylphenidate is structurally similar to the amphetamines but produces a milder CNS stimulation. Pemoline is structurally dissimilar from the amphetamines but produces the same pharmacologic actions. Pemoline predominantly affects the dopamine system and therefore has less effect on the sympathetic nervous system. Psychostimulants should be used very cautiously in individuals who have a history of substance abuse.

Although the stimulant effects of these medications may seem logically indicated for narcolepsy, a disorder in which the individual frequently and abruptly falls asleep, the indications for childhood ADHD seem less obvious. The etiology and neurobiology of ADHD remain unclear, but psychostimulants produce a paradoxic calming of the increased motor activity characteristic of ADHD. Studies show that medication decreases disruptive activity during school hours, reduces noise and verbal activity, improves attention span and short-term memory, improves ability to follow directions, and decreases distractibility and impulsivity. Although these improvements have been well documented in the literature, the diagnosis of ADHD and subsequent use of psychostimulants with children remain matters of controversy (see Chapter 29).

Modafinil (Provigil) is a new wake-promoting agent used for treating excessive daytime sleepiness (EDS) associated with narcolepsy and other health states. Patients with EDS cannot stay awake in the daytime, even after getting enough nighttime sleep. They fall asleep when they want to stay awake. Although modafinil is FDA approved only for treating narcolepsy, it is being used for people with EDS and general fatigue found in many diverse disorders, including fibromyalgia and major depression. This off-label use is a matter of controversy, and more research is needed.

Pharmacokinetics

Psychostimulants are rapidly absorbed from the gastrointestinal tract and reach peak plasma levels in 1 to 3 hours. Considerable individual variations occur between the drugs in terms of bioavailability, plasma levels, and half-life. Table 8.12 compares the primary psychostimulants used in psychiatry. Some of these differences are age dependent because children metabolize these medications more rapidly, producing shorter elimination half-lives. Methylphenidate (Ritalin) is available in a sustained-release form for slower absorption; this form of the drug should not be chewed or crushed.

The psychostimulants appear to be unaffected by food in the stomach and should be given after meals to reduce the appetite-suppressant effects when indicated. How-

Table 8.12 Psychostimulant Medications

Generic (Trade) Drug Name and Half-Life	Usual Dosage Range (mg/d)	Side Effects
Dextroamphetamine (Dexedrine); 6–7 h	5–40	• Overstimulation • Restlessness • Dry mouth • Palpitations • Cardiomyopathy (with prolonged use or high dosage) • Possible growth retardation (greatest risk); risk reduced with drug holidays
Methylphenidate (Ritalin); 2–4 h	10–60	• Nervousness • Insomnia • Anorexia • Tachycardia • Impaired cognition (with high doses) • Moderate risk for growth suppression
Pemoline (Cylert); 12 h (mean)	37.5–112.5	• Insomnia • Anorexia with weight loss • Elevated liver function tests (ALT, AST, LDH) • Jaundice • Least risk for growth suppression

ALT, alanine aminotransferase; AST, aspartate aminotransferase; LDH, lactic dehydrogenase

ever, changes in urine pH may affect the rates of excretion. Excessive sodium bicarbonate alkalizes the urine and reduces amphetamine secretion. Increased vitamin C or citric acid intake may acidify the urine and increase its excretion. Starvation from appetite suppression may have a similar effect. All of these drugs are highly lipid soluble, crossing easily into the CNS and the placenta. Pemoline (PemADD) has higher protein binding and lower bioavailability than do the others but also exhibits less potential for abuse. Psychostimulants undergo metabolic changes in the liver, where they may affect, or be affected by, other drugs. They are primarily excreted through the kidneys; therefore, renal dysfunction may interfere with excretion.

The precise action of modafinil (Provigil) in promoting wakefulness is unknown. It does appear to have wake-promoting actions similar to sympathomimetic agents such as amphetamine and methylphenidate, although the pharmacologic profile is not identical. It is absorbed rapidly and reaches peak plasma concentration in 2 to 4 hours. Absorption of modafinil mabe delayed by 1 to 2 hours if taken with food. Modafinil is eliminated via liver metabolism with subsequent excretion of metabolites through renal excretion. Modafinil may interact with drugs that inhibit, induce, or are metabolized by CYP450 isoenzymes, including phenytoin, diazepam, and propranolol. Concurrent use of modafinil and other drugs metabolized by the CYP450 isoenzyme system may lead to increased circulating blood levels of the other drugs.

Psychostimulants are usually begun at a low dose and increased weekly, depending on improvement of symptoms and occurrence of side effects. Initially, children with ADHD are given a morning dose so that their school performance may be compared from morning to afternoon. Rebound symptoms of excitability and over-talkativeness may occur when use of the medication is withdrawn or after dose reduction. These symptoms also begin about 5 hours after the last dose of medication, which may affect the dosing regimen for some individuals. The return of symptoms in the afternoon for children with ADHD may require that a second dose be given at school. Prescribers should work with parents to implement other interventions after school and on weekends when the psychostimulants are not used. Severity of symptoms may require that the medications be continued during these times, but this dosing schedule should be determined after careful evaluation on an individual basis. Use of these medications should not be stopped abruptly, especially with higher doses because the rebound effects may last for several days.

Side Effects, Adverse Reactions, and Toxicity

Side effects associated with psychostimulants typically arise within 2 to 3 weeks after use of the medication begins. From most to least common, these side effects include appetite suppression, insomnia, irritability, weight loss, nausea, headache, palpitations, blurred vision, dry mouth, constipation, and dizziness. Because of the effects on the sympathetic nervous system, some individuals experience blood pressure changes (both hypertension and hypotension), tachycardia, tremors, and irregular heart rates. Blood pressure and pulse should be monitored initially and after each dosage change. Pemoline is associated with elevated liver enzymes and produces hepatotoxicity in 1% to 3% of children taking the medication; therefore, liver function tests should be obtained at least every 6 months. Liver function returns to normal when use of the medication is discontinued.

Rarely, psychostimulants suppress growth and development in children. These effects are a matter of controversy, and research has produced conflicting results. Although suppression of height seems unlikely to some researchers, others have indicated that psychostimulants may have an effect on cartilage. More reports of suppressed growth have occurred with dextroamphetamine (Dexedrine) than methylphenidate (Ritalin), and both of these drugs are associated with greater growth suppression than is pemoline. Height and weight should be monitored several times annually for children taking these medications and compared with prior history of growth. Weight should be monitored especially closely during the initial phases of treatment. These effects also may be minimized by drug "holidays," such as during school vacations.

Rarely, individuals may experience mild dysphoria, social withdrawal, or mild to moderate depression. These symptoms are more common at higher doses and may require discontinuation of use of medication. Abnormal movements and motor tics may also increase in individuals who have a history of Tourette's syndrome. Psychostimulants should be avoided by patients with Tourette's symptoms or a positive family history of the disorder. In addition, dextroamphetamine has been associated with an increased risk for congenital abnormalities. Because there is no compelling reason for a pregnant woman to continue to take these medications, patients should be informed and should advise their prescriber immediately if they plan to become pregnant or if pregnancy is a possibility.

Death is rare from overdose or toxicity of the psychostimulants, but a 10-day supply may be lethal, especially in children. Symptoms of overdose include agitation, chest pain, hallucinations, paranoia, confusion, and dysphoria. Seizures may develop, along with fever, tremor, hypertension or hypotension, aggression, headache, palpitations, rashes, difficulty breathing, leg pain, and abdominal pain. Toxic doses of dextroamphetamine are above 20 mg, with potential death resulting from a 400-mg dose. Parents should be warned regarding the potential lethality of these medications and take preventive measures by keeping the medication in a safe place.

Side effects associated with modafinil include nausea, nervousness, headache, dizziness, and trouble sleeping. If the effects continue or are bothersome, patients should consult the prescriber. Modafinil is generally well tolerated with few clinically significant side effects. It is potentially habit forming and must be used with great caution in individuals with a history of substance abuse or dependence.

HERBAL SUPPLEMENTS

Many individuals are turning to dietary herbal preparations to address psychiatric symptoms. If these supplements were classified as drugs, their efficacy and safety would have to be approved by the FDA before marketing. However, herbal supplements are regulated like foods, not medications, and thus are exempt from the FDA efficacy and safety standards. Lack of regulation does not mean that these herbal supplements are effective and safe. These substances often have adverse effects and interact with prescribed medications. Nurses need to include an assessment of these agents into their overall patient assessment to understand the total picture.

Herbal supplements popular for psychiatric disorders include St. John's Wort and Kava. St. John's Wort (SJW), derived from *hypericum perforatum* L, is used for depression, pain, anxiety, insomnia, and premenstrual syndrome. SJW is believed to modulate serotonin, dopamine, and norepinephrine. The risk of developing serotonin syndrome is increased when taken with other serotonergic drugs. It is recognized as a potent inducer of CYP3A4 (Hume & Strong, 2006) and has the potential to interact with substrates of this enzyme. It should not be taken with prescribed antidepressants.

Kava, derived from the *Piper methysticum* plant, is used for anxiety reduction. Kava interacts with dopaminergic transmission, inhibits the MAO-B enzyme system, and modulates the GABA receptor. It may also inhibit uptake of noradrenaline. Kava is widely used by Pacific Islanders as a social and ceremonial tranquilizing drink. In 2002, the FDA issued warnings about the risk of severe liver injury associated with kava. Several countries have restricted its use. Thrombocytopenia, leukopenia, and hearing impairment have been reported with kava (Clouatre, 2004).

NUTRITIONAL THERAPIES AND SUPPLEMENTS

The neurotransmitters necessary for normal healthy functioning are produced from chemical building blocks taken in with the foods we eat. Many nutritional deficiencies may produce symptoms of psychiatric disorders. Fatigue, apathy, and depression are caused by deficiencies in iron, folic acid, pantothenic acid, magnesium, vitamin C, or biotin. Logically, treating these deficiencies with nutritional supplements should improve the psychiatric symptoms. The question becomes: Can nutritional supplements improve psychiatric symptoms that are not the result of such deficiencies?

Tryptophan, the dietary precursor for serotonin, has been most extensively investigated as it relates to low serotonin levels and increased aggression. Individuals who have low tryptophan levels are prone to have lower levels of serotonin in the brain, resulting in depressed mood and aggressive behavior (Neumeister et al., 2006).

Nutritional supplements such as melatonin, 2-dimethylaminoethanol (DMAE), and lecithin target CNS functioning. Melatonin, a naturally occurring hormone secreted from the pineal gland, is used for treatment of insomnia and prevention of "jet lag" in air travelers. DMAE is promoted for the treatment of attention deficit hyperactivity disorder, Alzheimer's disease, Huntington's chorea, and tardive dyskinesia. DMAE is similar to a former prescription medication removed from the market in 1983 for lack of efficacy. Lecithin, a precursor to acetylcholine, is used to improve memory and treat dementia. The extent to which the levels of acetylcholine is raised by ingestion of lecithin is not known (McQueen, 2006).

Medications may also influence the development of nutritional deficiencies that may worsen psychiatric symptoms. For example, drugs with strong anticholinergic activity often produce impaired or enhanced gastric motility, which may lead to generalized malabsorption of vitamins and minerals. In addition, many nutritional supplements have toxicities of their own when given in excess. For example, daily ingestion of more than 100 mg pyridoxine (vitamin B_6) can produce neurotoxic symptoms, photosensitivity, and ataxia. More research is needed to identify the underlying mechanisms and relationships of dietary supplements and dietary precursors of the bioamines to mood and behavior and psychopharmacologic medications. For now, it is important for the psychiatric–mental health nurse to recognize that these issues may be potential factors in improvement of the patient's mental status and target symptoms.

OTHER BIOLOGIC TREATMENTS

Although the primary biologic interventions remain pharmacologic, other somatic treatments have gained acceptance, remain under investigation, or show promise for the future. These include neurosurgery, electroconvulsive therapy (ECT), phototherapy, and most recently, transcranial magnetic stimulation (rTMS) and vagus nerve stimulation (VNS). The use of neurosurgery is very limited and outside the scope of this text.

Electroconvulsive Therapy (ECT)

For hundreds of years, seizures have been known to produce improvement in some psychiatric symptoms. Camphor-induced seizures were used in the 16th century to reduce psychosis and mania. With time, other substances, such as inhalants, were tried, but most were difficult to control or produced adverse reactions, sometimes even fatalities. Electroconvulsive therapy (ECT) was formally introduced in Italy in 1938. It is one of the oldest medical treatments available and remains safely in use today. It is one of the most effective treatments for severe depression but has been used for other disorders, including mania and schizophrenia, when other treatments have failed.

With ECT, a brief electrical current is passed through the brain to produce generalized seizures lasting 25 to 150 seconds. The patient does not feel the stimulus or recall the procedure. A short-acting anesthetic and a muscle relaxant are given before induction of the current. A brief pulse stimulus, administered unilaterally on the nondominant side of the head, is associated with less confusion after ECT. However, some individuals require bilateral treatment for effective resolution of depressive symptoms. Induction of a seizure is necessary to produce positive treatment outcomes. Because individual seizure thresholds vary, the electrical impulse and treatment method also may vary. In general, the lowest possible electrical stimulus necessary to produce seizure activity is used. Blood pressure and the ECG are monitored during the procedure. This procedure is repeated two or three times a week, usually for a total of 6 to 12 treatments. Because there is no particular difference in treatment efficacy and a twice-weekly regimen produces less accumulative memory loss, this treatment course is often chosen. After symptoms have improved, antidepressant medication may be used to prevent relapse. Some patients who cannot take or do not experience response to antidepressant treatment may continue to have ECT treatment. Usually, once-weekly treatments are gradually decreased in frequency to once monthly. The number and frequency vary depending on the individual's response.

Although ECT produces rapid improvement in depressive symptoms, its exact mechanism of antidepressant action remains unclear. It is known to down-regulate β-adrenergic receptors in much the same way as antidepressant medications. However, unlike antidepressant therapy, ECT produces an up-regulation in serotonin, especially 5-HT_2. ECT also has several other actions on neurochemistry, including increased influx of calcium and effects on second messenger systems.

Brief episodes of hypotension or hypertension, bradycardia or tachycardia, and minor arrhythmias are among the adverse effects that may occur during and immediately after the procedure but usually resolve quickly. Common after-effects from ECT include headache, nausea, and muscle pain. Memory loss is the most troublesome long-term effect of ECT. Many patients do not experience amnesia, whereas others report some memory loss for months or even years (Abrams, 2002). Evidence is conflicting on the effects of ECT on the formation of memories after the treatments and on learning, but most patients experience no noticeable change. Memory loss occurring as part of the symptoms of untreated depression presents a confounding factor in determining the exact nature of the memory deficits from ECT. It is important to remember that patient surveys are positive, with most individuals reporting that they were helped by ECT and would have it again (Hirose, 2002).

Electroconvulsive therapy is contraindicated in patients with increased intracranial pressure. Risk also increases in patients with recent myocardial infarction, recent cerebrovascular accident, retinal detachment, or pheochromocytoma (a tumor on the adrenal cortex) and in patients at high risk for complications from anesthesia. Although ECT should be considered cautiously because of its specific side effects, added risks of general anesthesia, possible contraindications, and substantial social stigma, it is a safe and effective treatment.

Psychiatric–mental health nurses are involved in many aspects of care for individuals undergoing ECT. Informed consent is required, and all treating professionals have a responsibility to ensure that the patient's and family's questions are answered completely. Available treatment options, risks, and consequences must be fully discussed. Sometimes memory difficulties associated with severe depression make it difficult for patients to retain information or ask questions. Nurses should be prepared to restate or explain the procedure as often as necessary. Whenever possible, the individual's family or other support systems should be educated and involved in the consent process. Videotapes are available, but they should not replace direct discussions. Language should be in terms the patient and family members can understand. Other nursing interventions involve preparation of the patient before treatment, monitoring immediately after treatment, and follow-up. Many of these considerations are listed in Box 8.5.

Light Therapy (Phototherapy)

Human circadian rhythms are set by time clues (zeitgebers) inside and outside the body. One of the most powerful regulators of these body patterns is the cycle of daylight and darkness.

BOX 8.5

Interventions for the Patient Receiving Electroconvulsive Therapy

- Discuss treatment alternatives, procedures, risks, and benefits with patient and family. Make sure that informed consent for electroconvulsive therapy (ECT) has been given in writing.
- Provide initial and ongoing patient and family education.
- Assist and monitor the patient who must take nothing by mouth (NPO) after midnight the evening before the procedure.
- Make sure that the patient wears loose, comfortable, nonrestrictive clothing to the procedure.
- If the procedure is performed on an outpatient basis, ensure that the patient has someone to accompany him or her home and stay with him or her after the procedure.
- Ensure that pretreatment laboratory tests are complete, including complete blood count, serum electrolytes, urinalysis, electrocardiogram, chest radiography, and physical examination.
- Teach the patient to create memory helps, such as lists and notepads, before the ECT.
- Explain that no foreign or loose objects can be in the patient's mouth during the procedure. Dentures will be removed, and a bite block may be inserted.
- Insert an intravenous line and provide oxygen by nasal cannula (usually 100% oxygen at 5 L/min).
- Obtain emergency equipment and be sure it is available and ready if needed.
- Monitor vital signs frequently immediately after the procedure, as in every postanesthesia recovery period.
- When the patient is fully conscious and vital signs are stable, assist him or her to get up slowly, sitting for some time before standing.
- Monitor confusion closely; patient may need reorientation to the bathroom and other areas.
- Maintain close supervision for at least 12 hours and continue observation for 48 hours after treatment. Advise family members to observe how patient manages at home, provide assistance as needed, and report any problems.
- Assist the patient to keep or schedule follow-up appointments.

Research findings indicate that some individuals with certain types of depression may experience disturbance in these normal body patterns or of circadian rhythms, particularly those who experience a seasonal variation in their depression. These individuals are more depressed during the winter months, when there is less light; they improve spontaneously in the spring (see Chapter 20). These individuals usually have symptoms that are somewhat different from classic depression, including fatigue, increased need to sleep, increased appetite and weight gain, irritability, and carbohydrate craving. Sometimes, the symptoms appear in the summer, and some individuals have only subtle changes without developing the full pattern. Administering artificial light to these patients during winter months has reduced these depressive symptoms.

Light therapy, sometimes called **phototherapy**, involves exposing the patient to an artificial light source during winter months to relieve seasonal depression. Artificial light is believed to trigger a shift in the patient's circadian rhythm to an earlier time. Research remains ongoing. The light source must be very bright, full-spectrum light, usually 2,500 lux, which is about 200 times brighter than normal indoor lighting. Harmful ultraviolet light is filtered out. Exposure to this light source has produced improvement and relief of depressive symptoms for significant numbers of seasonally depressed individuals. It produces no change for individuals who are not seasonally depressed.

Studies have shown that morning phototherapy produces a better response than either evening or morning and evening timing of the phototherapy session. Light banks with full-spectrum light may be put together by the individual or obtained from various companies now producing these light sources. Light visors (visors containing small, full-spectrum light bulbs that shine on the eyelids) have also been developed. The patient is instructed to sit in front of the lights at a distance of about 3 feet, engaging in a variety of other activities, but glancing directly into the light every few minutes. This should be done immediately on arising and is most effective before 8 AM. The duration of administration may begin with as little as 30 minutes and increase to 2 to 5 hours. One to 2 hours is usually sufficient, and the antidepressant response begins in 1 to 4 days, with the full effect usually complete after 2 weeks. Full antidepressant effect is usually maintained with daily sessions of 30 minutes.

Side effects of phototherapy are rare, but eye strain, headache, and insomnia are possible. An ophthalmologist should be consulted if the patient has a pre-existing eye disorder. In rare instances, phototherapy has been reported to produce an episode of mania. Irritability is a more common complaint. Follow-up visits with the prescriber or therapist are needed to help manage side effects and assess positive results. Phototherapy should be implemented only by a provider knowledgeable in its use.

Transcranial Magnetic Stimulation (rTMS)

Transcranial magnetic stimulation was introduced in 1985 as a noninvasive, painless method to stimulate the cerebral cortex. Undergirding this procedure is the hypothesis that a time-varying magnetic field will induce an electrical field, which, in brain tissue, activates inhibitory and excitatory neurons (Kanno, Matsumoto, Togashi, Yoshioka, & Mano, 2003), thereby modulating neuroplasticity in the brain. The low-frequency electrical stimulation from rTMS triggers lasting anticonvulsant effects in rats, and the therapeutic benefits of rTMS in humans are thought to be related to action similar to that produced by anticonvulsant medication. The rTMS has been used for both clinical and research purposes. The rTMS stimulation of the brain's prefrontal cortex may help some depressed patients in much the same way as ECT but without its side effects (Martis et al., 2003). Thus, it has been proposed as an alternative to ECT in managing symptoms of depression. The rTMS treatment is administered daily for at least a week, much like ECT, except that subjects remain awake. Although proven effective for depression, rTMS does have some side effects, including mild headaches.

Vagus Nerve Stimulation

Vagus nerve stimulation (VNS) is the newest of the currently available somatic treatments. For years, scientists have been interested in identifying how autonomic functions modulate activity in the limbic system and higher cortex. The vagus nerve has traditionally been considered a parasympathetic efferent nerve that was responsible only for regulating autonomic functions, such as heart rate and gastric tone. However, the vagus nerve (cranial X) also carries sensory information to the brain from the head, neck, thorax, and abdomen, and research has identified that the vagus nerve has extensive projections of its sensory afferent connections to many brain areas (Armitage, Husain, Hoffmann, & Rush, 2003). Although the basic mechanism of action of VNS is unknown, incoming sensory, or afferent, connections of the left vagus nerve directly project into many of the very same brain regions implicated in neuropsychiatric disorders. These connections help us to understand how VNS is helpful in treating psychiatric disorders. Vagus nerve stimulation changes levels of several neurotransmitters implicated in the development of major depression, including serotonin, norepinephrine, GABA, and glutamate in the same way that antidepressant medications produce their therapeutic effect (Forbes, Macdonald, Eljamel, & Roberts, 2003).

Approved by the FDA for the adjunctive treatment of severe depression for adults who are unresponsive to four or more adequate antidepressant treatments, VNS is a permanent implant. VNS is not a cure for depression and patients must be seen regularly for assessment of mood states and suicidality.

THE ISSUE OF COMPLIANCE

Medications and other biologic treatments work only if they are used. On the surface, **compliance** or **adherence** to a therapeutic routine seems amazingly simple. However, following therapeutic regimens, self-administering medications as prescribed, and keeping appointments are amazingly complex activities that often prevent successful treatment. Compliance exists on a continuum and can be conceived of as full, partial, or nil. Partial compliance, whereby a patient either attempts to take medications but misses doses or takes more than prescribed is by far the most common. Recent estimates indicate that on the average, 50% or more of the individuals with schizophrenia taking antipsychotic medications stop taking the medications or do not take them as prescribed. It should be remembered that problems with adherence are an issue with many chronic health states, including diabetes and arthritis, not just psychiatric disorders. Box 8.6 lists some of the common reasons for nonadherence. Psychiatric–mental health nurses should be aware that a number of factors influence individuals to stop taking their medication.

The most often cited reasons for noncompliance are related to side effects of the medication. Improved functioning may be observed by health care professionals but not felt by the patient. Side effects may interfere with work performance or other important aspects of the individual's life. For example, a construction worker cannot afford to be drowsy and sedated while operating a crane at a construction site, or a woman in an intimate relationship may find anorgasmia intolerable. Nurses need to be sensitive to the patient's ability to tolerate side effects and to the impact that side effects have on the patient's life. Medication choice, dosing schedules, and prompt treatment of side effects may be crucial factors in helping patients to continue their treatment, even if the symptoms for which they initially sought help have improved.

Cognitive deficits associated with some psychiatric disorders may make it difficult for the individual to self-monitor, develop insight, make choices, remember to fill prescriptions, or keep appointments. Forgetfulness, cost, and confusion regarding dosage or timing may also contribute to noncompliance.

Family members may have similar difficulties that influence the individual not to take the medication. They may misunderstand or deny the illness; for example, "My

BOX 8.6

Common Reasons for Noncompliance With Medication Regimens

- Uncomfortable side effects and those that interfere with quality of life, such as work performance or intimate relationships
- Lack of awareness of or denial of illness
- Stigma
- Feeling better
- Confusion about dosage or timing
- Difficulties in access to treatment
- Substance abuse

wife's better, so she doesn't need that medicine anymore." Family members may be distressed when observable side effects occur. Akinesia, which has been linked to suicidal thoughts as a way to relieve the subjective discomfort, may be the most distressing side effect for family members of individuals who have schizophrenia (Fischer, Ferger, & Kuschinsky, 2002; Meltzer, 2000).

Compliance concerns must not be dismissed as the patient's or family's problem. Psychiatric nurses should actively address this issue. A positive therapeutic relationship between the nurse and patient and family must provide a strong sense of trust that side effects and other difficulties in treatment will be addressed and minimized. When individuals report experiencing distressing side effects, the nurse should immediately respond with assessment and interventions to reduce these effects. It is important to assess compliance often, asking questions in a nonthreatening, nonjudgmental manner. It also may be helpful to seek information from others who are involved with the patient.

Compliance can be improved by psychoeducation. This approach is most helpful if it addresses the individual's specific symptoms and concerns. For example, if the patient is having difficulty with understanding the purpose of the medication, it may be helpful to link taking it to reduction of specific unwanted symptoms or improved functioning, such as continuing to work. Family members should also be included in these discussions.

Other factors that interfere with adherence should also be assessed and plans developed to minimize their effect. For example, an individual who is being considered for clozapine therapy may have missed a number of appointments in the past. On assessment, the nurse may discover that it takes the individual 2 hours on three different buses each way to reach the clinic. The nurse can then assist with arranging for a home health nurse to visit the patient's apartment, draw blood samples for analysis, and assess side effects, thus decreasing the number of trips the patient must make to the clinic.

SUMMARY OF KEY POINTS

- Target symptoms and side effects of medications should be clearly identified. The FDA approves the use of medications for specific disorders and symptoms.
- Psychiatric medications primarily act on CNS receptors, ion channels, enzymes, and carrier proteins. Agonists mimic the action of a specific neurotransmitter; antagonists block the response.
- A drug's ability to interact with a given receptor type depends on three qualities: selectivity—the ability to interact with specific receptors while not affecting other tissues and organs; affinity—the degree of strength of the bond between drug and receptor; and intrinsic activity—the ability to produce a certain biologic response.
- Pharmacokinetics refers to how the human body processes the drug, including absorption, distribution, metabolism, and excretion. Bioavailability describes the amount of the drug that actually reaches circulation throughout the body. The wide variations in the way each individual processes any medication often are related to physiologic differences caused by age, genetic makeup, other disease processes, and chemical interactions.
- Antipsychotic medications are drugs used in treating psychotic disorders, such as schizophrenia. They act primarily by blocking dopamine or serotonin postsynaptically. In addition, they have a number of actions on other neurotransmitters. Older typical antipsychotic drugs work on positive symptoms, are inexpensive, but produce many side effects. Newer atypical antipsychotic drugs work on positive and negative symptoms, are much more expensive, but have far fewer side effects and are better tolerated by patients.
- Medication-related movement disorders are a particularly serious group of side effects that principally occur with the typical antipsychotic medications and that may be acute syndromes, such as dystonia, pseudoparkinsonism, and akathisia, or chronic syndromes, such as tardive dyskinesia.
- The mood stabilizers, or antimania medications, are drugs used to control wide variations in mood related to mania, but these agents may also be used to treat other disorders. Lithium and the anticonvulsants are chemically unrelated and act in different ways to stabilize mood.
- Antidepressant medications are drugs used primarily for treating symptoms of depression. They act by blocking reuptake of one or more of the bioamines, especially serotonin and norepinephrine. These medications vary considerably in their structure and action. Newer antidepressants, such as the SSRIs, have fewer side effects and are less lethal in overdose than the older tricyclic antidepressants.
- Antianxiety medications also include several subgroups of medications, but benzodiazepines and nonbenzodiazepines are those principally used in psychiatry. Benzodiazepines act by enhancing the effects of GABA, whereas the nonbenzodiazepine buspirone acts on serotonin. Benzodiazepines can be used on a PRN basis, whereas buspirone, the one available nonbenzodiazepine, must be taken regularly.
- Psychostimulants enhance neurotransmitter activity, acting at a number of sites in the nerve. These med-

ications are most often used for treating symptoms related to attention deficit hyperactivity disorder and narcolepsy.

■ Electroconvulsive therapy uses the application of an electrical pulsation to induce seizures in the brain. These seizures produce a number of effects on neurotransmission that result in the rapid relief of depressive symptoms.

■ Repetitive transcranial magnetic stimulation and vagus nerve stimulation are two emerging somatic treatments for psychiatric disorders. They are both means to directly affect brain function through stimulation of the nerves that are direct extensions of the brain.

■ Phototherapy involves the application of full-spectrum light in the morning hours, which appears to reset circadian rhythm delays related to seasonal affective disorder and other forms of depression. Nutritional therapies are in various stages of investigation.

■ Compliance refers to the ability of an individual to self-administer medications as prescribed and to follow other instructions related to medication treatment. It can be either full, partial, or nil. Noncompliance is related to factors such as medication side effects, stigma, and family influences. Nurses play a key role in educating patients and helping them to improve adherence.

CRITICAL THINKING CHALLENGES

1. Discuss how you would go about identifying the target symptoms for a specific patient for the following medications: antipsychotic, antidepressant, and antianxiety drugs.
2. Track the approval process from identification of a potential substance to marketing a medication. Compare at least three psychiatric medications that are in phase III trials (hint: www.FDA.gov).
3. Obtain the PIs for the three atypical antipsychotics, two SSRIs, and one SNRI. Compare their boxed warnings, pharmacodynamics, pharmacokinetics, indications, side effects, and dosage.
4. Compare the oral and intramuscular dose of lorazepam. Why are these doses similar?
5. Mr. J. has schizophrenia and was just prescribed an antipsychotic. His family wants to know the risk–benefits of the medication. How would you answer?
6. Identify the CYP450 enzyme that metabolizes the following medications: risperidone, olanzapine, quetiapine, clozapine, fluoxetine, venlafaxine, trazodone, nefazodone, bupropion.
7. Find the four medications or substances that induce or inhibit the following CYP450 enzymes: 2D6, 2C19, 3A4, 1A2.
8. Obtain the PI for clozapine, risperidone, quetiapine and Risperdal Consta. Compare the half-lives of each drug. Discuss the relationship of the drug's half-life to the dosing schedule. When is steady state reached in each of these medications?
9. Explain the health problems associated with anticholinergic side effects of the antipsychotic medications.
10. Compare the type of movements that characterize tardive dyskinesia with those that characterize akathisia and dystonia and explore which one is easier for a patient to experience.
11. One patient is prescribed the MAOI Emsam, 6 mg per day, and another is taking another MAOI, Nardil, 15 mg per day. Are the dietary restrictions different?
12. A patient who is taking an MAOI asks you to explain what will happen if she eats pizza. Prepare a short teaching intervention beginning with the action of the medication and its consequences.
13. Explain how your nursing care would be different for a male patient taking lithium carbonate than for a female patient.
14. Patient A is taking depakote for mood stabilization and Patient B is taking lamictal. After comparing notes with each other, they ask you why Patient A has to have drug blood levels and Patient B does not. How are these two drugs alike? How are they different?
15. Two patients are getting their blood drawn. One patient is getting lithium and the other clozapine. What laboratory tests are being ordered?
16. A patient who is depressed has been started on sertraline. During the assessment, she tells you that she is also taking St. John's Wort, lecithin, and a multiple vitamin. What is your next step?
17. Compare different approaches that you might use with a patient with schizophrenia who has decided to stop taking his or her medication because of intolerance to side effects.

REFERENCES

Abrams, H. (2002). Does brief-pulse ECT cause persistent or permanent memory impairment? *The Journal of ECT, 18*(2), 71–73.

Arana, G. W. (2000). An overview of side effects caused by typical antipsychotics. *Journal of Clinical Psychiatry, 61* (Suppl. 8), 5–13.

Armitage, R., Husain, M., Hoffmann, R., & Rush, A. J. (2003). The effects of vagus nerve stimulation on sleep EEG in depression. A preliminary report. *Journal of Psychosomatic Research, 54*(5):475–482.

Bachmann, J. (2002). Genotyping and phenotyping the cytochrome p-450 enzymes. *American Journal of Therapeutics, 9*(4), 309–316.

Bilici, M., Tekelioglu, Y., Efendioglu, S., Ovali, E., & Ulgen, M. (2003). The influence of olanzapine on immune cells in patients with schizophrenia. *Progress in Neuro-psychopharmacology and Biological Psychiatry, 27*(3), 483–485.

Bschor, T., Baethge, C., Adli, M., Lewitzka, U., Eichmann, U., & Bauer, M. (2003). Hypothalamic-pituitary-thyroid system activity during lithium augmentation therapy in patients with unipolar major depression. *Journal of Psychiatry Neuroscience, 28*(3), 210–216.

Clouatre, D. (2004). Kava: examining new reports of toxicity. *Toxicology Letter, 150*, 85–96.

de Leon, J., Armstrong, S. C., & Cozza, K. L. (2006). Clinical guidelines for psychiatrists for the use of pharmacogenetic testing for CYP450 2D6 and CyP450 2C19. *Psychosomatics, 47*(1), 75–85.

Ferry, L., & Johnston, J. A. (2003). Efficacy and safety of bupropion SR for smoking cessation: Data from clinical trials and five years of postmarketing experience. *International Journal of Clinical Practice, 57*(3), 224–230.

Fischer, D. A., Ferger, B., & Kuschinsky, K. (2002). Discrimination of morphine- and haloperidol-induced muscular rigidity and akinesia/catalepsy in simple tests in rats. *Behavioural Brain Research, 21*;134(1–2): 317–321.

Forbes, R. B., Macdonald, S., Eljamel, S., & Roberts, R. C. (2003). Cost-utility analysis of vagus nerve stimulators for adults with medically refractory epilepsy. *Seizure, 12*(5), 249–256.

Goodwin, F. K., & Ghaemi, S. N. (2000). The impact of mood stabilizers on suicide in bipolar disorder: A comparative analysis. *CNS Spectrums, 5*(2), 12–19.

Hirose, S. (2002). ECT for depression with amnesia. *The Journal of ECT, 18*(1), 60.

Hume, A. L., & Strong, K. M. (2006). Botanical medicines. In R. R. Berardi, L. A. Kroon, J. H. McDermott, G. D. Newton, M. A. Oszko, N. G. Popovich, T. L. Remington, C. J. Rollins, L. A. Shimp, K. J. Tietze (Eds.), *Handbook of nonprescription drugs. An interactive approach to self-care* (pp. 1103–1136). American Pharmacists Association: Washington, DC.

Juran, B. D., Egan, L. J., & Lazaridis, K. N. (2006). The AmpliChip CYP450 test: principles, challenges, and future clinical utility in digestive disease. *Clinical Gastroenterology & Hepatology, 4*(7), 822–830.

Kava-containing dietary supplements may be associated with severe liver injury. Consumer Advisory Center for Food Safety and Applied Nutrition, March 25, 2002. www.cfsan.fda.gov. Retrieved April 6, 2007.

Kanno, M., Matsumoto, M., Togashi, H., Yoshioka, M., & Mano, Y. (2003). Effects of repetitive transcranial magnetic stimulation on behavioral and neurochemical changes in rats during an elevated plus-maze test. *Journal of the Neurological Sciences, 211*(1–2), 5–14.

Kennedy, S. H., Segal, Z. V., Cohen, N. L., Levitan, R. D., Gemar, M., & Bagby, R. M. (2003). Lithium carbonate versus cognitive therapy as sequential combination treatment strategies in partial responders to antidepressant medication: An exploratory trial. *Journal of Clinical Psychiatry, 64*(4), 439–444.

Kulkarni, S. K., & Naidu, P. S. (2003). Pathophysiology and drug therapy of tardive dyskinesia: Current concepts and future perspectives. *Drugs Today (Barc), 39*(1), 19–49.

Levy, G., Schupf, N., Tang, M. X., Cote, L. J., Louis, E. D., Mejia, H., Stern, Y., & Marder, K. (2002). Combined effect of age and severity on the risk of dementia in Parkinson's disease. *Annals of Neurology, 51*(6), 722–729.

Loscher, W. (2002). Basic pharmacology of valproate: A review after 35 years of clinical use for the treatment of epilepsy. *CNS Drugs, 16*(10), 669–694.

Kutscher, E.C., & Carnahan, R. (2006). CYP450 drug interactions with psychiatric medicines: A brief review for the primary care physician. *South Dakota Journal of Medicine*, 59(1), 5–9.

Martis, B., Alam, D., Dowd, S. M., Hill, S. K., Sharma, R. P., Rosen, C., et al. (2003). Neurocognitive effects of repetitive transcranial magnetic stimulation in severe major depression. *Clinical Neurophysiology, 114*(6), 1125–1132.

McQueen, C. E. (2006). Nonbotanical natural medicines. In R. R. Berardi, L. A. Kroon, J. H. McDermott, G. D. Newton, M. A. Oszko, N.G. Popovich, et al., *Handbook of nonprescription drugs. An interactive approach to self-care* (pp. 1137–1166). American Pharmacists Association: Washington, DC.

Meltzer, H. Y. (2000). Introduction. Side effects of antipsychotic medications: Physician's choice of medication and patient compliance. *Journal of Clinical Psychiatry, 61* (Suppl. 8), 3–4.

Nasrallah, H. A. (2002). Pharmacoeconomic implications of adverse effects during antipsychotic drug therapy. *American Journal of Health-System Pharmacy, 59*(22 Suppl 8), S16–S21.

Neumeister, A., Hu, X., Luckenbaugh, D. A., Schwarz, M., Nugent, A. C., et al. (2006). Differential effects of 5-HTTLPR genotypes on the behavioral and neural responses to tryptophan depletion in patients with major depression and controls. *Archives of General Psychiatry, 63*(9), 963–978.

O'Hara, R., Thompson, J. M., Kraemer, H. C., et al. (2002). Which Alzheimer patients are at risk for rapid cognitive decline? *Journal of Geriatric Psychiatry Neurology, 15*(4), 233–238.

Pandolfi, A., Grilli, A., Cilli, C., Patruno, A., Giaccari, A., DiSilvestre, S., et al. (2003). Phenotype modulation in cultures of vascular and smooth muscle cells from diabetic rats: Association with increased nitric oxide synthase expression and superoxide anion generation. *Journal of Cellular Physiology, 196*(2), 378–385.

Sandson, N. B. (2003). *Drug interactions casebook. The cytochrome P450 system and beyond.* American Psychiatric Publishing, Inc.: Washington, DC.

Sajatovic, M. (2000). Clozapine for elderly patients. *Psychiatric Annuals, 30*(3), 170–174.

Taylor, D. (2003). Ziprasidone in the management of schizophrenia: The QT interval issue in context. *CNS Drugs, 17*(6), 423–430.

Yeung, P. P., Tariot, P. N., Schneider, L. S., Salzman C., Rak, L. W. (2000). Quetiapine for elderly patients with psychotic disorders. *Psychiatric Annuals, 30*(3), 197–201.

Zhou, H. (2003). Pharmacokinetic strategies in deciphering atypical drug absorption profiles. *Journal of Clinical Pharmacology, 43*(3), 211–227.

Zullino, D., Delacrausaz, P., & Baumann, P. (2002). The place of SSRIs in the treatment of schizophrenia. *Encephale, 28*(5 Pt 1), 433–438.

UNIT III

Contemporary Psychiatric Nursing Practice

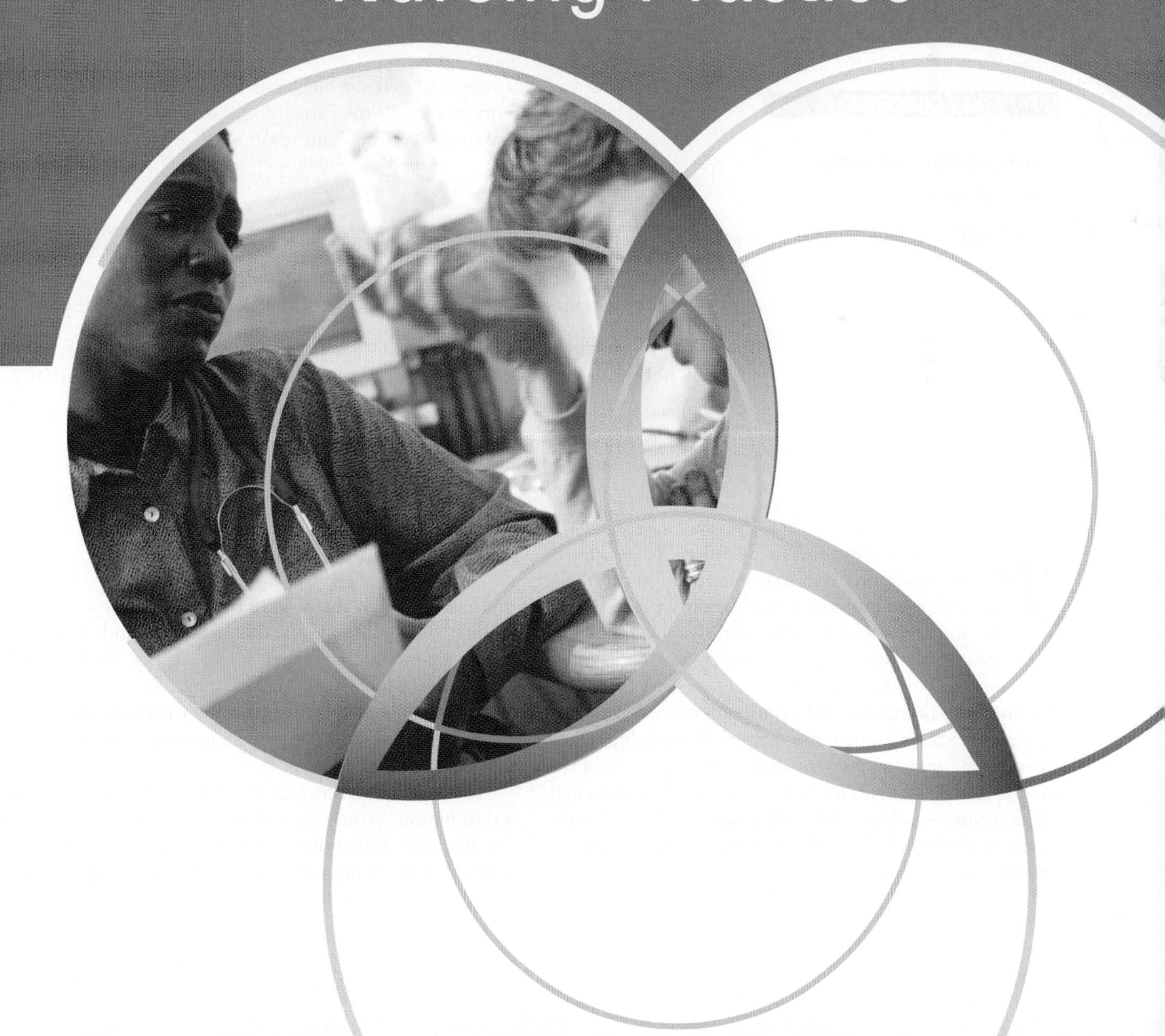

CHAPTER 9

Communication and the Therapeutic Relationship

Cheryl Forchuk and Mary Ann Boyd

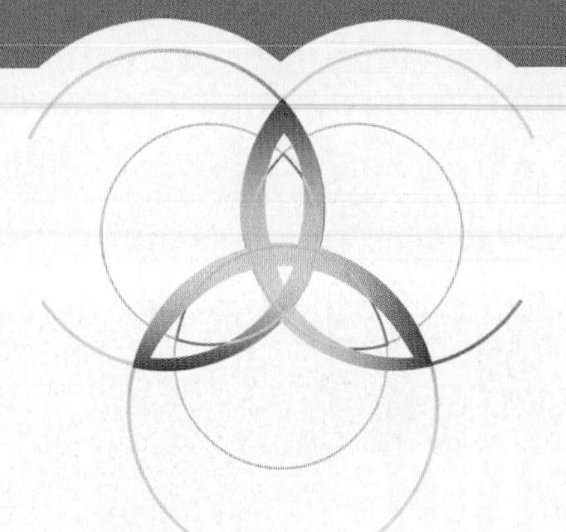

KEY CONCEPTS

- nurse–patient relationship
- self-awareness
- therapeutic communication

LEARNING OBJECTIVES

After studying this chapter, you will be able to:

- Identify the importance of self-awareness in nursing practice.
- Develop a repertoire of verbal and nonverbal communication skills.
- Develop a process for selecting effective communication techniques.
- Explain how the nurse can establish a therapeutic relationship with patients by using rapport and empathy.
- Explain the physical, emotional, and social boundaries of the nurse–patient relationship.
- Discuss the significance of defense mechanisms.
- Explain what occurs in each of the three phases of the nurse–patient relationship: orientation, working, and resolution.

KEY TERMS

• active listening • boundaries • communication blocks • content themes • defense mechanisms • empathy • empathic linkages • introspective • nontherapeutic relationships • nonverbal communication • orientation phase • passive listening • process recording • rapport • resolution • self-disclosure • symbolism • verbal communication • working phase

Patients with psychiatric disorders have special communication needs that require advanced therapeutic communication skills. In psychiatric nursing, the nurse–patient relationship is an important intervention tool that is used to reach treatment goals. The purposes of this chapter are (1) to help the nurse develop self-awareness and communication techniques needed for a therapeutic nurse–patient relationship; (2) to examine the specific stages or steps involved in establishing the relationship; (3) to explore the specific factors that make a nurse–patient relationship successful and therapeutic; and (4) to differentiate therapeutic from nontherapeutic relationships.

SELF-AWARENESS

Self-awareness is the process of understanding one's own beliefs, thoughts, motivations, biases, and limitations and recognizing how they affect others. Without self-awareness, nurses will find it impossible to establish and maintain therapeutic relationships with patients. "Know thyself" is a basic tenet of psychiatric–mental health nursing (Box 9.1).

To come to self-awareness, nurses can carry out self-examination, which can provoke anxiety and is rarely comfortable, either alone or with help from others. Self-examination without the benefit of another's perspective

BOX 9.1

"Know Thyself"

- What physical problems or illnesses have you experienced?
- What significant traumatic life events (e.g., divorce, death of significant person, abuse, disaster) have you experienced?
- What prejudiced or embarrassing beliefs and attitudes about groups different from yours can you identify from your family, significant others, and yourself?
- Which sociocultural factors in your background could contribute to being rejected by members of other cultures?
- How would the above experiences affect your ability to care for patients?

can lead to a biased view of self. Conducting self-examinations with a trusted individual who can give objective but realistic feedback is best. The development of self-awareness requires a willingness to be **introspective** and to examine personal beliefs, attitudes, and motivations.

KEY CONCEPT Self-awareness is the process of understanding one's own beliefs, thoughts, motivations, biases, and limitations, and recognizing how they affect others.

The Biopsychosocial Self

Each nurse brings a biopsychosocial self to nursing practice. The patient perceives the biologic dimension of the nurse in terms of physical characteristics: age, gender, body weight, height, ethnic or racial background, and any other observed physical characteristics. The nurse, too, can have a certain genetic composition, chronic illness, or unobservable physical disability that may influence the quality or delivery of nursing care. The nurse's psychological state also influences how he or she analyzes patient information and selects treatment interventions. An emotional state or behavior can inadvertently influence the therapeutic relationship. For example, a nurse who has just learned that her child is using illegal drugs and who has a patient with a history of drug use, may inadvertently project a judgmental attitude toward her patient, which would interfere with the formation of a therapeutic relationship. The nurse needs to examine underlying emotions, motivations, and beliefs and determine how these factors shape behavior.

The nurse's social biases can be particularly problematic for the nurse–patient relationship. Although the nurse may not verbalize these values to patients, some are readily evident in the nurse's behavior and appearance, such as how the nurse acts or appears at work. Other sociocultural values may not be immediately obvious to the patient; for example, the nurse's religious or spiritual beliefs or feelings about death, divorce, abortion, or homosexuality. These beliefs and thoughts can influence how the nurse interacts with a patient who is dealing with such issues.

Understanding Personal Feelings and Beliefs and Changing Behavior

Nurses must understand their own personal feelings and beliefs and try to avoid projecting them onto patients. The development of self-awareness will enhance the nurse's objectivity and foster a nonjudgmental attitude, which is so important in building and maintaining trust throughout the nurse–patient relationship. Soliciting feedback from colleagues and supervisors about how personal beliefs or thoughts are being projected onto others is a useful self-assessment technique. One of the reasons that ongoing clinical supervision is so important is that the supervisor really knows the nurse and can continually observe for inappropriate communication and question assumptions that the nurse may hold. Clinical supervision is different from administrative supervision in that the focus is on the therapeutic development of the helper and it does not generally involve a direct line reporting relationship.

Once a nurse has identified and analyzed personal beliefs and attitudes, behaviors that were driven by prejudicial ideas may change. The change process requires introspective analysis that may result in viewing the world differently. Through self-awareness and conscious effort, the nurse can change learned behaviors to engage effectively in therapeutic relationships with patients. Nevertheless, sometimes a nurse realizes that some attitudes are too ingrained to support a therapeutic relationship with a patient with different beliefs. In such cases, the nurse should refer the patient to someone who can be therapeutic.

COMMUNICATION

Effective communication skills, including verbal and nonverbal techniques, are the building blocks for all successful relationships. The nurse–patient relationship is built on therapeutic communication, the ongoing process of interaction through which meaning emerges (Box 9.2). **Verbal communication,** which is principally achieved by spoken words, includes the underlying emotion, context, and connotation of what is actually said. **Nonverbal communication** includes gestures, expressions, and body

BOX 9.2

Principles of Therapeutic Communication

1. The patient should be the primary focus of the interaction.
2. A professional attitude sets the tone of the therapeutic relationship.
3. Use self-disclosure cautiously and only when the disclosure has a therapeutic purpose.
4. Avoid social relationships with patients.
5. Maintain patient confidentiality.
6. Assess the patient's intellectual competence to determine the level of understanding.
7. Implement interventions from a theoretic base.
8. Maintain a nonjudgmental attitude. Avoid making judgments about patient's behavior.
9. Avoid giving advice. By the time the patient sees the nurse, he or she has had plenty of advice.
10. Guide the patient to reinterpret his or her experiences rationally.
11. Track the patient's verbal interaction through the use of clarifying statements. Avoid changing the subject unless the content change is in the patient's best interest.

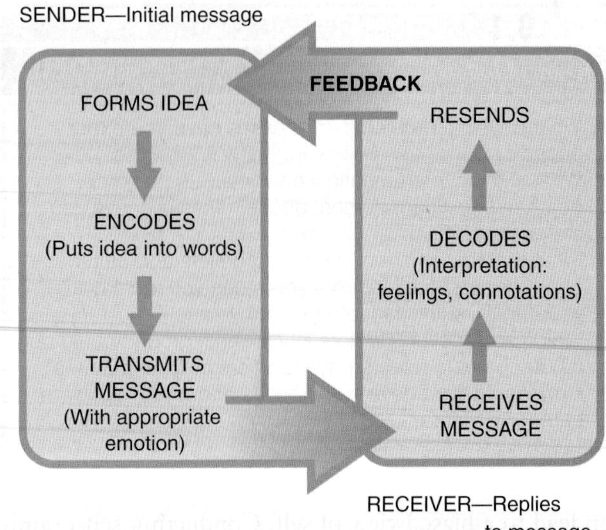

FIGURE 9.1. The communication process adapted from Boyd, M. [1995]. Communication with patients, families, healthcare providers, and diverse cultures. In M. Strader, & P. Decker [Eds.]. *Role transition to patient care management* [p. 431]. Norwalk. CT: Appleton & Lange.

language. Both the patient and the nurse use verbal and nonverbal communication. **Empathic linkages** are the direct communication of feelings. To respond therapeutically in a nurse–patient relationship, the nurse is responsible for assessing and interpreting all forms of patient communication.

• NCLEXNOTE

In analyzing patient–nurse communication, nonverbal behaviors and gestures are communicated first. If a patient's verbal and nonverbal communications are contradictory, priority should be given to the nonverbal behavior and gestures.

KEY CONCEPT Therapeutic communication is the ongoing process of interaction through which meaning emerges.

Therapeutic and social relationships are very different. In a therapeutic relationship, the nurse focuses on the patient and patient-related issues, even when engaging in social activities with that patient. For example, a nurse may take a patient shopping and out for lunch. Even though the nurse is engaged in a social activity, that trip should have a definite purpose, and conversation should focus only on the patient. The nurse must not attempt to meet his or her own social or other needs during the activity.

Using Verbal Communication

The process of verbal communication involves a sender, a message, and a receiver. The patient is often the sender, and the nurse is often the receiver (Figure 9.1), but communication is always two way. The patient formulates an idea, encodes a message (puts ideas into words), and then transmits the message with emotion. The patient's words and their underlying emotional tone and connotation communicate the individual's needs and emotional problems. The nurse receives the message, decodes it (interprets the message, including its feelings, connotation, and context), and then responds to the patient.

On the surface, this interaction is deceptively simple; unseen complexities lie beneath. Is the message the nurse receives consistent with the patient's original idea? Did the nurse interpret the message as the patient intended? Is the verbal message consistent with the nonverbal flourishes that accompany it? Validation is essential to ensure that the nurse has received the information accurately.

Self-Disclosure

One of the most important principles of therapeutic communication for the nurse to follow is to focus the interaction on the patient's concerns. **Self-disclosure,** telling the patient personal information, generally is not a good idea. The conversation should focus on the patient, not the nurse. If a patient asks the nurse personal questions, the nurse should elicit the underlying reason for the request. The nurse can then determine how much personal information to disclose, if any. In revealing personal information, the nurse should be purposeful and have identified therapeutic outcomes. For example, a male patient who was struggling with the implications of marriage and fidelity asked a male nurse if he had ever had an extramarital affair. The nurse interpreted the patient's statement as seeking role-modeling behavior for an adult

Table 9.1 Self-Disclosure in Therapeutic vs. Social Relationships

Situation	Appropriate Therapeutic Response	Inappropriate Social Response With Rationale
A patient asks the nurse if she had fun over the weekend.	"The weekend was fine. How did you spend your weekend?"	"It was great. My boyfriend and I went to dinner and a movie." *(This self-disclosure has no therapeutic purpose. The response focuses the conversation on the nurse, not the patient.)*
A patient asks a student nurse if she has ever been to a particular bar.	"Many people go there. I'm wondering if you have ever been there?"	"Oh yes—all the time. It's a lot of fun." *(Sharing information about outside activities is inappropriate.)*
A patient asks a nurse if mental illness is in the nurse's family.	"Mental illnesses do run in families. I've had a lot of experience caring for people with mental illnesses."	"My sister is being treated for depression." *(This self-disclosure has no purpose, and the nurse is missing the meaning of the question.)*
While shopping with a patient, the nurse sees a friend, who approaches them.	To her friend: "I know it looks like I'm not working, but I really am. I'll see you later."	"Hi, Bob. This is Jane Doe, a patient." *(Introducing the patient to the friend is very inappropriate and violates patient confidentiality.)*

man and judged self-disclosure in this instance to be therapeutic. He honestly responded that he did not engage in affairs and redirected the discussion back to the patient's concerns.

Nurses sometimes may feel uncomfortable avoiding patients' questions for fear of seeming rude. Sometimes they disclose too much personal information because they are trying to be "nice." However, being nice is not necessarily therapeutic. As appropriate, redirecting the patient, giving a neutral or vague answer, or saying, "Let's talk about you" may be all that is necessary to limit self-disclosure. In some instances, nurses may need to tell the patient directly that the nurse will not share personal information (Table 9.1).

Verbal Communication Techniques

Psychiatric nurses use many verbal techniques in establishing relationships and helping patients focus on their problems. Asking a question, restating, and reflecting are examples of such techniques. These techniques may at first seem artificial, but with practice, they can be useful.

Silence and Listening

One of the most difficult but often most effective techniques is the use of silence during verbal interactions. By maintaining silence, the nurse allows the patient to gather thoughts and to proceed at his or her own pace. It is important that the nurse not interrupt silences due to his or her own anxiety or concern of "not doing anything" if sitting quietly with a patient.

Listening is another valuable tool. Silence and listening differ in that silence consists of deliberate pauses to encourage the patient to reflect and eventually respond. Listening is an ongoing activity by which the nurse attends to the patient's verbal and nonverbal communication. The art of listening is developed through careful attention to the content and meaning of the patient's speech. There are two types of listening: passive and active. **Passive listening** involves sitting quietly and letting the patient talk. A passive listener allows the patient to ramble and does not focus or guide the thought process. Passive listening does not foster a therapeutic relationship. Body language during passive listening usually communicates boredom, indifference, or hostility (Fig. 9.2).

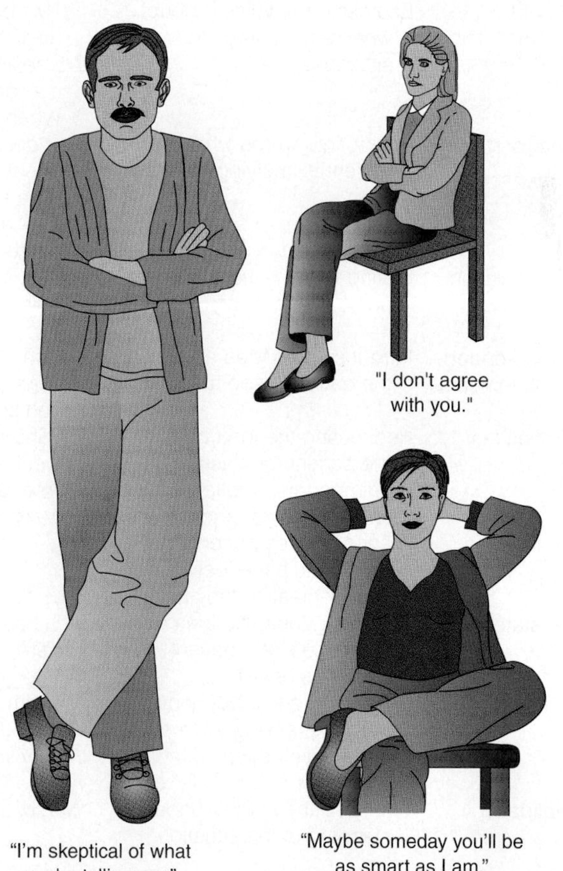
"I don't agree
with you."
"I'm skeptical of what
you're telling me."
"Maybe someday you'll be
as smart as I am."

FIGURE 9.2. Negative body language.

Through **active listening,** the nurse focuses on what the patient is saying to interpret and respond to the message objectively. While listening, the nurse concentrates only on what the patient says and the underlying meaning. The nurse's verbal and nonverbal behaviors indicate active listening. The nurse usually responds indirectly, using techniques such as open-ended statements, reflection (Table 9.2), and questions that elicit additional responses from the patient. In active listening, the nurse should avoid changing the subject and instead follow the patient's lead, although at times it is necessary to respond directly to help a patient focus on a specific topic or to clarify thoughts and beliefs.

• NCLEXNOTE

Self-disclosure can be used in very specific situations, but self-disclosure is not the first intervention to consider. In prioritizing interventions, active listening is one of the first to use.

Some verbal techniques block interactions and inhibit therapeutic communication (Table 9.3).

One of the biggest blocks to communication is giving advice, particularly that which others have already given. Giving advice is different from supporting a patient through decision making. The therapeutic dialogue pre-

Table 9.2 Verbal Communication Techniques

Technique	Definition	Example	Use
Acceptance	Encouraging and receiving information in a nonjudgmental and interested manner	*Pt:* I have done something terrible. *Nurse:* I would like to hear about it. It's OK to discuss it with me.	Used in establishing trust and developing empathy
Confrontation	Presenting the patient with a different reality of the situation	*Pt:* My best friend never calls me. She hates me. *Nurse:* I was in the room yesterday when she called.	Used cautiously to immediately redefine the patient's reality. However, it can alienate the patient if used inappropriately. A nonjudgmental attitude is critical for confrontation to be effective.
Doubt	Expressing or voicing doubt when a patient relates a situation.	*Pt:* My best friend hates me. She never calls me. *Nurse:* From what you have told me, that does not sound like her. When did she call you last?	Used carefully and only when the nurse feels confident about the details. It is used when the nurse wants to guide the patient toward other explanations.
Interpretation	Putting into words what the patient is implying or feeling	*Pt:* I could not sleep because someone would come in my room and rape me. *Nurse:* It sounds like you were scared last night.	Used in helping patient identify underlying thoughts or feelings
Observation	Stating to the patient what the nurse is observing	*Nurse:* You are trembling and perspiring. When did this start?	Used when a patient's behaviors (verbal or nonverbal) are obvious and unusual for that patient
Open-ended statements	Introducing an idea and letting the patient respond	*Nurse:* Trust means. . . . *Pt:* That someone will keep you safe.	Used when helping patient explore feelings or gain insight
Reflection	Redirecting the idea back to the patient for classification of important emotional overtones, feelings, and experiences. Gives patients permission to have feelings they may not realize they have.	*Pt:* Should I go home for the weekend? *Nurse:* Should you go home for the weekend?	Used when patient is asking for the nurse's approval or judgment. Use of reflection helps nurse maintain a nonjudgmental approach.
Restatement	Repeating the main idea expressed; lets patient know what was heard	*Pt:* I hate this place. I don't belong here. *Nurse:* You don't want to be here.	Used when trying to clarify what patient has said
Silence	Remaining quiet, but nonverbally expressing interest during an interaction	*Pt:* I am angry!! *Nurse:* (Silence) *Pt:* My wife had an affair.	Used when patient needs to express ideas but may not know quite how to do it. With silence, patient can focus on putting thoughts together.
Validation	Clarifying the nurse's understanding of the situation	*Nurse:* Let me see if I understand.	Used when nurse is trying to understand a situation the patient is trying to describe

Table 9.3 Techniques That Inhibit Communication

Technique	Definition	Example	Problem
Advice	Telling a patient what to do	*Pt:* I can't sleep. It is too noisy. *Nurse:* Turn off the light and shut your door.	Nurse solves the patient's problem, which may not be the appropriate solution, and encourages dependency on the nurse.
Agreement	Agreeing with a particular viewpoint of a patient	*Pt:* Abortions are sinful. *Nurse:* I agree.	Patient is denied opportunity to change view now that the nurse agrees.
Challenges	Disputing patient's beliefs with arguments, logical thinking, or direct order	*Pt:* I'm a cowboy. *Nurse:* If you are a cowboy, what are you doing in the hospital?	Nurse belittles the patient, and decreases self-esteem. Patient will avoid relating to the nurse who challenges.
Reassurance	Telling a patient that everything will be OK	*Pt:* Everyone thinks I'm bad. *Nurse:* You are a good person.	Nurse makes a statement that may not be true. Patient is blocked from exploring feelings.
Disapproval	Judging patient's situation and behavior	*Pt:* I'm so sorry. I did not mean to kill my mother. *Nurse:* You should be. How could anyone kill their mother?	Nurse belittles the patient. The patient will avoid the nurse.

sented in Box 9.3 differentiates between advice (telling the patient what to do or how to act) from therapeutic communication, by which the nurse and patient explore alternative ways of viewing the patient's world. The patient then can reach his or her own conclusions about the best approaches to use.

Using Nonverbal Communication

Gestures, facial expressions, and body language actually communicate more than verbal messages. Under the best circumstances, body language mirrors or enhances what is verbally communicated. However, if verbal and nonverbal messages conflict, the listener will believe the nonverbal message. For example, if a patient says that he feels fine but has a sad facial expression and is slumped in a chair away from others, the message of sadness and depression will be accepted, rather than the patient's words. The same is true of a nurse's behavior. If a nurse tells a patient, "I am happy to see you," but the nurse's facial expression communicates indifference, the patient will receive the message that the nurse is bored.

BOX 9.3

Therapeutic Dialogue: Giving Advice Versus Recommendations

Ms. J has just received a diagnosis of phobic disorder and been given a prescription for fluoxetine (Prozac). She was referred to the home health agency because she does not want to take her medication. She is fearful of becoming suicidal. Two approaches are given below.

Ineffective Communication (Advice)

Nurse: Ms. J, the doctor has ordered the medication because it will help you.

Ms. J: I don't want to take the medication because I am afraid of becoming suicidal. I heard that some of this psychiatric medication does that. I haven't had any attacks for 2 weeks.

Nurse: This medication has rarely had that side effect. You should try it and see if you have any suicidal thoughts.

Ms. J: OK.

(The nurse leaves and Ms. J does not take the medication. Within a week, Ms. J is taken to the emergency room with a panic attack.)

Effective Communication

Nurse: Ms. J, how have you been doing?

Ms. J: So far, so good. I haven't had any attacks for 2 weeks.

Nurse: I understand that the doctor gave you a prescription for medication that may help with the panic attacks.

Ms. J: Yes, but I don't want to take it because I am afraid of becoming suicidal. I heard that some of this psychiatric medication does that.

Nurse: Have you ever had feelings of hurting yourself?

Ms. J: Not really.

Nurse: If you took the medication and had thoughts like that what would you do?

Ms. J: I don't know.

Nurse: I think I see your dilemma. This medication may help your panic attacks, but the suicidal thoughts are a real fear. Is that it?

Ms. J: Yeah, that's it.

Nurse: What are the circumstances under which you would be able to try the medication?

Ms. J: If I knew that I would not have suicidal thoughts.

Nurse: I can't guarantee that, but I could call you every few days to see if you are having any of these thoughts and help you deal with them.

Ms. J: Oh, that will be OK.

(Ms. J successfully took the medication.)

Critical Thinking Challenge

- Contrast the communication in the first scenario with that in the second.
- What therapeutic communication techniques did the second nurse employ that may have contributed to a better outcome?
- Are there any cues in the first scenario that indicate that the patient will not follow the nurse's advice? Explain.

Because people with psychiatric problems often have difficulty verbally expressing themselves and interpreting the emotions of others, nurses need to assess continually the nonverbal communication needs of patients. Eye contact (or lack thereof), posture, movement (shifting in chair, pacing), facial expressions, and gestures are nonverbal behaviors that communicate thoughts and feelings. A patient who is pacing and restless may be upset or having a reaction to medication. A clenched fist usually indicates that a person feels angry or hostile.

Nonverbal behavior is culturally specific. The nurse must therefore be careful to understand his or her own cultural context as well as that of the patient. For example, in some cultures it is considered disrespectful to look a person straight in the eye. In other cultures, not looking a person in the eye may be interpreted as "hiding something" or low self-esteem. Whether one points with the finger, nose, or eyes and how much hand gesturing to use, are other examples of nonverbal communication that may vary considerably among cultures.

Nurses should use positive body language, such as sitting at the same eye level as the patient with a relaxed posture that projects interest and attention. Leaning slightly forward helps engage the patient. Generally, the nurse should not cross arms or legs during therapeutic communication because such postures erect barriers to interaction. Uncrossed arms and legs project openness and a willingness to engage in conversation (Fig. 9.3). Any verbal response should be consistent with nonverbal messages.

Recognizing Empathic Linkages

Empathic linkages are the communication of feelings (Peplau, 1952). This commonly occurs with anxiety. For example, a nurse may be speaking with a patient who is highly anxious, and the nurse may notice his or her own speech becoming more rapid in tandem with the patient's. The nurse may also become aware of subjective feelings of anxiety. It may be difficult for the nurse to determine if the anxiety was communicated interpersonally, or if the nurse is personally reacting to some of the content of what the patient is communicating. However, being aware of one's own feelings and analyzing them is crucial to determining the source of the feeling.

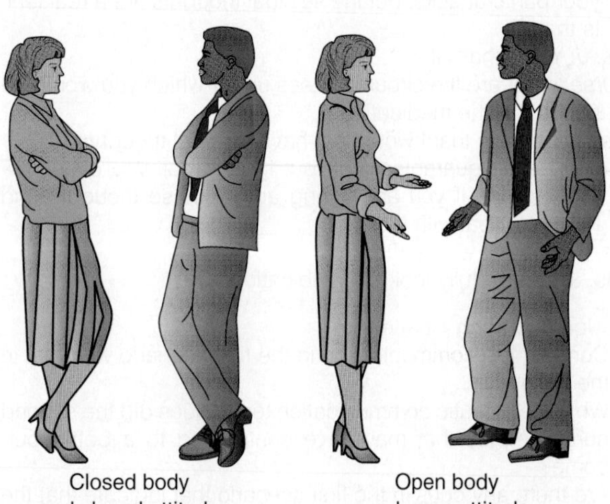

FIGURE 9.3. Open and closed body language.

Selecting Communication Techniques

In therapeutic communication, the nurse chooses the best words to say and uses nonverbal behaviors that are consistent with these words. If a patient is angry and upset, should the nurse invite the patient to sit down and discuss the problem, walk quietly with the patient, or simply observe the patient from a distance and not initiate conversation? Choosing the best response begins with assessing and interpreting the meaning of the patient's communication—both verbal and nonverbal.

Nurses should not necessarily take verbal messages literally, especially when a patient is upset or angry. For example, one nurse walked into the room of a newly admitted patient who accused, "You locked me up and threw away the key." The nurse could have responded defensively that she had nothing to do with the patient being admitted; however, that response could have ended in an argument, and communication would have been blocked. Fortunately, the nurse recognized that the patient was communicating frustration at being in a locked psychiatric unit and did not take the accusation personally.

The next step is identifying the desired patient outcome. To do so, the nurse should engage the patient with eye contact and quietly try to interpret the patient's feelings. In this example, the desired outcome was for the patient to clarify the hospitalization experience. The nurse responded that, "It must be frustrating to feel locked up." The nurse focused on the patient's feelings, rather than the accusations, which reflected an understanding of the patient's feelings. The patient knew that the nurse accepted these feelings, which led to further discussion. It may seem impossible to plan reactions for each situation, but with practice, the nurse will begin to respond automatically in a therapeutic way.

APPLYING COMMUNICATION CONCEPTS

When the nurse is interacting with patients, additional considerations can enhance the quality of communication. This section describes the importance of rapport, validation, empathy, and the role of boundaries and body space in nurse–patient interactions.

Rapport

Rapport, interpersonal harmony characterized by understanding and respect, is important in developing a trusting, therapeutic relationship. Nurses establish rapport through interpersonal warmth, a nonjudgmental attitude, and a demonstration of understanding. A skilled nurse will establish rapport that will alleviate the patient's anxiety in discussing personal problems.

People with psychiatric problems often feel alone and isolated. Establishing rapport helps lessen feelings of being alone. When rapport develops, a patient feels comfortable with the nurse and finds self-disclosure easier. The nurse also feels comfortable and recognizes that an interpersonal bond or alliance is developing. All these factors—comfort, sense of sharing, and decreased anxiety—are important in establishing and building the nurse–patient relationship.

Validation

Validation is explicitly checking out one's own thoughts or feelings with another person. To do so, the nurse must own his or her own thought or feeling by using "I" statements (Orlando, 1961). The validation generally refers to observation, thoughts, or feelings and seeks explicit feedback. For example, a nurse who sees a patient pacing the hallway before a planned family visit may conclude that the patient is anxious. Validation may occur with a statement such as, "I notice you pacing the hallway. I wonder if you are feeling anxious about the family visit?" The patient may agree, "Yes. I keep worrying about what is going to happen!" or disagree, "No. I have been trying to get into the bathroom for the last 30 minutes, but my roommate is still in there!"

Empathy

The use of empathy in a therapeutic relationship is central to psychiatric–mental health nursing. Empathy is sometimes confused with sympathy, which is the expression of compassion and kindness. **Empathy** is the ability to experience, in the present, a situation as another did at some time in the past. It is the ability to put oneself in another person's circumstances and feelings. The nurse does not actually have to have had the experience but has to be able to imagine the feelings associated with it. For empathy to develop, there must be a giving of self to the other individual and a reciprocal desire to know each other personally. The process involves the nurse receiving information from the patient with open, nonjudgmental acceptance and communicating this understanding of the experience and feelings so that the patient feels understood.

Biopsychosocial Boundaries and Body Space Zones

Boundaries are the defining limits of individuals, objects, or relationships. Boundaries mark territory or what is "mine" or "not mine." Human beings have many different types of boundaries. Material boundaries, such as fences around property, artificially imposed state lines, and bodies of water define territory as well as provide security and order. Personal boundaries can be conceptualized within the biopsychosocial model as including physical, psychological, and social dimensions. Physical boundaries are those established in terms of physical closeness to others—whom we allow to touch us or how close we want others to stand near us.

Psychological boundaries are established in terms of emotional distance from others—how much of our innermost feelings and thoughts we want to share. Social boundaries, such as norms, customs, and roles, help us establish our closeness and place within the family, culture, and community. Boundaries are not fixed, but dynamic. When boundaries are involuntarily transgressed, the individual feels threatened and responds to the perceived threat. The nurse must elicit permission before implementing interventions that invade personal space and boundaries.

Personal Boundaries

Every individual is surrounded by four different body zones that provide varying degrees of protection against unwanted physical closeness during interactions (Figure 9.4). The actual sizes of the different zones vary according to culture. Some cultures define the intimate zone narrowly and the personal zones widely. Thus, friends in these cultures stand and sit close while interacting.

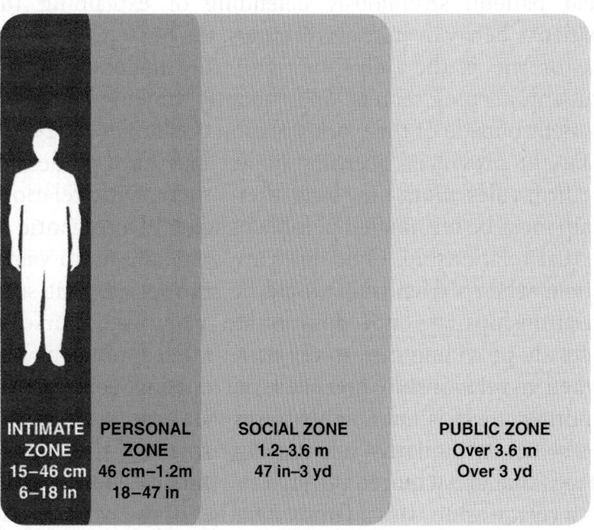

FIGURE 9.4. Body space zones.

People of other cultures define the intimate zone widely and are uncomfortable when others stand close to them. The variability of intimate and personal zones has implications for nursing. For a patient to be comfortable with a nurse, the nurse needs to protect the intimate zone of that individual. The patient usually will allow the nurse to enter the personal zone but will express discomfort if the nurse breaches the intimate zone. For the nurse, the difficulty lies in differentiating the personal zone from the intimate zone for each patient.

The nurse's awareness of his or her own need for intimate and personal space is another prerequisite for therapeutic interaction with the patient. It is important that a nurse feels comfortable while interacting with patients. Establishing a comfort zone may well entail fine-tuning the size of body zones. Recognizing this will help the nurse understand occasional inexplicable reactions to the proximity of patients.

Professional Boundaries and Ethics

For nurses, professional boundaries are also essential to consider in the context of the nurse–patient relationship. Patients often enter such relationships at a very vulnerable point, and nurses need to be aware of professional boundaries to avoid exploitation of the patient. For example, in a friendship there is a two-way sharing of personal information and feelings, but as mentioned previously, the focus is on the patient's needs, and the nurse generally does not share personal information or attempt to meet his or her own needs through the relationship. The patient may seek a friendship or sexual relationship with the nurse (or vice versa), which would be inconsistent with the professional role.

Indicators that the relationship may be moving outside the professional boundaries are gift-giving on either party's part, spending more time than usual with a particular patient, strenuously defending or explaining the patient's behavior in team meetings, the nurse feeling that he or she is the only one who truly understands the patient, keeping secrets, or frequently thinking about the patient outside of the work situation (Gallop et al., 2002). State or provincial licensing bodies may have guidelines or firm rules about how long after a therapeutic relationship must be terminated before engaging in a romantic or sexual relationship. Guidelines are generally more vague about when a friendship would be appropriate, but such relationships are not appropriate when the nurse is actively providing care to the patient. Exceptions may be when a relationship preceded the nursing context and another nurse is unavailable to provide care, such as in a rural area. Similarly, relationships to meet the nurse's needs that are acquired through the nursing context, such as a relationship with a family member of the patient, also breach professional boundaries. When concerns arise related to therapeutic boundaries, the nurse must seek clinical supervision or transfer the care of the patient immediately.

Defense Mechanisms

Defense mechanisms or coping styles are the automatic psychological processes protecting the individual against anxiety and from the awareness of internal or external dangers or stressors (Table 9.4). Individuals often are unaware of these processes, although they mediate reactions to emotional conflicts and to internal and external stressors (American Psychiatric Association, 2000). Some defense mechanisms (e.g., projection, splitting, and acting out) are almost invariably maladaptive. Others, such as suppression and denial, may be either maladaptive or adaptive, depending on their severity and the context in which they occur.

As nurses develop therapeutic relationships, they will recognize their patients using defense mechanisms. With experience, the nurse will evaluate the purpose of a defense mechanism and then determine whether or not it should be discussed with the patient. For example, if a patient is using humor to alleviate an emotionally intense situation, that may be very appropriate. On the other hand, if someone continually rationalizes antisocial behavior, the use of the defense mechanism should be discussed.

• NCLEXNOTE

NCLEXNOTE

When studying defense mechanisms, focus on those mechanisms and coping styles that are similar. For example, displacement *versus* devaluation *versus* projection should be differentiated. Identify these mechanisms in your process recordings.

COMMUNICATION ISSUES RELATED TO SPECIFIC MENTAL HEALTH CHALLENGES

It is important to consider also the individual's specific mental health challenges when selecting specific communication strategies. For example, patients may frequently be experiencing increased levels of anxiety. The nurse who understands that focal attention decreases as anxiety increases, will use shorter and simpler statements or questions when the patient exhibits higher levels of anxiety.

Patients who are experiencing depression may have difficulty articulating their feelings or may feel their thinking and responses are slowed. The nurse will frequently employ silence and empathic techniques throughout the interaction. The person who is depressed may also use communication styles such as over-generalizing ("This always happens to me….everything always turns out for

Table 9.4 Specific Defense Mechanisms and Coping Styles

The following defense mechanisms and coping styles are identified in the *DSM-IV, TR,* as being used when the individual deals with emotional conflict or stressors (either internal or external).

Defense Mechanism	Definition	Example
Acting out	Using actions rather than reflections or feelings during periods of emotional conflict	A teenager gets mad at parents and begins staying out late at night.
Affiliation	Turning to others for help or support (sharing problems with others without implying that someone else is responsible for them)	An individual has a fight with spouse and turns to best friend for emotional support.
Altruism	Dedicating life to meeting the needs of others (receives gratification either vicariously or from the response of others)	After being rejected by boyfriend, a young girl joins the Peace Corps.
Anticipation	Experiencing emotional reactions in advance or anticipating consequences of possible future events and considering realistic, alternative responses or solutions	A parent cries for 3 weeks before the last child leaves for college. On the day of the separation, the parent spends the day with friends.
Autistic fantasy	Excessive daydreaming as a substitute for human relationships, more effective action, or problem solving	A young man sits in his room all day and dreams about being a rock star instead of attending a baseball game with a friend.
Denial	Refusing to acknowledge some painful aspect of external reality or subjective experience that would be apparent to others (*psychotic denial* used when there is gross impairment in reality testing)	A teenager's best friend moves away, but the adolescent says he does not feel sad.
Devaluation	Attributing exaggerated negative qualities to self or others	A boy has been rejected by his long-time girlfriend. He tells his friends that he realizes that she is stupid and ugly.
Displacement	Transferring a feeling about, or a response to, one object onto another (usually less threatening), substitute object	A child is mad at her mother for leaving for the day, but says she is really mad at the sitter for serving her food she does not like.
Dissociation	Experiencing a breakdown in the usually integrated functions of consciousness, memory, perception of self or the environment, or sensory and motor behavior	An adult relates severe sexual abuse experienced as a child, but does it without feeling. She says that the experience was as if she were outside her body watching the abuse.
Help-rejecting complaining	Complaining or making repetitious requests for help that disguise covert feelings of hostility or reproach toward others, which are then expressed by rejecting the suggestions, advice, or help that others offer (complaints or requests may involve physical or psychological symptoms or life problems)	A college student asks a teacher for help after receiving a bad grade on a test. Every suggestion the teacher has is rejected by the student.
Humor	Emphasizing the amusing or ironic aspects of the conflict or stressor	A person makes a joke right after experiencing an embarrassing situation.
Idealization	Attributing exaggerated positive qualities to others	An adult falls in love and fails to see the negative qualities in the other person.
Intellectualization	Excessive use of abstract thinking or the making of generalizations to control or minimize disturbing feelings	After rejection in a love relationship, the rejected explains about the relationship dynamics to a friend.
Isolation of affect	Separation of ideas from the feelings originally associated with them	The individual loses touch with the feelings associated with a rape while remaining aware of the details.
Omnipotence	Feeling or acting as if one possesses special powers or abilities and is superior to others	An individual tells a friend about personal expertise in the stock market and the ability to predict the best stocks.
Passive aggression	Indirectly and unassertively expressing aggression toward others. There is a facade of overt compliance masking covert resistance, resentment, or hostility.	Passive aggression often occurs in response to demands for independent action or performance, or the lack of gratification of dependent wishes but may be adaptive for individuals in subordinate positions who have no other way to express assertiveness more overtly.
Projection	Falsely attributing to another one's own unacceptable feelings, impulses, or thoughts	A child is very angry at a parent, but accuses the parent of being angry.

(Continued on following page)

Table 9.4 Specific Defense Mechanisms and Coping Styles (Continued)

Defense Mechanism	Definition	Example
Projective identification	Falsely attributing to another one's own unacceptable feelings, impulses, or thoughts. Unlike simple projection, the individual does not fully disavow what is projected. Instead, the individual remains aware of his or her own affect or impulses but misattributes them as justifiable reactions to the other person. Not infrequently, the individual induces the very feelings in others that were first mistakenly believed to be there, making it difficult to clarify who did what to whom first.	A child is mad at a parent, who in turn becomes angry at the child, but may be unsure of why. The child then feels justified at being angry with the parent.
Rationalization	Concealing the true motivations for one's own thoughts, actions, or feelings through the elaboration of reassuring or self-serving but incorrect explanations.	A man is rejected by his girlfriend, but explains to his friends that her leaving was best because she was beneath him socially and would not be liked by his family.
Reaction formation	Substituting behavior, thoughts, or feelings that are diametrically opposed to one's own unacceptable thoughts or feelings (this usually occurs in conjunction with their repression).	A wife finds out about her husband's extramarital affairs and tells her friends that she thinks his affairs are perfectly appropriate. She truly does not feel, on a conscious level, any anger or hurt.
Repression	Expelling disturbing wishes, thoughts, or experiences from conscious awareness (the feeling component may remain conscious, detached from its associated ideas).	A woman does not remember the experience of being raped in the basement, but does feel anxious when going into that house.
Self-assertion	Expressing feelings and thoughts directly in a way that is not coercive or manipulative.	An individual reaffirms to another that going to a ball game is not what he or she wants to do.
Self-observation	Reflecting feelings, thoughts, motivation, and behavior and responding to them appropriately.	An individual notices an irritation at his friend's late arrival and decides to tell the friend of the irritation.
Splitting	Compartmentalizing opposite affect states and failing to integrate the positive and negative qualities of the self or others into cohesive images.	Self and object images tend to alternate between polar opposites: exclusively loving, powerful, worthy, nurturing, and kind — or exclusively bad, hateful, angry, destructive, rejecting, or worthless. One friend is wonderful and another former friend, who was at one time viewed as being perfect, is now believed to be an evil person.
Sublimation	Channeling potentially maladaptive feelings or impulses into socially acceptable behavior.	An adolescent boy is very angry with his parents. On the football field, he tackles someone very forcefully.
Suppression	Intentionally avoiding thinking about disturbing problems, wishes, feelings, or experiences.	A student is anxiously awaiting test results, but goes to a movie to stop thinking about it.
Undoing	Words or behavior designed to negate or to make amends symbolically for unacceptable thoughts, feelings, or actions.	A man has sexual fantasies about his wife's sister. He takes his wife away for a romantic weekend.

Adapted from the American Psychiatric Association. (2000). *Diagnostic and statistical manual of mental disorders* (4th ed., text revision, pp 811–814). Washington, DC: Author.

the worse…"). The nurse can assist the patient to be more specific, for example, asking about a specific time or a specific exception.

When patients are experiencing schizophrenia, they may have hallmark symptoms such as hallucinations or delusions. If a person is having auditory hallucinations (hearing sounds that are imagined), the nurse's voice may be one of several the patient is hearing. Clear short sentences may assist in getting the patient's attention on the nurse's voice. A person experiencing delusions may use pronouns vaguely ("they" did it) or other forms of vague or unclear communication. Clarifying and assisting the patient to be more specific may assist the patient's thinking as well as communication.

As you read through the chapters on various mental challenges, consider how the signs and symptoms of each illness could have an impact on communication and the evolving therapeutic relationship.

Analyzing Interactions

Many patients with psychiatric disorders have difficulty communicating. For example, perceptual, cognitive, and information-processing deficits, typical of people with schizophrenia, can interfere with the patient's ability to express ideas, understand concepts, and accurately perceive the environment. Because of the complexity of communication, mental health professionals monitor their interactions with patients using various methods, including audio recording, video recording, and **process recordings,** which entail writing a verbatim transcript of the interaction. A video or audio recording of an interaction provides the most accurate monitoring but is cumbersome to use. Process recording, one of the easiest methods to use, is adequate in most situations. Nurses should use it when first learning therapeutic communication and during times when communication becomes a problem. In a process recording, the nurse records, from memory, the verbatim interaction immediately after the communication (Box 9.4).

The nurse then analyzes the content of the interaction in terms of the words and their meaning for both the patient and the nurse. The analysis is especially important because the ability to communicate verbally is often compromised in people with mental disorders. Because words may not have the same meaning for the patient as they do for the nurse, clarification of meaning becomes especially important. The analysis can identify symbolic meanings, themes, and blocks in communication. **Symbolism,** the use of a word or phrase to represent an object, event, or feeling, is used universally. For example, automobiles are named for wild animals that represent speed, prowess, and beauty. In people with mental disorders, the use of words to symbolize events, objects, or feelings is often idiosyncratic, and they cannot explain their choices. For example, a person who is feeling scared and anxious may tell the nurse that bombs and guns are exploding. It is up to the nurse to make the connection between the bombs and guns and the patient's feelings and then validate this with the patient. Because of the patient's cognitive limitations, the individual may express feelings only symbolically. Another example is found in Box 9.5.

Some patients, for example some with developmental handicaps or organic brain difficulties, may have difficulty with abstract thinking and symbolism. Conversations may be interpreted literally. For example, in response to the question "What brings you to the hospital?" a patient might reply, "the ambulance." In these situations the nurse must be cautious to avoid using symbols or metaphors. Concrete language, that is, language reflecting what can be observed through the senses, will be more easily understood.

Verbal behavior is also interpreted by analyzing **content themes.** Patients often express concerns or feelings

BOX 9.4

Process Recording

Setting: The living room of Mr. S's home. Mr. S. is 23 years old and was hospitalized for 2 weeks. His diagnosis is a bipolar mood disorder and he is recovering from a depressive episode. His parents are in the room but cannot hear the conversation. Mr. S is sitting on the couch and the nurse is sitting on a chair. This is the nurse's first visit after Mr. S's discharge from the hospital.

Patient	Nurse	Interpretation/Analysis
	How are you doing, Mr. S? (smiles and offers hand to shake)	*Plan:* Initially develop a sense of trust and initiate a therapeutic relationship.
I'm fine. It's good to be home. (looking at floor, takes nurse's hand to briefly shake) I really don't like the hospital. (shakes his head while still looking at floor)	You didn't like the hospital?	*Interpretation:* Validating assumption that Mr. S does not want to return to hospital. Nonverbal communication may indicate sadness or low self-esteem. This needs further exploration. Patient validates assumption regarding hospital, but nonverbal behavior indicates there may be further concerns.
NO. The nurses lock you up. (maintains eye contact with nurse, frowning, arms crossed) Are you a nurse?	I'm a nurse. I'm wondering if you think that I will lock you up? (maintains eye contact and open posture)	*Interpretation:* Mr. S may be wondering what my role is and whether I will put him back in the hospital. This assumption needs to be validated, and my role needs clarification.
You could tell my mom to put me back in the hospital. (maintains eye contact with nurse)	Any treatment that I recommend will be thoroughly discussed with you first. I am here to help you stay out of the hospital. I will not discuss anything with your mother unless you give me permission to do so. (nurse maintains eye contact and open posture)	Use interpretation to clarify Mr. S's thinking. Mr. S is wondering about my relationship with his mother. Explain my role and confidentiality.
(Patient maintains eye contact and uncrosses arms.)		Patient's nonverbal communication appears to indicate he is more comfortable with this clarification.

BOX 9.5

Use of Symbolism

Setting: Mr. A has been diagnosed with schizophrenia and expresses himself through the use of television characters. A nurse observed another patient shoving him against the wall. As the nurse approached the two patients, the other patient ran, leaving Mr. A. noticeably shaking. The nurse checked to see if Mr. A. was all right.

Patient	Nurse	Interpretation/Analysis
Robin Hood saved the day. (trembling, arms crossed)	Mr. A, are you OK? (approaches patient)	Mr. A. could not say "thank you for helping me."
It's a glorious day in Sherwood Forest! (trembling decreases, smiles at nurse)	You feel that you are saved?	Instead, he could only describe a fictional character's response.
	Mr. A, are you hurting anywhere? (eyes scan over patient, using concerned tone of voice)	
The angel of mercy put out the fire (continues to smile and extends hand to shake hands with nurse)		The nurse focused on what Mr. A. must be feeling if he felt that he had been rescued. He seems to be happy now. The nurse wanted to check whether the patient had been hurt when pushed against the wall. The patient is apparently not hurting now.

repeatedly in several different ways. After a few sessions, a common theme emerges. Themes may emerge symbolically, as in the case with the patient who constantly talks about the "guns and bombs." Alternatively, a theme may simply be identified as a recurrent thread of a story that a patient retells at each session. For example, one patient always explained his early abandonment by his family. This led the nurse to hypothesize that he had an underlying fear of rejection. The nurse was then able to test whether there was an underlying fear and to develop strategies to help the patient explore the fear (Box 9.6). It is important to involve patients in analyzing themes so that they may learn this skill. Within the therapeutic relationship, the person who does the work is the one who develops the competencies, so the nurse must be careful to share this opportunity with the patient (Peplau, 1952).

Communication blocks are identified by topic changes that either the nurse or the patient makes. Topics are changed for various reasons. A patient may change the topic from one that does not interest him to one that he finds more meaningful. However, an individual usually changes the topic because he or she is uncomfortable with a particular subject. Once a topic change is identified, the nurse or patient hypothesizes the reason for it. If the nurse changes the topic, he or she needs to determine why. The nurse may find that he or she is uncomfortable with the topic or may not be listening to the patient. Novice mental health nurses who are uncomfortable with silences or trying to elicit specific information from the patient often change topics.

The nurse must also record and interpret the patient's nonverbal behavior in light of the verbal behavior. Is the patient saying one thing verbally and another nonverbally? The nurse must consider the patient's cultural background. Is the behavior consistent with cultural norms? For example, if a patient denies any problems but is affectionate and physically demonstrative (which is antithetical to her naturally stoic cultural beliefs and behaviors), the nonverbal behavior is inconsistent with what is normal behavior for that person. Further exploration is needed to determine the meaning of the culturally atypical behavior.

BOX 9.6

Themes and Interactions

Session 1	Patient discusses the death of his mother at a young age.
Session 2	Patient explains that his sister is now married and never visits him.
Session 3	Patient says that his best friend in the hospital was discharged and he really misses her.
Session 4	Patient cries about a lost kitten.
Interpretation:	Theme of loss is pervasive in several sessions.

The Nurse–Patient Relationship

The nurse–patient relationship is a dynamic process that changes with time. It can be viewed in steps or phases with characteristic behaviors for both patient and nurse. This text uses an adaptation of Hildegarde Peplau's model that she introduced in her seminal work, *Interpersonal Relations in Nursing* (1952, 1992). There is emerging evidence that a nurse–patient relationship positively affects patient care (Box 9.7).

BOX 9.7

Research For Best Practice: Therapeutic Relationships: From Psychiatric Hospital to Community

Forchuk, C., Martin, M. L., Chan, Y.C., & Jensen, E. (2005). Therapeutic relationships: from psychiatric hospital to community. Journal of Psychiatric and Mental Health Nursing, 12(5), 556–564.

The Question: This study questioned the effectiveness of a transitional discharge model (TDM) based on sustaining therapeutic relationships over the discharge process. The therapeutic relationships included staff and peer relationships.

Methods: The authors provided a history and overview of TDM. The current study included 26 tertiary care psychiatric wards that were matched into 13 pairs of similar wards. Of these, one half implemented TDM (intervention group) and the other half continued with usual care (control group). There were 390 research subjects who were followed for 1 year post-discharge. Comparisons of quality of life and use of services (costs) were made between the intervention and control groups.

Findings: The quality-of-life and post-discharge costs were not significantly different between the intervention and control groups. However, the intervention group subjects were able to leave the hospital an average of 116 days sooner. This is equal to a savings of more than 12 million Canadian dollars.

Implications for Nursing: Strategies focusing on developing and sustaining therapeutic relationships have the potential for significant health cost savings.

The nurse–patient relationship is conceptualized in three overlapping phases that evolve with time: orientation phase, working phase, and resolution phase.

The **orientation phase** is the phase during which the nurse and patient get to know each other. During this phase, which can last from a few minutes to several months, the patient develops a sense of trust in the nurse. The second is the **working phase**, in which the patient uses the relationship to examine specific problems and learn new ways of approaching them. The final stage, **resolution,** is the termination stage of the relationship and lasts from the time the problems are actually resolved to the close of the relationship. The relationship does not evolve as a simple linear relationship. Instead, the relationship may be predominantly in one phase, but reflections of all phases can be seen in each interaction (Table 9.5).

KEY CONCEPT The **nurse–patient relationship** is a dynamic process that changes with time. It can be viewed in steps or phases with characteristic behaviors for both the patient and the nurse.

Orientation Phase

The orientation phase begins when the nurse and patient meet and ends when the patient begins to identify problems to examine. During the orientation phase, the nurse discusses the patient's expectations, explains the purpose of the relationship and its boundaries, and facilitates the development of the relationship. It is natural for the nurse to be nervous during the first few sessions. The goal of the orientation phase is to develop trust and security within the nurse–patient relationship. During this initial phase, the nurse listens intently to the patient's history and perception of problems and begins to understand the patient and identify themes. The use of empathy facilitates the development of a positive therapeutic relationship.

First Meeting

During the first meeting, outlining both nursing and patient responsibilities is important. The nurse is responsible for providing guidance throughout the therapeutic

Table 9.5 Phases of the Nurse–Patient Relationship

	Orientation	Working	Resolution
Patient	Seeks assistance Identifies needs Commits to a therapeutic relationship Later part, begins to test relationship	Discusses problems underlying needs Uses emotional safety of relationship to examine personal issues Tests new ways of solving problems Feels comfortable with nurse May use transference	May express ambivalence about the relationship and its termination Uses personal style to say "good-bye"
Nurse	Actively listens Establishes boundaries of the relationship Clarifies expectations Uses empathy Establishes rapport	Supports development of healthy problem solving Identifies countertransference issues	Avoids returning to patient's initial problems Encourages patient to prepare for the future Encourages independence Promotes positive family interactions

relationship, protecting confidential information, and maintaining professional boundaries. The patient is responsible for attending agreed-upon sessions, interacting during the sessions, and participating in the nurse–patient relationship. The nurse should also explain clearly to the patient meeting times, handling of missed sessions, and the estimated length of the relationship. Issues related to recording information and how the nurse will work within the interdisciplinary team should also be made explicit.

Usually, both the nurse and the patient feel anxious at the first meeting. The nurse should recognize the anxieties and attempt to alleviate them before the meeting. The patient's behavior during this first meeting may indicate to the nurse some of the patient's problems in interpersonal relationships. For example, a patient may talk nonstop for 15 minutes or may brag of sexual conquests. What the patient chooses to tell or not to tell is significant. What a patient first does or says may not accurately indicate his or her true feelings or the situation. In the beginning, patients may deny problems or choose not to discuss them as defense mechanisms or to prevent the nurse from getting to know them. The patient is usually nervous and insecure during the first few sessions and may exhibit behavior reflective of these emotions, such as rambling. Usually, by the third session, the patient can focus on a topic.

Confidentiality in Treatment

Ideally, nurses include people who are important to the patient in planning and implementing care. The nurse and patient should discuss the issue of confidentiality in the first session. The nurse should be clear about any information that is to be shared with anyone else. Usually, the nurse shares significant assessment data and patient progress with a supervisor and a physician. Most patients expect the nurse to communicate with other mental health professionals and are comfortable with this arrangement.

Testing the Relationship

This first part of the orientation phase, called the "honeymoon phase," is usually pleasant. However, the therapeutic team typically hits rough spots before completing this phase. The patient begins to test the relationship to become convinced that the nurse will really accept him or her. Typical "testing behaviors" include forgetting a scheduled session or being late. Patients may also express anger at something a nurse says or accuse the nurse of breaking confidentiality. Another common pattern is for the patient to first introduce a relatively superficial issue as if it is the major problem. The nurse must recognize that these behaviors are designed to test the relationship and establish its parameters, not to express rejection or dissatisfaction with the nurse. The student nurse often feels personally rejected during the patient's testing and may even become angry with the patient. If the nurse simply accepts the behavior and continues to be available and consistent to the patient, these behaviors usually subside. Testing needs to be understood as a normal way that human beings develop trust.

Working Phase

When the patient begins identifying problems to work on, the working phase of the relationship has started. Problem identification can yield a wide range of issues, such as managing symptoms of a mental disorder, coping with chronic pain, examining issues related to sexual abuse, or dealing with problematic interpersonal relationships. Through the relationship, the patient begins to explore the identified problems and develop strategies to resolve them. By the time the working phase is reached, the patient has developed enough trust that he or she can examine the identified problems within the security of the therapeutic relationship. In the working phase, the nurse can use various verbal and nonverbal techniques to help the patient examine problems.

Transference (unconscious assignment to others of the feelings and attitudes that the patient originally associated with important figures) and countertransference (the provider's emotional reaction to the patient based on personal unconscious needs and conflicts) become important issues in the working phase. For example, a patient could be hostile to a nurse because of underlying resentment of authority figures; the nurse, in turn, could respond defensively because of earlier experiences of anger. The patient uses transference to examine problems. During this phase, the patient is psychologically vulnerable and emotionally dependent on the nurse. The nurse needs to recognize countertransference and prevent it from eroding professional boundaries.

Many times, nurses are eager to implement rehabilitation plans. However, this cannot be done until the patient trusts the nurse and identifies what issues he or she wishes to work on in the context of the relationship.

Resolution Phase

The final stage of the nurse–patient relationship is **resolution,** which begins when the actual problems are resolved and ends with the termination of the relationship. During this phase, the patient is redirected toward a life without this specific therapeutic relationship. The patient connects with community resources, solidifies a newly found understanding, and practices new behaviors. The patient takes responsibility for follow-up appointments and interacts with significant others in new ways. New problems are not addressed during this phase, except in terms of what was learned during the working stage. The nurse assists the client in strengthening relationships, making referrals, and recognizing and understanding signs of future relapse.

Termination begins the first day of the relationship, when the nurse explains that this relationship is time limited and was established to resolve the patient's problems and help him or her handle them. Because a therapeutic relationship is dependent, the nurse must constantly evaluate the patient's level of dependence and continually support the patient's move toward independence. Termination is usually stressful for the patient, who must sever ties with the nurse who has shared thoughts and feelings and given guidance and support over many sessions.

Depending on previous experiences with terminating relationships, some patients may not handle their emotions well during termination. Some may not show up for the last session at all to avoid their feelings of sadness and separation. Many patients display anger about the relationship ending. Patients may express anger toward the nurse or displace it onto others. For example, a patient may shout obscenities at another patient after being told that his therapeutic relationship with the nurse would end in a few weeks. One of the best ways to handle the anger is to help the patient acknowledge it, to explain that anger is a normal emotion when a relationship is ending, and to reassure the patient that it is acceptable to feel angry. The nurse should also reassure the patient that anger subsides once the relationship is over.

Another typical termination behavior is raising old problems that have already been resolved. The nurse may feel frustrated if patients in the termination phase present resolved problems as if they were new. The nurse may feel that the sessions were unsuccessful. In reality, patients are attempting to prolong the relationship and avoid its ending. Nurses should avoid addressing these problems. Instead, they should reassure patients that they already covered those issues and learned methods to control them. They should explain that the patient may be feeling anxious about the relationship ending and redirect the patient to newly found skills and abilities in forming new relationships, including support groups and social groups. The final meeting should focus on the future (Box 9.8). The nurse can reassure the patient that the nurse will remember him or her, but the nurse should not agree to see the patient outside the relationship.

Nontherapeutic Relationships

Although it is hoped that all nurse–patient relationships will go through the phases of the relationship described earlier, this is not always the case. Nontherapeutic relationships also go through predictable phases (Forchuk et al., 2000). These relationships also start in the *orientation* phase. However, trust is not established, and the relationship moves to a phase of *grappling and struggling*. The nurse and patient both feel very frustrated and keep varying their approach with each other in an attempt to establish a meaningful relationship. This is different from a prolonged orientation phase in that the efforts are not sustained; they vary constantly.

The nurse may try longer meetings, shorter meetings, being more or less directive, and varying the therapeutic stance from warm and friendly to aloof. Patients in this phase may try to talk about the past but then change to discussions of the "here and now." They will try talking about their family and in the next meeting talk about their work goals. Both grapple and struggle to come to a

BOX 9.8

Therapeutic Dialogue: The Last Meeting

Ineffective Approach

Nurse: Today is my last day.
Patient: I need to talk to you about something important.
Nurse: What is it?
Patient: I have been hearing voices again.
Nurse: Oh, how often?
Patient: Every night. You are the only one I'm going to tell.
Nurse: I think you should tell the new nurse.
Patient: She is too new. She won't understand. I feel so bad about your leaving. Is there any way you can stay?
Nurse: Well, I could check on you tomorrow?
Patient: Oh, would you? I would really appreciate it if you would give me your new telephone number.
Nurse: I don't know what the number will be but it will be listed in the telephone book.

Effective Approach

Nurse: Today is my last day.
Patient: I need to talk to you about something important.
Nurse: We talked about that. Anything "important" needs to be shared with the new nurse.
Patient: But, I want to tell you.
Nurse: Saying good-bye can be very hard.
Patient: I will miss you.
Nurse: Your feelings are very normal when relationships are ending. I will remember you in a very special way.
Patient: Can I please have your telephone number?
Nurse: No, I can't give that to you. It is important that we say good-bye today.
Patient: OK. Good-bye. Good luck.
Nurse: Good-bye.

Critical Thinking Challenge

- What were some of the mistakes the nurse in the first scenario made?
- In the second scenario, how does therapeutic communication in the termination phase differ from effective communication in the working phase?

common ground, and both become increasingly frustrated with each other.

Eventually the frustration becomes so great that the pair gives up on each other and moves to a phase of *mutual withdrawal*. The nurse may schedule seeing this patient at the end of the shift and "run out of time" so the meeting never happens. The patient will leave the unit or otherwise be unavailable during scheduled meeting times. If a meeting does occur, the nurse will try to keep it short. "What's the point—we just cover the same old ground anyway." The patient will attempt to keep it superficial and stay on safe topics. "You can always ask about your medications—nurses love to health teach, you know." Obviously no therapeutic progress can be made in such a relationship. The nurse may be hesitant to ask for a therapeutic transfer, assuming that a relationship would similarly fail with another nurse. However, each relationship is unique, and difficulties in one relationship do not predict difficulties in the next. Clinical supervision early on may assist the development of the relationship, but often a therapeutic transfer to another nurse is required.

SUMMARY OF KEY POINTS

- To deal therapeutically with the emotions, feelings, and problems of patients, nurses must understand their own cultural values and beliefs and interpersonal strengths and limitations.
- The nurse–patient relationship is built on therapeutic communication, including verbal and nonverbal interactions between the nurse and the patient. Some communication skills include active listening, positive body language, appropriate verbal responses, and ability of the nurse to interpret appropriately and analyze the patient's verbal and nonverbal behaviors.
- Two of the most important communication concepts are empathy and rapport.
- In the nurse–patient relationship, as in all types of relationships, certain physical, emotional, and social boundaries and limitations need to be observed.
- The therapeutic nurse–patient relationship consists of three major and overlapping stages or phases: the orientation phase, in which the patient and nurse meet and establish the parameters of the relationship; the working phase, in which the patient identifies and explores problems; and the resolution phase, in which the patient learns to manage the problems and the relationship is terminated.
- The nontherapeutic relationship also consists of three major and overlapping phases: the orientation phase, the grappling and struggling phase, and the phase of mutual withdrawal.

CRITICAL THINKING CHALLENGES

1 Describe how you would do a suicide assessment on a distraught patient who comes to the physician's office expressing concerns about her ability to cope with her current situation. Describe how you would approach this patient if you determined she was suicidal. How might this assessment look different depending on the phase of the therapeutic relationship?

2 Describe how you would communicate with a patient who is concerned that the diagnosis of bipolar disorder will negatively affect his or her social and work relationships.

3 Your depressed patient does not seem inclined to talk about the depression. Describe the measures you would take to initiate a therapeutic relationship with him or her.

4 Think of a time that you worked with a patient that you did not like. What was behind the dislike? How did you handle the therapeutic relationship? What could you do differently?

Good Will Hunting: 1997. Robin Williams plays a therapist to Will Hunting, a janitor identified as a mathematical genius, played by Matt Damon. Through a strong relationship, Will begins to realize his potential.

VIEWING POINTS: Watch closely how the relationship develops between the characters played by Williams and Damon. How does the relationship change as the characters move through different stages of their relationship?

Analyze That: 2002. In this comedy sequel to *Analyze This* (1999), Billy Crystal plays psychiatrist Dr. Ben Sobel. The patient is Paul Vitti (Robert De Niro), a mobster who has been sent to prison. Vitti is either having a psychotic break or is faking one, and his former psychiatrist is called back to assess the situation. Vitti is sent to Sobel's home for treatment. Both the psychiatrist and patient have unresolved feelings related to the deaths of their fathers.

VIEWING POINTS: The issue of therapeutic boundaries is a source of comedy in this film. What normal therapeutic boundaries are being violated? Whose needs are being met throughout the film? What would be appropriate if a patient evoked personal unresolved issues for the therapist?

Manhood: 2003. Jack is a reformed womanizer who is experiencing numerous family problems. He is also a single father raising a son. His sister asks him to take care of her son for a while so that she can sort out her marital situation. His brother-in-law also ends up moving in with him. The movie stars Nestor Carbonell, John Ritter, and Jeanine Garofalo.

VIEWING POINTS: Several different encounters with mental health professionals are depicted. Jack is seeing a therapist regularly, but it appears the therapist may be interested in him romantically. How does this affect the therapeutic relationship? What is appropriate if one feels attracted to a patient? Jack's brother-in-law receives psychiatric help, but the psychiatrist does not listen to Jack's concerns regarding discharge. What communication strategies might help in this situation?

REFERENCES

American Psychiatric Association. (2000). *Diagnostic and statistical manual of mental disorders* (4th ed., text revision). Washington, DC: Author.

Boyd, M. (1995). Communication with patients, families, healthcare providers, and diverse cultures. In M. Strader & P. Decker (Eds.), *Role transition to patient care management* (p. 431). Norwalk, CT: Appleton & Lange.

Forchuk, C., Westwell, J., Martin, M. L., Bamber-Azzapardi, W., Kosterewa-Tolman, D., & Hux, M. (2000). The developing nurse–client relationship: Nurses perspectives. *Journal of the American Psychiatric Nurses Association, 6*(1), 3–10.

Gallop, R., Choiniere, J., Forchuk, C., Golea, G., Jonston, N., Levac, A. M.,et al. (2002). *Nursing best practice guideline: Establishing therapeutic relationships.* Toronto, Canada: Registered Nurses Association of Ontario.

Orlando, I. (1961). *Orlando's Dynamic Nurse-Patient Relationship: Function, process and principles.* New York: Putnam.

Peplau, H. E. (1952, 1992). *Interpersonal relations in nursing*. New York: J. P. Putnam's Sons.

CHAPTER 10

The Nursing Process: Assessment, Diagnoses, Outcomes, Interventions, Evaluation

Mary Ann Boyd, Doris Bell, and Lorraine Williams

KEY CONCEPTS

- assessment
- mental status examination
- nursing diagnosis and defining characteristics
- outcomes
- nursing interventions

LEARNING OBJECTIVES

After studying this chapter, you will be able to:

- Define the nursing process in psychiatric–mental health nursing.
- Conduct a biopsychosocial psychiatric nursing assessment.
- Develop nursing diagnoses following a psychiatric nursing assessment.
- Develop patient outcomes from a nursing diagnosis.
- Apply psychiatric nursing interventions for persons with mental health problems and mental disorders.

KEY TERMS

• affect • behavior modification • behavior therapy • bibliotherapy • body image • chemical restraint • cognition • conflict resolution • containment • counseling • cultural brokering • de-escalation • distraction • dysphoric • euphoric • euthymic • guided imagery • home visits • insight • judgment • labile • milieu therapy • mood • NIC taxonomy • observation • open communication • outcome indicators • personal identity • physical restraint • psychoeducation • reminiscence • seclusion • self-concept • self-esteem • simple relaxation techniques • spiritual support • structured interaction • token economy • validation • win-win

The nursing process is the model of care used in psychiatric nursing. In this text, the nursing process is organized around the areas of assessment, diagnosis and outcome development, intervention, and evaluation.

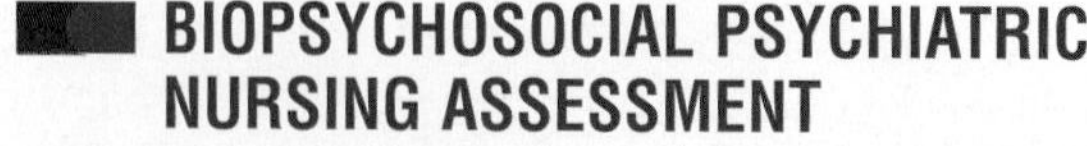

BIOPSYCHOSOCIAL PSYCHIATRIC NURSING ASSESSMENT

Assessment is the collection and interpretation of biopsychosocial information to determine health, functional

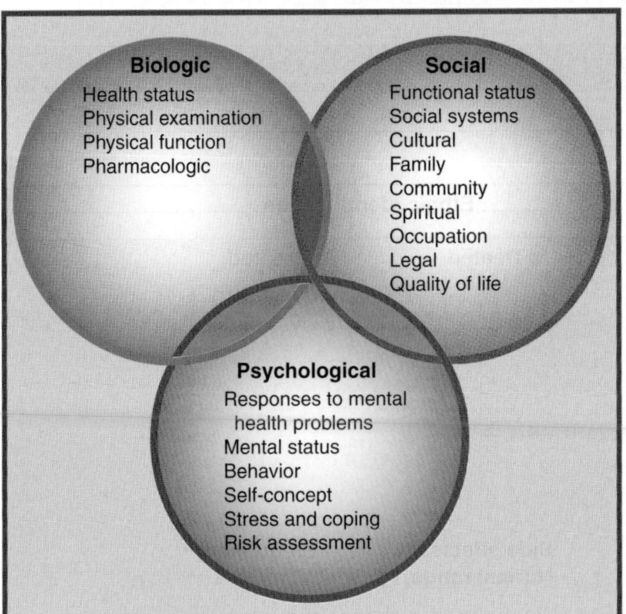

FIGURE 10.1. Biopsychosocial nursing assessment.

status, and human responses to mental health problems. These responses are expressed through biologic, psychological, and social manifestations (Fig. 10.1).

Assessment is not an isolated activity. It is a systematic and ongoing process that occurs throughout the nurse's care of the patient. The Biopsychosocial Psychiatric Nursing Assessment (Box 10.1) is a basic guide to collecting assessment data. Assessment information is entered into the patient's written or computerized record, which may be presented in several different formats, including forms, checklists, narratives, and problem-oriented notes.

KEY CONCEPT Assessment is the deliberate and systematic collection and interpretation of biopsychosocial information or data to determine current and past health, functional status, and human responses to mental health problems, both actual and potential.

Assessment begins with the first contact with the patient and is based on the establishment of rapport with the patient. Legal consent must be given by the patient and the nurse must follow the Health Insurance Portability and Accountability Act of 1996 (HIPAA) guidelines (see Chapter 3). The patient must develop a sense of trust before he or she will be comfortable revealing intimate life details. It is of paramount importance that the nurse has a healthy knowledge of self as well (Box 10.2). The nurse's own biases and values, which may be different from those of the patient, can influence the nurse's interpretation of assessment data. A careful self-assessment helps the nurse interpret the data objectively.

Patient Interviews

An assessment interview usually involves direct questions to obtain facts, clarify perceptions, validate observations, interpret the meanings of groups of facts, or compare information. The specific questions may take different forms. The nurse must clearly state the purpose of the interview and, if necessary, modify the interview process so that both patient and nurse agree on its purpose. The nurse may choose to use open-ended questions or closed-ended questions to complete the assessment. Open-ended questions are most helpful when beginning the interview because they allow the nurse to observe how the patient responds verbally and nonverbally. They also convey caring and interest in the person's well-being, which helps to establish rapport. Nurses should use closed-ended questions when they need specific information. For example, "How old are you?" asks for specific information about the patient's age. These types of questions limit the individual's response but often serve as good follow-up questions for clarification of thoughts or feelings expressed.

Questions such as "How did you come to this clinic today?" allow patients to describe their experience in their own way. Some patients may answer this question concretely by saying, "I took a taxi" or "I came by car." Others may address this question by responding, "My family thought I should come so they brought me" or "Well, I got up this morning . . . I took a shower, got dressed . . . and then, well you know, it's difficult sometimes to decide." Each of these answers helps the nurse assess the patient's thinking process as well as evaluate the content of the response.

Clarification is extremely important during the assessment process. Words do not have the same meaning to all people. Education, language, culture, history, and experience may influence the meaning of words. Sometimes, simple and direct questioning provides clarification. In other situations, the nurse may clarify by providing a specific example for a more global thought the patient is trying to express. For example, a patient may say, "Things have been so strange since the children left." The nurse may respond with, "Sometimes, parents feel sad and empty when their children leave home. They don't know what to do with their time." Frequently summarizing what has been said allows the patient the opportunity to correct the nurse's interpretation. For example, verbalizing a sequence of events that the patient has reported may help to identify omissions or inconsistencies. Restating information or reflecting feelings that the patient has described also allows opportunity for clarification. It is essential that nurses understand exactly what patients are attempting to communicate before beginning to intervene. Box 10.3 provides a summary of other

BOX 10.1

Biopsychosocial Psychiatric Nursing Assessment

I. **Major reason for seeking help** ______

II. **Initial information**

Name ______

Age ______ **Marital status** ______ **Gender** ______ **Ethnic identification** ______

III. **Present and past health status** ______

	Normal	Treated	Untreated
Physical functions: System review	□	□	□
Elimination	□	□	□
Activity/exercise	□	□	□
Sleep	□	□	□
Appetite and nutrition	□	□	□
Hydration	□	□	□
Sexuality	□	□	□
Self-care	□	□	□
Existing physical illnesses	□	□	□

Medications (prescription and over-the-counter)	**Dosage**	**Side effects**	**Frequency**
Significant laboratory tests	**Values**	**Normal range**	

IV. **Responses to mental health problems**

Major concerns regarding mental health problem ______

Major loss/change in past year: No ______ Yes ______

Fear of violence: No ______ Yes ______

Strategies for managing problems/disorder ______

V. **Mental status examination**

General observations (appearance, psychomotor activity, attitude) ______

Orientation (time, place, person) ______

Mood, affect, emotions ______

Speech (verbal ability, speed, use of words correctly) ______

Thought processes (tangential, logic, repetition, rhyming of words, loose connections, disorganized) ______

Cognition and intellectual performance ______

Attention and concentration ______

Abstract reasoning and comprehension ______

Memory (recall, short-term, recent, and remote) ______

Judgment and insight ______

VI. **Significant behaviors (psychomotor, agitation, aggression, withdrawn)** ______

VII. **Self-concept (body image, self-esteem, personal identity)** ______

VIII. **Stress and coping patterns** ______

IX. **Risk assessment**

Suicide: High ______ Low ______ Assault/homicide: High ______ Low ______

Suicide thoughts or ideation: No ______ Yes ______

Current thoughts of harming self ______

Plan ______

Means ______

Means available ______

Assault/homicide thoughts: No ______ Yes ______

What do you do when angry with a stranger? ______

What do you do when angry with family or partner? ______

Have you ever hit or pushed anyone? No ______ Yes ______

Have you ever been arrested for assault? No ______ Yes ______

Current thoughts of harming others ______

X. **Functional status**

GAF score (see Chapter 2) ______

XI. **Social systems**

Cultural assessment

Cultural group ______

Cultural group's view of health and mental illness ______

What cultural rules do you try to live by? ______

Important cultural foods ______

(Continued on following page)

BOX 10.1

Biopsychosocial Psychiatric Nursing Assessment (continued)

Family assessment
Family members ______
Members important to patient ______
Decision makers, family roles, supportive members ______
Community resources ______
XII. **Spiritual assessment**
XIII. **Economic status**
XIV. **Legal status**
XV. **Quality of life**
Summary of significant data that can be used in formulating a nursing diagnosis
SIGNATURE/TITLE ______ Date ______

behaviors that enhance the effectiveness of an assessment interview.

Many psychiatric symptoms are beyond a patient's awareness. Family members, friends, and other health care professionals are important sources of information. Before seeking information about the patient, the nurse must obtain permission from the patient. The nurse needs to provide the patient with a clear explanation of why the information is needed and how it will be used.

BOX 10.2

Self-Concept Awareness

Self-awareness is important in any interaction. To understand a patient's self-concept, the nurse must be aware of his or her own self-concept. By answering these questions, nurses can evaluate self-concept components and increase their self-understanding. The more comfortable the nurse is with himself or herself, the more effective the nurse can be in each and every patient interaction.

Body Image
How do I feel about my body?
How important is my physical appearance?
How does my body measure up to my ideal body? (How would I like to appear?)
What is positive about my body?
What would I like to change about my body?
How does my body image affect my self-esteem?

Self-Esteem
When do I feel confident and good about myself?
When do I feel unimportant?
What do I do when I feel good about myself? (Call friends, socialize?)
What do I do when I have negative feelings about myself? (Withdraw, dress poorly?)
When do I make negative statements?
Am I able to correct my negative self-statements?

Personal Identity
How do I describe myself?
What three adjectives describe who I am?
Do I identify with a particular cultural group, family role, or place of residence?
What would I like to have on my tombstone?

Biologic Domain

Many psychiatric disorders produce physical symptoms, such as the lack of appetite and weight loss associated with depression. A person's physical condition may also affect mental health, producing a recurrence or increase in symptoms. Many physical disorders may present first with symptoms considered to be psychiatric. For example, hypothyroidism often presents with feelings of lethargy, decreased concentration, and depressed mood. For these reasons, biologic information about the patient is always considered.

BOX 10.3

Assessment Interview Behaviors

The following behaviors carried out by the nurse will enhance the effectiveness of the assessment interview:

- Exhibiting empathy—to show empathy to the patient, the nurse uses phrases such as, "That must have been upsetting for you" or "I can understand your hurt feelings."
- Giving recognition—the nurse gives recognition by listening actively: verbally encouraging the patient to continue, and nonverbally presenting an open, interested demeanor.
- Demonstrating acceptance—note that acceptance does not mean agreement or nonagreement with the patient, but is a neutral stance that allows the patient to continue.
- Restating—the nurse tries to clarify what the patient is trying to say by restating it.
- Reflecting—the nurse presents the patient's last statement as a question. This gives the patient a chance to expand on the information.
- Focusing—the nurse attempts to bring the conversation back to the questions at hand when the patient goes off on a tangent.
- Using open-ended questions—general questions give the patient a chance to speak freely.
- Presenting reality—the nurse presents reality when the patient makes unrealistic or exaggerated statements.
- Making observations—the nurse says aloud what patient behaviors are observed, to give the patient a chance to speak to those behaviors. For example, the nurse may say, "I notice you are twisting your fingers; are you nervous about something?"

Current and Past Health Status

Beginning with a history of the patient's general medical condition, the nurse should consider the following:

- Availability of, frequency of, and most recent medical evaluation, including test results
- Past hospitalizations and surgical operations
- Cardiac problems, including cerebrovascular accidents (strokes), myocardial infarctions (heart attacks), and childhood illnesses
- Respiratory problems, particularly those that result in a lack of oxygen to the brain
- Neurologic problems, particularly head injuries, seizure disorders, or any losses of consciousness
- Endocrine disorders, particularly unstable diabetes or thyroid or adrenal dysfunction
- Immune disorders, particularly human immunodeficiency virus (HIV) and autoimmune disorders
- Use, exposure, abuse, or dependence on substances, including alcohol, tobacco, prescription drugs, illicit drugs, and herbal preparations.

Physical Examination

Body Systems Review

Once the nurse obtains historical information, he or she should examine physiologic systems to evaluate the patient's current physical condition. The physician or nurse practitioner usually conducts the physical examination, but the psychiatric nurse should pay special attention to various systems that treatment may affect. For example, if a patient is being treated with antihypertensive medication, the dosage may need to be adjusted if an antipsychotic medication is prescribed. If a patient is overweight or has diabetes, some psychiatric medications can affect these conditions. Those patients with compromised immune function (HIV, cancer) may experience mood alterations.

Neurologic Status

Particular attention is paid to recent head trauma, episodes of hypertension, and changes in personality, speech, or ability to handle activities of daily living. Also noted are any movement disorders.

Laboratory Results

Available laboratory data are reviewed for any abnormalities and documented. Particular attention is paid to any abnormalities of hepatic, renal, or urinary function because these systems metabolize or excrete many psychiatric medications. In addition, abnormal white blood cell and electrolyte levels should be noted. Laboratory data are especially important, particularly if the nurse is the only person in the mental health team who has a "medical" background (Table 10.1).

Physical Functions

Elimination

The patient's daily urinary and bowel habits should be elicited and documented. Various medications can affect bladder and bowel functioning, so a baseline must be noted. For example, diarrhea and frequency of urination can occur with the use of lithium carbonate. Anticholinergic effects of antipsychotic medication can cause constipation and urinary hesitancy or retention. Any history of eating disorders should also be noted in elimination patterns.

Activity and Exercise

The patient's daily methods and levels of activity and exercise must be queried and documented. Activities are important interventions, and baseline information is needed to determine what the patient already enjoys or dislikes and whether he or she is getting sufficient exercise or adequate recreation. A patient may have altered activity or exercise in response to medication or therapies. In addition, many psychiatric medications cause weight gain, and nurses need to develop interventions that assist the patient to increase activities to counteract the weight gain.

Sleep

Changes in sleep patterns often reflect changes in a patient's emotions and are symptoms of disorders. If the patient responds positively to a question about changes in sleep patterns, it is important to clarify just what those changes are. For example, "difficulty falling asleep" means different things to different people. For the person who usually falls right to sleep, it could mean that it takes 10 extra minutes to fall asleep. For the person who normally takes 35 minutes to fall asleep, it could mean that it takes 90 minutes to do so.

Appetite and Nutrition

Questions that ascertain changes in the patient's appetite and nutritional intake can uncover how a patient's everyday patterns are changing as mentation changes. For example, a patient who is depressed may not notice hunger or even that he or she does not have the energy to prepare food. Others may handle stressful emotions through eating more than usual. This information also provides valuable clues to possible eating disorders and problems with body image.

Hydration

Gaining perspective on how much fluid patients normally drink and how much they are drinking now provides

Table 10.1 Selected Hematologic Measures and Their Relevance to Psychiatric Disorders

Test	Possible Results	Possible Cause or Meaning
Complete Blood Count (CBC)		
Leukocyte count (WBC)	Leukopenia—decrease in leukocytes (white blood cells) Agranulocytosis—decrease in number of granulocytic leukocytes	May be produced by: Phenothiazines Clozapine Carbamazepine
	Leukocytosis—increase in leukocyte count above normal limits	Lithium causes a benign mild-to-moderate increase (11,000-17,000/mcl). Neuroleptic malignant syndrome (NMS) can be associated with increases of 15,000 to 30,000/mm^3 in about 40% of cases.
WBC differential	"Shift to the left"—from segmented neutrophils to band forms	Shift often suggests a bacterial infection, but has been reported in about 40% of cases of NMS.
Red blood cell count (RBC)	Polycythemia—increased RBCs	Primary form—true polycythemia caused by several disease states Secondary form—compensation for decreased oxygenation, such as in chronic pulmonary disease Blood is more viscous, and the patient should not become dehydrated.
	Decreased RBCs	Decrease may be related to some types of anemia, which requires further evaluation.
Hematocrit (Hct)	Elevations	Elevation may be due to dehydration.
	Decreased Hct	Anemia may be associated with a wide range of mental status changes, including asthenia, depression, and psychosis. 20% of women of childbearing age in the United States have iron-deficiency anemia.
Hemoglobin (Hb)	Decreased	Another indicator of anemia, further evaluation of source requires review of erythrocyte indices.
Erythrocyte indices, such as red cell distribution width (RDW)	Elevated RDW	Finding suggests a combined anemia as in that from chronic alcoholism, resulting from both vitamin B_{12} and folate acid deficiencies and iron deficiency. Oral contraceptives also decrease vitamin B_{12}.
Other Hematologic Measures		
Vitamin B_{12}	Deficiency	Neuropsychiatric symptoms such as psychosis, paranoia, fatigue, agitation, marked personality change, dementia, and delirium may develop.
Folate	Deficiency	The use of alcohol, phenytoin, oral contraceptives, and estrogens may be responsible.
Platelet count	Thrombocytopenia—decreased platelet count	Some psychiatric medications, such as carbamazepine, phenothiazines, or clozapine, or other nonpsychiatric medications, may cause thrombocytopenia. Several medical conditions are other causes.
Serum Electrolytes		
Sodium	Hyponatremia—low serum sodium	Significant mental status changes may ensue. Condition is associated with Addison's disease, the syndrome of inappropriate secretion of antidiuretic hormone (SIADH), and polydipsia (water intoxication) as well as carbamazepine use.
Potassium	Hypokalemia—low serum potassium	Produces weakness, fatigue, electrocardiogram (ECG) changes; paralytic ileus and muscle paresis may develop. Common in individuals with bulimic behavior or psychogenic vomiting and use or abuse of diuretics; laxative abuse may contribute; can be life-threatening.
Chloride	Elevation	Chloride tends to increase to compensate for lower bicarbonate.
	Decrease	Binging–purging behavior and repeated vomiting may be causes.
Bicarbonate	Elevation	Causes may be binging and purging in eating disorders, excessive use of laxatives, or psychogenic vomiting.
	Decrease	Decrease may develop in some patients with hyperventilation syndrome and panic disorder.

(Continued on following page)

Table 10.1 Selected Hematologic Measures and Their Relevance to Psychiatric Disorders (Continued)

Test	Possible Results	Possible Cause or Meaning
Renal Function Tests		
Blood urea nitrogen (BUN)	Elevation	Increase is associated with mental status changes, lethargy, and delirium. Cause may be dehydration. Potential toxicity of medications cleared via the kidney, such as lithium and amantadine, may increase.
Serum creatinine	Elevation	Level usually does not become elevated until about 50% of nephrons in the kidney are damaged.
Serum Enzymes		
Amylase	Elevation	Level appears to increase after binging and purging behavior in eating disorders and declines when these behaviors stop.
Alanine aminotransferase (ALT)—formerly serum glutamic pyruvic transaminase (SGPT)	ALT > AST	Disparity is common in acute forms of viral and drug-induced hepatic dysfunction.
Aspartate aminotransferase (AST)—formerly serum glutamic oxaloacetic transaminase (SGOT)	Elevation	Mild elevations are common with use of sodium valproate.
	AST > ALT	Severe elevations in chronic forms of liver disease and post-myocardial infarction may develop.
Creatine phospho-kinase (CPK)	Elevations of the isoenzyme related to muscle tissue	Muscle tissue injury is the cause. Level is elevated in neuroleptic malignant syndrome (NMS). Level is also elevated by repeated intramuscular injections (e.g., antipsychotics).
Thyroid Function		
Serum triiodothyronine (T_3)	Decrease	Hypothyroidism and nonthyroid illness cause decrease. Individuals with depression may convert less T_4 to T_3 peripherally, but not out of the normal range. Medications such as lithium and sodium valproate may suppress thyroid function, but clinical significance is unknown.
	Elevations	Hyperthyroidism, T_3, toxicosis, may produce mood changes, anxiety, and symptoms of mania
Serum thyroxine (T_4)	Elevations	Hyperthyroidism is a cause.
Thyroid stimulating hormone (TSH)—called *thyrotropin*	Elevations	Hypothyroidism—symptoms may appear very much like depression, except for additional physical signs of cold intolerance, dry skin, hair loss, bradycardia, etc. Lithium—may also cause elevations.
	Decrease	Considered nondiagnostic—may be hyperthyroidism, pituitary hypothyroidism, or even euthyroid status.

important data. Some medications can cause retention of fluids, and others can cause diuresis; thus, the patient's current fluid status must be understood.

Sexuality

Questioning a patient on issues involving sexuality requires comfort with one's own sexuality. Changes in sexual activity as well as comfort with sexual orientation are important to assess. Issues involving sexual orientation that are unsettled in a patient or between a patient and family member may cause anxiety, shame, or discomfort. It is necessary to explore how comfortable the patient is with his or her sexuality and sexual functioning. These questions should be asked in a matter-of-fact, but gentle and nonjudgmental, manner. Initiating the topic of sexuality may begin with a question such as "Are you sexually active?" Birth control medications may also alter mood.

Self-Care

Often, a patient's ability to care for self or carry out activities of daily living, such as washing and dressing, are indicative of his or her psychological state. For example, a depressed patient may not have the energy to iron a shirt before wearing it. This information may also help the nurse to determine actual or potential obstacles to a patient's compliance with a treatment plan.

Pharmacologic Assessment

If the patient will receive psychopharmacologic therapy, the review of systems will serve as a baseline from which the nurse may judge whether the medication exacerbates symptoms or causes new ones to develop. It is important to determine which medications the patient takes now or has taken in the past. This includes over-the-counter

(OTC), herbal or nonprescription medications, as well as those prescribed. This assessment is important for reasons other than serving as a baseline. It helps target possible drug interactions, determines whether the patient has already used medications that are being considered, and identifies whether medications may be causing psychiatric symptoms.

Psychological Domain

The psychological domain is the traditional focus of the psychiatric nursing assessment. By definition, psychiatric disorders are manifested through psychological symptoms related to mental status, moods, thoughts, behaviors, and interpersonal relationships. This domain also includes data related to psychological growth and development. Assessing this domain is important in developing a comprehensive picture of the patient.

Responses to Mental Health Problems

Individual concerns regarding the mental health problem or its consequences are included in the mental health assessment. A mental disorder, like any other illness, affects patients and families in many different ways. It is safe to say that a mental illness changes a person's life, and the nurse should identify what the changes are and their meaning to the patient and family members. Many patients experience specific fears, such as losing their job, family, or safety. Included in this part of the assessment is identification of current strategies or behaviors in dealing with the disorder. A simple question such as "How do you deal with your voices when you are with other people?" may initiate a discussion about responses to the mental disorder or emotional problem.

Mental Status Examination

The mental status examination establishes a baseline, provides a snapshot of where the patient is at a particular moment, and creates a written record. Areas of assessment include general observations, orientation, mood and affect, speech, thought processes, cognition, and insight. Box 10.4 provides a narrative note of the results from a patient's mental status examination.

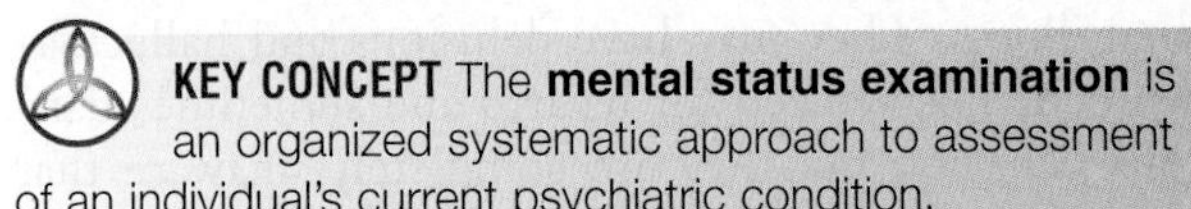

KEY CONCEPT The **mental status examination** is an organized systematic approach to assessment of an individual's current psychiatric condition.

General Observations

At the beginning of the interview, the nurse should record his or her initial impressions of the patient. These general observations include the patient's appearance, affect, psychomotor activity, and overall behavior. How is the patient dressed? Is the dress appropriate for weather and setting? What is the patient's affect (emotional expression)? What behaviors is the patient displaying? For example, the same nurse assessed two male patients with depression. At the beginning of the mental status examination, the differences between these two men were very clear. The nurse described the first patient as "a large, well-dressed man who is agitated and appears angry, shifts in his seat, and does not maintain eye contact. He interrupts often in the initial explanation of mental status." The nurse described the other patient as a "small, unshaven, disheveled man with a strong body odor who appears withdrawn. He shuffles as he walks, speaks very softly, appears sad, and avoids direct eye contact."

BOX 10.4

Narrative Mental Status Examination Note

The patient is a 65-year-old widowed man who is slightly disheveled. He is cooperative with the interviewer and judged to be an adequate historian. His mood and affect are depressed and anxious. He becomes tearful throughout the interview when speaking about his wife. His flow of thought is hesitant when speaking about his wife, but coherent. He is oriented to time, place, and person. He shows good recent and remote memory. He is able to recall several items given him by the interviewer. The patient shows poor insight and judgment regarding his sadness since the loss of his wife. He repeatedly says, "Mary wouldn't want me to be sad. She would want me to continue with my life."

Orientation

The nurse can determine the patient's orientation to date, day, time, place, and person by asking the date, time, and current location of the interview setting. If a patient knows the year, but not the exact date, the interviewer can ask the season. A person's orientation tells the nurse the extent of confusion. If a patient does not know the year or the place of the interview, he or she is exhibiting considerable confusion.

Mood and Affect

Mood refers to the prominent, sustained, overall emotions that the person expresses and exhibits. Mood may be sustained for days or weeks, or it may fluctuate during the course of a day. For example, some patients with depression have a diurnal variation in their mood. They experience their lowest mood in the morning, but as the day progresses, their depressed mood lifts and they feel somewhat better in the evening. Terms used to describe mood include **euthymic** (normal), **euphoric** (elated), **labile** (changeable), and **dysphoric** (depressed, disquieted, restless).

Affect refers to the person's capacity to vary outward emotional expression. Affect fluctuates with thought content and can be observed in facial expressions, vocal fluctuations, and gestures. During the assessment, the patient may exhibit anger, frustration, irritation, apathy, and helplessness while his or her overall mood remains unchanged.

Affect can be described in terms of range, intensity, appropriateness, and stability. Range can be full or restricted. An individual who expresses several different emotions consistent with the stated feelings and content being expressed is described as having a *full range* of affect that is congruent with the situation. An individual who expresses few emotions has a restricted affect. For example, a patient could be describing the recent, tragic death of a loved one in a monotone with little expression. In determining whether this response is normal, the nurse compares the patient's emotional response with the cultural norm for that particular response. *Intensity* can be increased, flat, or blunted. A patient may show an extreme reaction to the death of the victims of the September 11 tragedy, as if the victims were personal friends. One patient said that his life stopped when the World Trade Center towers came down. He could not eat or sleep for weeks afterward. *Stability* can be mobile (normal) or labile. If a patient reports feeling happy one minute and reduced to tears the next, the person probably has an unstable mood. During the interview, the nurse should look for rapid mood changes that indicate lability of mood. A patient who exhibits intense, frequently shifting emotional extremes has a labile affect.

Speech

Speech provides clues about thoughts, emotional patterns, and cognitive organization. The speech may be pressured, fast, slow, or fragmented. Speech patterns reflect thought patterns the patient is experiencing. To check the patient's comprehension, the nurse can ask the patient to name objects. During conversation, the nurse assesses the fluency and quality of the patient's speech. The nurse listens for repetition or rhyming of words.

Thought Processes

The nurse assesses the patient for rapid change of ideas; inability or taking a long time to get to the point; loose or no connections among ideas or words; rhyming or repetition of words, questions, or phrases; or use of unheard of words. Any of these observations indicates abnormal thought patterns. The content of what the patient says is also important. What thought is the patient expressing? The nurse listens for unreal stories and fears; for example, "The FBI is tracking me." He or she also listens for phobias, obsessions, and suicidal or homicidal thoughts.

Cognition and Intellectual Performance

To assess the patient's **cognition,** that is, the ability to think and know, the nurse uses memory, calculation, and reasoning tests to identify specific areas of impairment. The cognitive areas include (1) attention and concentration, (2) abstract reasoning and comprehension, (3) memory, and (4) insight and judgment.

Attention and Concentration

To test attention and concentration, the nurse asks the patient, without pencil or paper, to start with 100 and subtract 7 until reaching 65 or to start with 20 and subtract 3. The nurse must decide which is most appropriate for the patient considering education and understanding. Subtracting 3 from 20 is the easier of the two tasks.

Abstract Reasoning and Comprehension

To test abstract reasoning and comprehension, the nurse gives the patient a proverb to interpret. Examples include "People in glass houses shouldn't throw stones," "A rolling stone gathers no moss," and "A penny saved is a penny earned."

Memory: Recall, Short-Term, Recent, and Remote

There are four spheres of memory to check: recall, or immediate, memory; short-term memory; recent memory; and long-term, or remote, memory. To check immediate and short-term memory, the nurse gives the patient three unrelated words to remember and asks him or her to recite them right after telling them and at 5-minute and 15-minute intervals during the interview. To test recent memory, the nurse may question about a holiday or world event within the past few months. The nurse tests long-term or remote memory by asking about events years ago. If they are personal events and the answers seem incorrect, the nurse may check them with a family member.

Insight and Judgment

Insight and judgment are related concepts that involve the ability to examine thoughts, conceptualize facts, solve problems, think abstractly, and possess self-awareness. **Insight** is a person's awareness of his or her own thoughts and feelings and ability to compare them with the thoughts and feelings of others. It involves an awareness of how others view one's behavior and its meaning. For example, many patients do not believe that they have mental illness. They may have delusions and hallucinations or be hospitalized for bizarre and sometimes dangerous behavior, but they are completely unaware that their behavior is unusual or abnormal. During an interview, a patient may adamantly proclaim that nothing is wrong or that he or she does not have a mental illness. Even if a problem is recognized, the patient may lack insight regarding issues related to care.

Judgment is the ability to reach a logical decision about a situation and to choose a course of action after examining and analyzing various possibilities. Throughout the interview, the nurse evaluates the patient's ability to make logical decisions. For example, some patients may continually choose partners who are abusive. The nurse could logically conclude that these patients have poor judgment in selecting partners. Another way to examine a patient's judgment is to give a simple scenario and ask the person to identify the best response. An example of such a scenario is "What would you do if you found a bag of money outside a bank on a busy street?" If the patient responds, "Run with it," his or her judgment is questionable.

Behavior

Throughout the assessment, the nurse observes any behavior that may have significance in understanding the patient's response or symptoms of the mental disorder or emotional problem. For example, a depressed patient may be tearful throughout the session, whereas an anxious patient may twist or pull hair, shift in the chair, or be unable to maintain eye contact. The nurse needs to connect the behavior with the assessment topic. The nurse may find that whenever a particular topic is addressed, the patient's behavior changes. Throughout the assessment, the nurse attempts to identify patterned behaviors to significant events. For example, a patient may change jobs frequently, causing family distress and financial problems. Exploration of the events leading up to job changes may elicit important data regarding the patient's ability to solve problems.

Self-Concept

Self-concept, which develops over a lifetime, represents the total beliefs about three interrelated dimensions of the self: body image, self-esteem, and personal identity. The importance of each of the three dimensions of self-concept varies among individuals. For some, beliefs about themselves are strongly tied to body image; for others, personal identity is most important. Still others develop personal identity from what others have told them over the years. The nurse carrying out an assessment must keep in mind that self-concept and its components are dynamic and variable. For example, a woman may have a consistent self-concept until her first pregnancy. At that time, the many physiologic changes of pregnancy may cause her body image to change. She may be comfortable and enjoy the "glow of pregnancy," or she may feel like a "bloated cow." Suddenly, her body image is the most important part of her self-concept, and how she handles it can increase or decrease her self-esteem or sense of personal identity. Thus, all the components are tied together, and each one affects the others.

Nurses can assess self-concept through eliciting patients' thoughts about themselves and their ability to navigate in the world. A patient's self-concept becomes evident during other parts of the assessment. Disheveled, sloppy physical appearance outside cultural norms is an indication of poor self-concept. Negative self-statements, such as "I could never do that," "I have no control over my life," and "I'm so stupid" reveal poor views of self. The nurse must be aware of his or her own self-concept and its influence on the patient during the assessment because it can shape the nurse's view of the patient. For example, a nurse who is self-confident and feels inwardly scornful of a patient who lacks such confidence may intimidate the patient through unconscious behaviors or inconsiderate comments.

A useful approach to measuring self-concept is asking the patient to draw a self-portrait. For many patients, drawing is much easier than writing and serves as an excellent technique for monitoring changes. Interpretation of self-concept from drawings focuses on size, color, level of detail, pressure, line quality, symmetry, and placement. Low self-esteem is expressed by small size, lack of color variation, and sparse details. Powerlessness and feelings of inadequacy are expressed through lack of head, mouth, arms, feet, or eyes. A lack of symmetry (placement of figure parts or entire drawings off-center) represents feelings of insecurity and inadequacy. As self-esteem builds, size increases, color tends to become more varied and brighter, and more detail appears. Figure 10.2 shows a self-portrait of a patient at the beginning of treatment for depression and another drawn 3 months later.

Body Image

Body image represents a person's beliefs and attitudes about his or her body and includes such dimensions as size (large or small) and attractiveness (pretty or ugly). People who are satisfied with their body have a more positive body image than those who are not satisfied. Generally, women attach more importance to their body image than do men and may even define themselves in terms of their body.

Patients express body image beliefs through statements about their bodies. Statements, such as "I feel so ugly," "I'm so fat," and "No one will want to have sex with me," express negative body images. Nonverbal behaviors indicating problems with body image include avoiding looking at or touching a body part, hiding the body in oversized clothing, or bandaging a particularly sensitive area, such as a mole on the face. Cultural differences must be considered when evaluating behavior related to body image. For example, the expectation of some cultures is

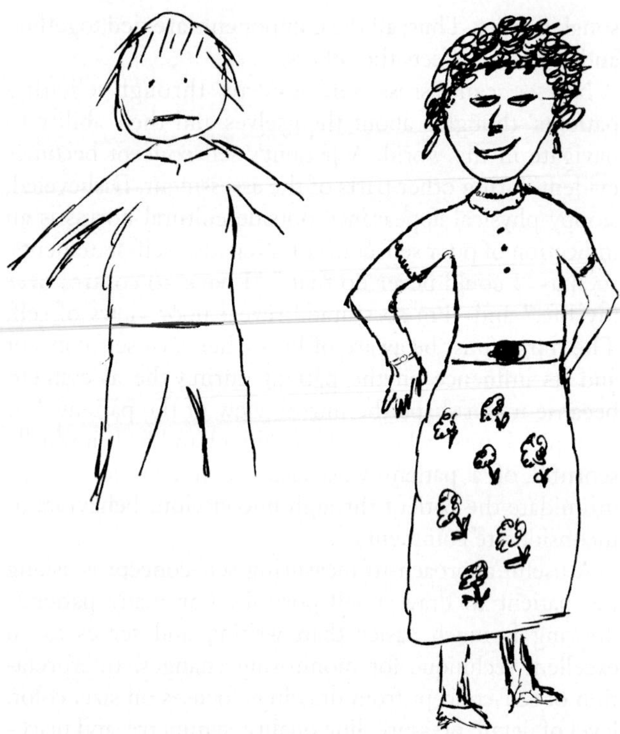

FIGURE 10.2. *Left:* Self-portrait of a 52-year-old woman at first group session following discharge from hospital for treatment of depression. *Right:* Self-portrait after 3 months of weekly group interventions.

that women and girls will keep their bodies completely covered and wear loose-fitting garments.

> **• NCLEXNOTE**
> Be prepared to assess reactions to a body image change (e.g., loss of vision, paralysis, colostomy, amputation).

Self-Esteem

Self-esteem is the person's attitude about the self. Self-esteem differs from body image because it concerns satisfaction with one's overall self. People who feel good about themselves are more likely to have the confidence to try new health behaviors. They are also less likely to be depressed. Negative self-esteem statements include "I'm a worthless person" and "I never do anything right."

Personal Identity

Personal identity is knowing "who I am" and is formed through meeting the numerous biologic, psychological, and social challenges and demands throughout the stages of life. Every life experience and interaction contributes to knowing oneself better. Personal identity allows people to establish boundaries and understand personal strengths and limitations. In some psychiatric disorders, individuals cannot separate themselves from others, which shows that their personal identity is not strongly developed. A problem with personal identity is difficult to assess. Statements such as, "I'm just like my mother and she was always in trouble," "I become whatever my current boyfriend wants me to be," and "I can't make a decision unless I check it out first" are all statements that require further exploration into the person's view of self.

Stress and Coping Patterns

Everyone has stress (see Chapter 14). Sometimes, the experience of stress contributes to the development of mental disorders. Identification of major stresses in a patient's life helps the nurse to understand the person and support the use of successful coping behaviors in the future. The nurse should explore with the patient past stresses and coping mechanisms (see Chapter 14) to discover coping mechanisms that are helpful and then, encourage their use. He or she also ascertains coping mechanisms that are not useful, such as use of drugs or alcohol.

> **• NCLEXNOTE**
> Each assessment should always focus on stress and coping patterns. Identifying how a patient copes with stress can be used as a basis of care in all nursing situations. Include content from Chapter 14 when studying these concepts.

Risk Assessment

Risk factors are those characteristics, conditions, situations, or events that increase the patient's vulnerability to threats to safety or well-being. Throughout this text, the sections concerning risk factors focus on the following:

- Risks to the patient's safety
- Risks for developing psychiatric disorders
- Risks for increasing, or exacerbating, symptoms and impairment in an individual who already has a psychiatric disorder.

Consideration of risk factors involving patient safety should be included in each assessment. Examples of these risks include the risk for suicide and violence toward others or the risk for events, such as falling, seizures, allergic reactions, or elopement (unauthorized absence from health care facility). Nurses must assess some of these risk factors on a priority basis. For example, they must assess the patient's risk for violence or suicide and take measures to prevent injury, such as implementing environmental constraints, before addressing other assessment factors.

Suicidal Ideation

During the assessment, the nurse needs to listen closely to whether the patient describes or mentions thinking about self-harm. If the patient does not openly express ideas of self-harm, it is necessary to ask in a straightforward and gentle manner, "Have you ever thought about injuring or killing yourself?" If the patient answers, "Yes, I am thinking about it right now," the nurse knows not to leave the patient unobserved and to institute suicide precautions as indicated by the facility protocols. General questions to ask to ascertain suicidal ideation follow:

- Have you ever tried to harm or kill yourself?
- Do you have thoughts of suicide at this time? If yes, do you have a plan? If yes, can you tell me the details of the plan?
- Do you have the means to carry out this plan? (If the plan requires a weapon, does the patient have it available?)
- Have you made preparations for your death (e.g., writing a note to loved ones, putting finances in order, giving away possessions)?
- Has a significant episode in your life caused you to think this way (e.g., recent loss of spouse or job)?

Assaultive or Homicidal Ideation

When assessing a patient, the nurse also needs to listen carefully to any delusions or hallucinations that the patient shares. If the patient gives any indication that he or she must or is being told to harm someone, the nurse must first think of self-safety and institute assaultive precautions as indicated by the facility protocols. General questions to ascertain assaultive or homicidal ideation follow:

- Do you intend to harm someone? If yes, who?
- Do you have a plan? If yes, what are the details of the plan?
- Do you have the means to carry out the plan? (If the plan requires a weapon, is it readily available?)

Social Domain

The assessment continues with examination of the patient's social domain. The nurse inquires about interactions with others in the family and community (work, church, or other organizations); the patient's parents and their marital relationship; the patient's place in birth order; names and ages of any siblings; and relationships with spouse, siblings, and children. The nurse also assesses work and education history and community activities. The nurse observes how the patient relates to any family or friends who may be in attendance. This component of the assessment helps the nurse anticipate how the patient may get along with other patients in an inpatient setting. It also allows the nurse to plan for any anticipated difficulties.

Functional Status

Assessment is necessary to understand how the patient functions in a social setting, whether with family or in the community. How the patient copes with strangers and those with whom he or she does not get along is important information. Many nurses use the Global Assessment of Functioning (GAF) scale (discussed in Chapter 2) as a single measure of functioning.

Social Systems

A significant component of the patient's life involves the social systems in which he or she may be enmeshed. The social systems to examine include the family, the culture to which the patient belongs, and the community in which he or she lives.

Family Assessment

How the patient fits in with and relates to his or her family is important to know. See Chapter 13 for a discussion of a comprehensive family assessment. General questions to ask include the following:

- Whom do you consider family?
- How important to you is your family?
- How does your family make decisions?
- What are the roles in your family and who fills them?
- Where do you fit in your family?
- With whom in your family do you get along best?
- With whom in your family do you have the most conflict?
- Who in your family is supportive of you?

Cultural Assessment

Culture can profoundly affect a person's world view. Culture helps a person frame beliefs about life, death, health and illness, and roles and relationships. During cultural assessment, the nurse must consider factors that influence the manifestations of the current mental disorder. For example, a patient mentions "speaking in tongues." The nurse may identify this experience as a hallucination when, in fact, the patient was having a religious experience common within some branches of Christianity. In this instance, knowing and understanding such religious practices will prevent a misinterpretation of the symptoms.

If the patient can respond, the nurse should ask the following questions:

- To what cultural group do you belong?
- Were you raised in an ethnic community?
- How do you define health?
- How do you define illness?
- How do you define good and evil?
- What do you do to get better when you are physically ill? Mentally ill?
- Whom do you see for help when you are physically ill? Mentally ill?
- By what cultural rules or taboos do you try to live?
- Do you eat special foods?

Community Support and Resources

Many patients are connected to community resources, and the nurse needs to assess what they are and the patterns of usage. For example, a homeless patient may know of a church where he or she can sleep but may go there only on cold nights. Or a patient may go to the community center daily for lunch to be with other people.

Spiritual Assessment

Among the many definitions of spirituality is one offered by Burkhardt and Nagai-Jacobson (1997, p. 42). Spirituality is "the unifying force of a person; the essence of being that shapes, gives meaning to, and is aware of one's self-becoming. Spirituality permeates all of life and is manifested in one's being, knowing, and doing. It is expressed and experienced uniquely by each individual through and within connection to God, Life Force, the Absolute, the environment, nature, other people, and the self." Nurses must be clear about their own spirituality to be sure it does not interfere with assessment of the patient's spirituality. General questions to ask include the following:

- What gives your life meaning?
- What is the purpose of your life?
- What do you do to bring joy into your life?
- What life goals have you set for yourself?
- Do you think that stress in any way has caused your illness?
- Can you forgive others?
- Can you forgive yourself?
- Is your faith helpful to you in stressful situations?
- Is worship important to you?
- Do you participate in any religious activities?
- Do any religious beliefs control your life?
- Do you believe in God or a higher power?
- Do you pray?
- Do you meditate?
- Do you feel connected with the world?

• NCLEXNOTE

NCLEXNOTE Identify emotional problems that are related to religion or spiritual beliefs such as conflict between recommended treatment and beliefs.

Occupational Status

The nurse should document the occupation the patient is now in as well as a history of jobs. If the patient has changed jobs frequently, the nurse should ask about the reasons. Perhaps the patient has faced such problems as an inability to focus on the job at hand or to get along with others. If so, such issues require further exploration.

Economic Status

Finances are very private for many people; thus, the nurse must ask questions about economic status carefully. What the nurse needs to ascertain is not specific dollar amounts, but whether the patient feels stressed by finances and has enough for basic needs.

Legal Status

Because of laws governing mentally ill people, ascertaining the patient's correct age, marital status, and any legal guardianship is important. The nurse may need to check the patient's medical records for this information.

Quality of Life

The patient's perspective on quality of life means how the patient rates his or her life. Does a patient feel his life is poor because he cannot purchase everything he wants? Does another patient feel blessed because the sun is shining today? Listening carefully to the patient's discussion of his or her life and how he or she measures the quality of that life provides important information about self-concept, coping skills, desires, and dreams.

NURSING DIAGNOSIS

After completing an assessment of the patient, the nurse generates nursing diagnoses based on the assessment data. With experience, the nurse can easily cluster the assessment data to support one nursing diagnosis over another. Nursing diagnoses are universally used in nursing practice and education. Because nursing diagnoses provide the basis for planning nursing interventions, they are used in diverse practice settings in multiple patient populations to assist patients to achieve positive health outcomes (Delaney, Herr, Maas, & Specht, 2000). In this text, the North American Nursing Diagnosis Association (NANDA) will be used. See Box 10.5 for more information. Each disorder will present data to support related nursing diagnoses.

KEY CONCEPT A **nursing diagnosis** is a clinical judgment about an identified problem or need that requires nursing interventions and nursing management. It is based on data generated from a nursing assessment. A formal nursing diagnosis statement includes **defining characteristics** and related factors (Carpenito-Moyet, 2005).

DEVELOPING PATIENT OUTCOMES

Mutually agreed-upon goals flow from the nursing diagnoses and provide guidance in determining appropriate interventions. Initial outcomes are determined and then are monitored and evaluated throughout the care process. Measuring outcomes not only demonstrates clinical effectiveness, but also helps to promote rational clinical decision making and is reflective of the nursing interventions.

KEY CONCEPT Outcomes are the patient's response to nursing care at a given point in time. An outcome is concise, stated in few words and in neutral terms. Outcomes describe a patient's state, behavior, or perception. Outcomes are variable and can be measured (Table 10.2)

Outcomes focus on the individual recipient of care (patient or family caregivers) and include patient statements, behaviors, or perceptions that are sensitive to or influenced by nursing interventions (Moorhead, Johnson, & Mass, 2004). Outcomes can also be nonspecific (i.e., not diagnosis-specific, meaning the outcome does not show resolution of the diagnosis). Indicators answer the question, "How close is the recipient moving toward the outcome?" The indicator represents the dimensions of the outcome. **Outcome indicators** repre-

BOX 10.5

Selected Nanda Nursing Diagnoses (2007–2008)

Activity intolerance
Risk for activity intolerance
Risk-Prone Health Behavior
Ineffective airway clearance
Latex allergy response
Risk for latex allergy response
Anxiety
Death anxiety
Risk for sudden infant death syndrome
Risk for aspiration
Risk for impaired parent/child/infant attachment
Autonomic dysreflexia
Risk for autonomic dysreflexia
Disturbed body image
Risk for imbalanced body temperature
Bowel incontinence
Effective breastfeeding
Ineffective breastfeeding
Interrupted breastfeeding
Ineffective breathing pattern
Decreased cardiac output
Caregiver role strain
Risk for caregiver role strain
Impaired verbal communication
Readiness for enhanced communication
Readiness for enhanced comfort
Decisional conflict
Parental role conflict
Acute confusion
Chronic confusion
Risk for acute confusion
Constipation
Perceived constipation
Risk for constipation
Contamination
Risk for contamination
Ineffective coping
Readiness for enhanced decision-making
Impaired dentition
Risk for delayed development
Diarrhea
Risk for disuse syndrome
Deficient diversional activity
Disturbed energy field
Impaired environmental interpretation syndrome
Adult failure to thrive
Risk for falls
Dysfunctional family processes: alcoholism
Interrupted family processes
Readiness for enhanced family processes
Fatigue
Fear
Deficient fluid volume
Excess fluid volume
Readiness for enhanced fluid volume
Risk for deficient fluid volume
Risk for unbalanced fluid volume
Risk for unstable blood glucose
Impaired gas exchange
Grieving
Complicated grieving
Risk for complicated grieving
Delayed growth and development
Risk for disproportionate growth
Ineffective health maintenance
Health-seeking behaviors (specify)
Impaired home maintenance
Hopelessness
Readiness for enhanced hope
Hyperthermia
Hypothermia
Disturbed personal identity
Bowel incontinence
Impaired urinary elimination
Functional urinary incontinence
Readiness for enhanced coping
Ineffective community coping
Readiness for enhanced community coping

(Continued on following page)

BOX 10.5

Selected Nanda Nursing Diagnoses (2007–2008) (continued)

Defensive coping
Compromised family coping
Disabled family coping
Readiness for enhanced family coping
Ineffective denial
Readiness for enhanced immunizations
Risk for compromised human dignity
Ineffective infant feeding pattern
Risk for infection
Risk for injury
Risk for perioperative-positioning injury
Decreased intracranial adaptive capacity
Deficient knowledge (specify)
Readiness for enhanced knowledge
Risk for impaired liver function
Sedentary lifestyle
Risk for loneliness
Impaired bed mobility
Impaired physical mobility
Impaired wheelchair mobility
Moral distress
Nausea
Unilateral neglect
Noncompliance
Imbalanced nutrition: less than body requirements
Imbalanced nutrition: more than body requirements
Risk for imbalanced nutrition: more than body requirements
Readiness for enhanced nutrition
Impaired oral mucous membrane
Acute pain
Chronic pain
Impaired parenting
Risk for impaired parenting
Readiness for enhanced parenting
Risk for peripheral neurovascular dysfunction
Risk for poisoning
Posttrauma syndrome
Risk for posttrauma syndrome
Powerlessness
Risk for powerlessness
Readiness for enhanced power
Ineffective protection
Rape-trauma syndrome
Rape-trauma syndrome: compound reaction
Rape-trauma syndrome: silent reaction
Relocation stress syndrome
Risk for relocation stress syndrome
Ineffective role performance
Bathing/hygiene self-care deficit
Dressing/grooming self-care deficit
Feeding self-care deficit
Toileting self-care deficit
Readiness for enhanced self-care
Readiness for enhanced self-concept
Chronic low self-esteem
Reflex urinary incontinence
Stress urinary incontinence
Total urinary incontinence
Urge urinary incontinence
Risk for urge urinary incontinence
Overflow urinary incontinence
Disorganized infant behavior
Risk for disorganized infant behavior
Readiness for enhanced organized infantbehavior
Situational low self-esteem
Risk for situational low self-esteem
Self-mutilation
Impaired religiosity
Risk for self-mutilation
Disturbed sensory perception (specify: visual, auditory, kinesthetic, gustatory, tactile, olfactory)
Sexual dysfunction
Ineffective sexuality pattern
Impaired skin integrity
Risk for impaired skin integrity
Sleep deprivation
Readiness for enhanced sleep
Insomnia
Impaired social interaction
Social isolation
Chronic sorrow
Spiritual distress
Risk for spiritual distress
Readiness for enhanced spiritual well-being
Stress overload
Risk for suffocation
Risk for suicide
Delayed surgical recovery
Impaired swallowing
Ineffective therapeutic regimen management
Ineffective family therapeutic regimen management
Ineffective community therapeutic regimen management
Readiness for enhanced therapeutic regimen management
Ineffective thermoregulation
Disturbed thought processes
Impaired tissue integrity
Ineffective tissue perfusion (specify type: renal, cerebral, cardiopulmonary, gastrointestinal, peripheral)
Impaired transfer ability
Risk for trauma
Impaired urinary elimination
Impaired spontaneous ventilation
Dysfunctional ventilatory weaning response
Risk for other-directed violence
Risk for self-directed violence
Impaired walking
Wandering

NANDA-I (2007) NANDA-I Nursing Diagnosis: Definitions & Classifications 2007–2008. Author: Philadelphia.

sent or describe patient status, behaviors, or perceptions evaluated during a patient's assessment. Indicators are a measurement of patient progress in relation to the patient outcomes and can serve as intermediate outcomes in a standardized care plan.

Nurses are accountable for documenting patient outcomes, nursing interventions, and any changes in diagnosis, care plan, or both. Patient responses to care are documented as changes in behavior or knowledge and can include the degree of satisfaction with the health care

Table 10.2 Example of Outcomes

Diagnosis	Outcome	Intervention
Impaired social Interaction (isolates self from others)	Social involvement **Indicators** a. Interact with other patients. b. Attend group meetings.	Using a contract format, explain role and responsibility of patients

provided (Kleinpell, 2003). Outcomes can be expressed in terms of the patient's actual responses (no longer reports hearing voices) or the status of a nursing diagnosis at a point in time after implementation of nursing interventions, such as Caregiver Role Strain resolved. This documentation is important for further research, cost, and continuity and quality of care studies.

NURSING INTERVENTIONS

Interventions can be either nurse-initiated treatment, which is an autonomous action in response to a nursing diagnosis, or physician-initiated treatment, which is a response to a medical diagnosis as a result of a "physician's order."

KEY CONCEPT Nursing interventions are nursing activities that promote and foster health, assess dysfunction, assist patients to regain or improve their coping abilities, or prevent additional disabilities (ANA et al., 2000).

The Nursing Interventions Classification (NIC) is an extensive system consisting of specific interventions, with discrete activities for each (Dochterman & Bulechek, 2004). This text uses many NIC interventions and those identified in the *Psychiatric-Mental Health Nursing: Scope and Standards of Practice.* (ANA et al., 2007) as well as others reported in the psychiatric nursing literature.

Interventions for the Biologic Domain

Biologic interventions focus on physical functioning and are directed toward the patient's self-care, activities and exercise, sleep, nutrition, relaxation, hydration, and thermoregulation as well as pain management and medication management. In the NIC taxonomy, these interventions are found within the physiologic basic and physiologic complex domains.

Promotion of Self-Care Activities

Self-care is the ability to perform activities of daily living (ADLs) successfully. Many patients with psychiatric–mental health problems can manage self-care activities such as bathing, dressing appropriately, selecting adequate nutrition, and sleeping regularly. Others cannot manage such self-care activities, either because of their symptoms or as a result of the side effects of medications.

In the inpatient setting, the psychiatric nurse structures the patient's activities so that basic self-care activities are completed. During acute phases of psychiatric disorders, the inability to attend to basic self-care tasks, such as getting dressed, is very common. Thus, ability to complete personal hygiene activities (e.g., dental care, grooming) is monitored, and patients are assisted in completing such activities. In a psychiatric facility, patients are encouraged and expected to develop independence in completing these basic self-care activities. In the community, monitoring these basic self-care activities is always a part of the nursing visit or clinic appointment.

Activity and Exercise Interventions

In some psychiatric disorders (e.g., schizophrenia), people become sedentary and appear to lack the motivation to complete ADLs. This lack of motivation is part of the disorder and requires nursing intervention. In addition, side effects of medication often include sedation and lethargy. Encouraging regular activity and exercise can improve general well-being and physical health. In some instances, exercise behavior becomes an abnormal focus of attention, as may be observed in some patients with anorexia nervosa.

When assuming the responsibility of direct care provider, the nurse can help patients identify realistic activities and exercise goals. As leader or manager of a psychiatric unit, the nurse can influence ward routine. Alternately, the nurse can delegate activity and exercise interventions to nurses' aides. Some institutions have other professionals (e.g., recreational therapists) available for the implementation of exercise programs. As a case manager, the nurse should consider the activity needs of individuals when coordinating care.

Sleep Interventions

Many psychiatric disorders and medications are associated with sleep disturbances. Sleep is also disrupted in patients with dementia; such patients may have difficulty falling asleep or may frequently awaken during the night. In dementia of the Alzheimer's type, individuals may reverse their sleeping patterns by napping during the day and staying awake at night.

Nonpharmacologic interventions are always used first because of the side-effect risks associated with the use of sedatives and hypnotics (see Chapter 8). Sleep interventions to communicate to patients include the following:

- Go to bed only when tired or sleepy.
- Establish a consistent bedtime routine.
- Avoid stimulating foods, beverages, or medications.
- Avoid naps in the late afternoon or evening.

- Eat lightly before retiring and limit fluid intake.
- Use bed only for sleep or intimacy.
- Avoid emotional stimulation before bedtime.
- Use behavioral and relaxation techniques.
- Limit distractions.

Nutrition Interventions

Psychiatric disorders and medication side effects can affect eating behaviors. For varying reasons, some patients eat too little, whereas others eat too much. For instance, homeless patients with mental illness have difficulty maintaining adequate nutrition because of their deprived lifestyle. Substance abuse also interferes with maintaining adequate nutrition, either through stimulation or suppression of appetite or neglecting nutrition because of drug-seeking behavior. Thus, nutrition interventions should be specific and relevant to the individual's circumstances and mental health. In addition, recommended daily nutritional allowances are important in the promotion of physical and mental health, and nurses should consider them when planning care.

Some psychiatric symptoms involve changes in perceptions of food, appetite, and eating habits. If a patient believes that food is poisonous, he or she may eat sparingly or not at all. Interventions are then necessary to address the suspiciousness as well as to encourage adequate intake of recommended daily allowances. Allowing patients to examine foods, participate in preparations, and test the safety of the meal by eating slowly or after everyone else may be necessary. For patients who are paranoid, it is sometimes helpful to serve prepackaged foods.

Relaxation Interventions

Relaxation promotes comfort, reduces anxiety, alleviates stress, eases pain, and prevents aggression. It can diminish the effects of hallucinations and delusions. The many different relaxation techniques used as mental health interventions range from simple deep breathing to biofeedback to hypnosis. Although some techniques, such as biofeedback, require additional training and, in some instances, certification, nurses can easily apply simple relaxation, distraction, and imagery techniques.

Simple relaxation techniques encourage and elicit relaxation to decrease undesirable signs and symptoms. **Distraction** is the purposeful focusing of attention away from undesirable sensations, and **guided imagery** is the purposeful use of imagination to achieve relaxation or direct attention away from undesirable sensations (Table 10.3) These interventions are helpful for people experiencing anxiety; guided imagery is especially useful in stress management.

Relaxation techniques that involve physical touch (e.g., back rubs) usually are not used for people with mental disorders. Touching and massaging usually are not appropriate, especially for those who have a history of physical or sexual abuse. Such patients may find touching too stimulating or misinterpret it as being sexual or aggressive.

Hydration Interventions

Assessing fluid status and monitoring fluid intake and output are often important interventions. Overhydration or underhydration can be a symptom of a disorder. For example, some patients with psychotic disorders experience chronic fluid imbalance. Many psychiatric medications affect fluid and electrolyte balance (see Chapter 8). For example, when taking lithium carbonate, patients must have adequate fluid intake and pay special attention to testing serum sodium levels. Interventions that help patients understand the relationship of medications to fluid and electrolyte balance are important in their overall care.

Thermoregulation Interventions

Many psychiatric disorders can disturb the body's normal temperature regulation. Thus, patients cannot sense temperature increases or decreases and consequently cannot protect themselves from extremes of hot or cold. This problem is especially difficult for people who are homeless or live outside the protected environments of institutions and boarding homes. In addition, many psychiatric medications affect the ability to regulate body temperature.

Interventions include educating patients about the problem of thermoregulation, identifying potential extremes in temperatures, and developing strategies to protect the patient from the adverse effects of temperature changes. For example, reminding patients to wear coats and sweaters in the winter or to wear loose, lightweight garments in the summer may prevent frostbite or heat exhaustion, respectively.

Pain Management

Psychiatric nurses are more likely to provide care to patients experiencing chronic pain than acute pain. However, a single intervention is seldom successful for relieving chronic pain. In some instances, pain is managed by medication; in other instances, nonpharmacologic strategies, such as simple relaxation techniques, distraction, or imagery, are used. Indeed, relaxation is one of the most widely used cognitive and behavioral approaches to pain. Education, stress management techniques, hypnosis, and biofeedback are also used in pain management. Physical agents include heat and cold therapy, exercise, and transcutaneous nerve stimulation.

Table 10.3 Relaxation Techniques: Descriptions and Implementation

Simple Relaxation Techniques	Distraction	Guided Imagery
• Create a quiet, nondisrupting environment with dim lights and a comfortable temperature. • Instruct the patient to assume a relaxed position, wearing loose and comfortable clothing. • Instruct the patient to relax and to let the sensations happen. • Use a low tone of voice with a slow, rhythmic pace of words. • Instruct the patient to take an initial slow, deep breath (abdominal breathing) while thinking about pleasant events. • Use soothing music (without words) to enhance relaxation. • Reinforce the use of relaxation by praising efforts and helping the patient to schedule time regularly for it. • Evaluate and document the patient's response to relaxation.	• Distraction techniques include music, counting, television, reading, play, and exercise. Help the patient choose a technique that will work for him or her. • Advise the patient to practice the distraction technique before he or she will need to use it. • Have the patient develop a specific plan for how and when he or she will use distraction. • Evaluate and document the patient's response to distraction.	• Help the patient choose a particular guided imagery technique (alone or with others). • Discuss an image the patient has experienced as pleasurable and relaxing, such as lying on a beach, watching snow fall, floating on a raft, or watching the sun set. • Individualize the images chosen, considering religious or spiritual beliefs, artistic interests, or other individual preferences. • Make suggestions to induce relaxation (e.g., peaceful images, pleasant sensations, or rhythmic breathing). • Use modulated voice when guiding the imagery experience. • Have the patient travel mentally to the scene, and assist in describing the setting in detail. • Use permissive directions and suggestions when leading the imagery, such as "perhaps," "if you wish," or "you might like." • Have the patient slowly experience the scene. How does it look? smell? sound? feel? taste? • Use words or phrases that convey pleasurable images, such as floating, melting, and releasing. • Develop cleansing or clearing portion of imagery (e.g., all pain appears as red dust and washes downstream in a creek as you enter). • Assist the patient in developing a method of ending the imagery technique, such as counting slowly while breathing deeply. • Encourage expression of thoughts and feelings regarding the experience. • Prepare the patient for unexpected (but often therapeutic) experiences, such as crying. • Evaluate and document the patient's response.

Adapted from Dochtermen, J., & Bulechek, G. (2004). *Nursing interventions classification (NIC)* (4th ed.). St. Louis: Mosby.

The key to managing pain is identifying how it disrupts the patient's personal, social, professional, and family life. Education focusing on the pain, use of medications for treatment, and development of cognitive skills are important pain management components. In some cases, redefining treatment success as improvement in functioning, rather than alleviation of pain, may be necessary. The interaction between stress and pain is important; that is, increased stress leads to increased pain. Patients can better manage their pain when stress is reduced.

Medication Management

The psychiatric–mental health nurse uses many medication management interventions to help patients maintain therapeutic regimens. Medication management involves more than the actual administration of medications. Nurses also assess medication effectiveness and side effects and consider drug–drug interactions. Monitoring the amount of lethal prescription medication is particularly important. For example, check if patients have old prescriptions of tricyclic antidepressants in their medicine cabinets. Treatment with psychopharmacologic agents can be lengthy because of the chronic nature of many disorders; many patients remain on medication regimens for years, never becoming free of medication. Thus, medication education is an ongoing intervention that requires careful documentation. Medication follow-up may include home visits as well as telephone calls.

Interventions for the Psychological Domain

A major emphasis in psychiatric–mental health nursing is on the psychological domain: emotion, behavior, and cognition. The nurse–patient relationship serves as the basis for interventions directed toward the psychological domain. Because the therapeutic relationship was extensively discussed in Chapter 9, it is not covered in this chapter. This section does cover counseling, conflict resolution, bibliotherapy, reminiscence, behavior therapy, psychoeducation, health teaching, and spiritual interventions. Cognitive interventions are presented in Chapter 11. Chapter 7 presents the theoretic basis for many of these interventions.

Counseling Interventions

Counseling interventions are specific, time-limited interactions between a nurse and a patient, family, or group experiencing immediate or ongoing difficulties related to their health or well-being. Counseling is usually short term and focuses on improving coping abilities, reinforcing healthy behaviors, fostering positive interactions, or preventing illness and disability. Counseling strategies are discussed throughout the text. Psychotherapy, which differs from counseling, is generally a long-term approach aimed at improving or helping patients regain previous health status and functional abilities. Mental health specialists, such as advanced practice nurses, use psychotherapy.

Conflict Resolution

A conflict involves an individual's perception, emotions, and behavior. In a conflict, a person believes that his or her own needs, interests, wants, or values are incompatible with someone else's. The individual experiences fear, sadness, bitterness, anger, hopelessness, or some combination of these emotions in response to the perceived threat. Consequently, the individual takes action to meet his or her own needs, a course of action that can potentially interfere with the other person's ability to do the same (Mayer, 2000).

Conflict resolution is a specific type of intervention through which the nurse helps patients resolve disagreements or disputes with family, friends, or other patients. Conflict can be positive if individuals see the problem as solvable and providing an opportunity for growth and interpersonal understanding. The nurse may be in the position of actually resolving a family conflict or teaching family members how to resolve their own conflicts positively. In addition, because nurses are in positions of leadership, they often need conflict resolution skills to settle employee conflicts.

Conflict Resolution Process

Calmness and objectivity are important in resolving any patient or family conflict. The desired outcome of conflict resolution is a "**win-win**" situation (in which the parties involved are satisfied with the outcomes). Conflict resolution includes the following steps:

1. Helping those involved identify the problem;
2. Developing expectations for a win-win situation;
3. Identifying interests;
4. Fostering creative brainstorming; and
5. Combining options into a win-win situation (Littlefield, Love, Peck, & Wertheim, 1993).

The first step in conflict management involves identifying the problem. Because the conflict exists, with each person thinking he or she has the solution, each must express a view of the problem and solution. During this phase, calming of emotions may be necessary. The next step involves developing expectations for a win-win situation by creating an atmosphere of mutual respect and trust. The nurse should avoid taking sides and reassure the involved parties that there may be a way to solve the problem and achieve an outcome about which everyone feels positive. Next, an exploration of underlying issues is important to elicit interest and response. Questions such as, "What do you really want?" or "What are you worried about?" often identify the real issues and target what could become acceptable outcomes. (Nurses need to determine whether they have any underlying issues by asking themselves the same questions.)

The next step, brainstorming creative options, can then occur. The nurse directs participants to create potential solutions. The nurse writes them down without allowing any criticism; deferring judgment of what has been said helps prevent premature rejection of good ideas. The final step involves combining the generated ideas into a win-win situation. The group develops solutions that meet many of the participants' key interests and usually represent new approaches that are acceptable to all (Littlefield et al., 1993).

Cultural Brokering in Patient–System Conflicts

At times, patients who are politically and economically powerless find themselves in conflict with the health care system. Differences in cultural values and languages between patients and health care organizations contribute to feelings of powerlessness. For example, migrant farm workers, people who are homeless, and people who need to make informed decisions under stressful conditions may be unable to navigate the health care system. The nurse can help to resolve such conflicts through **cultural brokering**, the act of bridging, linking, or mediating messages, instructions, and belief systems between groups of people of differing cultural systems to reduce conflict or produce change (Esperat, Inouye, Gonzalez, Owen, & Feng, 2004).

For the "nurse-as-broker" to be effective, he or she establishes and maintains a sense of connectedness or relationship with the patient. In turn, the nurse also establishes and cultivates networks with other health care facilities and resources. Cultural sensitivity enables the nurse to be aware of and sensitive to the needs of patients from a variety of cultures. Cultural competence is necessary for the brokering process to be effective.

Bibliotherapy

Bibliotherapy, sometimes referred to as bibliocounseling, is the reading of selected written materials to express feelings or gain insight under the guidance of a health care provider. The provider assigns and discusses with the patient a book, story, or article. The provider makes the assignment because he or she believes that the patient can receive therapeutic benefit from the reading. (It is assumed that the provider who assigned the reading has also read it.) The provider needs to consider the patient's reading level before making an assignment. If a patient has limited reading ability, the provider should not use bibliotherapy.

Literary works serve as a projective screen through which people see themselves in the story. Literature can help patients identify with characters and vicariously experience their reality. It can also expose patients to situations that they have not personally experienced—the vicarious experience allows growth in self-knowledge and compassion. Through reading, patients can enrich their lives in the following ways:

- *Catharsis:* expression of feelings stimulated by parallel experiences
- *Problem solving:* development of solutions to problems in the literature from practical ideas about problem solving
- *Insight:* increased self-awareness and understanding as the reader explores personal meaning from what is read
- *Anxiety reduction:* self-help written materials can reduce concerns about a diagnosed problem and treatment (Jones, 2002).

Reminiscence

Reminiscence, the thinking about or relating of past experiences, is used as a nursing intervention to enhance life review in older patients. Reminiscence encourages patients, either in individual or group settings, to discuss their past and review their lives. Through reminiscence, individuals can identify past coping strategies that can support them in current stressful situations. Patients can also use reminiscence to maintain self-esteem, stimulate thinking, and support the natural healing process of life review. Activities that facilitate reminiscence include writing an account of past events, making a tape recording and playing it back, explaining pictures in old family albums, drawing a family tree, and writing to old friends.

Behavior Therapy

Behavior therapy interventions focus on reinforcing or promoting desirable behaviors or altering undesirable ones. The basic premise is that, because most behaviors are learned, new functional behaviors can also be learned. Behaviors—not internal psychic processes—are the targets of the interventions. The models of behavioral theorists serve as a basis for these interventions (see Chapter 6).

Behavior Modification

Behavior modification is a specific, systematized behavior therapy technique that can be applied to individuals, groups, or systems. The aim of behavior modification is to reinforce desired behaviors and extinguish undesired ones. Desired behavior is rewarded to increase the likelihood that patients will repeat it, and over time, replace the problematic behavior with it. Behavior modification is used for various problematic behaviors, such as dysfunctional eating, addictions, anger management, impulse control, and often is used in the care of children and adolescents.

Token Economy

Used in inpatient settings and in group homes, a **token economy** applies behavior modification techniques to multiple behaviors. In a token economy, patients are rewarded with tokens for selected desired behaviors. They can use these tokens to purchase meals, leave the unit, watch television, or wear street clothes. In less restrictive environments, patients use tokens to purchase additional privileges, such as attending social events. Token economy systems have been especially effective in reinforcing positive behaviors in people who are developmentally disabled or have severe and persistent mental illnesses. The strategy also works with aggressive inpatients (Silverstein, Hatashita-Wong, & Bloch, 2002).

• NCLEXNOTE

NCLEXNOTE

Focus on helping patient achieve and maintain self-control of behavior (e.g., contract, behavior modification.)

Psychoeducation

Psychoeducation uses educational strategies to teach patients the skills they lack because of a psychiatric disorder. The goal of psychoeducation is a change in knowledge and behavior. Nurses use psychoeducation to meet the educational needs of patients by adapting teaching strategies to their disorder-related deficits. As patients gain skills, functioning improves. Some patients may need to learn how to maintain their morning hygiene. Others may need to understand their illness and cope with hearing voices that others do not hear.

Specific psychoeducation techniques are based on adult learning principles, such as beginning at the point the learner is currently at and building on his or her current experiences. Thus, the nurse assesses the patient's current skills and readiness to learn. From there, the nurse individualizes a teaching plan for each patient. He or she can conduct such teaching in a one-to-one situation or a group format.

Psychoeducation is a continuous process of assessing, setting goals, developing learning activities, and evaluating for changes in knowledge and behavior. Nurses use it with individuals, groups, families, and communities. Psychoeducation serves as a basis for psychosocial rehabilitation, a service-delivery approach for those with severe and persistent mental illness (see Chapter 18).

• NCLEXNOTE

Apply knowledge from social sciences to help patients manage responses to a psychiatric disorder and emotional problems.

Health Teaching

Health teaching is one of the standards of care for the psychiatric nurse (ANA et al., 2007). Teaching methods should be appropriate to the patients development level, learning needs, readiness, ability to learn, language preference, and culture. Based on principles of learning, health teaching involves transmitting new information to the patient and providing constructive feedback and positive rewards, practice sessions, homework, and experimental learning. Health teaching is the integration of principles of teaching and learning with the knowledge of health and illness (Fig. 10.3).

Thus, in health teaching, the psychiatric nurse attends to potential health care problems other than mental disorders and emotional problems. For example, if a person has diabetes mellitus and is taking insulin, the nurse provides health care teaching related to diabetes and the interaction of this problem with the mental disorder.

Spiritual Interventions

Spiritual care is based on an assessment of the patient's spiritual needs. A nonjudgmental relationship and just "being with" (not doing for) the patient are key to pro-

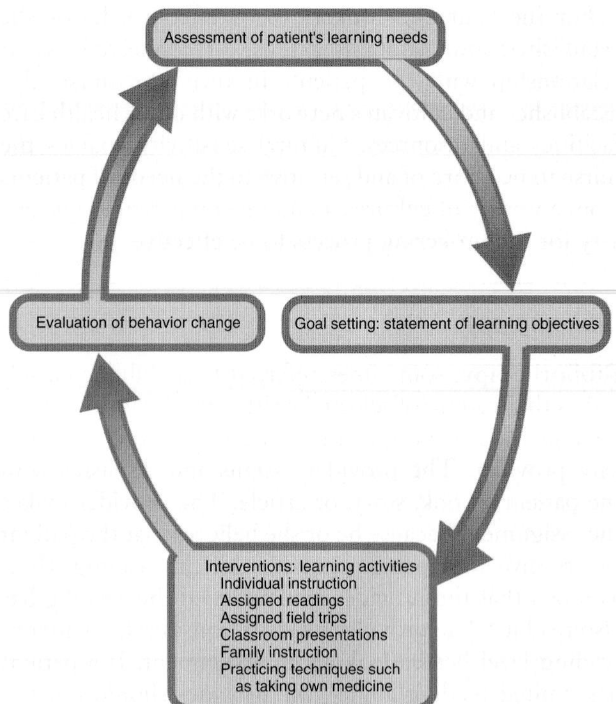

FIGURE 10.3. Teaching evaluation model. (Adapted from Rankin, S., & Stallings, K. [1990]. *Patient education* [p. 252]. Philadelphia: J. B. Lippincott.)

viding spiritual intervention. In some instances, patients ask to see a religious leader. Nurses should always respect and never deny these requests. To assist people in spiritual distress, the nurse should know and understand the beliefs and practices of various spiritual groups. **Spiritual support**, assisting patients to feel balance and connection within their relationships, involves listening to expressions of loneliness, using empathy, and providing patients with desired spiritual articles.

Interventions for the Social Domain

The social domain includes the individual's environment and its effect on his or her responses to mental disorders and distress. Interventions within the social domain are geared toward couples, families, friends, and large and small social groups, with special attention given to ethnicity and community interactions. In some instances, nurses design interventions that affect a patient's environment, such as helping a family member decide to place a loved one in long-term care. In other instances, the nurse actually modifies the environment to promote positive behaviors. Group and family interventions are discussed in Chapters 12 and 13, respectively.

Social Behavior and Privilege Systems in Inpatient Units

In psychiatric units, unrelated strangers who have problems interacting live together in close quarters. For this reason, most psychiatric units develop a list of behavioral expectations, called *unit rules* that staff members post and explain to patients upon admittance. Their purpose is to facilitate a comfortable and safe environment; they have little to do with the patients' reasons for admission. Getting up at certain times, showering before breakfast, making the bed, and not visiting in others' rooms are typical expectations. It is usually the nurse manager who oversees the operation of the unit and implementation of privilege systems.

Most psychiatric facilities use a privilege system to protect patients and to reinforce unit rules and other appropriate behavior (also see the previous section discussing a token economy). The more appropriate the behavior, the more privileges of freedom the person has. Privileges are based on the assessment of a patient's risk to harm himself or herself or others and ability to follow treatment regimens. For example, a patient with few privileges may be required to stay on the unit and eat only with other patients. A patient with full privileges may have freedom to leave the unit and go outside the hospital and into the community for short periods.

Milieu Therapy

Milieu therapy provides a stable and coherent social organization to facilitate an individual's treatment. (The terms *milieu therapy* and *therapeutic environment* are often used interchangeably.) In milieu therapy, the design of the physical surroundings, structure of patient activities, and promotion of a stable social structure and cultural setting enhance the setting's therapeutic potential. A therapeutic milieu facilitates patient interactions and promotes personal growth. Milieu therapy is the responsibility of the nurse in collaboration with the patient and other health care providers. The key concepts of milieu therapy include containment, validation, structured interaction, and open communication.

Containment

Containment is the process of providing safety and security and involves the patient's access to food and shelter. In a well-contained milieu, patients feel safe from their illnesses and protected against social stigma. The physical surroundings are also important in this process and should be clean and comfortable, with special attention paid to promoting a noninstitutionalized environment. Pictures on walls, comfortable furniture, and soothing colors help patients relax. Most facilities encourage patients and nursing staff to wear street clothes, which helps decrease the formalized nature of hospital settings and promotes nurse–patient relationships.

Therapeutic milieus emphasize patient involvement in treatment decisions and operation of the unit; nurses should encourage freedom of movement within the contained environment. Patients participate in maintaining the quality of the physical surroundings, assuming responsibility for making their own beds, attending to their own belongings, and keeping an acceptable living area. Families are viewed as a part of the patient's life, and ties are maintained. In most inpatient settings, specific times are set for family interaction, education, and treatment. Family involvement is often a criterion for admission for treatment, and the involvement may include regular family attendance at therapy sessions.

Validation

In a therapeutic environment, **validation** is another process that affirms patient individuality. Staff–patient interactions should constantly reaffirm the patient's humanity and human rights. Any interaction a staff member initiates with a patient should reflect his or her respect for that patient. Patients must believe that staff members truly like and respect them.

Structured Interaction

One of the most interesting milieu concepts is **structured interaction**: purposeful interaction that allows patients to interact with others in a useful way. For instance, the daily community meeting provides structure to explain unit rules and consequences of violations. Ideally, patients who are either elected or volunteer for the responsibility assume leadership for these meetings. In the meeting, the group discusses behavioral expectations, such as making beds daily, appropriate dress, and rules for leaving the unit. Usually, there are other rules, such as no fighting or name calling (Table 10.4).

In some instances, the treatment team assigns structured interactions to specific patients as part of their treatment. Specific attitudes or approaches are directed toward individual patients who benefit from a particular type of interaction. Nurses consistently assume indulgence, flexibility, passive or active friendliness, matter-of-fact attitude, casualness, watchfulness, or kind firmness when interacting with specific patients. For example, if a patient is known to overreact and dramatize events, the staff may provide a matter-of-fact attitude when the patient engages in dramatic behavior.

Open Communication

In **open communication,** staff and patient willingly share information. Staff members invite patient self-disclosure within the support of a nurse–patient relationship. In addition, they provide a model of effective communication when interacting with one another as well as with patients. They arrange an environment to facilitate optimal interaction and resocialization. Support, attention, praise, and reassurance given to patients improve self-esteem and increase confidence. Patient education is

Table 10.4 Patient-Staff Community Meeting

Goal	Implementation
Plan ahead.	• Designate leader and several deputy leaders. • Hold brief meeting with staff.
Operate the meeting.	• Establish rules and norms. • Announce the purpose, format, and rules (include patients who know the routine). • Keep meeting brief. • Refer treatment questions to outside of meeting.
Get everyone involved.	• Ask everyone to introduce themselves. • Address individuals by name. • Use structured exercises to engage all patients. • Delegate tasks of meeting to individuals.
Infuse energy.	• Use exercises to mobilize energy. • Use humor and empathy. • Maintain a lively and interesting approach.
Choose relevant topics.	• Focus on discussion of issues that affect all. • Deal with difficult issues calmly and frankly. • Affirm rules and norms.
Address unit process.	• Discuss needs of unit each meeting: containment, structure, support, involvement, validation. • Discuss strategies.

From Kahn, F. (1994). The patient-staff community meeting: Old tools, new rules. *Journal of Psychosocial Nursing, 32*(8), 23–26.

also a part of this support, as are directions to foster coping skills.

Milieu Therapy in Different Settings

Milieu therapy is applied in various settings. In long-term care settings, the therapeutic milieu becomes essential because patients may reside there for months or years. These patients typically have schizophrenia or developmental disabilities. Structure in daily living is important to the successful functioning of the individuals and the overall group but must be applied within the context of individual needs. For example, if a patient cannot get up one morning in time to complete assigned tasks (e.g., showering or making a bed) because of a personal crisis the night before, the nurse should consider the situation compassionately and flexibly, not applying the "consequences" rule or taking away the patient's privileges. In turn, the nurse must weigh individual needs against the collective needs of all the patients. For the patient who is consistently late for treatment activities, the nurse should apply the rules of the unit, even if it means taking away privileges.

Recently, concepts of milieu therapy have been applied to short-term inpatient and community settings. In acute-care inpatient settings, nursing actions provide limits to and controls on patient behavior and provide structure and safety for the patients. Milieu treatments are based on the individual needs of the patients and include relaxation groups, discussion groups, and medication groups. Spontaneous and planned activities are possible on a short-term unit as well as in a long-term setting. In the community, it is possible to apply milieu therapy approaches in day treatment centers, group homes, and single dwellings.

Promotion of Patient Safety

Although the use of social rules of conduct and privilege systems can enhance smooth operation of a unit, some potentially serious problems can be associated with these practices. A most critical aspect of psychiatric–mental health nursing is the promotion of patient safety, especially in inpatient units.

Observation

Observation is the ongoing assessment of the patient's mental status to identify and subvert any potential problem. An important process in all nursing practice, observation is particularly important in psychiatric nursing. In psychiatric settings, patients are ambulatory and thus more susceptible to environmental hazards. In addition, judgment and cognition impairment are symptoms of many psychiatric disorders. Often, patients are admitted because they pose a danger to themselves or others. In psychiatric nursing, observation is more than just "seeing" patients. It means continually monitoring them for any indication of harm to themselves or others.

All patients who are hospitalized for psychiatric reasons are continually monitored. The intensity of the observation depends on their risk to themselves and others. Some patients are merely asked to "check in" at different times of the day, whereas others have a staff member assigned to only them, such as in instances of potential suicide. Often "sharps," such as razors, are locked up and given to patients at specified times. Mental health facilities and units all have policies that specify levels of observation for patients of varying degrees of risk.

De-escalation

De-escalation is an interactive process of calming and redirecting a patient who has an immediate potential for violence directed toward self or others. This intervention involves assessing the situation and preventing it from escalating to one in which injury occurs to the patient, staff, or other patients. Once the nurse has assessed the situation, he or she calmly calls to the patient and asks the individual to leave the situation. The nurse must avoid rushing toward the patient or giving orders (see Chapter 38). Nurses can use various interventions in this situation, including distraction, conflict resolution, and cognitive interventions.

Seclusion

Seclusion is the involuntary confinement of a person in a room or an area where the person is physically prevented from leaving (Centers for Medicare & Medicaid Services [CMS], 2007). A patient is placed in seclusion for purposes of safety or behavioral management. The seclusion room has no furniture except a mattress and a blanket. The walls usually are padded. The room is environmentally safe, with no hanging devices, electrical outlets, or windows from which the patient could jump. Once a patient is placed in seclusion, he or she is observed at all times.

There are several types of seclusion arrangements. Some facilities place seclusion rooms next to the nurses' stations. These seclusion rooms have an observation window. Other facilities use a modified patient room and assign a staff member to view the patient at all times. Seclusion is an extremely negative patient experience; consequently, its use is seriously questioned and many facilities have completely abandoned its practice (Box 10.6). Patient outcomes may actually be worse if seclusion is used.

Restraints

The most restrictive safety interventions are restraints, which are used only in the most extreme circumstances. All other methods used for maintaining safety and control must be employed before and documented prior to the use of restraints. **Chemical restraint** is the use of medication to control patients or manage their behavior. Chemical restraints are added to the patient's regular drug regimen. A **physical restraint** is any manual method or physical or mechanical device attached or adjacent to the patient's body that restricts freedom of movement or normal access to one's body, material, or equipment and cannot be easily removed. Holding a patient in a manner that restricts movement constitutes restraint for that patient (CMS, 2002).

Different types of physical restraints are available. Wrist restraints restrict arm movement. Walking restraints, or ankle restraints, are often used if a patient cannot resist the impulse to run from a facility but is safe to go outside and to activities. Three-point and four-point restraints are applied to the wrist and ankles in bed. When five-point restraints are used, all extremities are secured, and another restraint is placed across the chest.

The use of both seclusion and restraints must follow the Medicare regulations contained in the *Patients' Rights Condition of Participation* (CoP) (CMS, 2002). Agencies that do not follow the regulations may lose their Medicare and Medicaid certification and, consequently, their funding. The application of physical restraints should also follow hospital policies. Nurses should document all the previously tried de-escalation interventions before the application of restraints. They should limit use of restraints to times when an individual is judged to be a danger to self or others; they should apply restraints only until the patient regains control over behavior. When a patient is in physical restraints, the nurse should closely observe the patient and protect him or her from self-injury.

BOX 10.6

Research for Best Practice: Evidence for Seclusion and Restraint Use

Sailas, E., & Fenton, M. (2005). Seclusion and restraint for people with serious mental illnesses. The Cochrane Library (Oxford) (ID #CD001163).

THE QUESTION: How effective are seclusion, restraint, or alternative controls for people with serious mental illness?

METHODS: A meta-analysis of the effectiveness of seclusion and restraint compared with the alternatives for persons with serious mental illnesses was conducted. Randomized controlled trials were included if they focused on the use of restraint or seclusion or strategies designed to reduce the need for restraint or seclusion in the treatment of serious mental illness. The search yielded 2,155 citations. Of these, 35 studies were obtained.

FINDINGS: No controlled studies exist that evaluate the value of seclusion or restraint in those with serious mental illness. There are reports of serious adverse effects for these techniques in qualitative reviews.

IMPLICATIONS FOR NURSING: Alternative ways of dealing with unwanted or harmful behaviors need to be developed. Continuing use of seclusion or restraint must therefore be questioned from within well-designed studies.

Home Visits

Patients usually have been hospitalized or have received treatment for acute psychiatric symptoms before being referred to psychiatric home service. The goal of **home visits**, the delivery of nursing care in the patient's living environment, is to maximize the patient's functional ability within the nurse–patient relationship and with the family or partner as appropriate. The psychiatric nurse who makes home visits needs to be able to work independently, is skilled in teaching patients and families, can administer and monitor medications, and uses community resources for the patient's needs.

Home visits are especially useful in several different situations, including helping reluctant patients enter therapy, conducting a comprehensive assessment, strengthening a support network, and maintaining patients in the community when their condition deteriorates. Home visits are also useful in helping individuals comply with taking medication. The home visit process consists of three steps: the previsit phase, the home visit, and the postvisit phase. During pre-visit planning, the nurse sets goals for the home visit based on data received from other health care providers or the patient. In addition, the nurse and patient agree on the time of the visit. As the nurse travels to the home, he or she should assess the neighborhood for access to services, socioeconomic factors, and safety.

The actual visit can be divided into four parts. The first is the greeting phase, in which the nurse establishes rapport with family members. Greetings, which are usually brief, establish the communication process and the atmosphere for the visit. Greetings should be friendly but professional. In cultures that consider greetings important, this phase may involve more formal interactions, such as taking food or tea with family members. The next phase establishes the focus of the visit. Sometimes the purpose of the visit is medication administration, health teaching, or counseling. The patient and family must be clear regarding the purpose. The implementation of the service is the next phase and should use most of the visit time. If the purpose of the visit is problem solving or decision making, the family's cultural values may determine the types of interaction and decision-making approaches. Closure is the last phase, the end of the home visit. It is a time to summarize and clarify important points. The nurse should also schedule any additional visits and reiterate patient expectations between visits. Usually, the nurse is the only provider to see the patient regularly. The nurse should acknowledge family members on leaving if they were not a part of the visit.

The postvisit phase includes documentation, reporting, and follow-up planning. This is also when the nurse meets with the supervisor and presents data from the home visit at the team meeting.

Community Action

Nurses have a unique opportunity to promote mental health awareness and support humane treatment for people with mental disorders. Activities range from being an advisor to support groups to participating in the political process through lobbying efforts and serving on community mental health boards. These unpaid activities are usually outside the realm of a particular job. However, an important role of professionals is to provide community service in addition to service through income-generating positions.

EVALUATING OUTCOMES

Evaluation of patient outcomes involves answering the following questions:

- What is the cost-effectiveness of the intervention?
- What benefits did the patient receive?
- What was the patient's level of satisfaction?
- Was the outcome diagnosis specific or nonspecific?

Outcomes can be measured immediately after the nursing intervention or after time passes. For example, a patient may be able to resolve the acute depression and demonstrate confidence and improved self-esteem during a hospital stay. In various cases, it may be several months before the person can engage in positive interpersonal relationships.

SUMMARY OF KEY POINTS

- Assessment is the deliberate and systematic collection of biopsychosocial information or data to determine current and past health and functional status and to evaluate present and past coping patterns.
- The biologic assessment includes current and past health status, physical examination with review of body systems, review of physical functions, and pharmacologic assessment.
- The psychological assessment includes the mental status examination, behavioral responses, and risk factor assessment.
- The mental status examination includes general observation of appearance, psychomotor activity, and attitude; orientations; mood; affect; emotions; speech; and thought processes.
- Behavioral responses are assessed, as are self-concept and current and past coping patterns.
- Risk factor assessment includes ascertaining whether the patient has any suicidal, assaultive, or homicidal ideation.

- The social assessment includes functional status; social systems; spirituality; occupational, economic, and legal status; and quality of life.
- The biopsychosocial assessment provides the data for nursing diagnoses and planning patient outcomes.
- Anticipated patient outcomes are the basis for psychiatric–mental health nursing interventions.
- Nursing interventions are implemented for each domain: biologic (self-care, activity and exercise, sleep, nutrition, thermoregulation, and pain and medication management); psychological (counseling, conflict resolution, bibliotherapy, reminiscence, behavior therapy, psychoeducation, health teaching, and spiritual interventions); and social (behavior therapy and modification, milieu therapy, and various home and community interventions).
- Evaluation of patient outcomes involves assessing cost-effectiveness of the interventions, benefits to the patient, and the patient's level of satisfaction. Outcomes should be measurable, either immediately following intervention or after some time passes.

CRITICAL THINKING CHALLENGES

1 A 23-year-old white woman is admitted to an acute psychiatric setting for depression and suicidal gestures. This admission is her first, but she has experienced bouts of depression since early adolescence. She and her fiancé have just broken their engagement and moved into separate apartments. She has not yet told anyone that she is pregnant. She said that her mother had told her that she was "living in sin" and that she would "pay for it." The patient wants to "end it all!" From this scenario, develop three assessment questions for each domain: biologic, psychological, and social.

2 Identify normal laboratory values for sodium, blood urea nitrogen (BUN), liver enzymes, leukocyte count and differential, and thyroid functioning. Why are these values important to know?

3 Write a paragraph on your self-concept, including all three components: body image, self-esteem, and personal identity. Explore the type of patient situations in which your self-concept can help your interactions with patients. Explore the types of patient situations in which your self-concept can hinder your interactions with patients.

4 Tom, a 25-year-old man with schizophrenia, lives with his parents, who want to retire to Florida. Tom goes to work each day but relies on his mother for meals, laundry, and reminders to take his medication. Tom believes that he can manage the home, but his mother is concerned. She asks the nurse for advice about leaving her son to manage on his own. Generate a nursing diagnosis, outcomes, and interventions that would meet some of Tom's potential responses to his changing lifestyle.

5 Joan, a 35-year-old married woman, is admitted to an acute psychiatric unit for stabilization of her mood disorder. She is extremely depressed but refuses to consider a recommended medication change. She asks the nurse what to do. Using a nursing intervention, explain how you would approach Joan's problem.

6 A nurse reports to work for the evening shift. The unit is chaotic. The television in the day room is loud; two patients are arguing about the program. Visitors are mingling in patients' rooms. The temperature of the unit is hot. One patient is running up and down the hall yelling, "Help me, help me." Using a milieu therapy approach, what would you do to calm the unit?

REFERENCES

American Nurses Association, American Psychiatric Nurses Association, & International Society of Psychiatric–Mental Health Nurses. (2007). *Scope and standards of psychiatric–mental health nursing practice*. Washington, DC: American Nurses Publishing.

Burkhardt, M. A., & Nagai-Jacobson, M. G. (1997). Spirituality and healing. In B. M. Dossey (Ed.), *Core curriculum for holistic nursing*, 42–51. Gaithersburg, MD: Aspen.

Carpenito-Moyet, L.J. (2005). *Nursing diagnosis: Application to clinical practice* (11th ed.).Philadelphia: Lippincott Williams & Wilkins.

Centers for Medicare & Medicaid Services. (2007). *Interpretive guidelines for hospital CoP for patient rights. Quality of care information, quality standards*. Retrieved from www.cms.hhs.gov/manuals. Retrieved April 16, 2007.

Delaney, C., Herr, K., Maas, M., & Specht, J. (2000). Reliability of nursing diagnoses documented in a computerized nursing information system. *Nursing Diagnosis, 11*(3), 121–135.

Dochterman, J., & Bulechek, G. M. (2004). *Nursing interventions classification (NIC)* (4th ed.). St. Louis: Mosby.

Esperat, M. C., Inouye, J., Gonzalez, E. W., Owen, D. C., & Feng, D. (2004). Health disparities among Asian Americans and Pacific Islanders. *Annual Review of Nursing Research, 22*, 135–159.

Jones, F. A. (2002). The role of bibliotherapy in health anxiety: An experimental study. *British Journal of Community Nursing*, 7(10), 498, 500–502.

Kleinpell, R. M. (2003). Measuring advanced practice nursing outcome, strategies and resources. *Critical Care Nurse, February* (Suppl), 6–10.

Littlefield, L., Love, A., Peck, C., & Wertheim, E. (1993). A model for resolving conflict: Some theoretical, empirical and practical implications. Special issue: The psychology of peace and conflict. *Australian Psychologist, 28*(2), 80–85.

Mayer, B. (2000). *The dynamics of conflict resolution*. San Francisco: Jossey-Bass.

Moorhead, S., Johnson, M., & Maas, M. L. (2004). *Nursing outcomes classification (NOC)* (3rd ed.). St. Louis: Mosby.

Rankin, S., & Stallings, K. (1990). *Patient education*. Philadelphia: JB Lippincott.

Silverstein, S. M., Hatashita-Wong, M., & Bloch, A. (2002). A second chance for people with "treatment-refractory" psychosis. *Psychiatric Services, 53*(4), 480.

CHAPTER 11

Cognitive Interventions in Psychiatric Nursing

Jeanne A. Clement

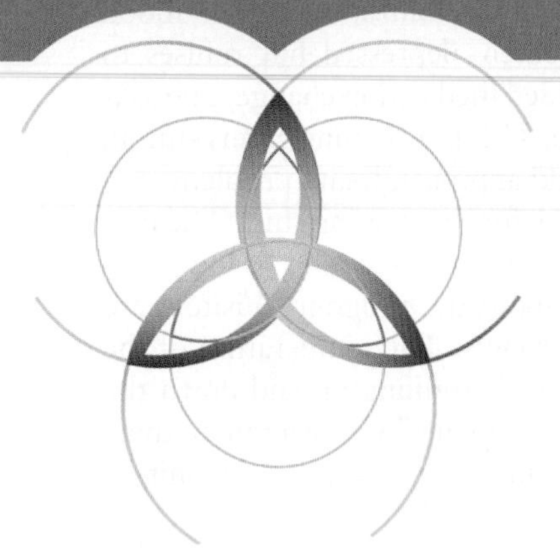

LEARNING OBJECTIVES

After studying this chapter, you will be able to:

- Discuss the history of cognitively based therapeutic interventions.
- Identify the concepts underlying cognitive interventions.
- Discuss three forms of cognitively based therapies.
- Apply cognitive interventions in a clinical setting.
- Describe the contexts in which psychiatric nurses use cognitive interventions.

KEY CONCEPTS

- cognitive behavioral therapy
- rational emotive behavior therapy
- solution-focused therapy

KEY TERMS

• ABCDE • activating event • belief system • cognitions • cognitive interventions • cognitive triad • cognitive distortions • compliments • dysfunctional consequences • exception questions • functional consequences • miracle questions • relationship questions • scaling questions • schema

The key to understanding evidence-based interventions used by psychiatric nurses in a variety of practice settings (inpatient and outpatient) is knowledge and skill in cognitive interventions. There is strong evidence regarding the effectiveness of cognitive interventions in a variety of psychiatric disorders, especially depression (see Chapter 20) and anxiety disorders (see Chapter 21). **Cognitive interventions** are based on the concept of cognition. **Cognition** can be defined as an internal process of perception, memory, and judgment through which an understanding of self and the world is developed. Cognitive interventions aim to change or reframe an individual's cognitions that result in a new view of self and environment.

Cognitive interventions had their beginnings in the long-term inpatient environment, but today they are a mainstay of psychiatric care in all settings and are used by all disciplines and at all levels of practice. Evidence from a number of studies in the past decade supports the use of cognitive therapies with a wide variety of psychological and psychiatric conditions, and it has been shown to be effective with diverse individuals in diverse settings. The Report of the Surgeon General notes that cognitive behavioral therapy (CBT) is considered a best practice in depression (U.S. Department of Health and Human Services, 1999).This chapter explains the theoretical perspectives and application of cognitive therapies.

DEVELOPMENT OF COGNITIVE THERAPIES

Cognitive therapy was first developed and implemented in the 1950s by Albert Ellis, a psychologist, who was uncomfortable with the nondirective Freudian and Neo-Freudian approaches. According to Ellis, cognition, emotions, and behavior are integrated and holistic. Since the 1950s, Ellis has continued to develop and refine his theory and therapeutic approach into what he calls rational emotive behavior therapy (Ellis, 2005).

Beginning in the 1960s, other cognitively based theories and therapeutic approaches were developed, the most prominent being CBT by Aaron Beck (see Chapter 6) (Beck, Thase, & Wright, 2003). Steven de Shazer and Insoo Kim Berg developed solution-focused brief therapy (SFBT), an approach that is useful with persons who have diagnoses such as depression, obsessive-compulsive disorder (OCD), schizophrenia, and other Axis I diagnoses (de Shazer et al., 2007; Trepper, Dolan, McCollum, & Nelson, 2006). All of these models will be discussed in this chapter.

COGNITIVE THERAPY MODELS

Psychiatric nurses have found that cognitive approaches are congruent with the standards of practice, and are particularly effective in the challenging care environments. Brief cognitive therapies offer approaches that can be applied within the therapeutic patient–nurse relationship and the biopsychosocial nursing process. Patients undergoing cognitively-based psychotherapy are frequently treated by an interdisciplinary team that supports this approach.

Cognitive Behavioral Therapy

KEY CONCEPT Cognitive behavioral therapy is a highly structured psychotherapeutic method used to alter distorted beliefs and problem behaviors by identifying and replacing negative inaccurate thoughts and changing the rewards for behaviors.

In CBT, thoughts, feelings, and behavior are not examined in isolation from each other. CBT operates on the following assumptions:

- People are disturbed not by an event, but by the perception of that event.
- Whenever and however a belief develops, the individual believes it.
- Work and practice can modify beliefs that create difficulties in living.

Figure 11.1 depicts the interaction of individual experiences, perception of these experiences, and the unique thoughts attached to these experiences that influence the development of beliefs (functional or dysfunctional). The person develops an explanation of their relationship to their environment and to other people from these beliefs. Dysfunctional thinking develops from a variety of human experiences and can become the predominant way the world is viewed. To quote from Shakespeare's *Hamlet:*

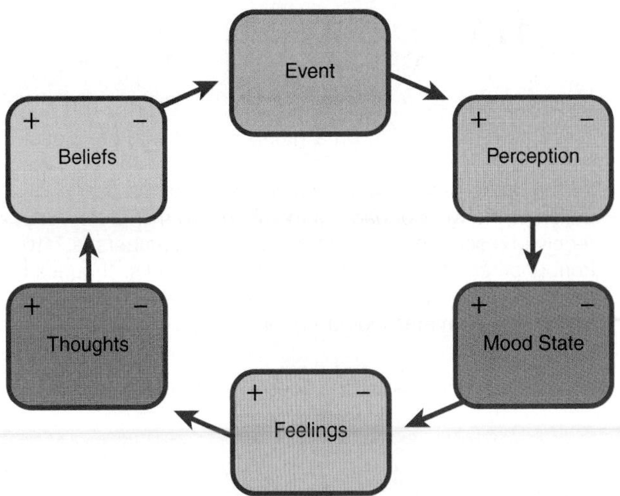

FIGURE 11.1. Model of perception, thoughts, and mood states: the cycle of cognition.

"For there is nothing either good or bad but thinking makes it so."

Thoughts have a powerful effect on emotion and behavior. By changing dysfunctional thinking, a person can alter their emotional reaction to a situation and reinterpret the meaning of an event. That is, by identifying, analyzing, and changing thoughts and behaviors that are counterproductive, feelings such as helplessness, anxiety, and depression can be reduced. The goal of CBT is to restructure how a person perceives events in his or her life to facilitate behavioral and emotional change.

Cognitive Processes

Three cognitive processes are involved in the development of common mental disorders such as depression. These processes include the cognitive triad, cognitive distortions, and schema.

The **cognitive triad** includes thoughts about oneself, the world, and the future. Accumulation of thoughts about oneself is reflected in spoken and unspoken beliefs and moods. Emotions and behavior reflect the strength of the accumulated beliefs. Dysfunctional thoughts about the self are usually overly negative or overly positive, whereas functional thoughts more closely reflect the reality of the perceived situation. For example, one student has the belief that learning is very difficult for him and that he will fail the examination no matter how hard he studies. He does not study for the examination because he believes that he will fail anyway. A second student believes that she is very bright, understands the material, and does not need to study. She attends a concert the night before the test. A third student believes that he has a grasp of the material to be covered on the test, but ensures this by studying notes and the text before the examination. The first two students fail the examination. Failure for the first

BOX 11.1

Clinical Vignette: Cognitive Distortions

Amy has been working on a group project with her classmates in a psychiatric nursing course. Part of the process for the group project was to provide anonymous peer evaluation of the work of each of the six group members. Amy received a score of 10/10 from four of the members, a 7/10 from another, and 5/10 from the 6th. Amy thinks, "I guess I didn't do a good job on this project. I never do anything right. My classmates look down on me."

What Do You Think?

- What cognitive distortions does Amy exhibit?

student reinforces the dysfunctional belief that no matter what, he will fail. The second student argues that the test was unfair, which also reinforces her dysfunctional belief that she is bright and understands the material. The third student earned a good grade. His functional thoughts and behaviors are also reinforced.

Students one and two above both hold distinctive views that are not supported by empirical evidence, but are generated automatically in response to a given situation. These automatic thoughts are called **cognitive distortions** and are generated by organizing distorted information and/or inaccurate interpretation of a situation. Cognitive distortions or "twisted thinking" occur in a variety of ways; however, there are some common distortions (Burns, 1999) (see Box 11.1).

Schema are the individual's life rules that act as a sieve or filter. They allow only information compatible with the internal picture of self and the world to be brought to the person's awareness. Schema develop in early childhood and become relatively fixed by middle childhood. They are the accumulation of both learning and experience from the individual's genetic makeup, family and school environments, peer relationships, and society as a whole. Ethnicity, culture, gender, and religious affiliation influence schema development. In the example, student number one believes that he is not intelligent. This schema increases vulnerability in a host of interpersonal situations, particularly those that relate to scholarly endeavors. Student number two was overly praised by parents and other relatives, and developed a schema of being more accomplished than most.

Implementing Cognitive Behavioral Therapy

The use of CBT is based on a collaborative therapeutic relationship in which a mutual trust develops through promoting patients' strengths and control over their own lives. CBT assumes that individuals have the innate ability to solve their own problems, thus the overarching treatment goal is for the patient to be able to engage in self-care, independent of professional assistance.

In CBT, goals are developed in partnership and supply a forward-looking focus for what "can be" in the future as opposed to "what happened" in the past. Movement toward goals is facilitated by strategies designed to engage the patient in the service of their own mental health. Strategies are developed when nurse and patient develop a working conceptualization of the issue or problem as the patient sees it. The nurse educates the patient about the therapeutic approach. An agenda is mutually established for each therapeutic interaction. Techniques that focus on both cognition and behavior are used to promote patient growth.

Engagement and Assessment

The first step in CBT is engagement and assessment. In this phase, the therapist establishes rapport with the patient and develops the theme that problems are manageable. The patient's definition of the problem that brought him or her into treatment is explored through a series of open-ended questions. A problem list is developed and reframed into manageable goals that are prioritized. The prioritized list forms the agenda for the treatment plan and structures the content of each individual session. A contract is developed for a number of sessions (frequently 10 to 12). The therapist seeks information about the patient's strengths and successes on which to base reframing of negative beliefs and to design interventions. During all sessions the therapist summarizes issues identified, and develops homework assignments that enhance and expand the work done during the sessions.

Interventions

Specific interventions used with CBT, in addition to the interaction that takes place in the therapy sessions, revolve around carefully crafted homework assignments that the patient works on in the time between sessions. Subsequently, sessions may be scheduled at bimonthly or monthly intervals. Typical homework assignments include evaluating the accuracy of automatic thoughts and beliefs. It is important for the therapist to realize that the thoughts a person has about a problem are not beliefs. In CBT the therapist helps the patient identify the underlying belief and then they

- Explore the evidence that supports or refutes the belief about the event.
- Identify alterative explanations for the event.
- Examine the real implications if the belief is true (e.g., "What is the worst thing that could happen?").

In the sessions, the therapist challenges negative beliefs and helps the patient examine the "self-talk" that helps to sustain these beliefs. Cognitive techniques focus on the patient's patterns of automatic thinking, first identifying what they are by examining the patient's recurrent patterns in everyday life and then testing the validity of these automatic thoughts.

Other tools that are used to help change the patient's self-perception include bibliotherapy (the use of books that offer alternative thoughts and responses), journaling, and keeping a diary focused on emotional and behavioral responses to upsetting situations that documents small changes that might otherwise go unnoticed. The patient is also encouraged to make note of positive events and positive thoughts about themselves and their ability to cope with negative events. These positive thoughts and effective coping responses are reinforced in interactions with the therapist. As goals are developed at the beginning of each therapy session, the last few minutes are spent reviewing the progress toward the goals for that day.

Evaluation and Termination

Evaluation and termination begins with the original contract when patient and therapist determined the number of sessions. The patient's progress toward treatment goals is continually evaluated and the patient is urged to become more self-reliant and independent. As progress is never a continuous upward process, therapists prepare the patient for setbacks by acknowledging that setbacks are normal and expected and crafting ways in which the patient can deal with them. It is not uncommon for the time between sessions to lengthen as the final session approaches. At the final session, the use of "booster" sessions is discussed, and frequently a session is scheduled in 6 months to do a quick "check up" and review continuing progress.

Strengths and Limitations of Cognitive Behavioral Therapy

One of the strengths of CBT lies in the body of empirical evidence supporting the effectiveness of these interventions (Mohr et al., 2005; Dinh-Zarr, 2004). Many studies show positive, sustained improvement in people treated with this form of intervention. Critics, however, identify some limitations. Chief among the limitations identified is the concern that the therapeutic relationship, long believed to be the main factor in patient improvement, may be forgotten in the rigid adherence to specific techniques. Others believe that change is dependent on the patient developing a clear understanding of their belief system and the origin of that system; thus CBT is not effective with persons who have thought disorders and other issues that interfere with the ability to do so.

Rational Emotive Behavior Therapy

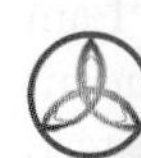

KEY CONCEPT: Rational emotive behavior therapy (REBT) is a psychotherapeutic approach which proposes that unrealistic and irrational beliefs cause many emotional problems. It is a form of CBT with a primary emphasis on changing irrational beliefs that cause emotional distress into thoughts that are more reasonable and rational.

REBT is based on the assumptions that people are born with the potential to be rational (self-constructive) and irrational (self-defeating). Ellis believes that highly cognitive, active, directive homework assignments and structured therapies are likely to be more effective in a shorter time than other therapies. Irrational thinking, self-damaging habituations, wishful thinking, and intolerance are exacerbated by culture and family groups (Ellis, 2005).

Rational Emotive Behavior Therapy Framework

The basic framework for REBT uses the acronym **ABCDE** (see Box 11.2)

The **activating event** may be either external or internal and not necessarily an actual event, but may be an emotion, or thought/expectation. For example, a person who is lonely and feels isolated but is uncomfortable in interpersonal situations may see a flyer advertising a gathering of people who are interested in discussing solutions to global warming and would really like to attend (**A**ctivating event). However, when this person thinks about going to the gathering he imagines going into the room where he does not know anybody and someone coming up to him and trying to engage him in conversation. His imagination provides a picture of not being able to respond, and leaving the room after suffering great embarrassment (**B**elief system: "I am a failure in social situations and everybody can see what a loser I am.") Of course, he decides not to go (**C**onsequences of his belief system).

Belief systems are shaped by rationality, which is self-constructive, and irrationality, which is self-defeating. Rational beliefs are flexible and lead to reasonable evalu-

BOX 11.2

The Rational EBT Framework

A activating event that triggers automatic thoughts and emotions
B beliefs that underlie the thoughts and emotions
C consequences of this automatic process
D dispute or challenge unreasonable expectations
E effective outlook developed by disputing or challenging negative belief systems.

ations of negative activating events. For example, after a low grade on an examination, instead of believing "I am stupid" or "that instructor is out to get me," student might conclude that "I earned a low grade on the test; I really need to work to develop a better understanding of the content" or "I think I need to get help with my test-taking skills." Other rational beliefs might be "I really didn't have time to study, so I can accept this grade and just move on." In other words, "I don't like it but I can live with it." Rational beliefs accept that human beings are fallible and reject absolutes such as always and never.

Irrational beliefs promote dysfunctional negative emotions that in turn lead to psychic pain and discomfort. Behaviors directed at relief of this pain tend to be self-defeating. "I can't fight the system; I will never succeed in this class." There are five themes common in irrational beliefs.

1. A demand: "This *must* happen.
2. Absolute thinking: "All or nothing at all."
3. Catastrophizing: exaggerating negative consequences of an event.
4. Low frustration tolerance: everything should be easy.
5. Global evaluations of human worth: "People can be rated and some are better than others."

Dysfunctional consequences of the interaction between A (activating event) and B (belief system) follow from absolute, rigid, irrational beliefs, whereas **functional consequences** follow from flexible, rational beliefs. For example, demands about self based on "musts" reinforce dysfunctional beliefs such as: "I must do well and be approved by significant others, and if I'm not, then it's awful." The consequences of these beliefs are often anxiety, depression, shame, and guilt that lead to the inability to develop or achieve life's goals, or to develop satisfying interpersonal relationships. Self-regard that is dependent on the approval of others demands that others "treat me fairly and considerately; it's terrible I can't bear it when you don't." Thus, when fairness and consideration is not forthcoming, passive-aggressiveness, anger, rage, and violence may erupt. Demands that the world or life be exactly as one wants can also lead to self-pity as well as problems of self-discipline and addictive behaviors.

Rational Emotive Behavior Therapy Interventions

REBT uses role-playing, assertion training, desensitization, humor, operant conditioning, suggestion, support, and other interventions. According to Ellis, there are two basic forms of REBT: general and preferential. General REBT is synonymous with cognitive behavioral therapy and teaches patients rational and healthy behavior. Preferential REBT includes general REBT, but also emphasizes a profound philosophic change. It teaches patients how to dispute irrational ideas and unhealthy behaviors and to become more creative, scientific, and skeptical thinkers (Ellis, 2005). The therapist uses the ABCDE model in a structured manner (Box 11.2). A major challenge for the therapist is to teach the patient the difference between thoughts and beliefs. Automatic thoughts are not irrational beliefs, but are inferences about the belief. The focus of interventions during the therapy sessions (frequently several weeks or months apart) is on developing rational beliefs to replace those that are irrational and interfere with the patient's quality of life. Figure 11.2 examines the sequence of treatment used in REBT.

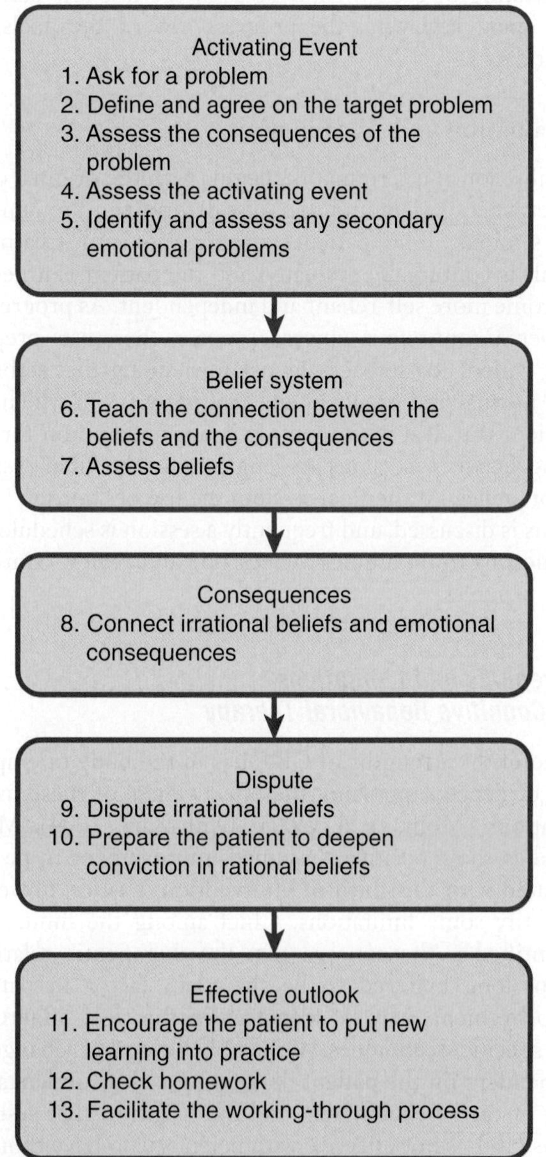

FIGURE 11.2. Rational emotive behavior therapy sequence of treatment.

Solution-Focused Brief Therapy

KEY CONCEPT: Solution-focused brief therapy focuses on solutions rather than problems. This approach does not challenge the existence of problems, but proposes that problems are best understood in relation to their solutions. Solution-focused therapy assists the client in exploring life without the problem (Miller & Berg, 1995).

Solution-focused brief therapy (SFBT), although basically a cognitive approach, differs in philosophy and approach from other cognitively based approaches. The primary difference is the de-emphasis on the patient's "problems," or symptoms, and an emphasis on what is functional and healthful. SFBT assists the patient in exploring life without the problem and it asserts that what is expected to happen influences what the patient does. By discovering what future the client sees as worth striving for, the present becomes important to that future. Otherwise, there is no sense in the patient doing something different or in seeing something in a different light.

Solution-focused theory views the patient as an individual with a collection of strengths and successes as opposed to a diagnosis and collection of symptoms. Solution-focused approaches emphasize the uniqueness of the individual and their capacity to make changes or to deal with their day-to-day lives despite what may seem to be predominant pathology (Iveson, 2002; Green et al., in press).

Solution-Focused Behavior Therapy Assumptions

SFBT assumes that change is constant and inevitable. Essentially, everyone changes constantly and is never the same from one minute to the next. A person interacts, if only in a minute way, with a constantly changing environment. Very small changes can lead to larger changes and the stimulus to change comes from a variety of sources. Constant change and its "ripple effect" direct the strategies and interventions used by the therapist. Both assumptions and strategies point the patient toward a positive, future-oriented change. Box 11.3 lists the assumptions that underlie this approach.

BOX 11.3

Solution-Focused Behavior Therapy Assumptions

1. People have the strengths and resources needed to solve their problems; therefore, the therapist's role is to recognize and emphasize these by amplifying them primarily through asking questions that enable a collaborative approach to co-constructing solutions.
2. It isn't necessary to know a lot about the complaint and its origins or functions in order to resolve it.
3. Define and dissect the "problem" from the perspective of the patient and look for exceptions to the "problem" in the patient's life.
4. Even long-standing issues can be resolved in a relatively short period of time.
5. There is no right or wrong way to see things.
6. Change is most likely to occur when the focus is on what is changeable.
7. The job of the therapist is to identify and amplify change; maintain a focus on the present and the future.
8. The therapist and patient co-create reality, utilizing what the patient perceives is "truth" and develop small, concrete, specific, and reality-based goals that are realistic in the context of the patient's life.
9. The therapist expects change and movement and that expectation is inherent in the questions used and the attitude of the therapist.

Adapted from O'Hanlon, W. H., & Weiner-Davis, M. (1989). *In search of solutions: A new direction in psychotherapy.* New York: W. W. Norton & Co.

Solution-Focused Behavior Therapy Interventions

In SFBT, the therapist takes a position of curiosity in learning about the patient, as opposed to an expert to whom the person has come to be helped. This curiosity is manifested in the questions and techniques that are integral to this approach, and enable the development of realistic goals at each session. Questions used in eliciting the "problem" (frequently referred to as the "issue"(s) to avoid focusing on the "problem") seek very specific information. Examples of questioning in the initial session might include:

1. "What brought you here today?" "What is going on that made you choose to seek help?"
2. "Give me a recent example of how that was demonstrated in your life?"
3. "Who was present when this happened, what did they say and do, and what did you say or do?" "And then what happened?"
4. "When does this kind of thing happen most often?"
5. "Where is it likely to occur?"
6. "Where is it least likely to occur?"
7. "Is there a particular time (of day, month, year) when this is **un**likely to happen?
8. "How does this interfere with your life, your relationships, self-image, etc.?"
9. If your spouse/significant other/coworker were here now, how would he or she say that you were trying to solve the issue or problem?

Interventions in SFBT focus on achievement of specific, concrete, and achievable goals developed in the collaboration of therapist and patient. These goals, formed using the patient's language, are specific, and focus on strengths. Primary techniques used to facilitate progress toward goal attainment are skillfully crafted questions that include the use of the "miracle question," exceptions, scaling, relationship, as well as the use of feedback,

BOX 11.4

Miracle Questions

"I want you to pretend that tonight after you go to bed and are soundly asleep a miracle occurs. The miracle is that the issues that have been bothering you and interfering in your life disappear. Since you have been asleep, you are not aware that the miracle has occurred when you wake up in the morning."

1. What would be your first clue that something was different for you?
2. How will your life be different?
3. What will you be doing instead of __________?
4. How will you be doing this?
5. Beside yourself, who will be the first to notice that there is something different about you?
6. What will that person say or do?
7. How will you respond differently than you might if the issue or problem was still present?

with an emphasis on complimenting any small, goal-oriented change the patient makes. Feedback conveys to the patient that the therapist has listened carefully and recognizes that working toward a goal of change is difficult and requires hard work.

In **miracle questions**, the therapist structures a scenario that the patient is asked to think about carefully (even though it sounds strange) and to use their imagination in crafting the response, again to very specific questions (see Box 11.4 for a sample scenario and questions).

Other ways of facilitating a similar focus on what the solution would look like are to ask the patient to keep track of what goes well in their life that he or she would like to see happen again. The patient is encouraged to keep a written list of what they have noticed and bring it to the next session.

Exception questions are rooted in the belief that nothing is constantly present at the same level of intensity, that there are fluctuations on how the patient experiences "the problem." Exception questions are used to help the patient identify times when whatever is bothering them is not present, or is present with less intensity, based on the underlying assumptions that during these times the patient is usually doing something to make things better. The role of the therapist is then to amplify these times for the patient. Questions used in order to elicit exceptions may be:

1. When do you not have that problem/issue?
2. How do you explain that the problem/issue doesn't happen then?
3. What is different in those times and what are you doing differently?
4. What has to happen for that to happen more often?

Scaling questions are useful in making the patient's problem or issue more specific, in quantifying exceptions noted in intensity, and in tracking change over time. Scaling questions ask the patient to rate the issue or problem on a scale of 1 to 10, with 1 being the worst, or greatest intensity, and 10 being the complete absence of the issue. The therapist notes any change on the scale toward 10, asking the patient what was done to make that happen.

Relationship questions are used to amplify and reinforce positive responses to the other questions (see Box 11.4). Patients are asked to consider the point of view of significant others in their lives. The use of relationship questions can expand the patient's world and help to develop and maintain empathic relationships with others.

Compliments are affirmations of the patient. They reinforce the patient's successes and the strengths needed to achieve those successes. For example, a patient who has frequently gotten into trouble because of a "bad" temper reports in a session that he almost got into an argument while standing in a supermarket checkout lane, but had instead walked away. An appropriate compliment by the therapist might be "Wow, that's great, that must have been very difficult for you." Compliments can create hope in the patient.

• NCLEXNOTE

NCLEXNOTE

Application of knowledge from the social sciences such as psychology will underlie many of the psychosocial questions. Familiarity with the basic cognitive therapy models will strengthen the application of these concepts to patient situations.

USE OF COGNITIVE THERAPIES IN PSYCHIATRIC NURSING

The context of practice has changed considerably for psychiatric nurses. Length of stay for patients in inpatient settings is becoming shorter each year. The patients admitted to inpatient settings are acutely ill and dealing with more complex issues than ever before. More psychiatric care occurs in prisons than in psychiatric hospitals. More and more the focus of practice is in the community, private homes, and primary care settings rather than in specialty hospitals.

Inpatient Settings

Solution-focused therapy is one of the brief cognitive therapies used by psychiatric nurses in acute inpatient psychiatric settings. The SFBT emphasis on strengths fits well with the values of psychiatric nurses, and the techniques used are well within their scope of practice (Hagen & Mitchell, 2001). Solution-focused approaches have been effective with hospitalized people who were

BOX 11.5

***Research for Best Practice:* Might Within Madness: Solution-Focused Therapy and Disordered Thought Clients**

Hagen, B. F., & Mitchell, D. S. (2001) Might within the madness: solution-focused therapy and thought disordered clients. Archives of Psychiatric Nursing 15(2), 86–93.

The Question: Is it possible to use SFBT with persons with thought disorders?

Methods: SFBT was tested with three persons with severe thought disorders.

Findings: The authors found that these three persons could identify their problems, respond to scaling questions, identify exceptions, identify strengths, and use homework. The "miracle question" did not work well. SFBT worked for these individuals.

Implications for Nursing: The result of these case studies indicate that persons with thought disorders can use elements of SFBT.

experiencing delusions, hallucinations, and/or loosening of associations (see Box 11.5).

Other cognitive therapeutic techniques used in inpatient settings include journaling and "homework" assignments that focus on education about diagnoses and medications, as well as on group process. These interventions seem to work well in conjunction with shortened length of stay in inpatient settings.

Community Settings

In community settings, cognitive approaches are used in combination with a broad array of interpersonal, behavioral, educational, and pharmacological interventions. These groups are usually time limited and encourage interaction among group members about their disorders, medications, coping techniques, resources, and services available. In community and clinic settings, CBT is used within a holistic evaluation of patients that includes a complete health history and physical examination, and evaluation of possible co-occurring disorders such as depression and alcohol and other drug use or abuse. In particular, the use of questioning such as that integral to solution-focused approaches elicits strengths in a relatively short time and can provide a means for the nurse to support positive coping. The focus on realistic goal development provides a means of evaluation of patient progress.

Home and primary care settings are also conducive to the implementation of cognitive techniques. Small, concrete, specific goals developed in a naturalistic setting such as the home can create significant change for the whole family. CBT and SFBT approaches are very useful in primary care settings where time with patients is very short. Goal setting, use of scaling questions, and compliments can be done in the course of a 15-minute interaction.

SUMMARY OF KEY POINTS

- Cognitive therapies have a long history in mental health care and have support as evidence-based interventions effective in several mental disorders.
- Psychiatric nurses use cognitive interventions in a variety of settings. Cognitive therapies serve as the framework for psychotherapy as well as interdisciplinary treatment.
- Cognitive behavioral therapy focuses on dysfunctional thinking through the examination of the cognitive triad, cognitive distortions, and schema.
- Rational emotive behavior therapy assumes that people are born with the tendency to be rational and irrational. Using the ABCDE framework, REBT focuses on identifying and changing irrational beliefs that lead to negative consequences.
- Solution-focused brief therapy identifies the possible solutions before addressing the problem.

CRITICAL THINKING CHALLENGES

1 Compare and contrast the three cognitive therapies in terms of assumptions and interventions.
2 A patient has recently been fired from her job, which is the third job that she has had within 1 year. She is depressed, but denies suicidal thoughts. She tells you that she is a failure and can never get and keep a job. Discuss how CBT, REBT, and SFBT would view and treat this patient.
3 A nurse manager plans to use CBT as a theoretical model for an inpatient unit. Discuss the interventions that should be used on an inpatient unit that applies the CBT model.

REFERENCES

Beck, A. T., Thase, M. D., & Wright, J. H. (2003). Cognitive therapy. In R. E. Hales and S. C. Yudofsky (Eds.), *Textbook of clinical psychiatry* (4th ed.), (pp. 1245–1283) Washington, DC: American Psychiatric Publishers, Inc.

Burns, D. D. (1999). *The Feeling Good Handbook.* New York: Penguin Group.

De Shazer, S., Dolan, Y., Korman, H., Trepper, T. S., McCollum, E. E., & Berg, I. K. (2007). *More than miracles: The state of the art in solution focused brief therapy.* New York: Haworth Press.

Dinh-Zarr, T., Goss, C., Heitman, E., Roberts, I. L., DiGuiseppi, D. (2004). Interventions for preventing injuries in problem drinkers. *The Cochrane Database of systematic Reviews.* Volume (2), 2006. Retrieved July 7, 2006. http://gateway.ut.ovid.com/gw3/ovidweb.cgi.

Ellis, A. (2005). Rational emotive behavior therapy. In R. J. Corsini, & D. Wedding (Eds.) (2005). *Current psychotherapies* (7th ed.), pp. 166–201. Belmont, CA: Thompson Brooks/Cole.

Greene, G. J., Kondrat, D. C, Lee, M. Y, Clement, J. A., Siebert, H., Mentzer, R. A., Pinnell, S. R. (2006). A solution focused approach to case management and recovery with consumers who have a severe mental disability. *Families in Society.*

Hagen, B. F., & Mitchell, D. S. (2001). Might within the madness: solution-focused therapy and thought disordered clients. *Archives of Psychiatric Nursing XV*(2), 86–93.

Iveson, C. (2002). Solution-focused brief therapy. *Advances in Psychiatric Treatment 8*, 149–157.

Miller, S. D., & Berg, I. K. (1995). *The miracle method: A radically new approach to problem drinking.* New York: Norton.

Mohr, D. C., Hart, S. L., Julian, L., Catledge, C., Honos-Webb, L., Vella, L., & Tasch, E. (2005). Telephone-administered psychotherapy for depression. *Archives of General Psychiatry, 62* (9), 1007–1014.

Trepper, T. S., Dolan, Y., McCollum, E. E., & Nelson, T. (2006). Steve de Shazer and the future of solution-focused therapy. *Journal of Marital and Family Therapy, 32* (2), 133–139.

U.S. Department of Health and Human Services. (1999). *Mental health: A report of the Surgeon General.* Washington, DC: U.S. Department of Health and Human Services, Substance Abuse and Mental Health Services Administration, Center for Mental Health Services, National Institutes of Health, National Institute of Mental Health.

CHAPTER 12

Interventions with Groups

Mary Ann Boyd

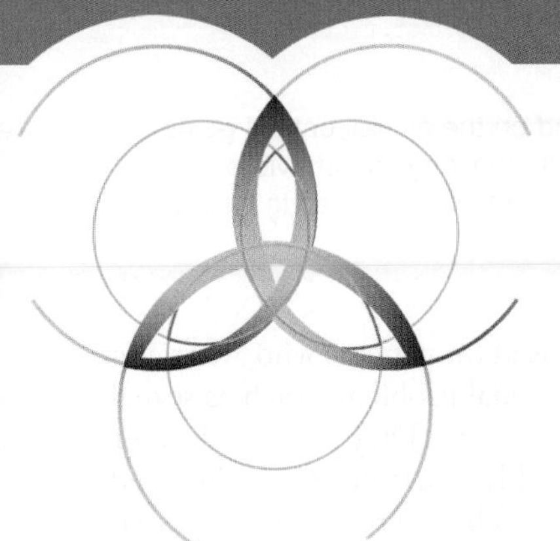

KEY CONCEPTS

- group
- group process

LEARNING OBJECTIVES

After studying this chapter, you will be able to:

- Discuss group concepts used in leading groups.
- Compare the roles that group members can assume.
- Identify important aspects of leading a group, such as member selection, leadership skills, seating arrangements, and ways of dealing with challenging behaviors of group members.
- Identify four types of groups: psychoeducation, supportive therapy, psychotherapy, and self-help.
- Describe common nursing intervention groups.

KEY TERMS

• closed group • direct leadership behavior • dyad • formal group roles • group cohesion • group dynamics • groupthink • indirect leader • individual roles • informal group roles • maintenance functions • open group • task functions • triad

Group interventions can have powerful treatment effects on patients who are trying to develop self-understanding, conquer unwanted thoughts and feelings, and change behaviors. They are efficient because several patients can receive treatment at once. For interventions to be effective, the nurse must possess leadership skills that can shape and monitor group interactions. The psychiatric–mental health nurse uses group interventions in all roles, including direct care provider, case manager, and unit leader. In addition, all nurses can use group interventions, such as when conducting patient education or leading support groups. This chapter presents relevant group concepts that the psychiatric nurse uses. It explores group leadership, with special emphasis on the groups that nurses commonly lead.

GROUP: DEFINITIONS AND CONCEPTS

There are many different definitions of a group. In the psychoanalytic tradition, a group is a collection of individuals who identify with the leader and then with one another but who act, for the most part, independently. According to systems theory, a group consists of parts or components that exist to perform some activity or purpose. As members of a group interact, subsystems form, which challenges the leader to understand the effect of these components on the total system and to improve channels of communication. A global, but rather simple, definition of a group is two or more people who are in an interdependent relationship with one another. The simplicity of the definition is misleading because interactions within groups, or **group dynamics,** are anything but simple. Group dynamics influence the group's development and process. In fact, it takes an astute observer to determine the real dynamics of a group and their effects on individuals. No matter the type of group, its theoretic orientation, or its purpose, group dynamics influence the success or failure of a group intervention.

In this text, a group is defined as two or more people who develop interactive relationships and share at least one common goal or issue. Groups can be further defined according to the number of people or the relationship of members. A **dyad** is a group of only two people who are usually related, such as a married couple, siblings, or parent and child. A **triad** is a group of three people who may or may not be related. A family is a special type of group and will be discussed in Chapter 13.

KEY CONCEPT A **group** is two or more people who develop interactive relationships and share at least one common goal or issue.

Open Versus Closed Groups

A group can be viewed as either an open or a closed system. In an **open group,** new members may join and old members may leave the group at different sessions. For example, a newly admitted patient may join an anger management group that is part of an ongoing program in an inpatient unit. As a new member, the individual is at a disadvantage because the other members already know one another and have established relationships. The advantage of an open group is that participants can join at any time and stay in the group for as long as they need. In addition, these groups can function on an ongoing basis and thus can be available to more people.

In a **closed group,** members begin the group at one time, and no new members are admitted. If a member of a closed group leaves, no replacement joins. Advantages of a closed group are that the participants get to know one another at the same time, the group is more cohesive, and members move through the group process concurrently. Most clinicians prefer closed groups because such groups facilitate the best treatment results. However, implementing closed-group interventions is often difficult because patients are not always available at the same time.

Group Size

Group size is an important consideration in forming group programs. Many mental health professionals favor small groups, but large groups can also be effective. Whether to form a large or small group depends on the purpose, abilities, and availability of the participants and the skills of the leader. Small groups (usually no more than eight to 10 members) become more cohesive, are less likely to form subgroups, and can provide a richer interpersonal experience than large groups. Small groups function nicely with one group leader, although many small groups are led by two people. An ideal small group is about seven to eight people in addition to the leader or leaders (Yalom with Leszcz, 2005).

• NCLEXNOTE

NCLEXNOTE Size of group will depend on the overall patient goals and abilities. Patients with challenging behaviors should be carefully screened and assigned to smaller groups.

Small groups often are used for patients who are trying to deal with complex emotional problems, such as sexual abuse, eating disorders, or trauma. They are also ideal for individuals who have special learning needs or who need much individual attention. These groups work best if they are closed to new members or if new members are gradually introduced. The disadvantage of small groups is that they cannot withstand the loss of members and can quickly dissolve if members leave. In addition, if places are unfilled, the group's dynamics change, which may interfere with the therapeutic process.

A large group (more than 10 members) can also be therapeutic, as well as cost-effective in clinical settings. Some research suggests that large treatment groups are effective for specific problems, such as smoking, or settings such as the workplace (Moher, Hey, & Lancaster, 2003). A large group can be ongoing and open-ended. It can be effective without the development of intense transference and countertransference issues. A disadvantage is that participants of large groups are more likely to feel alienated from one another.

Leading a large group is more complex than leading a small group because of the number of potential interactions and relationships that can form. The leader needs both presentation and group leadership skills. In a large group, determining the feelings and thoughts of the participants can be difficult. The leader of a large group usually views the group as a system and identifies the various subgroups that form. If subgroups form, the leader changes the structure and function of communication within the subgroups by rearranging seating and encouraging the subgroup to interact with the rest of the group.

Group Development

In the same way that the development of the therapeutic relationship is a process, so is the development of a group (see Chapter 9). Many researchers view group development as a sequence of phases, particularly in small groups (Table 12.1). Although models of group development dif-

Table 12.1 Comparison of Models of Group Development

Robert Bales (1955)	William Schutz (1960)	Bruce Tuckman (1965)
• *Orientation:* What is the problem? • *Evaluation:* How do we feel about it? • *Control:* What should we do about it?	• *Inclusion:* Deal with issues of belonging and being in and out of the group. • *Control:* Deal with issues of authority (who is in charge?), dependence, and autonomy. • *Affection:* Deal with issues of intimacy, closeness, and caring, versus dislike and distancing.	• *Forming:* Get to know one another and form a group. • *Storming:* Tension and conflict occur; subgroups form and clash with one another. • *Norming:* Develop norms of how to work together. • *Performing:* Reach consensus and develop cooperative relationships.

fer, most follow a pattern of a beginning, middle, and ending phase (Alvarez, 2002). These stages should be thought of not as a straight line with one preceding another, but as a dynamic process that is constantly revisiting and re-examining group interactions and behaviors, as well as progressing forward.

KEY CONCEPT Group process is the culmination of the session-to-session interactions of the members that move the group toward its goals.

Beginning Stage

The beginning of a group is when group members get to know one another and the group leader. The length of the beginning stage depends on, among other variables, the purpose of the group, the number of members, and the skill of the leader. It may last for only a few sessions or several. "Honeymoon" behavior characterizes this stage in the beginning, but "conflict" dominates at the end. During the initial sessions, members usually display polite, congenial behavior typical of those in new social situations. They are "good patients" and often intellectualize their problems; that is, these patients deal with emotional conflict or stress by excessively using abstract thinking or generalizations to minimize disturbing feelings. Members are usually anxious and sometimes display behavior that does not truly represent their feelings. In the first few sessions, members test whether they can trust one another. Sometime after the initial sessions, group members usually experience a period of conflict, either among themselves or with the leader. This conflict is a normal part of group development, and many believe that conflict is necessary to move into any working phase. Sometimes, one or more group members become the scapegoat. Such situations challenge the leader to guide the group during this period by avoiding taking sides and treating all members respectfully.

Working Stage

The working stage of groups involves a real sharing of ideas and the development of closeness. A group personality may emerge that is distinct from the individual personalities of its members. The group develops its own rules and rituals and has its own behavioral norms; for example, groups develop regular patterns of seating and interaction. During this stage, the group realizes its purpose. If the purpose is education, the participants engage in learning new content or skills. If the aim of the group is to share feelings and experiences, these activities consume group meetings. During this phase, the group starts on time, and the leader often needs to remind members when it is time to stop.

Termination Stage

Termination can be difficult for a group, especially a successful one. During the final stages, members begin to grieve for the loss of the group's closeness and begin to re-establish themselves as individuals. Individuals terminate from groups as they do from any relationship. One person may not show up at the last session, another person may bring up issues that the group has already addressed, and others may demonstrate anger or hostility. Most members of successful groups are sad as the group terminates. During the last meetings, members may make arrangements for meeting after group. These plans rarely materialize or continue. Leaders should recognize these plans as part of the farewell process—saying good-bye to the group.

Roles of Group Members

There are two official or **formal group roles,** the leader and the members; however, in small groups members often assume **informal group roles** or positions in the group with rights and duties that are directed toward one or more group members. These roles can either help or hinder the group's process. One of the first and oldest models is Benne and Sheats' (1948) list of task, maintenance, and individual roles. **Task functions** involve the business of the group or "keeping things focused." Individuals who provide this function keep the group focused on a main purpose. For any group to be successful, it must have members who assume some of these task roles, such as *information seeker* (asks for clarification), *coordinator* (spells out relationships between ideas), and *recorder* (keeper of the minutes). **Maintenance functions** help the group stay together by ensuring it starts on time, assisting individuals to compromise, and determining membership. These individuals are more interested in maintaining the group's cohesiveness than focusing on the group's tasks. The *harmonizer, compromiser*, and *standard setter* are examples of maintenance roles. In a successful group, members assume both group task and maintenance functions (Table 12.2).

Individual roles are those member roles that either enhance or detract from the group's functioning. These roles have nothing to do with the group's purpose or cohesion; for example, someone who monopolizes the group inhibits the group's work. People who are participating in the group may be meeting personal needs, such as feeling important or being an expert on a subject. However, when individual roles predominate, the risk is that dominant individuals may contribute to neither the task nor the maintenance of the group.

In selecting members and analyzing the progress of the group, the leader must pay attention to the balance between the task and maintenance functions. If too many group members assume task functions and too few assume maintenance functions, the group may have difficulty developing cohesion. If too many members assume maintenance functions, the group may never finish its work. Although it is usually impossible to select individuals only because of their group role, tracking the group in terms of how well it functions and how much it actually gets done is important.

Group Communication

One of the responsibilities of the group leader is to facilitate both verbal and nonverbal communication to meet the treatment goals of the individual members and the entire group. Because of the number of people involved, developing trusting relationships within groups is more complicated than is developing a single relationship with a patient. The communication techniques used in estab-

Table 12.2 Roles and Functions of Group Members

Task Roles	Maintenance Roles	Individual Roles
Initiator-contributor suggests or proposes new ideas or a new view of the problem or goal.	*Encourager* praises, agrees with, and accepts contributions of others.	*Aggressor* deflates the status of others; expresses disapproval of the values, acts, or feelings of others; attacks the group or problem; jokes aggressively; tries to take credit for the work.
Information seeker asks for clarification of the values pertinent to the group activity.	*Harmonizer* mediates differences among members and relieves tension in conflict situations.	*Blocker* tends to be negative and resistant, disagrees and opposes without or beyond "reason," and attempts to bring back an issue after group has rejected it.
Information giver offers "authoritative" facts or generalizations or gives own experiences.	*Compromiser* operates from within a conflict and may yield status or admit error to maintain group harmony.	*Recognition-seeker* calls attention to self through such activities as boasting, reporting on personal achievements, acting in unusual ways.
Opinion giver states belief or opinions with emphasis on what should be the group's values.	*Gate-keeper* attempts to keep communication channels open by encouraging or facilitating the participation of others or proposes regulation of the flow of communication through limiting time.	*Self-confessor* uses group setting to express personal, non–group-oriented feelings or insights.
Elaborator spells out suggestions in terms of examples, develops meanings of ideas and rationales, tries to deduce how an idea would work.	*Standard setter* expresses standards for the group to achieve.	*Playboy* makes a display of lack of involvement in group's processes.
Coordinator shows or clarifies the relationships among various ideas and suggestions.	*Group observer* keeps records of various aspects of group processes and interprets data to group.	*Dominator* tries to assert authority or superiority in manipulating the group or certain members of the group through flattery, being directive, interrupting others.
Orienter defines the position of the group with respect to its goals.	*Follower* goes along with the movement of the group.	*Help-seeker* attempts to call forth sympathy from other group members through expressing insecurity, personal confusion, or depreciation of self beyond reason.
Evaluator-critic measures the outcome of the group against some standard.		*Special interest pleader* speaks for a special group, such as "grass roots," usually representing personal prejudices or biases.
Energizer attempts to stimulate the group to action or decision.		
Procedural technician expedites group movement by doing things for the group such as distributing copies, arranging seating.		
Recorder writes suggestions, keeps minutes, serves as group memory.		

lishing and maintaining individual relationships are the same for groups, but the leader also attends to the communication patterns among the members.

Verbal Communication

Group interaction can be viewed as a communication network that becomes patterned and predictable. In a group, verbal comments are linked in a chain formation.

Communication Network

Asking a colleague to observe and record the content and interaction is a useful technique in determining the interaction pattern within a group; the leader may also use an audio or video recorder. In some groups, one person may always change the subject when another raises a sensitive topic. One person may always speak after another. People who sit next to each other tend to communicate among themselves. By analyzing the content and patterns, the leader can determine the existence of communications pathways—who is most liked in the group, who occupies a position of power, what subgroups have formed, and who is isolated from the group. Moreno's (1953) sociometric diagrams of interpersonal choice provide a way to identify stars, isolates, and overchosen and underchosen group members. Usually, those who are well liked or display leadership abilities tend to be chosen for interactions more often than do those who are not (Fig 12.1). In one study of communication networks, members who exhibited more dominant behaviors or who the group perceived as being dominant emerged as more central to the group's communication networks and both sent and received more messages. The study also found that the task at hand affects the communication network. Groups that worked on low-complexity tasks had more centralized communication than when they worked on high-complexity tasks (Brown & Miller, 2000).

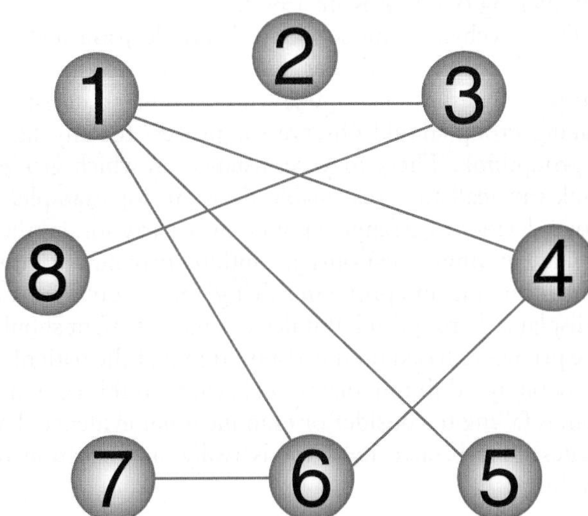

FIGURE 12.1. Sociometric analysis of group behavior. In this sociometric structure, response pattern was recorded during member interaction. Group members interacted with number 1 the most. Therefore, number 1 is the overchosen person. Numbers 5 and 7 are underchosen. Number 2 is never chosen and is determined to be the isolate.

Group Themes

Group themes are the collective conceptual underpinnings of a group and express the members' underlying concerns or feelings, regardless of the group's purpose. Themes that emerge in groups help members to understand group dynamics. Different groups have different themes. For example, three themes emerged for a support group for grieving children, including their vulnerability, the importance of maintaining memories, and the contribution of the group to the process of grieving (Graham & Sontag, 2001). Although some predictable themes occur in groups, the obvious or assumed themes at the beginning may actually wind up differing from reality as the process continues. In one hospice support group, the members seemed to be focusing on the memories of their loved ones. However, upon examination of the content of their interactions, discussions were revolving around financial planning for the future (Box 12.1).

BOX 12.1

Group Themes

A large symptom-management group is ongoing at a psychiatric facility. It is co-led by two nurses who are skilled in directing large groups and knowledgeable about the symptoms of mental disorders. Usually 12 people attend. The usual focus of the group is on identifying symptoms that indicate an impending re-emergence of psychotic symptoms, medication side effects, and managing the numerous symptoms that medication is not controlling.

The nurses identified the appearance of the theme of powerlessness based on the following observations:

Session 1: T. L. expressed his frustration at being unable to keep a job because of his symptoms. The rest of the group offered their own experiences of being unable to work.

Session 2: C. R. is late to group and announces that she was late because the bus driver forgot to tell her when to get off, and she missed her stop. She is irritated with the new driver.

Session 3: N. T. is out of medication and says that he cannot get more because he is out of money again. He asks the nurses to lend him some money and make arrangements to get free medication.

Session 4: G. M. relies on his family for all transportation and refuses to use public transportation.

In all these sessions, participants expressed feelings that are consistent with loss of power.

Nonverbal Communication

Nonverbal communication is important to understanding group behavior. All members, not just the group leader, observe the eye contact, posture, and body gestures of the participants. What is expressed is the result of individual and group, as well as internal and external, processes. For example, if one member is explaining a painful experience and another member looks away and tries to engage still another, the self-disclosing member may feel devalued and rejected because he or she interprets the disruptive behavior as disinterest. However, if the leader interprets the disruptive behavior as anxiety over the topic, he or she may try to engage the other member in discussing the source of the anxiety.

The leaders should monitor the nonverbal behavior of group members during each session. Often, one or two people can set the overall mood of the group. Someone who comes to a session very sad or angry can set a tone of sadness or anger for the whole group. An astute group leader recognizes the effects of an individual's mood on the total group. If the purpose of the group is to deal with emotions, the group leader may choose to discuss the members' problem at the beginning of the session. The leader thus limits the mood to the one person experiencing it. If the group's purpose is inconsistent with self-disclosure of personal problems, the nurse should acknowledge the individual members' distress and offer a private session after the group. In this instance, the nurse would not encourage repeated episodes of self-disclosure from that member or others.

Group Norms and Standards

Groups develop norms or rules and standards that establish acceptable group behaviors. Some norms are formalized, such as beginning group on time, but others are never really formalized. These standards encourage conformity of behavior among group members. The group discourages deviations from these established norms. A member must quickly learn the norms or be ostracized.

Group Cohesion

One of the goals of most group leaders is to foster **group cohesion,** the forces that act on the members to stay in a group. Leaders can encourage cohesiveness by placing participants in situations that promote social interaction with minimal supervision, such as refreshment periods and through team-building exercises. Cohesiveness is especially important in groups that focus on health maintenance behaviors such as exercise and weight control. These groups typically have high dropout rates, but members are more likely to attend when a group is cohesive (Fraser & Spink, 2002).

Without cohesiveness, the group's true existence is questionable. In cohesive groups, members are committed to the existence of the group. In large groups, cohesiveness tends to be decreased, with subsequent poorer performance among group members in completing tasks. When members are strongly committed to completing a task and the leader encourages equal participation, cohesiveness promotes job satisfaction and higher performance (Steinhardt, Dolbier, Gottlieb, & McCalister, 2003). However, cohesiveness can be a double-edged sword. In very cohesive groups, members are more likely to transgress personal boundaries. Dysfunctional relationships may develop that are destructive to the group process and ultimately not in the best interests of individual members.

Groupthink and Decision Making

Groupthink is the tendency of many groups to avoid conflict and adopt a normative pattern of thinking that is often consistent with the ideas of the group leader (Janis, 1972, 1982). In groupthink, striving for unanimity overrides the motivation of members to appraise realistically alternative courses of action. Many catastrophes, such as the *Challenger* explosion and Bay of Pigs invasion, have been attributed to groupthink, but the empiric evidence of groupthink's negative implications in organizations is small. Studies have shown that closed leadership style and external threat, particularly time pressure, appear to promote symptoms of groupthink and defective decision making (Neck & Moorhead, 1995). Groupthink can also have positive effects on the group. In one study, groupthink was positively associated with group activities and team performance and negatively associated with concurrence (pressure for everyone to agree) and defective decision making (Choi & Kim, 1999).

The psychiatric nurse often leads decision-making groups that decide activities, unit governance issues, and learning materials. The nurse who is leading a decision-making group should observe the process for any signs of groupthink. There may be instances in which groupthink can lead to a reasonable decision: for example, a group decides to arrange a going-away party for another patient. In other situations, groupthink may inhibit individual thinking and problem solving: for example, a team is displaying groupthink if it decides that a patient should lose privileges based on the assumption that the patient is deliberately exhibiting bizarre behaviors. In this case, the team is failing to consider or examine other evidence that suggests the bizarre behavior is really an indication of psychosis.

GROUP LEADERSHIP

In the beginning, the group leader establishes the presence of each member, constructs a working environment, builds a working relationship with the group and among participants, and clarifies outcomes, processes, and skills related to the group's purpose (Alf & Wilson, 2001). To carry out these functions, the leader must process the group interactions by staying objective and viewing what occurs as well as participating in the group. The leader reflects on, evaluates, and responds to just-completed interactions. The use of various techniques enhances the leader's ability to lead the group effectively and to help the group meet its goals (Table 12.3).

One of the most important leadership skills is listening. A leader who practices active listening provides group members with someone who is responsive to what they say. A group leader who listens also models listening behavior for others, helping them improve their skills. Listening enables the leader to process events and track interactions. The leader should be able to listen to the group members and formulate responses based on an understanding of the discussion. Members may

Table 12.3 Techniques in Leading Groups

Technique	Purpose	Example
Support: giving feedback that provides a climate of emotional support	Helps a person or group continue with ongoing activities Informs group about what the leader thinks is important Creates a climate for expressing unpopular ideas Helps the more quiet and fearful members speak up	"We really appreciate your sharing that experience with us. It looked like it was quite painful."
Confrontation: challenging a participant (needs to be done in a supportive environment)	Helps individuals learn something about themselves Helps reduce some forms of disruptive behavior Helps members deal more openly and directly with one another	"Tom, this is the third time that you have changed the subject when we have talked about spouse abuse. Is something going on?"
Advice and suggestions: sharing expertise and knowledge that the members do not have	Provides information that members can use once they have examined and evaluated it Helps focus group's task and goals	"The medication that you are taking may be causing you to be sleepy."
Summarizing: statements at the end of sessions that highlight the session's discussion, any problem resolution, and unresolved problems	Provides continuity from one session to the next Brings to focus still-unresolved issues Organizes past in ways that clarify; brings into focus themes and patterns of interaction	"This session we discussed Sharon's medication problems, and she will be following up with her physicians."
Clarification: restatement of an interaction	Checks on the meanings of the interaction and communication Avoids faulty communication Facilitates focus on substantive issues rather than allowing members to be sidetracked into misunderstandings	"What I heard you say was that you are feeling very sad right now. Is that correct?"
Probing and questioning: a technique for the experienced group leader that asks for more information	Helps members expand on what they were saying (when they are ready to) Gets at more extensive and wider range of information Invites members to explore their ideas in greater detail	"Could you tell us more about your relationship with your parents?"
Repeating, paraphrasing, highlighting: a simple act of repeating what was just said	Facilitates communication among group members Corrects inaccurate communication or emphasizes accurate communication	*Member:* "I forgot about my wife's birthday." *Leader:* "You forgot your wife's birthday."
Reflecting feelings: identifying feelings that are being expressed	Orients members to the feelings that may lie behind what is being said or done Helps members deal with issues they might otherwise avoid or miss	"You sound upset."
Reflecting behavior: identifying behaviors that are occurring	Gives members an opportunity to see how their behavior appears to others and to evaluate its consequences Helps members to understand others' perceptions and responses to them	"I notice that when the topic of sex is brought up, you look down and shift in your chair."

Adapted from Sampson, E.,& Marthas, M. (1990). *Group process for the health professions* (pp. 222–224). Albany, NY: Delmar.

need to learn to listen to one another, track discussions without changing the subject, and not speak while others are talking.

The leader tracks the verbal and nonverbal interactions throughout the group. Depending on the group's purpose, the leader may keep this information to him or herself to understand the group process or may share the observations with the group. For example, if the purpose of the group is psychoeducation, the leader may use the information to facilitate the best learning environment. If the purpose of the group is to improve the self-awareness and interaction skills of members, the leader may point out the observations. The leader needs to be clear about the purpose of the group and tailor leadership strategies accordingly.

The leader maintains a neutral, nonjudgmental style and avoids showing preference to one member over another. This may be difficult because some members may naturally seek out the leader's attention or ask for special favors. These behaviors are divisive to the group, and the leader should discourage them. Other important skills include providing everyone with an opportunity to contribute and respecting everyone's ideas. A leader who truly wants group participation and decision making does not reveal his or her beliefs.

Some generally accepted guidelines in leading groups include setting start and stop times, arranging for the introduction of new members, and listening while other people talk. Leaders should explain these rules at the first group meeting and re-emphasize them at different points. A group should always begin at its scheduled time; otherwise, members who tend to be late will not change their behavior, and those who are on time will resent waiting for the others. A group should also end on time. Members should understand from the beginning that either new people can attend without the group knowing about it or that the group will discuss the introduction of new members before their attendance. Whatever the group decides, the leader must also follow the rules.

Choosing Leadership Styles

A group is led within the context of the group leader's theoretic background and the group's purpose. For example, a leader with training in cognitive-behavioral therapy may focus on treating depression by asking members to think differently about situations, which in turn leads to feeling better. A leader with a psychodynamic orientation may focus on the feelings of depression by examining situations that generate the same feelings. Whatever the leader's theoretic background, his or her leadership behavior can be viewed on a continuum of direct to indirect. **Direct leadership behavior** enables the leader to control the interaction by giving directions and information and allowing little discussion. The leader literally tells the members what to do. On the other end of the continuum is the **indirect leader,** who primarily reflects the group members' discussion and offers little guidance or information to the group. Sometimes the group needs more direct leadership; other times it needs a leader who is indirect. The challenge of providing leadership is to give sufficient direction that the group can meet its goals and develop its own group process but enough freedom that members can make mistakes and recover from their thinking errors in a supportive, caring, learning environment.

Selecting the Members

Individuals can refer themselves or be referred to groups by treatment teams or clinicians. The leader is responsible for assessing the individual's suitability to the group. In instances when a new group is forming, the leader selects and invites members so that the group can be well functioning and successful. The leader should consider the following criteria when selecting members:

- Does the purpose of the group match the needs of the potential member?
- Does the potential member have the social skills to function comfortably in the group?
- Will the other group members accept the new group member?
- Can the potential member make a commitment to attending group meetings?

Arranging Seating

Spatial and seating arrangements contribute to group communication. Group members tend to sit in the same places. Those who sit close to the group leader are more likely to have more power in the group than those who sit far away. Communication flows better when no physical barriers, such as tables, are between members. Arranging a group in a circle with chairs comfortably close to one another without a table enhances group work. No one should sit outside the group. If a table is necessary, a round table is better than a rectangular one, which implicitly increases the power of those who sit at the ends.

The session should be held in a quiet, pleasant room with adequate space and privacy. Holding a session in too large or too small a room inhibits communication. Group sessions should not be held in rooms to which nonparticipants have access because of compromised confidentiality and potential distractions.

Dealing with Challenging Group Behaviors

Problematic behaviors occur in all groups. They can be challenging to the most experienced group leaders and frustrating to new leaders. In dealing with any problematic behavior or situation, the leader must remember to support the integrity of the individual members and the group as a whole.

Monopolizer

Some people tend to monopolize a group by constantly talking or interrupting others. This behavior is common in the beginning stages of group formation and usually represents anxiety that the member displaying such behavior is experiencing. Within a few sessions, this person usually relaxes and no longer attempts to monopolize the group. However, for some people monopolizing discussions is part of their normal personality and will continue. Other group members usually find the behavior mildly irritating in the beginning and extremely annoying as time passes. Members may drop out of the group to avoid that person. The leader needs to decide if, how, and when to intervene. The best case scenario is when savvy group members remind the monopolizer to let others speak. The leader can then support the group in establishing rules that allow everyone the opportunity to participate. However, the group often waits for the leader to manage the situation. There are a couple of ways to deal with the situation. The leader can interrupt the monopolizer by acknowledging the member's contribution but redirecting the discussion to others, or the leader can become more directive and limit the discussion time per member.

"Yes, But..."

Some people have a patterned response to any suggestions from others. Initially, they agree with suggestions others offer them, but then they add "yes, but" and give several reasons why the suggestions will not work for them. Leaders and members can easily identify this patterned response. In such situations, it is best to avoid problem solving for the member and encourage the person to develop his or her own solutions. The leader can serve as a role model of the problem-solving behavior for the other members and encourage them to let the member develop a solution that would work specifically for him or her.

Disliked Member

In some groups, members clearly dislike one particular member. This situation can be challenging for the leader because it can result in considerable tension and conflict. This person could become the group's scapegoat. The group leader may have made a mistake by placing the person in this particular group, and another group may be a better match. One solution may be to move the person to a better-matched group. Whether the person stays or leaves, the group leader must stay neutral and avoid displaying negative verbal and nonverbal behaviors that indicate that he or she too dislikes the group member or that he or she is displeased with the other members for their behavior. Often, the group leader can manage the situation by showing respect for the disliked member and acknowledging his or her contribution. In some instances, getting supervision from a more experienced group leader is useful. Defusing the situation may be possible by using conflict resolution strategies and discussing the underlying issues.

The Silent Member

The engagement of a member who does not participate in group discussion can be challenging. This member has had a lifetime of being "the quiet one" and is usually comfortable in the silent role. The leader should respect the person's silent nature. Like all the other group members, the silent member often gains a considerable amount of information and support without verbally participating. It is best for the group leader to get to know the member and understand the meaning of the silence before encouraging interaction.

Group Conflict

Most groups experience periods of conflict. The leader first needs to decide whether the conflict is a natural part of the group process or whether the group needs to address some issues. Member-to-member conflict can be handled through the previously discussed conflict resolution process (see Chapter 10). Leader-to-member conflict is more complicated because the leader has the formal position of power. In this instance, the leader can use conflict resolution strategies but should be sensitive to the power differential between the leader's role and the member's role.

TYPES OF GROUPS

Psychoeducation Groups

Psychoeducation groups include task groups that focus on completion of specific activities, such as planning a week's menu, and teaching groups used to enhance knowledge, improve skills, or solve problems. Learning how to manage a medication regimen or control angry outbursts is often the aim of teaching groups. Psychoeducation groups are formally planned, and members are purposefully selected. Members are asked to join specific groups because of the focus of the group. The group leader develops a lesson plan for each session that includes objectives, content outline, references, and evaluation tools. These groups are time-limited and last for only a few sessions.

Supportive Therapy Groups

Supportive therapy groups are usually less intense than psychotherapy groups and focus on helping individuals cope with their illnesses and problems. Implementing supportive therapy groups is one of the basic functions of the psychiatric nurse. In conducting this type of group, the nurse focuses on helping members cope with situations that are common for other group members. Counseling strategies are used. For example, a group of patients with bipolar illness whose illness is stable may discuss at a monthly meeting how to tell other people about the illness or how to cope with a family member who seems insensitive to the illness. Family caregivers of persons with mental illnesses benefit from the support of the group, as well as additional information about providing care for an ill family member.

Psychotherapy Groups

Psychotherapy groups treat individuals' emotional problems and can be implemented from various theoretic perspectives, including psychoanalytic, behavioral, and cognitive. These groups focus on examining emotions and helping individuals face their life situations. At times, these groups can be extremely intense. Psychotherapy groups provide an opportunity for patients to examine and resolve psychological and interpersonal issues within a safe environment. Mental health specialists who have a minimum of a master's degree and are trained in group psychotherapy lead such groups. Patients can be treated in psychotherapy and still be members of other nursing groups. Communication with the therapists is important for continuity of care.

One of the most respected approaches is Irvin D. Yalom's model of group psychotherapy. According to Yalom, there are 11 primary factors through which therapeutic changes occur (see Box 12.2). In this model, interpersonal relationships are very important because change occurs through a corrective emotional experience within the context of the group, The group is viewed as a social microcosm of the patients' psychosocial environment (Yalom with Leszcz, M., 2005).

Self-Help Groups

Self-help groups are led by people who are concerned about coping with a specific problem or life crisis. These groups do not explore psychodynamic issues in depth. Professionals usually do not attend these groups or serve as consultants. Alcoholics Anonymous, Overeaters Anonymous, and One Day at a Time (a grief group) are examples of self-help groups.

BOX 12.2

Yalom's Therapeutic Factors

Therapeutic Factors	Definition
• Instillation of hope	Hope is required to keep patient in therapy
• Universality	Finding out that others have similar problems
• Imparting information	Didactic instruction about mental health, mental illness, etc.
• Altruism	Learning to give to others
• Corrective recapitulation of the primary family group	Reliving and correcting early family conflicts within the group
• Development of socializing techniques	Learning basic social skills
• Imitative behavior	Assuming some of the behaviors and characteristics of the therapist
• Interpersonal learning	Analogue of therapeutic factors in individual therapy, such as insight, working through the transference, and corrective emotional experience
• Group cohesiveness	Group members' relationship to therapist and other group members
• Catharsis	Open expression of affect to purge or "cleanse" self
• Existential factors	Patients' ultimate concerns of existence: death, isolation, freedom, and meaninglessness.

Age-Related Groups

Group interventions for specific age groups require attention to the developmental needs of the group members, any physical and mental impairments, social ability, and cognitive level. Children's groups should be structured to accommodate their intellectual and developmental functioning. Groups for older people should be adapted for age-related changes of the members (Box 12.3).

COMMON NURSING INTERVENTION GROUPS

Common intervention groups that nurses lead include medication, symptom management, anger management, and self-care groups. In addition, nurses lead many other groups, including stress management, relaxation groups, and women's groups. The key to being a good leader is to

BOX 12.3

Working With Older People in Groups

Self-Assessment
Because most group leaders do not have personal experience with the issues faced by the older adult, the leaders should sensitize themselves to the positive and negative aspects of aging and the developmental issues facing the older adult. Leaders need to be aware of their own negative reactions to aging and how this might affect their work.

Cohort Experiences
There is a wide variation in the experiences and history of the older adult. The 80- to 90-year-old adults grew up in the Great Depression of the 1930s, the 65- to 80-year-old adults commonly experienced growing up during World War II, and the Baby Boomers (aged 55 to 65) were teenagers or young adults during the political and sexual revolution of the 1960s.

Typical Themes in Group Meetings
- Continuity with the past: Older adults enjoy recalling, reliving, and reminiscing about past accomplishments.
- Understanding the modern world: They often use groups to understand and adapt to the modern world.
- Independence: They worry about becoming dependent. Physical and cognitive impairments are threats to independence. Loss of family members and friends are also threats. Leaders should be familiar with the grieving processes.
- Changes in family relationships: Family relationships, especially with children and grandchildren, are increasingly important as social roles change.
- Changes in resources and environment: Living on a fixed income focuses older people on the importance of their disposable income. They are more vulnerable to community and neighborhood changes because of physical and financial limitations.

Group Leadership
Pace of group meetings should be slowed
Greater emphasis on using wisdom and experience rather than learning new information
Encourage group to use life review strategies such as autobiography and reminiscence
Teaching new coping skills should be placed within the context of previous attempts to resolve issues and problems (Toseland & Rizzo, 2004).

integrate group leadership, knowledge, and skills with nursing interventions that fit a selected group.

Medication Groups

Nurse-led medication groups are common in psychiatric nursing. Not all medication groups are alike, so the nurse must be clear regarding the purpose of each specific medication group (Box 12.4). A medication group can be used primarily to transmit information about medications, such as action, dosage, and side effects, or it can focus on issues related to medications, such as compliance, management of side effects, and lifestyle adjustments. Many nurses incorporate both perspectives.

BOX 12.4

Medication Group Protocol

Purpose: Develop strategies that reinforce a self-medication routine.

Description: The medication group is an open, ongoing group that meets once a week to discuss topics germane to self-administration of medication. Members will not be asked to disclose the names of their medications.

Member Selection: The group is open to any person taking medication for a mental illness or emotional problem who would like more information about medication, side effects, and staying on a regimen. Referrals from mental health providers are encouraged. Each person will meet with the group leader before attending the group to determine if the group will meet the individual's learning needs.

Structure: Format is a small group, with no more than eight members and one psychiatric nurse group leader facilitating a discussion about the issues. Topics are rotated.

Time and Location: 2:00–3:00 PM, every Wednesday at the Mental Health Center

Cost: No charge for attending

Topics:
- How Do I Know If My Medications Are Working?
- Side Effect Management: Is It Worth It?
- Hints for Taking Medications Without Missing Doses!
- Health Problems That Medications Affect
- (Other topics will be developed to meet the needs of group members.)

Evaluation: Short pretest and posttest for instructor's use only

Assessing a member's medication knowledge is important before he or she joins the group to determine what the individual would like to learn. People with mental illness may have difficulty remembering new information, so assessment of cognitive abilities is important. Assessing attention span, memory, and problem-solving skills gives valuable information that nurses can use in designing the group. The nurse should determine the members' reading and writing skills to select effective patient education materials.

An ideal group is one in which all members use the same medication. In reality, this situation is rare. Usually, the group members are using various medications. The nurse should know which medications each member is taking, but to avoid violating patient confidentiality, the nurse needs to be careful not to divulge that information to other patients. If group members choose, they can share the names of their medications with one another. A small group format works best, and the more interaction, the better. Using a lecture method of teaching is less effective than involving the members in the learning process. The nurse should expose the members to various audio and visual educational materials, including workbooks, videotapes, and handouts. The nurse should ask members to write down information to help them remember and learn through various modes. Evaluation of the learning outcomes begins with the first class. Nurses can develop and give pretests and posttests, which in combination can measure learning outcomes.

Symptom Management Groups

Nurses often lead groups that focus on helping patients deal with a severe and persistent mental illness. Handling hallucinations, being socially appropriate, and staying motivated to complete activities of daily living are a few common topics. In symptom management groups, members also learn when a symptom indicates that relapse is imminent and what to do about it. Within the context of a symptom management group, patients can learn how to avoid relapse.

Anger Management Groups

Anger management is another common topic for a nurse-led group, often in the inpatient setting. The purposes of an anger management group are to discuss the concept of anger, identify antecedents to aggressive behavior, and develop new strategies to deal with anger other than verbal and physical aggression (see Chapter 38). The treatment team refers individuals with histories of being verbally and physically abusive, usually to family members, to these groups to help them better understand their emotions and behavioral responses. Impulsiveness and emotional lability are problems for many of the group members. Anger management usually includes a discussion of associated stressful situations, events that trigger anger, feelings about the situation, and unmet personal needs.

Self-Care Groups

Another common nurse-led psychiatric group is a self-care group. People with psychiatric illnesses often have self-care deficits and benefit from the structure that a group provides. These groups are challenging because members usually know how to perform these daily tasks (e.g., bathing, grooming, performing personal hygiene), but their illnesses cause them to lose the motivation to complete them. The leader not only reinforces the basic self-care skills, but also, more importantly, helps identify strategies that can motivate the patients and provide structure to their daily lives.

Reminiscence Groups

Reminiscence therapy has been shown to be a valuable intervention for elderly clients. In this type of group, members are encouraged to remember events from past years. Such a group is easily implemented. Usually, a simple question about an important family event will spark memories. Reminiscence groups are usually associated with patients who have dementia who are having difficulty with recent memory. Recalling distant memories is comforting to patients and improves well-being. Reminiscence groups can also be used in caring for patients with depression (Jones & Beck-Little, 2002).

SUMMARY OF KEY POINTS

- The definition of group can vary according to theoretic orientation. A general definition is that a group is two or more people who have at least one common goal or issue. Group dynamics are the interactions within a group that influence the group's development and process.
- Groups can be open, with new members joining at any time, or closed, with members admitted only once. Either small or large groups can be effective, but dynamics change in different size groups.
- The process of group development occurs in phases: beginning, middle, and termination. These stages are not fixed but dynamic. The process challenges the leader to guide the group. During the working stage, the group addresses its purpose.
- Although there are only two formal group roles, leader and member, there are many informal group roles. These roles are usually categorized according to purpose—task functions, maintenance functions, and individual roles. Members who assume task functions encourage the group members to stay focused on the group's task. Those who assume maintenance functions worry more about the group working together than the actual task itself. Individual roles can either enhance or detract from the work of the group.
- Verbal communication includes the communication network and group themes. Nonverbal communication is more complex and involves eye contact, body posture, and mood of the group. Decision-making groups can be victims of groupthink, which can have positive or negative outcomes. Groupthink research is ongoing.
- Leading a group involves many different functions, from obtaining and receiving information to testing and evaluating decisions. The leader should explain the rules of the group at the beginning of the group.
- Seating arrangements can affect group interaction. The fewer physical barriers there are, such as tables, the better the communication. Everyone should be a part of the group, and no one should sit outside of it. In the most interactive groups, members face one another in a circle.
- Leadership skills involve listening, tracking verbal and nonverbal behaviors, and maintaining a neutral, nonjudgmental style.

■ The leader should address behaviors that challenge the leadership, group process, or other members to determine whether to intervene. In some instances, the leader redirects a monopolizing member; at other times the leader lets the group deal with the behavior. Group conflict occurs in most groups.

■ There are many different types of groups. Psychiatric nurses lead psychoeducation and supportive therapy groups. Mental health specialists who are trained to provide intensive therapy lead psychotherapy groups. Consumers lead self-help groups, and professionals assist only as requested. Leading age-related groups requires attention to developmental, physical, social, and intellectual abilities of the participants. Themes of older adult groups include continuity with the past, understanding the modern world, independence, and changes in family and resources. Group leadership for older adult groups builds on participants' previous experiences and coping abilities in developing new coping skills.

■ Medication, symptom management, anger management, and self-care groups are common nurse-led groups.

CRITICAL THINKING CHALLENGES

1 Group members are very polite to one another and are superficially discussing topics. You would assess the group as being in which phase? Explain your answer.
2 After three sessions of a supportive therapy group, two members begin to share their frustration with having a mental illness. The group is moving into which phase of group development? Explain your answer.
3 Define the roles of the task and maintenance functions in groups. Observe your clinical group and identify classmates who are assuming task functions and maintenance functions.
4 Observe a patient group for at least five sessions. Discuss the seating pattern that emerges. Identify the communication network and the group themes. Then identify the group's norms and standards.
5 Discuss the conditions that lead to groupthink. When is groupthink positive? When is groupthink negative? Explain.
6 List at least six behaviors that are important for a group leader including one for age-related groups. Justify your answers.
7 During the first meeting, one member seems very anxious and tends to monopolize the conversation. Discuss how you would assess the situation and whether you would intervene.
8 At the end of the fourth meeting, one group member angrily accuses another of asking too many questions. The other members look on quietly. How would you assess the situation? Would you intervene? Explain

12 Angry Men: 1998. In this excellent film, a young man stands accused of fatally stabbing his father. A jury of his "peers" is deciding his fate. This jury is portrayed by an excellent cast, including Jack Lemmon, George C. Scott, Tony Danza, and Ossie Davis. At first, the case appears to be "open and shut." This film depicts an intense struggle to reach a verdict and is an excellent study of group process and group dynamics.

VIEWING POINTS: Identify the leaders in the group. How does leadership change throughout the film? Do you find any evidence of groupthink? How does the group handle conflict?

REFERENCES

Alf, L., & Wilson, K. (2001). Facilitating group beginnings 1: A practice model. *Groupwork, 13*(1), 6–30.

Alvarez, A. (2002). Pitfalls, pratfalls, shortfalls and windfalls: Reflection on forming and being formed by groups. *Social Work With Groups, 25*(1), 93–105.

Benne, K., & Sheats, P. (1948). Functional roles of group members. *Journal of Social Issues, 4*(2), 41–49.

Brown, T., & Miller, C. (2000). Communication networks in task-performing groups: Effects of task complexity, time, pressure, and interpersonal dominance. *Small Group Research, 31*(2), 131–157.

Choi, J., & Kim, M. (1999). The organizational application of groupthink and its limitations in organizations. *Journal of Applied Psychology, 84*(2), 297–306.

Fraser, S. N., & Spink, K. S. (2002). Examining the role of social support and group cohesion in exercise compliance. *Journal of Behavior Medicine, 25*(3), 233–249.

Graham, M., & Sontag, M. (2001). Art as an evaluative tool: A pilot study. *Art Therapy, 18*(1), 37–43.

Janis, I. (1972). *Victims of groupthink.* Boston: Houghton Mifflin.

Janis, I. (1982). *Groupthink* (2nd ed.). Boston: Houghton Mifflin.

Jones, E. D., & Beck-Little, R. (2002). The use of reminiscence therapy for the treatment of depression in rural-dwelling older adults. *Issues in Mental Health Nursing, 23,* 279–280.

Moher,M., Hey, K., & Lancaster,T. (2003). Workplace interventions for smoking cessation. *Cochrane Database Syst Rev* 2003;(2):CD003440.

Moreno, J. (1953). *Who shall survive?* Beacon, NY: Beacon House.

Neck, C. P., & Moorhead, G. (1995). Groupthink remodeled: The importance of leadership, time pressure, and methodical decision-making procedures. *Human Relations, 48*(5), 537–557.

Steinhardt, M. A., Dolbier, C. L., Gottlieb, N. H., & McCalister, K. T. (2003). The relationship between hardiness, supervisor support, group cohesion, and job stress as predictors of job satisfaction. *American Journal of Health Promotion, 17*(6), 382–389.

Toseland, R.W. & Rizzo, V.M. (2004). What's different about working with older people in groups? *Journal of Gerontological Social Work, 44*(1/2), 5–23.

Yalom, I., with Leszcz, M. (2005). *The theory and practice of group psychotherapy.* New York: Basic Books.

CHAPTER 13

Family Assessment and Interventions

Mary Ann Boyd

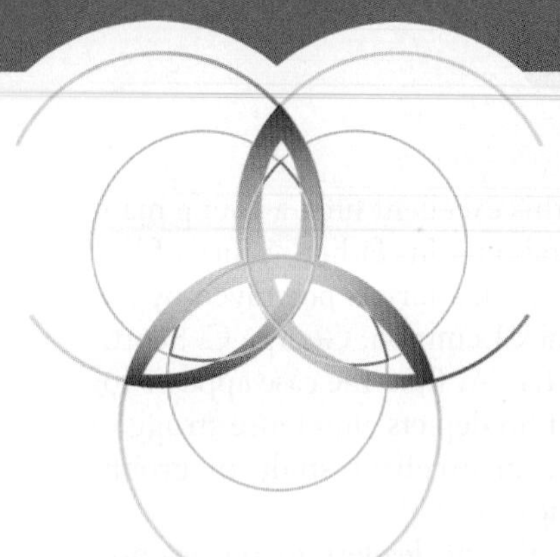

LEARNING OBJECTIVES

After studying this chapter, you will be able to:

- Discuss the balance of family mental health with family dysfunction.
- Develop a genogram that depicts the family history, relationships, and mental disorders across at least three generations.
- Develop a plan for a comprehensive family assessment.
- Apply family nursing diagnoses to families who need nursing care.
- Discuss nursing interventions that are useful in caring for families.

KEY CONCEPTS

- comprehensive family assessment
- family

KEY TERMS

boundaries • differentiation of self • dysfunctional family • emotional cutoff • extended family • family development • family life cycle • family projection process • family structure • genogram • multigenerational transmission process • nuclear family • nuclear family emotional process • sibling position • subsystems • transition times • triangles time • triangles

A family is a group of people connected emotionally, or by blood, or in both ways that has developed patterns of interaction and relationships. Family members have a shared history and a shared future (Carter & McGoldrick, 2005). **A nuclear family** is two or more people living together and related by blood, marriage, or adoption. An **extended family** is several nuclear families whose members may or may not live together and function as one group. Families are unique in that, unlike all other organizations, they incorporate new members only by birth, adoption, or marriage, and members can leave only by divorce or death.

> **KEY CONCEPT Family** is a group of people connected by emotions, or blood, or both, that has developed patterns of interaction and relationships. Family members have a shared history and a shared future (Carter & McGoldrick, 2005).

The psychiatric nurse interacts with families in various ways. Because of the interpersonal and chronic nature of many mental illnesses, psychiatric nurses often have frequent and long-term contact with families. Involvement may range from meeting family members only once or twice to treating the whole family as a patient. Unlike a therapeutic group (see Chapter 12), the family system has a history and continues to function when the nurse is not there. The family reacts to past, present, and anticipated future relationships within at least a three-generation family system. This chapter explains how to integrate important family concepts into the nursing process when providing psychiatric nursing care to families experiencing mental health problems.

FAMILY MENTAL HEALTH AND FAMILY DYSFUNCTION

In a mentally healthy family, members live in harmony among themselves and within society. Ideally, these families support and nurture their members throughout their lives. However, dysfunction and mental illness can affect a family's overall mental health.

A family becomes **dysfunctional** when interactions, decisions, or behaviors interfere with the positive development of the family and its individual members. Most families have periods of dysfunction such as during a crisis or stressful situation when the coping skills are not available. Families usually adapt and regain their mentally healthy balance. A family can be mentally healthy and at the same time have a member who has a mental illness. Conversely, a family can be dysfunctional and have no member with a diagnosable mental illness.

Effects of Mental Illness on Family Functioning

Families of people with persistent mental disorders have special needs. Many mentally ill adults live with their parents well into their 30s and beyond. For these adults with persistent mental illness, the family serves several functions that those without mental illness do not need. Such functions include the following:

Providing support. People with mental illness have difficulty maintaining nonfamilial support networks and may rely exclusively on their families.

Providing information. Families often have complete and continuous information about care and treatment over the years.

Monitoring services. Families observe the progress of their relative and report concerns to those in charge of care.

Advocating for services. Family groups advocate for money for residential care services.

Conflicts can occur between parents and mental health workers who place a high value on independence. Members of the mental health care system may criticize families for being overly protective when, in reality, the patient with mental illness may face real barriers to independent living. Housing may be unavailable; when available, quality may be poor. The patient may fear leaving home, may be at risk for relapse if he or she does leave, or may be too comfortable at home to want to leave. When long-term caregivers, usually the parents, die, patients with mental illness experience housing disruptions and potentially traumatic transitions. Siblings who have other responsibilities expect to be less involved than their parents in the care and oversight of the mentally ill brother or sister. Few families actually plan for this difficult eventuality (Hatfield & Lefley, 2005).

Nurses must use an objective and rational approach when discussing independence and dependence with the family. Family emotions often obscure the underlying issues, but nurses can diffuse such emotions so that everyone can explore the alternatives comfortably. Although separation must eventually occur, the timing and process vary according to each family's particular situation. Parents may be highly anxious when their adult children first leave home and need reassurance and support.

Influence of Cultural Beliefs and Values on Family Functioning

Conceptualizations of normal family functioning vary among different cultural groups. For example, some Asian cultures expect a mother-in-law to move in with her married child and his or her spouse to help care for the couple's children. In some families of European descent, a mother-in-law's presence is construed as unusual or an interference with family functioning. One challenge of psychiatric nursing is to avoid classifying certain family patterns as pathologic just because they deviate from either dominant cultural norms or the nurse's theoretically based or theoretically driven values. On the other hand, the nurse must be careful not to overattribute symptoms and dysfunctional patterns to culture when such difficulties reflect actual problems. For instance, the nurse might overlook a patient's withdrawal as a symptom of depression if he or she attributes such behavior to a "cultural" tendency.

Beliefs about seeking help for mental health problems are also culturally based and vary among groups. General help-seeking patterns include the following:

- African American and Latino families tend to seek support from extended family and other community members, rather than from health or mental health professionals in the initial stages of a family problem (Celano & Kaslow, 2000).
- Although most families experience some discomfort in sharing family problems with outsiders, uneasiness with disclosure is particularly prominent in families from ethnic minority groups (Celano & Kaslow, 2000).
- African Americans may fear misdiagnosis, the prescribing of medication for behavioral and population control, and governmental abuse (Hines & Boyd-Franklin, 2005).

COMPREHENSIVE FAMILY ASSESSMENT

A comprehensive family assessment is the collection of all relevant data related to family health, psychological well-being, and social functioning to identify problems for which the nurse can generate nursing diagnoses. The assessment consists of a face-to-face interview with family members and can be conducted during several sessions. Nurses conduct a comprehensive family assessment when they care for patients and their families for an extended period. They also use them when a patient's

BOX 13.1

Family Mental Health Assessment

I. Family members present

Name	**Age**	**Relationship**

II. Health status

Member	**Disorder and current treatment**

III. Mental health status

Member	**Disorder and current treatment**

IV. Impact of mental illness on family function
Describe the changes that occur in the family as a result of the family member's disorder:

V. Family life cycle
Describe the family life cycle stage and any transitions that are occurring.

VI. Communication patterns
Describe the family communication patterns in terms of usual times of communication (morning, dinner etc.), which family members talk to each other, who communicates the family rules, who carries out discipline. Identify triangulated messages.

VII. Stress and coping
Identify current family stressful events and family coping mechanisms.

VIII. Problem-solving skills
Determine who solves problems in the family. Are the problem-solving skills of the family able to manage most family problems?

IX. Family system (from the genogram)
Family composition

Health and illness patterns

Relationship patterns

(Continued on following page)

BOX 13.1

Family Mental Health Assessment (continued)

Social functioning patterns__________

Financial and legal status__________

Formal and informal network__________

X. Nursing diagnoses

mental health problems are so complex that family support is important for optimal care (Box 13.1).

KEY CONCEPT A comprehensive family assessment is the collection of all relevant data related to family health, psychological well-being, and social functioning to identify problems for which the nurse can generate nursing diagnoses.

Relationship Building

In preparing for a family assessment, nurses must concentrate on developing a relationship with the family. Although necessary when working with any family, relationship development is particularly important for families from ethnic minority cultures. Developing a relationship takes time, so the nurse may need to complete the assessment during several meetings, rather than just one.

To develop a positive relationship with a family, nurses must establish credibility with the family and address its immediate intervention needs. To establish credibility, the family must see the nurse as knowledgeable and skillful. Possessing culturally competent nursing skills and projecting a professional image are crucial to establishing credibility. With regard to immediate intervention needs, a family who needs shelter or food is not ready to discuss a member's medication regimen until the first needs are met. The nurse will make considerable progress in establishing a relationship with a family when he or she helps members meet their immediate needs.

Genograms

Families possess various structural configurations (e.g., single-parent, multigenerational, same-gender relationships). The nurse can facilitate taking the family history by completing a **genogram**, which is a multigenerational schematic diagram that lists family members and their relationships. The genogram is a skeleton of the family that the nurse can use as a framework for exploring relationships and patterns of health and illness.

A genogram includes the age, dates of marriage and death, and geographic location of each member. Squares represent men and circles represent women; ages are listed inside the squares and circles. Horizontal lines represent marriages with dates; vertical lines connect parents and children. Genograms can be particularly useful in understanding family history, composition, relationships, and illnesses (Fig. 13.1).

Genograms vary from simple to elaborate. The patient's and family's assessment needs guide the level of detail. In a small family with limited problems, the genogram can be rather general. In a large family with multiple problems, the genogram should reflect these complexities. Thus, depending on the level of detail, nurses collect various data. They can study important events such as marriages, divorces, deaths, and geographic movements. They can include cultural or religious affiliations, education and economic levels, and the nature of the work of each family member. Psychiatric nurses should always include mental disorders and other significant health problems in the genogram.

Analyzing and Using Genograms

For a genogram to be useful in assessment, the nurse needs to analyze the data for family composition, relationship problems, and mental health patterns. Nurses can begin with composition. How large is the family?

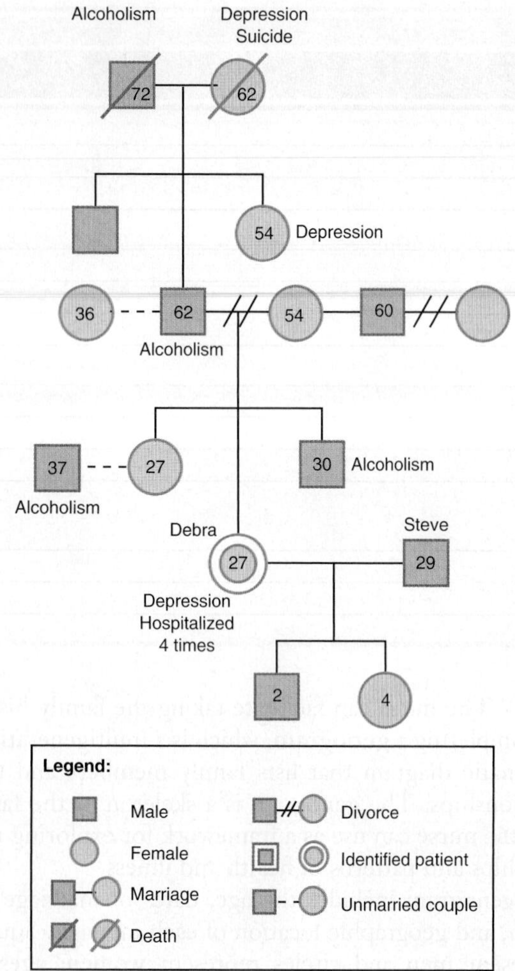

FIGURE 13.1. Analysis of genogram for Debra. Illness patterns are depression (paternal aunt, grandmother [suicide]) and alcoholism (brother, father, grandfather). Relationship patterns show that parents are divorced and neither sibling is married.

Where do family members live? A large family whose members live in the same city is more likely to have support than a family in which distance separates members. Of course, this is not always the case. Sometimes even when family members live geographically close, they are emotionally distant from one another.

The nurse should also study the genogram for relationship and illness patterns. For instance, in terms of relationship patterns, the nurse may find a history of divorces or family members who do not keep in touch with the rest of the family. The nurse can then explore the significance of these and other relationships. In terms of illness patterns, alcoholism, often seen across several generations, may be prevalent in men on one side of a family. The nurse can then hypothesize that alcoholism is one of the mental health risks for the family and design interventions to reduce the risk. Or the nurse may find via a genogram that members of a family's previous generation were in "state hospitals" or had "nerve problems."

Family Biologic Domain

In the family biologic domain, the family assessment includes a thorough picture of physical and mental health status and how the status affects family functioning. The family with multiple health problems, both physical and mental, will be trying to manage these problems as well as obtain the many financial and health care resources it needs.

Physical Health Status

The family health status includes the physical illnesses and disabilities of all members; the nurse can record such information on the genogram and also include the physical illnesses and disabilities of other generations. Illnesses of family members are an indication not only of their physical status, but also of the stress currently being placed on the family and its resources. The nurse should pay particular attention to any physical problems that affect family functioning. For example, if a member requires frequent visits to a provider or hospitalizations, the whole family will feel the effects of focusing excessive time and financial resources on that member. The nurse should explore how such situations specifically affect other members.

Mental Health Status

Detecting mental disorders in families may be difficult because these disorders often are hidden or the "family secret." Very calmly, the nurse should ask family members to identify anyone who has had or has a mental illness. He or she should record the information on the genogram as well as in the narrative. If family members do not know if anyone in the family had or has a mental illness, the nurse should ask if anyone was treated for "nerves" or had a "nervous breakdown." Overall, a good family history of mental illness across multiple generations helps the nurse understand the significance of mental illness in the current generation. If one family member has a serious mental illness, the whole family will be affected. Usually, siblings of the mentally ill member receive less parental attention than the affected member.

Family's Psychological Domain

Assessment of the family's psychological domain focuses on the family's development and life cycle, communication patterns, stress and coping abilities, and problem-solving skills. One aim of the assessment is to understand the relationships within the family. Although family roles and structures are important, the true value of the family is in its relationships, which are irreplaceable. For example, if a parent leaves or dies, another person (e.g., stepparent, grandparent) can assume some parental functions but can never really replace the emotional relationship with the missing parent.

Family Development

Family development is a broad term that refers to all the processes connected with the growth of a family, including changes associated with work, geographic location, migration, acculturation, and serious illness. In optimal family development, family members are relatively differentiated (capable of autonomous functioning) from one another, anxiety is low, and the parents have good emotional relationships with their own families of origin.

Family Life Cycles

The concept of **family life cycle** refers to stages that evolve based on significant events related to the arrival and departure of members, such as birth or adoption, child rearing, departure of children from home, occupational retirement, and death. The family life cycle is a process of expansion, contraction, and realignment of relationship systems to support the entry, exit, and development of family members in a functional way (Carter & McGoldrick, 2005) (Table 13.1). A family's life cycle is conceptualized in terms of stages throughout the years. To move from one stage to the next, the family system undergoes changes. Structural and potential structural changes within stages can usually be handled by rearranging the family system (first-order changes), whereas transition from one stage to the next requires changes in the system itself (second-order changes). An example of a first-order change is when all the children are finally in school and the stay-at-home parent returns to work. The system is rearranged, but the structure remains the same. In second-order changes, the family structure does change, such as when a member moves away from the family home to live independently.

• NCLEXNOTE

NCLEXNOTE

Apply family life cycle stages to a specific family with a member who has a psychiatric disorder. Identify the emotional transitions and the required family changes.

The nurse should not view this model as the "normal" life cycle for every family and should limit its use to those families it clearly fits. As second marriages, career changes in midlife, and other phenomena occur with increasing frequency, this traditional model is being challenged, modified, and redesigned to address such contemporary structural and role changes. This model also may not fit many cultural groups. Variations of the family life cycle are presented for the divorced family (Table 13.2) and the remarried family (Table 13.3).

Table 13.1 Stages of the Family Life Cycle

Family Life Cycle Stage	Emotional Transition	Required Family Changes
1. Leaving home: single young adults	Accepting emotional and financial responsibility for self	Differentiation of self in relation to family of origin Development of intimate peer relationships Establishment of self regarding work and financial independence
2. The joining of families through marriage: the new couple	Commitment to new system	Formation of marital system Realignment of relationships with extended families and friends to include spouse
3. Families with young children	Accepting new members into the system	Adjusting marital system to make space for children Joining in child rearing, financial, and household tasks Realignment of relationships with extended family to include parenting and grandparenting roles
4. Families with adolescents	Increasing flexibility of family boundaries to include children's independence and grandparents frailties	Shifting of parent–child relationships to permit adolescent to move in and out of system Refocus on midlife marital and career issues Beginning shift toward joint caring for older generation
5. Launching children and moving on	Accepting multitude of exits from and entries into the family system	Renegotiation of marital system as a dyad Development of adult–adult relationships between grown children and their parents Realignment of relationships to include in-laws and grandchildren Dealing with disabilities and death of parents (grandparents)
6. Families in later life	Accepting the shifting of generational roles	Maintaining own and couple functioning interests in face of physiologic decline, exploration of new familial and social role options Support for a more central role of middle generation Making room in the system for the wisdom and experience of the elderly, supporting the older generation without overfunctioning for them Dealing with loss of spouse, siblings, and other peers and preparation for own death.

From Carter B. & McGoldrick, M. (2005). Overview: The expanded family life cycle. In B. Carter & M. McGoldrick (Eds.), *The expanded family life cycle* (p. 2). New York: Allyn & Bacon.

Table 13.2 The Divorcing Family

Family Life Cycle Stage	Prerequisite Attitude	Developmental Issues
Divorce		
1. Decision to divorce	Acceptance of inability to resolve marital tensions sufficiently to continue relationship	Acceptance of one's own part in the failure of the marriage
2. Planning the breakup of the system	Supporting viable arrangements for all parts of the system	Working cooperatively on problems of custody, visitation, and finances Dealing with extended family about the divorce
3. Separation	Willingness to continue cooperative coparental relationship and joint financial support of children Work on resolution of attachment to spouse	Mourning loss of intact family Restructuring marital and parent–child relationships and finances; adaptation to living apart Realignment of relationships with extended family staying connected with spouse's extended family
4. The divorce	More work on emotional divorce: Overcoming hurt, anger, guilt, etc.	Mourning loss of intact family: giving up fantasies of reunion Retrieval of hopes, dreams, expectations from the marriage Staying connected with extended families
Postdivorce Family		
1. Single-parent (custodial household or primary residence)	Willingness to maintain financial responsibilities, continue parental contact with ex-spouse, and support contact of children with ex-spouse and his or her family.	Making flexible visitation arrangements with ex-spouse and his family Rebuilding own financial resources Rebuilding own social network
2. Single-parent (noncustodial)	Willingness to maintain parental contact with ex-spouse and support custodial parent's relationship with children.	Finding ways to continue effective parenting relationship with children Maintaining financial responsibilities to ex-spouse and children Rebuilding own social network

From Carter, B., & McGoldrick, M. (1999a). The divorce cycle: A major variation in the American family life cycle. In B. Carter & M. McGoldrick (Eds.), *The expanded family life cycle* (p. 375). New York: Allyn & Bacon.

Transition times are the addition, subtraction, or change in status of family members. During transitions, family stresses are more likely to cause symptoms or dysfunction. Significant family events, such as the death of a member or the introduction of a new member, also affect the family's ability to function. During transitions, families may seek help from the mental health system.

Cultural Variations

In caring for families from diverse cultures, the nurse should examine whether the underlying assumptions and frameworks of the dominant life-cycle models apply. Even the concept of "family" varies among cultures. For example, the dominant Caucasian middle-class culture's definition of family refers to the intact nuclear family. For Italian Americans, the entire extended network of aunts, uncles, cousins, and grandparents may be involved in family decision making and share holidays and life-cycle transitions. For African Americans, the family may include a broad network of kin and community that includes long-time friends who are considered family members (Hines & Boyd-Franklin, 2005).

Cultural groups also differ in the importance they give to certain life-cycle transitions. For example, Irish American families may emphasize the wake, viewing death as an important life-cycle transition. African American families may emphasize funerals, going to considerable expense and delaying services until all family members arrive. Italian American and Polish American families may place great emphasis on weddings (McGoldrick, Giordano, & Garcia-Preto, 2005).

Families in Poverty

The family life cycle of those living in poverty may vary from those with adequate financial means. People living in poverty struggle to make ends meet, and members may face difficulties in meeting their own or other members' basic developmental needs. To be poor does not mean that a family is automatically dysfunctional. But poverty is an important factor that can force even the healthiest families to crumble. In studying African American families living in poverty, Hines (1999) observed four distinguishing characteristics: condensed life cycle, female-headed households of the extended-family type, chronic stress and untimely losses, and reliance on institutional supports.

When the life cycle is condensed, family members leave home, mate, have children, and become grandpar-

Table 13.3 Remarried Family Formulations

Family Life Cycle Stage	Prerequisite Attitude	Developmental Issues
1. Entering the new relationship	Recovery from loss of first marriage (adequate "emotional divorce")	Recommitment to marriage and to forming a family with readiness to deal with the complexity and ambiguity
2. Conceptualizing and planning new marriage and family	Accepting one's own fears and those of new spouse and children about remarriage and forming a stepfamily. Accepting need for time and patience for adjustment to complexity and ambiguity of multiple new roles Boundaries: space, time, membership, and authority. Affective issues: guilt, loyalty conflicts, desire for mutuality, unresolvable past hurts	Work on openness in the new relationships to avoid pseudomutuality Plan for maintenance of cooperative financial and co-parental relationships with ex-spouses Plan to help children deal with fears, loyalty conflicts, and membership in two systems Realignment of relationships with extended family to include new spouse and children Plan maintenance of connections for children with extended family of ex-spouses
3. Remarriage and reconstitution of family	Final resolution of attachment to previous spouse and ideal of "intact" family Acceptance of a different model of family with permeable boundaries.	Restructuring family boundaries to allow for inclusion of new spouse-stepparent Realignment of relationships and financial arrangement throughout subsystems to permit interweaving of several systems Making room for relationships of all children with biologic (noncustodial) parents, grandparents, and other extended family Sharing memories and histories to enhance stepfamily integration

From Carter, B., & McGoldrick, M. (1999a). The divorce cycle. A major variation in the American family life cycle. In B. Carter & M. McGoldrick (Eds.), *The expanded family life cycle* (p. 377). New York: Allyn & Bacon.

ents at much earlier ages than their working-class and middle-class counterparts. Consequently, many individuals in such families assume new roles and responsibilities before they are developmentally capable.

The condensed life cycle can be loosely divided into three overlapping stages: adolescence and unattached adulthood, family with young children, and family in later life. In the African American family living in poverty, members may either push male adolescents out of the home or cling to them desperately as a source of assistance. Education subsequently becomes a low priority, and these teens often drop out of school. Peer relationships are powerful and can conflict with expectations at home. Male adolescents cannot differentiate themselves from either family or peers. They often cannot find employment, except for menial work. They may assert their masculinity in transient heterosexual relationships. Both family burdens and peer pressure leave them ill-equipped to handle later stages. They quickly move into the next stage of family with young children but often cannot assume parental roles.

The second characteristic that Hines observed is female-headed households of the extended-family type, in which a woman, her children, and her daughter's children often live together without clear delineation of their respective roles. This scenario can create economic and emotional burdens for the older women and difficulty for the younger women in assuming parental responsibilities.

Often, the role of women living in poverty is conscripted to child rearing as pregnancies interrupt their education and they eventually become dependent on public support. Then, older family members (usually the baby's grandmother) become the primary sources of assistance. Subsequent pregnancies may increase the burden of caregiving. The next stage, the family in later life, does not signal a decrease in daily responsibilities or a shift into concerns about retirement. Instead, despite possible poor health, elderly family members continue to work to support their children and grandchildren (Hines, 1999).

The third characteristic is chronic stress and untimely losses. Families living in poverty are subject to family disruption via abrupt loss of members, loss of unemployment compensation, illness, death, imprisonment, or alcohol or drug addiction. Men may die relatively young compared with their middle-class counterparts. Ordinary problems, such as transportation or a sick child, can become major crises because of a lack of resources to solve them.

Reliance on institutional supports is the final distinguishing characteristic. Poor families are often forced to seek public assistance, which ultimately can result in additional stress in having to deal with a governmental agency.

Communication Patterns

Family communication patterns develop over a lifetime. Some family members communicate more openly and honestly than others. In addition, family subgroups develop from communication patterns. Just as in any assessment interview, the nurse should observe the verbal and nonverbal communication of the family members. Who sits next to each other? Who talks to whom? Who answers most questions? Who volunteers information? Who changes the subject? Which subjects seem acceptable to discuss? Which topics are not discussed? Can spouses be intimate with each other? Are any family secrets revealed? Does the nonverbal communication match the verbal communication? Nurses can use all this information to help identify family problems and communication issues.

Nurses should also assess the family for its daily communication patterns. Identifying which family members confide in one another is a place to start examining ongoing communication. Other areas include how often children talk with parents, which child talks to the parents most, and who is most likely to discipline the children. Another question considers whether family members can express positive and negative feelings. In determining how open or closed the family is, the nurse explores the type of information the family shares with nonfamily members. For example, one family may tell others about a member's mental illness, whereas another family may not discuss any illnesses with those outside the family.

Stress and Coping Abilities

One of the most important assessment tasks is to determine how family members deal with major and minor stressful events and their available coping skills. Some families seem able to cope with overwhelming stresses, such as the death of a member, major illness, or severe conflict, whereas other families seem to fall apart over relatively minor events. It is important for the nurse to listen to which situations a family appraises as stressful and help the family identify usual coping responses. The nurse can then evaluate these responses. If the family's responses are maladaptive (e.g., substance abuse, physical abuse), the nurse will discuss the need to develop coping skills that lead to family well-being (see Chapter 14).

• NCLEXNOTE

NCLEXNOTE Identifying stressful events and coping mechanisms should be a priority in a family assessment.

Problem-Solving Skills

Nurses assess family problem-solving skills by focusing on the more recent problems the family has experienced and determining the process that members used to solve them. For example, a child is sick at school and needs to go home. Does the mother, father, grandparent, or babysitter receive the call from the school? Who then cares for the child? Underlying the ability to solve problems is the decision-making process. Who makes and implements decisions? How does the family handle conflict? All these data provide information regarding the family's problem-solving abilities. Once these abilities are identified, the nurse can build on these strengths in helping families deal with additional problems.

Family Social Domain

An assessment of the family's social domain provides important data about the operation of the family as a system and its interaction within its environment. Areas of concern include the system itself, social and financial status, and formal and informal support networks.

Family Systems

Just as any group can be viewed as a system, a family can be understood as a system with interdependent members. Family system theories view the family as an open system whose members interact with their environment as well as among themselves. One family member's change in thoughts or behavior can cause a ripple effect and change everyone else's. For example, a mother who decides not to pick up her children's clothing from their bedroom floors anymore forces the children to deal with cluttered rooms and dirty clothes in a different way than before.

One common scenario in the mental health field is the effect of a patient's improvement on the family. With new medications and treatment, patients are more likely to be able to live independently, which subsequently changes the responsibilities and activities of family caregivers. Although on the surface members may seem relieved that their caregiving burden is lifted, in reality, they must adjust their time and energies to fill the remaining void. This transition may not be easy because it is often less stressful to maintain familiar activities than to venture into uncharted territory. Families may seem as though they want to keep an ill member dependent, but in reality they are struggling with the change in their family system.

Several system models are used in caring for families: the Wright Leahey Calgary model, Bowen's family system, and Minuchin's structural family system.

Calgary Family Model

Lorraine M. Wright and Maureen Leahey developed the Calgary Family Assessment Model (CFAM) and the Calgary Family Intervention Model (CFIM). These nursing models are based on systems, cybernetics, and communication and change theories (Wright and Leahey, 2000). Families seek help when they have family health and illness problems, difficulties, and suffering. These two models are multidimensional frameworks that conceptualize the family into structural, developmental, and functional categories. Each assessment category contains several subcategories. Structure is further categorized into internal (family, gender, sexual orientation, etc.), external (extended family and larger systems), and context (ethnicity, race, social class, religion, spirituality, environment). Family developmental assessment is organized according to stages, tasks, and attachments. Functional assessment areas include instrumental (activities of daily living) and expressive (communication, problem-solving roles, beliefs, etc.).

The CFAM and CFIM are built around four stages: engagement, assessment, intervention, and termination. The *engagement* stage is the initial stage in which the family is greeted and made comfortable. In the *assessment* stage, problems are identified and relationships between family and health providers develop. During this stage, the nurse opens space for the family to tell its story. The *intervention* stage is the core of the clinical work and involves providing a context in which the family can make changes (see Intervention section in this chapter). The *termination* phase refers to the process of ending the therapeutic relationship (Wright and Leahey, 2000).

Family Systems Therapy Model

Bowen recognized the power of a system and believed that there is a balance between the family system and the individual. Bowen developed several concepts that professionals often use today when working with families (Bowen, 1975, 1976; Knauth, 2003; Miller, Anderson, & Kaulana, 2004):

Differentiation of self involves two processes: intrapsychic and interpersonal. Intrapsychic differentiation means separating thinking from feeling: a differentiated individual can distinguish between thoughts and feelings and can consequently think through behavior. For example, a person who has experienced intrapsychic differentiation, even though angry, will think through the underlying issue before acting. However, the feeling of the moment will drive the behavior of an undifferentiated individual. Interpersonal differentiation is the process of freeing oneself from the family's emotional chaos. That is, the individual can recognize the family turmoil but avoid re-entering arguments and issues. For Bowen, the individual must resolve attachment to this chaos before he or she can differentiate into a mature, healthy personality. Nursing research is currently investigating the use of assessment tools to measure differentiation (see Box 13.2).

Triangles: According to Bowen, the triangle is a three-person system and the smallest stable unit in human relations. Cycles of closeness and distance characterize a two-person relationship. When anxiety is high during periods of distance, one party "triangulates" a third person or thing into the relationship. For example, two partners may have a stable relationship when anxiety is low. When anxiety and tension rise, one partner may be so uncomfortable that he or she confides in a friend instead of the other partner. In these cases, triangulating reduces the tension but freezes the conflict in place. In families, triangulating occurs when a husband and wife diffuse tension by focusing on the children. To maintain the status quo and avoid the conflict, one of the parents develops an overly intense relationship with one of the children, which tends to produce symptoms in the child (e.g., bed wetting, fear of school).

Family projection process: Through this process, the triangulated member becomes the center of the family conflicts; that is, the family projects its conflicts onto the child or other triangulated person. Projection is anxious, enmeshed concern. For example, a husband and wife are having difficulty deciding how to spend money. One of their children is having difficulty with interpersonal relationships in school. Instead of the parents resolving their differences over money, one parent focuses on the child's needs and becomes intensely involved in the child's issues. The other parent then relates coolly and distantly to the involved parent.

Nuclear family emotional process: This concept describes patterns of emotional functioning in a family in a single generation. This emotional distance is a patterned reaction in daily interactions with the spouse.

BOX 13.2

***Research for Best Practice:* Psychometric Evaluation of the Differentiation of Self Inventory for Adolescents**

Knauth, D. G., & Skowron, E. A. (2004). Psychometric evaluation of the Differentiation of Self Inventory for adolescents. Nursing Research, 53(3), 163–171.

The Question: What is the reliability and validity of the self-report instrument, Differentiation of Self Inventory (DSI) for use with adolescents?

Methods: The DSI was administered to an ethnically diverse sample of 363 adolescents 14 to 19 years of age.

Findings: The DSI scale had good internal consistency reliability (Cronbach alpha of 0.84). The results of the study support the use of the DSI in the adolescent population.

Implications for Nursing: The DSI can be used with the adolescent population in determining the ability to differentiate between emotional and intellectual functioning. This tool is appropriate if the Bowen Family Theory model is guiding practice.

Multigenerational transmission process: Bowen believed that one generation transfers its emotional processes to the next generation. Certain basic patterns between parents and children are replicas of those of past generations, and generations to follow will repeat them as well. The child who is the most involved with the family is least able to differentiate from his or her family of origin and passes on conflicts from one generation to another. For example, a spouse may stay emotionally distant from his partner, just as his father was with his mother.

Sibling position: Children develop fixed personality characteristics based on their **sibling position** in their families. For example, a first-born child may have more confidence and be more outgoing than the second-born child, who has grown up in the older child's shadow. Conversely, the second-born child may be more inclined to identify with the oppressed and be more open to other experiences than the first-born child. These attitudinal and behavioral patterns become fixed parts of both children's personalities. Knowledge of these general personality characteristics is helpful in predicting the family's emotional processes and patterns. These theoretical ideas of Bowen have not been supported by research, but the more general principle that a child's position in the family origin affects the child's personality has significant empirical support (Miller et al., 2004).

Emotional cutoff: If a member cannot differentiate from his or her family, that member may just flee from the family, either by moving away or avoiding personal subjects of conversation. Yet a brief visit from parents can render these individuals helpless.

In using this model, the nurse can observe family interactions to determine how differentiated family members are from one another. Are members autonomous in thinking and feeling? Do triangulated relationships develop during periods of stress and tension? Are family members interacting in the same manner as their parents or grandparents? How do the personalities of older siblings compare with those of younger siblings? Who lives close to one another? Does any family member live in another city? The Bowen model can provide a way of assessing the system of family relationships.

Family Structure Model

Salvador Minuchin emphasizes the importance of family structure. In his model, the family consists of three essential components: structure, subsystems, and boundaries (Minuchin, Lee, & Simon, 1996).

Family structure is the organized pattern in which family members interact. As two adult partners come together to form a family, they develop the quantity of their interactions, or how much time they spend interacting. For example, a newly married couple may establish their evening interaction pattern by talking to each other during dinner but not while watching television. The quality of the interactions also becomes patterned. Some topics are appropriate for conversation during their evening walk (e.g., reciting daily events), whereas controversial or emotionally provocative topics are relegated to other times and places.

Family rules are important influences on interaction patterns. For example, "family problems stay in the family" is a common rule. Both the number of people in the family and its development also influence the interaction pattern. For instance, the interaction between a single mother and her children changes when she remarries and introduces a stepfather. Over time, families repeat interactions, which develop into enduring patterns. For example, if a mother tells her son to straighten his room and the son refuses until his father yells at him, the family has initiated an interactional pattern. If this pattern continues, the child will come to see the father as the disciplinarian and the mother as incompetent. However, the mother will be more affectionate to her son, and the father will remain the disciplinarian on the "outside."

Subsystems develop when family members join together for various activities or functions. Minuchin views each member, as well as dyads and other larger groups that form, as a subsystem. Obvious groups are parents and children. Sometimes, there are "boy" and "girl" systems. Such systems become obvious in an assessment when family members talk about "the boys going fishing with dad" and "the girls going shopping with mother." Family members belong to several different subgroups. A mother may also be a wife, sister, and daughter. Sometimes, these roles can conflict. It may be acceptable for a woman to be very firm as a disciplinarian in her role as mother. However, in her sister, wife, or daughter role, similar behavior would provoke anger and resentment.

Boundaries are invisible barriers with varying permeabilities that surround each subsystem. They regulate the amount of contact a person has with others and protect the autonomy of the family and its subsystems. If family members do not take telephone calls at dinner, they are protecting themselves from outside intrusion. When parents do not allow children to interrupt them, they are establishing a boundary between themselves and their children. According to Minuchin, the spouse subsystem must have a boundary that separates it from parents, children, and the outside world. A clear boundary between parent and child enables children to interact with their parents but excludes them from the spouse subsystem.

Boundaries vary from rigid to diffuse. If boundaries are too rigid and permit little contact from outside subsystems, disengagement results, and disengaged individuals are relatively isolated. On the other hand, rigid boundaries permit independence, growth, and mastery within the subsystem, particularly if parents do not hover over their children, telling them what to do or fighting their battles for them. Enmeshed subsystems result when boundaries are diffuse. That is, when boundaries are too relaxed, parents may become too involved with their children, and the children learn to rely on the parents to make decisions, resulting in decreased independence. According to Minuchin, if children see their parents as friends and treat them as they would peers, then, enmeshment exists.

Indeed, autonomy and interdependence are key concepts, important both to individual growth and family system maintenance. Relationship patterns are maintained by universal rules governing family organization (especially power hierarchy) and mutual behavioral expectations. In the well-functioning family, boundaries are clear, and a hierarchy exists with a strong parental subsystem. Problems result when there is a malfunctioning of the hierarchical arrangement or boundaries or a maladaptive reaction to changing developmental or environmental requirements. Minuchin believes in clear, flexible boundaries by which all family members can live comfortably.

In the family structural theory, what distinguishes normal families is not the absence of problems but a functional family structure to handle them. Normal husbands and wives must learn to adjust to each other, rear their children, deal with their parents, cope with their jobs, and fit into their communities. The types of struggles change with developmental stages and situational crises. The psychiatric nurse assesses the family structure and the presence of subsystems or boundaries. He or she uses these data to determine how the subsystems and boundaries affect the family's functioning. Helping family members change a subsystem, such as including girls in the boys' activities, may improve family functioning.

Social and Financial Status

Social status is often linked directly to financial status. The nurse should assess the occupations of the family members. Who works? Who is primarily responsible for the family's financial support? Families of low social status are more likely to have limited financial resources, which can place additional stresses on the family. Nurses can use information regarding the family's financial status to determine whether to refer the family to social services.

Cultural expectations and beliefs about acceptable behaviors may cause additional stress. For example, in one qualitative study of 12 black West Indian depressed women who emigrated to Canada or were first-born Canadians, the women rarely sought professional help because of the strong culturally defined stigma against mental disorders. Instead, they managed depression by "being strong," which meant that they tried not to dwell on their feelings, focused on diversions, tried to regain composure, or used other approaches. The researchers concluded that "being strong" may be a factor in inducing depression or slowing or preventing recovery for some women (Schreiber, Noerager Stern, & Wilson, 2000).

Formal and Informal Support Networks

According to balance theory (see Chapter 6), both formal and informal networks are important in providing support to individuals and families. These networks are the link among the individual, families, and the community. Assessing the extent of formal support (e.g., hospitals, agencies) and informal support (e.g., extended family, friends, neighbors) gives a clearer picture of the availability of support. In assessing formal support, the nurse should ask about the family's involvement with government institutions and self-help groups such as Alcoholics Anonymous. Assessing the informal network is particularly important in cultural groups with extended family networks or close friends because these individuals can be major sources of support to patients. If the nurse does not ask about the informal network, these important people may be missed. Nurses can inquire whether family members volunteer at schools, local hospitals, or nursing homes. They can also ask whether the family attends religious services or activities.

FAMILY NURSING DIAGNOSES

From the assessment data, nurses can choose several possible nursing diagnoses. Interrupted Family Processes; Ineffective Therapeutic Regimen Management; or Compromised, Disabling, or Ineffective Family Coping are all possibilities. Nurses choose Interrupted Family Processes if a usually supportive family is experiencing stressful events that challenge its previously effective functioning. They choose Ineffective Family Therapeutic Regimen Management if the family is experiencing difficulty integrating into daily living a program for the treatment of illness and the sequela of illness that meets specific health goals. They select Ineffective Family Coping when the primary supportive person is providing insufficient, ineffective, or compromised support, comfort, or assistance to the patient in managing or mastering adaptive tasks related to the individual's health challenge (Carpenito-Moyet, 2006).

The assessment data may also reveal other nursing diagnoses of individual family members, such as Caregiver Role Strain, Ineffective Denial, or Complicated Grieving. If the nurse finds that any other nursing diagnosis is appropriate, the individual family member should have an opportunity to explore ways of managing the problem.

FAMILY INTERVENTIONS

Family interventions focus on supporting the biopsychosocial integrity and functioning of the family as defined by its members. Although family therapy is reserved for mental health specialists, the generalist psychiatric–mental health nurse can implement several biopsychosocial interventions, such as counseling, promotion of self-care activities, supportive therapy, education and health teaching, and the use of genograms.

In implementing any family intervention, flexibility is essential, particularly when working with culturally diverse groups. To implement successful, culturally competent family interventions, nurses need to be open to modifying the structure and format of the sessions. Longer sessions are often useful, especially when a translator or interpreter is used. Nurses also need to respect and work with the changing family composition of family and nonfamily participants (e.g., extended family members, intimate partners, friends and neighbors, community helpers) in sessions. Because of the stigma that some cultural groups associate with seeking help, nurses may need to hold intervention sessions in community settings (e.g., churches and schools) or at the family's home. If adequate progress is made, it is time to decrease the frequency of sessions and move toward termination. Families may move toward termination if they recognize that improvement has been made (Wright & Leahey, 2004).

Counseling

Nurses often use counseling when working with families because it is a short-term problem-solving approach that addresses current issues. If the assessment reveals complex, longstanding relationship problems, the nurse needs to refer the family to a family therapist. If the family is struggling with psychiatric problems of one or more family members or the family system is in a life-cycle transition, the nurse should use short-term counseling. The counseling sessions should focus on specific issues or problems using sound group process theory. Usually, a problem-solving approach works well once an issue has been identified (see Chapter 10).

Promoting Self-Care Activities

Families often need support in changing behaviors that promote self-care activities. For example, families may inadvertently reinforce a family member's dependency out of fear of the patient being taken advantage of in work or social situations. A nurse can help the family explore how to meet the patient's need for work and social activity and at the same time help alleviate family fears.

Caregiver distress or role strain can occur in families who are responsible for the care of members with long-term illness. Family interventions can help families deal with the burden of caring for members with psychiatric disorders. An analysis of 16 studies indicated that family interventions can affect relatives' burden, psychological distress, and the relationship between patient and relative and family functioning. Family intervention may decrease the frequency of relapse (in persons with schizophrenia) and encourage compliance with medication (Pharoah, Rathbone, Mari, & Streiner, 2005).

Supporting Family Functioning and Cohesiveness

Supporting family functioning involves various nursing approaches. In meeting with the family, the nurse should identify and acknowledge its values. In developing a trusting relationship with the family, the nurse should confirm that all members have a sense of self and self-worth. Supporting family subsystems, such as encouraging the children to play while meeting with the spouses, reinforces family boundaries. Based on assessment of the family system's operation and communication patterns, the nurse can reinforce open, honest communication.

In communicating with the family, the nurse needs to observe boundaries constantly and avoid becoming triangulated into family issues. An objective, empathic leadership style can set the tone for the family sessions.

Providing Education and Health Teaching

One of the most important family interventions is education and health teaching, particularly in families with mental illness. Families have a central role in the treatment of mental illnesses. Members need to learn about mental disorders, medications, actions, side effects, and overall treatment approaches and outcomes. For example, families are often reluctant to have members take psychiatric medications because they believe the medications will "drug" the patient or become addictive. The family's beliefs about mental illnesses and treatment can affect whether patients will be able to manage their illness.

Using Genograms

Genograms not only are useful in assessment, but also can be used as intervention strategies. Nurses can use genograms to help family members understand current feelings and emotions as well as the family's evolution over several generations. Genograms allow the family to examine relationships from a factual, objective perspec-

BOX 13.3

John and Judy Jones

John and Judy Jones were married 3 years ago, after their graduation from a small liberal arts college in the Midwest. Judy's career choice required that she live on the East Coast, where she should be near her large family. John willingly moved with her and quickly found a satisfying position. After about 6 months of marriage, John became extremely irritable and depressed. He kept saying that his life was not his own. Judy was very concerned but could not understand his feelings of being overwhelmed. His job was going well, and they had a very busy social life, mostly revolving around her family, whom John loved. They decided to seek counseling and completed the following genogram:

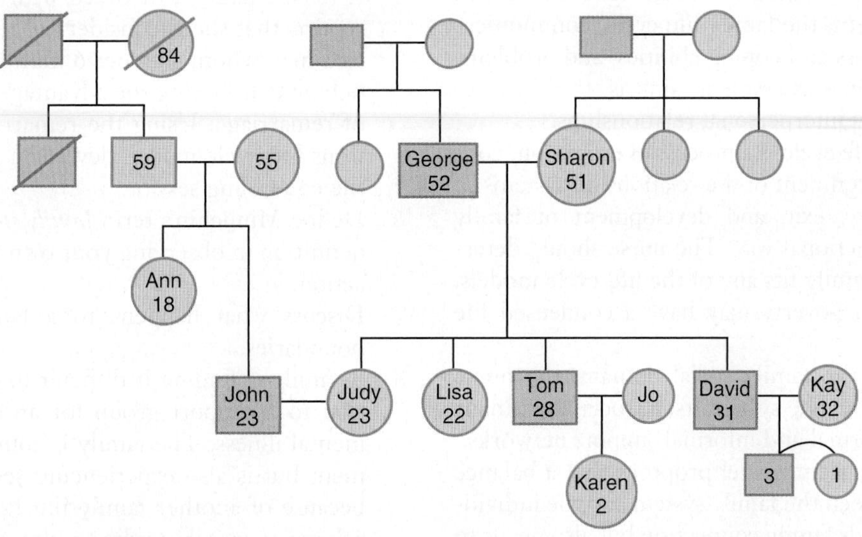

After looking at the genogram, both John and Judy began to realize that part of John's discomfort had to do with the number of family members who were involved in their lives. Judy and John began to redefine their social life, allowing more time with friends and each other.

tive. Often, family members gain new insights and can begin to understand their problems within the context of their family system. For example, families may begin to view depression in an adolescent daughter with new seriousness when they see it as part of a pattern of several generations of women who have struggled with depression. A husband, raised as an only child in a small Midwestern town, may better understand his feelings of being overwhelmed after comparing his family structure with that of his wife, who comes from a large family of several generations living together in the urban Northeast (Box 13.3).

Using Family Therapy

Family therapy is useful for families who are having difficulty maintaining family integrity. Various theoretic perspectives are used in family therapy, but the Minuchin and Bowen models discussed in the assessment section serve as the basis for most approaches. Family therapy can be short term or long term and is conducted by mental health specialists, including advanced practice psychiatric–mental health nurses.

SUMMARY OF KEY POINTS

- A family is a group of people who are connected emotionally, by blood, or in both ways that has developed patterns of interactions and relationships. Families come in various compositions, including nuclear, extended, multigenerational, single-parent, and same-gender families. Cultural values and beliefs define family composition and roles.
- Nurses complete a comprehensive family assessment when they care for families for extended periods or if a patient has complex mental health problems.
- In building relationships with families, nurses must establish credibility and competence with the family. Unless the nurse addresses the family's immediate needs first, the family will have difficulty engaging in the challenges of caring for someone with a mental disorder.
- The genogram is an assessment and intervention tool that is useful in understanding health problems, relationship issues, and social functioning across several generations.

- In assessing the family biologic domain, the nurse determines physical and mental health status and their effects on family functioning.
- Family members are often reluctant to discuss the mental disorders of family members because of the stigma associated with mental illness. In many instances, family members do not know whether mental illnesses were present in other generations.
- The family psychological assessment focuses on family development, the family life cycle, communication patterns, stress and coping abilities, and problem-solving skills. One assessment aim is to begin to understand family interpersonal relationships.
- The family life cycle is a process of expansion, contraction, and realignment of the relationship systems to support the entry, exit, and development of family members in a functional way. The nurse should determine whether a family fits any of the life-cycle models. Families living in poverty may have a condensed life cycle.
- In assessing the family social domain, the nurse compiles data about the system itself, social and financial status, and formal and informal support networks.
- The family system model proposes that a balance should exist between the family system and the individual. A person needs family connection but also needs to be differentiated as an individual. Important concepts include triangles, family projection process, nuclear family emotional process, multigenerational transmission, sibling position, and emotional cutoff.
- The family structure model explains patterns of family interaction. Subsystems develop that also influence interaction patterns. Boundaries can vary from rigid to relaxed. The rigidity of the boundaries affects family functioning.
- Family interventions focus on supporting the family's biopsychosocial integrity and functioning as defined by its members. Family psychiatric nursing interventions include counseling, promotion of self-care activities, supportive therapy, education and health teaching, and the use of genograms. Mental health specialists, including advanced practice nurses, conduct family therapy.
- Education of the family is one of the most useful interventions. Teaching the family about mental disorders, life cycles, family systems, and family interactions can help the family develop a new understanding of family functioning and the effects of mental disorders on the family.

CRITICAL THINKING CHALLENGES

1 Differentiate between a nuclear and extended family. How can a group of people who are unrelated by blood consider themselves a family?

2 Interview a family with a member who has a mental illness and identify who provides support to the individual and family during acute episodes of illness.

3 Interview someone from another culture regarding family beliefs about mental illness. Compare them to your own.

4 Develop a genogram for your family. Analyze the genogram in terms of its pattern of health problems, relationship issues, and social functioning.

5 A female patient, divorced with two small children, reports that she is considering getting married again to a man whom she met 6 months ago. She asks for help in considering the advantages and disadvantages of remarriage. Using the remarried family formulations life-cycle model, develop a plan for structuring the counseling session.

6 Define Minuchin's term *family structure* and use that definition in observing your own family and its interaction.

7 Discuss what happens to a family that has rigid boundaries.

8 A family is finding it difficult to provide transportation to a support group for an adult member with mental illness. The family is committed to his treatment but is also experiencing severe financial stress because of another family illness. Using a problem-solving approach, outline a plan for helping the family explore solutions to the transportation problem.

American Beauty: 1999. This film depicts the life of a family undergoing structural change. Lester and Carolyn Burnham are a seemingly ordinary couple in an anonymous suburban neighborhood whose lives and marriage are slowly unraveling. Their lack of communication and anger toward each other set the stage for a cascade of events that estranges their daughter and psychologically damages everyone. Lester's behavior shows how a family member can lose his or her good sense while undergoing the stresses of a dysfunctional marriage.

VIEWING POINTS: Identify the life cycle phase of the Burnham family. Identify the triangulation that occurs within the family. How does Lester's attraction to his daughter's friend represent a violation of boundaries among family members? How would you describe the communication between Lester and Carolyn?

The Godfather: 1972. The film is the first of a trilogy (*The Godfather*, Part 2, 1974; and *The Godfather*, Part 3, 1990) depicting the violent lives and times of Mafia patriarch Vito Corleone and his son (and successor) Michael. Violence, corruption, and crime in America are examined within the context of family loyalties. In this film, the family dynamics and cultural practices are the basis for decisions in all aspects of life.

VIEWING POINTS: Identify how beliefs about family affect its functioning. Who are the important family members? How are decisions made? Look for triangulation in interactions that occur throughout the film. If this film were made today, how do you think it would be different?

What's Eating Gilbert Grape: 1993. Gilbert has the weighty responsibility of assuming the role of father-figure in a very complex family with dysfunctional interaction patterns. His father died several years ago, the victim of suicide. His mother is morbidly obese and incapable of moving off the sofa. Arnie is Gilbert's brain-damaged younger brother who has to be constantly watched because he will climb the watertower and throw himself off. Gilbert works at the local grocery store, hangs out with his friends and carries on an affair with the wife of a local salesman. When Gilbert falls in love, his lack of freedom and claustrophobic existence impacts the relationship.

VIEWING POINTS: Using Minuchin and Bowen's models, discuss the family's structure and functioning. Identify the stresses the family is experiencing and the coping skills that are needed. If Arnie were your patient, how would you support the family in order for Arnie to be safe?

REFERENCES

Bowen, M. (1975). Family therapy after twenty years. In S. Arieti, D. Freedman, & J. Dyrud (Eds.), *American handbook of psychiatry* (2nd ed., vol. 5, pp. 379–391). New York: Basic Books.

Bowen, M. (1976). Theory in the practice of psychotherapy. In P. Guerin (Ed.), *Family therapy: Theory and practice* (pp. 42–90). New York: Gardner Press.

Carpenito-Moyet, L. (2006). *Nursing diagnosis: Application to clinical practice* (10th ed.). Philadelphia: Lippincott Williams & Wilkins.

Carter, B., & McGoldrick, M. (1999a). The divorce cycle: A major variation in the American family life cycle. In B. Carter & M. McGoldrick (Eds.), *The expanded family life cycle* (pp. 373–398). New York: Allyn & Bacon.

Carter, B., & McGoldrick, M. (2005). Overview: The expanded family life cycle. Individual, family, and social perspectives. In B. Carter & M. McGoldrick (Eds.), *The expanded family life cycle* (pp. 1–24). New York: Allyn & Bacon.

Celano, M., & Kaslow, N. (2000). Culturally competent family interventions: Review and case illustrations. *American Journal of Family Therapy, 28*(3), 217–228.

Cuellar, N., & Butts, J. (1999). Caregiver distress: What nurses in rural settings can do to help. *Nursing Forum, 34*(3), 24–30.

Hatfield, A. B., & Lefley, H. P. (2005). Future involvement of siblings in the lives of persons with mental illness. *Community Mental Health Journal, 41*(3), 327–338.

Hines, P. M. (1999). The family life cycle of African American families living in poverty. In B. Carter & M. McGoldrick (Eds.), *The expanded family life cycle* (pp. 327–345). New York: Allyn & Bacon.

Hines, P.M., & Boyd-Franklin, N. (2005). African American families. In M. McGoldrick, J. Giordano, & N. Garcia-Preto (Eds.), *Ethnicity & Family Therapy* (3rd ed. pp. 87–116). New York: The Guilford Press.

Knauth, D. (2003). Family secrets: An illustrative clinical case study guided by Bowen family systems theory. *Journal of Family Nursing, 9*, 331–344.

Knauth, D. G., & Skowron, E. A. (2004). Psychometric evaluation of the Differentiation of Self Inventory for adolescents. *Nursing Research, 53* (3), 163–171.

McGoldrick, M., Giordano, F., & Garcia-Preto, N. (Eds.), (2005). *Ethnicity and family therapy*. New York: The Guilford Press.

Miller, R. B., Anderson, S. K., Kaulana, D. (2004). Is Bowen theory valid? A review of basic research. *Journal of Marital & Family Therapy, 30*(4), 453–466.

Minuchin, S., Lee, W., & Simon, G. (1996). *Mastering family therapy: Journey of growth and transformation*. New York: John Wiley & Sons.

Pharoah, F. M., Rathbone, J., Mari, J. J., Streiner, D. (2005). Family intervention for schizophrenia. *Cochrane Database of Systematic Reviews*. Retrieved January 23, 2005 from http://gateway.ut.ovid.com/gw1/ovidweb.chi.

Schreiber, R., Noerager Stern, P., & Wilson, C. (2000). Being strong: How Black West-Indian Canadian women manage depression and its stigma. *Journal of Nursing Scholarship, 32*(1), 39–45.

Wright, L. M., & Leahey, M. (2004). How to conclude or terminate with families. *Journal of Family Nursing Care, 10*(3), 379–401.

Wright, L. M., & Leahey, M. (2000). *Nurses and families: A guide to family assessment and intervention*. Philadelphia: F. A. Davis Company.

UNIT IV
Mental Health Promotion

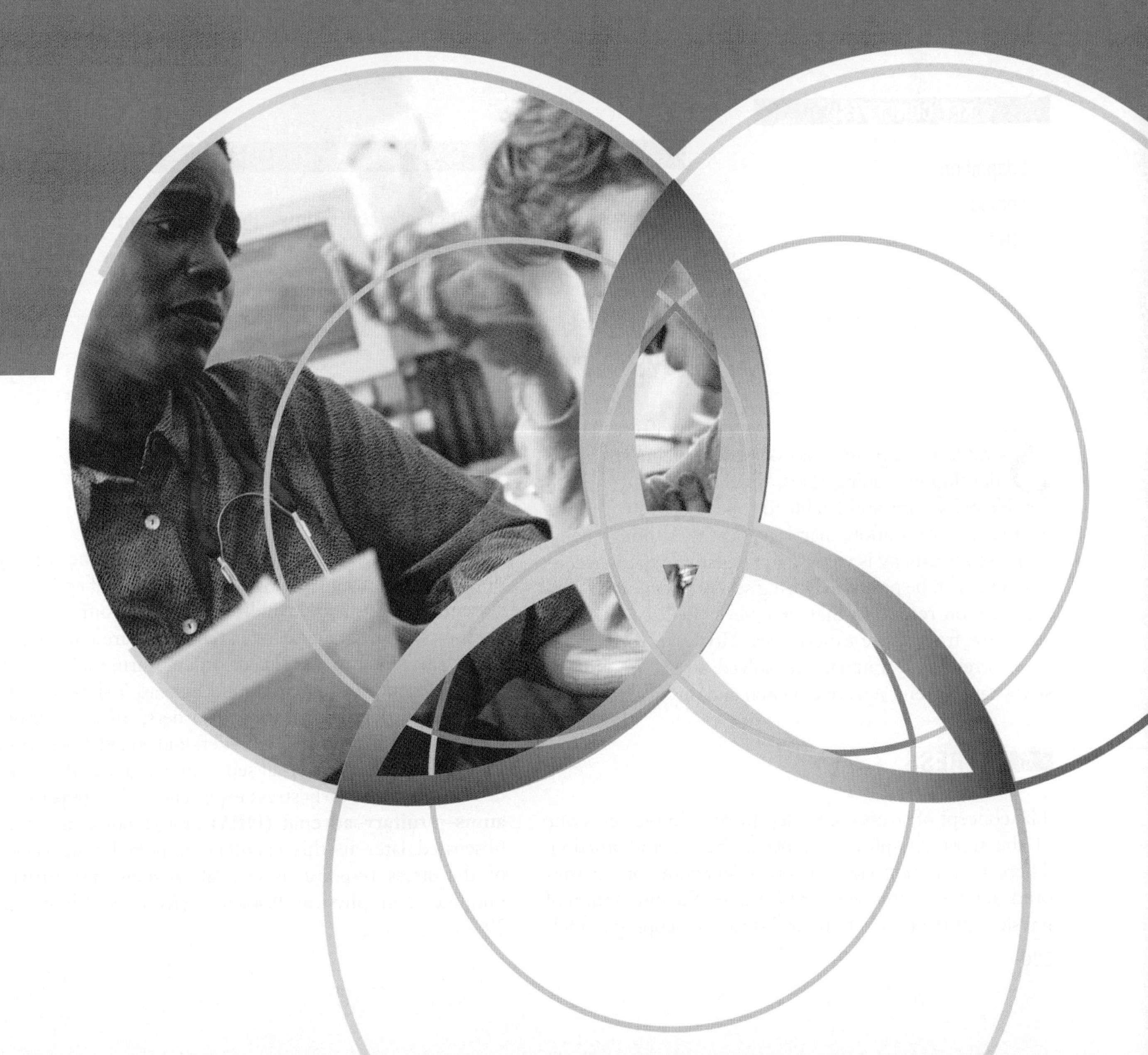

CHAPTER 14

Stress and Mental Health

Mary Ann Boyd and Rita Canfield

LEARNING OBJECTIVES

After studying this chapter, you will be able to:

- Discuss the concept of stress related to mental health and mental illness.
- Discuss evidence that supports theoretical models of stress.
- Evaluate person–environment factors that contribute to the stress experience.
- Discuss the importance of cognitive appraisal in experiencing stress.
- Determine when problem-focused and emotion-focused coping should be used.
- Define adaptation in terms of health, psychological well-being, and social function.

KEY CONCEPTS

- adaptation
- coping
- stress

KEY TERMS

• allostasis • cognitive appraisal • constraints • demands • diathesis • emotion-focused coping • emotions • homeostasis • life events • person–environment relationship • problem-focused coping • reappraisal • social functioning • social network • social support • stress response

Stress and coping are a natural part of life. When children are protected from experiencing stress and developing coping skills, they are likely to be vulnerable in later life and unable to cope effectively with **life events** (e.g., relocation, marriage, death). Although being under stress usually is viewed as a negative experience, its outcomes can be positive. During severe stress, some people draw on resources that they never realized they had and grow from those experiences. However, early childhood stress and trauma, unresolved stress, or chronic stress can portend negative mental and physical health.

STRESS

The concept of stress seems deceptively simple yet is one of the most complex concepts in health and nursing. There are different views of stress depending on the theoretical model. This chapter focuses on the integration of physiological and psychological stress and coping models useful in mental health promotion and prevention of mental illness.

Stress in Mental Health and Illness

Stress during early life can profoundly affect the healthy developing brain and alter life-long function of endocrine systems. For instance, children who have suffered psychological neglect, abuse, or parental loss are more likely to display mood or anxiety disorders during adulthood. Adverse events during childhood increase risk of alcohol and drug dependence, eating disorders, affective disorders, posttraumatic stress disorder, and suicidal behavior. In animal models, maternal separation and abandonment demonstrate that early stress experiences alter **hypothalamus–pituitary–adrenal (HPA)** axis response to stress (discussed later in this chapter). Impaired functioning of the stress response is central to many psychiatric, immune, and physical disorders (Kaye & Lightman, 2005).

Stress has long been associated with the development or exacerbation of symptoms of mental illness. For example, psychiatric disorders are prevalent in caregivers of persons with chronic illnesses. Many caregivers of family members with dementia, AIDS, and other long-term illnesses experience severe and chronic stress leading to depression. The caregiver must monitor the family member, cope with illness-related behaviors and, in many of the disabilities, witness deterioration of their significant other. In addition, the caregiver's own activities are curtailed (De Frias, Tuokko, & Rosenberg, 2005; Knussen, Tolson, Swan, Stott, & Brogan, 2005; Stetz & Brown, 2004).

The *diathesis-stress model* proposes that emotional and psychiatric disorders arise from interaction of negative life events with pre-existing vulnerabilities that can be psychological and biological, specific or general. Certain genes or genetic combinations produce a **diathesis**, or constitutional predisposition to a disorder. Events interacting with the vulnerability result in emotional distress, which predisposes an individual to mental ill health and psychiatric disorders. The diathesis-stress model suggests that for a mental disorder to develop both the diathesis and stress must interact, that is, an individual with a predisposition toward a disorder must be "challenged" by a stressor.

Acute Vs. Chronic Stress

Stress responses occur at physiological, behavioral, and cognitive levels. Psychological stressors can potentiate physiological responses, although the physiological response to each type of stressor varies (McEwen, 2005; Levine, 2005). Stress has its potentially most deleterious health effects when it becomes chronic. Although there are severe stressors that would distress everyone, less-severe stressors that persist over a long period of time weaken the ability to cope. If coping ability is exhausted, more stress and distress follow (Linden, 2005; Stanley & Burrows, 2005).

The present views of the physiology of stress can be traced primarily to the contributions of Walter Cannon (1914, 1932) and Hans Selye (1956, 1974). Both found a physiological stress response, but Cannon described an *acute stress response*, while Selye was more concerned with a *chronic challenge*. Cannon focused primarily on the sympathetic nervous system and the role of the hormones, epinephrine and noradrenaline, labeled the "fight or flight" response that creates a mobilization of energy (increased heart rate, blood pressure, blood sugar, etc.) which potentiates physical action. Selye expanded the understanding of the stress response by identifying the role of the HPA in stress, which included the end-product cortisol (in humans) among others. Selye's notion was that the body attempted to maintain **homeostasis** or internal equilibrium by adjusting its physiological processes and resisting physiological change.

Homeostasis Versus Allostasis

It is now known that the brain and body are in two-way communication via the autonomic nervous system and the endocrine and immune systems. Homeostasis applies only to a few physiological functions with narrow ranges such as body pH, temperature, and oxygen. Most of the other regulatory systems have wider ranges of functioning (such as blood pressure, heart rate, etc.) and achieve stability through adaptation or change. This process is called **allostasis.** Critical to survival, allostasis involves the autonomic nervous system, the HPA axis, and the cardiovascular, metabolic, and immune systems, which act to protect the body by responding to internal and external stimuli (McEwen, 2005). Hormones are released in varying magnitudes and act as mediators of the stress response. Differences in magnitude of response are dependent on individual psychological factors and the context in which the stressor occurs. Responses are also influe8. by genetic makeup, early life experiences, and specific characteristics of the individual, together with situational and environmental differences (Kaye & Lightman, 2005).

Paradoxically, these same systems, when activated by chronic stress, can also damage the body. The sympathetic nervous system, HPA axis, cardiovascular, metabolic, and immune systems are at risk for damage in conditions of chronic or repeated stressors. In chronic stress, the continuous sustained activation of these systems contributes to a hormonal overload that can lead to impairment in memory, immunity, cardiovascular, and metabolic function (McEwen, 2000, 2005).

BIOPSYCHOSOCIAL MODEL: STRESS, COPING, AND ADAPTATION

When one understands the complex role of stress on the physiologic, cognitive, psychological, and behavioral systems, together with the potential risks for mental and physical illness, then the ability to intervene in the stress response becomes a primary focus for the nurse and health care provider. The potential to mediate or moderate the stress response is best understood in the light of the cognitive process of stress appraisal and coping. By focusing on cognitive processes, the nurse can develop interventions based on individual responses (See Box 14.1).

In 1984, Lazarus and Folkman published the classic work, *Stress, Appraisal and Coping*. They offered a new approach to understanding stress, arguing that stress is much more complicated than a stimulus response. They

BOX 14.1

Research for Best Practice

Moneyham, L., Murdaugh, C., Phillips, K., Jackson, K., Tavakoli, A., Boyd, M., et al. (2005). Patterns of risk of depressive symptoms among HIV-positive women in the Southeastern United States. Journal of the Association of Nurses in Aids Care, 16(4), 25–38.

The Question: What factors contribute to depression among rural women with HIV/AIDS?

Methods: This study used the Lazarus stress theory for the framework to identify potential risk factors of depressive symptoms in women with HIV/AIDS. A sample of 278 HIV-infected women was interviewed in rural areas of South Carolina, Georgia, and Alabama. HIV symptoms, function, social support, coping, and depressive symptoms were measured.

Findings: The researchers were able to identify factors that correlated with the development of depression. The frequency of HIV symptoms, feeling sadness and hopeless in the past 12 months, and coping with HIV by isolation/withdrawal and denial/avoidance were all associated with depressive symptoms. Availability of social support and coping by living positively with HIV were both negatively associated with less depression.

Implications for Nursing: Results can guide the development of interventions in preventing depression in this population Assessing women with HIV/AIDS for depressive symptoms is important in the care of these patients. Developing interventions that increase social support and teaching patients how to live positively with HIV are useful in reducing the likelihood of developing depressive symptoms.

focused on what happens inside a person's mind, defining stress as a relationship between the person and the environment that is appraised by the person as taxing or exceeding biopsychosocial resources and endangering his or her well-being (Lazarus, 1999; Yeager & Roberts, 2003). The experience of stress, the person's responses, and the effects of the stress are presented in the stress, coping, and adaptation model depicted in Figure 14.1. This systems model has four components: (1) antecedents to the stress, (2) stress, (3) coping, and (4) adaptation. This model, which is consistent with the biopsychosocial approach of psychiatric mental health nursing practice, is used as a framework in this chapter for understanding stress.

KEY CONCEPT Stress is the relationship between the person and the environment that is appraised as exceeding the person's resources and endangering the person's well-being.

Antecedents to Stress

Two important antecedents or precursors to the stress response are the person–environment relationship, which involves many factors, and the person's cognitive appraisal of the risks and benefits of the situation, which mediates or moderates the interpretation of its meaning. The appraisal of the relationship determines the manifestation of stress and the potential for coping.

Person–Environment Relationship

The **person–environment relationship** can be defined as the interaction between the individual and the environment that changes throughout the stress experience. A person brings to any interaction a set of values and beliefs that he or she has developed throughout a lifetime. These values are based on cultural, ethnic, family, and religious traditions that form the person's beliefs about the world. A person's underlying values and beliefs shape his or her decision about the significance of any particular situation. Therefore, what is important to one person may not be to another; for example, one person may value a college education, whereas another may value living with neighbors in a small, isolated community.

Values and Commitment

When a person values a particular outcome, he or she is likely to be committed to activities directed toward that outcome. The commitment to a goal is an important factor in the stress response. The following example illustrates the relationship between values and commitment.

Students who earn mostly or all As often feel more stress and worry about examinations than do students who earn Bs and Cs. Before they take a test, the former often express fear that they will flunk. These high-achieving students are devastated if they earn a B or C, whereas other students are often relieved to receive a B or C. Although it seems illogical that students who consistently earn higher grades are more stressed than those who perform less well, the test-taking situation is actually more threatening to the better students, who place a higher value on the A grade than do the other students.

Personality and Behavior Patterns

People bring not only their values, beliefs, and goals to any situation, but also their own behavioral characteristics. Each person develops ways of interacting with the world from early childhood. These behaviors form patterns during a lifetime, so that people automatically respond to events with a particular behavior pattern. For example, the preschool-aged child who refuses to attend nursery school often fears going to kindergarten and may later have difficulty leaving home for college.

The importance of behavior patterns is demonstrated by type A and B personalities. In the mid-1970s, cardiol-

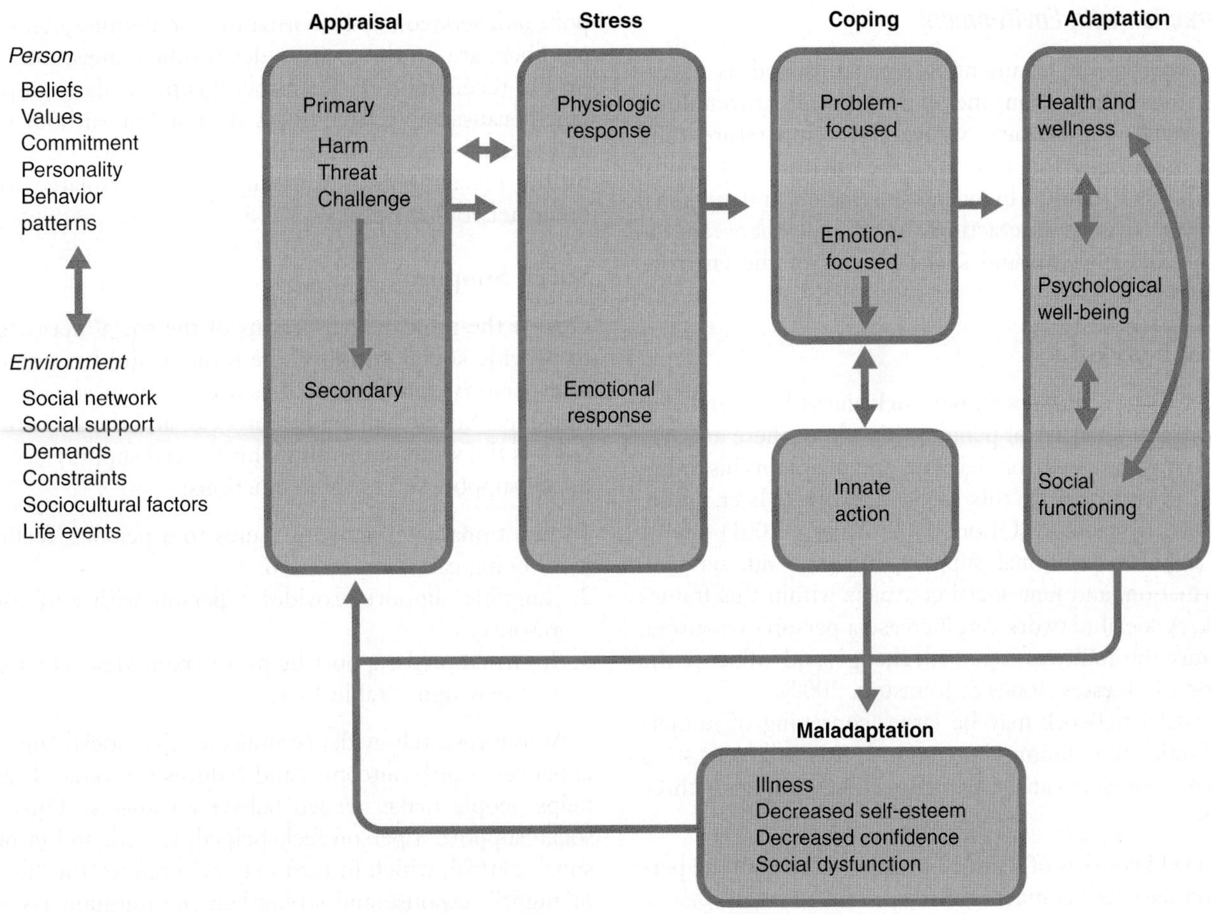

FIGURE 14.1. Stress, coping, and adaptation model.

ogists Meyer Friedman and Ray Rosenman observed that their patients' personalities and lifestyles seemed to be related to the development of cardiovascular disease. From their work, the widely known conceptualization of type A and B personality behavior patterns evolved (Frei, Racicot, & Travagline, 1999; Friedman & Rosenman, 1974).

Type A people are characterized as competitive, aggressive, ambitious, and impatient. Alert, tense, and restless, they think, speak, and act at an accelerated pace. They reflect an aggressive, hostile, and time-urgent style of living that is often associated with increased psychophysiologic arousal. In contrast, type B people do not exhibit these chronic behaviors and generally are more relaxed, easy-going, and easily satisfied. They have an accepting attitude about trivial mistakes and a problem-solving approach to major problems. Rarely do type B people push themselves to obtain excesses from the environment or try to accomplish too much in too little time (Rosenman & Chesney, 1985).

These two behavior patterns have been studied extensively in relation to the development of cardiovascular illnesses. The initial studies supported a link between type A personality and atherosclerosis leading to coronary heart disease. More recent studies suggest that type A behavior and coronary disease are evident primarily in people with middle-class occupations and lifestyles, not in people with low-status occupations (Donker, 2000; Woodward, Oliphant, Lowe, & Tunstall-Pedoe, 2003).

Two other personality types have received less attention than types A or B. Type C persons are described as having difficulty expressing emotion, introverted, respectful, conforming, compliant, and eager to please and avoid conflict. They respond to stress with depression and hopelessness. This personality type was initially associated with the development of cancer, specifically breast cancer in women, but there has been no clear evidence that stress has a role in the etiology of cancer (Bryant-Lukosius, 2003).

There is interest in the risk of myocardial infarction in persons with type D (distressed) personality. These individuals experience increased negative emotions (depression), pessimism, and do not share emotions. Recent medical studies support an association between type D personality and the occurrence of adverse events in patients with ischemic heart disease (Pedersen et al., 2004; Denollet & Brutsaert, 2001). More studies are needed to provide a strong evidence-based support for this hypothesized relationship.

Interaction with Environment

The external environment is conceptualized as everything outside a person, including physical surroundings and social interactions. Crowding, temperature, and noise are all physical aspects of the environment. Social aspects also include living arrangements and personal contacts. Unique interactions occur daily between the person and physical and social aspects of the environment.

Social Networks

People live within a **social network** consisting of linkages among a defined set of people with whom there are personal contacts. A person develops and maintains his or her social identity within this social network (Majer, Jason, Ferrarie, Venable, & Olson, 2002; Moran, 2001). He or she acquires emotional support, material aid, services, information, and new social contracts within this framework. A social network can increase a person's resources, enhance the ability to cope with change, and influence the course of illnesses (Jones & Johnston, 2000).

A social network may be large, consisting of numerous family and community contacts, or small, consisting of few. Contacts can be categorized according to three levels:

1. Level I consists of six to 12 people with whom the person has close contact.
2. Level II consists of a larger number of contacts, generally 30 to 40 people whom the person sees regularly.
3. Level III consists of the large number of people with whom a person has direct contact, such as the grocer and mail carrier, and can represent several hundred people.

Each person's social network is slightly different. These multiple contacts allow several networks to interact. Generally, the larger the network is, the more support that is available to the person. An ideal network structure is fairly dense and interconnected; people within the network are also in contact with one another. Dense networks are better able to respond in times of stress and crisis and to provide emotional support to a person in distress.

Two concepts, intensity and reciprocity, relate to social networks. *Intensity* is the degree of closeness of a relationship. Some relationships are naturally more intense than others. Ideally, a person's social network reflects a balance between intense and less intense relationships. Intense relationships can restrict a person's opportunity to interact with other network members, but without at least a few intense relationships, a person becomes isolated. *Reciprocity* is the extent to which there is give and take. Network members both provide and receive support, aid, services, and information. Sometimes, network members are on the giving side; at other times, they are on the receiving side. Reciprocity is particularly important because most friendships do not last without give and take of support and services. A person who is always on the receiving end eventually becomes isolated from other network members.

Social Support

One of the important functions of the social network is to provide **social support**, the positive and harmonious interpersonal interactions that occur within social relationships. Social support is a process, and the social network is the structure within which social support occurs. Social support serves three functions:

1. Emotional support contributes to a person's feelings of being cared for or loved.
2. Tangible support provides a person with additional resources.
3. Informational support helps a person view situations in a new light (Table 14.1).

Ample research evidence indicates that social support enhances health outcomes and reduces mortality. It also helps people make needed behavior changes. Through social support, a person feels helped, valued, and in personal control, which in turn may help reduce the "fight-or-flight" response and strengthen the immune system. Social support also either directly or indirectly buffers stressful life events in two ways. First, during stressful events, network members collect and analyze information, offer guidance, and help the person under stress interpret the world. Second, by treating the person under stress as a unique, special human being, members of the social network provide comfort and a sanctuary or place of refuge.

People who are relatively healthy are more likely to have a stronger support system and to be able to prevent undesirable life events than are those who are physically

Table 14.1 Examples of Functions of Social Support

Function	Example
Emotional support	Attachment, reassurance, being able to rely on and confide in a person
Tangible support	Direct aid such as loans or gifts, services such as taking care of someone who is ill, doing a job or chore
Informational support	Providing information or advice, and giving feedback about how a person is doing

From Schaefer, C., Coyne, J., & Lazarus, R. (1982). The health-related functions of social support. *Journal of Behavioral Medicine, 44*, 381–406.

or mentally ill. In addition, some life events, such as marriage, divorce, and bereavement, actually change the level of social support by adding to or subtracting from a person's social network. For example, if a person loses a spouse and the spouse was the main source of support, the stress is greater because not only the spouse, but also the support, is lost. Therefore, social support should be viewed as a dynamic process that is in constant flux and varies with life events and health status (Yeager & Roberts, 2003). Not all interpersonal interactions within a network are supportive. A person can have a large, complex social network but little social support.

Demands and Constraints

Within the social network are external and internal demands and personal and environmental constraints. Internal **demands** are generated by physiologic and psychological needs. The physical environment imposes some external demands, such as crowding, crime, noise, and pollution; the social environment imposes others, such as behavioral and role expectations. In contrast to demands, **constraints** are limitations that are both personal and environmental. Personal constraints include internalized cultural values and beliefs that dictate actions or feelings and psychological deficits that are products of the person's unique development. Environmental constraints are finite resources, such as money and time, that are available to people.

These demands and constraints vary with the individual and contribute to or initiate a stress response (Lazarus, 2001; Yeager & Roberts, 2003). They also interact with one another (Box 14.2); for example, work demands, such as changing shifts, may interact with physical demands, such as a need for sleep, creating a high-risk situation in which stress is likely to occur.

BOX 14.2

The Meaning of a Loss of Job

Incident: Two women lost their jobs at a local company. One was a single parent who was the sole supporter of two small children, and the other had no children but lived with a man who paid most of their expenses. Both women were being treated at the mental health center for depression. The single parent was devastated, but the other woman seemed almost relieved that she no longer had to work. The nurse was confused about the different reactions of the two women.

Reflection: Upon reflection, the nurse understood the variation in reactions to the job loss. Because the demands and constraints of the environment are different for the two women, the meaning of the job loss is different for each. The job loss significantly affects the single parent's ability to support her children, whereas it is merely an inconvenience for the other woman because her partner helps share expenses. The economic demands on the single parent are greater, and thus she is likely to experience greater stress.

Sociocultural Factors

Cultural expectations and role strain serve as both demands and constraints in the experience of stress. If a person violates cultural group values to meet role expectations, stress occurs; for example, a person may stay in an abusive relationship to avoid the stress of violating a cultural norm that values life-long marriage, no matter what the circumstances. The potential guilt associated with norm violation and the anticipated isolation from being ostracized are worse for that person than the physical and psychological pain caused by the abusive situation.

Employment is a highly valued cultural norm and provides social, psychological, and financial benefits. In all cultures, work is assigned significance beyond economic compensation. It is often the central focus of adulthood and, for many, a source of personal identity. Even if a person's employment brings little real happiness, being employed implies that a person's or family's financial needs are being met. Work offers status, regulates life activities, permits association with others, and provides a meaningful life experience. Although work is demanding, unemployment can actually be more stressful because of the associated isolation and loss of social status.

Gender expectations often become a source of demands and constraints for women, who assume multiple roles. In most cultures, women who work outside the home are expected to assume primary responsibility for care of the children and household duties. Most women are adept at separating these roles and can compartmentalize problems at work from those at home. When there is a healthy balance between work and home, women experience a low level of psychological stress. However, when the balance is disturbed, daily stressors contribute to health problems (Stuart & Garrison, 2002; Tang, Lee, Tang, Cheung, & Chan, 2002).

Life Events

In 1967, Holmes and Rahe presented a psychosocial view of illness by pointing out the complex relationship between life changes and the development of illnesses (Holmes & Rahe, 1967). They hypothesized that people become ill after they experience life event changes. The more frequent the changes are, the greater is the possibility of becoming sick. The investigators cited the events that they believed partially accounted for the onset of illnesses and began testing whether these life changes were actual precursors to illness. It soon became clear that not all events have the same effects. For example, the death of a spouse is usually much more devastating and stressful than a change in residence. From their research, the investigators were able to assign relative weights to various life events according to the degree of associated stress. Rahe devised the Recent Life Changes Questionnaire (Table 14.2) to evaluate the frequency and significance of life change events (Rahe, 1994; 1997). Numerous research studies subsequently demonstrated the relationship between a recent life change and the severity of near-future illness (Rahe, 1994; Rahe et al., 2002). If several life changes occur within a short period, the likelihood of an illness appearing is even greater.

Appraisal

All stress responses are affected by the personal meaning of the situation; for example, chest pain is stressful to a person not only because of the immediate pain and incapacitation it causes, but also because it may mean that the person is having a heart attack. The fear of having a heart attack and dying is part of the stress of chest pain. Thus, the significance of the event actually determines the importance of the person–environment relationship (Lazarus, 2001; Moran, 2001).

Table 14.2 Recent Life Changes Questionnaire

Social Area	Life Changes	LCU Values*
Family	Death of spouse	105
	Marital separation	65
	Death of close family member	65
	Divorce	62
	Pregnancy	60
	Change in health of family member	52
	Marriage	50
	Gain of new family member	50
	Marital reconciliation	42
	Spouse begins or stops work	37
	Son or daughter leaving home	29
	In-law trouble	29
	Change in number of family get-togethers	26
Personal	Jail term	56
	Sex difficulties	49
	Death of a close friend	46
	Personal injury or illness	42
	Change in living conditions	39
	Outstanding personal achievement	33
	Change in residence	33
	Minor violations of the law	32
	Begin or end school	32
	Change in sleeping habits	31
	Revision of personal habits	31
	Change in eating habits	29
	Change in church activities	29
	Vacation	29
	Change in school	28
	Change in recreation	28
	Christmas	26
Work	Fired at work	64
	Retirement from work	49
	Trouble with boss	39
	Business readjustment	38
	Change to different line of work	38
	Change in work responsibilities	33
	Change in work hours or conditions	30
Financial	Foreclosure of mortgage or loan	57
	Change in financial state	43
	Mortgage (e.g., home, car)	39
	Mortgage or loan less than $10,000 (e.g., stereo)	26

Directions: Sum the LCUs for your life change events during the past 12 months.

250 and 400 LCUs per year: Minor life crisis

Over 400 LCUs per year: Major life crisis

*LCU, Life change unit. The number of LCUs reflects the average degree or intensity of the life change.

(From Rahe, R. H. (2000). Recent Life Changes Questionnaire [RLCQ] (1997). Holmes, T. H. in American Psychiatric Association. Task Force for the Handbook of Psychiatric Measures. *Handbook of psychiatric measures*. Washington, DC: American Psychiatric Association, pp. 235–237.)

A given event or situation may be extremely stressful to one person but not to another. Lazarus attributes this variation in response to stress to the significance of the outcome of the situation to the person involved. The person who regards the outcome as important is naturally worried, concerned, or anxious. That person is also more likely to be stressed by the situation than another. The more important or meaningful the outcome, the more vulnerable the person is to stress.

The meaning of the person–environment situation is evaluated or appraised for its risks and benefits. Lazarus uses the term **cognitive appraisal** to refer to the process of examining the demands, constraints, and resources of the environment and negotiating them with personal goals and beliefs. During this appraisal process, the person integrates his or her personality and environmental factors into a relational meaning based on the relevance of what is happening to the person's well-being (Aguilera, 1998; Lazarus, 2001; Yeager & Roberts, 2003).

Box 14.3 demonstrates the relationship between personal meaning and stress. An analysis of this scenario makes it clear that even though both students took the same test, Susan was less stressed than Joanne. The critical factor is the risk involved: For Susan, a failed test meant a retake; for Joanne, a failed test meant not returning to school.

BOX 14.3

Clinical Vignette: Stress Responses to an Examination

Two students are preparing for the same examination. Susan is genuinely interested in the subject, prepares by studying throughout the semester, and reviews the content 2 days before test day. The night before the examination, she goes to bed early, gets a good night's sleep, and wakes refreshed but is slightly nervous about the test. She wants to do well and expects a difficult test but knows that she can retake it at a later date if she does poorly.

In contrast, Joanne is not interested in the subject matter and does not study throughout the semester. She "crams" 2 days before the test date and does an "all nighter" the night before. This is the last time that Joanne can take the examination, but she believes that she will pass because she has already taken it twice and is familiar with the questions. If she does not pass, she will not be able to return to school. On entering the room, Joanne is physically tired and somewhat fearful of not passing the test. As she looks at the test, she instantly realizes that it is not the examination she expected. The questions are new. She begins hyperventilating and tremoring. After yelling obscenities at the teacher, she storms out of the room. She is very distressed and describes herself as "being in a panic."

What Do You Think?

- How are the students' experiences different? Are there any similarities?
- Are there any nursing diagnoses that apply to Joanne's situation?

The appraisal process has two levels: primary and secondary. In a primary appraisal, a person evaluates the events occurring in his or her life as a threat, harm, or challenge. During primary appraisal of a goal, the person determines whether (1) the goal is relevant, (2) the goal is consistent with his or her values and beliefs, and (3) a personal commitment is present. In the vignette, Susan's commitment to the goal of doing well on the test was consistent with her valuing the content, which in turn motivated her to study regularly and prepare carefully for the examination. She believed that the test would be difficult. Joanne had a commitment to pass the test but did not value the content. Unlike Susan, Joanne believed that the test would be relatively easy because she expected the questions to be the same as those on the previous examination.

In a secondary appraisal, the person explains the outcome of events. There may be blame or credit given for the outcome. In the example, Susan was nervous but took the test. Joanne's secondary appraisal of the test-taking situation began with the realization that she might not pass the test because the questions were different. She acted impulsively by blaming the teacher for giving a different examination and by storming out of the room. She clearly did not cope effectively with a difficult situation.

Stress is initiated not by a single stressor but by an unfavorable person–environment relationship that is meaningful in terms of the risks or benefits to that person's well-being. The person's commitment to the goal influences the stress response as well as the meaning of the situation. The more committed the person is to a specific goal, the greater his or her vulnerability to stress.

Stress Responses

Once a person–environment relationship is established and the person appraises it as threatening, harmful, or challenging, an internal stress response occurs. The person has simultaneous physiologic and emotional responses.

• NCLEXNOTE

NCLEXNOTE

Stress and coping are key concepts in nursing practice and are emphasized in NCLEX questions. The stress and coping models should be considered in all patients including those with mental illnesses. Nursing assessment should focus on the patient's appraisal of the stressful event. Understanding a person's beliefs, values, commitment, and personality patterns will help the nurse support the patient's coping skills.

Physiologic Responses

Physiologic changes are automatic and differ based on type of stress, duration, and intensity, which will depend on the appraised risk of the situation. *The riskier the situation, the more intense the response.* The immune system, sympathetic nervous system, HPA, cardiovascular, and metabolic systems are a part of the stress response.

In acute stress, the locus ceruleus in the brain initiates the stress response by responding to the appraisal with the release of norepinephrine, which in turn stimulates the sympathetic nervous system centers located in the hypothalamus. If the person experiences fear or pain, the sympathetic nervous system responds by discharging almost as a complete unit, causing excitatory effects in some organs and inhibitory effects in others (See Chapter 7). This "mass discharge" activates large portions of the system, *sympathetic alarm reaction*, or the fight-or-flight response, and the body is physically prepared to perform vigorous muscle activity because of the following sympathetic responses:

The sympathetic nervous system activates the HPA axis. That is, the hypothalamus secretes corticotropin-releasing hormone (CRH), which causes a marked increase in adrenocorticotropic hormone (corticotropin) secretion by the pituitary gland, which in turn stimulates the adrenocortical secretion of cortisol. The benefits of the increase in circulating cortisol to the human body are initially adaptive, but if it continues can be quite damaging to both mental (depression) and physical health (immune, cardiovascular, and metabolic). The connection between the immune and sympathetic nervous systems is immune cells, which have receptors for cortisol and catecholamines that have the capacity to bind with lymphatic cells and suppress the immune system. Cortisol is primarily immunosuppressive and contributes to reduction in lymphocyte numbers and function (primarily T-lymphocyte and monocyte subsets) and natural killer activities. Therefore, during stress, when the production of both cortisol and norepinephrine increases, the immune system is negatively affected.

Other neurobiologic reactions occur during a stress response. For example, CRH is secreted into the amygdala and hippocampus, a process important for memory retrieval and emotional analysis. The locus ceruleus has connections with the cerebrum, which has dopamine-producing neurons that project into the mesolimbic and mesocortical dopamine tracts, helping to control motivation, reward, and reinforcement.

Chronic unfavorable person–environment relationships such as academic examinations, job strain, caregiving for a family member with dementia, marital conflict, and daily stressors elevate white blood cell counts and lower those for T, B, and natural killer (NK) cells. Negative moods (chronic hostility, depression, and anxiety), social isolation, and marital disagreement also alter many parameters of immune function. Antibody titers to Epstein-Barr and herpes simplex viruses are elevated in stressed populations. If the stress is long term, the immune alteration continues (Kiecolt-Glaser, et al., 2005; Silberman, Wald, & Genaro, 2002; Yeager & Roberts, 2003). With time, biologic responses to stress compromise a person's health status.

Emotional Responses

After cognitively appraising a situation, a person experiences specific emotions along with physiologic changes. Lazarus defines **emotions** as organized psychophysiologic reactions. The emotion the person experiences depends on the significance of the person–environment event to his or her personal well-being. The person's mental state is one of excitement or distress, marked by strong feelings and usually accompanied by an impulse toward definite action. If the emotion is intense, a disturbance in intellectual functions occurs.

For an emotion to occur, an individual must subjectively evaluate a situation or person–environment relationship as having certain harms or benefits. The significance or meaning of the evaluation depends on the person's goals and beliefs and the environmental context (family conflict has a different meaning than does stranger conflict). Some emotions are evaluated as being negative and others as positive. The person is more likely to experience positive emotions when he or she views the situation as a challenge. Conversely, negative emotions are elicited if the person evaluates the episode as threatening or harmful. According to Lazarus, emotions are categorized as follows:

- *Negative emotions* occur when there is a threat to, delay in, or thwarting of a goal or a conflict between goals: anger, fright, anxiety, guilt, shame, sadness, envy, jealousy, and disgust.
- *Positive emotions* occur when there is movement toward or attainment of a goal: happiness, pride, relief, and love.
- *Borderline emotions* are somewhat ambiguous: hope, compassion, empathy, sympathy, and contentment.
- *Nonemotions* connote emotional reactions but are too ambiguous to fit into any of the preceding categories: confidence, awe, confusion, and excitement.

Each emotion is expressed as a theme that summarizes the personal harms and benefits of each person–environment relationship. This core relational theme is unique and specific to each emotion. For instance, physical danger stimulates fear in a person. A loss produces feelings of sadness (Table 14.3). Each emotion also has its own innate response that is automatic and unique to a particular person; for example, anger may automatically provoke tremors in one person but both tremors and perspiration in another. Sadness may provoke tears in one person but not in another. Emotions often provoke an automatic tendency (impulse) to act. For example, fear

Table 14.3 Core Relational Themes for Each Emotion

Emotion	Relational Meaning
Anger	A demeaning offense against me and mine
Anxiety	Facing an uncertain, existential threat
Fright	Facing an immediate, concrete, and overwhelming physical danger
Guilt	Having transgressed a moral imperative
Shame	Having failed to live up to an ego ideal
Sadness	Having experienced an irrevocable loss
Envy	Wanting what someone else has
Jealousy	Resenting a third party for the loss of or a threat to another's affection
Disgust	Taking in or being too close to an indigestible object or idea (metaphorically speaking)
Happiness	Making reasonable progress toward the realization of a goal
Pride	Enhancement of one's ego-identity by taking credit for a valued object or achievement, either our own or that of someone or a group with whom we identify
Relief	A distressing goal-incongruent condition that has changed for the better or gone away
Hope	Fearing the worst but yearning for better
Love	Desiring or participating in affection, usually but not necessarily reciprocated
Compassion	Being moved by another's suffering and wanting to help

Adapted from Lazarus, R. S. (1999). *Stress and emotion: A new synthesis.* New York: Springer.

produces an impulse to escape to safety. The first impulse of a young musician facing his first performance at Carnegie Hall who experiences stage fright is to run home. As he resists this impulse, he begins coping with his fears in order to perform.

COPING

Coping is a deliberate, planned, and psychological effort to manage stressful demands. The coping process may inhibit or override the innate urge to act. Positive coping leads to adaptation, which is characterized by a balance between health and illness, a sense of well-being, and maximum social functioning. When a person does not cope positively, maladaptations occur that can shift the balance toward illness, a diminished self-concept, and deterioration in social functioning.

KEY CONCEPT Coping is a deliberate, planned, and psychological effort to manage stressful demands.

There are two types of coping: problem focused, which actually changes the person–environment relationship, and emotion focused, which changes the meaning of the situation. In **problem-focused coping**, the person attacks the source of stress by eliminating it or changing its effects. In **emotion-focused coping**, the person reinterprets the situation, reducing the stress and the need for additional coping without changing the actual person–environment relationship (Table 14.4; see Box 14.4).

The situation is reappraised following completion of the coping process. Reappraisal is important because of the changing nature of the person–environment relationship. **Reappraisal**, which is the same as appraisal except that it happens after coping, provides feedback about the

Table 14.4 Ways of Coping: Problem-Focused Versus Emotion-Focused

Problem-Focused Coping	Emotion-Focused Coping
When noise from the television interrupts a student's studying and causes the student to be stressed, the student turns off the television and eliminates the noise.	A husband is adamantly opposed to visiting his wife's relatives because they keep dogs in their house. Even though the dogs are well cared for, their presence in the relative's home violates his need for an orderly, clean house and causes the husband sufficient stress that he copes by refusing to visit. This becomes a source of marital conflict. One holiday, the husband is given a puppy and immediately becomes attached to the dog, who soon becomes a valued family member. The husband then begins to view his wife's relatives differently and willingly visits their house more often.
An abused spouse is finally able to leave her husband because she realizes that the abuse will not stop, even though he promises never to hit her again.	A mother is afraid that her teenaged daughter has been in an accident because she did not come home after a party. Then the woman remembers that she gave her daughter permission to stay at a friend's house. She immediately feels better.

BOX 14.4

Research for Best Practice

Ahmad, M. M., Musil, C. M., Zauszniewski, J. A., & Resnick, M. I. (2005). Prostate cancer: appraisal, coping, and health status. Journal of Gerontological Nursing, 31(10), 34–43.

The Question: Do men use emotion- or problem-focused coping when appraising a health threat?

Methods: A convenience sample of 131 men with prostate cancer was surveyed to identify how cognitive appraisal and types of coping affected their health status.

Findings: Men who appraised more harm or loss experienced worse physical and mental health. When the men perceived their diagnosis as posing more harm or loss or greater threat, they were more likely to use emotion-focused coping. When the diagnosis was perceived as a challenge, men were more likely to use problem-focused coping.

Implications for Nursing: Patients will respond differently to the same medical diagnosis depending on how they appraise the threat of the diagnosis. Problem-focused coping is more likely to be used if the diagnosis is viewed as a challenge ("I can beat it"), rather than a threat ("I will die"). Assessing the coping style will provide important assessment data for planning interventions.

outcomes and allows for continual adjustment to new information. Thus, the stress response becomes part of the dynamic relationship between the person and the environment.

No one coping strategy is best for all situations. Coping strategies work best in particular situations. These strategies become automatic and develop into patterns for each person. Some situations require a combination of strategies and activities. Ideally, a person can cope with a stressful situation by matching the resources that are needed with the events that are unfolding. Social support can be critical in helping people cope with difficult situations. Successful coping with life stresses is linked to quality of life, as well as to physical and mental health (Lazarus, 2001).

ADAPTATION

Adaptation can be conceptualized as a person's capacity to survive and flourish (Lazarus, 1999). Adaptation or lack of it affects three important areas: health, psychological well-being, and social functioning. A period of stress may compromise any or all of these areas. If a person copes successfully with stress, he or she returns to a previous level of adaptation. Successful coping results in an improvement in health, well-being, and social functioning. Unfortunately, at times, maladaptation occurs.

KEY CONCEPT Adaptation is the person's capacity to survive and flourish. Adaptation affects three important areas: health, psychological well-being, and social functioning.

It is impossible to separate completely the adaptation areas of health, well-being, and social functioning. A maladaptation in any one area can negatively affect the others. For instance, the appearance of psychiatric symptoms can cause problems in performance in the work environment that in turn elicit a negative self-concept. Although each area will be discussed separately, the reader should realize that when one area is affected, most likely all three areas are affected (Fig. 14.2).

Health and Illness

Health can be negatively affected when coping is ineffective. When the damaging condition or situation is not ameliorated or the emotional distress is not regulated, stress occurs that in turn affects a person's health. If emotion-focused coping is used when a problem-focused approach is appropriate, stress is not relieved. In addition, if a coping strategy violates cultural norms and lifestyle, stress is often exaggerated. Some coping strategies actually increase the risk for mortality and morbidity, such as the excessive use of alcohol, drugs, or tobacco. Many people use overeating, smoking, or drinking to reduce stress. They may feel better temporarily but are actually increasing their risk for illness. For people whose behaviors exacerbate their illnesses, learning new behaviors becomes important. Healthy coping strategies such as exercising and obtaining adequate sleep and nutrition

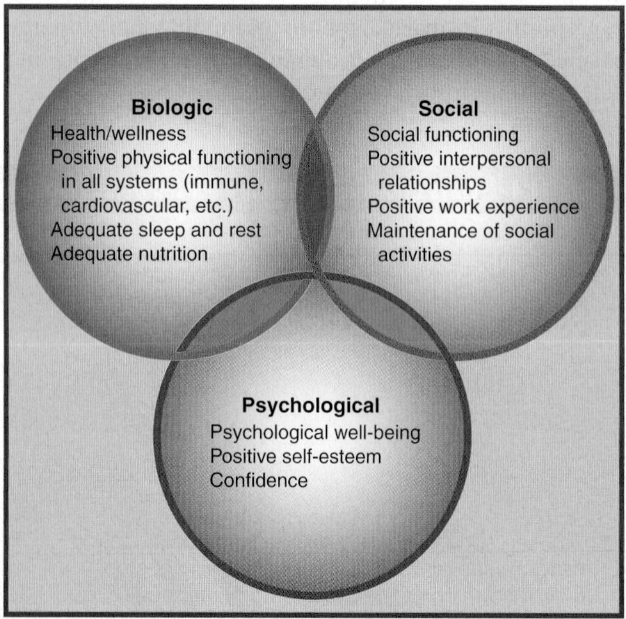

FIGURE 14.2. Biopsychosocial adaptation.

contribute to stress reduction and the promotion of long-term health.

Psychological Well-Being

An ideal outcome is feeling good. Outcome satisfaction for one person does not necessarily represent outcome satisfaction for another. For instance, suppose that two students receive the same passing score on an examination. One may feel a sense of relief, but the other may feel anxious because this student appraises the score as too low. Understanding a person's emotional response to an outcome is essential to analyzing its personal meaning. People who consistently have positive outcomes from stressful experiences are more likely to have positive self-esteem and self-confidence. Unsatisfactory outcomes from stressful experiences are associated with negative mood states, such as depression, anger, guilt leading to decreased self-esteem, and feelings of helplessness. If the situation was appraised as challenging, rather than harmful or threatening, increased self-confidence and a sense of well-being are likely to follow. If the situation was accurately appraised as harmful or threatening but viewed as manageable, the outcome may also be positive.

Social Functioning

Social functioning, the performance of daily activities within the context of interpersonal relations and family and community roles, can be seriously impaired during stressful episodes. For instance, a person who is experiencing the stress of a divorce may not be able to carry out job responsibilities satisfactorily. If successful coping with a stressful encounter leads to a positive outcome, social functioning returns to normal or is improved. Social functioning will continue to be impaired if the person views the outcome as unsuccessful and experiences negative emotions.

NURSING MANAGEMENT: HUMAN RESPONSE TO STRESS

The overall goals for those with acute stress responses are to change the stressful person–environment situations (when possible), reduce the stress response, and develop positive coping skills. The goals for those who are at high risk for stress (experiencing recent life changes, vulnerable to stress, or have limited coping mechanisms) are to recognize the potential for stressful situations and strengthen positive coping skills. These people benefit from education and practice of new coping skills.

Stress responses vary from one person to another. Patients recognize acute stress easier than chronic stress. In many instances, living with chronic stress has become a way of life and is no longer recognized as a source of physical and psychosocial problems. From the assessment data, the nurse can determine any illnesses, the intensity of the stress response, and the effectiveness of coping strategies. Nurses typically identify stress responses in people or family members who are receiving treatment for other health problems.

Individuals experiencing stress may or may not have a psychiatric disorder diagnosis. If an existing Axis I or II disorder is present, the stress responses are usually conceptualized within the particular diagnosis. If there are significant emotional or behavioral symptoms in response to an identifiable stressful situation, but the psychiatric disorder does not account for the response or there is no existing disorder, a diagnosis of adjustment disorder may be made (American Psychiatric Association [APA], 2000) (Table 14.5).

Biologic Domain

Biologic Assessment

The nurse should include a careful health history, focusing on past and present illnesses and traumas. If a psychiatric disorder is present, psychiatric symptoms may spontaneously reappear even when no alteration has occurred in the patient's medication regimen. Nurses should also pay special attention to disorders of the endocrine system, such as hypothyroidism.

Gender Differences

It is now known that people experience stressors differently depending on their gender. Males are more likely to respond to stressors with a fight or flight response, whereas females have less aggressive responses; they "tend and befriend." There is a difference in perception of and behavioral response to the stressor, as well as a difference in the physiology of the stress response (McEwen 2005).

Review of Systems

A systems review can elicit the person's own unique response to stress and can also provide important data on the effect of chronic illnesses. These data are useful for understanding the person–environment situation and the person's stress reactions, coping responses, and adaptation.

Physical Functioning

Physical functioning usually changes during a stress response. Typically, sleep is disturbed, appetite either increases or decreases, body weight fluctuates, and sexual activity changes. Physical appearance may be uncharacteristically disheveled—a projection of the

Table 14.5  Key Diagnostic Characteristics of Adjustment Disorder 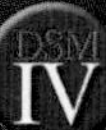

Diagnostic Criteria	Target Symptoms and Associated Findings
• Emotional or behavioral symptoms in response to an identifiable stressor occurring within 3 months of the onset of the stressors. • Clinically significant symptoms or behaviors (1) are characterized by distress that is in excess of what would be expected from exposure to the stressor, or (2) cause a significant impairment in social or occupational (academic) functioning. • Stress-related disturbance does not meet the criteria for another specific Axis I disorder and is not merely an exacerbation of a pre-existing Axis I or Axis II disorder. • Symptoms do not represent bereavement. • Symptoms do not persist for more than 6 months after the stressor has terminated. Acute: disturbance lasts more than 6 months Chronic: disturbance lasts for 6 months or longer 309.0 With depressed mood 309.24 With anxiety 309.28 With mixed anxiety and depressed mood 309.3 With disturbance of conduct 309.4 With mixed disturbance of emotions and conduct 309.9 Unspecified	• Subjective distress or impairment in functioning • Decreased performance at work or school • Temporary changes in relationships *Associated Physical Examination Findings* • Decreased compliance with recommended medical regimen

person's feelings. Body language expresses muscle tension, which conveys a state of anxiety not usually present. Because exercise is an important strategy in stress reduction, the nurse should assess the amount of physical activity, tolerance for exercise, and usual exercise patterns. Sometimes, a person was exercising regularly until changes in daily activities interrupted the routine. Determining the details of the person's exercise pattern can help in formulating reasonable interventions.

Pharmacologic Assessment

In assessing a person's coping strategies, the nurse needs to ask about the use of alcohol, tobacco, marijuana, and any other addictive substances. Many people begin or increase the frequency of using these substances as a way of coping with stress. In turn, substance abuse contributes to the stress behavior. Knowing details about the person's use of these substances (number of times a day or week, amount, circumstances, side effects) helps in determining the role these substances play in overall stress reduction or management. The more important the substances are in the person's handling of stress, the more difficult it will be to change the addictive behavior.

Stress often prompts people to use antianxiety medication without supervision. Use of over-the-counter and herbal medications is common. The nurse should carefully assess the use of any drugs to manage stress symptoms. If drugs are the primary coping strategy, further evaluation is needed with a possible referral to a mental health specialist. If a psychiatric disorder is present, the nurse should assess medication compliance, especially if the psychiatric symptoms are reappearing.

Nursing Diagnoses f or the Biologic Domain

Several nursing diagnoses may be generated from an assessment of the biologic domain. For patients with changes in eating, sleeping, or activity, nursing diagnoses of Imbalanced Nutrition, Disturbed Sleep Pattern, and Impaired Mobility may be appropriate. Ineffective Therapeutic Regimen may also be used for patients using excessive over-the-counter medications. For patients who discontinued use of their regularly prescribed medication, Noncompliance may be appropriate.

Interventions for the Biologic Domain

People under stress can usually benefit from several biologic interventions. Their activities of daily living are usually interrupted, and they often feel that they have no time for themselves. The stressed patient who is normally fastidiously groomed and dressed may appear disheveled and unkempt. Simply reinstating the daily routine of shaving (for a man) or applying makeup (for a woman) can improve the person's outlook on life and ability to cope with the stress (see Chapter 10).

Stress is commonly manifested in the areas of nutrition and activity. During stressful periods, a person's eating patterns change. To cope with stress, a person may either overeat or become anorexic. Both are ineffective coping behaviors and actually contribute to stress. Educating the patient about the importance of maintaining an adequate diet during the period of stress will highlight its importance. It will also allow the nurse to help the person decide how eating behaviors can be changed.

Exercise can reduce the emotional and behavioral responses to stress. In addition to the physical benefits of exercise, a regular exercise routine can provide structure to a person's life, enhance self-confidence, and increase feelings of well-being. People who are stressed are often not receptive to the idea of exercise, particularly if it has not been a part of their routine. Exploring the patient's personal beliefs about the value of activity will help to determine whether exercise is a reasonable activity for that person.

The person under stress tends to be tense, nervous, and on edge. Simple relaxation techniques help the person relax and may improve coping skills. If these techniques do not help the patient relax, the nurse may teach distraction or guided imagery to the patient (see Chapter 10). Nurses should consider referral to a mental health specialist for hypnosis or biofeedback for patients who have severe stress responses.

Psychological Domain

Psychological Assessment

Unlike assessment for other mental health problems, psychological assessment of the person under stress does not ordinarily include a mental status examination. Instead, psychological assessment focuses on the person's emotions and their severity, as well as his or her coping strategies. The assessment elicits the person's appraisal of risks and benefits, the personal meaning of the situation, and the person's commitment to a particular outcome. The nurse can then understand how vulnerable the person is to stress.

Using therapeutic communication techniques, the nurse assesses a person's emotional state in a nurse–patient interview. By beginning the interview with a statement such as, "Let's talk about what you have been feeling," the nurse can elicit the feelings that the person has been experiencing. Identifying the person's emotions can be helpful in assessing the intensity of the stress being experienced. Negative emotions (anger, fright, anxiety, guilt, shame, sadness, envy, jealousy, and disgust) are usually associated with an inability to cope and severe stress.

After identifying the person's emotions, the nurse determines how the person reacts initially to them. For example, does the person who is angry respond by carrying out the innate urge to attack someone whom the person blames for the situation? Or does that person respond by thinking through the situation and overriding the initial innate urge to act? The person who tends to act impulsively has few real coping skills. For the person who can resist the innate urge to act and has developed coping skills, the focus of the assessment becomes determining their effectiveness.

In an assessment interview, the nurse can determine whether the person uses problem-focused or emotion-focused coping strategies effectively. Problem-focused coping is effective when the person can accurately assess the situation. In this case, the person sets goals, seeks information, masters new skills, and seeks help as needed. Emotion-focused coping is effective when the person has inaccurately assessed the situation and coping corrects the false interpretation.

Nursing Diagnoses for the Psychological Domain

The nurse should consider a nursing diagnosis of Ineffective Coping for patients experiencing stress who do not have the psychological resources to effectively manage the situation. Other useful nursing diagnoses include Disturbed Thought Processes, Disturbed Sensory Perception, Low Self-esteem, Fear, Hopelessness, and Powerlessness.

Interventions for the Psychological Domain

Numerous interventions help reduce stress and support coping efforts. All the interventions are best carried out within the framework of a supportive nurse–patient relationship. Assisting patients to develop appropriate problem-solving strategies based on personal strengths and previous experiences is important in understanding and coping with stressful situations. Encouraging patients to examine times when coping has been successful and examine aspects of that situation can help in identifying strengths and strategies for the current problem. For example, a young mother was completely overwhelmed with feelings of inadequacy following the birth of her third child. Further assessment revealed that the patient's mother had helped during the 6 weeks after the other children had been born. The patient's mother was not available for the third birth. First, the nurse validated that having three children could be overwhelming for anyone. The nurse also explained the postpartum hormonal changes that were occurring validating that the patient's feelings were typical of many mothers. Finally, together, the nurse and the patient identified resources in her environment that could support her during the postpartum period.

It is important to have the patient discuss the person–environment situation and develop alternative coping strategies. Some aspects of any situation cannot be changed, such as a family member's illness or a death of a loved one, but usually there are areas within the patient's control that can be changed. A caregiver cannot reverse the family member's disability, but she can arrange for short-term respite.

Social Domain

Social Assessment

Social assessment data are invaluable in determining the person's resources. The ability to make healthy lifestyle changes is strongly influenced by the person's health beliefs and family support system. Even the expression of stress is related to social factors, particularly cultural expectations and values.

Assessment should include use of the Recent Life Changes questionnaire to determine the number and importance of life changes that the patient has experienced within the past year. If several recent life changes have occurred, the person–environment relationship has changed. The person is likely to be either at high risk for or already experiencing stress.

Social assessment also includes identification of the person's social network. Because employment is the mainstay of adulthood and the source of many personal contacts, assessment of any recent changes in employment status is important. If a person is unemployed, the nurse should determine the significance of the unemployment and its effects on the person's social network. For children and adolescents, nurses should note any recent changes in their attendance at school. The nurse should elicit the following data:

- Size and extent of the network, both relatives and nonrelatives, professional and nonprofessional, and how long known
- Functions that the network serves (e.g., intimacy, social integration, nurturance, reassurance of worth, guidance and advice, access to new contacts)
- Degree of reciprocity between the patient and other network members; that is, who provides support to the patient and who the patient supports
- Degree of interconnectedness; that is, how many of the network members know one another and are in contact

Nursing Diagnoses for the Social Domain

The nurse can generate several nursing diagnoses from the social assessment data that involve the person–environment interaction. The challenge of generating nursing diagnoses is to make sure that they are based on the person's appraisal of the situation. Some possible nursing diagnoses include Ineffective Role Performance, Impaired Parenting, Impaired Social Interaction, Social Isolation, and Disabled Family Coping.

Interventions for the Social Domain

Because the experience of stress and the ability to cope are a result of the appraisal of the person–environment relationship, interventions that affect the environment are important. People who are coping with stressful situations can often benefit from interventions that facilitate family unit functioning and promote the health and welfare of family members. For the nurse to intervene with the total family, the stressed person must agree for the family members to be involved. If the data gathered from the assessment of supportive and dissupportive factors indicate that the family members are not supportive, the nurse should assist the patient to consider expanding his or her social network. If the family is the major source of support, the nurse should design interventions that support the functioning of the family unit. Parent education can also be effective in supporting family unit functioning. If family therapy is needed, the nurse should refer the family to an advanced practice specialist.

Evaluation and Treatment Outcomes

The treatment outcomes established in the initial plan of care guide the evaluation. Individual outcomes relate to improved health, well-being, and social function. Depending on the level of intervention, there can also be family and network outcomes. Family outcomes may be related to improved communication or social support; for instance, caregiver stress is reduced once other members of the family help in the care of the ill member. Social network outcomes focus on modifying the social network.

SUMMARY OF KEY POINTS

- Stress affects everyone. Coping with stress can produce positive and negative outcomes. The person can learn and grow from the experience or maladaptation can occur.
- The concept of homeostasis applies to a limited number of biologic functions, whereas the concept of allostasis applies to many of the physiologic regulatory mechanisms affected by stressful events including the hormonal, immune, cardiovascular, and HPA axis.
- Acute stress can lead to physiologic overload which in turn can have a negative impact on a person's health, well-being, and social functioning. Chronic stress is clearly associated with negative health outcomes.
- Stress is defined as a person–environment relationship that is appraised as being unfavorable. Stress responses are simultaneously emotional and physiologic, leading to an innate tendency to act.

- Many personal factors, such as personality patterns, beliefs, values, and commitment to an outcome interact with environmental demands and constraints that produce a person–environment relationship.
- Within the social network, social support can help a person cope with stress.
- Effective coping can be either problem focused or emotion focused. The outcome of successful coping is enhanced health, psychological well-being, and social functioning.

CRITICAL THINKING CHALLENGES

1 Compare and contrast the concepts of homeostasis and allostasis.
2 Discuss the impact of acute stress versus chronic stress. Why is chronic stress of more concern than acute stress?
3 Explain why one person may experience the stress of losing a job differently from another.
4 Explain the HPA response to stress.
5 A woman at the local shelter announced to her group that she was returning to her husband because it was partly her fault that her husband beat her. Is this an example of problem-focused or emotion-focused coping? Justify your answer.

Schindler's List: 1993. The film presents the true story of Oskar Schindler, member of the Nazi party, womanizer, and war profiteer, who saved the lives of more than 1,000 Jews during the Holocaust. The movie shows how, during long periods of political turmoil and terror, life can become somewhat normalized. Yet, fear underlies people's daily lives. Crises erupt at different times during the very long period of chronic stress.

VIEWING POINTS: Differentiate the periods of chronic stress from crisis in this film. Observe the reactions of different characters under stress. Is the behavior different from what you would expect? Observe your own feelings throughout the movie. Did you experience stress?

REFERENCES

Aguilera, D. C. (1998). *Crisis intervention: Theory and methodology*, St. Louis: Mosby.

American Psychiatric Association (APA). (2000). *Diagnostic and statistical manual of mental disorders* (4th ed., text revision). Washington, DC: Author.

Bryant-Lukosius, D. (2003). Review: Limited evidence exists on the effect of psychological coping styles on cancer survival or recurrence. *Evidence Based Nursing, 6*(3), 88.

Cannon W. B. (1932). *The wisdom of the body*. New York: Norton.

Cannon W. B. (1914). The emergency function of the adrenal medulla in pain and the major emotions. *Am J Physiol, 33*, 356–372,.

De Frias, C. M., Tuokko, H., & Rosenberg, T. (2005). Caregiver physical and mental health predicts reactions to caregiving. *Aging & Mental Health, 9*(4), 331–336.

Denollet, J., & Brutsaert, D. L. (2001). Reducing emotional distress improves prognosis in coronary heart disease: 9-year mortality in a clinical trial of rehabilitation. *Circulation, 104*(17), 2018–2023.

Donker, F. J. (2000). Cardiac rehabilitation: A review of current developments. *Clinical Psychology Review, 20*(7), 923–943.

Frei, R. L., Racicot, B. R., & Travagline, A. (1999). The impact of monochromic and type A behavior patterns on research productivity and stress. *Journal of Managerial Psychology, 14*(5), 374–387.

Friedman, M., & Rosenman, R. (1974). *Type A and your heart*. New York: Knopf.

Holmes, T., & Rahe, R. (1967). The Social Readjustment Patient Scale. *Journal of Psychosomatic Research, 11*(2), 213–218.

Jones, M. C., & Johnston, D.W. (2000). Reducing distress in first level and student nurses: A review of the applied stress management literature. *Journal of Advanced Nursing, 32*(1),66–74.

Kaye, J. M., & Lightman, S. L. (2005). Psychological stress and endocrine axes. In K. Vedhara, M. R. Irwin (Eds.). *Human Psychoneuroimmunology*. New York: Oxford University Press.

Kiecolt-Glaser, J. K., Loving, T. J., Stowell, J. R., Malarkey, W. B., Lemeshow, S., Dickinson, S. L., & Glaser, R. (2005). Hostile marital interactions, proinflammatory cytokine production, and wound healing. *Archives of General Psychiatry, 62*(12), 1377–1384.

Knussen, C., Tolson, D., Swan, I. R. C., Stott, D. J., & Brogan, C. A. (2005). Stress proliferation in caregivers: the relationships between caregiving stressors and deterioration in family relationships. *Psychology and Health, 20*(2), 207–221.

Lazarus, R., & Folkman, S. (1984). *Stress, appraisal and coping*. New York: Springer.

Lazarus, R. S. (2001). Relational meaning and discrete emotions. In K. R. Scherer, A. Schorr, & T. Johnstone (Eds.), *Appraisal processes in emotion: Theory, methods, research* (pp. 37–67). New York: Oxford University Press.

Lazarus, R. S. (1999). *Stress and emotion: A new synthesis*. New York: Springer.

Levine, S. (2005). *Stress: an historical perspective*. In T. Steckler, N. H. Kalin, J. M. H. M. Reul (Eds.), *Handbook of Stress and the Brain*. Boston: Elsevier.

Linden, L. (2005). *Stress Management: From basic science to better practice*. Thousand Oaks, California: Sage Publications.

Majer, J. M., Jason, L. A., Ferrarie, J. R., Venable, L. B., & Olson, B.D. (2002). Social support and self-efficacy for abstinence: Is peer identification an issue? *Journal of Substance Abuse Treatment, 23*(3), 209–215.

McEwen, B. S. (2005). Stressed or stressed out: What is the difference? *Journal of Psychiatry Neuroscience, 30*(5), 315–318.

McEwen, B. S. (2000). Allostasis and allostatic load: Implications for neuropsychopharmacology. *Neuropsychopharmacology, 22*, 108–124.

Moneyham, L., Murdaugh, C., Phillips, K., Jackson, K., Tavakoli, A., Boyd, M., et al. (2005). Patterns of risk of depressive symptoms among HIV-positive women in the Southeastern United States. *Journal of the Association of Nurses in Aids Care, 16*(4), 25–38.

Moran, C. C. (2001). Personal predictions of stress and stress reactions in firefighter recruits. *Disaster Prevention & Management 10*(5), 356–365.

Pedersen, S. S., Lemos, P. A., van Vooren, P. R., Liu, T. K. K., Daemen, J., Erdman, R. A.) M., et al. (2004). Type D personality predicts death or myocardial infarction after bare metal stent or sirolimus-eluting stent implantation. *Journal of the American College of Cardiology, 44*(5), 997–1001.

Rahe, R. (1994). The more things change. *Psychosomatic Medicine, 56*(4), 306–307.

Rahe, R. H. (2000). Recent Life Changes Questionnaire [RLCQ].

Rahe, R. H., Taylor, C., Tolles, R. L., Newhall, L. M., Veach, T. L., & Bryson, S. (2002). A novel stress and coping workplace program reduces illness and healthcare utilization. *Psychosomatic Medicine, 64*(2), 278–286.

Rosenman, R., & Chesney, M. (1985). Type A behavior pattern: Its relationship to coronary heart disease and its modification by behavioral and pharmacological approaches. In M. Zales (Ed.), *Stress in health and disease* (pp. 206–241). New York: Brunner/Mazel.

Selye, H. (1956). *The stress of life*. New York: McGraw-Hill.

Selye, H. (1974). *Stress without distress*. Philadelphia: J. B. Lippincott.

Silberman, D. V., Wald, M., & Genaro, A. M. (2002). Effects of chronic mild stress on lymphocyte proliferative response: Participation of serum thyroid hormones and corticosterone. *International Immunopharmacology, 2*(4), 487–497.

Stanley, R. O., & Burrows, G. D. (2005). The role of stress in mental illness: the practice. In C. L. Cooper (Ed.). *Handbook of Stress Medicine and Health (second edition)*. New York: CRC Press.

Stetz, K. M., & Brown, M. (2004). Physical and psychosocial health in family caregiving: a comparison of AIDS and cancer caregivers. *Public Health Nursing, 21*(6), 533–540.

Stuart, T. D., & Garrison, M. E. (2002). The influence of daily hassles and role balance on health status: A study of mothers of grade school children. *Women's Health, 36*(3), 1–11.

Tang, C. S., Lee, A. M., Tang, T., Cheung, F. M., & Chan, C. (2002). Role occupancy, role quality, and psychological distress in Chinese women. *Women's Health, 36*(1), 49–66.

Woodward, M., Oliphant, J., Lowe, G., & Tunstall-Pedoe, H. (2003). Contribution of contemporaneous risk factors to social inequality in coronary heart disease and all causes mortality. *Preventive Medicine, 36*(5), 561–568.

Yeager, K. R., & Roberts, A. R. (2003). Differentiating among stress, acute stress disorder, crisis episodes, trauma, and PTSD: Paradigm and treatment goals. *Brief Treatment and Crisis Intervention, 3*(1), 3–26.

CHAPTER 15

Cultural and Spiritual Issues Related to Mental Health Care

Mary Ann Boyd

KEY CONCEPTS

- culture
- cultural competence
- spirituality

LEARNING OBJECTIVES

After studying this chapter, you will be able to:

- Identify various cultural groups in the United States.
- Describe the beliefs about mental health and illness in different cultural groups.
- Differentiate concepts of religion and spirituality.
- Discuss the role of spirituality in persons with mental illness.
- Discuss the beliefs of major religions and their role in shaping views on mental illnesses.
- Discuss the changing family structure and the mental health implications.

KEY TERMS

• cultural competence • culture of poverty • religiousness

All cultural groups have sets of values, beliefs, and patterns of accepted behavior, and it is often difficult for those of one culture to understand those of another. This is especially true regarding mental illness—some cultures view it as a condition for which the ill person must be punished and ostracized from society, whereas other cultures are more tolerant and believe that family and community members are key to the care and treatment of the mentally ill. Nurses' and patients' religious backgrounds and cultural heritages may be different, so it is important for nurses to understand clearly the thinking and perspectives of other cultures and groups.

This chapter examines cultural and social mores of various cultural and religious groups and the overall changing profile of today's American family structure. Understanding cultural and religious beliefs and the significance of spirituality is especially important when caring for people with mental health problems. These beliefs and practices can define and shape the experience of being mentally ill and influence the willingness to seek care. Treating mental disorders is intertwined with peoples' attitudes about themselves, their beliefs, values, and ways of interacting with their families and communities.

> **KEY CONCEPT Culture** is not only a way of life for people who identify or associate with one another on the basis of some common purpose, need, or similarity of background but also the totality of learned, socially transmitted beliefs, values, and behaviors that emerge from its members' interpersonal transactions.
>
> **Cultural competence** is developed through cultural awareness, acquisition of cultural knowledge, development of cultural skills, and engagement of numerous cultural encounters.
>
> **Cultural competence** is a process in which the "healthcare professional continually strives to achieve the ability and availability to work effectively within the cultural context of the client (family, individual or community)" (Campinha-Bacote, 2002).

BOX 15.1

Mental Health Care within Latino Communities

- Major depression is the most common form of depression
- Latinos tend to express depression in the form of bodily aches and pains that persist in spite of medical treatment
- Less than one in 11 contacts a mental health specialist; fewer than one in five contacts a general health care provider.
- Latinos are likely to seek treatment for mental health problems in a primary care setting
- There are fewer than 20 Latino mental health specialists for every 100,000 Latinos
- Mental health concerns appear to increase among Latino immigrants as they acculturate

NCLR/California State University, Long Beach Center for Latino Community Health & Leadership Training and the National Council of La Raza (NCLR) (2005). Critical Disparities in Latino Mental Health: Transforming Research Into Action. White Paper. Institute for Hispanic Health.
www.nclr.org/files/34795_file_WP_**Latino_Mental**_Health_FNL.pdf, retrieved 4/10/07.

CULTURAL BELIEFS ABOUT MENTAL ILLNESS

African Americans

In 2004, the estimated population of African Americans, including those of more than one race, was 39.2 million or 13% in the United States population (U.S. Census Bureau, 2006a). Although African Americans share many beliefs, attitudes, values, and behaviors, there are also many subcultural and individual differences based on social class, country of origin, occupation, religion, educational level, and geographic location. Many African Americans have extensive family networks in which members can be relied on for moral support, help with child rearing, financial aid, and help in crises, and in most African American families, elderly members are treated with great respect. But African Americans with mental illness suffer from the stresses of double stigma—not only from their own cultural group but also from long-time racial discrimination. To make matters worse, racial discrimination may come from within the health community itself. Several studies show that diagnoses and treatment for African Americans often are racially biased (Dixon, et al., 2001a; Dixon et al., 2001b).

Latino Americans

The number of Latino Americans living in the United States has been gradually increasing, and this group is now the largest minority in the United States. From 1980 to 2000, there was a 122% increase in population, from 14.6 to 32.5 million. In 2004, the estimated number of Latino Americans was 40.5 or 14.2% of the U.S. population. Countries of origin include Mexico (64%), Puerto Rico (10%), and Cuba (4%). Latino populations are largest in urban areas, such as New York, Chicago, Los Angeles, San Francisco, and Miami–Fort Lauderdale (U.S. Census Bureau, 2006b).

Studies indicate that Latino Americans tend to use all other resources before seeking help from mental health professionals. Reasons for this include (1) many Latino patients believe that mental health facilities do not accommodate their cultural needs (e.g., language, beliefs, values), and (2) many still seek help through supportive home care and counseling from the church. If bilingual, bicultural mental health facilities are available, Latino patients will seek care. An analysis of a household survey from 3,000 respondents in California of immigrants and U.S.-born Mexican Americans found that both groups were more likely to use the general medical sector for treating mental health problems (Vega, Kolody, & Aguilar-Gaxiola, 2001). (See Box 15.1).

Asian Americans, Polynesians, and Pacific Islanders

In 2004, more than 12 million (4.2%) Asian Americans, Polynesians, and Pacific Islanders lived in the United States. This large multicultural group includes Chinese, Filipino, Japanese, Asian Indian, Korean, Vietnamese, Laotian, Cambodian, Hawaiian, Samoan, and Guamanian people. Most Chinese, Japanese, Korean, Asian Indian, and Filipino immigrants have migrated to urban areas, whereas the Vietnamese have settled throughout the United States (U.S. Census Bureau, 2006c).

Generally, Asian cultures have a tradition of denying or disguising the existence of mental illnesses. In many of these cultures, it is an embarrassment to have a family member treated for mental illness, which may explain the extremely low utilization of mental health services. Only 17% of those experiencing problems seek care. Asian Americans may experience culture-bound syndrome, such as neurasthenia, which is characterized by fatigue, weakness, poor concentration, memory loss, irritability, aches and pains, and sleep disturbances or hwa-byung, "suppressed anger syndrome" (see Chapter 2). Research regarding specific mental health problems in Asian cultures is sparse, but various data suggest rates of suicide within Native Hawaiian adolescents are higher than those of other adolescents in Hawaii, and older Asian American women have the highest suicide rate of all women over age 65 in the United States (U.S. Department of Health and Human Services, 2006).

BOX 15.2

***Research for Best Practice:* Depression in Korean Immigrant Wives**

Um, C., & Dancy, B. (1999). Relationship between coping strategies and depression among employed Korean immigrant wives. Issues in Mental Health Nursing, 20, 485–494.

The Question: What is the correlation of stress and coping strategies in depression among immigrant women?

Methods: Korean immigrant wives volunteered to participate in a research study that looked at their coping strategies and the development of depression. The study group consisted of 282 women ranging in age from 25 to 55 years (mean age, 41.7 years). Most of these women (92%) arrived in the United States with at least a high school education. Most (86%) had children. All of the women were employed outside the home and worked from 20 to 84 hours per week.

Findings: The researchers found that depression was positively correlated to the management of stress by working harder at cleaning the house. Depression was negatively correlated to negotiation (discussion with husband).

Women of Minority Groups

Women within minority groups may experience more conflicting feelings and psychological stressors than do men in trying to adjust to both their defined role in the minority culture and a different role in the larger predominant society (see Box 15.2). For men, who usually earn a living and work within the cultural neighborhood, the socioeconomic status and social position remain the same. In a qualitative study comparing work and family domains of Caucasian working women with minority working women, researchers found that the groups differed in their perceptions of work. Caucasian women view work as a "choice," rather than an "obligation," whereas minority women compartmentalized their work and family lives (Robinson & Swanson, 2002).

Native Americans

In 2004, the estimated population of Native Americans was over 2 million people, less than 1% of the U.S. population. Native American cultures emphasize respect and reverence for the earth and nature, from which come survival and comprehension of life and one's relationships with a separate, higher spiritual being and with other human beings. Shamans, or medicine men, are central to most cultures. They are healers believed to possess psychic abilities. Healing treatments rely on herbal medicines and healing ceremonies and feasts. Self-understanding derives from observing nature; relationships with others emphasize interdependence and sharing.

Traditional views about mental illnesses vary among the tribes. In some, mental illness is viewed as a supernatural possession, as being out of balance with nature. In certain Native American groups, people with mental illnesses are stigmatized. However, the degree of stigmatization is not the same for all disorders. In tribal groups that make little distinction between physical and mental illnesses, there is little stigma. In other groups, a particular event, such as suicide, is stigmatized. Different illnesses may be encountered in different Native American cultures and gene pools.

Culture of Poverty

Culture of poverty is a term that describes the norms and behaviors of people living in poverty. Poverty affects all cultural groups and other groups, such as the elderly, disabled, psychiatrically impaired, and single-parent families. In the United States, one third of people living below the poverty line are single mothers and their children; 27% of African Americans live below the poverty level, as do 23% of Latino Americans and 12% of Americans of European descent. Currently in the United States, the poverty guidelines for a family of four is a yearly income of $20,000 or less in the 48 mainland states; $25,000 or less in Alaska; and $23,000 or less in Hawaii (Federal Register, 2005).

Families living in poverty are under tremendous financial and emotional stress, which may trigger or exacerbate mental problems. Along with the daily stressors of trying to provide food and shelter for themselves and their families, the lack of time, energy, and money prevents them from attending to their psychological needs. Often, these families become trapped in a downward economic spiral, as tension and stress mount. The inability to gain employment and the lack of financial independence only add to the feelings of powerlessness and low self-esteem. Being self-supporting gives one a feeling of control over life and bolsters self-esteem. Dependence on others or the government causes frustration, anger, apathy, and feelings of depression and meaninglessness. Alcoholism, depression, and child and partner abuse may become a means of coping with such hopelessness and despair. The homeless population is the group most at risk for being unable to escape this spiral of poverty.

Rural Cultures

Most mental health services are located in urban areas because most people live near cities. *All* age groups in rural areas have limited access to health care. The lack of resources is particularly problematic for children and elderly people, who have specialized needs. Rural areas are diverse in both geography and culture. For example, access to mental health for those in the deep South is different from access for those with the same problems in the Northwest. Also, treatment approaches may be accepted in one part of the country but not in another.

SPIRITUALITY

KEY CONCEPT Spirituality can be defined as thinking about one's self as a part of a spiritual force such as a God, a spirit, nature and a feeling of connectedness/relationship/oneness with God, spirit, nature, or unifying force (Corrigan, McCorkle, Schell, & Kidder, 2003; Hill et al., 2000). It is a connection to life, a way of interpreting life events and a source of hope, joy, comfort, and guidance on life's journey (O'Reilly, 2004).

People with mental illness benefit from spiritual assessment and interventions (see Chapter 10). Perception of well-being and health in persons with severe mental illness has been positively associated with spirituality and **religiousness** (the participation in a community of people who gather around common ways of worshiping; see Box 15.3). To carry out spiritual interventions, the nurse enters a therapeutic relationship with the patient and uses the self as a therapeutic tool. Examples of spiritual interventions include meditation, guided imagery, and, where appropriate, prayer to connect with inner sources of solace and hope (O'Reilly, 2004; see Box 15.4).

RELIGION AND MENTAL ILLNESS

Religious beliefs often define an individual's relationship within a family and community. Many different religions are practiced throughout the world. Judeo-Christian thinking tends to dominate Western societies. Other religions, such as Islam, Hinduism, and Buddhism, dominate Eastern and Middle Eastern cultures (Table 15.1). Because religious beliefs often influence approaches to mental health, it is important to understand the basis of various religions that appear to be growing in the United States. Both religion and spirituality can provide support and strength in dealing with mental illnesses and emotional problems.

BOX 15.3

Research for Best Practice

Corrigan, P., McCorkle, B., Schell, B., & Kidder, K. (2003). Religion and spirituality in the lives of people with serious mental illness. Community Mental Health Journal, 39(6), 487–499.

The Question: How does religiousness and spirituality affect outcomes in people with psychiatric disabilities?

Methods: In this study, 1,824 people with serious mental illness completed self-report measures of religiousness and spirituality. Three health outcomes measures were self-perceived well-being, psychiatric symptoms, and life goal achievement.

Findings: Both religiousness and spirituality were significantly associated with reports of well being and psychiatric symptoms, but not goal achievement. Over 90% of the participants identified themselves as religious.

Implications for Nursing: Patients should be assessed for their cultural and religious background. The importance of religion and its relationship to the mental illness should be established. Patients' spiritual experiences should be assessed and considered while interventions are formulated.

BOX 15.4

Using Reflection: Facilitating Spiritual Connections

Incident: A young gay man with severe depression, psychosis, and HIV was shunned by his family and church. He is homeless and sleeps at a shelter each night, roaming the streets during the day. As a veteran, he seeks health services at a local Veterans Administration. He is reluctant to seek out mental health care. In an interview, he asks the nurse if God is punishing him for being gay.

Reflection: The nurse's immediate thought was to assure him that he was not being punished. As the nurse reflected on the situation, she realized that he might be asking for help in understanding the meaning of his situation and how he could understand his connection to his God. She initiated a therapeutic relationship with him and then conducted a spiritual assessment.

CHANGING FAMILY STRUCTURE 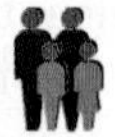

Although families may be defined differently within various cultures, they all play an important role in the life of the individual and influence who and what we are. Traditionally, families are considered a source of guidance, security, love, and understanding. This is also true for people who have mental illnesses and emotional problems. It is often the family who assumes primary care for the person with mental illness and supports that individual throughout treatment. For patients, the family unit may provide their only constant support throughout their lives. Although the nuclear family remains the basic unit of social organization, its structure and size have changed drastically in recent times and so have the functions and roles of family members.

Family Size

Family size in the United States has decreased. In 1790, about one third of all households, including servants, slaves, and other people not related to the head, consisted of seven people or more. By 1960, only one household in 20 was this size. Few households contained members not

Table 15.1 World's Major Religions or Belief Forms

Source of Power or Force (Deity)	Historical Sacred Texts or Beliefs	Key Beliefs or Ethical Life Philosophy
Christianity		
God, a unity in tripersonality; Father, Son, and Holy Ghost	Bible Teachings of Jesus through the apostles and the church fathers	God's love for all creatures is a basic belief. Salvation is gained by those who have faith and show humility toward God. Brotherly love is emphasized in acts of charity, kindness, and forgiveness.
Islam		
Allah (the only God) Has two major sects: *Sunni* (orthodox), traditional and simple practices are followed, human will is determined by outside forces *Shiite*, practices are rapturous and trancelike; human beings have free will	Koran (the words of God delivered to Mohammed by the angel Gabriel) Hadith (commentaries by Mohammed) Five Pillars of Islam (religious conduct) Islam was built on Christianity and Judaism	God is just and merciful; humans are limited and sinful. God rewards the good and punishes the sinful. Mohammed, through the Koran, guides people and teaches them truth. Peace is gained through submission to Allah. The sinless go to Paradise, and the evil go to Hell. A "good" Muslim obeys the Five Pillars of Islam.
Hinduism		
Brahma (the Infinite Being and Creator that pervades all reality) Other gods: Vishnu (preserver) Shiva (destroyer) Krishna (love)	Vedas (doctrine and commentaries)	All people are assigned to castes (permanent hereditary orders, each having different privileges in society; each was created from different parts of Brahma): 1. *Brahmans:* includes priests and intellectuals 2. *Kshatriyas:* includes rulers and soldiers 3. *Vaisya:* includes farmers, skilled workers, and merchants 4. *Sudras:* includes those who serve the other three castes (servants, laborers, peasants) 5. *Untouchables:* the outcasts, those not included in the other castes
Buddhism		
Buddha Individual responsibility and logical or intuitive thinking Buddhist subjects include: *Lamaism* (Tibet), in which Buddhism is blended with spirit worship *Mantrayana* (Himalayan area, Mongolia, Japan), in which intimate relationship with a guru and recitations of secret mantras are emphasized; belief in sexual symbolism and demons *Ch'an* (China) *Zen* (Japan), in which self-reliance and awareness through intuitive understanding are stressed. *Satori* (enlightenment) may come from "sudden insight" or through self-discipline, meditation, and instruction	Tripitaka (scripture) Middle Path (way of life) The Four Noble Truths Eightfold Path (guides for life) The Texts of Taoism (include the Tao Te Ching of Lao Tzu and The Writings of Chuang Tzu) Sutras (Buddhist commentaries) Sangha (Buddhist Community)	Buddhism attempts to deal with problems of human existence such as suffering and death. Life is misery, unhappiness, and suffering with no ultimate reality in the world or behind it. The cause of all human suffering and misery is desire. The "middle path" of life avoids the personal extremes of self-denial and self-indulgence. Visions can be gained through personal meditation and contemplation; good deeds and compassion also facilitate the process toward nirvana, the ultimate mode of existence. The end of suffering is the extinction of desire and emotion, and ultimately the unreal self. Present behavior is a result of past deed.
Confucianism		
No doctrine of a god or gods or life after death Individual responsibility and logical and intuitive thinking	Five Classics (Confucian thought) Analects (conversations and sayings of Confucius)	A philosophy or a system of ethics for living, rather than a religion that teaches how people should act toward one another. People are born "good." Moral character is stressed through sincerity in personal and public behavior. Respect is shown for parents and figures of authority. Improvement is gained through self-responsibility, introspection, and compassion for others.

(Continued on following page)

Table 15.1 World's Major Religions or Belief Forms (Continued)

Source of Power or Force (Deity)	Historical Sacred Texts or Beliefs	Key Beliefs or Ethical Life Philosophy
Shintoism		
Gods of nature, ancestor worship, national heroes	Tradition and custom (the way of the gods) Beliefs were influenced by Confucianism and Buddhism	Reverence for ancestors and traditional Japanese way of life is emphasized. Loyalty to places and locations where one lives or works and purity and balance in physical and mental life are major motivators of personal conduct.
Taoism		
All the forces in nature	Tao-te-Ching ("The Way and the Power")	Quiet and happy harmony with nature is the key belief. Peace and contentment are found in the personal behaviors of optimism, passivity, humility, and internal calmness. Humility is an especially valued virtue. Conformity to the rhythm of nature and the universe leads to a simple, natural, and ideal life.
Judaism		
God	Hebrew Bible (Old Testament) Torah (first five books of Hebrew Bible) Talmud (commentaries on the Torah)	Jews have a special relationship with God: obeying God's law through ethical behavior and ritual obedience earns the mercy and justice of God. God is worshiped through love, not out of fear.
Tribal Beliefs		
Animism: Souls or spirits embodied in all beings and everything in nature (trees, rivers, mountains) Polytheism: Many gods, in the basic powers of nature (sun, moon, earth, water)	Passed on through ceremonies, rituals, myths, and legends. Oral history, rather than written literature, is the common medium.	All living things are related. Respect for powers of nature and pleasing the spirits are fundamental beliefs to meet basic and practical needs for food, fertility, health, and interpersonal relationships and individual development. Harmonious living is comprehension and respect of natural forces.

Summary of Other Belief Forms

- *Atheism:* the belief that no God exists, as "God" is defined in any current existing culture of society.
- *Agnosticism:* the belief that whether there is a God and a spiritual world or any ultimate reality is unknown and probably unknowable.
- *Scientism:* the belief that values and guidance for living come from scientific knowledge, principles, and practices; systematic study and analysis of life, rather than superstition, lead to true understanding and practice of life.
- *Maoism:* the faith that is centered in the leadership of the Communist Party and all the people; the major belief goal is to move away from individual personal desires and ambitions, toward viewing and serving all people as a whole.

Adapted from Axelson, J. A., & McGrath, P. (1998, 1993, 1985). *Counseling and development in a multicultural society.* Pacific Grove, CA: Brooks/Cole Publishing Company, a division of International Thomson Publishing Inc. Used with permission of the publisher.

related to the head (Taeuber, 1968). The average family household in 2004 was 2.60 people (U.S. Bureau of the Census, 2006c).

Changing Roles

A woman's role in the family has changed drastically in the past years. Today, most women, including those who are mothers, work—both in dual-income families and single-parent families. Women make up 46% of the American civilian work force. There are 117 million women age 16 years and over in the United States and 69 million work or are looking for work. More than half of the female work force is married. Half the single, never-married women have children younger than 18 years. More than 75% of divorced, widowed, or separated women have children, and more than 70% of married women have children (U.S. Bureau of the Census, 2006d). Although the traditional roles for men and women have changed somewhat by women entering the work force, working women still bear the bulk of responsibility for child care and household duties. They report feeling guilty and stressed from trying to be everything—a good parent and a success at a demanding job. Women often become emotionally exhausted, particularly during periods of personal conflict. They are at high risk for depression.

Mobility and Relocation

Families are more mobile and may change residences more often than ever before. Leaving familiar environments and readjusting to new surroundings and lifestyles stresses family members. Moreover, these moves impose separation from the extended family, which traditionally has been a stabilizing force and a much-needed support system.

Unmarried Couples

More unmarried couples are cohabitating before or instead of marrying. And some elderly couples, most often widowed, find it economically practical to cohabitate without marrying. In 2003, unmarried couples accounted for 5.5 million households. The lifestyles chosen as an alternative to the traditional male-female, two-parent, nuclear families are often stigmatized.

Single-Parent Families

It is estimated that 50% to 60% of all American children will reside at some point in a single-parent home. In the past, one-parent families usually were the result of the death of a spouse. Now, one-parent families are mostly the result of divorce. Of the nation's 76 million family households in 2004, married couples (with or without children) accounted for 57 million; there were 18 million single-person family households (U.S. Bureau of the Census, 2006d). The divorce rate has been steadily rising in the United States since the 1960s; by 1997, more than one of four children lived with only one parent. Of all children in one-parent homes, 84% live with their mother. Because women maintaining families tend to have considerably lower incomes than do their male counterparts, they now make up a disproportionate share of the poor population in the United States.

Stepfamilies

Remarried families or stepfamilies have a unique set of problems that are not completely understood. Many parents find that step-parenting is much more difficult than parenting a biologic child. The bonding that occurs with biologic children rarely occurs with the stepchildren, whose natural bond is with a parent not living with them. However, it is the step-parent who often assumes a measure of financial and parental responsibility. The care and management of children often become the primary stressor to the marital partners. In addition, the children are faced with multiple sets of parents whose expectations may differ. They may also compete for the children's attention. It is not unusual for second marriages to fail because of the stressors inherent in a remarried family.

Childless Families

Couples can be involuntarily childless because of infertility or voluntarily childless by choice. Approximately 15% of all couples in the reproductive age are involuntarily childless. There is evidence that this group experiences grief over being childless (Johansson & Berg, 2005). As the opportunities for women increased, many people chose not to have children. Research on childlessness is sparse, but it appears that middle and old age childless adults are not more vulnerable to loneliness and depression than those with children (Korokpeckyj-Cox, 1998).

Same-Sex Families

Among the most stigmatized people are those who are gay or lesbian. It is estimated that most lesbian and gay populations have encountered some form of verbal harassment or violence in their lives. The exact number of people who are gay or lesbian is believed to be undercounted as much as 62%. In the 2000 U.S. Census, over 601,000 gay or lesbian families were identified (Smith & Gates, 2001; U.S. Bureau of the Census, 2000). Higher smoking and drinking rates are present in this population and may indicate higher rates of depression, stress, low self-esteem, and complications of childhood abuse (O'Hanlan, Dibble, Hagan, & Davids, 2004).

Although at one time people believed that being gay or lesbian was a result of faulty parenting or personal choice, it is generally accepted that sexual orientation is determined early in life by a combination of factors, including genetic predisposition, biologic development, and environmental events. In the past, it was also believed that sexual preference could be changed through counseling by making a concerted effort to establish new relationships. However, no evidence supports the hypothesis that change in sexual orientation is possible.

SUMMARY OF KEY POINTS

- The term *culture* is defined as a way of life that manifests the learned beliefs, values, and accepted behaviors that are transmitted socially within a specific group.
- Cultural competence consists of cultural awareness, cultural knowledge, cultural skills, and cultural encounters. Developing cultural competence in psychiatric nursing practice is an ongoing process in caring for patients within the context of their culture.
- Spirituality can be a source of strength and support for both the patient with mental illness and the nurse providing the care.

- Religious beliefs are closely intertwined with beliefs about health and mental illness.
- Mental illnesses are stigmatized in most cultural groups. A variety of cultural and religious beliefs underlie the stigmatization.
- Access to mental health treatment is particularly limited for those living in rural areas or those within the culture of poverty.
- The family is an important societal unit that often is responsible for the care and coordination of treatment of members with mental disorders. The family structure, size, and roles are rapidly changing. Traditional health care services will have to adapt to meet the mental health care needs of these families.

CRITICAL THINKING CHALLENGES

1 Assess your cultural competence with groups who have the following heritage: African, Asian, Latino, and Native American.
2 Compare beliefs about mental illnesses within African and Asian American groups.
3 Discuss the differences between spirituality and religiousness. Is it possible that someone can be spiritual and not religious?
4 Identify the religious groups that are associated with the following sacred texts: Bible, Koran, Vedas, Texts of Taoism, Talmud.
5 Compare the access to mental health services in your state or county in rural areas versus urban areas.
6 Define the culture of poverty and discuss how powerlessness affects the life of people living in poverty.
7 Trace the structure of the changing family through the 1900s to the present.
8 Discuss how nontraditional family units, such as single-parent families, stepfamilies, and single-sex families, are stigmatized by society.

House of Sand and Fog (2003). Colonel Massoud Amir Behrani, an Iranian immigrant played by Ben Kingsley, has spent most of his savings trying to enhance his daughter's chances of a good marriage. The rest of his funds were spent at an auction on a repossessed house owned by Kathy Nicoli (Jennifer Connelly), an emotionally unstable, depressed young woman who failed to pay property taxes. The struggle for the house ensues with tragic results.

VIEWING POINTS: Identify the cultural differences between the Behrani and Nicoli families. Discuss the role of prejudice and discrimination in the outcome of the movie. How did Kathy's mental illness and relationship with the police officer influence the negotiation for the house?

Brokeback Mountain (2005). This movie is a powerful story of two young men, a Wyoming ranch hand and a rodeo cowboy, who meet in the summer of 1963 sheep-herding in the harsh, high grasslands and have an unorthodox, yet life-long bond. At the end of the summer, a long affair begins that the two of them desperately try to hide from those around them.

VIEWING POINTS: Observe your feelings as you watch this movie. Identify the cultural mores that prevent Jack and Ennis from being open about their relationship. Discuss the social settings in which a homosexual relationship would be accepted.

REFERENCES

Campinha-Bacote, J. (2002). *A culturally competent model of care.* Transcultural C.A.R.E. Associates. Available: www.transcultural.net.

Corrigan, P., McCorkle, B., Schell, B., & Kidder, K. (2003). Religion and spirituality in the lives of people with serious mental illness. *Community Mental Health Journal, 39*(6), 487–499.

Dixon, L., Green-Paden, L., Delahanty, J., Lucksted, A., Postrado, L., & Hall, J. (2001a). Variables associated with disparities in treatment of patients with schizophrenia and comorbid mood and anxiety disorders. *Psychiatric Services, 52*(9), 1216–1222.

Dixon, L., Lyles, A., Smith, C., Hoch, J. S., Fahey, M., Postrado, L., et al. (2001b). Use and costs of ambulatory care services among Medicare enrollees with schizophrenia. *Psychiatric Services, 52*(6), 786–792.

2006 HHS Poverty Guidelines, 71(15) Federal Register 3848–3849 (2005).

Hill, P. C., Pargament, K. I., Hood, R. W., McCullough, M. D., Swyers, J.P., Larson, D.B., et al. (2000). Conceptualizing religion and spirituality: Points of commonality, points of departure. *Journal for Theory of Social Behaviour, 30*, 51–77.

Johansson, M., & Berg, M. (2005). Women's experiences of childlessness 2 years after the end of in vitro fertilization treatment. *Scandinavian Journal of Caring Sciences, 19*(1), 58–63.

Koropeckyj-Cox, T. (1998). Loneliness and depression in middle and old age: Are the childless more vulnerable? *Journals of Gerontology-Series B: Psychological Sciences & Social Sciences, 53*(6), S303–S312.

O'Hanlan, K. A., Dibble, S. L., Hagan, H. J. J., & Davids, R. (2004). Advocacy for women's health should include lesbian health. *Journal of Women's Health, 13*(2), 227–234.

O'Reilly, M. D. (2004). Spirituality and mental health clients. *Journal of Psychosocial Nursing, 42*(7), 44–55.

Robinson, J. W., & Swanson, N. (2002). Psychological well-being of working women: A cross-cultural perspective. *Current Women's Health Report, 2*(3), 214–218.

Smith, D. M., & Gates, G. (2001). Gay and Lesbian Families in the United States: Same-Sex Unmarried Partner Households: A Preliminary Analysis of 2000 United States Census Data. A Human Rights Campaign Report. www.hrc.org. Retrieved April 10, 2007.

Taeuber, C. (1968). Population trends and characteristics. In E. Sheldon & W. Moore (Eds.), *Indication of social change: Concepts and Measurements* (pp. 27–74). New York: Russell Sage Foundation.

Um, C., & Dancy, B. (1999). Relationship between coping strategies and depression among employed Korean immigrant wives. *Issues in Mental Health Nursing, 20*, 485–494.

U.S. Bureau of the Census. (2000). *Statistical abstract of the United States.* Washington, DC: U.S. Government Printing Office.

U.S. Census Bureau. (2006a). Facts for Features African-American History Month: February 2006. Retrieved June 21, 2006, from www.census.gov/Press-Release.

U.S. Census Bureau. (2006b). American FactFinder. Hispanic or Latino origin by specific origin. 2004 American Community Survey: February 2006. Retrieved June 21, 2006, from www.census.gov/Press-Release.

U.S. Census Bureau. (2006c). American FactFinder. 2004 American Community Survey, Data Profile Highlights. http://www.census.gov/Press-Release. Retrieved June 21, 2006, from www.census.gov/Press-Release.

U.S. Census Bureau. (2006d). Statistical Abstracts of the United States. Retrieved from www.census.gov/prod/www/statistical-abstract.html.

U.S. Department of Health and Human Services. (2006). Fact Sheets Asian Americans/Pacific Islanders *Mental Health: Culture, Race, Ethnicity-Fact Sheets.* Retrieved June 21, 2006, from www.mentalhealth.samhsa.gov/cre/fact2.asp.

Vega, W. A., Kolody, B., & Aguilar-Gaxiola, S. (2001). Help seeking for mental health problems among Mexican Americans. *Journal of Immigrant Health, 3*(3), 133–140.

CHAPTER 16

Mental Health Promotion of the Young and Middle-Aged Adult

Richard Yakimo

KEY CONCEPTS

- young adulthood
- middle-age adulthood

LEARNING OBJECTIVES

After studying this chapter, you will be able to:

- Describe psychosocial problems common to young and middle-aged adults.
- Describe protective factors in the mental health promotion of young and middle-aged adults.
- Identify risk factors related to psychopathology in young and middle-aged adults.
- Analyze the role of the nurse in mental health promotion with young and middle-aged adults.

KEY TERMS

• risk factors • sandwich generation • empty nest • peak marriage age • informal caregivers • protective factors

Concepts of young and middle-age adulthood are relatively new in American culture.

KEY CONCEPTS The generally accepted range for **young adulthood** is from 18 to 44 years. **Middle-age adulthood** spans the period from approximately 45 to 65 years.

These concepts do not necessarily exist across nations and cultures due to the differences in the chronological lifespan of other societies. Western families have achieved unprecedented economic stability that provides for long periods of development. Technological advances such as economic development, improved nutrition, public health control of infectious diseases, access to health care, and other modern developments have resulted in the lengthening of the lifespan chronologically in the developed world. Such advances do not exist worldwide. In many nondeveloped areas, the lifespan is characterized by a brief childhood, followed by a mature adulthood that evolves quickly into old age.

Psychological changes in adulthood occur slowly and subtly with age and experience, not in a fixed stepwise manner. Until recently, adult development was viewed as a relatively stationary plateau with the rapid and complex changes of childhood and adolescence forming one steep side and the declining changes of old age the other. However, this oversimplifies young and middle-aged development. Today, young and middle-aged development is viewed as dynamic and multifaceted.

The developmental concepts of identity, intimacy, and generativity are recurrent and continue to be renegotiated in the face of life stresses such as job loss, career change, relocation, illness, divorce, and widowhood (see Chapter 6). Chronological age is losing its customary social meaning, resulting in a more fluid life cycle. Traditional notions of young adulthood as a time of leaving the parental home and establishing an independent career and family life, of college education taking place during late adolescence, or of the middle-aged parents facing the **"empty nest"** —a home devoid of children and caregiving responsibilities—are being replaced with fewer age-defined life roles.

The timing of life events such as education, marriage, childrearing, career development, and retirement is becoming less regular and more alternatives are tolerated by society. Some people never marry and others retire very early. Many young adults now remain in their parents' home while they pursue their professional education rather than strike out on their own as was customary in previous generations. Their middle-aged parents are often already caring for their own parents, creating the **sandwich generation**, with its responsibilities toward the elder generation above and two generations of children below them. Many women choose to marry and establish a family and then return to finish their college education when their children start school.

PSYCHOSOCIAL PROBLEMS IN YOUNG AND MIDDLE-AGED ADULTS

Unemployment

Young and middle-aged adults seek and maintain employment that maintains their lifestyle and provides for their children. In a society that is consumer driven, the ability to generate resources becomes critical. In addition, shifts in the ownership and organizational structure of companies, downsizing, and the job market's ever-changing demands for workers with particular skills make current employment stability questionable. Career changes and the continuing necessity of training for new positions are now the norm.

In the United States, the unemployment rate has remained relatively low (6.5% at the end of 2005); however, this figure represents only those persons looking for employment. In 2005, the percentage of Americans who have been out of work for 1 year or longer was 13%, which has doubled since 2001. These data suggest that a growing minority of Americans who have lost jobs are finding it more difficult to find another job.

Disparities in unemployment rates exist by race, gender, and ethnic groups. African Americans are faring the worst, with a falling employment rate. By the first quarter of 2005, the overall African American unemployment rate was 10.6%. Rural Hispanic populations tend to have larger families and are significantly younger than rural white families. For them, resources are stretched and opportunities limited. Non-skilled workers are at special risk for unemployment and low wages (Economic Policy Institute, 2005).

Single mothers are another group at high risk for low wages and unemployment. The proportion of single mothers who were employed increased in the mid and late 1990s, but has fallen in the past few years. The employment rate among single mothers fell from 73% in 2000 to 69.8% in 2003—a larger decline than among other parents or the population overall (Sherman, Fremstad, & Parrott, 2004).

Employment is an important societal value and thus serves as a source of economic, social, and emotional stability and self-esteem. The unemployed have at least double the rate of psychiatric disorders (with the exception of drug abuse) compared with those employed (Keyes, 2002; Outram, Mishra, & Schofield, 2004; Tohen, Bromet, Murphy, & Tsuang, 2000).

Changes in Family Structure

The young and middle-aged years are characterized by changes in family structures. Older adolescents finish school and often leave home, which alters the primary family structure. Marriage establishes new roles for adults who previously lived by themselves or their parents. The arrival of children changes the structure and dynamics of the newly formed family. These are all normal developmental events but they can also lead to mental distress, physical problems, and social alienation.

Middle-aged adults are most likely to be married compared with younger adults and adults 65 years or older. There appears to be a **"peak marriage age"** in the mid-twenties. People who get married between the age of 23 and 27 are more likely to remain married than those who marry as teens (DiCaro, 2005; see Table 16.1).

Married adults are healthier than those in other non-married groups. They are least likely to experience health problems and least likely to engage in risky health behaviors. They are also less likely to experience serious psychological distress. Prevalence of physical inactivity in leisure time, current cigarette smoking, and heavier drinking of alcohol are also lower for married couples (Schoenborn, 2004). However, middle-aged married men have the highest rate of overweight or obesity.

Table 16.1 Marital Status of the U.S. Adult Population

Marital Status	Percent of Adult Population
Married	52.8
Widowed	6.0
Divorced, separated	11.9
Never married	29.4

U.S. Census Bureau (2007). America's Families and Living Arrangements: 2006. Household Economic Statistics Division, Fertility and Family Branch. www.census.gov/population. Retrieved April 10, 2007.

Middle-aged adults are also twice as likely as younger and older adults to be divorced or separated. Nearly half of marriages in which the woman is 18 or younger divorce or separate within 10 years (Schoenborn, 2004). Rates of separation or divorce are at least twice as high for those with almost any psychiatric disorder as for those without a disorder. The exceptions are drug abuse and cognitive impairment (Keyes, 2002; Tohen, Bromet, Murphy, & Tsuang).

Caring for Others

In 2002, 72 million children (under the age of 18) resided in the United States, up from 64 million in 1990 (see Table 16.2). These children represent 26% of the U.S. noninstitutionalized population. There are variations in ethnic groups. Over half (53%) of African American children live with a single parent. Twenty-three percent live with their mother and 4% with their single fathers (U.S. Census Bureau, 2007).

Parents working out of the home must provide for the care and safety of their children during their absence. Childcare outside the home is often disproportionately expensive compared with income and often is not available for parents working evenings, nights, holidays, or weekends, and during periods of illness and other crises. Federal support to single-parent families is limited. In the past, working parents could rely on their own parents and other family members to assist with childcare, but today, many parents have no family available locally or are also serving as caretakers to family members in addition to their children.

Informal caregivers, unpaid individuals who provide care, are the largest source of long-term care services in the United States. It is estimated that more than 50 million people provide care for a chronically ill, disabled, or aged family member or friend during any given year. Although men are increasingly becoming more involved in caregiving, women comprise the majority and perform the more difficult tasks of caregiving. The average caregiver is age 46, female, married, working outside the home, and earning an annual income of $35,000 (Family Caregiver Alliance, 2006). Duration of caregiving spans from less than a year to more than 40 years, with an average time of 4 to 5 years (National Alliance for Caregiving and AARP, 2004; Donelan et al., 2002).

Caregivers are under considerable stress and often neglect their physical and mental health needs. Caregivers also report higher levels of loneliness, anxiety, depressive symptoms, and other mental health problems than noncaregiving peers. In turn, altered physical and mental health reduces the quality, satisfaction, and ability to cope with daily stresses related to caregiving (Beeson, 2003; De Frias, Tuokko, & Rosenberg, 2005).

Table 16.2 Living Arrangements of U.S. Children

Arrangements	Percent of U.S. Children
Living with two parents	67.4
Living with mother	23
Living with father	4
Households with neither parent	4

U.S. Census Bureau (2007). America's Families and Living Arrangements: 2006. Housing and Household Economic Statistics Division. Fertility and Family Branch. www.census.gov/population. Retrieved April 10, 2007.

MENTAL DISORDERS IN YOUNG AND MIDDLE-AGED ADULTS

The great majority of people experience their first symptoms of mental illness when they are adolescents or early in the young adult stage. By far, the highest rates of mental disorder occur among young adults. Late-life onset of mental disorder (over age 40) is relatively rare, with the exception of cognitive impairment, which typically occurs past the age of 70. Recent research suggests that 46% of people will experience a mental disorder in their lifetime and that the average age of onset for anxiety and impulse control disorders is 11 years and substance use disorders is 20 years. Mood disorders are an exception to this early trend, with onset occurring at the average age of 30 (Hasin, Goodwin, Stinson, & Grant, 2005; Kessler, Berglund, Demler, Jin, Merikangas, & Walters, 2005).

Changes in the biological, psychological, and social domains can create the matrix of stress that may foster mental disorder. The vast majority of people with mental disorders do not come to the attention of the mental health system. In fact, less than half of those who are afflicted with a mental disorder receive any kind of treatment from mental health professionals (Wang, Lane, Olfson, Pincus, Wells, & Kessler, 2005).

RISK FACTORS OF YOUNG AND MIDDLE-AGED ADULTS

Mental health promotion and illness prevention is driven by cultivating awareness of personal risk factors for mental illness and modifying those that can be changed. Specific **risk factors**, or characteristics that increase the likelihood of developing a disorder, can contribute to poor mental health and influence the development of a mental disorder. Risk factors do not cause the disorder or problem, and are not symptoms of the illness, but are factors that influence the likelihood that the symptoms will appear. The existence of a risk factor does not always mean the person will get the disorder or disease; it just increases the chances. There are many different kinds of risk factors, including genetic, biologic, environmental, cultural, and occupational. Even gender is a risk factor for some disorders (e.g., more women experience depression than men; see Chapter 2). In general, gender, age, unemployment, and lower education are risk factors associated with mental illness.

Biological Risk Factors

The biological functioning of young versus middle-aged adults is a contrast between optimally running physiological systems and those showing definite signs of wear and inefficiency. Of course, there are wide variations in the health of the various systems within each stage, with some young adults more physiologically and functionally compromised than their middle-aged counterparts. Most physical and mental systems have completed development by the time an individual reaches young adulthood. In general, the optimal health state of young adults begins to show changes around the age of 30. The perception of these physical changes often makes individuals aware of their aging process and may result in threats to bodily integrity and self-esteem.

Skin

The most obvious change in physical appearance starts with the skin. While the young adult's skin is smooth and taut, by late young adulthood, the skin begins to lose moisture and tone and wrinkles develop. Self-esteem issues can erupt as the skin ages, especially for women.

Cardiovascular and Respiratory Systems

Maximum cardiac output is reached between 20 and 30 years of age. Thereafter, blood pressure and cholesterol levels gradually increase. Although men are especially prone to cardiovascular disease in middle age due to testosterone levels, women are not exempt from risk of heart disease. In a parallel manner, respiratory function also decreases with age. After the age of 30, maximum breathing capacity slowly decreases and may be reduced up to 75% compared with young adulthood. Such changes are compounded if the individual smoked throughout adulthood. Alterations in cardiac and respiratory efficiency may result in limited energy for daily tasks and preference for lower activity levels, which makes exercise less of an enjoyable activity.

Sensory Function

Sensory functions are also compromised as the individual moves from young adulthood into middle age. While the visual sense is at its peak in early young adulthood, the lenses of the eyes gradually lose their elasticity around age 30 and corrective lenses may be necessary. Such changes may result in issues regarding physical appearance that may affect self-esteem. While hearing is optimal in young adulthood, middle age brings changes in the bones of the inner ear and auditory nerve, which result in the gradual inability to hear high-pitched tones and detect certain consonants. Such alterations in hearing may also present issues related to body integrity.

Neurological System

In middle age, brain structural changes are minimal. Although neurons are gradually being lost, changes in cognition are not evident. There may be some slowing of speed of reflexes due to small changes in nerve conduction speed during middle age.

Basal Metabolic Rate

Basal metabolic rate is at maximum functional capacity at age 30 and then gradually decreases at a rate of 2% per decade, related to a gradual loss in highly physiologically active muscle mass. The ratio of fat tissue to lean body mass gradually increases, which may result in weight gain if calories are not restricted. There is currently an epidemic of obesity within the Unites States due to poor nutrition and low activity levels. Weight gain also raises concerns about physical attractiveness, especially in women. It is also related to decreased cardiac and respiratory efficiency, which makes exercise less of a preferred activity.

Sexual and Reproductive Functioning

Concerns about changing physical appearance may also be tied to reactions to changes in sexual functioning. In middle-aged men, testosterone production decreases, resulting in lower sex drive, more time needed to achieve erection, and production of fewer sperm cells. Men whose sense of self was dependent on the level of sexual functioning typical of young adulthood may experience anxiety over such changes. Diminishing estrogen levels in middle-aged women results in the cessation of menses and capacity for pregnancy. The beginning of menopause may bring unpleasant symptoms such as hot flashes, night sweats, fatigue, and nausea. However, most women experience menopause as a relief from menses, fluctuating hormone levels, and the possibility of pregnancy. Women whose view of self was based on sexual characteristics may also be prone to anxiety due to these changes.

Psychosocial Risk Factors

Any of the psychosocial problems of adulthood previously discussed such as unemployment, changing family structure, and caregiving may serve as risks factors for mental disorders. These more general problems reveal underlying risk factors that have been shown to be common in the development of mental disorders. Also, risk factors rarely occur in isolation but tend to cluster because one may bring about another and they influence each other.

Age

The majority of mental disorders occur among young adults and appear to be less common with increasing age. The first symptoms may occur in childhood but are usually evident in late adolescence and early middle adulthood. Such symptoms may be partially tied to the increasing demands for independence and social responsibility that Western society places on developing individuals. As adults get older, they may experience decreasing stress because they have learned to cope more efficiently (Hasin, Goodwin, Stinson, & Grant, 2005; Kessler, Berglund, Demler, Jin, Merikangas, & Walters, 2005).

Marital Status

Individuals who are married experience higher rates of both physical and mental health compared with those who are single, separated, or divorced. Marriage may serve as a general marker for psychological health and the ability to connect with larger social networks. Those remaining unmarried may be more isolated and do not enjoy the supportive effects of contact with the larger social system (Berkman & Glass, 2000; Schoenborn, 2004).

Unemployment

In this consumer-oriented society, economic stability is a major value. Unemployment is a larger indicator of such socioeconomically related variables such as poverty, lack of education, and the ability to obtain economic power within the larger social system. This creates an environment of stress that may contribute to the development of a mental disorder or may indicate the negative effect that a mental disorder has had on obtaining the education and independence necessary for obtaining job security and advancement (Outram, Mishra, & Schofield, 2004; Tohen, Bromet, Murphy, & Tsuang, 2000).

Job Stresses

Employment has its own set of stresses. Many in low-paying jobs work two jobs, often literally going from one job to another. Changes in hours or expectations in one job can impact the ability to work the second job, which is often needed to meet financial obligations. Shift work causes changes in circadian rhythms and sleep patterns leading to increase in stress (Lee, Smith, & Eastman, 2006; see Box 16.1). Interpersonal problems with coworkers can lead to emotional distress.

> **BOX 16.1**
>
> ***Research for Best Practice:* Physical and Mental Health of Middle-Aged Nurses**
>
> *Letvack, S. (2005). Health and safety of older nurses. Nursing Outlook, 53, 66–72.*
>
> **The Question:** What is the relationship between job characteristics and the physical and mental health of working nurses over the age of 50?
>
> **Methods:** 308 employed registered nurses (RNs) over the age of 50 from the Southeastern United States completed a survey regarding demographic variables, job attributes, physical and mental health, and job-related injuries and health disorders during the past 5 years.
>
> **Findings:** The average age of the respondents was 57 years. The majority were married and worked full-time. About half worked in a hospital and two-thirds worked the day shift. About 88% reported that they were highly or generally satisfied with their jobs.
>
> The number of years respondents worked as an RN was associated with better mental health.
>
> Those nurses reporting higher job satisfaction, higher control over their practice, and lower job demands experienced increased levels of physical health.
>
> About 23% of nurses reported a job-related injury within the past 5 years.
>
> Nurses with higher job demands and those in hospital settings were more likely to experience an injury.
>
> About 36% of nurses indicated physical and mental health problems attributable to their jobs.
>
> **Implications for Nursing:** Retention of experienced RNs is important because the current recruitment rate of new RNs will not solve the nursing shortage problem. Middle-aged RNs also have developed the expertise needed to ensure quality care. Job redesign and improvements in the work environment are necessary to prevent related illnesses and injuries that may prompt nurses to leave the workforce. Recent legislation enforcing minimum staffing levels and limiting mandatory overtime may also result in improved work environments.

Gender

Women come to the attention of the mental health system because of their greater awareness of health issues and willingness to seek health care. However, women also differ in the types of mental disorders that they show. Women are more prone to anxiety and depression, whereas men tend to show problems with impulse control that result in problems such as alcohol and drug abuse (Outram, Mishra, & Schofield, 2004; Tohen, Bromet, Murphy, & Tsuang, 2000). Women are more likely to seek help, especially in the general medical area, than men (Kessler et al., 2005c).

History of Child Abuse

Being abused as a child increases the risk of a mental disorder as an adult. In the MIDUS study (Box 16.2), data indicated that there are long-term consequences of early childhood abuse. Reported emotional abuse was associated with lower personal control, which in turn leads to lower health ratings (Irving & Ferraro, 2006).

Prior Mental Disorder

Mental illness tends to be a chronic disorder whose symptoms manifest fairly early in life. Research has shown that mental illness arising in childhood and adolescence predicts further disorder in later years. Because most mental disorders are never cured, the existence of prior symptoms or a full-blown disorder is a risk for mental illness at later periods in life. Increased stress provides the foundation for the current emergence of symptoms of mental disorders that may have appeared to be in remission (Hasin, Goodwin, Stinson, & Grant, 2005; Kessler, Berglund, Demler, Jin, Merikangas, & Walters, 2005).

Coping

Although the quality of coping is important in the reduction of stress, little is known about the continuity and changes in coping styles over the lifespan. Because past behavior is the best predictor of future behavior, it would appear that coping styles used in the past would be repeated in the present time. The quality of such coping would determine how well stress is handled in the present and sets the stage for continued positive outcomes or more problems in the future (Cohen, 2000). There is initial epidemiologic evidence that coping is a process that improves in quality as life continues (see Box 16.2).

BOX 16.2

Research for Best Practice: *The MIDUS (MIDUS) National Survey: An Overview*

Brim, O. G., Ryff, C. D., & Kessler, R. C. (2004). The MIDUS National Survey: An overview. In O. G. Brim, C. D. Ryff, & R. C. Kessler (Eds.), How healthy are we? A national study of well-being at midlife (pp. 1–34). Chicago: University of Chicago Press.

The Question: The John D. and Catherine T. MacArthur Foundation established the Research Network on Successful Midlife Development to generate new knowledge related to the challenges faced by those in the middle years. The network created and implemented a national survey of midlife Americans. The major purposes were to determine the well-being of those in the middle of their life. The goals were to develop indicators (physical, psychological, social) for assessing midlife development, establish an empirical basis of what happens in midlife, and identify factors that influence midlife development, including illness, life stresses, work, and family.

Methods: This study involved surveying over 7,000 subjects aged between 25 and 74 years to compare those at midlife (defined as 40–60 years) with those in young and older adulthood. Demographics, psychosocial factors, mental health, physical illnesses, and health-related beliefs were surveyed.

Findings: There are many findings being generated from this large data set. One set of findings suggests that coping is a process that improves in quality as life continues and is shown in increasing satisfaction with life. Initial findings of the study are that mood in mid-life is more contextually determined, influenced by work and social relationships, compared with younger and older adults. Self-reported quality of life improves with age but increases do not significantly start until middle age (around age 40), with the strongest predictors being quality of the marital relationship and finances. Only a quarter of middle-aged adults report having a midlife crisis, and the majority of middle-aged Americans report that they are healthy and in control of their lives.

Implications for Nursing: From this study, nurses can appreciate that most people in midlife are able to cope as long as they have a good quality of life, including social relationships and financial security. By assessing coping skills, nurses can identify strengths that can be supported in times of emotional turmoil and exacerbation of illnesses. Because work and social relationships are very important to this group, these areas should always be assessed.

Sad, Blue, or Depressed Days

Depression is a major public health problem that is related to disability and impaired quality of life; however, little is known about lesser symptoms of feeling sad or blue that may not meet the diagnostic criteria for a mood disorder. As part of the Behavioral Risk Factor Surveillance System, a national survey that monitors behaviors that place individuals at risk for health problems, respondents were asked how many days in the past month they experienced sad, blue, or depressed days (SBDD). Such symptoms were common, with respondents reporting a mean of 3 days in which they experienced SBDD within the past month. Women reported more SBDD than men, while young adults reported the highest number and older adults the fewest. The difference between men and women's SBDD decreased with increasing age (Kobau, Safran, Zack, Moriarty, & Chapman, 2004).

The number of reported SBDD was highly associated with problems in health maintenance. Those who reported more SBDD also engaged in more unhealthy behaviors such as smoking, binge drinking, and physical inactivity. These findings suggest the link between depressive symptoms and lack of health-promoting activities and the need for interventions that increase positive feelings, self-efficacy, and the motivation to engage in health-promoting behaviors (Kobau, Safran, Zack, Moriarty, & Chapman, 2004).

Lack of Health Promotion Behaviors

People with mental disorders in young adult and middle-age appear to lack basic health promotion behaviors. This results in high rates of physical illness and premature mortality compared with the general population. This includes low levels of awareness about physical and mental health issues, smoking, lack of exercise, lack of leisure activities and contact with friends, negative attitudes toward help-seeking, and stigma associated with mental health problems (Barry, Doherty, Hope, Sixsmith, & Kelleher, 2000; Crone, Heaney, Herbert, Morgan, Johnston, & McPherson, 2004; Grzywacz & Keyes, 2004; Outram, Mishra, & Schofield, 2004).

• NCLEXNOTE

People with mental disorders frequently neglect their physical health and have premature mortality. Assessment of physical health and health-promoting activities is important in the care of people with mental disorders due to their high rate of smoking, lack of physical activity, and resistance to seeking help for physical concerns.

Parenting Stress

Young adults often find that the addition of children to the family, and particularly the birth of the second child, tends to insulate the nuclear family from larger social networks. The responsibilities and time constraints involved in rearing small children may limit the couple's worldview to the home and definitions of self may be constricted to the activities of the nuclear family. However, as children grow and create their own lives, the social connectedness of the parents tends to expand. By middle age, the couple is anticipating the emancipation of their children and may entertain more options for socializing with other people (Alessi, 2000).

Factors Associated With Suicide

Despite a dramatic increase in treatment, no significant decrease has been found in rates of suicidal thoughts, plans, or gestures in the United States from 1990 to 2003 (Kessler, Berglund, Borges, Nock, & Wange, 2005; see Box 16.3). Few studies have examined gender differences among young adults who attempt rather than complete suicide (see Chapter 17).

BOX 16.3

***Research for Best Practice:* Trends in Suicide Ideation, Plans, Gestures, and Attempts in the United States, 1990–1992 to 2001–2003.**

Kessler, R. C., Berglund, P., Borges, G., Nock, M., & Wang, P. S. (2005). JAMA, 293, 2487–2495.

The Question: The purpose of this study was to analyze nationally representative data on suicidal ideation, plans, gestures, attempts, and their treatment.

Methods: Data from the 1990–1992 National Co-morbidity Survey and the 2001–2003 National Comorbidity Survey Replication were compared. These surveys asked identical questions to 9,708 people aged 18 to 54 years about the past year's occurrence of suicidal ideation, plans, gestures, attempts, and treatment. Self-report instruments were used.

Findings: No significant changes occurred between 1990 and 1992 and 2001 and 2003 in suicidal ideation, plans, and gestures. The risk of suicide-related behaviors is consistently elevated in several vulnerable subgroups including the young, women, individuals with low education, and individuals lacking stable relationships or employment. Treatment increased dramatically among those who made gestures and attempts, but treatment did not reduce the disparities in risk of suicide-related behaviors associated with these vulnerable subgroups.

Implications for Nursing: The meaning of these results is unclear, but nurses should be aware that suicide continues to be a problem in the United States, despite more reported treatment, especially for vulnerable populations. Nurses have an opportunity to assess the risk of suicide in all of their patients.

PROTECTIVE FACTORS

Protective factors are those characteristics that reduce the probability that a person will develop a mental health disorder or problem or decrease the severity of existing problems. There is strong evidence that some people are genetically less susceptible to mental disorders than others. Physical activity and exercise are also protective factors against symptoms of anxiety and depression (Brown, Ford, Burton, Marshall, & Dobson, 2005; Grzywacz & Keyes, 2004).

Common psychosocial protective factors are older age, education, marriage, and social support (Tohen, Bromet, Murphy, & Tsuang, 2000). Self-development, personal growth, and purposeful engagement in aging women are associated with less daily salivary cortisol, proinflammatory cytokines, cardiovascular risk, and longer duration of rapid eye movement (REM) sleep when compared with those with lower levels of these characteristics (Ryff, Singer, & Love, 2004). A person's mental health can be challenged by a variety of factors, e.g., biologic changes or illnesses, psychological pressures, and interpersonal tensions. Developing coping strategies to eliminate or reduce the impact of these potentially destructive factors is a part of normal growth and development. In addition, sustaining positive health behaviors such as relaxation, proper nutrition, adequate sleep, regular exercise, and forming a network of trusting relationships can support one's mental health. Mental health promotion focuses on increasing the individual's physical, mental, emotional, and social competencies in order to increase well-being and actualize potential.

NURSING INTERVENTIONS

Mental Health Promotion

The psychiatric–mental health nurse supports the young and middle-aged adult through the developmental journey of life. Stresses associated with balancing the psychosocial demands and the adjustment to changes in the biological, psychological, and social domains can be overwhelming. Validation and education are important interventions in helping these individuals cope with these changes (see Chapter 14).

Social Support During Life Transitions

The young and middle-aged adults are prone to many life transitions: entrance into the work force, job loss, career change, separation, divorce, the birth of children and their eventual leaving home, and changes in health status. Middle-aged adults are also subject to watching their parents age and possibly lose independence. Both young and middle-aged adults can benefit from education about coping with the stresses involved with such transitions, linking with sources of social support, and anticipating the changes in role and adjustment (Box 16.4).

BOX 16.4

Using Reflection: A Need for Coping Skills

Incident: The young woman kept repeating that she was scared and not ready for marriage. The elaborate wedding was the following week. The nurse assured her that everything would be fine and her concerns were normal. The following week, the local newspaper reported that this bride had run away the day of the wedding.

Reflection: Upon reflection, the nurse realized that the young woman had been raised by a single parent who had several short-term romantic relationships and had no exposure to a successful marriage. The young woman was clearly telling the nurse that she did not have the coping skills that are needed for marriage.

Lifestyle Support

Although health may be at its maximum during the young adult years, changes in bodily appearance and function become evident by age 30 and are more pronounced as middle age begins. While such changes are inevitable, their magnitude can be tempered by health promotion activities such as attention to regular exercise, good nutrition, adequate sleep, health screening, relaxation, leisure, and other forms of stress management. The young adult years are times of learning positive coping strategies for the stresses inherent to personal, marital, family, and occupational life. Such learning can be enhanced by a social support network consisting of people who are currently undergoing such stresses as well as older people who have the perspective and experience in handling these domains of life. These networks can be informal, such as regular contact with a circle of friends, or more formal, such as support groups sponsored by social, occupational, and religious organizations. Research has consistently shown the crucial importance of the sense of belonging and availability of social support for the maintenance of health and recovery from illness of all kinds (Berkman & Glass, 2000).

Self-Care Enhancement

The latter part of young adulthood and middle age are times when chronic illnesses such as hypertension, heart disease, and arthritis may become evident. Symptoms of mental disorders may have arisen earlier in life but require continuous care due to their chronic and episodic nature. It is important for both young and middle-aged adults to be educated about the physiological aspects of such disorders, the advances in medications used in treating them, possible side effects, the importance of medication adherence, lifestyle changes that can be instituted to control such disorders, and the possible use of complementary healing methods (e.g., massage, meditation). Such strategies require a good relationship with a health care provider as well as initiative from individuals to contribute to their own care through seeking and evaluating information available from the press, on the Internet, or from advocacy groups.

Prevention of Depression and Suicide

Although suicide is highest among older adults and adolescents, it still poses a major mental health issue for young and middle-aged adults. Symptoms of most psychiatric disorders have made their appearance by the time an individual enters young adulthood. In particular, mood disorders may first arise during the young adult years and continue through middle age and older adulthood. Because depression is a significant precipitating factor for suicide, early detection and intervention is critical for managing mood disorders and preventing suicide; see Chapter 16.

Reducing the Stigma of Mental Health Treatment

Mental disorders are common within the community, and the rate of treatment has risen over the past 20 years; however, over half of people do not receive mental health treatment of any kind. Part of this lack of attention is certainly due to the lack of available treatment in many communities (such as rural areas), but another major factor is the stigma that continues to be associated with mental illness and seeking help for mental health problems. Organizations such as the National Alliance for the Mentally Ill (NAMI) have spearheaded the movement toward viewing mental disorders as biologically based and devoid of moral implications, putting them on par with physical disorders. NAMI is an important organization for obtaining information, support, and referrals for treatment for individuals with mental disorders as well as their families.

The periods of adult development known as young adulthood and middle age can be some of the most productive in life. They can also be the most stressful and debilitating due to the rapid rate of social change that society is currently experiencing. The division of adulthood into young and middle-aged stages and the interest in adult development have paved the way for examining the challenges unique to these stages in which individuals spend the majority of their lives. More needs to be known about the stresses of these stages, the ways that individuals cope, the changes that bring about increased life satisfaction, and the ways in which nurses can support adaptation and ensure health promotion. Such health-promoting interventions may serve as the foundation for future mental health.

SUMMARY OF KEY POINTS

- Western families have achieved unprecedented economic stability that provides for long periods of development. The periods of young and middle adulthood do not exist in less developed countries; a brief childhood progresses quickly into old age.
- Western society has recently shown greater tolerance for the timing of life events such as education, marriage, and childrearing.
- Unemployment is a growing common problem in adulthood, particularly for single mothers and African Americans.
- The periods of youth and middle-age are characterized by changes in family structure due to leaving home, marriage, and divorce.
- Caregiving for both children and older parents is a problem faced by both young and middle-aged adults.
- Mental disorders are most common in young adults, with the first symptoms evident in late adolescence and young adulthood (with the exception of depression and cognitive impairment).
- As individuals progress from young to middle-aged adulthood, they experience changes from optimally running physiological systems to those showing wear and inefficiency.
- Important psychosocial risk factors for mental disorder include unemployment, poverty, lack of education, prior mental disorder, depressive symptoms, and stresses related to parenting. Despite changes in the physiological functioning, young and middle-aged adults often lack health-promoting behaviors, especially if they have mental disorders.
- Suicide remains a problem in young and middle adulthood and requires early detection and treatment.
- Social support and stress management are important in helping people to cope with the stresses involved in life transitions.
- Less than half of individuals receive treatment for their mental health problems and stigma remains toward mental health problems.

CRITICAL THINKING CHALLENGES

1 What are your assumptions about the psychosocial tasks that should be accomplished by an individual in American society who is young versus middle-aged? Describe the challenges that each age group faces in terms of education, marriage, career, children, financial stability, and health, and the expected outcomes for each of these challenges. Then compare your answers to another person's. In which areas do you agree and disagree? Why does the perception of the tasks of young and middle adulthood differ from person to person?

2 Describe the modifiable risk factors for mental disorders for young and middle-aged adults and suggest mental health promotion activities that can be used to address these risk factors.

***The Family Stone.* 2005.** This is a film about the annual holiday gathering of a family in New England and the changing relationships among its members. Diane Keaton and Craig T. Nelson play a middle-aged mother and father whose children are at various stages of young adulthood. The movie illustrates the two sides of young adult and midlife in issues such as leaving home, establishing marriages, becoming parents and grandparents, the potential empty nest, and the stress brought about by the disclosure of the serious illness of the mother.

VIEWING POINTS: Identify the life transitions faced by each of the family members in the film. How does each member cope with the stresses they are experiencing? How did the mother's illness and death change the dynamics in this family?

REFERENCES

Alessi, G. (2000). The family and parenting in the 21st century. *Adolescent Medicine, 11*(1), 35–49.

Barry, M. M., Doherty, A., Hope, A, Sixsmith, H., & Kelleher, C. C. (2000). A community needs assessment for rural mental health promotion. *Health Education Research, 15*, 293–304.

Beeson, R. A. (2003). Loneliness and depression in spousal caregivers of those with Alzheimer's disease versus non-caregiving spouses. *Archives of Psychiatric Nursing, 17*, 135–143.

Berkman, L. F., & Glass, T. (2000). Social integration, social networks, social support, and health. In I. Kawachi & L. F. Berkman (Eds.), *Social Epidemiology* (pp. 137–173). New York: Oxford.

Brim, O. G., Ryff, C. D., & Kessler, R. C. (2004). The MIDUS National Survey: An overview. In O. G. Brim, C. D. Ryff, & R. C. Kessler (Eds.), *How healthy are we? A national study of well-being at midlife* (pp. 1–34). Chicago: University of Chicago Press.

Brown, W. J., Ford, J. H., Burton, N. W., Marshall, A. L., & Dobson, A. J. (2005). Prospective study of physical activity and depressive symptoms in middle-aged women. *American Journal of Preventive Medicine, 29*, 265–272.

Cohen, J. I. (2000). Stress and mental health: A biobehavioral perspective. *Issues in Mental Health Nursing, 21*, 185–202.

Crone, D., Heaney, L., Herbert, R., Morgan, J., Johnston, L., & Macpherson, R. (2004). *Journal of Mental Health Promotion, 3*(4), 19–25.

DiCaro, V. (2005). NFI Releases report on national marriage survey. *Fatherhood Today, 10*(3), 4–5.

De Frias C. M,. Tuokko H., & Rosenberg, T. (2005). Caregiver physical and mental health predicts reactions to caregiving. *Aging & Mental Health, 9*, 331–336.

Donelan, K., Hill, C. A., Hoffman, C., Scoles, K., Feldman, P. H., Levine, C., & Gould, D. (2002). Challenged to care: Informal caregivers in a changing health system. *Health Affairs, 21*, 222–231.

Economic Policy Institute. (2005). Economic snapshots. www.epinet.org. Retrieved January 6, 2006, from http://www.ers.usda.gov/publications/aer826/aer826.pdf

Family Caregiver Alliance (2006). Selected caregiver statistics. Family Caregiver Alliance. Retrieved January 6, 2006 , from www.caregiver.org/caregiver/jsp/content_node.jsp:nodeid=439.

Grzywacz, J. G., & Keyes, C. L. M. (2004). Toward health promotion: Physical and social behaviors in complete health. *American Journal of Health Behavior, 28*, 99–111.

Hasin, D. S., Goodwin, R. D., Stinson, F. S., & Grant, B. F. (2005). Epidemiology of major depressive disorder. *Archives of General Psychiatry, 62*, 1097–1106.

Irving, S. M., & Ferraro, K. F. (2006). Reports of abusive experiences during childhood and adult health ratings: personal control as a pathway? *Journal of Aging & Health, 18*(3), 458–485.

Kessler, R. C., Berglund, P., Borges, G., Nock, M., & Wang, P. S. (2005a). Trends in suicide ideation, plans, gestures, and attempts in the Unitead States, 1990–1992 to 2001–2003. *JAMA, 293*, 2487–2495.

Kessler, R. C., Berglund, P., Demler, O., Jin, R., Merikangas, K. R., & Walters, E. E. (2005b). Lifetime onset and age-of-onset distributions for DSM-IV disorders in the National Comorbidity Survey Replication. *Archives of General Psychiatry, 62*, 593–602.

Kessler, R. C., Demler, O, Frank, R. G., Olfson, M., Pincus, H. A., Walters, E.E., et al. (2005c). Prevalence and treatment of mental disorders, 1990–2003. *The New England Journal of Medicine, 352*(24), 2515–2523.

Keyes, C. L. (2002). The mental health continuum: From languishing to flourishing in life. *Journal of Health and Social Behavior, 43*, 207–222.

Kobau, R., Safran, M. A., Zack, M. M., Moriarty, D. G., & Chapman, D. (2004). Sad, blue, or depressed days, health behaviors and health-related quality of life, Behavioral Risk Factor Surveillance System, 1995–2000. *Health and Quality of Life Outcomes, 2*, 40–53.

Lee, C., Smith, M. R., Eastman, C. I. (2006). A compromise phase position for permanent night shift workers: circadian phase after two night shifts with scheduled sleep and light/dark exposure. *Chronobiology International, 23*(4), 859 *Health and Quality of Life Outcomes* 875. National Alliance for Caregiving and AARP. (2004), *Caregiving in the U.S.* Bethesda: National Alliance for Caregiving, Washington, DC: AARP.

Outram, S., Mishra, G. D., & Schofield, M. J. (2004). Sociodemographic and health related factors associated with poor mental health in midlife Australian women. *Women and Health, 39*, 97–115.

Ryff, C. D., Singer, B. H., & Dienberg Love, G. (2004), Positive health: connecting well-being with biology. Philosophical transactions of the Royal Society of London. Series B: Biological Sciences, *359*(1449), 1383–1394.

Schoenborn, C. A. (2004). Marital status and health: United States, 1999–2002. *Advance Data from Vital and Health Statistics.* U.S. Department of Health and Human Services, Centers for Disease Control and Prevention, National Center for Health Statistics, No 351.

Sherman, A., Fremstad, S., & Parrott, S. (2004). Employment rates for single mothers fell substantially during recent period of labor market weakness. Center on Budget and Policy Priorities. Retrieved January 6, 2006, from http://www.cbpp.org/6-22-04ui.htm

Tohen, M., Bromet, E., Murphy, J. M., & Tsuang, M. T. (2000). Psychiatric epidemiology. *Harvard Review of Psychiatry, 8*, 111–125.

U.S. Cemsus Bureau (2007). America's Families and Living Arrangements: 2006. Housing and Household Economic Statistics Division, Fertility and Family Branch. www.census.gov/population.

Wang, P. S., Lane, M., Olfson, M., Pincus, H. A., Wells, K.B., & Kessler, R. C. (2005). Twelve-month use of mental health services in the United States. *Archives of General Psychiatry, 62*, 629–640.

CHAPTER 17

Suicide: A Major Mental Health Problem

Emily J. Hauenstein and Mary Ann Boyd

LEARNING OBJECTIVES

After studying this chapter, you will be able to:

- Identify suicide as a major mental health problem in the United States.
- Define suicide, suicidality, suicide attempt, parasuicide, and suicidal ideation.
- Describe population groups that have high rates of suicide.
- Describe risk factors associated with suicide completion.
- Describe the nursing management of short- and long-term promotion of recovery in suicidal patients.

KEY CONCEPTS

- suicide
- hopelessness
- lethality

KEY TERMS

• case finding • commitment to treatment statement • no-suicide contract • suicidality • parasuicide • suicide attempt • suicide contagion • suicidal ideation

Suicide is highly stigmatized in contemporary society, even more so than mental illness. The fear of being stigmatized prevents individuals with strong suicidal thoughts from seeking treatment. Speaking about or attempting suicide makes a mental illness obvious to others, especially if the person requires medical intervention or psychiatric hospitalization. The subsequent visibility of the mental disorder discredits the person, leaving him or her open to stigmatization (Joachim & Acorn, 2000). Reports and portrayals of suicide in the popular press and television contribute to the stigmatization of those who consider or attempt suicide (Coverdale, Naim, & Claasen, 2002). Society's unwillingness to talk openly about suicide also contributes to the common misperception that firearms are used more often to commit murder than suicide. There are many other myths regarding suicide (see Box 17.1).

Nurses can do much to demystify suicide and destigmatize those at risk through individual and public education. Because those at risk frequently seek help in health care settings prior to their attempt, nurses are in a unique position to prevent suicides. All practicing nurses will come into contact with patients who are thinking about suicide. It is critical that nurses are comfortable with assessing patients for suicide and implementing preventive interventions.

This chapter contains tools that nurses can use to reduce the broad effects of suicide and provide appropriate care for suicidal patients.

SUICIDE AND ITS CONCEPTS

Suicide is not a new phenomenon, but today it is one of the major mental health problems in the United States. Not easily understood, suicide is preventable. Most suicidal individuals want to live. They are just unable to see alternatives to their problems. People commit suicide when they and those in the patient's environment do not recognize the signs or fail to initiate treatment of the

BOX 17.1

Myths and Facts about Suicide

Myth: People who talk about suicide do not complete suicide.
Fact: Many people who die by suicide have given definite warnings of their intentions. Always take any comment about suicide seriously.
Myth: Suicide happens without warning.
Fact: Most suicidal people give many clues and warning signs regarding their suicidal intention.
Myth: Suicidal people are fully intent on dying.
Fact: Most suicidal people are undecided about living or dying. A part of them wants to live; however, death seems like the only way out of their pain or situation. They may allow themselves to "gamble" with death, leaving it up to others to save them.
Myth: Males are more likely to be suicidal.
Fact: Males complete suicide more often than females. However, females attempt suicide three times more often than men. Females tend to choose less lethal methods than males.
Myth: Improvement following a suicide crisis means that the risk is over.
Fact: Most suicides occur within 3 months of "improvement" when the individual has the energy and motivation to actually follow through with his or her suicidal thoughts.

Adapted from the Baton Rouge Crisis Intervention Center web site (www.brcic.org).

underlying depression. There are approximately 30,000 suicides each year in the United States, and 650,000 people per year are seen in the emergency rooms after attempting suicide (Goldsmith, Pellmar, Kleinman, & Bunney, 2002; Minino, Arias, Kochanek, Murphy, & Smith, 2002).

KEY CONCEPT Suicide is defined as the voluntary act of killing oneself. It is a fatal, self-inflicted destructive act with explicit or inferred intent to die. It is sometimes called suicide completion. This behavioral definition of suicide is limited and does not consider the complexity of the underlying depressive illness, personal motivations, and situational and family factors that provoke the suicide act.

Except for the very young, suicide occurs in all age groups, social classes, and cultures (see Figure 17.1). More than 90% of suicides in the United States are associated with mental illness or alcohol and substance abuse. About 56% of people complete suicide in their first attempt, and about 25% of people hospitalized for a failed suicide attempt kill themselves within 3 months after discharge (Isometsa & Lonnqvist, 1998).

The term **suicidality** refers to all suicide-related behaviors and thoughts of completing or attempting suicide and suicide ideation. **Suicidal ideation** is thinking about and planning one's own death. It also includes excessive or unreasoned worrying about losing a significant other. Suicidal ideation occurs in approximately 14% of people during their lifetimes (Kessler, Borges, & Walters, 1999). Of those who experience suicidal ideation, 34% form a plan; 72% of those who form a plan attempt suicide (Kessler et al., 1999).

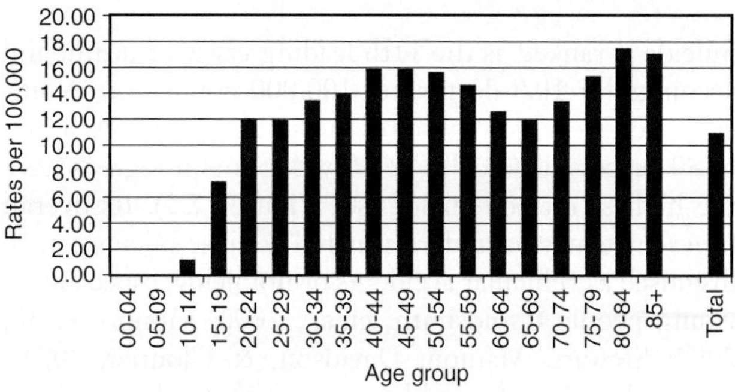

FIGURE 17.1. Suicide rates for all ages. Reporting on Suicide: Recommendations for the Media. February 22, 2006. Retrieved September 3, 2006, from www.suicidology.com.

A **suicide attempt** is a nonfatal, self-inflicted destructive act with explicit or implicit intent to die. The person believes that the choice of method will result in death (Goldsmith, Pellmar, Kleinman, Bunney, 2002). No official data are compiled about suicide attempts in the United States. Still, it is estimated that 734,000 suicide attempts are made annually, and that more than 5 million living Americans (5%) have attempted suicide at some point in their life (Minino Arias, Kochanek, Murphy, & Smith, 2002). Women make three attempts to every male attempt. As many as 20% of men and 40% of women attempt suicide and fail in the year preceding a completed suicide (Isometsa & Lonnqvist, 1998). Most completed suicides occur during the first year after hospitalization for a failed suicide attempt. Adolescents make more attempts than do adults, but they generally are less successful. One of the best predictors for suicide is a previous attempt (Nemeroff, Compton, & Berger, 2001).

Parasuicide is a voluntary, apparent attempt at suicide, commonly called a suicidal gesture, in which the aim is not death (e.g., taking a sublethal drug). Parasuicidal behavior varies by intent. Some people truly wish to die, but others simply wish to feel nothing for awhile. Still others want to send a message about their emotional state. Parasuicide behavior is never normal and should always be taken seriously. Parasuicide occurs frequently in younger age groups but declines after the age of 44 years.

KEY CONCEPT Lethality refers to the probability that a person will successfully complete suicide. Lethality is determined by the seriousness of the person's intent and the likelihood that the planned method of death will succeed. A plan to use an accessible firearm to commit suicide has greater lethality than a suicide plan that involves superficial cuts of the wrist.

EPIDEMIOLOGY OF SUICIDE

Suicide is ranked as the 11th leading cause of death, and accounts for 10.8 deaths per 100,000 population. A suicide occurs every 17 minutes in the United States: a rate of 80 successful suicides per day. Mountain regions have the highest rate of suicide (see Figure 17.2). Its overall prevalence may be underestimated because suicide can be disguised as vehicular accidents or homicide, especially in young people (Goldsmith, et al., 2002; Minino, et al., 2002; Stewart, Manion, Davidson, & Cloutier, 2001). The public health problem of suicidal behavior is so important that several goals stated in Healthy People 2010 directly target the reduction of deaths by suicide (United States Department of Health and Human Services [U.S. DHHS], 2000) (see Chapter 2).

Risk Factors Associated with Suicide

Mental illness, especially depressive disorder, is the primary factor contributing to suicide in adults. Most young adults who commit suicide also have a depressive disorder, and many have personality disorders (Brieger, Ehrt, Bloeink, & Marneros, 2002). Recent purchase of a handgun increases the risk of self-harm. Substance abuse increases the likelihood that suicidal ideation will result in parasuicide. Adolescents who have panic attacks are particularly at risk for suicide (Kishi, Robinson, & Kosier, 2001; Vilhjalmsson, Kristjansdottir, & Sveinbjarnardottir, 1998; Pilowsky, Wu, & Anthony, 1999; (see Box 17.2).

BOX 17.2

Factors Enhancing Suicide Risk

Vulnerability
Primary family member who has completed suicide
Psychiatric disorder
Previous attempt by the patient
Loss (e.g., death of significant other, divorce, job loss)
Unrelenting physical illness

Risk
White man
Elderly man
Adolescent male
Gay, lesbian, or bisexual orientation
Access to firearm

Intent
Suicide plan and means of executing it
Inability to enter into a no-suicide contract

Disinhibition
Impulsivity
Isolation
Psychotic thoughts
Drug or alcohol use

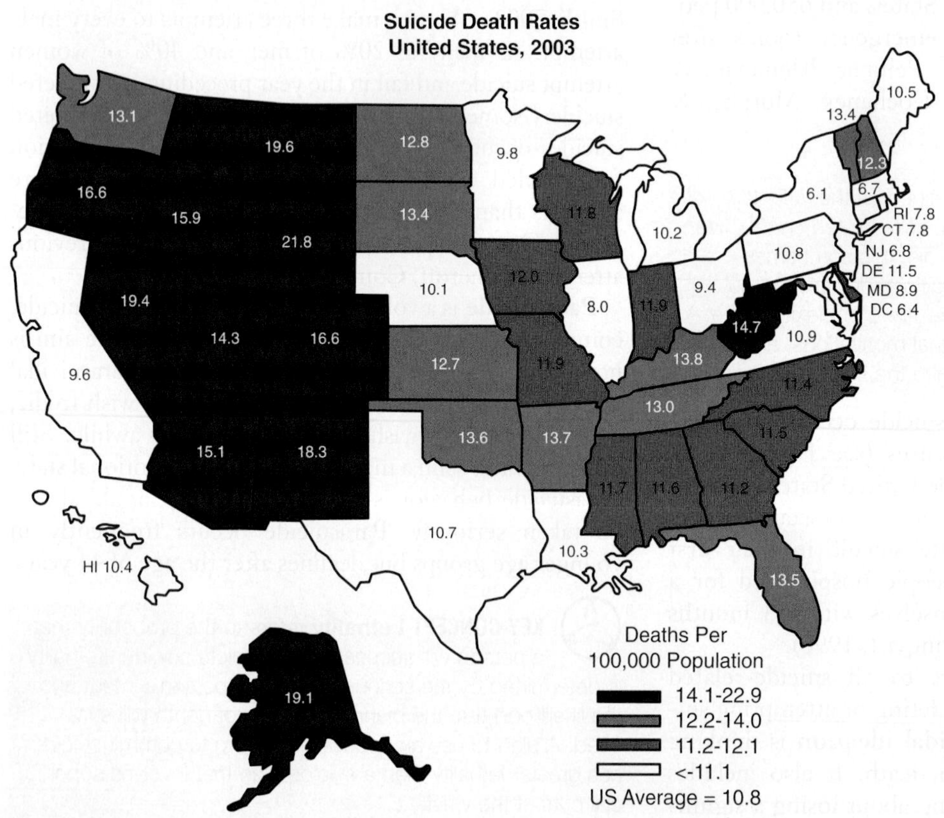

FIGURE 17.2. Suicide death rates in the United States, 2003. Retrieved on September 3, 2006 from www.thebethfoundation.com (National Center for Health Statistics).

Medical illnesses are also risk factors for suicide and likely contribute to the increased rate of suicide in people over the age of 65 (Erlangsen, Vach, & Jeune; 2005; Heisel, 2006). Medical illness increases the likelihood of chronic depression and, hence, long term-suicide risk (Gilmer, Trivedi, Rush, et al., 2005). Additionally, symptoms of comorbid illnesses often are similar to that of depressive disorder, making recognition of depressive disorder difficult. For example, in the month before an elderly person commits suicide, 75% will have consulted their primary care physician (Hendin, 1999).

Psychological Risk Factors

Internal distress, low self-esteem, and interpersonal distress have long been associated with suicide. Cognitive risk factors include problem-solving deficits and hopelessness (D'Zurilla, Chang, Nottingham, & Faccini, 1998). Childhood physical and sexual abuse has been linked to suicide, suicide ideation, and parasuicide (Molnar, Berkman, & Buka, 2001). Among children reporting neglect or physical or sexual abuse, 51% attempt suicide (Lipschitz et al., 1999).

In contrast to those who carefully prepare to take their own lives are those who decide impulsively to end their lives. Impulsivity and disinhibition increase the risk of suicide. An impulsive act during a moment of depression can lead to deadly consequences. Poor judgment and lowered inhibitions because of psychosis or substances (drugs and alcohol) are temporary. Patients with psychoses who act impulsively to "voices" that direct them to kill themselves are at considerable risk because of their inability to separate their psychotic thinking from reality. Keeping a person alive is possible if others are around to protect the patient.

Social Risk Factors

Many victims of suicide are socially isolated. They generally cannot name anyone in their immediate environment with whom they can stay while they are acutely suicidal. They often wish to be alone or are unwilling to ask anyone for help. Patients at high risk for suicide may not subscribe to the rules and mores of any social group. Frequently, they can enter into a no-suicide agreement, but the lack of supportive people in their environment may indicate that they cannot safely remain in the community.

Social isolation, financial hardship, legal stress, family difficulties, and poor social support contribute to the risk of suicide (Vilhjalmsson et al., 1998). Other risk factors include family discord, neglect, physical abuse, adolescent unemployment, residential transience, chronic behavior problems, and recent interpersonal stress. Economic deprivation and unemployment have been shown to precipitate suicide in men, but unemployed women are also at serious risk for suicide (Hawton, Harriss, Hodder, Simkin, & Gunnell, 2001).

Gender

Males have a higher suicide completion rate than females. For men, suicide is the eighth leading cause of death, with a rate of 17.5 per 100,000, more than four times the rate in women (Minino et al., 2002). Caucasian men complete 73% of all suicides; 80% of these deaths are by firearms. Men are more likely to use means that have a higher rate of success, such as firearms and hanging (Denning, Conwell, King, & Cox, 2000). Recent data show that rural men have a much higher risk of suicide than urban men, and that gap is widening, perhaps attributable to the higher rates of gun ownership in rural areas (Singh & Siahpush, 2002).

Substance abuse, aggression, hopelessness, emotion-focused coping, social isolation, and having little purpose in life have been associated with suicidal behavior in men (Edwards & Holden, 2001; Alexander, 2001). Unmarried, unsociable men between the ages of 42 and 77 years with minimal social networks and no close relatives have a significantly increased risk for committing suicide (Eng, Rimm, Fitzmaurice, & Kawachi, 2002). For women, current or previous exposure to violence, sexual assault, or both increases women's risk for suicide (Koplin & Agathen, 2002; Nelson et al., 2002) and having a small child reduces it (Qin, Agerbo, Westergård-Nielson, Eriksson, & Mortenson, 2000).

Homosexual men who attempt suicide are more likely to have experienced harassment because of their sexual orientation. Other risk factors include early disclosure of their sexual orientation and early onset of homosexual activity (Paul et al., 2002).

Race and Ethnicity

In all racial groups, men commit suicide at much higher rates than do women. However, there is considerable variation in the profile of suicide rates across racial groups, including the age when rates are at their peak and the duration of high rates across several age groups. For example, Caucasian males have high rates from the age of 15 years onward, but the peak suicide rate is among those older than 75 years. Recent data show exceptional suicide risk in young recently widowed Caucasian men between the ages of 20 and 34 years: the suicide risk was 17 times that of married men in that same age group; the risk was nine times greater for African American men (Luoma & Pearson, 2002). There also are significant differences in rates among those of Spanish heritage. Mexican Americans have a very low suicide rate, whereas that of Cuban Americans is two times higher (Oquendo et al., 2001).

The reasons for racial and ethnic variations are not clear. The rates of depressive disorder, a major risk factor for suicide, vary across racial groups; however, a recent study using nationally representative databases concluded that suicide rates do not vary with depression rates (Oquendo et al., 2001). These findings suggest that differences in suicide rates may be related to social and cultural risk factors for suicide within racial groups (Gutierrez, Rodriguez, & Garcia, 2001).

For Caucasian males, social isolation and access to firearms play important roles in suicide risk (Eng et al., 2002; Miller, Azrael, & Hemenway, 2002b). Although the overall suicide rate for African Americans is low, young African American men take their lives at a rate considerably above that of other age groups. Family cohesion and social support in African American families contribute to the low rates in this group (Harris & Molock, 2000). High rates of suicide in young men may be attributable to alienation from family and access to firearms (King et al., 2001; Miller, Azrael, & Hemenway, 2002a; "Suicide among black youths," 1998). Although the suicide risk is high among older Hispanic women and men, little appears in the literature about possible risk factors. More is written about Native Americans, whose suicide rates are the highest in the nation. Exposure to suicide and access to firearms contributed to suicide rates for Native Americans, whereas family support and cultural and tribal orientation were protective (Borowsky, Resnick, Ireland, & Blum, 1999; Garroutte, Goldberg, Beals, Herrell, & Manson, 2003; Wissow, Walkup, Barlow, Reid, & Kane, 2001).

Suicide in Special Populations

Children and Adolescents

Suicide is rare among children who are younger than 10 years of age. Among children 10 to 14 years of age, suicide is the third leading cause of death in the United States, accounting for 7.2% of all deaths in this age group (Anderson, 2002). Boys commit 79% of suicides in this age group; 82% of these boys are Caucasian. Suicide is the second leading cause of death among Native American boys 10 to 14 years of age, accounting for 15.2% of deaths in this age group.

Adolescents and young adults are successful in completing suicide once for every 100 to 200 attempts (Minino et al., 2002). More teenagers die of suicide than of cancer, heart disease, birth defects, stroke, pneumonia, influenza, and chronic lung disease combined. Suicide is the third leading cause of death among people 15 to 19 years old, accounting for 12% of all deaths (Anderson, 2002). As in the younger age group, boys are more likely to commit suicide than are girls; 83% of all suicides in this age group were boys.

For Caucasian males 15 to 19 years of age, suicide is the second leading cause of death, accounting for 70% of all deaths in this group. Although still the third leading cause of death among African American youth, suicide is less common than for Caucasians. Suicide accounts for only 6.3% of African American deaths; 87% of these are boys. Suicide is the second leading cause of death among Native American boys in this age range; 28.4 boys per 100,000 died of suicide in the year 2000. Suicide attempts are most common among Hispanics/Latinos (2.8%) and teenage girls (3.3%) of all ethnic groups.

Adults

Suicide is the third leading cause of death for individuals 20 to 24 years old, accounting for 13.4% of deaths in this age group (Anderson, 2002). Suicide is the second leading cause of death for those in the 25- to 34-year age group. Young adults are more likely to commit suicide than are middle-aged adults. By age 55 to 64 years, suicide is the ninth leading cause of death. Suicidal behavior is often associated with substance abuse, especially among men. For men, substance abuse may be the primary psychiatric disorder and depression a side effect of it. For women, depression commonly is the primary psychiatric disorder, and substance abuse results from attempts to medicate the underlying depressive condition.

Elderly

Suicide rates are high in the elderly population. Although people older than 65 years comprised only 13% of the U.S. population in 2000, 18% of all suicides are in this age group. Nationally, the rate of suicide attempts to completion is about 25:1; among the elderly the rate is 4:1. The elderly generally have a stronger intent to die, plan their suicide more carefully, and are more likely to use lethal means of killing themselves than are younger persons (Conwell & Duberstein, 2001). In one study, only 2.6% of elderly suicides had a previous attempt (Bennet & Collins, 2001). Their often frail health contributes to the rate of successful suicides in the elderly. Because many elderly live alone, the chance of thwarting a suicide often is less than among younger people. Although highly stigmatized in other age groups, suicide often is viewed as more acceptable for the elderly.

Among the highest rates are suicide deaths for Caucasian men older than 85 years, who in 2000 had a rate of 59 suicides per 100,000 people. These men are more likely to be single, live in rural areas, and use a gun to commit suicide (Dresang, 2001). As in other age groups, depressive disorder is a significant contributor to suicide deaths. Physical illness and financial difficulties also are important precipitants to suicide in the elderly (Conwell & Duberstein, 2001; Kishi et al., 2001). For elderly men and women, suicide is associated with less education, widowhood, previous attempts, depressive disorder, and substance abuse (Conwell & Duberstein, 2001; Conwell et al., 2000).

ETIOLOGY OF SUICIDAL BEHAVIOR

Although suicidal behavior occurs in a variety of situations and with various means, it is usually triggered by stressors that are unmanageable and exceed typical coping efforts. The convergence of biological, psychological, and social factors can be directly linked to suicidal behavior (see Fig. 17.3). Depressive disorder, with its physiological, psychological, and social antecedents, appears to be a powerful predictor of suicide. Firearms are the most common method of suicide (AAS, 2006).

Biologic Theories

Most people who attempt or complete suicide have severe depression, either alone or in conjunction with another major acute psychiatric disturbance. Severe depression tends to develop when a person is subjected to repeated or sustained stress, which changes neurotransmitter and hormonal functioning (see Chapter 14). These neurochemical changes directly contribute to suicidal behavior. Those who complete suicide have extremely low levels of the neurotransmitter serotonin, or 5-hydroxytryptamine (5-HT). The cerebrospinal fluid of people who exhibit suicidal behavior contains extremely low levels of the 5-HT metabolite 5-hydroxyindoleacetic acid (5-HIAA) (Samuelsson, Jokinen, Nordström, & Nordström, 2006). Recent evidence also shows that people who make near-lethal suicide attempts have much lower levels of the neurotransmitter dopamine (Pitchot et al., 2001). Low levels of omega-3 proportions of a lipid profile are also associated with suicidal behavior in depressed people (Sublette, Hibbeln, Galfalvy, Oquendo, & Mann, 2006). Two other important vulnerabilities for suicidal behavior are genetics and the experience of severe childhood trauma.

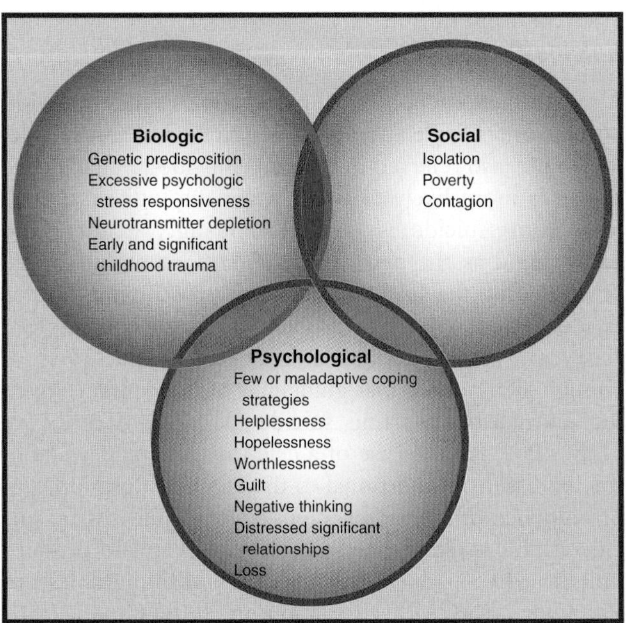

FIGURE 17.3. Biopsychosocial etiologies of suicide.

Genetic Factors

Considerable evidence exists showing that suicide runs in families (McGuffin, Marusic, & Farmer, 2001; Qin, Agerbo, & Mortenson, 2003). First-degree relatives of individuals who have completed suicide have two to eight times higher risk for suicide than do individuals in the general population (McGuffin, Marusic, & Farmer, 2001). Suicide of a first-degree relative is highly predictive of a medically serious suicide attempt in another first-degree relative (Modai et al., 1999). This risk is slightly heightened in females (Qin et al.). The children of depressed mothers with a history of suicide attempts have higher rates of suicidal behavior (Klimes-Dougan et al., 1999). The genetic link to suicide is evident in studies of twins. Qin and colleagues (2003) showed that suicidal behavior in one monozygotic twin increased the risk 11-fold for suicidal behavior in the co-twin.

Physiological Effects of Child Abuse

Child abuse has been described as a specific vulnerability for psychopathology and suicide. Enhanced vulnerability to depressive disorder and suicide associated with child abuse apparently are attributable to changes in the hypothalamic–pituitary–adrenal axis caused by intractable stress and altered serotonin and dopamine metabolism (Skodol, Siever, & Livesley, 2002). Evidence from twin studies suggests that the link between childhood sexual abuse and biological alterations contributing to psychopathology may be independent of other environmental influences. Several studies show that adult psychopathology is greater in abused twins when compared with nonabused co-twins (Bulik, Prescott, & Kendler, 2001; Kendler et al., 2000; Nelson et al., 2002).

Psychological Theories

The negativity, pessimism, and feelings of hopelessness, helplessness, and worthlessness associated with depression lead to suicide ideation, planning, and acts (King et al., 2001; Sourander, Helstelä, Haavisto, & Bergroth, 2001; Weinberger, Sreenivasan, Sathyavagiswaran, & Markowitz, 2001; Brådvik & Berglund, 2000; Brown,

Beck, Steer, & Grisham, 2000; Nemeroff et al., 2001; see Chapter 20). Emotional factors associated with suicide are low self-esteem, guilt, and shame. Loss and grief are also important considerations (see Chapter 14).

Hopelessness has long been shown to play an important role in mediating suicidal behavior (Beck, Schuyler, Herman, 1974).

KEY CONCEPT Hopelessness is a state of despair characterized by feelings of inadequacy, isolation, and inability to act on one's own behalf. It is connected with the belief that one's situation is unlikely to improve.

Depressed persons who are hopeless are more likely to consider suicide than those who are depressed, but hopeful about the future. Furthermore, it appears that lack of positive thoughts about the future is more likely to predict suicidal behavior than negative thoughts, even though both contribute to hopelessness (MacLeod, Tata, Tyrer, Schmidt, Davidson, & Thompson, 2005).

Theoretical Explanations

Most psychological theories presented throughout this text have explanations for suicide. Freud argued that suicide is hostility turned against self (1917). Adler viewed suicide as an interpersonal act of hurting others by hurting self (1958). Jungian analysts think that suicide represents a desire for rebirth (Wahl, 1957). Cognitive-behaviorists emphasize the interaction of the cognitive, affective, behavioral, and emotional schemas (Rudd, Joiner, & Rajab, 2004). The dialectical cognitive-behavioralists argue that suicidal behaviors are learned maladaptive efforts to cope with low distress tolerance and limited coping resources (see Chapter 22).

Reaction to Surviving Suicide

A well-known risk factor for suicide completion is a previous suicide attempt. Now we are beginning to understand that the survivors' reactions to surviving a suicide may be a predictor of future suicides. In one study, 393 suicide attempters were evaluated according to their reaction to surviving a suicide attempt. They were followed for 5 to 10 years. Those who wished they had died after a suicide attempt were 2.5 times more likely to commit suicide than those who were glad they survived or were ambivalent about the attempt (Henriques, Wenzel, Brown, & Beck, 2005).

Social Theories

Many contend that suicide is an outcome of the individual's social context. Socioeconomic status (SES) is recognized as important because it affects the physical structures that surround an individual and the social structures that are available to him or her (Cohen, Mason, & Bedimo, 2003).

Poverty

Poverty represented by substandard housing affects other important neighborhood social structures, such as schools, voluntary organizations, and jobs. Poverty also reduces exposure to opportunities for individual advancement. Health outcomes are directly affected by environmental hazards or indirectly through inadequate access to health care.

Substantial data exist that implicates poverty and its consequences as contributing to suicide. The percentage of boarded-up buildings in a neighborhood was positively associated with suicide (Cohen, Mason, & Bedimo, 2003). Socioeconomic deprivation and unemployment were found to be associated with suicide in several studies (Cubbin, LeClere, & Smith, 2000; Goodman, 1999; Hawton et al., 2001; Kposowa, 2001; Steenland, Halperin, Hu, & Walker, 2003). Using nationally representative data, Cubbin and colleagues found a strong relationship between unemployment and suicide; risk increased twofold in the unemployed when compared with employed, white-collar workers. Steenland and colleagues, in a study of 261,723 deaths, found enhanced risk for suicide in all but the highest income level. Men in the lowest income level had more than twice the risk of men with the most income; the same association was weaker for women. The relationship between income and suicidal behavior also was seen for adolescents (Goodman, 1999). Social policy also can affect suicide rates; Zimmerman (2002) found a strong association between diminished state spending for welfare and suicide.

Suicide Contagion

A social phenomenon seen among adolescents is **suicide contagion:** suicide attempts that imitate a recent suicide. These are also referred to as cluster suicides. Suicide contagion is more likely to occur when the individual contemplating suicide is of the same age, gender, and background as the person who died. Contagion can be prompted by the suicide of a friend, an acquaintance, or an idolized celebrity. The problem of suicide contagion or "copycat suicide" following a celebrity's suicide is of enough significance that guidelines have been developed for journalists reporting suicide (Moskos, Achilles, & Gray, 2004). In the case of a celebrity, the magnitude of the increase is proportional to the amount, duration, and prominence of media coverage. Celebrity deaths by suicide are more likely than noncelebrity deaths to produce imitation (American Academy of Child and Adolescent Psychiatry [AACAP] Official Action, 2001; Gould, 2001; Poijula, Wahlberg, & Dyregrov, 2001; Stack, 2003).

INTERDISCIPLINARY TREATMENT

Prevention of suicide and promotion of mental health involves the whole health team. Suicide behavior is related to a variety of different underlying problems such as depression, substance abuse, stress, and grieving. A solid support network of health care professionals, family and friends, and community resources (suicide hotlines) is needed for the individual who is at high risk for suicide.

Emergency! Priority Care 

Acutely suicidal behavior is a true psychiatric emergency. Immediate action is needed to prevent the patient's death. By considering the patient's balance of stressors and resources, the nurse can determine whether the patient has sufficient resources to manage his or her suicidal impulses. The first priority is to provide for the patient's safety while initiating the *least* restrictive care possible. In contrast, an example of the *most* restrictive care would be an outpatient who is admitted to a locked unit with one staff member who is assigned to observe the person at all times. This type of care should be reserved for those whose safety cannot be otherwise ensured.

Ensuring Safety

During the early part of a hospitalization, the most important way to reduce stress is to help the patient feel more secure and hopeful. Nurses can do so by ensuring the patient's safety with as little intrusion as possible on the person's exercise of free will. Achieving this goal can be difficult because the major deterrent to patients committing suicide in psychiatric hospitals is their continual observation by nurses. Hospital policy will dictate the specific procedures to follow. In a national study of all suicides reported during a 2-year period, the rate of suicide while hospitalized was 16% (Appleby et al., 1999). Each hospital has its own specific protocol for maintaining patients' safety.

Maintaining a safe environment includes observing the patient regularly for suicidal behavior, removing dangerous objects, and providing outlets for expression of the patient's feelings. Part of ensuring patient safety is helping patients to re-establish personal control by including them in decisions about their care and restricting their behavior only as necessary. In this vein, the nurse must reassure patients, inquire how they are feeling, and ask what they have been doing to manage their feelings and keep safe since the last observation period.

Patients often feel shaky in the first hours of psychiatric hospitalization, and it is comforting to know that a caring person is nearby. Observational periods can be used to help the patient express a broad range of feelings and strengthen their belief in their own abilities to keep themselves safe. The nurse can help the patient who is not skilled in self-expression or self-management skills to describe feelings more effectively and cite ways of managing safety needs. Then, at the next observation time, the nurse may have the opportunity to reinforce the patient's own safety behavior. Thus, the observation period can be transformed from something negative ("The patient can't be trusted," "I am out of control") to something positive ("The patient is becoming safer," "Maybe I can keep myself safe after all") (Cardell & Pitula, 1999). As the patient becomes more confident in being able to control his or her behavior, the frequency of observation periods can be reduced.

FAMILY RESPONSE TO SUICIDE 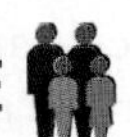

One suicide is estimated to leave six survivors, which means 4.4 million Americans are estimated to be survivors (Minino et al., 2002). Suicide has devastating effects on everyone it touches, especially family and close friends. Undue and prolonged suffering can be caused by the sudden shock, the unanswered questions of "why," and potentially the discovery of the body (Knieper, 1999). Suicide bereavement is different than that experienced by families whose loved one's death is not self-inflicted. The grieving over the way the death occurred, the social processes affecting the survivor, and the effect of the suicide on the family converge to establish a grieving process that is unique (Jordan, 2001). One study showed that it takes 3 to 4 years after a child's suicide for parents to put the death in perspective, but often these parents do so more quickly than parents of children lost to homicide or accident (Murphy, Johnson, Wu, Fan, & Lohan, 2003).

Coping abilities do mediate grief responses. Although recovery from a loved one's suicide is an ongoing task, survivors who are emotionally healthy before the suicide act and who have social support are able to manage the psychological trauma associated with suicide (Mitchell, Gale, Garand, & Wesner, 2003).

NURSING MANAGEMENT: PREVENTION OF SUICIDE AND PROMOTION OF MENTAL HEALTH

Suicidal behaviors are seriously underreported and often unrecognized by health care professionals. Estimates are that approximately 40% of people who commit suicide have visited a health care provider within 1 to 6 months of a suicide attempt (Link, Phelan, Bresnahan, Stueve, & Pescosolido, 1999). In one study of 76 patients who committed suicide, almost 80% met the criteria for severe anxiety or agitation during the week prior to the suicide (Busch, Fawcett, & Jacobs, 2003). Nurses can play important roles in suicide prevention because they practice in diverse health care settings and thus work with many different kinds of patients. Further, the proximity of nurses to patients relative to other professionals often allows them to identify changes in patient behavior that may signal suicidal intent.

Case Finding

Case finding refers to identifying people who are at risk for suicide to initiate proper treatment. Identification of depression and risk factors associated with suicide are essential nursing roles that should be incorporated into routine health care of patients. This is true for nurses practicing in primary care settings as well as for those who care for patients in mental health specialty settings.

The nurse first identifies people who are experiencing extreme stress, anxiety, agitation, have little social support, or have insufficient coping skills to manage the stressors that are affecting them. The nurse asks the patient about emotional symptoms, specifically suicidal thoughts. Many nurses are concerned that asking patients about their suicidal thoughts will provoke a suicide attempt. This belief simply is not true. The suicidal patient usually has been considering suicide for some time and will often be relieved that someone understands the seriousness of their situation. When a nurse identifies a person at risk for suicide, he or she should conduct an individual assessment (see Box 17.3 for the warning signs developed by the American Association of Suicidology [2006]; the mnemonic, IS PATH WARM, can serve as a useful memory aide for these signs).

BOX 17.3

Warning Signs

I Ideation	Expressed or communicated ideation Threatening to harm or kill self, or talking of wanting to hurt or kill self Looking for ways to kill self: seeking access to firearms, available pills, or other means Talking or writing about death, dying or suicide
S Substance Abuse	Increased substance (alcohol or drug) use
P Purposelessness	No reason for living; no sense of purpose in life
A Anxiety	Anxiety, agitation, unable to sleep or sleeping all the time
T Trapped	Feeling trapped (like there is no way out)
H Hopelessness	Hopelessness
W Withdrawal	Withdrawal from friends, family and society
A Anger	Rage, uncontrolled anger, seeking revenge
R Recklessness	Acting reckless or engaging in risky activities, seemingly without thinking
M Mood Change	Dramatic mood changes

These warning signs were derived at a consensus meeting held under the auspices of the American Association of Suicidology, November, 2003.

Individual Suicide Risk Assessment

The goals of a suicide risk assessment are identification of suicide ideation, elicitation of a plan, determination of the severity of intent, and evaluation of availability of means. Specific assessment questions are found in Chapter 10 and discussion of their relationship to depression in Chapter 20. For adolescents, a key question is whether any family member has attempted or completed suicide (Cerel, Fristad, Weller, & Weller, 1999; Klimes-Dougan et al., 1999). Under no circumstances should the nurse promise a patient secrecy about suicidal thoughts, plans, or acts. To protect the patient, any suicidal thoughts should be communicated to other team members. Box 17.4 lists some questions that the nurse might ask in assessing the risk for suicide. However, the denial of suicidal ideation is insufficient evidence to determine the absence of suicide risk. This is evident in the results of one retrospective study of 76 suicides that occurred during inpatient hospitalization or immediately after discharge (Busch, Fawcett, & Jacobs, 2003). These investigators reported that 78% of the patients had denied suicidal ideation before completing the act (see Box 17.5).

The nurse should assess all related events (a death of a loved one; major financial crisis) and behaviors (giving things away) when determining suicide risk. Behaviors that should raise suspicion about potential suicidal behavior include giving possessions away, getting legal affairs in order, and any apparently normal act that says "good-bye" to family and friends.

Alcoholism is another prominent factor in suicide. Patients with alcoholism accounted for 25% of completed suicides in one study (Berglund & Ojehagen, 1998). The destabilizing effects of alcohol and other drugs increases suicidal risk sufficiently that recent use of these substances should be included as a routine component of suicide assessment.

There are many different means of suicide ranging from overdoses of illegal or legal substances to using firearms to purposeful fatal accidents. Circumstances

BOX 17.4

Assessment of Suicidal Episode

Intent to Die
1. Have you been thinking about hurting or killing yourself?
2. How seriously do you want to die?
3. Have you attempted suicide before?
4. Are there people or things in your life who might keep you from killing yourself?

Severity of Ideation
1. How often do you have these thoughts?
2. How long do they last?
3. How much do the thoughts distress you?
4. Can you dismiss them or do they tend to return?
5. Are they increasing in intensity and frequency?

Degree of Planning
1. Have you made any plans to kill yourself? If yes, what are they?
2. Do you have access to the materials (e.g., gun, poison, pills) that you plan to use to kill yourself?
3. How likely is it that you could actually carry out the plan?
4. Have you done anything to put the plan into action?
5. Could you stop yourself from killing yourself?

also vary from an isolated attempt to seeking assistance with suicide for ending a terminal illness. In the assessment, the nurse makes a judgment about the lethality of the method. Guns, hanging, jumping off tall structures are more lethal than a slight overdose of minimally toxic medications (e.g., NSAIDs). No matter how slight the gesture, however, all suicidal plans and acts should be taken seriously.

• NCLEXNOTE

Suicide assessment is always considered a priority. Practice by asking patients about suicidal thoughts and plans. Develop a plan with a suicidal patient that focuses on resisting the suicidal impulse. Apply the assessment process that delineates the (1) intent to die, (2) severity of ideation, (3) availability of means, and (4) degree of planning.

BOX 17.5

Using Reflection: An Inpatient Suicide Attempt

Incident: An inpatient attempted to hang himself in the shower during the change of shift report. This patient had denied any suicidal thoughts or intentions 20 minutes earlier.

Reflection: Upon reflection, the nurse realized that the patient knew the hospital routine and could attempt suicide at the change of shift, the time when most of the nursing staff were busy. In retrospect, she identified several behaviors (feeling better, giving personal items away) that indicated suicidal intentions even though there was verbal denial.

What makes some patients more likely to kill themselves than others? A successful suicide requires intent, a plan, knowledge of how to carry out the act, and few obstacles to completing it. Patients who successfully complete suicide have developed a workable method of killing themselves. They are less likely to have young children or other immediate responsibilities and may not be concerned with religious prohibitions on the act. The relationship between the availability of a method of suicide and suicide completion is strong (Cantor & Baume, 1998). Any patient without specific social or other inhibitions should be considered at higher risk for suicide; patients who are psychotic or who have rapidly cycling bipolar illness, for example, may be especially likely to attempt suicide.

To determine how serious a patient is about dying, the nurse must ask about what thought the patient has put into the decision and why the patient views suicide as a solution. The nurse needs to determine whether the patient has considered other solutions to his or her difficulties, whether the patient has a specific plan for committing suicide, and the patient's means of completing the suicide. People who have developed a plan and the means to carry it out and who have executed some parts of the plan are serious about their intent to kill themselves. Inquiring about suicidal ideation and access to firearms has the potential to reduce successful suicides substantially (see Box 17.6).

Nursing Diagnoses and Outcome Identification

Several nursing diagnoses may be useful when dealing with a suicidal patient, including Risk for Suicide, Interrupted Family Processes, Anxiety, Ineffective Health Maintenance, Risk for Self-Directed Violence, Impaired Social Interaction, Ineffective Coping, Chronic Low Self-Esteem, Insomnia, Social Isolation, and Spiritual Distress.

Documentation and Reporting

The nurse must thoroughly document encounters with suicidal patients. This action is for the patient's ongoing treatment and the nurse's protection. Lawsuits for malpractice in psychiatric settings often involve completed suicides. The medical record must reflect that the nurse took every reasonable action to provide for the patient's safety.

The record should describe the patient's history, assessment, and interventions agreed upon by the patient and nurse. The nurse should document the presence or absence of suicidal thoughts, intent, plan, and available means to illustrate current and on-going suicide risk. If

BOX 17.6

Therapeutic Dialogue: Suicide

When Caroline sought medical care for a cold from her nurse practitioner, the nurse observed more than a cough and runny nose. Caroline appeared downcast and unusually sad. As the nurse and patient talked, the subject of family life came up, whereupon Caroline began to cry softly. As words tumbled out, she said that she had been unhappy at home for a long time. When she was very young, she recalled being happy, but things changed when her brother was born, 4 years after her. Her father began to abuse her sexually, starting when Caroline was 5 years old and continuing until he moved out of the house when she was 12 years old. Caroline suspects her mother knew of the abuse, although she did nothing about it.

Two years ago, Caroline's father committed suicide. Caroline feels relieved about his death but frustrated that she never got a chance to tell him how angry she was with him. Caroline's relationship with her mother has not improved. Caroline says that her mother favors her brother and is always telling her she won't amount to anything. Caroline begins to cry harder.

Ineffective Approach

Nurse: Clearly, many things are troubling you. Don't you think that things seem worse now because you have a cold?

Caroline: Well, that could be. What are you going to do to make me feel better?

Nurse: Give you some medicine to help you sleep and clear your nose. I think you should see a psychiatrist, too.

Caroline: I don't need a psychiatrist. I came here for my cold.

Nurse: I know you did, but you seem to be depressed.

Caroline: What are you, some kind of social worker? I am just tired.

Nurse: I am a nurse, and you seem down to me. Are you thinking about suicide?

Caroline: I don't think you know what you're talking about. I want to go now. Could you give me my medicine?

Effective Approach

Nurse: It seems as though many things have been piling up on you. Does it seem that way to you, too?

Caroline: It sure does. I've just been trying to get through one day at a time, but now with this cold and no sleep, I feel like I can't go on.

Nurse: When you say you can't go on, what does that mean to you?

Caroline: Lately, I have been thinking about running away to some place where I can't be found and maybe starting over. But then I think, where would I go? Where would I stay? Who would take care of me?

Nurse: When you think that your plan for escape won't work, what happens?

Caroline: (Starting to cry again.) Then I think that maybe it would be better if I just did what my father did. I really don't think anyone would miss me.

Nurse: So you think you might take your life, like your Dad did?

Caroline: Yeah, and what really scares me is lately I have been thinking about that a lot. I keep saying to myself, "You're just tired," but I am so exhausted now that I can't chase the thoughts away.

Nurse: So, do you think about suicide every day?

Caroline: It seems like I never stop thinking about it.

Nurse: Is there anything you can do to make the thoughts go away?

Caroline: Nothing. (Silence.)

Nurse: What would you do?

Caroline: I think I would get as many pills as I could find, drink a lot of alcohol, and maybe smoke some pot and just go to sleep.

Nurse: Do you have enough pills at home to kill yourself?

Caroline (wan smile): I was hoping that the sleeping medicine you would give me might do the job.

Nurse: It sounds like you need some help getting through this time in your life. Would you like some?

Caroline: I honestly don't know—I just want to sleep for a long time.

Critical Thinking Challenge

- In the first interaction, the nurse made two key blunders. What were they? What effect did they have on the patient? How did they interfere with the patient's care?
- What did Caroline do that might have contributed to the nurse's behavior in the first interaction?
- In the second interaction, the nurse did several things that ensured reporting of Caroline's suicidal ideation. What were they? What differences in attitude might differentiate the nurse in the first interaction from the nurse in the second?

the patient denies any suicidal ideation, it is important that the denial is documented. Documentation must include any use of drugs, alcohol, or prescription medications by the patient during the 6 hours before the assessment. It should include the use of antidepressants that are especially lethal (e.g., tricyclics), as well as any medication that might impair the patient's judgment (e.g., a sleep medication). Notes should reflect the level of the patient's judgment and ability to be a partner in treatment.

The notes should include the agreed-on interventions. For example, if a no-suicide contract has been instituted, the record must contain specific aspects of the contract. It should include factors influencing the decision to use the contract, including the patient's behaviors that led providers to believe that the patient could be safely cared for as an outpatient. The documentation should reflect if any medication was prescribed, the dosage, and the number of pills dispensed. The record must also contain the provider's part in the contract, including information given to the patient about how to re-enter the health care system during the term of the contract. Significant others who will care for the patient during the term of the no-suicide contract should also be mentioned.

Nursing Interventions

The routine hospitalization of patients with suicidal intent is a thing of the past. Civil law requires the patient to be hospitalized only when he or she cannot make reasoned decisions to ensure his or her safety (see Chapter 3). Safety in such cases is commonly determined by whether a patient may be a threat to self or others. If the nurse and another professional determine that the patient is acutely suicidal and at considerable risk for completing suicide, he or she must decide whether to hospitalize the patient for the patient's safety.

Until the nurse has determined a patient's safety needs and implemented a plan to ensure the patient's safety, the nurse must not leave the acutely suicidal person alone for any reason, not even briefly. As the initial suicidal crisis subsides, the nurse's responsibility changes to assisting the patient to reduce his or her responsiveness to stress and to strengthen existing supports and resources. Nurses coach patients in self-care and coping skills, symptom management, identification of depressive symptoms, and relapse prevention.

Interventions for the Biologic Domain

For patients who are suicidal, but have not yet made an attempt, interventions should focus on safety, alleviation of the immediate crisis, and referral to an appropriate clinician. For patients who have survived a suicide attempt, they often need physical care of their self-inflicted injury. Overdose, gunshot wounds, and skin wounds are common. For both groups, there will be biologic interventions for the underlying psychiatric disorder (see Unit 5).

Medication Management

The objective of medication for suicidal behavior is to raise serotonin rapidly to a level that reduces suicide risk (Nemeroff et al., 2001). To that end, third-generation and newer antidepressant medications should be used for those who are in imminent danger of harming themselves. These include fluoxetine (Prozac), sertraline (Zoloft), paroxetine (Paxil), bupropion (Wellbutrin), venlafaxine (Effexor), citalopram (Celexa), and escitalopram (Lexapro) (see Chapter 20).

Electroconvulsive Therapy

ECT may be useful for selected inpatients with intractable suicidal ideation and severe depression. ECT often eliminates suicidal behavior in people who do not respond to medication. This treatment also is useful for people who do not tolerate antidepressant medications, such as elderly people and those with comorbid medical disorders. In those cases, ECT can stabilize the patient sufficiently to permit a return to the community (see Chapter 7).

Interventions for the Psychological Domain

Assisting the patient to make behavior changes is an immediate priority. Nurses can use the brief hospitalization period to find out what may have precipitated or contributed to the suicidal crisis. A suicide threat should always be taken seriously. Often, the precipitating factors and how the patient's coping process began to break down are evident. After identifying extreme stressors experienced by the patient, the nurse and patient can help determine ways for the patient to avoid those stressors in the future or, if they cannot be avoided, to manage them more effectively.

Changing Negative Thought Patterns

The hospitalization is a good time for the nurse to evaluate the patient's ways of thinking about problems and generating solutions. Some patients, by virtue of their depressive illness or social learning, have an unusually pessimistic view of life. They often think such thoughts as, "I am no good," "Everything I do is useless," "I have no future," or "Nobody has ever liked me, and nobody ever will." The nurse can point out negative thinking and invite the patient to begin to note instances in conversation when he or she is being pessimistic. Most patients can do so and are often surprised at the extent of their negativity. Once a patient is aware of this pessimistic outlook, the nurse can suggest that the patient "play detective" and try to figure out whether the negative views are true. For example, the nurse can ask the patient who feels that he or she is "no good" to write down on a piece of paper anything that the patient did that day that can be construed as "good." The nurse can help with that process by also keeping a list of "good" things that the patient does during that day. Then, if the patient says, "I did nothing good; I am no good," the nurse can counter with, "But I saw you helping Mrs. Barnes with her lunch. Why did you help her if you are no good?" The nurse and patient can then address these logical inconsistencies in a straightforward manner (see Chapter 11).

No-Suicide Contract

The **no-suicide contract** is an agreement between the patient and nurse in which patients agree not to harm themselves and to seek help when they are in a situation where they cannot honor the commitment. The contract specifies a certain length of time, usually until the next time of contact. In the hospital the agreement may be made from shift to shift; whereas in the community, the specified time may be in hours or days, depending on the patient's ability to engage in suicide prevention efforts, but should not exceed a week. A rule of thumb is that these contracts should be somewhat shorter than the longest period of time that the patient feels they can keep themselves safe. Included in the contract is an explicit statement (written or verbal) agreeing not to harm or kill oneself (Drew, 2001; Rudd, Mandrusiak, & Joiner, 2006). To date, there has been little research to support the effectiveness of these contracts, but the majority of inpatient and outpatient clinicians working with high-risk patients use some form of a no-suicide contract. Patients who can make such contracts may be at a lower risk for suicide than those who cannot. Moreover, they have a greater chance of being cared for in the community. Patients who make no-suicide contracts sometimes break them, but the frequency has not been adequately studied.

The nurse should consider a no-suicide contract only after a thorough assessment of the patient. The nurse must consider several factors in making a no-suicide contract with a patient. The patient must be competent to enter into such a contract. Patients under the influence of drugs or alcohol or experiencing psychoses are not competent to make no-suicide contracts. Patients who have made previous suicide attempts or who are extremely isolated are not good risks for no-suicide contracts. Legal and professional scholars disagree on the ability of children and adolescents to make decisions of this gravity on their own behalf. Involving parents in the decision about the appropriate mode of environment for their suicidal child is important.

In making a no-suicide contract, the nurse must first help the patient dismantle the suicide plan. If the patient has a gun, it must be locked up in a room or cabinet to which the patient does not have access. If the patient's suicide plan involves taking medication, a family member must remove medications from the patient. If the plan involves the use of a motor vehicle, the patient must give the keys to that vehicle to someone for safekeeping. This facet of the no-suicide contract requires careful consideration because the determined patient may not disclose alternative methods. Isometsa and Lonnqvist (1998) showed that people completing suicide often have tried different methods in the past. A patient's cooperation in dismantling a suicide plan is an important indicator of his or her ability to maintain the no-suicide contract. Uncooperativeness at this stage may indicate that the patient cannot be safely cared for at home.

Patients often cannot keep contracts if they are isolated from family or friends. They are much more likely to keep their part of the contract if they have support and some assistance in making their environment safe. Thus, it is critical that patients identify someone who can stay with them or be nearby during the suicidal crisis. If they are unable or unwilling to do so, this may be sufficient reason for emergency hospital admittance.

Commitment to Treatment

An alternative to the no-suicide contract is the **Commitment to Treatment Statement** (CTS), an agreement between the patient and clinician in which the patient agrees to make a commitment to treatment (Rudd et al., 2006). CTS agreements are also sometimes referred to as advance directives. Different from the no-suicide contract, the CTS does not restrict the patient's rights regarding the option of suicide. Instead, the patient makes a commitment to live by engaging in treatment and accessing emergency service if needed. Underlying CTS is cognitive-behavioral theory with the expectation that the patient will communicate openly and honestly about all aspects of treatment including suicide. This commitment is written and signed by the patient (Rudd et al., 2006).

Removal of any firearms or permit to purchase a gun is a priority commitment. Family members should be made aware of the importance of removing firearms and any other lethal means including sedating prescriptions. It is important to note, however, that a recent study reported that less than 25% of parents of adolescents with serious suicidal intent removed guns from the household despite repeated requests from their children's mental health providers (Brent, Baugher, Brimaher, Kolko, & Bridge, 2000, cited in Moskos et al., 2004, pg. 177). It may be necessary to hospitalize adolescents under these circumstances until they can be sufficiently stabilized to return to a home with an accessible gun.

Developing a Contingency Plan

The nurse and patient must also devise ways to prevent future suicidal behavior. Patients are likely to have periods of suicidal ideation throughout treatment. They must have a plan ready to manage these thoughts when they appear. The plan may include recalling that suicidal thoughts are caused by a biochemical imbalance and will go away. The plan may also include methods of distraction from suicidal thoughts. Exercise, such as taking walks or engaging in some other pleasurable activities, should be part of the plan to help diminish the frequency and intensity of suicidal thoughts.

Psychoeducation

The objectives of patient and family education are to increase the patient's understanding of the underlying mental disorder and the biochemical origins of suicidal behavior and prevention of future suicide attempts. Through education, patients can learn to identify thoughts and behaviors that lead to suicidal ideation and action. Teaching positive coping skills for stress

BOX 17.7

Psychoeducation Checklist Suicide Prevention

When teaching the patient and family about suicide and its prevention, be sure to address the following topics:

- Importance of talking to someone
- Suicidal behavior
- Identification of stressors
- Coping mechanisms
- Positive self-talk
- Information about medications and treatments of underlying mental disorders

management is critical in suicide education and prevention (see Box 17.7 and 17.8).

Interventions for the Social Domain

Poor social skills may interfere with the patient's ability to engage others. The nurse should assess the patient's social capability early in the hospitalization and make necessary provisions for social skills training. The nurse must gently make the patient aware of any behaviors that may interfere with interpersonal relationships including family and friends and suggest alternative behaviors.

Developing Support Networks

In many cases, although patients can identify family and friends who are willing to help, they are usually concerned about burdening these people or do not feel comfortable sharing their concerns with others. Helping the suicidal patient express these concerns and arrive at ways of reducing them is important. While hospitalized, the patient may be able to convey to the significant other how much he or she needs the other person's help and how difficult it is to ask for it. If patients can make that step, they and their significant others can develop a plan for managing those times when patients feel most isolated. Different friends and family members can use the plan at various times so that no one person is asked to assume too much of the patient's social care. In addition to engaging family and friends in the patient's ongoing care, finding sources of help in the community, such as church groups, clubhouses, drop-in centers, or other social groups, is a necessary task. A patient's inability to name any significant others or social groups or entertain plans to engage socially often means a poor outpatient course.

Stigma Reduction

A final concern may be the patient's embarrassment about the hospitalization and his or her emotional state. Through education, the nurse can do much to destigmatize the situation for both the patient and significant others. Before discharge, the patient should be able to name people who can act as a support. The nurse should encourage the patient to invite supportive friends and family to visit the patient. When visitors are present, with the patient's permission, the nurse can work with them to begin to develop a network for the patient to rely on to remain safe. They also should have a plan to contact another person, either a confidante or a mental health care provider, when they have distressing thoughts or feel unable to control their behavior.

BOX 17.8

Educational Resources for Suicidal Patients

Aarons, L. (1996). *Prayers for Bobby: A mother's coming to terms with the suicide of her gay son.* San Francisco: Harper.

Biebel, D. B. & Foster, S. L. (2005). *Finding your way after the suicide of someone you love.* Grand Rapids, MI: Zondervan Publishing Company.

Blauner, S. R., & Siegel, B. S. (2002). *How I stayed alive when my brain was trying to kill me: One person's guide to suicide prevention.* New York: Harper Collins Publishers.

Cobain, B., & Verdick, E. (Eds.). (1998). *When nothing matters anymore: A survival guide for depressed teens.* Free Spirit Publishing.

Cox, D., & Arrington, R. N. (2003). *Aftershock: help, hope, and healing in the wake of suicide.* Nashville: Broadman & Holman Publishers.

Fine, C. (1999). *No time to say goodbye: Surviving the suicide of a loved one.* New York: Doubleday.

Hays, H. (2005). *Surviving suicide: Help to heal your heart.* Dallas: Brown Books Publishing Group.

Jamison, K. R. (1999). *Night falls fast: Understanding suicide.* New York: Knopf.

Joiner, T. (2005). *Why people die by suicide.* Cambridge: Harvard University Press.

Miller, S. S. (2000). *An empty chair: Living in the wake of a sibling's suicide.* Lincoln, Nebraska: IUniverse, Inc.

Rubel, B. (2000). *But I didn't say goodbye: For parents and professionals helping child suicide survivors.* Kendall Park, NJ: Griefwork Center, Inc.

Thompson, T. (1995). *The beast: A reckoning with depression.* New York: Putnam.

Evaluation and Treatment Outcomes

Evidence has shown that many suicidal patients persist in their attempts to commit suicide, and that 25% are successful within 3 months of discharge from hospitalization for a suicide attempt (Appleby et al., 1999; Isometsa & Lonnqvist, 1998).

The most desirable treatment outcome is the patient's return to the community with no future suicide attempts.

Short-term outcomes include maintaining the patient's safety, averting suicide, and mobilizing the patient's resources. Whether the patient is hospitalized or cared for in the community, his or her emotional distress must be reduced. Long-term outcomes must focus on maintaining the patient in psychiatric treatment, enabling the patient and family to identify and manage suicidal crises effectively, and widening the patient's support network.

Continuum of Care

Objectives of hospitalization are to maintain the patient's safety, reduce or eliminate the suicidal crisis, decrease the level of suicidal ideation, initiate treatment for the underlying disorder, evaluate for substance abuse, and reduce the patient's level of social isolation. At the time of discharge, the patient is still considered very ill. Most suicides occur during the first week after discharge, and many happen within the first 24 hours (Appleby et al., 1999). Before the patient's release, a specific, concrete plan for outpatient care must be in place. The care plan includes scheduling an appointment for outpatient treatment, providing for continuing medication until the first outpatient treatment visit, ensuring postrelease contact between the patient and significant other, providing for access to emergency psychiatric care, and arranging the patient's environment so that it provides both structure and safety.

At discharge, the patient should have enough medication on hand to last until the first outpatient provider visit. At that time, the community provider can assess the patient's level of stability and determine whether a full prescription can be given safely to the patient. At that visit, the patient and community provider can establish a plan of care that specifies the intensity of outpatient care. Very unstable patients may need frequent supervision (e.g., telephone and/or face-to-face meetings) in the early days after hospitalization to maintain their safety in the community. These contacts often can be short; their purpose is to convey the ongoing concern and caring of professionals involved in the patient's care. In arranging outpatient care, the nurse must be certain to refer the patient to a community provider who can provide the intensity of care the patient may need.

The patient's outpatient environment should be made as safe as possible before discharge. The nurse must share the care plan with family members so that they can remove any objects in the patient's environment that could be of assistance in committing suicide. The nurse must explain this measure to the patient to reinforce his or her sense of self-control. It is important to be reasonable in deciding what to remove from the environment. Patients who are truly determined to kill themselves after discharge will succeed in doing so, using whatever means are available.

NURSES' SELF-EVALUATION

Caring for suicidal patients is highly stressful and often leads to secondary trauma, which is the nurse's emotional reaction to certain circumstances of patients or to the repeated stress of coping with suicidal crises. Few other situations in nursing exist in which misinterpreting data that are often subjective can contribute to a preventable death. The nurse who experiences secondary trauma may begin to have symptoms that reflect the early stage of posttraumatic stress disorder (PTSD) (see Chapter 39). These symptoms include fatigue, dysphoria, tearfulness without provocation, sleep disturbances or nightmares, preoccupation with the stressful situation or morbid thoughts, inability to be distracted from the stressor, anxiety, and cynicism. The nurse may begin to avoid the stress through absenteeism. These symptoms signal that a nurse's mental health is at risk. All nurses are vulnerable to this syndrome. Their vulnerability to secondary trauma increases when nurses manage crises similar to those in their own present or past. Caring for suicidal patients who are close to their own age or having a history of being abused or neglected in childhood enhances the risks. The suicidal behavior of a patient with whom the nurse can particularly identify can be especially upsetting.

To care successfully for suicidal patients or others prone to crises, the nurse must engage in an active program of self-care. Such a program begins with proper rest, exercise, and nutrition so that the nurse can better manage stress physiologically. Self-monitoring of symptoms is the next step. Nurses should be alert to fatigue, crying spells, and other symptoms of PTSD. Like their patients, nurses need to develop cognitive coping skills and engage in stress-reduction exercises. An important component of developing these skills is debriefing. Nurses who care for suicidal patients must regularly share their experiences and feelings with one another. Talking about how the situations or actions of patients make them feel will help alleviate symptoms of stress. Some nurses find outpatient therapy helpful because it enhances their understanding of what situations are most likely to trigger secondary trauma. By demonstrating how to manage effectively the stressors in their own lives, nurses can be powerful role models for their patients.

SUMMARY OF KEY POINTS

- Suicide is a common and major public health problem.
- Suicide completion is more common in Caucasian men, especially elderly men.

- Rising rates of adolescent suicide correspond with the increasing availability of firearms and alcohol.
- Parasuicide is more common among women than men.
- People who attempt suicide and fail are likely to try again without treatment.
- Suicidal behavior has genetic and biologic origins.
  - A suicide assessment focuses on the intention to die, severity of ideation, available means, and degree of planning.
- Patients who are in crisis, depressed, or use substances are at risk for suicide.
- The no-suicide contract and commitment to treatment statement are means of increasing the suicidal patient's safety in the community.
- The major objectives of brief hospital care are to maintain the patient's safety, re-establish the patient's biologic equilibrium, strengthen the patient's cognitive coping skills, and develop an outpatient support system.
- The nurse who cares for suicidal patients is vulnerable to secondary trauma and must take steps to maintain personal mental health.

CRITICAL THINKING CHALLENGES

1. A religious African American woman who lives with her three children, husband, and mother comes to her primary care provider. She is tearful and very depressed. What factors should be investigated to determine her risk for suicide and need for hospitalization?
2. A poor woman with no insurance is hospitalized after her third suicide attempt. Antidepressant medication is prescribed. What issues must be considered in providing medication for this woman?
3. A young man enters his workplace inebriated and carrying a gun. He does not threaten anyone but says that he must end it all. Assuming that he can be disarmed, what civil rights must be considered in taking further action in managing his suicidal risk?
4. You are a nurse in a large outpatient primary care setting responsible for an impoverished population. You want to implement a case-finding program for suicide prevention. Discuss how you would proceed and some potential problems you might face.

Night Mother: 1986. Sissy Spacek stars as Jessie Cates, who has decided to end her desperately unhappy life by shooting herself with her father's gun. While putting her house in order, she tries to explain her decision to her mother Thelma, played by Anne Bancroft. Thelma tries to talk Jessie out of suicide.

VIEWING POINTS: What factors have contributed to Jessie's decision to end her life? What approach would you have taken to help Jessie?

Daughter of a Suicide: 1996 (Documentary). This personal documentary is the story of a woman whose mother committed suicide when the daughter was 18 years old. The daughter recounts the emotional struggle and depression left as the lifelong legacy of suicide and explores her efforts to heal. Combining digital video, 16-mm, and super-8 film, *Daughter of a Suicide* uses interviews with family and friends to tell the story of both mother and daughter.

VIEWING POINTS: How does this movie show that the effects of suicide do not end with a person's death?

REFERENCES

Adler, A. (1958). *What life should mean to you.* New York: Capricorn.

Alexander, J. (2001). Depressed men: An exploratory study of close relationships. *Journal of Psychiatric & Mental Health Nursing, 8*(1), 67–75.

American Academy of Child and Adolescent Psychiatry (AACAP) Official Action. (2001). Practice parameter for the assessment and treatment of children and adolescents with suicidal behavior. *Journal of the American Academy of Child and Adolescent Psychiatry, 40*(7, Suppl.), 24S–51S.

American Association of Suicidology. (2006). Understanding and helping the suicidal individual. Fact Sheet. Retrieved September 4, 2006, from www.suicidology.

Anderson, R. N. (2002). Deaths: Leading causes. *National Vital Statistics Reports, 50*(16), 1–86.

Appleby, L., Shaw, J., Amos, T., McDonnell, R., Harris, C., McKann, K., et al. (1999). Suicide within 12 months of contact with mental health services: national clinical survey. *British Medical Journal, 318*(7193), 1235–1239.

Beck, A. T., Schuyler, D., & Herman, I. (1974). Development of suicidal intent scales, in the prediction of suicide. In A. T. Beck, H. L. Resnick, D. J. Lettieri (Eds.), *The prediction of suicide* (pp. 45–56). Bowie, Maryland: Charles Press.

Bennet, A. T., & Collins, K. A. (2001). Elderly suicide: A 10 year retrospective study. *The American Journal of Forensic Medicine and Pathology, 22*(2), 169–172.

Berglund, M., & Ojehagen, A. (1998). The influence of alcohol drinking and alcohol use disorders on psychiatric disorders and suicidal behavior. *Alcoholism: Clinical & Experimental Research, 22*(Suppl. 7), 3335–3455.

Borowsky, I. W., Resnick, M. D., Ireland, M., & Blum, R. W. (1999). Suicide attempts among American Indian and Alaska native youth. *Archives of Pediatric and Adolescent Medicine, 153,* 573–580.

Brådvik, L., & Berglund, M. (2000). Treatment and suicide in severe depression: A case control study of antidepressant therapy at last contact before suicide. *The Journal of ECT, 16*(4), 399–408.

Brieger, P., Ehrt, U., Bloeink, R., & Marneros, A. (2002). Consequences of comorbid personality disorders in major depression. *Journal of Nervous and Mental Disease, 190*(5), 304–309.

Brown, G. K., Beck, A. T., Steer, R. A., & Grisham, J. R. (2000). Risk factors for suicide in psychiatric outpatients: A 20 year prospective study. *Journal of Counseling and Clinical Psychology, 68*(3), 371–377.

Bulik, C. M., Prescott, C. A., & Kendler, K. S. (2001). Features of childhood sexual abuse and the development of psychiatric and substance abuse disorders. *British Journal of Psychiatry, 179,* 444–449.

Busch, K. A., Fawcett, J., & Jacobs, D. G. (2003). Clinical correlates of inpatient suicide. *Journal of Clinical Psychiatry, 64*(1), 14–19.

Cantor, C. H., & Baume, P. J. (1998). Access to methods of suicide: What impact? *Australian & New Zealand Journal of Psychiatry, 32*(1), 8–14.

Cardell, R., & Pitula, C. R. (1999). Suicidal inpatients' perceptions of therapeutic and non-therapeutic aspects of constant observation. *Psychiatric Services, 50*(8), 1066–1070.

Cerel, J., Fristad, M. A., Weller, E. B., & Weller, R. A. (1999). Suicide-bereaved children and adolescents: A controlled longitudinal examination. *Journal of the American Academy of Child and Adolescent Psychiatry, 38*(6), 672–679.

Cohen, D. A., Mason, K., & Bedimo, T. A. (2003). Neighborhood physical conditions and health. *American Journal of Public Health, 93*(3), 467–471.

Conwell, Y., & Duberstein, P. R. (2001). Suicide in elders. *Annals of the New York Academy of Sciences, 932,* 132–150.

Conwell, Y., Lyness, J. M., Duberstein, P., et al. (2000). Completed suicide among older patients in primary care practices: A controlled study. *Journal of the American Geriatric Society, 48*(1), 23–29.

Coverdale, J., Naim, R., & Claasen, D. (2002). Depictions of mental illness in print media: A prospective study. *Australian & New Zealand Journal of Psychiatry, 36*(5), 697–700.

Cubbin, C., LeClere, F. B., & Smith, G. S. (2000). Socioeconomic status and the occurrence of fatal and non-fatal injury in the United States. *American Journal of Public Health, 90*(1), 70–77.

D'Zurilla, T. J., Chang, E. C., Nottingham, E. J., & Faccini, L. (1998). Social problem-solving deficits and hopelessness, depression, and suicidal risk in college students and psychiatric inpatients. *Journal of Clinical Psychology, 54*(8), 1091–1107.

Denning, D. G., Conwell, Y., King, D., & Cox, C. (2000). Method, choice, intent, and gender in completed suicide. *Suicide & Life Threatening Behavior, 30*(3), 282–288.

Dresang, L. T. (2001). Gun deaths in rural and urban settings: Recommendations for prevention. *The Journal of the American Board of Family Practice, 14*(2), 107–115.

Drew, B. L (2001). Self-harm behavior and no-suicide contracting in psychiatric inpatient settings. *Archives of Psychiatric Nursing 15*(3), 99–106.

Edwards, M. J., & Holden, R. R. (2001). Coping, meaning in life, and suicidal manifestations: Examining gender differences. *Journal of Clinical Psychology, 57*(12), 1517–1534.

Eng, P. M., Rimm, E. B., Fitzmaurice, G., & Kawachi, I. (2002). Social ties and change in social ties in relation to subsequent total and cause-specific mortality and coronary heart disease incidence in men. *American Journal of Epidemiology, 155*(8), 700–709.

Erlangsen, A., Vach, W. & Jeune, B. (2005). The effect of hospitalization with medical illnesses on the suicide risk in the oldest old: A population based register study. *Journal of the American Geriatric Society, 53,* 771–776.

Freud, S. (1917). Mourning and Melancholia. In Strachey, J., et al., *The Complete Works of Sigmund Freud* (vol. 14). (1957). London: Hogarth Press.

Garroutte, E. M., Goldberg, J., Beals, J., Herrell, R., & Manson, S. M. (2003). Spirituality and attempted suicide among American Indians. *Social Science & Medicine, 56,* 1571–1579.

Gilmer, W. S., Trivedi, M. H., Rush, A. J., Wisniewski, S. R., Luther, J., Howland, R. H., et al. (2005). Factors associated with chronic depressive episodes: a preliminary report from the STAR-D project. *Acta Psychiatric Scandinavica,* 112, 425–433.

Goldsmith, S. K., Pellmar, T. C., Kleinman, A. M., & Bunney, W. E. (Eds.). (2002). Reducing suicide: A national imperative. Institute of Medicine. The National Academies Press: Washington, DC.

Goodman, E. (1999). The role of socioeconomic status gradients in explaining differences in US adolescents' health. *American Journal of Public Health, 89*(10), 1522–1528.

Gould, M. S. (2001). Suicide and the media. *Annals of the New York Academy of Science, 932,* 200–224.

Gutierrez, P. M., Rodriguez, P. J., & Garcia, P. (2001). Suicide risk factors for young adults: Testing a model across ethnicities. *Death Studies, 25,* 319–340.

Harris, T. L., & Molock, S. D. (2000). Cultural orientation, family cohesion, and family support in suicide ideation and depression among African American college students. *Suicide and Life-Threatening Behavior, 30*(4), 341–353.

Hawton, K., Harriss, L., Hodder, K., Simkin, S., & Gunnell, D. (2001). The influence of economic and social environment on deliberate self-harm and suicide: An ecological and person-based study. *Psychological Medicine, 31*(5), 826–836.

Heisel, M. J. (2006). Suicide and its prevention among older adults. *Canadian Journal of Psychiatry, 51*(3), 143–154.

Hendin, H. (1999). Suicide, assisted suicide, and medical illness. *Journal of Clinical Psychiatry, 60*(Suppl. 2), 46–50.

Henriques, G., Wenzel, A., Brown, G. K., & Beck, A. T. (2005). Suicide attempters' reaction to survival as a risk factor for eventual suicide. *American Journal of Psychiatry,* 162(11), 2180–2182.

Isometsa, E. T., & Lonnqvist, J. K. (1998). Suicide attempts preceding completed suicide. *British Journal of Psychiatry, 173,* 531–535.

Joachim, G., & Acorn, S. (2000). Stigma of visible and invisible chronic conditions. *Journal of Advanced Nursing, 32*(1), 243–248.

Jordan, J. R. (2001). Is suicide bereavement different? A reassessment of the literature. *Suicide and Life Threatening Behavior, 31*(1), 91–102.

Kendler, K. S., Bulik, C. M., Silberg, J., Hettema, J. M., Myers, J., & Prescott, C. A. (2000). Childhood sexual abuse and adult psychiatric and substance use disorders: an epidemiological and cotwin control analysis. *Archives of General Psychiatry, 57,* 953–959.

Kessler, R. C., Borges, G., & Walters, E. (1999). Prevalence of and risk factors for lifetime suicide attempts in the National Comorbidity Survey. *Archives of General Psychiatry, 56*(7), 617–626.

King, R. A., Schwab-Stone, M., Flisher, A. J., Greenwald, S., Kramer, P. A., Goodman, S. H., et al. (2001). Psychosocial and risk correlates of youth suicide attempts and suicidal ideation. *Journal of American Child and Adolescent Psychiatry, 40*(7), 837–846.

Kishi, Y., Robinson, R. B., & Kosier, J. (2001). Suicidal ideation among patients during the rehabilitation period after life threatening physical illness. *Journal of Nervous and Mental Disease, 189*(9), 623–628.

Klimes-Dougan, B., Free, K., Rounsaville, D., et al. (1999). Suicidal ideation and attempts: A longitudinal investigation of children of depressed and well mothers. *Journal of American Academy of Child & Adolescent Psychiatry, 38*(6), 651–659.

Knieper, A. J. (1999). The suicide survivor's grief and recovery. *Suicide and Life Threatening Behavior, 29*(4), 353–364.

Koplin, B., & Agathen, J. (2002). Suicidality in children and adolescents: A review. *Current Opinion in Pediatrics, 14,* 713–717.

Kposowa, A. J. (2001). Unemployment and suicide: A cohort analysis of social factors predicting suicide in the US National Longitudinal Mortality Study. *Psychological Medicine, 31*(1), 127–138.

Link, B. G., Phelan, J. C., Bresnahan, M., Stueve, A., & Pescosolido, B. (1999). Public conceptions of mental illness: Labels, causes, dangerousness, and social distance. *American Journal of Public Health, 89*(9), 1328–1333.

Lipschitz, D. S., Winegar, R. K., Nicolaou, A. L., et al. (1999). Perceived abuse and neglect as risk factors for suicidal behavior in adolescent inpatients. *Journal of Nervous & Mental Disease, 187*(1), 32–39.

Luoma, J., & Pearson, J. L.(2002). Suicide and marital status in the United States, 1991-1996: Is widowhood a risk factor? *American Journal of Public Health, 92*(9), 1518–1522.

MacLeod, A. K., Tata, P., Tyrer, P., Schmidt, U., Davidson, K., Thompson, S. (2005). Hopelessness and positive and negative future thinking in parasuicide. *British Journal of Clinical Psychology, 44* (Part 4): 495–504.

McGuffin, P., Marusic, A., & Farmer, A. (2001). What can psychiatric genetics offer suicidology. *Journal of Crisis Intervention and Suicide, 22*(2), 62–65.

Miller, M., Azrael, D., & Hemenway, D. (2002a). Firearm availability and unintentional firearm deaths, suicide, and homicide among 5–14 year olds. *The Journal of Trauma, Injury, Infection, and Critical Care, 52*(2), 267–275.

Miller, M., Azrael, D., & Hemenway, D. (2002b). Household firearm ownership and suicide rates in the United States. *Epidemiology, 13*(5), 517–524.

Minino, A. M., Arias, E., Kochanek, K. D., Murphy, S. L., & Smith, B. L. (2002). Deaths: Final data for 2000. *National Vital Statistics Reports,* 50–15, 1–120.

Mitchell, A. M., Gale, D. D., Garand, L., & Wesner, S. (2003). The use of narrative data to inform the psychotherapeutic process with suicide survivors. *Issues in Mental Health Nursing, 24,* 91–106.

Modai, I., Valevski, A., Solomish, A., et al. (1999). Neural network detection of files of suicidal patients and suicidal profiles. *Medical Informatics, 24*(4), 249–256.

Molnar, B., Berkman, L. F., & Buka, S. L. (2001). Psychopathology, childhood sexual abuse and other childhood adversities: Relative links to subsequent suicidal behavior in the U.S. *Psychological Medicine, 31*(6), 965–977.

Moskos, M. A., Achilles, J., & Gray, D. (2004). Adolescent suicide myths in the United States. *Crisis, 25*(4), 176–182.

Murphy, S. A., Johnson, L. C., Wu, L., Fan, J. J., & Lohan, J. (2003). Bereaved parents' outcomes 4 to 60 months after their children's death by accident, suicide, or homicide. A comparative study demonstrating differences. *Death Studies*, 39–61. Retrieved on September 3, 2006.

National Center for Health Statistics. (2002). *Health, United States.* www.cdc.gov/nchs. Retrieved on September 3, 2006.

Nelson, E. C., Heath, A. C., Madden, P. A., Cooper, M. L., Dinwiddie, S. H., Pucholz, K. K., et al. (2002). Association between self-reported childhood sexual abuse and adverse psychosocial outcomes: Results from a twin study. *Archives of General Psychiatry, 59*, 139–145.

Nemeroff, C. B., Compton, M. T., & Berger, J. (2001). The depressed suicidal patient: Assessment and treatment. *Annals of the New York Academy of Sciences, 932*, 1–23.

Oquendo, M. A., Ellis, S. P., Greenwald, S., Malone, K. M., Weissman, M. M., & Mann, J. J. (2001). Ethnic and sex differences in suicide rates relative to major depression in the United States. *American Journal of Psychiatry, 158*(10), 1652–1658.

Paul, J. P., Catania, J., Pollack, L., Moskowitz, J., Conchola, J., Mills, T., et al. (2002). Suicide attempts among gay and bisexual men: Lifetime prevalence and antecedents. *American Journal of Public Health, 92*(8), 1338–1345.

Pilowsky, D. J., Wu, L. T., & Anthony, J. C. (1999). Panic attacks and suicide attempts in mid-adolescence. *American Journal of Psychiatry, 156*(10), 1545–1549.

Pitchot, W., Hansenne, M., Gonzalez Moreno, A., Pinto, E., Reggers, J., Fuchs, S., et al. (2001). Reduced dopamine function in depressed patients is related to suicidal behavior but not its lethality. *Psychoneuroendocrinology, 26*, 689–696.

Poijula, S., Wahlberg, K. E., & Dyregrov, A. (2001). Adolescent suicide and suicide contagion in three secondary schools. *International Journal of Emergency Mental Health, 3*(3), 163–168.

Qin, P., Agerbo, E., Westergård-Nielson, N., Eriksson, T., & Mortenson, P. B. (2000). Gender differences in risk factors for suicide in Denmark. *British Journal of Psychiatry, 177*, 546–550.

Qin, P., Agergbo, E., & Mortensen, P. B. (2003). Suicide risk in relationship to socioeconomic, demographic, psychiatric, and familial factors: A national register-based study of all suicides in Denmark, 1981–1997. *American Journal of Psychiatry, 160*(4), 765–772.

Rudd, M. D., Joiner, T. E., & Rajab, J. H. (2004). *Treating suicidal behavior* (2nd ed.). New York: Guilford Press.

Rudd, M. D., Mandrusiak, M., Joiner, T. E. (2006). The case against no-suicide contracts: The commitment to treatment statement as a practice alternative. *Journal of Clinical Psychology: In Session, 62*(2), 243–251.

Samuelsson, M., Jokinen, J., Nordström, A-L., Nordström, P. (2006). CSF 5-HIAA, suicide intent and hopelessness in the prediction of early suicide in male high-risk suicide attempters. *Acta Psychiatr Scand, 113*, 44–47.

Singh, G. K., & Siahpush, M. (2002). Increasing rural-urban gradients in US suicide mortality, 1970–1997. *American Journal of Public Health, 92*(7): 1161–1167.

Skodol, A. E., Siever, L. J., & Livesley, W. J. (2002). The borderline diagnosis II: Biology, genetics, and clinical course. *Biological Psychiatry, 51*, 951–963.

Sourander, A., Helstelä, L., Haavisto, A., & Bergroth, L. (2001). Suicidal thoughts and attempts among adolescents: A longitudinal 8-year follow-up study. *Journal of Affective Disorders, 63*, 59–66.

Stack, S. (2003). Media coverage as a risk factor in suicide. *Journal of Epidemiology and Community Health, 57*, 238–240.

Steenland, K., Halperin, W., Hu, S., & Walker, J. T. (2003). Deaths due to injuries among employed adults: The effects of socioeconomic class. *Epidemiology, 14*(1), 74–79.

Stewart, S. E., Manion, I. G., Davidson, S., & Cloutier, P. (2001). Suicidal children and adolescents with first emergency room presentations: Predictors of six-month outcome. *Journal of the American Academy of Child and Adolescent Psychiatry, 40*(5), 580–587.

Sublette, M. D., Hibbeln, J. R., Galfalvy, H., Oquendo, M. A., Mann, J. J. (2006). Omega-3 polyunsaturated essential fatty acid status as a predictor of future suicide risk. *The American Journal of Psychiatry, 163*, 1100–1102.

Suicide among black youths—United States, 1980–1995. (1998). *Morbidity and Mortality Weekly Report, 47*(10), 193–195.

United States Department of Health and Human Services (U.S. DHHS). (2000). *Healthy people 2010* (Conference Edition). Washington, DC: Author.

Vilhjalmsson, R., Kristjansdottir, G., & Sveinbjarnardottir, E. (1998). Factors associated with suicide ideation in adults. *Social Psychiatry and Psychiatric Epidemiology, 33*(3), 97–103.

Wahl, C. (1957). Suicide as a magical act. *Bulletin of Menninger Clinic, 21*, 91–98.

Weinberger, L. E., Sreenivasan, S., Sathyavagiswaran, L., & Markowitz, E. (2001). Child and adolescent suicide in a large, urban area: Psychological, demographic and situation factors. *Journal of Forensic Sciences, 46*(4), 902–907.

Wissow, L. S., Walkup, J., Barlow, A., Reid, R., & Kane, S. (2001). Cluster and regional influences on suicide in an American Indian tribe. *Social Science and Medicine, 53*, 1115–1124.

Zimmerman, S. L. (2002). States' spending for public welfare and their suicide rates, 1960 to 1995. What is the problem? *The Journal of Nervous and Mental Disease, 190*(6), 349.

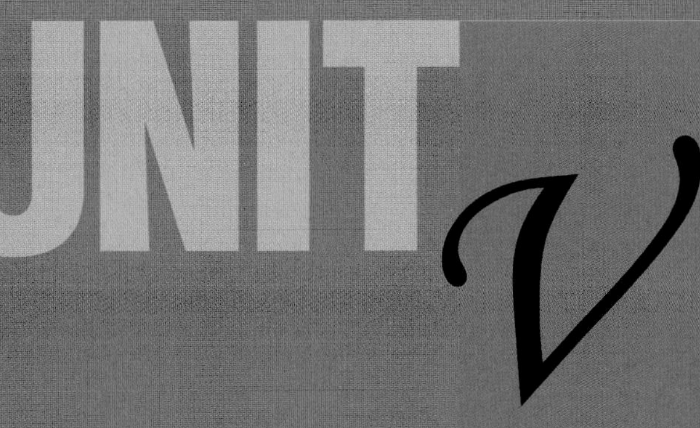

UNIT V

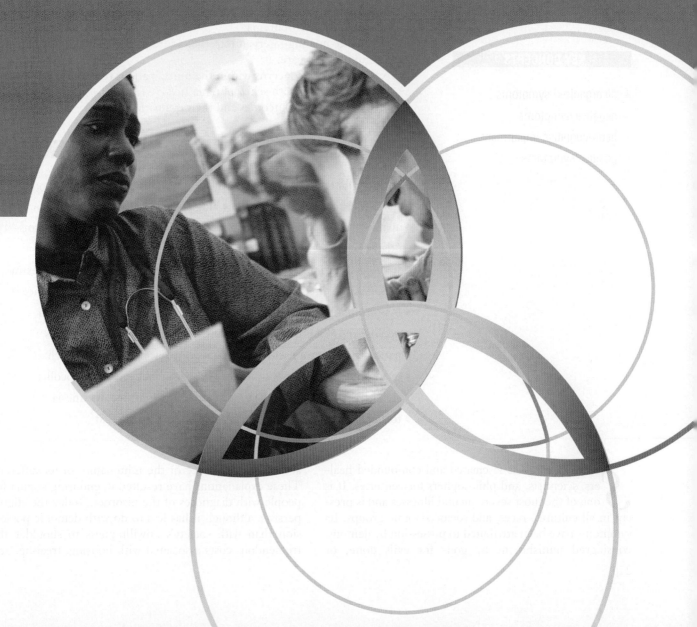

Care of Persons with Psychiatric Disorders

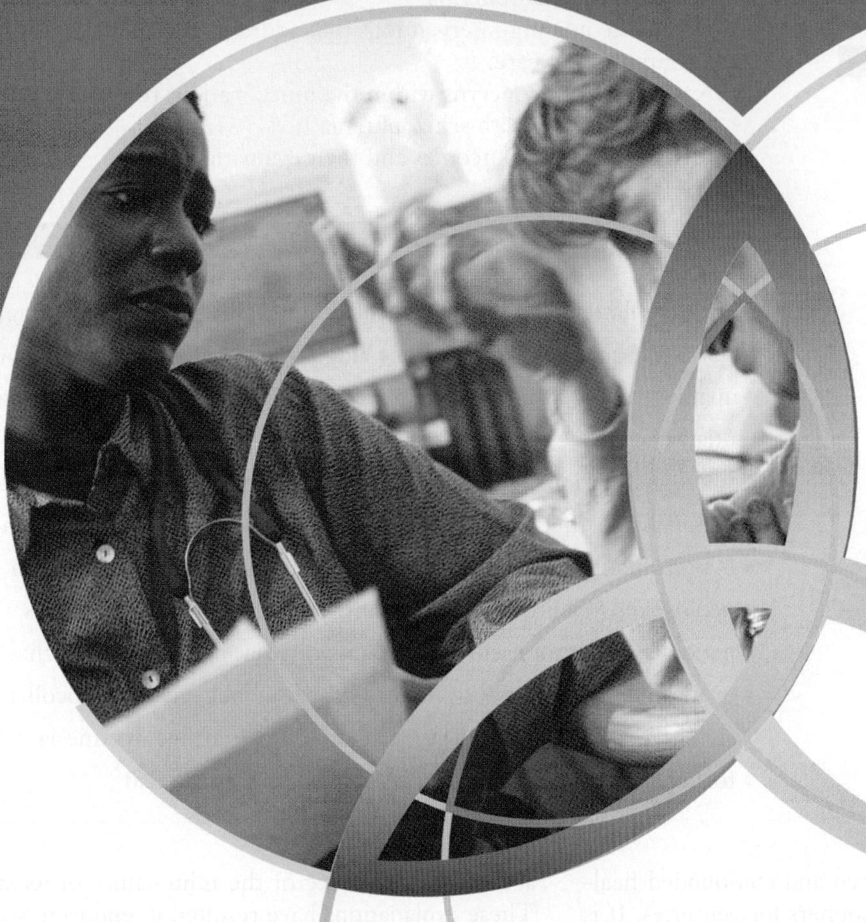

CHAPTER
18

Schizophrenia: Management of Thought Disorders

Andrea C. Bostrom and Mary Ann Boyd

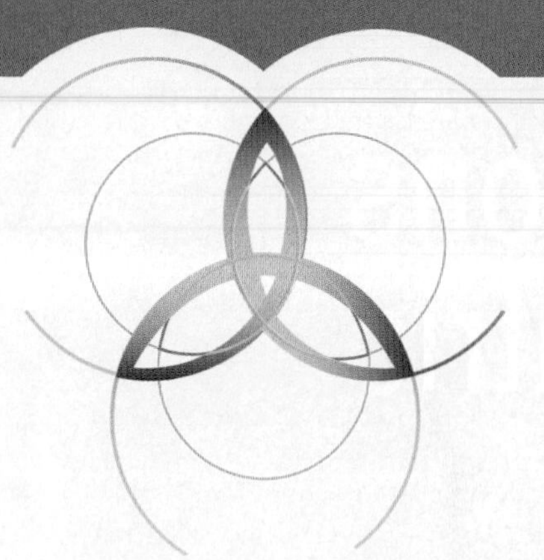

KEY CONCEPTS

- disorganized symptoms
- negative symptoms
- neurocognitive impairment
- positive symptoms

LEARNING OBJECTIVES

After studying this chapter, you will be able to:

- Distinguish key symptoms of schizophrenia.
- Analyze the prevailing biologic, psychological, and social theories that are the basis for understanding schizophrenia.
- Analyze the human response to schizophrenia, with emphasis on hallucinations, delusions, and social isolation.
- Formulate nursing diagnoses based on a biopsychosocial assessment of people with schizophrenia.
- Formulate nursing interventions that address specific diagnoses based on a continuum of care.
- Analyze special concerns within the nurse–patient relationship common to treating those with schizophrenia.
- Identify expected outcomes and their evaluation.

KEY TERMS

• affective flattening or blunting • affective lability • aggression • agitation • agranulocytosis • akathisia • alogia • ambivalence • anhedonia • apathy • autistic thinking • avolition • catatonic excitement • circumstantiality • clang association • concrete thinking • confused speech and thinking • delusions • echolalia • echopraxia • expressed emotion • extrapyramidal side effects • flight of ideas • hallucinations • hypervigilance • hypofrontality • illusions • loose associations • metonymic speech • neologisms • neuroleptic malignant syndrome • oculogyric crisis • paranoia • paranoid schizophrenia • polyuria • pressured speech • prodromal • referential thinking • regressed behavior • retrocollis • stereotypy • stilted language • tangentiality • tardive dyskinesia • torticollis • verbigeration • waxy flexibility • word salad

Schizophrenia has fascinated and confounded healers, scientists, and philosophers for centuries. It is one of the most severe mental illnesses and is present in all cultures, races, and socioeconomic groups. Its symptoms have been attributed to possession by demons, considered punishment by gods for evils done, or accepted as evidence of the inhumanity of its sufferers. These explanations have resulted in enduring stigma for people with diagnoses of the disorder. Today the stigma persists, although it has less to do with demonic possession than with society's unwillingness to shoulder the tremendous costs associated with housing, treating, and rehabilitating patients with schizophrenia. All nurses need to understand this disorder.

CLINICAL COURSE

In the late 1800s, Emil Kraepelin first described the course of the disorder he called *dementia praecox*. In the early 1900s, Eugen Bleuler renamed the disorder *schizophrenia*, meaning *split minds*, and began to determine that there was not just one type of schizophrenia, but rather a group of schizophrenias. More recently, Kurt Schneider differentiated behaviors associated with schizophrenia as "first rank" symptoms (psychotic delusions, hallucinations) and "second rank" symptoms (all other experiences and behaviors associated with the disorder). These pioneering physicians had a great influence on the current diagnostic conceptualizations of schizophrenia that emphasize the heterogeneity of the disorder in terms of symptoms, course of illness, and positive and negative symptoms.

Overview of Schizophrenia

The natural progression of schizophrenia is usually described as deteriorating with time, with an eventual plateau in the symptoms. Only for elderly patients with schizophrenia has it been suggested that improvement might occur. In reality, no one really knows what the course of schizophrenia would be if patients were able to adhere to a treatment regimen throughout their lives. Only recently have medications been relatively effective, with manageable side effects. The clinical picture of schizophrenia is complex, individuals differ from one another, and the experience for a single individual may be different from episode to episode.

Acute Illness Period

Initially, the illness behaviors may be both confusing and frightening to the patient and the family. The changes may be subtle; however, at some point, the changes in thought and behavior become so disruptive or bizarre that they can no longer be overlooked. These might include episodes of staying up all night for several nights, incoherent conversations, or aggressive acts against self or others. For example, one patient's parents reported their son walking around the apartment for several days holding his arms and hands as if they were a machine gun, pointing them at his parents and siblings, and saying "rat-a-tat-tat, you're dead." Another father described his son's first delusional–hallucination episode as so convincing that it was frightening. His son began visiting cemeteries and making "mind contact" with the deceased. He saw his deceased grandmother walking around in the home and was certain that there were pipe bombs in objects in his home. Another patient believed he had been visited by space aliens who wanted to unite their world with earth and assured him that he would become Speaker of the House and then President following the deaths of the President and Vice President.

As symptoms progress, patients are less and less able to care for basic needs, such as eating, sleeping, and bathing. Substance use is common. Functioning at school or work deteriorates. Dependence on family and friends increases and those individuals recognize the need for treatment. In the acute phase, these individuals with schizophrenia are at high risk for suicide. Patients usually are hospitalized to protect themselves or others.

The initial treatment focuses on alleviation of symptoms through initiation of medications, decreasing the risk of suicide through safety measures, normalizing sleep, and reducing substance use. Functional deficits persist during this period, and the patient and family must begin to learn to cope with these. Emotional blunting diminishes the ability and desire to engage in hobbies, vocational activities, and relationships. Limited participation in social activities spirals into numerous skill deficits, such as difficulty engaging others interpersonally. Cognitive deficits lead to problems recognizing patterns in situations and transferring learning and behaviors from one circumstance to another similar one.

Stabilization Period

After the initial diagnosis of schizophrenia and initiation of treatment, stabilization of symptoms becomes the focus. Symptoms become less acute but may be present. Treatment is intense during this period as medication regimens are established and patients and their families begin to adjust to the idea of a family member having a long-term severe mental illness. Ideally, the use of substances is eliminated. Socialization with others begins to increase, and rehabilitation begins.

Maintenance and Recovery Period

After the patient's condition is stabilized, the patient focuses on regaining the previous level of functioning and quality of life. Medication treatment of schizophrenia has generally contributed to an improvement in the lifestyle of people with this disorder; however, no medication has cured it. Faithful medication management tends to make the impairments in functioning less severe when they occur and to diminish the extremes an individual might experience. As with any chronic illness, stresses of life and major crises can contribute to exacerbations of symptoms.

Clearly family support and involvement are extremely important at this time. Once the initial diagnosis is made, patients and families must be educated to anticipate and expect relapse and know how to cope with it. This is one of the important themes throughout the nursing process for people with schizophrenia.

Relapses

Relapses can occur at any time during treatment and recovery. Relapse is not inevitable; however, it occurs with sufficient regularity to be a major concern in the treatment of schizophrenia. Relapses can occur and are very detrimental to the successful management of this disorder. With each relapse, there is a longer period of time to recover. Combining medications and psychosocial treatment greatly diminishes the severity and frequency of recurrent relapses (van Meijel, van der Gaag, Kahn, & Grypdonck, 2003).

One of the major reasons for relapse is noncompliance with the medication regimen. Even with newer medications, noncompliance leading to relapse continues to be a problem (Leucht et al, 2003). Stopping use of medications almost certainly leads to a relapse and may actually be a stressor that causes a severe and rapid relapse (Baldessarini, 2002). Lower relapse rates are, for the most part, among groups who were following a treatment regimen.

Many other factors trigger relapse: the degree of impairment in cognition and coping that leaves patients vulnerable to stressors; the accessibility of community resources, such as public transportation, housing, entry-level and low-stress employment, and social services; income supports that buffer the day-to-day stressors of living; the degree of stigmatization that the community holds for mental illness that attacks the self-concept of patients; and the responsiveness of family members, friends, and supportive others (such as peers and professionals) when patients need help.

Diagnostic Criteria

The current definition outlined in the American Psychiatric Association's *Diagnostic and Statistical Manual of Mental Disorders*, 4th edition, text revision (*DSM-IV-TR*) (APA, 2000) states that schizophrenia is a mixture of positive and negative symptoms that present for a significant portion of a 1-month period but with continuous signs of disturbance persisting for at least 6 months.

Positive symptoms can be thought of as symptoms that exist but should not, and negative symptoms as ones that should be there but are not.

KEY CONCEPT Positive symptoms reflect an excess or distortion of normal functions, including delusions and hallucinations.

KEY CONCEPT Negative symptoms reflect a lessening or loss of normal functions, such as restriction or flattening in the range and intensity of emotion (affective flattening or blunting); reduced fluency and productivity of thought and speech (alogia); withdrawal and inability to initiate and persist in goal-directed activity (avolition); and inability to experience pleasure (anhedonia).

The *DSM-IV-TR* criteria for diagnosing schizophrenia include necessary symptomatology, duration of symptoms, evaluation of functional impairment, and elimination of alternate hypotheses that might account for the symptoms (APA, 2000). Several schizophrenia subtypes are currently recognized: paranoid, disorganized, catatonic, undifferentiated, and residual. There is a growing belief that this subtyping is not useful for predicting the course and response to treatment. The diagnostic criteria and current subtypes are listed in Table 18.1 and Box 18.1, respectively. The Scale for the Assessment of Positive Symptoms (SAPS) (Box 18.15), and the Scale for the Assessment of Negative Symptoms (SANS) (Box 18.16) are presented later in this chapter.

BOX 18.1

Key Diagnostic Characteristics of Schizophrenia Subtypes

Paranoid Type: *DSM-IV-TR* 295.30
- Preoccupation with delusions or auditory hallucinations
- Disorganized speech, disorganized or catatonic behavior, or flat or inappropriate affect is not prominent

Disorganized Type: *DSM-IV-TR* 295.10
- Disorganized speech, disorganized behavior, and flat or inappropriate affect

Catatonic Type: *DSM-IV-TR* 295.20

At least two of the following characteristics present:
- Motor immobility or stupor
- Excessive purposeless motor activity
- Extreme negativism
- Posturing, stereotyped movements, prominent mannerisms, or prominent grimacing
- Echolalia or echopraxia

Undifferentiated Type: *DSM-IV-TR* 295.90
- Only characteristic symptoms present, but does not meet criteria for other subtypes

Residual Type: *DSM-IV-TR* 295.60
- Absence of prominent delusions, hallucinations, disorganized speech, and grossly disorganized or catatonic behavior
- Negative symptoms persist or two or more positive symptoms are present in attenuated form such as odd beliefs or unusual perceptual experiences.

Table 18.1  **Key Diagnostic Characteristics of Schizophrenia** 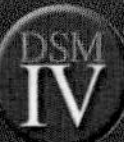

Diagnostic Criteria and Target Symptoms	Associated Findings
Diagnostic Criteria • Two or more of the following characteristic symptoms present for a significant portion of time during a 1-month period: delusions; hallucinations; disorganized speech; grossly disorganized or catatonic behavior; negative symptoms • One or more major areas of social or occupational functioning (such as work, interpersonal relations, self-care) markedly below previously achieved level • Continuous signs persisting for at least 6 months • Absence or insignificant duration of major depressive, manic, or mixed episodes occurring concurrently with active symptoms • Not a direct physiologic effect of a substance or medical condition • Prominent delusions or hallucinations present when a prior history of autistic disorder or another pervasive developmental disorder exists	• Disturbed sleep patterns • Lack of interest in eating or refusal of food • Difficulty concentrating • Some cognitive dysfunction, such as confusion, disorientation, memory impairment • Lack of insight • Depersonalization, derealization, and somatic concerns • Motor abnormalities ***Associated Physical Examination Findings*** • Physically awkward • Poor coordination or mirroring • Motor abnormalities • Cigarette-related pathologies, such as emphysema and other pulmonary and cardiac problems
Target Symptoms and Associated Findings • Inappropriate affect • Loss of interest or pleasure • Dysphoric mood (anger, anxiety, or depression)	***Associated Laboratory Findings*** • Enlarged ventricular system and prominent sulci in the brain cortex • Decreased temporal and hippocampal size • Increased size of basal ganglia • Decreased cerebral size • Slowed reaction times • Abnormalities in eye tracking

Positive Symptoms of Schizophrenia

Delusions are erroneous fixed, false beliefs that cannot be changed by reasonable argument. They usually involve a misinterpretation of experience. For example, the patient believes someone is reading his or her thoughts or plotting against him or her. Various types of delusions include the following:

- *Grandiose:* the belief that one has exceptional powers, wealth, skill, influence, or destiny
- *Nihilistic:* the belief that one is dead or a calamity is impending
- *Persecutory:* the belief that one is being watched, ridiculed, harmed, or plotted against
- *Somatic:* beliefs about abnormalities in bodily functions or structures

BOX 18.2

Signs and Symptoms of Hyponatremia

Chronic Hyponatremia
Generalized weakness, giddiness, headache, irritability, loss of appetite, muscle cramps, nausea, restlessness, slight confusion, and vomiting.

Acute Hyponatremia
Coma, confusion, decreased serum osmolality, decreased urine osmolality, increased urinary volume, lethargy, muscle twitching, seizures, specific urine gravity < 1.010, and weakness.

Hallucinations are perceptual experiences that occur without actual external sensory stimuli. They can involve any of the five senses, but they are usually *visual* or *auditory*. Auditory hallucinations are more common than visual ones. For example, the patient hears voices carrying on a discussion about his or her own thoughts or behaviors.

Negative Symptoms of Schizophrenia

Negative symptoms are not as dramatic as positive symptoms, but they can interfere greatly with the patient's ability to function day to day. Because expressing emotion is difficult for them, people with schizophrenia laugh, cry, and get angry less often. Their affect is flat, and they show little or no emotion when personal loss occurs. They also suffer from **ambivalence**, which is the concurrent experience of equally strong opposing feelings so that it is impossible to make a decision. The avolition may be so profound that simple activities of daily living, such as dressing or combing hair, may not get done. Anhedonia prevents the person with schizophrenia from enjoying activities. People with schizophrenia have limited speech and difficulty saying anything new or carrying on a conversation. These negative symptoms cause

FAME AND FORTUNE

Vincent Van Gogh (1853–1890)

Dutch Artist

Public Persona

One of the world's most renowned artists, Vincent van Gogh, is unique in the history of Western art. Although he sold only one painting in his lifetime, his works command millions of dollars today and bring millions of people enjoyment and enrichment via prints and exhibits. Van Gogh was a prolific painter and produced more than 2,000 paintings and drawings despite a long history of mental and emotional problems.

Personal Realities

Like many people with mental illness, van Gogh's symptoms do not easily fit a diagnostic category. Historians argue that van Gogh suffered from depression, schizophrenia, bipolar disorder, digitalis toxicity, temporal epilepsy, or personality disorders. The son of a preacher, he had been a theology student and lay preacher before turning to art. His adulthood included periods of hypersexuality, hyposexuality, bisexuality, and homosexuality. His stormy homosexual relationship with the painter Paul Gauguin ended in one of van Gogh's most dramatic moments. In 1888, following the breakup of the relationship, van Gogh, thought to be plagued with a hallucination, cut off one of his ears. He was admitted to a mental hospital, where he was allowed to paint outdoors; after discharge, he painted more than 80 pictures. In 1890, van Gogh shot himself.

the person with schizophrenia to withdraw and suffer feelings of severe isolation.

Neurocognitive Impairment

Neurocognitive impairment exists in schizophrenia and may be independent of positive and negative symptoms. Neurocognition includes memory (short- and long-term), vigilance or sustained attention, verbal fluency or the ability to generate new words, and executive functioning, which includes volition, planning, purposive action, and self-monitoring behavior. Working memory is a concept that includes short-term memory and the ability to store and process information.

KEY CONCEPT **Neurocognitive impairment in** memory, vigilance, and executive functioning is related to poor functional outcome in schizophrenia (Green, Kern, Braff, & Mintz, 2000).

This impairment is independent of the positive symptoms. That is, cognitive dysfunction can exist even if the positive symptoms are in remission. Not all areas of cognitive functioning are impaired. Long-term memory and intellectual functioning are not necessarily affected. However, many people with the disorder appear to have low intellectual functioning, which may be related to lack of educational opportunities, which is common for people with mental illnesses. Neurocognitive dysfunction often is manifested in disorganized symptoms.

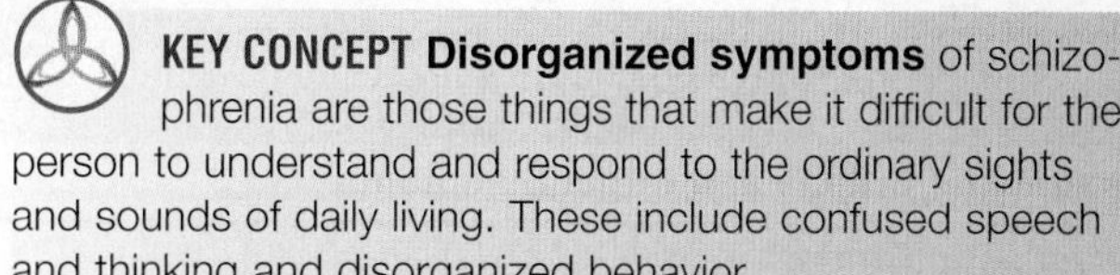

KEY CONCEPT **Disorganized symptoms** of schizophrenia are those things that make it difficult for the person to understand and respond to the ordinary sights and sounds of daily living. These include confused speech and thinking and disorganized behavior.

Disorganized Thinking

The following are examples of confused speech and thinking patterns:

- **Echolalia**—repetition of another's words that is parrot-like and inappropriate
- **Circumstantiality**—extremely detailed and lengthy discourse about a topic
- **Loose associations**—absence of the normal connectedness of thoughts, ideas, and topics; sudden shifts without apparent relationship to preceding topics
- **Tangentiality**—the topic of conversation is changed to an entirely different topic that is a logical progression but causes a permanent detour from the original focus
- **Flight of ideas**—the topic of conversation changes repeatedly and rapidly, generally after just one sentence or phrase
- **Word salad**—string of words that are not connected in any way
- **Neologisms**—words that are made up that have no common meaning and are not recognized
- **Paranoia**—suspiciousness and guardedness that are unrealistic and often accompanied by grandiosity
- **Referential thinking**—belief that neutral stimuli have special meaning to the individual, such as the television commentator speaking directly to the individual
- **Autistic thinking**—restricts thinking to the literal and immediate so that the individual has private rules of logic and reasoning that make no sense to anyone else
- **Concrete thinking**—lack of abstraction in thinking; inability to understand punch lines, metaphors, and analogies
- **Verbigeration**—purposeless repetition of words or phrases
- **Metonymic speech**—use of words interchangeably with similar meanings
- **Clang association**—repetition of words or phrases that are similar in sound but in no other way, for example, right, light, sight, might
- **Stilted language**—overly and inappropriately artificial formal language
- **Pressured speech**—speaking as if the words are being forced out

Disorganized perceptions often create oversensitivity to colors, shapes, and background activities. **Illusions** occur when the person misperceives or exaggerates stimuli that actually exist in the external environment. This is in contrast to hallucinations, which are perceptions in the absence of environmental stimuli. Ancillary symptoms that may accompany schizophrenia include anxiety, depression, and hostility.

Disorganized Behavior

Disorganized behavior (which may manifest as very slow, rhythmic, or ritualistic movement) coupled with disorganized speech make it difficult for the person to partake in daily activities. Examples of disorganized behavior include the following:

- **Aggression**—behaviors or attitudes that reflect rage, hostility, and the potential for physical or verbal destructiveness (usually comes about if the person believes someone is going to do him or her harm)
- **Agitation**—inability to sit still or attend to others, accompanied by heightened emotions and tension
- **Catatonic excitement**—a hyperactivity characterized by purposeless activity and abnormal movements such as grimacing and posturing
- **Echopraxia**—involuntary imitation of another person's movements and gestures
- **Regressed behavior**—behaving in a manner of a less mature life stage; childlike and immature
- **Stereotypy**—repetitive, purposeless movements that are idiosyncratic to the individual and to some degree outside of the individual's control
- **Hypervigilance**—sustained attention to external stimuli as if expecting something important or frightening to happen
- **Waxy flexibility**—posture held in odd or unusual fixed position for extended periods of time

Schizophrenia in Special Populations

Children

The diagnosis of schizophrenia is rare in children before adolescence. When it does occur in children aged 5 or 6 years, the symptoms are essentially the same as in adults. In this age group, hallucinations tend to be visual and delusions less developed. Because disorganized speech and behavior may be explained better by other disorders that are more common in childhood, those disorders should be considered before applying the diagnosis of schizophrenia to a child (APA, 2000).

However, new studies suggest that the likelihood of children later experiencing schizophrenia can be predicted. Developmental abnormalities in childhood, including delays in attainment of speech and motor development, problems in social adjustment, and poorer academic and cognitive performance have been found to be present in individuals who experience schizophrenia in adulthood. Specific factors that appear to predict schizophrenia in adulthood include problems in motor and neurologic development, deficits in attention and verbal short-term memory, poor social competence, positive formal thought disorder-like symptoms, and severe instability of early rearing environment (Niemi, Suvisaari, Tuulio-Henriksson, & Lonnqvist, 2003).

Elderly People

People with schizophrenia do grow old. The 1-year prevalence for schizophrenia among those 65 years of age and older was estimated in the Surgeon General's report (U.S. Department of Health and Human Services [U.S. DHHS], 1999) to be 0.6% (about half the percentage for adults 18 to 54 years of age). For elderly patients who have had schizophrenia since young adulthood, this may be a time in which they experience some improvement in symptoms or relapse fluctuations. However, their lifestyle probably is dependent on the effectiveness of earlier treatment, the support systems that are in place (including relationships with family members and professionals), and the interaction between environmental stressors and the patient's functional impairments.

In late-onset schizophrenia, the diagnostic criteria are met after age 45 years. Women are affected more than men. The presentation of late-onset schizophrenia is most likely to include positive symptoms, particularly paranoid or persecutory delusions. Cognitive deterioration and affective blunting occur less frequently. Social functioning is more intact. Many individuals with diagnoses of late-onset schizophrenia have disturbances in sensory functions, primarily hearing and vision losses (APA, 2000). The cost of caring for elderly patients with schizophrenia remains high because many are no longer cared for in an institution, and community-based treatment has developed more slowly for this age group than for younger adults. We have little information regarding the effects of gender and ethnicity (Reeves, Stewart, & Howard, 2002).

EPIDEMIOLOGY

Schizophrenia occurs in all cultures and countries. The incidence and prevalence rates are similar across studies, with variations explained by the definition of schizophrenia and the sampling method used. It occurs in about 1.3% of the population, or more than 3 million people in the United States (Goldner, Hsu, Waraich, & Somers, 2002). Its economic costs are enormous. Direct costs include treatment expenses, and indirect costs include lost wages, premature death, and incarceration. In addition, employment among people with schizophrenia is one of the lowest of any group with disabilities (New

Freedom Commission on Mental Health, 2003). The costs of schizophrenia in terms of individual and family suffering probably are inestimable.

People with schizophrenia tend to cluster in the lowest social classes in industrialized countries and urban communities. The symptoms of the illness are so pervasive that it is difficult for these individuals to maintain any type of gainful employment. Homelessness is a problem for the severely mentally ill (e.g., people with schizophrenia or bipolar illness). People with schizophrenia may make up 11% to 14% of the homeless population, compared with 1% to 1.3% of the general population (U.S. DHHS, 2001). See also Chapter 33.

Risk Factors

Risk factors for schizophrenia include stresses in the perinatal period (starvation, poor nutrition, infections), obstetrical complications, and genetic and family susceptibility. There has been recent evidence that parental age may also be a risk factor (Byrne, Agerbo, Ewald, Eaton, & Mortensen, 2003). Birth cohort studies suggest that the incidence may be higher among individuals born in urban settings than those born in rural ones and may be somewhat lower in later-born birth cohorts (Harrison et al., 2003). Infants affected by these maternal stressors may have conditions that create their own risk, such as low birth weight, short gestation, and early developmental difficulties. In childhood, stressors may include central nervous system infections.

Age of Onset

Most people who experience schizophrenia have the disorder diagnosed in late adolescence and early adulthood. A sex difference exists for age of onset. Men tend to be diagnosed between the ages of 18 and 25. Women are diagnosed most frequently between the ages of 25 and 35 (APA, 2000). When schizophrenia begins earlier than age 25 years, symptoms seem to develop more gradually, and negative symptoms predominate throughout the course of the disease. People with early-onset schizophrenia experienced a greater number of neuropsychological problems. Finally, disruptions occur in milestone events of early adulthood, such as achieving in education, work, and long-term relationships (Csernansky, 2003).

Gender Differences

The difference in the age of onset for men and women suggests other outcomes and issues. Men tend to have a poorer prognosis than women. This may be a sex-linked outcome, but it may also reflect the poorer prognosis for any individual who develops the disorder at an early age. In addition, these gender differences have received attention because of hypotheses about sex-linked genetic etiologies. For instance, estrogen may play a protective role against the development of schizophrenia that disappears as estrogen levels drop during menopause (Hafner, 2003). This would account for the higher median age of onset and a more favorable treatment outcome in women.

Ethnic and Cultural Differences

Increasingly, efforts are being made to consider culture and ethnic origin when diagnosing the disorder and treating individuals with symptoms of schizophrenia (APA, 2000; U.S. DHHS, 1999). Although symptoms of schizophrenia appear to be clearly defined, it is possible to find cultures in which what appears to be a hallucination may be considered a vision or a religious experience. In addition, behaviors such as averting eyes during a conversation or minimizing emotional expression may be culturally bound yet easily misinterpreted by clinicians of a different cultural or ethnic background.

Individuals of various racial groups may have varying diagnosis rates of schizophrenia. However, it is not clear if these findings represent correct diagnosis or misdiagnosis of the disorder based on a cultural bias of the clinician. For instance, schizophrenia has been consistently overdiagnosed among African Americans. African American and Hispanic individuals with bipolar disorder are more likely to have misdiagnoses of schizophrenia than are Caucasian individuals. Serious mental disorders may be unrecognized in Asian Americans because of stereotypical beliefs that they are "problem free" (U.S. DHHS, 2001).

Treatment variables also may differ (U.S. DHHS, 2001). For instance, clinicians prescribe higher doses of antipsychotic medications to African Americans. Evidence also supports that African American patients receive more antipsychotic medications than do Caucasians. Physiologically, African Americans may represent a higher percentage of slow metabolizers. The combination of these factors may lead to faster rates of response to medication effects and to side effect sensitivity. Another example suggests that because Mexican American beliefs attribute the cause of schizophrenia to a combination of physical and emotional ailments, families are more likely to tolerate or compensate for a family member with schizophrenia.

Familial Differences 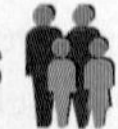

First-degree biologic relatives (children, siblings, parents) of an individual with schizophrenia have a 10 times greater risk for schizophrenia than the general population (APA, 2000). Other relatives may have an increased risk for disorders within the "schizophrenia spectrum" (a group of disorders with some similarities of behavior, such as schizoaffective disorder and schizotypal personality disorder) (APA, 2000).

Comorbidity

Several somatic and psychological disorders coexist with schizophrenia. It is estimated that nearly 50% of patients with schizophrenia have a comorbid medical condition, but many of these illnesses are misdiagnosed or undiagnosed (Goldman, 1999). Recently, more attention has been paid to the causes of mortality among people with schizophrenia. Several physical disorders have been identified, including vision and dental problems, hypertension, diabetes, and sexually transmitted diseases (U.S. DHHS, 1999).

Substance Abuse and Depression

Among the behavioral comorbidities, substance abuse is common. Depression may also be observed in patients with schizophrenia. This is an important symptom for several reasons. First, depression may be evidence that the diagnosis of a mood disorder is more appropriate (see Chapters 20 and 25). Second, depression is not unusual in chronic stages of schizophrenia and deserves attention. Third, the suicide rate (10%) among individuals with schizophrenia is higher than that of the general population. Risk factors for suicide are male gender, chronic illness with frequent relapses, frequent short hospitalizations, a negative attitude toward treatment, impulsive behavior, parasuicide (nonfatal self-harm or gesture), psychosis, and depression (De Hert, McKenzie, & Peuskens, 2001). More recently, periods of untreated psychosis exceeding 1 year and treatment with older conventional antipsychotic drugs also have been associated with a higher risk of suicide attempts (Altamura, Bassetti, Bignotti, Pioli, & Mundo, 2003).

Diabetes Mellitus

There is a renewed interest in the relationship of diabetes mellitus and schizophrenia. Years ago, an association was established between glucose regulation and psychiatric disorders (Franzen, 1970; Schimmelbusch, Mueller, & Sheps, 1971). In fact, insulin shock therapy was used in treating severe disorders. Also of growing concern is the possibility that people with schizophrenia may be more prone to type II diabetes than is the general public. Some suggest (Ryan, Collins, & Thakore, 2003) that this may be attributable to inherent characteristics. Evidence that supports this view includes a higher rate of type II diabetes in first-degree relatives of people with schizophrenia and higher rates of impaired glucose tolerance and insulin resistance among people with schizophrenia. However, obesity, which is associated with type II diabetes, is a growing problem in the United States in general and is complicated in schizophrenia treatment by the tendency of individuals to gain weight once their disease is managed with medications. Weight gain in some individuals may be attributed to a return to a healthier living situation in which regular meals are available and symptoms that interfere with obtaining food regularly (e.g., delusions) are decreased. For other individuals, weight gain may result from the antipsychotic drug (either typical or atypical) selected for treatment.

Disordered Water Balance

Patients with schizophrenia, particularly of early onset, may experience disordered water balance. Often this takes the form of water intoxication characterized by abnormally high water intake, followed by a rapid drop in serum sodium levels. The alteration in sodium level leads to diverse neurologic signs, ranging from ataxia to coma and possibly death. The prevalence rate of disordered water balance reportedly ranges around 6% (Mercier-Guidez & Loas, 2000).

The cause of water intoxication is unknown. Research studies, conducted primarily in the 1990s, suggest multiple physiologic or behavioral causes (Boyd and Lapierre, 1996). Disordered water balance generally precedes water intoxication. Symptoms of chronic hyponatremia are shown in Box 18.2. Often a benign condition, disordered water balance may go undetected for months to years; however, ingesting large amounts of water over a prolonged period may lead to complications, such as renal dysfunction, urinary incontinence, cardiac failure, malnutrition, or permanent brain damage (Boyd and Lapierre, 1996).

Water intoxication, a complication that is life-threatening, occurs when unusually large volumes of ingested water overwhelm the kidneys' capacity to excrete water. As a result, serum sodium levels rapidly fall below the normal range of 135 to 145 mEq/L to a level of 120 mEq/L or less (acute hyponatremia; see Box 18.2). This rapid decrease in sodium produces muscle twitching and irritability and puts the patient at risk for seizures or coma. The physiologic signs and symptoms of disordered water balance and its progression are presented in Box 18.3.

Behaviorally, these patients seem to be "driven to drink" (polydipsia) and may consume between 4 and 10 liters of fluid a day. They carry soda cans and water bottles with them, hoard cups or other water containers, and drink frequently from fountains and showers and sometimes from toilets. They make frequent trips to the bathroom because of the excessive need to urinate (**polyuria**). Generally the amount of urine excreted reflects the amount of fluid ingested. The patient's urine becomes

BOX 18.3

Physiologic Signs and Symptoms of Disordered Water Balance

Mild Disordered Water Balance
- Increased diurnal weight gain
- Specific urine gravity (1.011–1.025)
- Normal serum sodium (135–145 mEq/L)

Moderate Disordered Water Balance
- Increased diurnal weight gain
- Specific urine gravity (1.010–1.003)
- Possible facial puffiness
- Periodic nocturia

Severe Disordered Water Balance
- Possible evidence of stomach or bladder dilation
- Specific urine gravity (1.003–1.000)
- Frequent signs of nausea, vomiting
- Possible history of major motor seizure
- Possible change in blood pressure or pulse
- Polyuria
- Polydipsia
- Urinary incontinence during the night

From Snider, K., & Boyd, M. (1991). When they drink too much: Nursing interventions for patients with disordered water balance. *Journal of Psychosocial Nursing, 29*(7), 13.

very dilute with a very low specific gravity, which may reflect a condition called hyposthenuria, in which the specific gravity falls below 1.008. Because of increased urgency and incontinence, especially at nighttime, the patient's clothing and room may smell like urine. Some patients may become highly agitated when efforts are made to limit access to water and other fluids. Other emotional/behavioral responses, such as increased psychotic symptoms, irritability, and lability, are caused by changes in sodium levels and the rapidity with which they occur.

ETIOLOGY

Since the 1970s, hypothetical causes of schizophrenia have changed dramatically. Purely psychological theories have been replaced by a neurobiologic model that says that patients with schizophrenia have a biologic predisposition or vulnerability that is exacerbated by environmental stressors (see the diathesis-stress model discussed in Chapter 6). Those with schizophrenia are thought to have a genetically or biologically determined sensitivity that leaves them vulnerable to an overwhelming onslaught of stimuli from without and within (U.S. DHHS, 1999). These inherent vulnerabilities include cognitive, psychophysiologic, social competence, and coping deficits that alter the individual's ability, both cognitively and emotionally, to manage life events and interpersonal situations (Box 18.4 and Fig. 18.1).

BOX 18.4

Deficits That Cause Vulnerability in Schizophrenia

Cognitive Deficits
- Deficits in processing complex information
- Deficits in maintaining a steady focus of attention
- Inability to distinguish between relevant and irrelevant stimuli
- Difficulty forming consistent abstractions
- Impaired memory

Psychophysiologic Deficits
- Deficits in sensory inhibition
- Poor control of autonomic responsiveness

Social Skills Deficits
- Impairments in processing interpersonal stimuli, such as eye contact or assertiveness
- Deficits in conversational capacity
- Deficits in initiating activities
- Deficits in experiencing pleasure

Coping Skills Deficits
- Overassessment of threat
- Underassessment of personal resources
- Overuse of denial

Adapted from McGlashan, T. H. (1994). Psychosocial treatments of schizophrenia: The potential relationships. In N. C. Andreasen (Ed.), *Schizophrenia: From mind to molecule* (pp. 189–215). Washington, DC: American Psychiatric Press.

Biologic Theories

Theories and research about the biologic vulnerability for schizophrenia focus on incorporating multiple observations into a coherent explanation. These observations

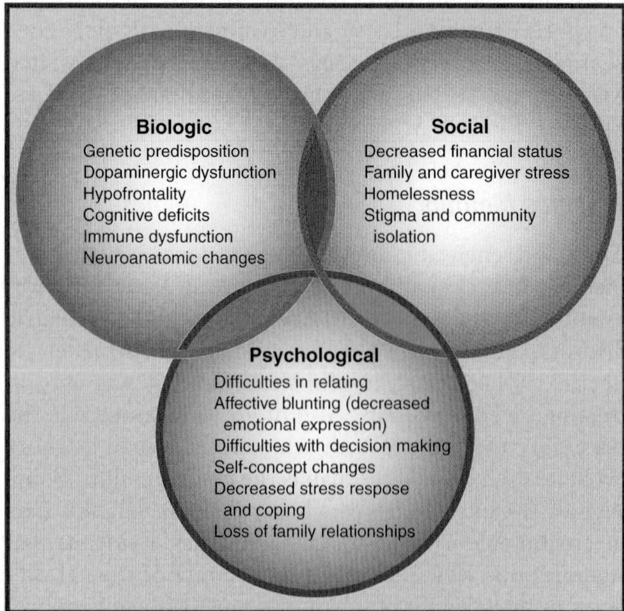

FIGURE 18.1. Biopsychosocial etiologies for patients with schizophrenia.

include the course of the illness already described, possible brain structure changes identified by postmortem and neuroimaging techniques, familial patterns, and pharmacologic effects on behavior and neurotransmitter functions in the brain. One of the more recent theories about the cause of schizophrenic vulnerability focuses on neurodevelopment of the brain from the prenatal period through adolescence. This section describes the various observations and current theories about the cause of schizophrenia. However, the exact cause of schizophrenia remains elusive.

Neuroanatomic Findings

Postmortem and neuroimaging brain studies of patients with schizophrenia show four consistent changes in brain anatomy:

- decreased blood flow to the left globus pallidus early in the disease
- absence of normal blood flow increase in frontal lobes during tests of frontal lobe functioning, such as working memory tasks
- thinner cortex of the medial temporal lobe and a smaller anterior portion of the hippocampus
- decreases in gray matter and enlarged lateral and third ventricles and widened sulci (Chance, Esiri, & Crow, 2003)

These findings are being used as a basis for exploring the influence of genetic loading, obstetric complications, and differences in familial and nonfamilial patients with schizophrenia (Falkai et al., 2003; McDonald et al., 2002).

Familial Patterns 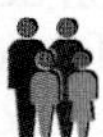

Evidence supports a familial or genetic base for schizophrenia. First-degree relatives (including siblings and children) are 10 times more likely to experience schizophrenia than are individuals in the general population (APA, 2000; U.S. DHHS, 1999). Concordance for schizophrenia is higher among monozygotic (identical) twins than among dizygotic (fraternal) twins, although the rate is not perfectly concordant.

Genetic researchers have sought to identify specific genes responsible for schizophrenia, but replicated results are emerging very slowly (Tsuang, Stone, & Faraone, 2001). The infrequency of reproducible results is likely attributable to the heterogeneity of the disorder, which may not be consistent with a single gene theory. A model that includes several genes is more likely to explain the development of schizophrenia (U.S. DHHS, 1999). Two possible locations are on the long arm of chromosome 22 and on chromosome 6 (Kandel, Schwartz, & Jessell, 2000).

Neurodevelopment

Current theory and research attempt to explain how genes or events early in life (especially perinatal events such as infections or obstetric irregularities) would cause schizophrenia yet manifest symptoms only after years—in adolescence or young adulthood. The neurodevelopmental theory explains and reconciles the inconsistent neuroanatomic brain changes that have been found and links them to early development.

Brain development from prenatal periods through adolescence requires several coordinated molecular activities, including cell proliferation, cell migration, axonal outgrowth, pruning of neuronal connections, programmed cell death, and myelination. All of these activities require coordinated development, usually through activation and inactivation of proteins by genes. Any of these processes could be disrupted by (1) inherited genes that place the individual at risk for schizophrenia, (2) a wild-type allele of this gene that is activated in adolescence or early adulthood, or (3) genetic sensitizing that leaves the individual susceptible to environmental causes or development of lesions during some adverse perinatal event. In addition, several maturational events normally occur during puberty that may affect brain development: (1) changes in dopaminergic, serotonergic, adrenergic, glutamatergic, gamma-aminobutyric acid (GABA)-ergic, and cholinergic neurotransmitter systems and substrates; (2) a complex combination of synaptic pruning along with substantial brain growth in some areas of the cortex; and (3) changes in the steroid-hormonal environment (Chou, Halldin, & Farde, 2003).

Neurotransmitters, Pathways, and Receptors

The *dopamine hypothesis* of schizophrenia arose from observations that first-generation antipsychotic drugs (Table 18.2), which so successfully ameliorate or reduce the positive symptoms of schizophrenia, act primarily by blocking postsynaptic dopamine receptors in the brain. In addition, other drugs that enhance dopamine function, such as amphetamines or cocaine, cause behavioral symptoms similar to those of **paranoid schizophrenia** in humans and bizarre stereotyped behavior in monkeys. Antipsychotic drugs stop these drug-induced behaviors. Based on these observations, researchers concluded that schizophrenia was a syndrome of hyperdopaminergic action in the brain.

This old, straightforward hypothesis of dopamine hyperactivity is clearly complicated by recent findings. Positron emission tomography (PET) scan findings suggest that in schizophrenia, there is a general reduction in brain metabolism, with a relative hypermetabolism in the left side of the brain and in the left temporal lobe. Abnormalities exist in specific areas of the brain, such as

Table 18.2 Selected Antipsychotic Drugs

Generic Name	Trade Name	Dosage Range for Adults (mg/d)
Atypical Antipsychotics		
Aripiprazole	Abilify	10–15
Clozapine	Clozaril	200–600
Risperidone	Risperdal	4–16
Olanzapine	Zyprexa	10–20
Paliperidone	Invega	3–12
Quetiapine	Seroquel	300–400
Ziprasidone	Geodon	40–160
Selected Conventional Antipsychotic Drugs Used to Treat Psychosis in the United States		
Chlorpromazine	Thorazine	30–800
Fluphenazine	Prolixin; Permitil	0.5–20
Haloperidol	Haldol	1–15
Loxapine	Loxitane	20–250
Mesoridazine	Serentil	100–300
Molindone	Moban	15–225
Perphenazine	Trilafon	4–32
Pimozide	Orap*	1–10
Prochlorperazine	Compazine†	15–25
Thiothixene	Navane	5–25
Trifluoperazine	Stelazine	5–25
Triflupromazine	Vesprin	60–150

*Approved in the United States for Tourette's syndrome.

†Adapted from Stahl, S. (2000). *Essential psychopharmacology: Neuroscientific basis and practical application* (2nd ed., p. 404). Cambridge, UK: Cambridge University Press.

in the left globus pallidus (Sedvall, 1994). These findings support further exploration of differential brain hemisphere function in schizophrenia (Fig. 18.2). Other PET studies show **hypofrontality**, or a reduced cerebral blood flow and glucose metabolism in the prefrontal cortex of people with schizophrenia and hyperactivity in the limbic area (Buchsbaum, 1990) (Figs. 18.3 and 18.4). In addition, several types of dopamine receptors (labeled D_1, D_2, D_3, D_4, and D_5) and dopamine are found in four pathways (mesolimbic, mesocortical, nigrostriatal, and tuberoinfundibular) that innervate different parts of the brain (Kandel et al., 2000) (see Chapter 7). Based on the current understanding of schizophrenia, the following discussion relates the neurobiologic changes to the clinical symptoms.

Positive Symptoms: Hyperactivity of Mesolimbic Tract

Positive symptoms of schizophrenia (hallucinations and delusions) are thought to be caused by dopamine *hyperactivity* in the mesolimbic tract, which regulates memory and emotion. It is hypothesized that this hyperactivity could result from overactive modulation of neurotransmission from the nucleus accumbens (Kandel et al., 2000). Another explanation for dopaminergic hyperactivity in the mesolimbic tract is hypoactivity of the mesocortical tract, which normally inhibits dopamine activity in the mesolimbic tract by some type of feedback mechanism. In schizophrenia, the primary defect may be in the mesocortical tract, where dopaminergic function is diminished, thereby decreasing the inhibitory effects on the mesolimbic tract. This disinhibition may be responsible for the overactivity of dopamine in the mesolimbic tract, resulting in the positive symptom cluster (Kandel et al.).

Support for this interconnection between mesocortical and mesolimbic tracts has been found in laboratory animals. Destruction of the mesocortical tract of animals resulted in increased activity in the mesolimbic tract, especially in the nucleus accumbens. A compensatory increase in mesolimbic neurons is a suggested mechanism by which this overactivity occurs.

Negative Symptoms and Cognitive Impairment: Hypoactivity of the Mesocortical Tract

Negative symptoms and cognitive impairment are thought to be related to hypoactivity of the mesocortical dopaminergic tract, which by its association with the prefrontal and neocortex contributes to motivation, planning, sequencing of behaviors in time, attention, and social behavior (Jibson & Tandon, 2000; Kandel et al., 2000). Negative symptoms, such as poor motivation and planning, and flat affect are remarkably similar to symptoms of patients who underwent lobotomy procedures in the late 1940s and early 1950s to disconnect the frontal cortex from the rest of the brain. Monkeys who have had

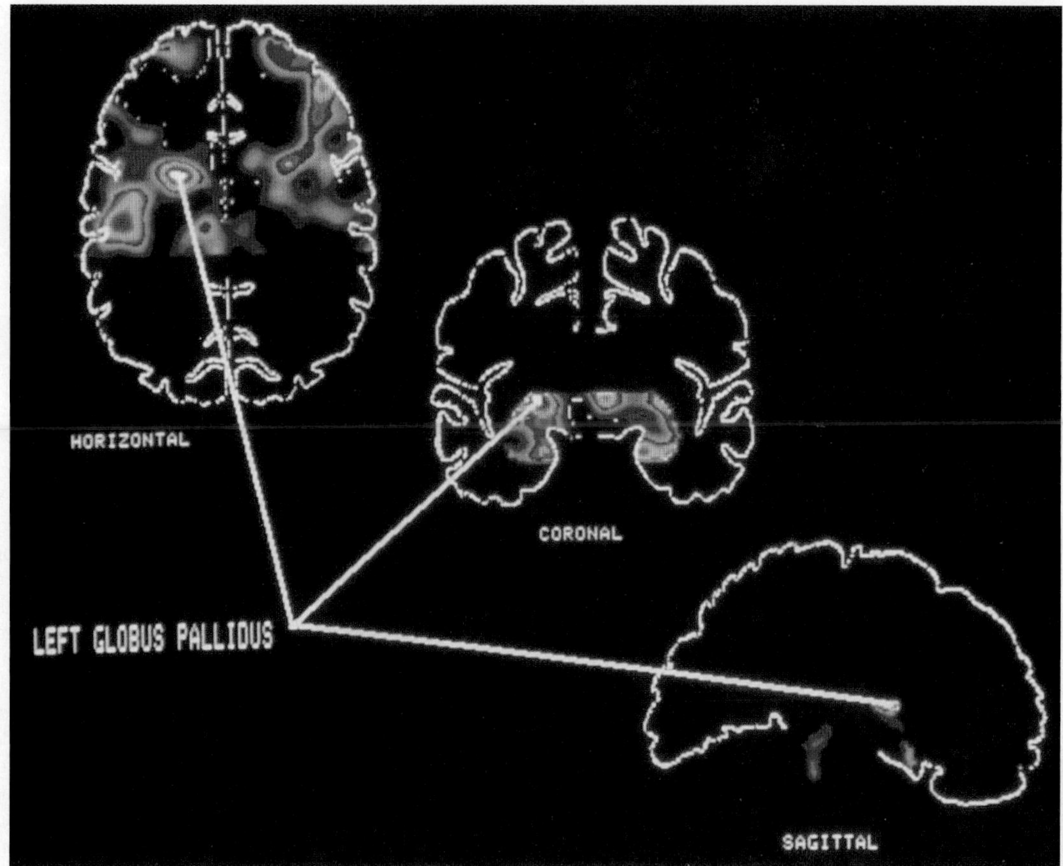

FIGURE 18.2. Area of abnormal functioning in a person with schizophrenia. These three views show the excessive neuronal activity in the left globus pallidus (portion of the basal ganglia next to the putamen). (Courtesy of John W. Haller, PhD, Departments of Psychiatry and Radiology, Washington University, St. Louis, MO.)

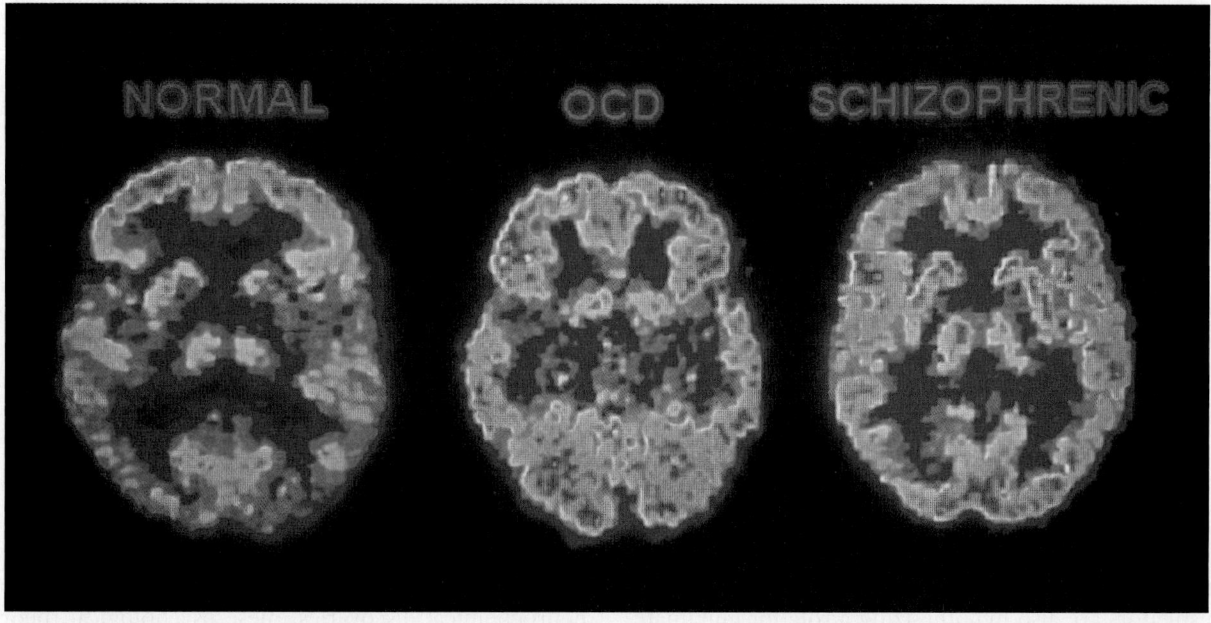

FIGURE 18.3. Metabolic activity in a control subject (*left*), a subject with obsessive-compulsive disorder (center), and a subject with schizophrenia (*right*). (Courtesy of Monte S. Buchsbaum, MD, The Mount Sinai Medical Center and School of Medicine, New York, NY.)

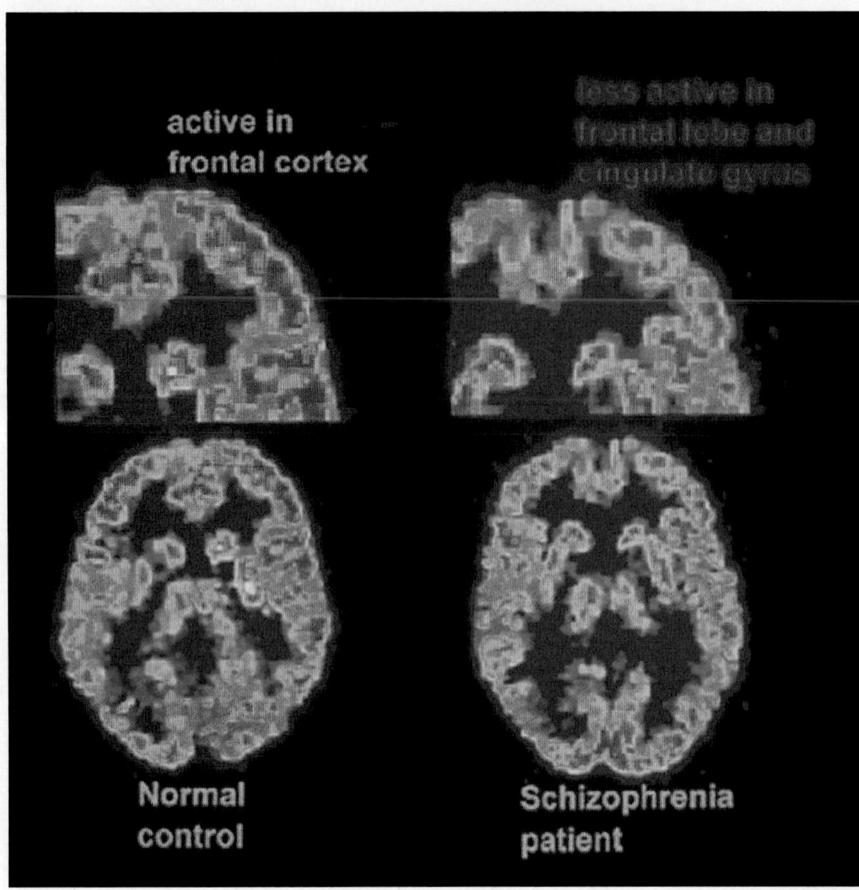

FIGURE 18.4. Positron emission tomography (PET) scan with 18F-deoxyglucose shows metabolic activity in a horizontal section of the brain in a control subject (*left*) and in an unmedicated patient with schizophrenia (*right*). Red and yellow indicate areas of high metabolic activity in the cortex; green and blue indicate lower activity in the white-matter areas of the brain. The frontal lobe is magnified to show reduced frontal activity in the prefrontal cortex of the patient with schizophrenia. (Courtesy of Monte S. Buchsbaum, MD, The Mount Sinai Medical Center and School of Medicine, New York, NY.)

dopamine in the prefrontal cortex depleted have difficulty with cognitive tasks. Finally, PET scans of energy metabolism suggest a reduced metabolism in frontal and prefrontal areas (Davidson & Heinrichs, 2003).

Role of Other Dopamine Pathways

The tuberoinfundibular dopaminergic tract is active in prolactin regulation and may be the source of neuroendocrine changes observed in schizophrenia. The nigrostriatal dopaminergic tract modulates motor activity and is believed to be the site of the **extrapyramidal side effects** of antipsychotic drugs, such as pseudoparkinsonism and tardive dyskinesia. This may also be the site of some motor symptoms of schizophrenia, such as stereotypical behavior.

Role of Other Receptors

Other receptors are also involved in dopamine neurotransmission, especially serotonergic receptors. It is becoming clear that schizophrenia does not result from dysregulation of a single neurotransmitter or biogenic amine (e.g., norepinephrine, dopamine, or serotonin). Investigators are also hypothesizing a role for glutamate and GABA (Ghose et al., 2004) because of the complex interconnections of neuronal transmission and the complexity and heterogeneity of schizophrenia symptoms. The N-methyl-D-aspartate (NMDA) class of glutamate receptors is being studied because of the actions of phencyclidine (PCP) at these sites and the similarity of the psychotic behaviors that are produced when someone takes PCP (see Figs. 18.2, 18.3, and 18.4).

Neural Connectivity

Manifestations of poor mental coordination include difficulty in a variety of functions, such as measuring time or space, making inferences about relationships, and coordinating the processing, priority setting, retrieval, and expression of information. It is now being hypothesized that there may be a basic developmental disorder of the neural connectivity involving multiple molecular mechanisms (Benes, 2000; Penn, 2001; Sallet et al., 2003).

Psychological Theories

Several psychological frameworks have been used to explain the etiology of schizophrenia. Before biologic and neurochemical discoveries, these psychological theories, held by the mental health community, viewed the primary cause of schizophrenia to be dysfunctional parenting in early childhood development. Families often were blamed and alienated by mental health professionals. These theories are no longer valid, and neurochemical-biologic theories have replaced them.

Social Theories

There are no social theories believed to explain schizophrenia, but some theories focus on patterns of family interaction that seem to affect the eventual outcome and social adjustment of individuals with schizophrenia. The theory of **expressed emotion** (EE) correlates certain family communication patterns with an increase in symptoms and relapse in patients with schizophrenia. Families are classified as high-EE families when they make comments about family members or there are aspects of speech that connote criticism, hostility, and negativity about the patient, and they are emotionally overly involved with the patient, such as overprotective or self-sacrificing. Low-EE families make fewer negative comments and show less overinvolvement with the patient. Families that rate high in the areas of criticism, hostility, and battles for control are hypothesized to be associated with increases in the patient's positive symptoms and relapse.

Research related to emotional expressiveness is contradictory. Although families categorized as low in EE have been shown to accept the patient as having a legitimate illness and have an understanding that interpersonal problems can exacerbate the illness (Weisman, Gomes, & Lopez, 2003), families high in EE have not been associated with either a greater family history of schizophrenia or the chronicity of the illness (Subotnik, Goldstein, Nuechterlein, Woo, & Mintz, 2002; Wuerker, Long, Haas, & Bellack, 2002).

Although this research might contribute to the understanding of how negative family interaction affects the patient, there are drawbacks to categorizing families in this manner. Professionals may tend to blame families for causing schizophrenia or limit the patient's contact with family, thus further alienating families who are so vital to the care and support of the patient.

There are numerous social barriers that prevent people with mental illness getting the care they need. One of the major ones is the social stigma that surrounds mental illnesses (see Chapter 1). Box 18.5 describes the impact of living with a stigmatized illness. Another obstacle, unfair treatment limitation and financial requirements placed on mental health benefits and private health insurance, inhibits quality and continuity of care. Finally, the mental health service delivery system is fragmented, and the quality and types of services vary from community to community (New Freedom Commission on Mental Health, 2003).

BOX 18.5

***Clinical Vignette:* Graduate Student in Peril**

Adapted from First Person Account: Graduate Student in Peril. (2002). Schizophrenia Bulletin, 28(4), 745–755.

BGW, born in 1973, spent most of his teenage years using drugs and alcohol, behavior that started when he was 11. He and his small group of friends spent their teenage years outside of school running around on bicycles. He failed 8th grade, repeated it, and made it to 10th grade. He was removed permanently from school at the age of 16 years. His dress included a dirty denim jacket or Army fatigues, torn tee shirts with rock band logos, and tight-fitting jeans. At age 16, he was hospitalized for a psychotic episode initiated by LSD; it was the scariest moment of his life. His mind had been getting fuzzier every day; he had dabbled with black magic and Satanism. Later, he admitted that for years he had been trapped in a fantasy land, only partially explained by his drug use.

Years of treatment followed, and even with abstinence from drugs, his mental status fluctuated. Once antipsychotic agents were prescribed, he began to feel like himself. He was motivated to complete his GED and entered college. He kept his mental illness a secret. While in graduate school, his thoughts, feelings, and behaviors began to change. His thinking became delusional, his moods unpredictable, and his behaviors illogical. Finally, he was hospitalized once again and his condition was stabilized with medication. Currently, he is reapplying to graduate school and this time vowing to keep people close to him aware of his mental status.

What Do you think?

- What role did stigma play in the treatment process?
- What information should BGN share with his social network about his mental illness and treatment?

INTERDISCIPLINARY TREATMENT

The most effective treatment approach for individuals with schizophrenia involves a variety of disciplines, including nursing (both generalist and advanced practice psychiatric nurses), psychiatry, psychology, social work, occupational and recreational therapy, and pastoral counseling. Pharmacologic management is the responsibility of the physicians and nurses; various psychosocial interventions can be implemented by all of the members of the mental health team. Individuals with general education in psychology, sociology, and social work often serve as case managers, nursing aids or technicians, and other support personnel in hospitals and community treatment agencies. These varied professionals and paraprofessionals are necessary because of the complex nature of the symptoms and chronic course of schizophrenia.

A considerable amount of overlap exists among these professionals and the therapeutic interventions and services they perform. Advanced practice nurses, along with psychiatrists, may monitor or prescribe psychoactive medications, depending on state nurse practice acts. Individual, group, and family counseling may be performed by advanced practice nurses, psychiatrists, psychologists, certified social workers, and pastoral counselors. Nurses, along with occupational and recreational therapists, can help patients with schizophrenia cope with the disruptions in their day-to-day functioning caused by cognitive and social deficits associated with negative symptoms. Teams of professionals working from all of these perspectives create the best environment for stabilizing and enhancing the lives of people who have schizophrenia. However, barriers to this type of treatment abound and include inadequate funding and reimbursements, staff shortages, huge caseloads, and insufficient community facilities to serve patients whose time in inpatient care facilities is all too brief.

Despite the barriers, nurses can play a central role in multidisciplinary teams because of nursing's emphasis on patients' responses to their illnesses, patients' functional adaptation, and patients' holistic needs, including their physical and psychosocial requirements.

PRIORITY OF CARE ISSUES

Several special concerns exist when working with people with schizophrenia. About 20% to 50% of people with the diagnosis of schizophrenia attempt suicide, and 10% commit suicide either as a result of psychosis in acute stages or in response to depression in the chronic phase (De Hert et al., 2001). Suicide assessment always should be done with a person who is experiencing his or her first psychotic episode. In an inpatient unit, patient safety concerns extend to potential aggressive actions toward staff and other patients during episodes of psychoses.

A priority of care during times of acute illness is treatment with antipsychotic medications. During the chronic phase of schizophrenia, patients need help in accepting their illness and developing expectations for their future that are realistic. They also need help to avoid social isolation through improved social and vocational skills and living arrangements that ensure contact with others (De Hert et al., 2001). Interventions that focus on these goals may address the hopelessness that leads to suicide.

FAMILY RESPONSE TO DISORDER 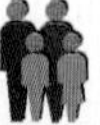

Few families have had the background to help them deal with the manifestations of schizophrenia. The initial episodes are often accompanied by mixed emotions of disbelief, shock, fear, and care and concern for the family member. Hope that this is an isolated or transient episode may also be present. Families initially may seek reasons, attributing the episode to taking illicit drugs or to extraordinary stress or fatigue. They do not know how to comfort their disturbed family member and may find themselves fearful of his or her behaviors. If the patient is hostile and aggressive toward family members, the family may respond with anger and hostility along with fear, confusion, and anxiety. During these episodes, some families seek help from police to help control the situation.

The initial period of illness for a patient and family who receive a diagnosis of schizophrenia is extraordinarily difficult. Families may deny the severity and chronicity of the illness, engage in the activities of their previous lifestyle, and only partially engage in treatment within the mental health system. Often, during the initial phase of treatment, explanation and education about the illness may be minimal. As families acknowledge the severity of the diagnosis and the long-term care and extensive rehabilitation required, they may feel overwhelmed, angry, and depressed (see Box 18.6).

NURSING MANAGEMENT: HUMAN RESPONSE TO SCHIZOPHRENIA

The nursing management of the patient with schizophrenia lasts many years. Different phases of the illness require various nursing interventions. During exacerbation of symptoms, many patients are hospitalized for stabilization. During periods of relative stability, the nurse helps the patient maintain a therapeutic regimen, develop positive mental health strategies, and cope with the stress of having a severe, chronic illness.

Because of the complexity of this major psychiatric disorder, the nursing management for each domain is discussed separately. In reality, the nursing process steps overlap in all domains. For example, medication management is a direct biologic intervention; however, the effects of medications also are seen in psychological functioning. In the clinical area, effective nursing management requires an integration of the assessment data from all domains into meaningful interventions. Nursing interventions should cover all aspects of functioning, including biologic, psychological, social, and family functioning (see Nursing Care Plan 18.1 and the Interdisciplinary Treatment Plan 18.1).

Many nursing diagnoses apply to a person with schizophrenia. This is particularly true given that schizophrenia affects so many aspects of an individual's functioning and that symptoms can be observed in cognitive, emotional, family, social, and physical functioning. The applicable diagnoses can be categorized into the phases in which they are most likely to appear. However, it is important to note that just because they have been sorted into these categories, they may still represent problems in other phases. It is also important

BOX 18.6

***Research for Best Practice:* Impact of Schizophrenia on Siblings**

Lively, S., Friedrich, R. M., & Rubenstein, L. (2004). The effect of disturbing illness behaviors on siblings of persons with schizophrenia. Journal of the American Psychiatric Nurses Association, 10, 222–232.

The Question: What is the impact of schizophrenia on well siblings?

Methods: This study is descriptive and uses a survey methodology. The relationship of type and severity of symptoms to family member stress is described. The authors were interested in the types of behaviors that caused the most stress for the family member. The literature supports a relationship between symptoms and caregiver burden. The authors adapted a conceptual model from the study of caregiver burden among family members of Alzheimer's patients.

Siblings were identified through the National Alliance for the Mentally Ill (NAMI). They completed the Friedrich-Lively Instrument to Assess the Impact of Schizophrenia on Siblings (FLI-ISS). Of 1,254 questionnaires sent to siblings, 761 (60.7%) returned. Respondent siblings' age ranged from 18 to 79; ill siblings ranged in age from 18 to 77. Respondent siblings were 20 years old on average when their sibling had been diagnosed with schizophrenia; they had lived with the ill sibling from 0 to 7 years. Over three quarters of the ill siblings had never married and over half had been hospitalized five times or more.

Findings: The ill siblings' behaviors that the respondents found the most disturbing included "nonsensical communication, disruption of the household, refusal to take medication, social isolation, lack of motivation, and verbal abuse" (p. 227). Three stress scores were calculated: total disturbing behavior, other-directed behavior, and self-directed behavior. The behaviors that contributed the most to the total disturbing behavior score were verbal abuse, disruption of household routine, mood swings, and property damage. For the other-directed score, verbal abuse, property damage, and disturbing neighbors contributed the most statistically. When the researchers explored the behaviors that contributed to the self-directed score, they found that the most disturbing behaviors were inability to care for living space, refusal to take medications, hygiene, and sleep patterns.

Implications for Nursing: The authors suggest that many of these behaviors are related to the chronic nature of schizophrenia. They also suggest that the stress of living with the behaviors of schizophrenia contributes to the physical and emotional illness of siblings. Nurses should develop community-based strategies that minimize the disturbing behaviors of schizophrenia while supporting the family's involvement with their ill member. Nurses should be especially sensitive to the signs of physical and emotional illness of siblings.

to note that the quieter periods between exacerbations of symptoms are actually very active and important phases for intervention.

Biologic Domain

Biologic Assessment

The following discussion highlights the important assessment areas for people with schizophrenia.

Current and Past Health Status and Physical Examination

It is important to conduct a thorough history and physical examination to rule out medical illness or substance abuse that could cause the psychiatric symptoms. It is also important to screen for comorbid medical illnesses that need to be treated, such as diabetes mellitus, hypertension, and cardiac disease or a family history of such disorders. People with schizophrenia have a higher mortality rate from physical illness and often have smoking-related illnesses, such as emphysema, and other pulmonary and cardiac problems. The nurse should determine whether the patient smokes or chews tobacco, which not only affects the patient's health but also can affect the metabolism of medications.

Physical Functioning

The negative symptoms of schizophrenia are often manifested in terms of impairment in physical functioning. Self-care often deteriorates, and sleep may be nonexistent during acute phases. Information regarding physical functioning may best be collected from family members.

• NCLEXNOTE

When assessing a patient with schizophrenia, the nurse should prioritize the severity of the current responses to the disorder. If hallucinations are impairing function, then managing hallucinations is a priority and medications are needed immediately. If hallucinations are not a problem, coping with the negative symptoms becomes a priority.

Nutritional Assessment

A nutritional history should be completed to determine baseline eating habits and preferences. Medications can alter normal nutrition, and the patient may need to limit calories or fat consumption.

Fluid Imbalance Assessment

The nurse should remain alert for signs of polydipsia and polyuria to identify disordered water balance.

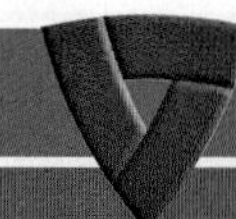

Nursing Care Plan 18.1

The Patient With Schizophrenia

JT is a 19-year-old African American man who was brought to the hospital following his return from college, where he had locked himself in his room for 3 days. He was talking to nonexistent people in a strange language. His room was covered with small pieces of taped paper with single words on them. His parents immediately made arrangements for him to be hospitalized.

Setting: Psychiatric Intensive Care Unit

Baseline Assessment: JT is a 6'1", 145-lb. young man whose appearance is disheveled. He has not slept for 4 days and appears frightened. He is hypervigilant, pacing, and mumbling to himself. He is vague about past drug use, but his parents do not believe that he has used drugs. He appears to be hallucinating, conversing as if someone is in the room. He is confused and unable to write, speak, or think coherently. He is disoriented to time and place. Lab values are within normal limits except hemoglobin, 10.2, and hematocrit, 32. He has not eaten for several days.

Associated Psychiatric Diagnoses

Axis I: Schizophrenia, paranoid
Axis II: None
Axis III: None
Axis IV: Educational problems (failing)
Social problems (withdrawn from peers)
Axis V: Current 25
Potential ?

Medications

Risperidone (Risperdal), 2 mg bid

Lorazepam (Ativan), 2 mg PO or IM for agitation PRN

Nursing Diagnosis 1: Disturbed Thought Processes

Defining Characteristics

- Delusional thinking (people are thinking his thoughts; CIA agents are searching for him because of the plan he has developed)
- Suspiciousness
- Hallucinations (responding to voices that are not heard by others)
- Cognitive impairment—attention, memory, and executive function impairments

Related Factors

- Uncompensated alterations in brain activity

Outcomes

Initial

- Decreased delusional thinking through accurate interpretation of environment
  - Conversations include fewer references to thought broadcasting and concerns about the CIA
- Expresses less suspiciousness about staff and other patients
- Decreased evidence of talking to people that others can't see (fewer vocalizations and observations of responding to sounds that others can't hear)
- Able to participate in activities of increasing length and complexity (e.g., sitting through group and group activities, able to make projects that require increased concentration and contain more steps)

Long-term

- Able to identify and monitor his own experiences of symptoms that indicate an increase in delusional thinking and hallucinations
- Able to use coping mechanisms that will help to minimize or control symptoms of delusions and hallucinations, particularly reaching out to peer, professional, and family support systems
- Able to participate in conversations with others that stay on topic and contain little delusional content
- Able to demonstrate stable cognitive functioning through self-care activities, participation in recreational and vocational activities, and support connections to important others

Continued

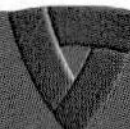

Nursing Care Plan 18.1 *(Continued)*

Interventions

Interventions	Rationale	Ongoing Assessment
• Initiate a nurse–patient relationship by using an accepting, nonjudgmental approach. • Be patient	• A therapeutic relationship will provide patient support as he begins to deal with a devastating disorder. • Be patient because his brain is not processing information normally.	• Determine the extent to which JT is willing to trust and engage in a relationship. • Determine the length of time JT can attend to conversation or activity with others.
• Administer risperidone as prescribed. Observe for affect, side effects, and adverse effects. Begin teaching about the medication and its importance, once symptoms subside.	• Risperidone is a D_2 and 5-HT_{2A} antagonist and is indicated for the treatment of schizophrenia.	• Make sure JT swallows pills. Monitor for relief of positive symptoms using a standardized measure such as the SAPS. Assess side effects, especially extrapyramidal. Monitor BP for orthostatic hypotension and body temperature increase (NMS).
• During hallucinations and delusional thinking, assess significance (what feelings is JT experiencing; what actions do the voices and/or his thoughts suggest he accomplish?). Reassure JT that you will keep him safe; that you are aware that his experiences are very real to him even though you may not be having the same experiences. (Do not try to convince JT that his hallucinations are not real or his delusions are not true.) Redirect JT to here-and-now activities and experiences.	• It is important to understand the experience and context of the hallucinations and delusions to be able to provide appropriate interventions and redirect the patient to more reality-based activities. By avoiding arguments about the content of the patient's delusional beliefs or the experiences of patient's hallucinations, the nurse will enhance communication. Arguing about delusional thoughts or hallucinatory experiences just places the patient in a position to defend his beliefs.	• Assess the meaning of the hallucinations or delusions of the patient. Determine whether he is a danger to himself or others. Determine whether patient can be directed to a more reality-based activity.
• Assess ability for self-care activities.	• Disturbed thinking may interfere with JT's ability to carry out ADLs.	• Continue to assess: Determine whether patient can manage own self-care.

Evaluation

Outcomes	Revised Outcomes	Interventions
• Hallucinations and delusions began to decrease within 3 days. • Is oriented to time, place, and person. Attention and memory improving.	• Participate in unit activities according to ITP. • Agree to continue to take antipsychotic medication as prescribed.	• Encourage attendance at treatment activities. • Teach JT about medications. • Teach JT about schizophrenia.

Nursing Diagnosis 2: Risk for Violence

Defining Characteristics	Related Factors
• Assaultive toward others, self, and environment • Presence of pathophysiologic risk factors: delusional thinking and auditory hallucinations	• Frightened, secondary to auditory hallucinations and delusional thinking • Poor impulse control • Dysfunctional communication patterns

Outcomes

Initial	Long-term
• Avoid hurting self or assaulting other patients or staff. • Decrease agitation and aggression.	• Control behavior with assistance from staff and parents.

Continued

Nursing Care Plan 18.1 (Continued)

Interventions

Interventions	Rationale	Ongoing Assessment
• Acknowledge patient's fear resulting from the experience of hallucinations and delusional thoughts.	• Hallucinations and delusions change an individual's experience of environmental stimuli.	• Assess patient's ability to hear you and respond appropriately to your comments and requests; assess patient's ability to concentrate on what is being said and happening around him.
• Be genuine and empathic.	• The patient will benefit from your ability to understand his experience and express that understanding while presenting reality.	• Assess for evidence that client is less frightened with less potential for striking out.
• Offer patient choices of maintaining safety, including helping patient to be less overwhelmed by the environment: minimize the noise and people around the patient.	• By having choices, he will begin to develop a sense of control over his behavior.	• Observe patient's nonverbal communication for evidence of increased agitation.
• Use medications to help patient relax and maintain more calm: administer lorazepam, 2 mg, for agitation. Oral route is preferable to injection, so offer the patient this choice long before he has lost control.	• Exact mechanisms of action are not understood, but medication is believed to potentiate the inhibitory neurotransmitter γ-aminobutyric acid, relieving anxiety and producing sedation. • Offering this to the patient early, as fear and agitation are beginning to become evident, prevents the potential for the patient to lose control.	• Observe for decrease in agitated behavior.

Evaluation

Outcomes	Revised Outcomes	Interventions
• JT gradually decreased agitated behavior. • Lorazepam was given regularly for first 2 days.	• Demonstrate control of behavior by resisting auditory command hallucinations and delusional thoughts that cause suspicion and fear of others.	• Teach JT about the effects of hallucinations and delusions. • Problem solve ways of controlling response to hallucinations when they occur. • Problem solve ways to refrain from discussing delusional beliefs with people who are unfamiliar with the patient. • Emphasize the importance of taking prescribed antipsychotic medication.

Patients with these symptoms make frequent trips to the water fountain or display other excessive water-drinking behaviors. Polydipsia is difficult to detect in patients who do not drink fluid more often than normal but simply consume large volumes (Boyd & Lapierre, 1996). Patients suspected of having disordered water balance should be assessed, at the least, using daily weights, urine specific gravity, serum sodium levels, and other physiological and observational measures of fluid volume changes.

Pharmacologic Assessment

Baseline information about initial psychological and physical functioning should be obtained before initiation of medication (or as early as possible). Side effects of medications should be assessed. Patients are often physically awkward and have poor coordination, motor abnormalities, and abnormal eye tracking. Before medication begins, standardized assessment of abnormal motor movements should be conducted using one of several assessment tools designed for that purpose, such as the Abnormal Involuntary Movement Scale (AIMS) (see Appendix D); the Dyskinesia Identification System (DISCUS) (Sprague & Kalachnik, 1991) (Table 18.3), or the Simpson-Angus Rating Scale (see Appendix C) (Simpson & Angus, 1970), which is designed for Parkinson's symptoms.

Nursing Diagnoses for Biologic Domain

Typical nursing diagnoses focusing on the biologic domain for the person during all phases of schizophre-

INTERDISCIPLINARY TREATMENT PLAN 18.1

Patient With Schizophrenia

Admission Date	Date of This Plan	Type of Plan: Check Appropriate Box
		☐ Initial ☐ Master ☐ 30 ☐ 60 ☐ 90 ☐ Other

Treatment Team Present:
A. Barton, MD; J. Jones, RNC; C. Anderson, CNS; B. Thomas, PhD; T. Toon, Mental Health Technician (MHT); J. Barker, MHT.

DIAGNOSIS (*DSM-IV-TR*):

AXIS I: Schizophrenia, paranoid
AXIS II: None
AXIS III: None
AXIS IV: Educational problems (failing)
Social problems (withdrawn from peers)
AXIS V: Current GAF: 25
Highest-Level GAF This Past Year: 90

ASSETS (MEDICAL, PSYCHOLOGICAL, SOCIAL, EDUCATIONAL, VOCATIONAL, RECREATIONAL):

1. First episode of psychosis. No evidence of drug use.
2. Premorbid functional level appears to be normal.
3. Maintained good grades in high school.
4. Has supportive family members.

				Change	
Prob. No.	*Date*	*Problem/Need*	*Code*	*Code*	*Date*
1	3/5/08	Is hallucinating and had delusional thoughts. Unable to communicate with parents or staff.		T	
2	3/5/08	Is aggressive and is striking out at staff and unfamiliar people.		T	
3	3/5/08	Dropped out of college because of thoughts and behaviors.		X	
4	3/5/08	Family members are very upset about their son's psychiatric symptoms.		T	

CODE T = Problem must be addressed in treatment.
N = Problem noted and will be monitored.
X = Problem noted, but deferred/inactive/no action necessary.
O = Problem to be addressed in aftercare/continuing care.
I = Problem incorporated into another problem.
R = Resolved.

INDIVIDUAL TREATMENT PLAN PROBLEM SHEET

#1 Problem/Need	*Date Identified*	*Problem Resolved Discontinuation Date*
	3/5/08	

Is hallucinating and has delusional thoughts. Unable to communicate with parents or staff.

Objective(s)/Short-Term Goals	*Target Date*	*Achievement Date*
1. Reduce report and observations of hallucinations and delusions.	3/15/08	

(Continued on following page)

INTERDISCIPLINARY TREATMENT PLAN 18.1 (Continued)

Treatment Interventions	Frequency	Person Responsible
1. Antipsychotic therapy for hallucinations and delusions. Administer and monitor for adherence, effect, and side effects.	As prescribed	MD/RN
2. Monitor frequency of hallucinations and delusions.	Close observation for 24–48 hours, then according to RN judgment	RN/MHT
3. Attend Symptom Management group as symptoms subside.	Daily	PhD, RN

#2 Problem/Need	Date Identified	Problem Resolved/Discontinuation Date
	3/5/08	

Is aggressive and is hitting out at staff and unfamiliar people.

Objective(s)/Short-Term Goals	Target Date	Achievement Date
1. De-escalate aggressive behavior.	3/15/08	

Treatment Interventions	Frequency	Person Responsible
1. Keep patient in a quiet, nonstimulating environment.Assign private room.	Ongoing	RN
2. Administer antianxiety medication as needed.	PRN	MD/RN
3. Use de-escalation techniques when approaching patient.	Ongoing	Everyone
4. Assign to anger management group if needed when psychotic symptoms decrease.	In 1 week	CNS

#3 Problem/Need	Date Identified	Problem Resolved/Discontinuation Date
	3/5/08	

Family members are very upset about their son's psychiatric symptoms.

Objective(s)/Short-Term Goals	Target Date	Achievement Date
Increase family's comfort levels with mental illness.	3/15/08	

Treatment Interventions	Frequency	Person Responsible
1. Meet with family each time they visit. Provide counseling and education to family.	Ongoing	CNS/RN/MD/PhD
2. Encourage to attend family support group.	Weekly	PhD
3. Provide community resources for the treatment of mental illness.	When visiting	CNS

Responsible QMHP		Client or Guardian		Staff Physician	
Signature	Date	Signature	Date	Signature	Date

nia include Self-Care Deficit and Disturbed Sleep Pattern. During a relapse, Ineffective Therapeutic Regimen Management, Imbalanced Nutrition, Excess Fluid Volume, and Sexual Dysfunction are possible diagnoses. Constipation may occur if the patient takes anticholinergic medications.

• NCLEXNOTE

Monitoring actions and side effects of medications are priority nursing interventions. Conventional antipsychotics are used with increasing frequency and should be easily recognized. The older medications will be used occasionally.

Interventions for Biologic Domain

Nursing interventions during the initial acute phase of schizophrenia include prompt, safe, and informed administration of antipsychotic medications. During any stage, attention to self-care needs and the patient's ability to maintain hygiene and adequate nutrition are important.

Promotion of Self-Care Activities

For many with schizophrenia, the plan of care will include specific interventions to enhance self-care,

Table 18.3 The Dyskinesia Identification System (DISCUS)

____

(facility)

Dyskinesia Identification System: Condensed User Scale (DISCUS)

CURRENT PSYCHOTROPICS/ANTI-CHOLINERGIC AND TOTAL MG/DAY

_______________ _____ mg

_______________ _____ mg

_______________ _____ mg

_______________ _____ mg

See Instructions on Other Side

NAME I.D.

EXAM TYPE (check one)
- □ 1. Baseline
- □ 2. Annual
- □ 3. Semi annual
- □ 4. D/C—1 mo
- □ 5. D/C—2 mo
- □ 6. D/C—3 mo
- □ 7. Admission
- □ 8. Other

COOPERATION (check one)
- □ 1. None
- □ 2. Partial
- □ 3. Full

SCORING
- 0—**Not present** (movements not observed or some movements observed but not considered abnormal)
- 1—**Minimal** (abnormal movements are difficult to detect or movements are easy to detect but occur only once or twice in a short nonrepetitive manner)
- 2—**Mild** (abnormal movements occur infrequently and are easy to detect)
- 3—**Moderate** (abnormal movements occur frequently and are easy to detect)
- 4—**Severe** (abnormal movements occur almost continuously **and** are easy to detect)
- NA—**Not assessed** (an assessment for an item is not able to be made)

ASSESSMENT
DISCUS Item and Score (circle one score for each item)

Area	Item	Score
FACE	1. Tics	0 1 2 3 4 NA
	2. Grimaces	0 1 2 3 4 NA
EYES	3. Blinking	0 1 2 3 4 NA
ORAL	4. Chewing/Lip Smacking	0 1 2 3 4 NA
	5. Puckering/Sucking/Thrusting Lower Lip	0 1 2 3 4 NA
LINGUAL	6. Tongue Thrusting/Tongue in Cheek	0 1 2 3 4 NA
	7. Tonic Tongue	0 1 2 3 4 NA
	8. Tongue Tremor	0 1 2 3 4 NA
	9. Athetoid/Myokymic/Lateral Tongue	0 1 2 3 4 NA
HEAD NECK/ TRUNK	10. Retrocollis/Torticollis	0 1 2 3 4 NA
	11. Shoulder/Hip Torsion	0 1 2 3 4 NA
UPPER LIMB	12. Athetoid/Myokymic Finger–Wrist–Arm	0 1 2 3 4 NA
	13. Pill Rolling	0 1 2 3 4 NA
LOWER LIMB	14. Ankle Flexion/Foot Tapping	0 1 2 3 4 NA
	15. Toe Movement	0 1 2 3 4 NA

COMMENTS/OTHER

____

____

____

____

____

TOTAL SCORE (items 1–15 only) ____

EXAM DATE

EVALUATION (see other side)

1. Greater than 90 days neuroleptic exposure?	:	YES	NO
2. Scoring/intensity level met?	:	YES	NO
3. Other diagnostic conditions? (if yes, specify)	:	YES	NO

____

____

____

4. Last exam date: ________
   Last total score: ________
   Last conclusion: ________

Preparer signature and title for items 1–4 (if different from physician):

5. Conclusion (circle one):
   - A. No TD (if scoring prerequisite met, list other diagnostic condition or explain in comments)
   - B. Probable TD
   - C. Masked TD
   - D. Withdrawal TD
   - E. Persistent TD
   - F. Remitted TD
   - G. Other (specify in comments)

6. Comments:

____

____

____

____

____

____

____

____

RATER SIGNATURE AND TITLE	NET EXAM DATE	CLINICIAN SIGNATURE	DATE

From Sprague, R. L., & Kalachnik, J. E. (1991). Reliability, validity, and a total score cutoff for the Dyskinesia Identification System, Condensed User Scale (DISCUS) with mentally ill and mentally retarded populations. *Psychopharmacology Bulletin, 27*(1), 51–58.

nutrition, and overall health knowledge. Negative symptoms commonly leave patients unable to initiate these seemingly simple activities. Developing a daily schedule of routine activities (such as showering and shaving) can help the patient structure the day. Most patients actually know how to perform self-care activities (e.g., hygiene, grooming) but are not motivated (avolition) to carry them out consistently. Interventions include developing a schedule with the patient for various hygiene activities and emphasizing the importance of maintaining appropriate self-care activities. Given the problems related to attention and memory in people with schizophrenia, education about these areas requires careful planning.

Activity, Exercise, and Nutritional Interventions

Encouraging activity and exercise is necessary, not only to maintain a healthy lifestyle, but also to counteract the side effects of psychiatric medications that cause weight gain. Because the diagnosis is usually made in late adolescence or early adulthood, it is possible to establish solid exercise patterns early.

During episodes of acute psychosis, patients are unable to focus on eating. Often when patients begin antipsychotic medication, normal satiety and hunger responses change, and overeating or weight gain can become a problem. Promoting healthy nutrition is a key intervention. Maintaining healthy nutrition and monitoring calorie intake also becomes important because of the effect many medications have on eating habits. Patients report that appetite increases and cravings for food develop when some medications are initiated.

Weight gain is one of the reasons some patients become resistant to taking medication. It also may be a contributing factor to the development of type II diabetes mellitus. Increased weight places patients at greater risk for several health complications and early death. Monitoring for diabetes and managing weight are important activities for all care providers (Stahl, 2002). Patients should be screened for risk factors of diabetes, such as family history, obesity as indicated by a body mass index (BMI) exceeding or equal to 27, and age older than 45 years. Patients' weight should be measured at regular intervals and the BMI calculated. Blood pressure readings should be taken regularly. Laboratory findings for triglycerides, HDL cholesterol, and glucose level should be monitored and reviewed regularly. All providers should be alert to the development of hyperglycemia, particularly in patients known to have diabetes who begin taking new antipsychotic agents. A program to address weight gain should be initiated at the earliest sign of weight gain (probably between 5 and 10 pounds over desired body weight). Reduced caloric intake may be accomplished by increasing the patient's access to affordable, healthful, and easy-to-prepare foods. Behavioral management of weight gain includes keeping a food diary, diet teaching, and support groups.

Thermoregulation Interventions

Patients with schizophrenia may have disturbed body temperature regulation. In winter, they may seem to be oblivious to cold weather. In the heat of summer, they may dress for winter. Observing patients' responses to temperatures helps in identifying problems in this area. In patients who are taking psychiatric medications, body temperature needs to be monitored, and the patient needs to be protected from extremes in temperature.

Promotion of Normal Fluid Balance and Prevention of Water Intoxication

Nursing interventions for disordered water balance include teaching and assisting the patient to develop self-monitoring skills. Fluid intake and weight gain should be monitored to control fluid intake and reduce the likelihood of developing water intoxication.

Patients can be classified as having mild, moderate, or severe disordered water balance based on the signs and symptoms outlined in Box 18.3. Patients with mild disordered water balance are easily treated in outpatient settings and benefit from educational programs that teach them to monitor their own urine specific gravity and daily weight gains. Patients classified with moderate disordered water balance may respond well to education but have a more difficult time controlling their own fluid intake. Using a targeted weight procedure, a baseline weight is established, a targeted weight is calculated, and the patient is regularly weighed throughout the day (Box 18.7). Patients are taught that a 5- to 7-pound weight gain in 1 to 3 hours indicates too much fluid. Exceeding the targeted weight places the patient at risk for water intoxication. Patients with severe disordered water balance require considerable assistance to restrict their continual water-seeking behavior. These patients may create considerable disruption in an inpatient setting but often are best managed by one-on-one observation to redirect their behavior.

Pharmacologic Interventions: Antipsychotics

Early in the 20th century, somatic treatment of schizophrenia included hydrotherapy (baths), wet-pack sheets, insulin shock therapy, electroconvulsive therapy, psychosurgery, and occupational and physical therapy. But in the early 1950s, treatment of schizophrenia drastically changed with the accidental discovery that a drug, chlorpromazine, used to induce anesthesia also calmed patients with schizophrenia. Following this dis-

BOX 18.7

Water Intoxication Protocol

I. Observation: evidence of polydipsia and polyuria
II. Assessment of fluid balance
   A. History of polydipsia and polyuria
   B. Hyponatremia: serum Na^+ <135 mEq/L
   C. Hyposthenuria: urine specific gravity <1.1005
III. Interventions:
   A. If the above symptoms are present, institute the following interventions
      1. Target weight procedure
      2. Assess behavioral changes daily
      3. Monitor urine specific gravity daily
      4. Identify specific interventions for helping patient develop control over fluid intake and learn self-monitoring skills
         a. Cognitive therapy approaches
         b. Individual or group therapy approaches
         c. Arrange access to sugarless candies, gum, and fruit to reduce feelings of thirst
         d. Limit access to fluids during the day
   B. If weight reaches or exceeds target weight, initiate the following:
      1. Prohibit fluid intake
      2. Restrict to program and residential area
      3. Assess vital signs q1h × 2
      4. Provide low-fluid diet after symptoms subside
   C. If more severe symptoms develop, notify physician and transfer patient to a medical unit.
IV. Evaluation
   A. Patient gains control over fluid balance as evidenced by developing strategies to stay under target weight.
   B. If there is no evidence of water intoxication and there is evidence that patient is gaining control over fluid balance, the target weight procedure and daily assessments of behavior and urine specific gravity can be discontinued.

covery, a new category of medication was developed: first-generation (or conventional) antipsychotics.

Antipsychotic drugs have the general effect of blocking dopamine transmission in the brain by blocking D_2 receptors to some degree (see Chapter 8). Some also block other dopamine receptors and receptors of other neurotransmitters to varying degrees. For the most part, the antidopamine effects are not specific to the mesolimbic and mesocortical tracts associated with schizophrenia, but instead travel to all the dopamine receptor sites throughout the brain. This results in desirable antipsychotic effects but also creates some unpleasant and undesirable side effects. The effects of these drugs on other neurotransmitter systems account for additional side effects.

The second-generation antipsychotic drugs risperidone (Risperdal) (Box 18.8), olanzapine (Zyprexa), quetiapine (Seroquel), paliperidone (Invega), ziprasidone (Geodon), and aripiprazole (Abilify) appear to be more efficacious and safer than conventional antipsychotics. They are available in a variety of formulations. Risperidone is also available in a long-acting injectable form (Consta). They are effective in treating negative and positive symptoms. These newer drugs also affect several other neurotransmitter systems, including serotonin. This is believed to contribute to their antipsychotic effectiveness (see Chapter 7).

Monitoring and Administering Medications

Antipsychotic medications are the treatment of choice for patients with psychosis. The use of conventional antipsychotics (e.g., haloperidol, chlorpromazine) decreased dramatically with the introduction of the second generation of antipsychotics. Generally, it takes about 1 to 2 weeks for antipsychotic drugs to effect a change in symptoms. During the stabilization period, the type of drug selected should be given an adequate trial, generally 6 to 12 weeks, before considering a change in the drug prescription. If treatment effects are not seen, another antipsychotic agent may be tried. Clozapine (Clozaril) is used when no other atypical antipsychotic is effective (see Box 18.9 for more information about clozaril).

Adherence to a prescribed medication regimen is the best approach to preventing relapse. Unfortunately, patient compliance with medication with atypical antipsychotic agents is not much different from that with conventional antipsychotic agents (Dolder, Lacro, Dunn, & Jeste, 2002). The use of long-acting injectables is expected to improve compliance outcomes (see Box 18.10).

Patients with schizophrenia generally face a lifetime of taking antipsychotic medications. Rarely is discontinuation of medications prescribed; however, many patients stop taking medications on their own. Some situations that require the cessation of medication use are neuroleptic malignant syndrome (see later) or agranulocytosis (dangerously low level of circulating neutrophils). Discontinuation is an option when tardive dyskinesia develops. Discontinuation of medications, other than in circumstances of a medical emergency, should be achieved by gradually lowering the dose over time. This diminishes the likelihood of withdrawal symptoms, which include withdrawal dyskinesias and withdrawal psychosis.

BOX 18.8

Drug Profile: Risperidone (Risperdal)

DRUG CLASS: Atypical antipsychotic

RECEPTOR AFFINITY: Antagonist with high affinity for D_2 and 5-HT_2, also histamine (H_1) and α_{1-}, α_2-adrenergic receptors, weak affinity for D_1 and other serotonin receptor subtypes; no affinity for acetylcholine or β-adrenergic receptors.

INDICATIONS: Treatment of schizophrenia, short-term treatment of acute manic or mixed episodes associated with bipolar I disorder, irritability associated with autistic disorder in children and adolescents, including symptoms of aggression towards others, deliberate self-injuriousness, temper tantrums, and quickly changing moods.

ROUTES AND DOSAGE: 0.25-, 0.5-, 1-, 2-, 3-, and 4-mg tablets and liquid concentrate (1 mg/mL). Orally disintegrating tablets, 0.5-, 1-, 2-, 3-, and 4-mg.

Adult: Schizophrenia: Initial dose: typically 1 mg bid. Maximal effect at 6 mg/d. Safety not established above 16 mg/d. Use lowest possible dose to alleviate symptoms.
Bipolar mania: 2 to 3 mg per day

Geriatric: Initial dose, 0.5 mg/d, increase slowly as tolerated.

Children: 0.25 mg per day for patients < 20 kg & 0.5 mg per day > 20 kg.

HALF-LIFE (PEAK EFFECT): mean, 20 h (1 h, peak active metabolite = 3–17 h).

SELECT ADVERSE REACTIONS: Insomnia, agitation, anxiety, extrapyramidal symptoms, headache, rhinitis, somnolence, dizziness, headache, constipation, nausea, dyspepsia, vomiting, abdominal pain, hypersalivation, tachycardia, orthostatic hypotension, fever, chest pain, coughing, photosensitivity, weight gain.

BOXED WARNING: Increased mortality in elderly patients with dementia-related psychosis

WARNING: Rare development of neuroleptic malignant syndrome. Observe frequently for early signs of tardive dyskinesia. Use caution with individuals who have cardiovascular disease; risperidone can cause ECG changes. Avoid use during pregnancy or while breastfeeding. Hepatic or renal impairments increase plasma concentration.

SPECIFIC PATIENT/FAMILY EDUCATION

- Notify prescriber if tremor, motor restlessness, abnormal movements, chest pain, or other unusual symptoms develop.
- Avoid alcohol and other CNS depressant drugs.
- Notify prescriber if pregnancy is possible or planning to become pregnant. Do not breastfeed while taking this medication.
- Notify prescriber before taking any other prescription or OTC medication.
- May impair judgment, thinking, or motor skills; avoid driving or other hazardous tasks.
- During titration, the individual may experience orthostatic hypotension and should change positions slowly.
- Do not abruptly discontinue.

BOX 18.9

Drug Profile: Clozapine (Clozaril)

DRUG CLASS: Atypical antipsychotic

RECEPTOR AFFINITY: D_1 and D_2 blockade, antagonist for 5-HT_2, histamine (H_1), α-adrenergic, and acetylcholine. These additional antagonist effects may contribute to some of its therapeutic effects. Produces fewer extrapyramidal effects than standard antipsychotics with lower risk for tardive dyskinesia.

INDICATIONS: Severely ill individuals who have schizophrenia and have not responded to standard antipsychotic treatment; reduction in risk of recurrent suicidal behavior in schizophrenia or schizoaffective disorders

ROUTES AND DOSAGE: Available only in tablet form, 25- and 100-mg doses.

Adult Dosage: Initial dose 25 mg PO bid or qid, may gradually increase in 25–50 mg/d increments, if tolerated, to a dose of 300–450 mg/d by the end of the second week. Additional increases should occur no more than once or twice weekly. Do not exceed 900 mg/d. For maintenance, reduce dosage to lowest effective level.

Children: Safety and efficacy with children under 16 years have not been established.

HALF-LIFE (PEAK EFFECT): 12 h (1–6 h).

SELECT ADVERSE REACTIONS: Drowsiness, dizziness, headache, hypersalivation, tachycardia, hypo/hypertension, constipation, dry mouth, heartburn, nausea/vomiting, blurred vision, diaphoresis, fever, weight gain, hematologic changes, seizures, tremor, akathisia.

BOXED WARNING: Agranulocytosis, defined as a granulocyte count of <500 mm^3 occurs at about a cumulative 1-year incidence of 1.3%, most often within 4–10 weeks of exposure, but may occur at any time. WBC count before initiation, and weekly WBC counts while taking the drug and for 4 weeks after discontinuation.
Seizures, myocarditis, and other adverse cardiovascular and respiratory effects (orthostatic hypotension)

WARNING: Increased mortality in elderly patients with dementia-related psychosis
Rare development of neuroleptic malignant syndrome. *Hyperglycemia and diabetes, tardive dyskinesia,* cases of sudden, unexplained death have been reported. Avoid use during pregnancy or while breastfeeding.

PRECAUTIONS: fever, pulmonary embolism, hepatitis, anticholinergic toxicity, and interference with cognitive and motor functions.

SPECIFIC PATIENT/FAMILY EDUCATION

- Need informed consent regarding risk for agranulocytosis. Weekly or biweekly blood draws are required. Notify

(Continued on following page)

BOX 18.9

Drug Profile: Clozapine (Clozaril) (Continued)

prescriber immediately if lethargy, weakness, sore throat, malaise, or other flu-like symptoms develop.
- You should not take Clozaril if taking other medicines that cause the same serious bone marrow side effects.
- Inform patient of risk of seizures, hyperglycemia and diabetes, and orthostatic hypotension. It may potentiate the hypotensive effects of antihypertensive drugs and anticholinergic effects of atropine-type drugs.
- Administration of epinephrine should be avoided in the treatment of drug-induced hypotension.
- Notify prescriber if pregnancy is possible or planning to become pregnant. Do not breastfeed while taking this medication.
- Notify prescriber before taking any other prescription or OTC medication. Avoid alcohol or other CNS depressant drugs.
- May cause drowsiness and seizures; avoid driving or other hazardous tasks.
- During titration, the individual may experience orthostatic hypotension and should change positions slowly.
- Do not abruptly discontinue.

Monitoring Side Effects

Extrapyramidal Side Effects. *Parkinsonism* that is caused by antipsychotic drugs is identical in appearance to Parkinson's disease and tends to occur in older patients. The symptoms are believed to be caused by the blockade of D_2 receptors in the basal ganglia, which throws off the normal balance between acetylcholine and dopamine in this area of the brain and effectively increases acetylcholine.

The symptoms are managed by re-establishing the balance between acetylcholine and dopamine by either reducing the dosage of the antipsychotic (thereby increasing dopamine activity) or adding an anticholinergic drug (decreasing acetylcholine activity), such as benztropine (Cogentin) or trihexyphenidyl (Artane).

Discontinuation of the use of anticholinergic drugs should never be abrupt, which can cause a cholinergic rebound and result in withdrawal symptoms, such as vomiting, excessive sweating, and altered dreams and nightmares. Thus, the anticholinergic drug dosage should be reduced gradually (tapered) over several days. If a patient experiences akathisia (physical restlessness), an anticholinergic medication may not be particularly helpful. Table 18.4 lists anticholinergic side

BOX 18.10

Research for Best Practice: ***Awareness of Illness and Medication Adherence***

Kozuki, Y., & Froelicher, E. S. (2003). Lack of awareness and nonadherence in schizophrenia. Western Journal of Nursing Research, 25, 57–74.

The Question: How does the awareness of illness and symptoms on the part of the patient with schizophrenia predict the success of taking prescribed medications as directed?

Methods: Patients with a schizophrenia spectrum disorder (based on the DSM-IV criteria) from three metropolitan hospitals with a total of seven acute psychiatric units were included in this cross-sectional descriptive study. These participants had been prescribed at least one oral psychotropic medication for the 3 weeks prior to admission to one of the psychiatric units in the study. A total of 134 participants agreed to participate. They were primarily men (64%) from a variety of ethnic backgrounds: 41.6% were Caucasian, 30.6% were African American, 18.7% were Asian/Pacific Islander, and 7.5% were Latino. Almost 50% were living in unstable surroundings; 19% were actually homeless. Participants were assessed with the Scale to Assess Unawareness of Mental Disorder (SUMD), which is an observer rating scale with three dimensions related to awareness of mental illness, necessity of medications, and social consequences and an assessment of specific psychiatric symptoms. Nonadherence with drug regimen was defined as taking less than 50% of the prescribed medications during the 3 weeks prior to admission. Participants were also asked the reasons for not taking medications using the Rating on Medication Influences Scale (ROMI). Clinician assessment of psychiatric symptoms was done on the Positive and Negative Syndrome Scale (PANSS).

Findings: The symptom that participants were most aware of was hallucinating; the symptoms for which they experienced the least awareness were delusional thinking and poor social judgment. In terms of awareness of illness, 41.7% were fully aware and accepting of their illness, 19.7% were somewhat aware, and 38.6% were unaware or in denial about their illness. The researchers found that almost a quarter of the sample had taken medications as prescribed prior to their hospitalization; 56.1% took no prescribed psychotropic medications prior to their hospitalization. The remaining participants had a variety of experiences with medication taking. The sample was divided into two groups (adherent and nonadherent) and statistical analyses were completed to examine the most contributory variables. Homelessness was the single variable that most affected the outcome of nonadherence to taking medications. The authors also found some support for their hypothesis in that symptom lack of awareness was also associated with nonadherence. Experiences of side effects from psychotropic medications also had an impact on taking prescribed medications.

Implications for Nursing: The authors suggest that maximizing patient awareness of symptoms and assisting patients with symptom self management are interventions that may enhance adherence to psychiatric medications. Clearly, advocating for patients to have the most stable living arrangements after discharge is suggested by the strong association of homelessness and nonadherence to medications.

Table 18.4 Nursing Interventions for Anticholinergic Side Effects

Effect	Intervention
Dry mouth	Sips of water; hard candies and chewing gum (preferably sugar free)
Blurred vision	Avoid dangerous tasks; teach patient that this side effect will diminish in a few weeks
Decreased lacrimation	Artificial tears if necessary
Mydriasis	May aggravate glaucoma; teach patient to report eye pain
Photophobia	Sunglasses
Constipation	High-fiber diet; increased fluid intake; laxatives as prescribed
Urinary hesitancy	Privacy; run water in sink; warm water over perineum
Urinary retention	Regular voiding (at least every 2–3 h) and whenever urge is present; catheterize for residual; record intake and output; evaluate benign prostatic hypertrophy
Tachycardia	Evaluate for pre-existing cardiovascular disease; sudden death has occurred with thioridazine (Mellaril)

effects of antiparkinson drugs and several antipsychotic medications and interventions to manage them.

Dystonic reactions are also believed to result from the imbalance of dopamine and acetylcholine, with the latter dominant. Young men seem to be more vulnerable to this particular extrapyramidal side effect. This side effect, which develops rapidly and dramatically, can be very frightening for patients as their muscles tense and their body contorts. The experience often starts with **oculogyric crisis**, in which the muscles that control eye movements tense and pull the eyeball so that the patient is looking toward the ceiling. This may be followed rapidly by **torticollis**, in which the neck muscles pull the head to the side, or **retrocollis**, in which the head is pulled back, or orolaryngeal-pharyngeal hypertonus, in which the patient has extreme difficulty swallowing. The patient may also experience contorted extremities. These symptoms occur early in antipsychotic drug treatment, when the patient may still be experiencing psychotic symptoms. This compounds the patient's fear and anxiety and requires a quick response. The immediate treatment is to administer benztropine (Cogentin), 1 to 2 mg, or diphenhydramine (Benadryl), 25 to 50 mg, intramuscularly or intravenously. This is followed by daily administration of anticholinergic drugs and, possibly, by a decrease in antipsychotic medication (see Box 18.11 for more information about benztropine).

Akathisia appears to be caused by the same biologic mechanism as other extrapyramidal side effects. Patients are restless and report they feel driven to keep moving. They are very uncomfortable. Frequently, this response is misinterpreted as anxiety or increased psychotic symptoms, and the patient may be inappropriately given increased dosages of antipsychotic drug, which only perpetuates the side effect. If possible, the dose of antipsychotic drug should be reduced. A beta-adrenergic blocker such as propranolol (Inderal), 20 to 120 mg, may be required. Failure to manage this side effect is a leading cause of patients ceasing to take antipsychotic medications. See Chapter 8.

Tardive dyskinesia, tardive dystonia, or tardive akathisia are less likely to appear in individuals taking atypical, rather than conventional, antipsychotics. Table 18.5 describes these and associated motor abnormalities. **Tardive dyskinesia** is late-appearing abnormal involuntary movements (dyskinesia). It can be viewed as the opposite of parkinsonism both in observable movements and in etiology. Whereas muscle rigidity and absence of movement characterize parkinsonism, constant movement characterizes tardive dyskinesia. Typical movements involve the mouth, tongue, and jaw and include lip smacking, sucking, puckering, tongue protrusion, the bonbon sign (where the tongue rolls around in the mouth and protrudes into the cheek as if the patient were sucking on a piece of hard candy), athetoid (worm-like) movements in the tongue, and chewing. Other facial movements, such as grimacing and eye blinking, also may be present.

Movements in the trunk and limbs are frequently observable. These include rocking from the hips, athetoid movements of the fingers and toes, jerking movements of the fingers and toes, guitar strumming movements of the fingers, and foot tapping. The long-term health problems for people with tardive dyskinesia are choking associated with loss of control of muscles used for swallowing and compromised respiratory function leading to infections and possibly respiratory alkalosis.

Because the movements resemble the dyskinetic movements of some patients who have idiopathic Parkinson's disease and who have received long-term treatment with L-dopa (a direct-acting dopamine agonist that crosses the blood–brain barrier), the suggested hypothesis for tardive dyskinesia includes the supersensitivity of the dopamine receptor in the basal ganglia.

There is no consistently effective treatment; however, antipsychotic drugs mask the movements of tardive dyskinesia and have periodically been suggested as a treatment. This is counterintuitive because these are the drugs that cause the disorder. Newer antipsychotic drugs, such as clozapine, may be less likely to cause the disorder. The best management remains prevention through using the lowest possible dose of antipsychotic

BOX 18.11

Drug Profile: ***Benztropine mesylate (Cogentin)***

DRUG CLASS: Antiparkinson agent

RECEPTOR AFFINITY: Blocks cholinergic (acetylcholine) activity, which is believed to restore acetylcholine/dopamine balance in the basal ganglia.

INDICATIONS: Used in psychiatry to reduce extrapyramidal symptoms (acute medication-related movement disorders), including pseudoparkinsonism, dystonia, and akathisia (not tardive syndromes) due to neuroleptic drugs such as haloperidol. Most effective with acute dystonia.

ROUTES AND DOSAGE: Available in tablet form, 0.5-, 1-, and 2-mg doses, also injectable 1 mg/mL.

Adult Dosage: For acute dystonia, 1–2 mg IM or IV usually provides rapid relief. No significant difference in onset of action after IM or IV injection. Treatment of emergent symptoms may be relieved in 1 or 2 days, with 1–2 mg orally 2–3 times/d. Maximum daily dose is 6 mg/d. After 1–2 weeks withdraw drug to see if continued treatment is needed. Medication-related movement disorders that develop slowly may not respond to this treatment.

Geriatric: Older adults and very thin patients cannot tolerate large doses.

Children: Do not use in children under 3. Use with caution in older children.

HALF-LIFE: 12–24 h, very little pharmacokinetic information is available.

SELECT ADVERSE REACTIONS: Dry mouth, blurred vision, tachycardia, nausea, constipation, flushing or elevated temperature, decreased sweating, muscular weakness or cramping, urinary retention, urinary hesitancy, dizziness, headache, disorientation, confusion, memory loss, hallucinations, psychoses, and agitation in toxic reactions, which are more pronounced in the elderly and occur at smaller doses.

WARNING: Avoid use during pregnancy or while breastfeeding. Give with caution in hot weather due to possible heatstroke. Contraindicated with angle-closure glaucoma, pyloric or duodenal obstruction, stenosing peptic ulcers, prostatic hypertrophy or bladder neck obstructions, myasthenia gravis, megacolon, or megaesophagus. May aggravate the symptoms of tardive dyskinesia or other chronic forms of medication-related movement disorder. Concomitant use of other anticholinergic drugs may increase side effects and risk for toxicity. Coadministration of haloperidol or phenothiazines may reduce serum levels of these drugs.

SPECIFIC PATIENT/FAMILY EDUCATION

- Take with meals to reduce dry mouth and gastric irritation.
- Dry mouth may be alleviated by sucking sugarless candies, adequate fluid intake, or good oral hygiene; increase fiber and fluids in diet to avoid constipation; stool softeners may be required. Notify prescriber if urinary hesitancy or constipation persists.
- Notify prescriber if rapid or pounding heartbeat, confusion, eye pain, rash, or other adverse symptoms develop.
- May cause drowsiness, dizziness, or blurred vision; use caution driving or performing other hazardous tasks requiring alertness. Avoid alcohol and other CNS depressants.
- Do not abruptly stop this medication because a flu-like syndrome may develop.
- Use caution in hot weather. Ensure adequate hydration. May increase susceptibility to heat stroke.

drug over time that minimizes the symptoms of schizophrenia (see Table 18.5).

Orthostatic hypotension is another side effect of antipsychotic drugs. Primarily an antiadrenergic effect, decreased blood pressure may be general or orthostatic. Patients may be protected from falls by teaching them to rise slowly and by monitoring blood pressure before giving the medication. The nurse should monitor and

Table 18.5 Extrapyramidal Side Effects of Antipsychotic Drugs

Side Effect	Period of Onset	Symptoms
Acute Motor Abnormalities		
Parkinsonism or pseudoparkinsonism	5–30 d	Resting tremor, rigidity, bradykinesia/akinesia, mask-like face, shuffling gait, decreased arm swing
Acute dystonia	1–5 d	Intermittent or fixed abnormal postures of the eyes, face, tongue, neck, trunk, and extremities
Akathisia	1–30 d	Obvious motor restlessness evidenced by pacing, rocking, shifting from foot to foot; subjective sense of not being able to sit or be still; these symptoms may occur together or separately
Late-Appearing Motor Abnormalities		
Tardive dyskinesia	Months to years	Abnormal dyskinetic movements of the face, mouth, and jaw; choreoathetoid movements of the legs, arms, and trunk
Tardive dystonia	Months to years	Persistent sustained abnormal postures in the face, eyes, tongue, neck, trunk, and limbs
Tardive akathisia	Months to years	Persisting, unabating sense of subjective and objective restlessness

Adapted from Casey, D.E. (1994). Schizophrenia: Psychopharmacology. In J. W. Jefferson & J. H. Greist (Eds.), *The Psychiatric Clinics of North America Annual of Drug Therapy* (Vol. 1, pp. 81–100). Philadelphia: W. B. Saunders.

document lying, sitting, and standing blood pressures when any antipsychotic drug therapy begins.

Hyperprolactinemia can occur. When dopamine is blocked in the tuberoinfundibular tract, it can no longer repress prolactin, the neurohormone that regulates lactation and mammary function. The prolactin level increases and, in some individuals, side effects appear. Gynecomastia (enlarged breasts) can occur among both sexes and is understandably distressing to individuals who may be experiencing delusional or hallucinatory body image disturbances. Galactorrhea (lactation) also may occur. Menstrual irregularities and sexual dysfunction are also possible. If these symptoms appear, the medication should be reduced or changed to another antipsychotic agent. Hyperprolactinemia is associated with the use of haloperidol and risperidone.

Weight gain is related to antipsychotic agents, especially olanzapine and clozapine. Patients may gain as much as 20 or 30 pounds within 1 year. Increased appetite and weight gain are distressing to patients. Diet teaching and monitoring may have some effect on this side effect. Another solution is to increase the accessibility of healthful, easy-to-prepare food.

Sedation is another possible side effect of antipsychotic medication. Patients should be monitored for the sedating effects of antipsychotic agents. In elderly patients, sedation can be associated with falls.

New-onset diabetes should be assessed in patients taking antipsychotic drugs. There is an association between new-onset diabetes mellitus and the administration of atypical antipsychotic agents, especially olanzapine and clozapine. Patients should be monitored for clinical symptoms of diabetes. Fasting blood glucose tests are commonly ordered for these individuals.

Cardiac arrhythmias may also occur. Prolongation of the QTc interval is associated with torsades de pointes (polymorphic ventricular tachycardia) or ventricular fibrillation. The potential for drug-induced prolonged QT interval is associated with many drugs. Ziprasidone (Geodon) is more likely than other atypical antipsychotics to prolong the QT interval and change the heart rhythm. For these patients, baseline electrocardiograms may be ordered. Nurses should observe these patients for cardiac arrhythmias.

Agranulocytosis is a reduction in the number of circulating granulocytes and decreased production of granulocytes in the bone marrow that limits one's ability to fight infection. Agranulocytosis can develop with the use of all antipsychotic drugs, but it is most likely to develop with clozapine use. Although laboratory values below 500 cells/mm^3 are indicative of agranulocytosis, often granulocyte counts drop to below 200 cells/mm^3 with this syndrome.

Patients taking clozapine should have regular blood tests. White blood cell and granulocyte counts should be measured before treatment is initiated and at least weekly or twice weekly after treatment begins. Initial white blood cell counts should be above 3,500 cells/mm^3 before treatment initiation; in patients with counts of 3,500 and 5,000 cells/mm^3, cell counts should be monitored three times a week if clozapine is prescribed. Any time the white blood cell count drops below 3,500 cells/mm^3 or granulocytes drop below 1,500 cells/mm^3, use of clozapine should be stopped, and the patient should be monitored for infection.

However, a faithfully implemented program of blood monitoring should not replace careful observation of the patient. It is not unusual for blood cell counts to drop precipitously in a period of 2 to 3 days. This may not be discovered when the patient is on a strict weekly blood monitoring schedule. Any reported symptoms that are reminiscent of a bacterial infection (fever, pharyngitis, and weakness) should be cause for concern, and immediate evaluation of blood count status should be undertaken. Because patients are frequently discharged before the critical period of risk for agranulocytosis, patient education about these symptoms is also essential so that they will report these symptoms and obtain blood monitoring. In general, granulocytes return to normal within 2 to 4 weeks after discontinuation of use of the medication.

Drug–Drug Interactions

Several potential drug–drug interactions are possible when administering antipsychotic medications. One of the cytochrome P450 enzymes responsible for the metabolism of olanzapine and clozapine is 1A2. If either olanzapine or clozapine is given with another medication that inhibits this enzyme, such as fluvoxamine (Luvox), the antipsychotic blood level could increase and possibly become toxic. On the other hand, cigarette smoking can also induce 1A2 and lower concentration of drugs metabolized by this enzyme, such as olanzapine and clozapine. Smokers may require a higher dose of these medications than do nonsmokers (Stahl, 2000).

Several atypical antipsychotic agents, including clozapine, quetiapine, and ziprasidone, are metabolized by the 3A4 enzyme. Weak inhibitors of this enzyme include the antidepressants fluvoxamine, nefazodone, and norfluoxetine (an active metabolite of fluoxetine). Potent inhibitors of 3A4 enzyme include ketoconazole (antifungal), protease inhibitors, and erythromycin. If these drugs are given with clozapine, quetiapine, or ziprasidone, the antipsychotic level will rise. In addition, the mood stabilizer carbamazepine (Tegretol) is a 3A4 inducer. When this drug is given with clozapine, quetiapine, or ziprasidone, the antipsychotic dose should be increased to compensate for the 3A4 induction. If the use of carbamazepine is discontinued, dosage of the antipsychotic agent needs to be adjusted (Stahl, 2000).

Risperidone, clozapine, and olanzapine are substrates for the enzyme 2D6. Theoretically, antidepressants (fluoxetine and paroxetine) that inhibit this enzyme could increase levels of these antipsychotics. However, this is not usually clinically significant (Stahl, 2000).

Pharmacologic Intervention: Anticholinergics

Anticholinergics are administered for parkinsonism and dystonia secondary to antipsychotic medication (see Chapter 8). There is also potential for abuse of anticholinergic drugs. Some patients may find the anticholinergic effects of these drugs on mood, memory, and perception pleasurable. Although at toxic dosages, patients may experience disorientation and hallucinations, lesser doses may cause patients to experience greater sociability and euphoria.

Teaching Points 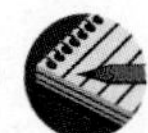

Nonadherence to the medication regimen is an important factor in relapse; the family must be made aware of the importance of the patient consistently taking medications. Medication education should cover the association between medications and the amelioration of symptoms, side effects and their management, and interpersonal skills that help the patient and family report medication effects.

Emergency! Neuroleptic Malignant Syndrome 

In neuroleptic malignant syndrome (NMS), severe muscle rigidity develops with elevated temperature and a rapidly accelerating cascade of symptoms (occurring during the next 48 to 72 hours), which can include two or more of the following: hypertension, tachycardia, tachypnea, prominent diaphoresis, incontinence, mutism, leukocytosis, changes in level of consciousness ranging from confusion to coma, and laboratory evidence of muscle injury (e.g., elevated creatinine phosphokinase). NMS occurs in about 1% of those who receive antipsychotic drugs, especially the conventional antipsychotics such as haloperidol (and other drugs that block dopamine, such as metoclopramide) (Montoya, Ocampo, & Torres-Ruiz, 2003). As many as one third of these patients may die as a result of the syndrome. NMS is probably underreported and may account for unexplained emergency room deaths of patients taking these drugs who do not have diagnoses because their symptoms do not seem serious. The presenting symptom is a temperature greater than 99.5°F (usually between 101°F and 103°F) with no apparent cause.

The most important aspects of nursing care for patients with NMS relate to recognizing symptoms early, holding any antipsychotic (any dopamine-blocking agent) medications, and initiating supportive nursing care (see Figure 18.5). In any patient with fever, fluctuating vital signs, abrupt changes in levels of consciousness, or any of the symptoms presented in Box 18.12, NMS should be suspected. The nurse should be especially alert for early signs and symptoms of NMS in high-risk patients, such as those who are agitated, physically exhausted, or dehydrated or who have an existing medical or neurologic illness. Patients receiving parenteral or higher doses of neuroleptic drugs or lithium concurrently must also be carefully assessed. The nurse should carefully monitor fluid intake and fluid and electrolyte status.

• NCLEXNOTE

NCLEXNOTE

Recognition of side effects, including movement disorders, tardive dyskinesia, and weight gain, should lead to interventions. Neuroleptic malignant syndrome is a medical emergency.

Medical treatment includes administering dopamine agonist drugs, such as bromocriptine (modest success), and muscle relaxants, such as dantrolene or benzodiazepine. Antiparkinsonism drugs are not particularly useful. Some patients experience improvement with electroconvulsive therapy.

The vital signs of the patient with symptoms of NMS must be monitored frequently. In addition, it is important to check the results of the patient's laboratory tests for increased creatine phosphokinase, elevated white blood cell count, elevated liver enzymes, or myoglobinuria. The nurse must be prepared to initiate supportive measures or anticipate emergency transfer of the patient to a medical-surgical or an intensive care unit.

Treating high temperature (which frequently exceeds 103°F) is an important priority for these patients. High body temperature may be reduced with a cooling blanket and acetaminophen. Because many of these patients experience diaphoresis, temperature elevation, or dysphagia, it is important to monitor fluid hydration. Another important aspect of care for patients with NMS is safety. Joints and extremities that are rigid or spastic must be protected from injury. The treatment of these patients depends on the facility and availability of medical support services. In general, patients in psychiatric inpatient units that are separated from general hospitals are transferred to medical-surgical settings for treatment.

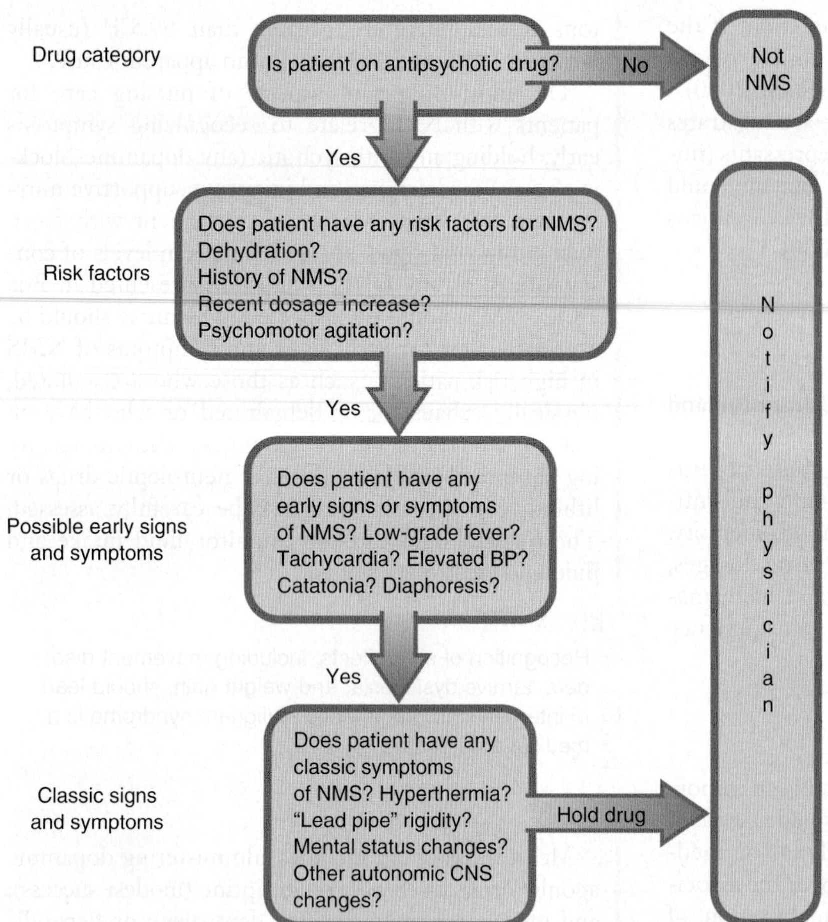
Drug category
Is patient on antipsychotic drug?
No
Not NMS
Yes
Risk factors
Does patient have any risk factors for NMS?
Dehydration?
History of NMS?
Recent dosage increase?
Psychomotor agitation?
Notify physician
Yes
Possible early signs and symptoms
Does patient have any early signs or symptoms of NMS? Low-grade fever? Tachycardia? Elevated BP? Catatonia? Diaphoresis?
Yes
Classic signs and symptoms
Does patient have any classic symptoms of NMS? Hyperthermia? "Lead pipe" rigidity? Mental status changes? Other autonomic CNS changes?
Hold drug

FIGURE 18.5. Action tree for "holding" an antipsychotic drug because of suspected neuroleptic malignant syndrome.

Emergency! Anticholinergic Crisis 

Anticholinergic crisis is a potentially life-threatening medical emergency caused by an overdose of or sensitivity to drugs with anticholinergic properties. This syndrome (also called anticholinergic delirium) may result from an accidental or intentional overdose of antimuscarinic drugs, including atropine, scopolamine, or belladonna alkaloids, which are present in numerous prescription drugs and over-the-counter medicines. The syndrome may also occur in psychiatric patients who are receiving therapeutic doses of anticholinergic drugs, especially when such agents are combined with other psychotropic drugs that produce anticholinergic side effects. Numerous drugs commonly prescribed in psychiatric settings produce anticholinergic side effects, including tricyclic antidepressants and some antipsychotics. As a result of either drug overdose or sensitivity, these anticholinergic substances may produce an acute delirium or a psychotic reaction resembling schizophrenia. More severe anticholinergic effects may occur in older patients, even at therapeutic levels (Stahl, 2000).

BOX 18.12

*Diagnostic Criteria for Neuroleptic Malignant Syndrome**

1. Treatment with antipsychotics within 7 days of onset (2–4 weeks for depot neuroleptic medications).
2. Hyperthermia
3. Muscle rigidity
4. Five of the following:
   - Change in mental status
   - Tachycardia
   - Hypertension or hypotension
   - Tachypnea or hypoxia
   - Diaphoresis or sialorrhea
   - Tremor
   - Incontinence
   - Creatinine phosphokinase elevation or myoglobinuria
   - Leukocytosis
   - Metabolic acidosis
5. Exclusion of other drug-induced, systemic, or neuropsychiatric illnesses

*All five items are required concurrently.

From Caroff, S., & Mann, S. (1993). Neuroleptic malignant syndrome. *Medical Clinics of North America, 77*, 185–202. Used with permission.

BOX 18.13

Signs and Symptoms of Anticholinergic Crisis

Neuropsychiatric signs: confusion; recent memory loss; agitation; dysarthria; incoherent speech; pressured speech; delusions; ataxia; periods of hyperactivity alternating with somnolence, paranoia, anxiety, or coma

Hallucinations: accompanied by "picking," plucking, or grasping motions; delusions; or disorientation

Physical signs: unreactive dilated pupils; blurred vision; hot, dry, flushed skin; facial flushing; dry mucous membranes; difficulty swallowing; fever; tachycardia; hypertension; decreased bowel sounds; urinary retention; nausea; vomiting; seizures; or coma

The signs and symptoms of anticholinergic crisis are dramatic and physically uncomfortable (Box 18.13). This disorder is characterized by elevated temperature; parched mouth; burning thirst; hot, dry skin; decreased salivation; decreased bronchial and nasal secretions; widely dilated eyes (bright light is painful); decreased ability to accommodate visually; increased heart rate; constipation; difficulty urinating; and hypertension or hypotension. The face, neck, and upper arms may become flushed because of a reflex blood vessel dilation. In addition to peripheral symptoms, patients with anticholinergic psychosis may experience neuropsychiatric symptoms of anxiety, agitation, delirium, hyperactivity, confusion, hallucinations (especially visual), speech difficulties, psychotic symptoms, or seizures. The acute psychotic reaction that is produced resembles schizophrenia. The classic description of anticholinergic crisis is summarized in the following mnemonic: "Hot as a hare, blind as a bat, mad as a hatter, dry as a bone."

In general, episodes of anticholinergic crisis are self-limiting, usually subsiding in 3 days. However, if untreated, the associated fever and delirium may progress to coma or cardiac and respiratory depression. Although rare, death is generally due to hyperpyrexia and brain stem depression. Once use of the offending drug is discontinued, improvement usually occurs within 24 to 36 hours.

A specific and effective antidote, physostigmine, an inhibitor of anticholinesterase, is frequently used for treating and diagnosing anticholinergic crisis. Administration of this drug rapidly reduces both the behavioral and physiologic symptoms. However, the usual adult dose of physostigmine is 1 to 2 mg intravenously, given slowly during a period of 5 minutes because rapid injection of physostigmine may cause seizures, profound bradycardia, or heart block. Physostigmine is relatively short acting, so it may need to be given several times during the course of treatment. This drug provides relief from symptoms for a period of 2 to 3 hours. In addition to receiving physostigmine, patients who intentionally overdose on large amounts of anticholinergic drugs are treated by gastric lavage, administration of charcoal, and catharsis. The dose may be repeated after 20 or 30 minutes.

It is important for the nurse to be alert for signs and symptoms of anticholinergic crisis, especially in elderly and pediatric patients, who are much more sensitive to the anticholinergic effects of drugs, and in patients who are receiving multiple medications with anticholinergic effects. If signs and symptoms of the syndrome occur, the nurse should discontinue use of the offending drug and notify the physician immediately.

Other Somatic Interventions

Electroconvulsive therapy is suggested as a possible alternative when the patient's schizophrenia is not being successfully treated by medication alone. There are recent reports of electroconvulsive therapy as an augmentation to antipsychotic therapy (Ota et al., 2003; Tang & Ungvari, 2003). For the most part, this is not indicated unless the patient is catatonic or has a depression that is not treatable by other means.

Psychological Domain

Although schizophrenia is a brain disorder, the psychological manifestations are the most difficult to assess and treat. Many of these psychological manifestations improve with the use of medications, but they are not necessarily eliminated.

Psychological Assessment

Several assessment scales have been developed to help evaluate positive and negative symptom clusters in schizophrenia. Box 18.14 lists standardized instruments used in assessing symptoms of patients with schizophrenia. These include the Scale for the Assessment of Positive Symptoms (SAPS) (Box 18.15), the Scale for the Assessment of Negative Symptoms (SANS) (Box 18.16), and the Positive and Negative Syndrome Scale (PANSS) (Kay, Fiszbein, & Opler, 1987), which assesses both symptom clusters in the same instrument. Tools that list symptoms, such as the Brief Psychiatric Rating Scale (see Appendix B), SANS, or SAPS can also be used to help patients self-monitor their symptoms.

Usually, information about prediagnosis experiences requires retrospective reporting by the patient or the family. This reporting is reliable for the frankly psychotic symptoms of delusions and hallucinations; however, negative symptoms are more difficult to date. In fact, negative symptoms vary from a slight deviation from normal to a clear impairment. Negative symp-

BOX 18.14

Rating Scales for Use With Schizophrenia

Scale for the Assessment of Negative Symptoms (SANS)
Available from Nancy C. Andreasen, MD, PhD, Department of Psychiatry, College of Medicine, The University of Iowa, Iowa City, IA 52242. Copyright 1984. *See Box 18–15.*

Scale for the Assessment of Positive Symptoms (SAPS)
Available from Nancy C. Andreasen (see above). *See Box 18–15.*

Positive and Negative Syndrome Scale (PANSS)
Kay, S. R., Fiszbein, A., & Opler, L. A. (1987). The Positive and Negative Syndrome Scale (PANSS) for Schizophrenia. *Schizophrenia Bulletin, 13,* 261–276. Available from first author.

Abnormal Involuntary Movement Scale (AIMS)
Guy, W. (1976), *ECDEU: Assessment manual for psychopharmacology* (DHEW Publication No. 76-338). Washington, DC: Department of Health, Education, and Welfare, Psychopharmacology Branch.

Brief Psychiatric Rating Scale (BPRS)
Overall, J. E., & Gorham, D. R. (1988). The Brief Psychiatric Rating Scale (BPRS): Recent developments in ascertainment and scaling. *Psychopharmacology Bulletin, 24,* 97–99.

Dyskinesia Identification System: Condensed User Scale (DISCUS)
Sprague, R. L., & Kalachnik, J. E. (1991). Reliability, validity, and a total score cutoff for the Dyskinesia Identification Scale System: Condensed User Scale (DISCUS) with mentally ill and mentally retarded populations. *Psychopharmacology Bulletin, 27*(1), *51–58. See Table 18–3.*

Simpson-Angus Rating Scale
Simpson, G. M., Angus, J. W. S. L. (1970). A rating scale for extrapyramidal side effects. *Acta Psychiatrica Scandinavica (Suppl), 212,* 11–19. Copyright 1970 Munksgaard International Publishers, Ltd.

toms probably occur earlier than positive symptoms but are less easily recognized (Box 18.17).

Responses to Mental Health Problems

Schizophrenia robs people of mental health and imposes social stigma. People with schizophrenia struggle to maintain control of their symptoms, which affect every aspect of their life. The person with schizophrenia displays a variety of interrelated symptoms and experiences deficits in several areas. More than half of patients report the following prodromal symptoms (in order of frequency): tension and nervousness, lack of interest in eating, difficulty concentrating, disturbed sleep, decreased enjoyment and loss of interest, restlessness, forgetfulness, depression, social withdrawal from friends, feeling laughed at, more religious thinking, feeling bad for no reason, feeling too excited, and hearing voices or seeing things.

Because schizophrenia is a disorder of thoughts, perceptions, and behavior, it is sometimes not recognized as an illness by the person experiencing the symptoms. Many people with thought disorders do not believe that they have a mental illness. Their denial of mental illness and the need for treatment poses problems for the family and clinicians. Ideally, in lucid moments, patients recognize that their thoughts are really delusions, that their perceptions are hallucinations, and that their behavior is disorganized. In reality, many patients do not believe that they have a mental illness but agree to treatment to please family and clinicians.

Mental Status and Appearance

The patient may look eccentric or disheveled or have poor hygiene and bizarre dress. The patient's posture may suggest lethargy or stupor.

Mood and Affect

Patients with schizophrenia often display altered mood states. In some cases, they may show heightened emotional activity; others may display severely limited emotional responses. Affect, the outward expression of mood, is categorized on a continuum: flat (emotional expression entirely absent), blunted (expression of emotions present but greatly diminished), and full range. Inappropriate affect is marked by incongruence between the emotional expression and the thoughts expressed. Other common emotional symptoms include the following:

- **Affective lability**—abrupt, dramatic, unprovoked changes in type of emotions expressed
- **Ambivalence**—the presence and expression of two opposing feelings, leading to inaction
- **Apathy**—reactions to stimuli are decreased, diminished interest and desire

Speech

Speech patterns may reflect obsessions, delusions, pressured thinking, loose associations, or flight of ideas and neologism. Speech is an indicator of thought content and other mental processes and is usually altered. An assessment of speech should note any difficulty articulating words (dysarthria) and difficulty swallowing (dysphagia) as indicators of medication side effects. In many instances, what an individual says is as important as how it is said. Both content and speech patterns should be noted.

Thought Processes and Delusions

Delusions can be distinguished from strongly held ideas by "the degree of conviction with which the belief

BOX 18.15

Scale for the Assessment of Positive Symptoms (SAPS)

0=None 1=Questionable 2=Mild 3=Moderate 4=Marked 5=Severe

Hallucinations

1 *Auditory Hallucinations* 0 1 2 3 4 5
The patient reports voices, noises, or other sources that no one else hears.

2 *Voices Commenting* 0 1 2 3 4 5
The patient reports a voice that makes a running commentary on his behavior or thoughts.

3 *Voices Conversing* 0 1 2 3 4 5
The patient reports hearing two or more voices conversing.

4 *Somatic or Tactile Hallucinations* 0 1 2 3 4 5
The patient reports experiencing peculiar physical sensations in the body.

5 *Olfactory Hallucinations* 0 1 2 3 4 5
The patient reports experiencing unusual smells that no one else notices.

6 *Visual Hallucinations* 0 1 2 3 4 5
The patient sees shapes or people that are not actually present.

7 *Global Rating of Hallucinations* 0 1 2 3 4 5
This rating should be based on the duration and severity of the hallucinations and their effect on the patient's life.

Delusions

8 *Persecutory Delusions* 0 1 2 3 4 5
The patient believes he is being conspired against or persecuted in some way.

9 *Delusions of Jealousy* 0 1 2 3 4 5
The patient believes his spouse is having an affair with someone.

10 *Delusions of Guilt or Sin* 0 1 2 3 4 5
The patient believes that he has committed some terrible sin or done something unforgivable.

11 *Grandiose Delusions* 0 1 2 3 4 5
The patient believes he has special powers or abilities.

12 *Religious Delusions* 0 1 2 3 4 5
The patient is preoccupied with false beliefs of a religious nature.

13 *Somatic Delusions* 0 1 2 3 4 5
The patient believes that somehow his body is diseased, abnormal, or changed.

14 *Delusions of Reference* 0 1 2 3 4 5
The patient believes that insignificant remarks or events refer to him or have some special meaning.

15 *Delusions of Being Controlled* 0 1 2 3 4 5
The patient feels that his feelings or actions are controlled by some outside force.

16 *Delusions of Mind Reading* 0 1 2 3 4 5
The patient feels that people can read his mind or know his thoughts.

17 *Thought Broadcasting* 0 1 2 3 4 5
The patient believes that his thoughts are broadcast so that he or others can hear them.

18 *Thought Insertion* 0 1 2 3 4 5
The patient believes that thoughts that are not his own have been inserted into his mind.

19 *Thought Withdrawal* 0 1 2 3 4 5
The patient believes that thoughts have been taken away from his mind.

20 *Global Rating of Delusions* 0 1 2 3 4 5
This rating should be based on the duration and persistence of the delusions and their effects on the patient's life.

Bizarre Behavior

21 *Clothing and Appearance* 0 1 2 3 4 5
The patient dresses in an unusual manner or does other strange things to alter his appearance.

22 *Social and Sexual Behavior* 0 1 2 3 4 5
The patient may do things considered inappropriate according to usual social norms (e.g., masturbating in public).

23 *Aggressive and Agitated Behavior* 0 1 2 3 4 5
The patient may behave in an aggressive, agitated manner, often unpredictably.

24 *Repetitive or Stereotyped Behavior* 0 1 2 3 4 5
The patient develops a set of repetitive actions or rituals that he must perform over and over.

25 *Global Rating of Bizarre Behavior* 0 1 2 3 4 5
This rating should reflect the type of behavior and the extent to which it deviates from social norms.

Positive Formal Thought Disorder

26 *Derailment* 0 1 2 3 4 5
A pattern of speech in which ideas slip off track onto ideas obliquely related or unrelated.

27 *Tangentiality* 0 1 2 3 4 5
Replying to a question in an oblique or irrelevant manner.

28 *Incoherence* 0 1 2 3 4 5
A pattern of speech that is essentially incomprehensible at times.

29 *Illogicality* 0 1 2 3 4 5
A pattern of speech in which conclusions are reached that do not follow logically.

30 *Circumstantiality* 0 1 2 3 4 5
A pattern of speech that is very indirect and delayed in reaching its goal idea.

31 *Pressure of Speech* 0 1 2 3 4 5
The patient's speech is rapid and difficult to interrupt; the amount of speech produced is greater than that considered normal.

32 *Distractible Speech* 0 1 2 3 4 5
The patient is distracted by nearby stimuli that interrupt his flow of speech.

33 *Clanging* 0 1 2 3 4 5
A pattern of speech in which sounds rather than meaningful relationships govern word choice.

34 *Global Rating of Positive Formal Thought Disorder* 0 1 2 3 4 5
This rating should reflect the frequency of abnormality and degree to which it affects the patient's ability to communicate.

Inappropriate Affect

35 *Inappropriate Affect* 0 1 2 3 4 5
The patient's affect is inappropriate or incongruous, not simply flat or blunted.

BOX 18.16

Scale for the Assessment of Negative Symptoms (SANS)

0=None 1=Questionable 2=Mild 3=Moderate 4=Marked 5=Severe

Affective Flattening or Blunting

1 *Unchanging Facial Expression* 0 1 2 3 4 5
The patient's face appears wooden, changes less than expected as emotional content of discourse changes.

2 *Decreased Spontaneous Movements* 0 1 2 3 4 5
The patient shows few or no spontaneous movements, does not shift position, move extremities, etc.

3 *Paucity of Expressive Gestures* 0 1 2 3 4 5
The patient does not use hand gestures, body position, etc., as an aid to expressing ideas.

4 *Poor Eye Contact* 0 1 2 3 4 5
The patient avoids eye contact or "stares through" interviewer even when speaking.

5 *Affective Nonresponsivity* 0 1 2 3 4 5
The patient fails to smile or laugh when prompted.

6 *Lack of Vocal Inflections* 0 1 2 3 4 5
The patient fails to show normal vocal emphasis patterns, is often monotonic.

7 *Global Rating of Affective Flattening* 0 1 2 3 4 5
This rating should focus on overall severity of symptoms, especially unresponsiveness, eye contact, facial expression, and vocal inflections.

Alogia

8 *Poverty of Speech* 0 1 2 3 4 5
The patient's replies to questions are restricted in amount; tend to be brief, concrete, and unelaborated.

9 *Poverty of Content of Speech* 0 1 2 3 4 5
The patient's replies are adequate in amount but tend to be vague, overconcrete, or overgeneralized, and convey little information.

10 *Blocking* 0 1 2 3 4 5
The patient indicates, either spontaneously or with prompting, that his train of thought was interrupted.

11 *Increased Latency of Response* 0 1 2 3 4 5
The patient takes a long time to reply to questions; prompting indicates that the patient is aware of the question.

12 *Global Rating of Alogia* 0 1 2 3 4 5
The core features of alogia are poverty of speech and poverty of content.

Avolition–Apathy

13 *Grooming and Hygiene* 0 1 2 3 4 5
The patient's clothes may be sloppy or soiled, and patient may have greasy hair, body odor, etc.

14 *Impersistence at Work or School* 0 1 2 3 4 5
The patient has difficulty seeking or maintaining employment, completing school work, keeping house, etc. If an inpatient, cannot persist at ward activities, such as OT, playing cards, etc.

15 *Physical Anergia* 0 1 2 3 4 5
The patient tends to be physically inert. May sit for hours and does not initiate spontaneous activity.

16 *Global Rating of Avolition–Apathy* 0 1 2 3 4 5
Strong weight may be given to one or two prominent symptoms if particularly striking.

Anhedonia–Asociality

17 *Recreational Interests and Activities* 0 1 2 3 4 5
The patient may have few or no interests. Both the quality and quantity of interests should be taken into account.

18 *Sexual Activity* 0 1 2 3 4 5
The patient may show a decrease in sexual interest and activity, or enjoyment when active.

19 *Ability to Feel Intimacy and Closeness* 0 1 2 3 4 5
The patient may display an inability to form close or intimate relationships, especially with the opposite sex and family.

20 *Relationships With Friends and Peers* 0 1 2 3 4 5
The patient may have few or no friends and may prefer to spend all of time isolated.

21 *Global Rating of Anhedonia–Asociality* 0 1 2 3 4 5
This rating should reflect overall severity, taking into account the patient's age, family status, etc.

Attention

22 *Social Inattentiveness* 0 1 2 3 4 5
The patient appears uninvolved or unengaged. May seem "spacey."

23 *Inattentiveness During Mental Status Testing* 0 1 2 3 4 5
Tests of "serial 7s" (at least five subtractions) and spelling "world" backward: Score: 2 = 1 error; 3 = 2 errors; 4 = 3 errors.

24 *Global Rating of Attention* 0 1 2 3 4 5
This rating should assess the patient's overall concentration, clinically and on tests.

From Nancy C. Andreasen, MD, PhD, Department of Psychiatry, College of Medicine, The University of Iowa, Iowa City, IA 52242.

is held despite clear contradictory evidence" (APA, 2000, p. 299). Culture must be considered when evaluating delusions. Delusional beliefs are those not sanctioned or held by a cultural or religious subgroup.

Bizarre delusions alone are sufficient to diagnose schizophrenia. It can often be difficult to distinguish between bizarre and nonbizarre delusions. Nonbizarre delusions generally have themes of jealousy and persecution and are derived from ordinary life experiences. For example, a woman believes that her husband, from whom she has recently separated, is trying to poison her, or a man believes that members of the Mafia are trying to kill him because, when he was in high school, he reported to the principal that several of his classmates were selling drugs at school (APA, 2000).

Bizarre delusions are those that are impossible, illogical, and not derived from ordinary life experiences. Bizarre delusions often include delusions of control (that some outside force controls thoughts and actions), thought broadcasting (that others can read or hear

BOX 18.17

Understanding A Son's Symptoms of Schizophrenia

Dr. Willick (1994) described his reactions and observations of his son diagnosed with schizophrenia:

...Struggling as he does with many of what we now call the "negative symptoms," he has lost that gleam in his eye, that joyous good humor, that zest for life which he once showed. Today, it is hard for him to feel things strongly, or to enjoy his music, sports, or being with his family....There has also been a significant cognitive impairment. Things that he was easily able to grasp when he was 14 years old are now much harder for him. He has lost considerable capacity for abstract thinking. His language is very concrete and has lost the richness and subtlety of expression it once had. He has a hard time following a moderately complicated plot of an article he reads or a movie he sees, and he can describe it only in a superficial and concrete way (pp. 8–9).

I know that I should be most proud of Gary, and I can often feel that. The problem is that it is not easy to see that he is displaying great courage in coping with what has happened to him. The symptoms of the illness make him appear lacking in motivation, initiative, and will, and even he accuses himself of not trying hard enough. It is hard for an observer to see how difficult it must be for him to get up every day, hoping to feel different, only to awake with the same feeling of anhedonia. In some ways, those admirable qualities that he possessed before he became ill are no doubt serving him well as he tries to fight an illness that none of us, let alone Gary himself, can really comprehend (pp. 11–12).

Willick, M. S. (1993). Schizophrenia: A parent's perspective—mourning without end. In N.C. Andreasen (Ed.), *Schizophrenia: From mind to molecule* (pp. 5–19). Washington, D.C.: American Psychiatric Press.

one's thoughts), thought insertion (that someone has placed thoughts into one's mind), and thought withdrawal (that someone is removing thoughts from one's mind) (APA, 2000). For example, a patient who has been with a hypnotist for 2 months reports that the hypnotist continued to read his mind and was "picking his brain away piece by piece." Another patient was convinced that a computer chip was placed in her vagina during a gynecologic examination and that this somehow directly influenced her physical movements and her thoughts.

Assessing and judging the content of the delusion and exploring other aspects of the delusional experience is helpful in understanding the significance of these false beliefs. The underlying feeling that accompanies the delusion should be identified. Other aspects to consider include the conviction with which the delusion is held; the extent other aspects of the individual's life are incorporated or affected by the delusion; the degree of internal consistency, organization, and logic evidenced in the delusion; and evaluating the amount of pressure (in terms of preoccupation and concern) individuals feel in their lives as a result of the delusion (see Box 18.18).

Hallucinations

Hallucinations are the most common example of disturbed sensory perception observed in patients with schizophrenia. Hallucinations can be experienced in all sensory modalities; however, auditory hallucinations are the most common in schizophrenia. Some specific hallucinations may be sufficient to diagnose schizophrenia, such as hearing voices conversing with each other or carrying on a discussion with someone who is not there. Because most individuals will not spontaneously share their hallucinatory experiences with an interviewer, the nurse may need to rely on indirect evidence in the patient's behavior, such as (1) pauses during conversations in which the individual seems preoccupied or appears to be listening to someone other than the interviewer, (2) looking toward the perceived source of a voice, or (3) responding to the voices in some manner. Although patients may not spontaneously share their hallucinations, many validate observations of the examiner or admit to a history of hallucinations when asked (see Box 18.19).

Disorganized Communication

The other aspect of thought content and processes that may be altered in schizophrenia is the organization of expressed thoughts. Impaired verbal fluency (ability to produce spontaneous speech) is commonly present. Abrupt shifts in the focus of conversation are a typical symptom of disorganized thinking. The most severe shifts in focus may occur after only one or two words (word salad), after one or two phrases or sentences (flight of ideas or loose associations), or somewhat less severely as a shift that occurs when a new topic is repeatedly suggested and pursued from the current topic (tangentiality).

Cognitive Impairments

Although cognitive impairments in schizophrenia vary widely from patient to patient, several primary problems have been identified:

- Attention may be increased and sustained on external stimuli over a period of time (hypervigilance)
- The ability to distinguish and focus on relevant stimuli may be diminished
- Familiar cues may go unrecognized or be improperly encoded
- Information processing may be diminished, leading to inappropriate or illogical conclusions from available observations and information (Cirillo &

BOX 18.18

Therapeutic Dialogue: The Patient With Delusions

John joined the nurse in a game of pool. The following conversation occurred as they played.

Ineffective Approach

John: The CIA put a transmitter in my molar, here (points to his right cheek).

Nurse: No one would put a transmitter in your tooth; come on, the CIA isn't looking for you.

John: You get the striped ones. Yeah, they want to monitor me while I'm here. I know that they have the real Jenna Bush here in the hospital. They are trying to get George Bush to intervene with the Michigan Militia. Mark from Michigan told me that.

Nurse: Jenna Bush can't possibly be here, I saw her on television this morning.

John: Maybe—she does have darker hair and has different colored contacts to disguise her eyes, but they're just trying to keep people from knowing what they're doing.

Nurse: John, Jenna Bush isn't in the hospital; if she were, I would know it because I work here.

John: (With anger) You don't know anything! You are probably from the CIA also. I have nothing else to say to you.

Effective Approach

John: The CIA put a transmitter in my molar, here (points to his right cheek).

Nurse: Oh. Which balls are mine?

John: You get the striped ones. Yeah, they want to monitor me while I'm here. I know that they have the real Jenna Bush here in the hospital. They are trying to get George Bush to intervene with the Michigan Militia. Mark from Michigan told me that.

Nurse: I suppose it could be Jenna Bush, but do you suppose that it could just be someone who looks like her?

John: Maybe—she does have darker hair and has different colored contacts to disguise her eyes. But they're just trying to keep people from knowing what they're doing.

Nurse: You sound a little overwhelmed with all the information you have.

John: No, no. I can handle it. The CIA can't do anything to me, I' ll never talk.

Nurse: I thought they could hear you when you talk to me.

John: Huh? Oh, that transmitter is so that they can send me misinformation. They send a tower of babble to my brain. They are trying to confuse me so that I stay away from Jenna Bush. They all think they can keep me from my mission.

Nurse: Who's they?

John: Everyone in the government. The CIA, FBI, ATF, IRS—all those alphabets.

Nurse: So everyone in the government is trying to get to you.

John: Well, maybe not everybody. Just the ones that care about money and the militia. I don't think they care about me much in commerce or health and human services. Although they'd care too if they knew.

Nurse: I would think that's pretty frightening to have all these people out looking for you. You must be scared a lot.

John: It's scary but I can handle it. I've handled it all my life.

Nurse: You've been in scary situations all your life?

John: Yeah. I don't know. Maybe not scary, just hard. I never seemed to be able to do as well as my parents wanted—or as I wanted.

Critical Thinking Challenge

- How did the nurse's argumentative responses cause the patient to react in the first scenario?
- What effective communication techniques did the nurse use in the second scenario?

Seidman, 2003; Hartman, Steketee, Silva, Lanning, & Andersson, 2003).

Cognitive impairments are not easy to recognize. By relying only on clinical assessment, the nurse can miss the extent of the impairment. Using a standardized instrument, such as the Mini-Mental Status Examination (MMSE) or the Cognitive Abilities Screening Instrument (CASI), can provide a screening measurement of cognitive function (see Chapter 10). If impairment exists, neuropsychological testing by a qualified psychologist may be necessary.

Memory and Orientation

Impairments in orientation, memory, and abstract thinking may be observed. Orientation to time, place, and person may remain relatively intact unless the patient is particularly preoccupied with delusions and hallucinations. Although all aspects of memory may be affected in schizophrenia, registration or the recall within seconds of newly learned information may be particularly diminished. This affects the individual's short-term and long-term memory. The ability to engage in abstract thinking may be impaired.

Insight and Judgment

Individuals display insight when they display evidence of knowing their own thoughts, the reality of external objects, and their relationship to these. Judgment is the ability to decide or act about a situation. Insight and judgment are closely related to each other and depend on cognitive functions that are frequently impaired in people with schizophrenia.

Behavioral Responses

During periods of psychosis, unusual or bizarre behavior often occurs. These behaviors can usually be under-

BOX 18.19

Therapeutic Dialogue: The Patient With Hallucinations

The following conversation took place in a dayroom with several staff in the room. The patient was potentially very violent. Although it is a good example of dealing with someone who is hallucinating it is not a situation that should be taken lightly. Always make certain that you have a means to leave a situation (i.e., that you are not in the corner of a room), that the patient does not have a potential weapon, and that you have sufficient staff close by so that you are safe.

Jason approached the nurse and asked to play pool. The nurse debated about playing but chose to play because Jason appeared distracted, and the game might give him something to focus on.

Ineffective Approach

Nurse: Shall I break?

Jason: (Had been looking off to his right, but turns and looks directly at the nurse.) Yeah, go ahead. (Looks at the table briefly and then turns to look out the door and down the hallway.)

Nurse: (Breaking the pool balls without putting any in a pocket.) It's your turn. You can hit any that you'd like.

Jason: (Turning back to the table.) Huh? (Shaking his head as he stared at the table.) What?

Nurse: You know, Jason, you really should pay attention.

Jason: (Hits a ball in and moves to the other side of the table. Stops in line with the next shot but doesn't bend down to take aim. Stands very still, then shakes his head slightly and quickly. Leans down to take aim and then stands up again.)

Nurse: Jason. (Looks at nurse.) Jason! Are you going to play or not, I don't have all day.

Jason: Oh yeah. (Leans down, takes aim, and misses.)

Nurse: (Moves to where the next shot is. Position is near where Jason is standing. Nurse watches him carefully, moving closer to him.) Please move over, Jason.

Jason: No. (Doesn't move. In peripheral vision, nurse sees Jason's lips move and he again looks to his right and shakes his head in a staccato motion, as if trying to shake something out of his head.)

Effective Approach

Nurse: Shall I break?

Jason: (Had been looking off to his right, but turns and looks directly at the nurse.) Yeah, go ahead. (Looks at the table briefly and then turns to look out the door and down the hallway.)

Nurse: (Breaking the pool balls without putting any in a pocket.) Your turn; you can hit any that you'd like.

Jason: (Turning back to the table.) Huh? (Shakes his head as he stares at the table.) What?

Nurse: You can hit any ball you like. I didn't get any.

Jason: (Hits a ball in and moves to the other side of the table. Stops in line with the next shot but doesn't bend down to take aim. Stands very still, then shakes his head slightly and quickly. Leans down to take aim and then stands up again.)

Nurse: Jason. (He looks at nurse.) Are you aiming at the 10 ball?

Jason: Oh yeah. (Leans down, takes aim, and misses.)

Nurse: (Moving to where her next shot is. The position is very close to where Jason is standing. Nurse watches him carefully while moving closer to him.) Here, let me take this shot.

Jason: Oh. (Moves back. In peripheral vision nurse sees Jason's lips move and again he looks to his right and shakes his head in a staccato motion, as if trying to shake something out of his head.)

Nurse: I missed again. (Moves away from table and turns to Jason, who moves up to the table. He leans down and then stands up again. His lips move again as he turns his head to the right and then looks over his back toward the doorway.) Jason. Jason. (He looks at the nurse.) You have the striped ones.

Jason: (Nods and leans down to take a shot, which he makes. He then misses the next shot. He stands up and moves back from the table, again looking back toward the doorway. He shakes his head.) No!

Nurse: (Watches him closely and moves to the opposite side of the table, making the next shot. Lining up the next shot, Jason leans the pool cue against the table, looks past the nurse, and turns and walks away toward the door. Looks down the hallway, takes a few steps, stops for a minute or so, turns back into the room, and again looks past the nurse. Sits down and shakes his head again. Holds his head in his hands, with his hands covering his ears. The nurse picks up his pool cue and places both against the wall, out of the way. The nurse sits next to another staff member at a vantage point from which Jason can still be watched.)

Critical Thinking Challenge

- How did the nurse's impatience translate into Jason's behavior in the first scenario?
- What effective communicating techniques did the nurse use in the second scenario?

stood within the context of the patient's disturbed thinking. The nurse needs to understand the significance of the behavior to the individual. One patient moved the family furniture into the yard because he thought that evil spirits were hiding in the furniture. His bizarre behavior was an attempt to protect his family. Another patient painted a sequence of numbers on his bedroom walls. He said that the numbers were the language of the angels. His delusional thoughts were at the basis of his behavior.

Because of the negative symptoms, specifically, avolition, patients may not seem interested or organized to complete normal daily activities. They may stay in bed most of the day or refuse to take a shower. Many times, they will agree to get up in the morning and go to work, but they never get around to it. Several specific behaviors are associated with schizophrenia, including stereotypy (idiosyncratic repetitive, purposeless movements), echopraxia (involuntary imitation of others' movements), and waxy flexibility (posture held in odd or unusual fixed positions for extended periods). In some cases, certain behaviors need to be evaluated carefully to distinguish them from movements that are associated with medication side effects, such as grimacing, stereotypical behavior, or agitation.

Self-Concept

In schizophrenia, self-concept is usually poor. Patients often are aware that they are hearing voices others do not hear. They recognize that they are different from others and are often scared of "going crazy." Many are aware of the loss of expectations for their future achievements. The pervasive stigma associated with having a mental illness contributes to the poor self-concept. Body image can be disturbed, especially during periods of hallucinations or delusions. One patient believed that her body was infected with germs and she could feel them eating away her insides.

Stress and Coping Patterns

Stressful events are often linked to psychiatric symptoms (see Chapter 17 for discussion of the diathesis-stress model). It is important to determine stresses from the patient's perspective because a stressful event for one may not be stressful for another (see Chapter 14). It is also important to determine typical coping patterns, especially negative coping strategies, such as the use of substances or aggressive behavior.

Risk Assessment

Because of high suicide and attempted suicide rates among patients with schizophrenia, the nurse needs to assess the patient's risk for self-injury: Does the patient speak of suicide, have delusional thinking that could lead to dangerous behavior, have command hallucinations telling him or her to harm self or others? Does the patient have homicidal ideations? Does the patient lack social support and the skills to be meaningfully engaged with other people or a vocation? Substance-related disorders are also common among patients with schizophrenia, and nurses should assess for substance abuse.

Nursing Diagnoses for Psychological Domain

Many nursing diagnoses can be generated from data collected assessing the psychological domain. Disturbed Thought Processes can be used for delusions, confusion, and disorganized thinking (see Figure 18.6). Disturbed Sensory Perception is appropriate for hallucinations or illusions. Other examples of diagnoses include Chronic Low Self-esteem, Personal Identity Disturbance, Risk for Violence, Ineffective Coping, and Knowledge Deficit.

Interventions for Psychological Domain

All of the psychological interventions, such as counseling, conflict resolution, behavior therapy, and cognitive

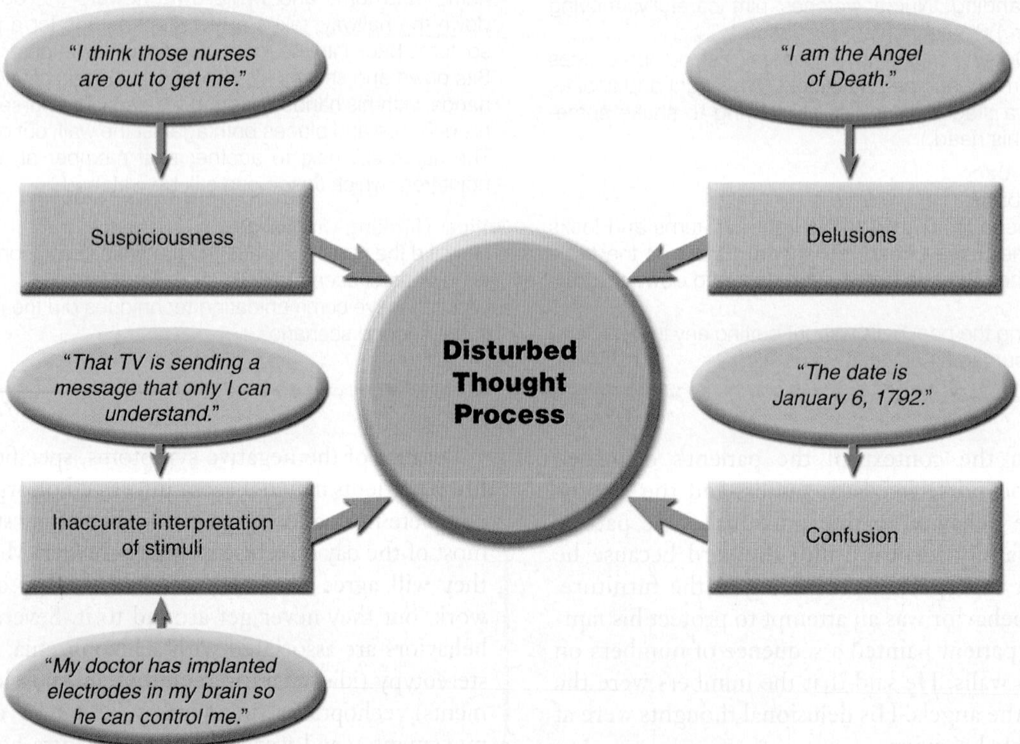
"I think those nurses are out to get me."
Suspiciousness
"That TV is sending a message that only I can understand."
Inaccurate interpretation of stimuli
"My doctor has implanted electrodes in my brain so he can control me."
Disturbed Thought Process
"I am the Angel of Death."
Delusions
"The date is January 6, 1792."
Confusion

FIGURE 18.6. Nursing diagnosis concept map: disturbed thought process.

interventions, are appropriate for patients with schizophrenia. The following discussion focuses on applying these interventions.

Special Issues in the Nurse–Patient Relationship

The development of the nurse–patient relationship with patients with schizophrenia centers on developing trust and accepting the person as a worthy human being. People with schizophrenia are often reluctant to engage in any relationship because of previous rejection and, in some instances, an underlying suspiciousness that is a part of the illness. If they are having hallucinations, their images of other people may be distorted and frightening. They are struggling to trust their own thoughts and perceptions, and engaging in an interaction with another human being may prove too overwhelming.

The nurse should approach the patient in a calm and caring manner. Engaging the patient in a relationship may take time. Short, time-limited interactions are best for a patient who is experiencing psychosis. Being consistent in interactions and following through on promises will help establish trust within the relationship.

Establishing a therapeutic relationship is crucial, especially with patients who deny that they are ill. Patients are more likely to agree to treatment if these recommendations are made within the context of a safe, trusting relationship. Even if some patients deny having mental illness, they may take medication and attend treatment activities because they trust the nurse (see Box 18.20).

Management of Disturbed Thoughts and Sensory Perceptions

Although antipsychotic medications may relieve positive symptoms, they do not always eliminate hallucinations and delusions. The nurse must continue helping the patient develop creative strategies for dealing with these sensory and thought disturbances. Information about the content of the hallucinations and delusions is needed, not only to determine whether the medications are effective, but also to assess safety and the meaning of these thoughts and perceptions to the patient. In caring for a patient who is experiencing hallucinations or delusions, nursing actions should be guided by three general patient outcomes:

- Decrease the frequency and intensity of hallucinations and delusions.
- Recognize that hallucinations and delusions are symptoms of a brain disorder.

BOX 18.20

A Brother's Perspective

A sibling describes his brother with schizophrenia and the importance of both medications and relationships.

At the age of 40, Robert was admitted to a psychiatric hospital in 1998. His brother was told at the time that he would never be able to live independently, and even if discharged, would only be repeatedly hospitalized. Robert had a long history of treatment and in 1998 had received all types of antipsychotic medications ... except he had not received any of the "new atypical variety." He was prescribed one of these drugs and within months, the staff who had predicted the most discouraging of outcomes told Robert's brother that he was in the midst of a miraculous recovery—his thinking was clear and free of delusions and they were preparing Robert's discharge.

A few weeks into the discharge planning, Robert called his brother distressed because his social worker, whom Robert had known for years from a prior hospitalization, was leaving. The social worker had been abruptly transferred to another hospital. Robert deteriorated rapidly into tantrums and hallucinations and dangerous behaviors. His discharge was put on hold. Robert's brother's rhetorical question was, what was the difference between Robert on the same medication on Monday, when he was alright, and Tuesday, when he no longer was? His answer for Robert was, the loss of an important relationship.

Robert is now living in a community-based home where the dedicated staff members have shown that they can keep rehospitalization rates below 3%.

Robert's brother has interviewed many former psychiatric patients for a book. He found that every one of his interviewees, while attributing their recovery to medications or finding God or a particular program, also identified an important relationship with one human being who believed in their ability to recover. Most of the time this person was a professional: a social worker, a nurse, a doctor. Sometimes it was a clergy or family member. A believing relationship...

Robert's brother concluded, "let's provide a range of medications, and let's study their effectiveness, but let's remember that the pill is the ultimate downsizing. Let's find resources to give people afflicted with mental illness what all of us need: fellow human beings upon whom we can depend to help us through our dark times and, once through, to emerge into gloriously imperfect lives."

For nurses, it is important to remember that it is not what we do to people, but rather, what we do with people: give hope, listen to their dreams, help them find ways to get as close as they can.

Adapted from: Neugeboren, J. (2006). Meds alone couldn't bring Robert back. *Newsweek*. Retrieved on January 31, 2006, from http://www.msnbc.msn.com/id/11077662/site/newsweek

- Develop strategies to manage the recurrence of hallucinations or delusions.

When interacting with a patient who is experiencing hallucinations or delusions, the nurse must remember that these experiences are real to the patient. The nurse should never tell a patient that these experiences are not real. Discounting the experiences blocks communication. It also is dishonest to tell the patient that you are having the same hallucinatory experience. It is best to validate the patient's experiences and identify the meaning of these thoughts and feelings to the patient. For example, a patient who believes that he or she is under surveillance by the Federal Bureau of Investigation probably feels frightened and suspicious of everyone. By acknowledging how frightening it must be to always feel like you are being watched, the nurse focuses on the feelings that are generated by the delusion, not the delusion itself. The nurse can then offer to help the patient feel safe within this environment. The patient, in turn, begins to feel that someone understands him or her (see Box 18.21).

Teaching Points 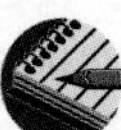

Teaching patients that hallucinations and delusions are part of the disorder becomes easier after the medication begins working. Once patients believe and acknowledge that they have a mental illness and that some of their thoughts are delusions and some of their perceptions are hallucinations, they can develop strategies to manage their symptoms.

Patients benefit greatly by learning techniques of self-regulation, symptom monitoring, and relapse prevention. By monitoring events, time, place, and stimuli surrounding the appearance of symptoms, the patient can begin to predict high-risk times for symptom recurrence. Cognitive behavioral therapy is often used in helping patients monitor and identify their emerging symptoms in order to prevent relapse (Gumley et al., 2003).

BOX 18.21

Using Reflection: Delusional Thinking

Incident: A patient was convinced that he married a famous movie star.

Reflection: At first the nurse discounted the delusion as being trivial and insignificant. Upon further analysis, the nurse realized that by being married to a famous person, the patient would also believe that he was an important, special person. The nurse developed a new perspective of the patient who was probably suffering from low self-esteem.

Another important nursing intervention is to help the patient identify to whom and where to talk about delusional or hallucinatory material. Because self-disclosure of these symptoms immediately labels someone as having a mental illness, patients should be encouraged to evaluate the environment for negative consequences of disclosing these symptoms. It may be fine to talk about it at home but not at the grocery store.

Enhancement of Cognitive Functioning

After identifying deficits in cognitive functioning, the nurse and patient can develop interventions that target specific deficits. The most effective interventions usually involve the whole treatment team. If the ability to focus or attend is an issue, patients can be encouraged to select activities that improve attention, such as computer games. For memory problems, patients can be encouraged to make lists and to write down important information.

Executive functioning problems are the most challenging for these patients. Patients who cannot manage daily problems may have planning and problem solving impairments. For these patients, developing interventions that closely simulate real-world problems may help. Through coaching, the nurse can teach and support the development of problem-solving skills. For example, during hospitalizations, patients are given medications and reminded to take them on time. They are often instructed in a classroom setting but rarely have an opportunity to practice self-medication and figure out what to do if their prescription expires, the medications are lost, or they forget their medications. Yet, when discharged, patients are expected to take medication at the prescribed dose at the prescribed time. Interventions designed to have patients actively engage in problem-solving behavior with real problems are needed.

Another approach to helping patients solve problems and learn new strategies for dealing with problems is solution-focused therapy, which focuses on the strengths and positive attributes that exist within each person. This is a therapy that involves years of training to master, but there are techniques that can be used. For example, patients can be asked to identify the most important problem from their perspective. This focuses the patient on an important issue for that patient (Box 18.22).

Behavioral Interventions

Behavioral interventions can be very effective in helping patients improve motivation and organize routine, daily activities, such as maintaining a regular schedule and completing activities. Reinforcement of positive behaviors (getting up on time, completing hygiene,

BOX 18.22

Research for Best Practice: Might Within the Madness

Hagen, B., & Mitchell, D. (2001). Might within the madness: Solution-focused therapy and thought-disordered clients. Archives of Psychiatric Nursing, 15(2), 86–93.

The Question: Can the use of solution-focused therapy (SFT) help thought-disordered patients better cope with some of their negative experiences and symptoms?

Methods: The authors provided an overview of SFT, focusing on how these techniques might be used in an inpatient psychiatry setting with patients experiencing disordered thoughts.

Three patient cases were presented: a 26-year-old man admitted to an inpatient hospital psychiatric unit with intrusive auditory and visual hallucinations; a 67-year-old woman who lived most of her life on a farm and managed her symptoms well until a recent move to the city; and a 49-year-old woman who was experiencing paranoid delusions about bombers and airplanes.

Findings: By using SFT, the nurses could see the individual as a person with hopes, dreams, and strengths. They also concluded that the SFT process was as important as the outcome.

Implications for Nursing: This study can have direct clinical application for those interested in developing solution-focused techniques. Using some of the SFT techniques can help the nurse see past the disorder and view the patient as a human being with strengths.

going to treatment activities) can easily be included in a treatment plan. In the hospital, patients gain unit privileges by following an agreed-on treatment plan.

Stress and Coping Skills

Developing skills to cope with personal, social, and environmental stresses is important to everyone, but particularly to those with a severe mental illness. Stresses can easily trigger symptoms that patients are trying to avoid. Establishing regular counseling sessions to support the development of positive coping skills is helpful for both the hospitalized patient and those in the community.

Patient Education 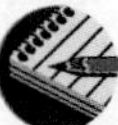

Cognitive deficits (difficulty in processing complex information, maintaining steady focus of attention, distinguishing between relevant and irrelevant stimuli, and forming abstractions), may challenge the nurse planning educational activities. Evidence indicates that people with schizophrenia may learn best in an errorless learning environment (O'Carroll, Russell, Lawrie, & Johnstone, 1999), that is, they are directly given correct information and then encouraged to write it down. Asking questions that encourage guessing is not as effective in helping them retain information. Trial-and-error learning is avoided. In one study, a group of people with schizophrenia who were taught using an errorless learning approach improved work skill in two entry-level job tasks (index card filing and toilet-tank assembly) and performed better than the group that was instructed with conventional trial-and-error instruction (Kern, Green, Mintz, & Liberman, 2003; Kern, Liberman, Kopelowicz, Mintz, & Green, 2002).

Teaching and explaining should occur in an environment with minimal distractions. Terminology should be clear and unambiguous. Visual aids can supplement verbal information, but these materials should have simple information stated in simple language. The nurse takes care not to overcrowd the visual material or incorporate images that draw attention away from important content. Teaching should occur in small segments with frequent reinforcement. Most important of all, teaching should occur when the patient is ready. Regular assessments of cognitive abilities with standardized instruments can help determine this readiness. These suggestions can be adapted for teaching during any phase of the illness.

Skill-training interventions should be designed to compensate for cognitive deficits. To help patients learn to process complex activities, such as catching a bus, preparing a meal, or shopping for food or clothing, nurses should break the activity into small parts or steps and list them for the patient's reference, for example:

- Leave apartment with keys in hand.
- Make sure you have correct bus fare in your pocket.
- Close the door.
- Walk to the corner.
- Turn right and walk three blocks to the bus stop.

Family Education 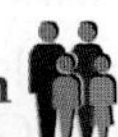

Because having a family member with schizophrenia is a life-changing event for the family and friends who provide care and support, educating patients and their families is crucial. It is a primary concern for the psychiatric–mental health nurse. Family support is crucial to help patients maintain treatment. Education should include information about the disease course, treatment regimens, support systems, and life management skills (see Box 18.23). The most important factor to stress during patient and family education is the consistent taking of medication.

Social Domain

Social Assessment

Several difficulties with social functioning occur in schizophrenia. As the disorder progresses, individuals

BOX 18.23

Psychoeducation Checklist: Schizophrenia

When caring for the patient with schizophrenia, be sure to include the caregiver as appropriate and address the following topic areas in the teaching plan:

- Psychopharmacologic agents, including drug action, dosage, frequency, and possible adverse effects. Stress importance of adherence to the prescribed regimen.
- Management of hallucinations
- Coping strategies such as self-talk, getting busy
- Management of the environment
- Use of contracts that detail expected behaviors, with goals and consequences
- Community resources

can become increasingly socially isolated. On a one-to-one basis, this occurs as the individual seems unable to connect with people in his or her environment. Several aspects of the symptoms already discussed can contribute to this. For example, emotional blunting and anhedonia (the inability to form emotional attachment and experience pleasure) result in an experience of not being engaged in activities and relationships.

Cognitive deficits that contribute to difficult social functioning include problems with face and affect recognition, deficiencies in recall of past interactions, problems with decision making and judgment in conflictual interactions, and poverty of speech and language. Poor functioning and the inability to complete activities of daily living are manifested in poor hygiene, malnutrition, and social isolation.

Functional Status

Functional status of patients with schizophrenia should be assessed initially and at regular periods. The usual assessment instrument is the Global Assessment of Functioning (GAF). If the GAF score is below 60, interventions should be designed to enhance social or occupational functioning.

Social Systems

In schizophrenia, support systems become very important in maintaining the patient in the community. The individual may become socially isolated if the treatment and management occur in long-term care facilities and group homes away from family and friends. One challenge in treating schizophrenia is to identify and maintain the patient's links with family and significant others. Assessment of the formal support (e.g., family, providers) and informal support (e.g., neighbors, friends) should be conducted (see Chapter 6 for discussion of the balance theory).

Quality of Life

People with schizophrenia often have a poor quality of life, especially older people, who may have spent many years in a long-term hospital. The nurse should assess the patient's quality of life and how it could be improved. Simple changes, such as arranging for a different roommate or improving access to social activities by meeting transportation needs, can greatly improve a patient's quality of life.

Family Assessment 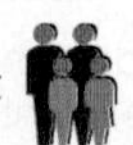

The assessment of the family could take many forms, and the family assessment guide presented in Chapter 13 can be used. In some instances, the patient will be young and living with his or her parents. Often, the nurse's first contact with the patient and family is in the initial phases of the disorder. The family is dealing with the shock and disbelief of seeing a child with a mental illness that has lifelong consequences. In this instance, the assessment process may be extended over several sessions to provide the family with support and education about the disorder.

Because women with schizophrenia generally have better treatment outcomes than do men, many will marry and have children. These women experience the same life stresses as other women and may find themselves single parents, raising children in poverty-stricken conditions. Managing a psychiatric illness and trying to be an effective parent in a socially stigmatizing society is almost an impossibility because of the lack of financial resources and social support. This family will need an extensive assessment of financial need and social support. The family life cycle model presented in Chapter 13 can also be used as a framework for the assessment.

Nursing Diagnoses for Social Domain

The nursing diagnoses generated from the assessment of the social domain are typically Impaired Social Interaction, Ineffective Role Performance, Disabled Family Coping, or Interrupted Family Processes. Outcomes will depend on the specific diagnostic area.

Interventions for Social Domain

Promoting Patient Safety

Although violence is not a consistent behavior of people with schizophrenia, it is always a concern during the initial phase when hallucinations or delusions may put patients at risk for harming themselves or others. Nonviolent patients who are experiencing hallucinations and delusions can also be at risk for victimization by more aggressive patients. The patient who is hallucinating needs to be protected. This protection may include increased staff monitoring and, if necessary, a safer environment in a secluded area.

The nurse's best approach to avoiding violence or aggression is to demonstrate respect for the patient and the patient's personal space, assess and monitor for signs of fear and agitation, and use preventive interventions before the patient loses control. Medications should be administered as ordered. Because most antipsychotic and antidepressant medications take 1 to 2 weeks to begin moderating behavior, the nurse must be vigilant during the acute illness.

Reducing environmental stimulation is particularly important for individuals who are experiencing hallucinations but can be helpful for all patients when signs of fear and agitation are observed. Allowing patients to use private rooms or seclusion for brief periods can be an important preventive method.

Other techniques of managing the environment (milieu management) have been found to be helpful in inpatient settings. One researcher who examined aggression and violence in psychiatric hospitals found violent behavior to be associated with the following predictors: history of violence, a coercive interaction style of using violence to obtain what is desired, and an environment in which violence is inadvertently rewarded, for example, by gaining staff attention (Morrison, 1992, 1993; Morrison & Carney-Love, 2003). Morrison proposed methods to help avoid acts of violence or aggression:

- Taking a thorough history that includes information about the patient's past use of violence
- Helping the patient to talk directly and constructively with those with whom they are angry, rather than venting anger to staff about a third person
- Setting limits with consistent and justly applied consequences
- Involving the patient in formulating a contract that outlines patient and staff behaviors, goals, and consequences
- Scheduling brief but regular time-outs to allow the patient some privacy without the attention of staff either before or after the time-out (these time-outs may be patient activated)

If the patient loses control and is a danger to self or others, restraints and seclusion may be used as a last resort. Health Care Financing Administration (HCFA) guidelines and hospital policy must be followed (see Chapter 3), and staff should be trained in the proper use of seclusion and restraints. In addition, staff need to have planned sessions after all incidents of violence or physical management in which the event is analyzed. These sessions allow staff to learn how better to manage these situations and evaluate patients' cues. With sensitive leadership, these sessions can help staff to learn more about the interaction of patient and staff characteristics that can contribute to these incidents.

Convening Support Groups

People with mental illness benefit from support groups that focus on daily problems and the stress of dealing with a mental illness. These groups are useful throughout the continuum of care and help reduce the risk of suicide. In the hospital setting, the focus of the group can be simply sharing the experience of living with a mental illness. In the community, a regular support group can provide interaction with people with similar problems and issues. Friendships often develop from these groups.

Implementing Milieu Therapy

Individuals with schizophrenia can be hospitalized or live in group homes for a long period of time. The challenge is helping people who are unable to live with family members to live harmoniously with strangers who have similar interpersonal difficulties. Arranging the treatment environment to maximize therapy is crucial to the rehabilitation of the patient.

Developing Psychiatric Rehabilitation Strategies

Rehabilitation strategies are used to support the individual's recovery and integration into the community (see Chapter 19). Community-based psychosocial rehabilitation programs usually offer long-term intensive case management services to adults with schizophrenia. Programs provide a continuum of services to meet the changing needs of people with psychiatric disabilities. Patients set rehabilitation goals, and services are then provided to help "clients" (most programs do not use the term "patients") reach their goals. Services range from daily home visits to providing transportation, occupational training, and group support.

Social skills training shows much promise for patients with schizophrenia, both individually and in groups. This is a method for teaching patients specific behaviors needed for social interactions. The skills are taught by lecture, demonstration, role playing, and homework assignments. Nurses may be team members and involved in case management or provision of services. These and other psychological treatment approaches, combined with breakthroughs in biologic therapy, continue to help improve the functioning and quality of life for patients with schizophrenia.

Family Interventions 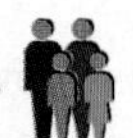

When schizophrenia first becomes apparent, the patient and family must negotiate the mental health system for the first time (in most cases), a challenge that almost equals that of confronting the family member's illness. In most states, the mental health system is huge and is usually ignored unless an adult foster care home moves into a neighborhood or a family member becomes seriously mentally ill. The system includes private inpatient and outpatient clinics supported by insurance and public community mental health clinics and hospitals supported by public funds. Because mental health coverage in most insurance packages is insufficient for someone with schizophrenia, most families eventually deal with the public mental health system. If the patient is aggressive, many private facilities encourage hospitalization in a public sector facility even for the first admission.

Family members should be encouraged to participate in support groups that help family members deal with the realities of living with a loved one with a mental illness (see Chapter 13). Family members should be given information about local community and state resources and organizations such as mental health associations and those that can help families negotiate the complex provider systems.

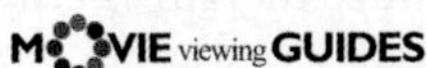

Evaluation and Treatment Outcomes

Outcome research related to schizophrenia has redefined previous ways of thinking about the course of the disorder. Schizophrenia was once considered to have a progressively long-term and downward course, but it is now known that schizophrenia can be successfully treated and managed. In one older, but significant study, the researchers interviewed patients 20 to 25 years after diagnosis and found that 50% to 66% experienced significant improvement or recovery (Harding, Zubin, & Strauss, 1987). This study is important because it occurred before the development of atypical antipsychotic agents. Today, we can be hopeful that even more people can experience improvement or recover from schizophrenia.

Continuum of Care

Continuity of care has been identified as a major goal of community mental health systems for patients with schizophrenia because they are at risk for becoming "lost" to services if left alone after discharge. Discharge planning encourages follow-up care in the community. In fact, many state mental health systems require an outpatient appointment before discharge. Treatment of schizophrenia occurs across a variety of settings. Not only inpatient hospitalization but also partial hospitalization, day treatment, and crisis stabilization can be used effectively.

Inpatient-Focused Care

Much of the previous discussion concerns care in the inpatient setting. Today, inpatient hospitalizations are brief and focus on patient stabilization. Many times, patients are involuntarily admitted for a short period (see Chapter 3). During the stabilization period, the status is changed to voluntary admission, whereby the patient agrees to treatment.

Emergency Care 

Emergency care ideally takes place in a hospital emergency room, but often the crisis occurs in the home. Patients are usually relapsing and do not recognize their bizarre or aggressive behaviors as symptoms. A specially trained crisis team is sent to assess the emergency and recommend further treatment. In the emergency room, patients are brought not only because of relapse but also because of medication side effects or water intoxication. Nurses should refer to the previous discussion for nursing management.

Community Care

Most of the care of patients with schizophrenia will be in the community through publicly supported mental health delivery systems. Community services include assertive community treatment, outpatient therapy, case management, and psychosocial rehabilitation, including clubhouse programs (Box 18.24). While the patient is in the community, his or her health care should be integrated with physical health care. Nurses should be especially vigilant that patients with mental illnesses receive proper primary and medical health care.

• NCLEXNOTE

NCLEXNOTE

Priorities in the patient with acute symptoms of schizophrenia include managing psychosis and keeping the patient safe and free from harming self or others. In the community, the priorities are preventing relapse, maintaining psychosocial functioning, engaging in psychoeducation, and improving quality of life.

Mental Health Promotion

In some cases, it is not the disorder itself that threatens the mental health of the person with schizophrenia, but the stresses of trying to receive care and services. Health care systems are complex and are often at the mercy of a system rule that is outdated. Development of assertiveness and conflict resolution skills can help the person in negotiating access to systems that will provide services. Developing a positive support system for stressful periods will help promote a positive outcome (see Fig. 18.7).

BOX 18.24

Research for Best Practice: The Concept of Home

Overmyer, C.A. (2005). *Home: A concept analysis with application of the concept to experiences of individuals with serious and persistent mental illness.* Unpublished master's thesis.

The Question: What is the best way to define the concept of home?

Methods: A concept analysis procedure was implemented. Theoretical and research literature from several disciplines was explored. These included social science, architecture, law, and history. Research and journalistic reports that described housing for people with SPMI were also reviewed. After defining attributes were determined, they were applied to the reports on housing for people with SPMI.

Findings: The defining attributes found in the literature are privacy, sense of safety and security, ability for some self-expression and development of one's personal identity, good social relationships, sense of continuity and ownership, sense of some control over one's space, warmth both in the physical and psychological sense, and a somewhat pleasing physical environment. The model case readily describes the "family home" in a safe neighborhood in which all members of the family have some space they can call their own and to which they return for acceptance and warmth after a day of work or school. No literature describing housing for individuals with SPMI met the defining attributes. The single project that described a system in England in which people with SPMI were placed in housing with the intention that they would stay there and return there following relapse should that occur came the closest to including all the defining attributes. This arrangement described a borderline case, in concept analysis terms. It also described the most successful housing situation for people with SPMI as they had more stability in their lives and in their illness.

Implications for Nursing: The defining attributes from this concept analysis suggest areas for assessment when housing placement is being planned for patients. They also suggest possible outcomes when advocating for people with schizophrenia.

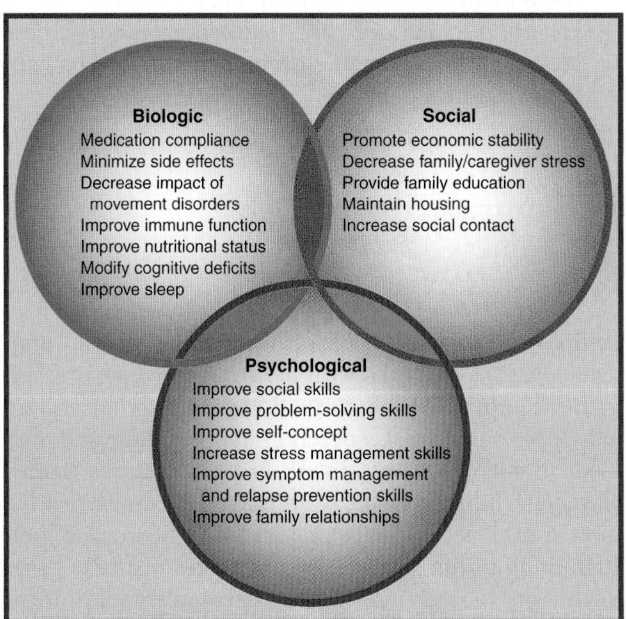

FIGURE 18.7. Biopsychosocial outcomes for patients with schizophrenia.

SUMMARY OF KEY POINTS

- The patient with schizophrenia displays a complex of myriad symptoms typically categorized as positive symptoms (those that exist but should not), such as delusions or hallucinations and disorganized thinking and behavior, and negative symptoms (characteristics that should be there but are lacking); these include alogia, avolition, anhedonia, and affective blunting.
- In the past, the diagnosis and treatment of schizophrenia focused on the more observable and dramatic positive symptoms (i.e., delusions and hallucinations), but recently scientists have shifted their focus to the disorganizing symptoms of cognition.
- The clinical presentation of schizophrenia occurs in three phases: phase 1 entails initial diagnosis and first treatment; phase 2 includes periods of relative calm between episodes of overt signs and symptoms but during which the patient needs sustained treatment; and phase 3 includes periods of exacerbation or relapse that require hospitalization or more frequent contacts with mental health professionals and increased use of resources.
- Biologic theories of what causes schizophrenia include genetic, neurodevelopment, and neurotransmission imbalances. The last is supported by the advanced technology of PET scan findings and the understanding of the mechanisms of antipsychotic medications.
- Biologic assessment of the patient with schizophrenia must include a thorough history and physical examination to rule out any medical illness or substance abuse problem that might be the cause of the patient's symptoms; assessment of risk for self-injury or injury to others; and creation of baseline health information before medications are administered. Several standardized assessment tools are available to help assess characteristic abnormal motor movements.

■ Several nursing interventions address the biologic domain—promotion of self-care activities, activity, exercise, nutritional, thermoregulation, and fluid balance interventions. In general the antipsychotic drugs used to treat schizophrenia block dopamine transmission in the brain but also cause some troublesome and sometimes serious side effects, primarily anticholinergic side effects and extrapyramidal side effects (motor abnormalities). Newer antipsychotic agents block serotonin as well as dopamine. The nurse should be familiar with these drugs, their possible side effects, and the interventions required to manage or control side effects.

■ The extrapyramidal side effects of antipsychotic drugs can appear early in drug treatment and include acute parkinsonism or pseudoparkinsonism, acute dystonia, and akathisia; or they can appear late in treatment after months or years. The primary example of late-appearing extrapyramidal side effects is tardive dyskinesia, which is a severe syndrome of abnormal motor movements of the mouth, tongue, and jaw.

■ Psychological assessment must include equal attention to manifestations of both positive and negative symptoms and a concentrated focus on the cognitive impairments that make it so difficult for these patients to manage their disorder. Several standardized assessment tools assess for positive and negative symptoms. Development of the nurse–patient relationship becomes key in helping patients manage the disturbed thoughts and sensory perceptions. Interventions should be designed to enhance cognitive functioning. Patient and family education are critical interventions for the person with schizophrenia.

■ Because schizophrenia is a lifetime disorder and patients require the continued support and care of mental health professionals and family or friends, one of the primary nursing interventions is ensuring that patients and families are properly educated regarding the course of the disorder, importance of drug maintenance, and need for consistent care and support. Research is demonstrating that interaction between patients and their families is key to the success of long-term treatments and outcomes.

CRITICAL THINKING CHALLENGES

1 Delusions are often based on beliefs not held by others. Occasionally delusions are based on cultural beliefs that are outside of those held by the majority of society. Describe steps that professional psychiatric caregivers should use to make sure their responses consider the cultural basis of a patient's delusions.

2 Delusions and hallucinations are based to varying degrees on patients' experiences and emotional responses to them. What experiences and emotions might form the basis of delusions that are grandiose or persecutory, etc.? What might form the basis of auditory hallucinations that tell patients of their importance or their need to harm themselves, etc.?

3 What steps might the nurse take to develop trust in a patient who has hallucinations and delusions and is frightened of other people?

4 Given that a patient with mental illness requires extra efforts at confidentiality, and that patients with schizophrenia are often suspicious of their family members, explain ways that you can help families and patients take advantage of the social support that may be available only from each other.

5 What steps can be taken in the community to enhance the living circumstances of people with schizophrenia?

6 Discuss how therapeutic communication might have to change when working with a person with schizophrenia who is displaying primarily negative symptoms. How will you deal with their diminished response to you (both verbally and emotionally) when you are teaching or giving instructions for activities? How will you help them compensate for some of their cognitive deficits?

Benny and Joon: 1993. Joon is a young woman with schizophrenia who lives with her overprotective brother. In an attempt to keep her safe, Joon's brother unsuccessfully hires one housekeeper after another. After winning a bet in a poker game, Joon's brother acquires Benny, played by Johnny Depp, who entertains and cares for Joon. A romance develops that results in Benny and Joon attempting to run away. Joon's symptoms reappear. After treatment, Joon struggles with becoming independent from both her brother and boyfriend.

VIEWING POINTS: How does Joon's brother's behavior interfere with her normal growth and development? When Joon's symptoms appeared, how would you classify them according to the DSM-IV-TR? What advice would you like to give to Joon and her brother?

Beautiful Mind: 2001. This academy award-winning movie starring Russell Crowe is based on the biography of the mathematician and Nobel Laureate John Nash by Sylvia Naasar. It presents the life and experiences of this man as he experienced schizophrenia. It shows how his life and work were altered and the effects on his relationships with family and colleagues. The movie depicts how this man came to terms with his illness.

VIEWING POINTS: How does the treatment John Nash received in the 1950s differ from treatment today? How would you classify his symptoms according to DSM-IV-TR? What is typical and/or problematic about Mr. Nash's relationship with the medications prescribed for him?

REFERENCES

Altamura, A. C., Bassetti, R., Bignotti, S., Pioli, R., & Mundo, E. (2003). Clinical variables related to suicide attempts in schizophrenic patients: A retrospective study. *Schizophrenia Research, 60*, 47–55.

American Psychiatric Association. (2000). *Diagnostic and statistical manual of mental disorders* (4th ed., text revision). Washington, DC: Author.

Baldessarini, R. J. (2002). Clinical psychopharmacology: Overview and recent advances. Symposium conducted at Cape Cod Symposia, Eastham, Massachusetts.

Benes, F. M. (2000). Emerging principles of altered neural circuitry in schizophrenia. *Brain Research Developmental Brain Research, 31* (2–3), 251–269.

Boyd, M., & Lapierre, E. (1996). Fluid imbalance and water intoxication: The elusive syndrome. In A. McBride & J. Austin (Eds.), *Psychiatric mental health nursing: Integration of the biological into behavioral* (pp. 396–424). Philadelphia: WB Saunders.

Buchsbaum, M. (1990). The frontal lobes, basal ganglia, and temporal lobes as a site for schizophrenia. *Schizophrenia Bulletin, 16*, 377–387.

Byrne, M., Agerbo, E., Ewald, H., Eaton, W. W., & Mortensen, P. B. (2003). Parental age and risk of schizophrenia: A case-control study. *Archives of General Psychiatry, 60* (7), 673–678.

Chance, S. A., Esiri, M. M., & Crow, T. J. (2003). Ventricular enlargement in schizophrenia: A primary change in the temporal lobe? *Schizophrenia Research, 62*, 123–131.

Chou, Y. H., Halldin, C., & Farde, L. (2003). Occupancy of 5HT(1A) receptors in clozapine in the primate brain: A PET study. *Psychopharmacology, 166* (3), 234–240.

Cirillo, M. A., & Seidman, L. J. (2003). Verbal declarative memory dysfunction in schizophrenia: From clinical assessment to genetics and brain mechanisms. *Neuropsychology Review, 13* (2), 43–77.

Csernansky, J. G. (2003). Treatment of schizophrenia: Preventing the progression of disease. *Psychiatric Clinics of North America, 26* (2), 367–379.

Davidson, L. L., & Heinrichs, R. W. (2003). Quantification of frontal and temporal lobe brain-imaging findings in schizophrenia: A meta-analysis. *Psychiatry Research, 122* (2), 69–87.

De Hert, M., McKenzie, K., & Peuskens, J. (2001). Risk factors for suicide in young people suffering from schizophrenia: A long-term follow-up study. *Schizophrenia Research, 47* (2–3), 127–134.

Dolder, C. R., Lacro, J. P., Dunn, L. B., & Jeste, D. V. (2002). Antipsychotic medication adherence: Is there a difference between typical and atypical agents? *American Journal of Psychiatry, 159* (1), 103–108.

Falkai, P., Schneider-Axmann, T., Honer, W. G., Vogeley, K., Schonell, H., Pfeiffer, U., et al. (2003). Influence on genetic loading, obstetric complications, and premorbid adjustment on brain morphology in schizophrenia: A MRI study. *European Archives of Psychiatry and Clinical Neuroscience, 253* (2), 92–99.

Franzen, G. (1970). Plasma free fatty acids before and after an intravenous insulin injection in acute schizophrenic men. *British Journal of Psychiatry, 116* (531), 173–177.

Ghose, S., Weickert, C. S., Colvin, S. M., Coyle, J. T., Herman, M. M., Hyde, T. M., & Kleinman, J. E. (2004). Glutamate carboxypeptidase II gene expression in the human frontal and temporal lobe in schizophrenia. *Neuropsychopharmacology, 29* (1), 117–125.

Goldman, L. S. (1999). Medical illness in patients with schizophrenia. *Journal of Clinical Psychiatry, 60* (Suppl 21), 1015.

Goldner, E. M., Hsu, L., Waraich, P., & Somers, J. M. (2002). Prevalence and incidence studies of schizophrenia disorders: A systematic review of the literature. *The Canadian Journal of Psychiatry, 47* (9), 833–843.

Green, M. F., Kern, R. S., Braff, D. L., & Mintz, J. (2000). Neurocognitive deficits and functional outcome in schizophrenia: Are we measuring the "right stuff"? *Schizophrenia Bulletin, 26* (1), 119–137.

Gumley, A., O'Grady, M., McNay, L., Reilly, J., Power, K., & Norrie, J. (2003). Early intervention for relapse in schizophrenia: Results of a 12-month randomized controlled trial of cognitive behavioural therapy. *Psychological Medicine, 33* (3), 419–431.

Hafner, H. (2003). Gender differences in schizophrenia. *Psychoneuroendocrinology, 23* (Suppl 2), 17–54.

Harding, C., Zubin, J., & Strauss, J. (1987). Chronicity in schizophrenia: Fact, partial fact or artifact? *Hospital and Community Psychiatry, 38* (5), 477–486.

Harrison, G., Fouskakis, D., Rasmussen, F., Tynelius, P., Sipos, A., & Gunnell, D. (2003). Association between psychotic disorder and urban place of birth is not mediated by obstetric complications or childhood socioeconomic position: A cohort study. *Psychological Medicine, 33* (4), 723–731.

Hartman, M., Steketee, M. C., Silva, S., Lanning, K., & Andersson, C. (2003). Wisconsin Card Sorting Test performance in schizophrenia: The role of working memory. *Schizophrenia Research, 63* (3), 201–217.

Jibson, M. D., & Tandon, R. (2000). Treatment of schizophrenia. In D. L. Dunner & J. E. Rosenbaum (Eds.), *The psychiatric clinics of North America annual of drug therapy* (Vol. 7, pp. 83–113). Philadelphia: WB Saunders.

Kandel, E. R., Schwartz, J. H., & Jessell, T. M. (2000). *Principles of neural science* (4th ed.). New York: McGraw-Hill.

Kay, S. R., Fiszbein, A., & Opler, L. A. (1987). The Positive and Negative Syndrome Scale (PANSS) for schizophrenia. *Schizophrenia Bulletin, 13*, 261–276.

Kern, R. S., Green, M. V., Mintz, J., & Liberman, R. P. (2003). Does errorless learning compensate for neurocognitive impairments in the work rehabilitation of persons with schizophrenia? *Psychological Medicine, 33* (3), 433–442.

Kern, R. S., Liberman, R. P., Kopelowicz, A., Mintz, J., & Green, M. F. (2002). Applications of errorless learning for improving work performance in persons with schizophrenia. *American Journal of Psychiatry, 159* (11), 1921–1926.

Kozuki, V., & Froelicher, E. S. (2003). Lack of awareness and nonadherence in schizophrenia. *Western Journal of Nursing Research, 25*, 57–74.

Leucht, S., Barnes, T. R., Kissling, W., Engel, R. R., Correll, C., & Kane, J. M. (2003). Relapse prevention in schizophrenia with new-generation antipsychotics: A systematic review and exploratory meta-analysis of randomized, controlled trials. *American Journal of Psychiatry, 160* (7), 1209–1222.

Lively, S., Friedrich, R. M., & Rubenstein, L. (2004). The effects of disturbing illness behaviors on siblings of persons with schizophrenia. *Journal of the Psychiatric Nurses Association, 10*, 222–232.

McDonald, C., Grech, A., Toulopoulou, T., Schulze, K., Chapple, B., Sham, P., et al. (2003). Brain volumes in familial and non-familial schizophrenia probands and their unaffected relatives. *American Journal of Medical Genetics, 114* (6), 616–625.

Mercier-Guidez, E., & Loas, G. (2000). Polydipsia and water intoxication in 353 psychiatric inpatients: An epidemiological and psychopathological study. *European Psychiatry, 15* (5), 306–311.

Montoya, A., Ocampo, M., & Torres-Ruiz, A. (2003). Neuroleptic malignant syndrome in Mexico. *The Canadian Journal of Clinical Pharmacology, 10* (3), 111–113.

Morrison, E. F. (1992). A coercive interactional style as an antecedent to aggression in psychiatric patients. *Research in Nursing and Health, 15*, 421–431.

Morrison, E. F. (1993). Toward a better understanding of violence in psychiatric settings: Debunking the myths. *Archives of Psychiatric Nursing, 7*, 328–335.

Morrison, E. F., & Carney Love, C. (2003). An evaluation of four programs for the management of aggression in psychiatric settings. *Archives in Psychiatric Nursing, 17* (4), 146–155.

Neugeboren, J. (2006). Meds alone couldn't bring Robert back. *Newsweek*. Retrieved January 31, 2006, from http://www.msnbc.msn.com/id/11077662/site/newsweek.

New Freedom Commission on Mental Health. (2003). *Achieving the promise: Transforming mental health care in America: Final report.* Department of Health and Human Services (DHHS) Publication No. SMA-0303831. Rockville, MD: DHHS.

Niemi, L. T., Suvisaari, J. M., Tuulio-Henriksson, A., & Lonnqvist, J. K. (2003). Childhood developmental abnormalities in schizophrenia: Evidence from high-risk studies. *Schizophrenia Research, 60* (2–3), 239–258.

O'Carroll, R., Russell, H., Lawrie, S., & Johnstone, E. (1999). Errorless learning and the cognitive rehabilitation of memory-impaired schizophrenic patients. *Psychological Medicine*, 29, 105–112.

Ota, M., Mizukami, K., Katano, T., Sato, S., Takeda, T., & Asada, T. (2003). A case of delusional disorder, somatic type with remarkable improvement of clinical symptoms and single photon emission computed tomography findings following modified electroconvulsive therapy. *Progress in Neuro-Psychopharmacology & Biological Psychiatry*, *27* (5), 881–884.

Overmeyer, C. (2005). Home: A concept analysis with application of the concept to experiences of individuals with serious and persistent mental illness. (Unpublished master's thesis). Grand Valley State University, Grand Rapids, MI.

Penn, A. A. (2001). Early brain wiring: Activity-dependent processes. *Schizophrenia Bulletin*, 27(3), 336–347.

Reeves, S., Stewart, R., & Howard, R. (2002). Service contact and psychopathology in very–late-onset schizophrenia-like psychosis: The effects of gender and ethnicity. *International Journal of Geriatric Psychiatry, 17* (5), 473–479.

Ryan, M. C. M., Collins, P., & Thakore, J. H. (2003). Impaired fasting glucose tolerance in first-episode, drug-naive patients with schizophrenia. *American Journal of Psychiatry, 160*, 284–289.

Sallet, P. C., Elkis, H., Alves, T. M., Oliveira, J. R., Sassi, E., Campi de Castro, C., et al. (2003). Reduced cortical folding in schizophrenia: An MRI morphometric study. *American Journal of Psychiatry, 160* (9), 1606–1613.

Schimmelbusch, W. H., Mueller, P. S., & Sheps, J. (1971). The positive correlation between insulin resistance and duration of hospitalization in untreated schizophrenia. *British Journal of Psychiatry, 118* (545), 429–36.

Sedvall, G. (1994). Positron-emission tomography as a metabolic and neurochemical probe. In N. C. Andreasen (Ed.), *Schizophrenia: From mind to molecule* (pp. 147–155). Washington, DC: American Psychiatric Press.

Simpson, G. M., & Angus, J. W. S. L. (1970). A rating scale for extrapyramidal side effects. *Acta Psychiatrica Scandinavica, 212* (Suppl), 11–19.

Sprague, R. L., & Kalachnik, J. E. (1991). Reliability, validity, and a total score cutoff for the Dyskinesia Identification Scale System: Condensed User Scale (DISCUS) with mentally ill and mentally retarded populations. *Psychopharmacology Bulletin*, 27, 51–58.

Stahl, S. (2000). *Essential psychopharmacology: Neuroscientific basis and practical application* (2nd ed.). Cambridge, United Kingdom: Cambridge University Press.

Stahl, S. M. (2002). The metabolic syndrome: Psychopharmacologists should weigh the evidence for weighing the patient. *Journal of Clinical Psychiatry*, 63, 1094–1095.

Subotnik, K. L., Goldstein, M. J., Nuechterlein, K. H., Woo, S. M., & Mintz, J. (2002). Are communication deviance and expressed emotion related to family history of psychiatric disorders in schizophrenia? *Schizophrenia Bulletin, 28* (4), 719–729.

Tang, W. K., & Ungvari, G. S. (2003). Efficacy of electroconvulsive therapy in treatment resistant schizophrenia: A prospective open trial. *Progress in Neuro-psychopharmacology and Biological Psychiatry, 27*, 373–379.

Tsuang, M. T., Stone, W. S., & Faraone, S. V. (2001). Genes, environment and schizophrenia. *British Journal of Psychiatry, 178* (Suppl 40), S18–S24.

United States Department of Health and Human Services (U.S. DHHS). (1999). *Mental health: A report of the Surgeon General*. Rockville, MD: Author.

United States Department of Health and Human Services (U.S. DHHS). (2001). *Mental health: Culture, race, and ethnicity—A supplement to mental health: A report of the Surgeon General*. Rockville, MD: Author.

van Meijel, B., van der Gaag, M., Kahn, R. S., & Grypdonck, M. H. (2003). Relapse prevention in patients with schizophrenia: The application of an intervention protocol in nursing practice. *Archives of Psychiatric Nursing, 17* (4), 165–172.

Weisman, A. G., Gomes, L. G., & Lopez, S. R. (2003). Shifting blame away from ill relatives: Latino families' reactions to schizophrenia. *Journal of Nervous and Mental Disease, 191* (9), 574–581.

Willick, M. S. (1994). Schizophrenia: A patient's perspective – journey without end. In N. C. Andressen (Ed.), *Schizophrenia: From mind to molecule* (pp. 5–19). Washington, DC: American Psychiatric Press.

Wuerker, A. K., Long, J. D., Haas, G. L., & Bellack, A. S. (2002). Interpersonal control, expressed emotion, and change in symptoms in families of persons with schizophrenia. *Schizophrenia Research, 58* (2–3), 281–292.

CHAPTER 19

Schizoaffective, Delusional, and Other Psychotic Disorders

Nan Roberts and Roberta Stock

KEY CONCEPTS

- Psychosis
- Nonbizarre delusions

LEARNING OBJECTIVES

After studying this chapter, you will be able to:

- Define schizoaffective disorder and distinguish the major differences among schizophrenia, schizoaffective, and mood disorders.
- Discuss the important epidemiologic findings related to schizoaffective disorder.
- Explain the primary etiologic factors regarding schizoaffective disorder.
- Explain the primary elements involved in assessment, nursing diagnoses, nursing interventions, and evaluation of patients with schizoaffective disorder.
- Define delusional disorder and explain the importance of nonbizarre delusions in diagnosis and treatment.
- Explain the important epidemiologic findings regarding delusional disorder.
- Discuss the primary etiologic factors of delusional disorder.
- Explain the various subtypes of delusional disorder.
- Explain the nursing care of patients with delusional disorder.

KEY TERMS

• delusional disorder • delusions • erotomania • misidentification • persecutory delusions • psychosis • schizoaffective disorder • thymoleptic

Psychiatric–mental health nurses care for patients who have psychiatric disorders involving underlying psychoses other than schizophrenia and mood disorders. This chapter introduces other psychotic disorders and describes the associated nursing care. Central to understanding the problems of these patients is the concept of **psychosis**, a term used to describe a state in which an individual experiences positive symptoms, also known as psychotic symptoms (hallucinations, delusions, or disorganized thoughts, speech, or behavior) (see Chapter 18). Other psychotic disorders defined by the presence of psychosis include schizophreniform, schizoaffective, delusional, brief psychotic, and shared psychotic disorders. Other psychotic disorders may be induced by drugs or alcohol.

Schizoaffective disorder is one of the more complex psychotic disorders but one of the more common diagnoses that the generalist psychiatric nurse is likely to encounter. The person with delusional disorder is more likely to be treated in a medical-surgical setting and is rarely seen by a psychiatrist. This disorder often remains undiagnosed; therefore, for nurses practicing in nonpsychiatric settings, recognizing and understanding it are crucial to providing meaningful care.

SCHIZOAFFECTIVE DISORDER

Clinical Course

Schizoaffective disorder (SCA) is a complex and persistent psychiatric illness. This disorder was recognized in 1933 by Kasanin, who described varying degrees of symptoms of both schizophrenia and mood disorders, beginning in youth. All of his patients were well adjusted before the sudden onset of symptoms that erupted after the occurrence of a specific environmental stressor. Since Kasanin's time, debate and controversy about the status of this disorder have been extensive, resulting in many different definitions and classifications that remain under consideration (Maj, Pirozzi, Formicola, Bartoli, & Bucci, 2000). Box 19.1 reflects the history of this debate.

SCA is characterized by intervals of intense symptoms alternating with quiescent periods, during which psychosocial functioning is adequate. The episodic nature of this disorder is characteristic. This disorder is at times marked by symptoms of schizophrenia; at other times, it appears to be a mood disorder. In other cases, both psychosis and pervasive mood changes occur concurrently.

• NCLEXNOTE

Patients with schizoaffective disorder have many similar responses to their disorder as people with schizophrenia, with one exception. These patients have many more "mood" responses and are very susceptible to suicide.

BOX 19.1

History of the Diagnosis: Schizoaffective

- 1933: Kasanin first coined the phrase *schizoaffective psychosis*.
- 1980: *DSM-III* did not include diagnostic criteria for schizoaffective disorder.
- 1987: Schizoaffective disorder was first recognized as a separate diagnosis in the *DSM-III-R;* the definition included length of time in relationship to symptoms.
- 1994: Schizoaffective disorder was maintained as a separate disorder in the *DSM-IV.*
- 2000: Schizoaffective disorder was maintained as a separate disorder in *DSM-IV-TR.*

Patients with SCA are more likely to exhibit persistent psychosis, with or without mood symptoms, than are patients with a mood disorder. They feel that they are on a "chronic roller coaster ride" of symptoms that are often more difficult to cope with than the individual problem of either schizophrenia or mood disorder (Marneros, 2003). The diagnosis of this disorder is made only after these course-related characteristics are considered.

The long-term outcome of SCA is generally better than that of schizophrenia but worse than that of mood disorder (Moller et al., 2002). This group of patients resembles the mood disorder group in work function and the schizophrenia group in social function. In one study, compared with patients with a bipolar mood disorder, schizoaffective patients were less likely to recover and more likely to have persistent psychosis, with or without mood symptoms. Patients with SCA also have poorer executive function than do control subjects or patients with nonpsychotic bipolar disorder schizophrenia (Gooding & Tallent, 2002; Reichenberg et al., 2002).

Diagnostic Criteria

Mental health providers find SCA difficult to conceptualize, diagnose, and treat because the clinical picture varies. Patients often have misdiagnoses of schizophrenia. The difficulty in conceptualizing SCA is reflected in the controversy regarding the diagnostic criteria. For example, it has been argued that this disorder should be named either *schizophrenia with mood symptoms or mood disorder with schizophrenic symptoms.* More than 50 years after SCA was first described, the diagnosis was finally officially confirmed by the psychiatric community and included in the American Psychiatric Association's (APA, 1980) *Diagnostic and Statistical Manual of Mental Disorders,* 3rd edition, Revision (*DSM-III-R*) (Table 19.1).

To receive a diagnosis of SCA, a patient must have an uninterrupted period of illness when there is a major depressive, manic, or mixed episode, along with two of the following symptoms of schizophrenia: delusions, hallucinations, disorganized speech, disorganized or catatonic behavior, or negative symptoms (e.g., affective flattening, alogia, or avolition). In addition, although the person experiences problems with mood most of the time, the positive symptoms (delusions or hallucinations) must be present without the mood symptoms at some time during this period (for at least 2 weeks) (Table 19.1). Those with permanent delusions or auditory hallucinations report more basic symptoms (Fabisch et al., 2001). To clarify this disorder further, two related subtypes of SCA have been identified. In the bipolar type, the patient exhibits manic symptoms alone or a mix of manic and depressive symptoms. Patients with the depressive type display only symptoms of a major depressive episode (APA, 2000). The most common disorders

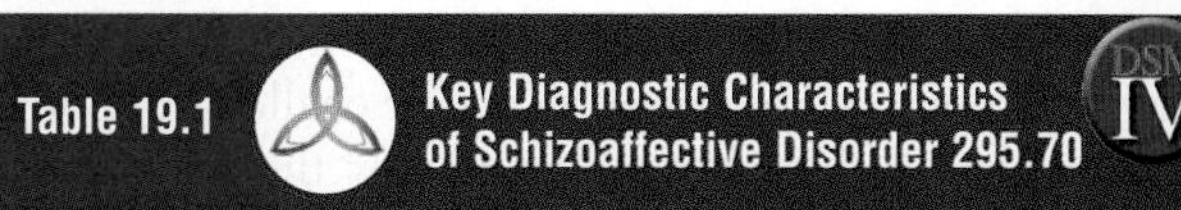

Table 19.1 Key Diagnostic Characteristics of Schizoaffective Disorder 295.70

Diagnostic Criteria and Target Symptoms

- Uninterrupted period of illness with concurrent major depressive episode, manic episode, or mixed episode
- Bipolar type: manic or mixed episode or manic or mixed episode and major depressive episode
- Depressive type: only major depressive episode
- Characteristic symptoms of schizophrenia (two or more) during a 1-month period
  - Delusions
  - Hallucinations
  - Disorganized speech
  - Grossly disorganized or catatonic behavior or negative symptoms
- Delusions or hallucinations for at least 2 weeks without prominent mood symptoms
- Symptoms of mood episode present for major portion of the active and residual periods of illness
- Not a direct physiologic effect of a substance or medical condition

Associated Findings

- Poor occupational functioning
- Restricted range of social contact
- Difficulties with self-care
- Increased risk for suicide

from which SCA must be differentiated include mood disorders of manic, depressive, or mixed types and schizophrenia.

Epidemiology and Risk Factors

The lifetime prevalence of SCA is estimated to be less than 1%, but there are no current studies (APA, 2000). This disorder occurs less commonly than does schizophrenia. The incidence of SCA is relatively constant across populations in varied geographic, climatic, industrial, and social environments. Environmental contributions are minimal.

Patients with schizoaffective disorder are at high risk for suicide. The risk for suicide in patients with psychosis is increased by the presence of depression. Risk for suicide is increased with the use of alcohol or substances, cigarette smoking, previous attempts at suicide, and previous hospitalizations (Potkin et al., 2003).

Lack of regular social contact may be a factor that confers a long-term risk for suicidal behavior, which may be reduced by treatments designed to enhance social networks and contact (Radomsky, Haas, Mann, & Sweeney, 1999) and help patients to protect themselves against environmental stressors (Huxley, Rendall, & Sederer, 2000). Cognition is more impaired with SCA than with nonpsychotic mood disorder (Evans et al., 1999).

Age of Onset

SCA can affect children and the elderly. In children, the disorder is rare and is often indistinguishable from schizophrenia. In the elderly, this disorder becomes complicated because of frequent comorbid medical conditions. The typical age of onset for this disorder is early adulthood, and the most common type presented is bipolar. Other studies have reported a relatively late onset of SCA of mainly the depressive type (APA, 2000). Earlier age of onset is associated with longer illness, more severe illness, and worse outcomes (APA).

Gender

This disorder is more likely to occur in women than in men, which may be accounted for by a greater incidence of the depressive type in women (APA, 2000).

Ethnicity and Culture

Most patients with diagnoses of SCA are Caucasian. Although some reports have indicated a connection between SCA and social class, others support no specific association with race, geographic area, or class. There is evidence that African Americans are more likely to receive a diagnosis of schizophrenia or schizoaffective disorder than a mood disorder (Mathews, Glidden, & Hargreaves, 2002).

Family

Relatives of patients with diagnoses of SCA appear to be at an increased risk for this disorder, schizophrenia, or bipolar disorder. There is some initial genome evidence that if there is a familial association, it is most likely related to the mother, not the father (DeLisi et al., 2002). There is also some evidence of an increased risk of development of SCA if a first-degree relative has some form of mental illness.

Comorbidity

SCA may be associated with substance abuse. Men may be likely to engage in antisocial behavior. Twenty-five percent of patients with diagnoses of SCA experience postpsychotic depression and panic attacks (APA, 2000).

Etiology

Biologic Theories

Although the etiologies of schizophrenia and mood disorder have been investigated extensively, the etiology of SCA remains unresolved. Research to locate a biologic marker has been limited. Variables may be structural, as well as neurochemical.

Neuropathologic

Magnetic resonance imaging (MRI) and computed tomography scans have been used in the study of SCA for more than 10 years (Crow & Harrington, 1994; Lewine, Hudgins, Brown, Caudle, & Risch, 1995; Scott, Price, George, Brillman, & Rothfus, 1993). Midline brain abnormalities, especially in women, have been found. In SCA, changes in brain structure appear to be similar to those seen in bipolar disorder (Getz et al., 2002). Whether midline structural abnormality is directly causal, indirectly contributory, or an intriguing phenomenon in SCA is unclear.

Genetic

The etiology is believed to be primarily genetic. Results from family, twin, and adoption studies vary but suggest that SCA may consist of phenotypic variations or expressions of a genetic interform between schizophrenia and affective psychoses (DeLisi et al., 2002).

Biochemical

Before 1999, the prevailing neurochemical hypothesis was overactivity of dopamine pathways. Whether this disturbance of dopaminergic transmission is primary remains unclear (Rietschel et al., 2000). In studies of deficit symptoms in SCA, altered patterns of glucose metabolism have been found that might cause neurobiologic and neurophysiologic impairments (Regenold, Thapar, Marano, Gavirneni, & Kondapavuluru, 2002).

Psychological and Social Theories

Psychological, psychodynamic, environmental, and interpersonal factors may have a precipitating role when they coincide with a biomedical diathesis that creates vulnerability to this disorder (see Chapter 6 for explanation of the diathesis-stress theory). No current psychodynamic behavioral, cognitive, or developmental theories of causation explain SCA. Family dynamics do not appear to affect the development of this disorder, except for the strong genetic predisposition, which is virtually unexplained.

Interdisciplinary Treatment

Patients with SCA benefit from comprehensive treatment. Because this disorder is persistent, these individuals are constantly trying to manage complex symptoms. Ideally, most of the treatment occurs within the patient's natural environment, and hospitalizations are limited to times of symptom exacerbation, when symptoms are so severe or persistent that extended care in a protected environment is necessary.

Pharmacologic intervention is always needed to stabilize the symptoms and presents specific challenges. Long-term atypical antipsychotic agents, now the mainstay of pharmacologic treatment, are as effective as the traditional combination of a standard antipsychotic agent and an antidepressant drug. Mood stabilizers, such as lithium or valproic acid (see Chapter 8), may also be used. A combination of antipsychotic and antidepressant agents is sometimes used.

After the patient's condition has stabilized (i.e., the patient exhibits a decrease in positive and negative symptoms), the treatment that led to remission of symptoms should be continued. Titrating antipsychotic agents to the lowest dose that provides suitable protection may enable optimal psychosocial functioning, while slowing recurrence of new episodes. Patients diagnosed with SCA are unlikely to be medication-free. Electroconvulsive therapy is considered when symptoms are refractory to other interventions or when the patient's life is at risk and a rapid response is required (Swoboda, Conca, Konig, Waanders, & Hansen, 2001).

The treatment plan is revised regularly, and symptoms are monitored to guide medication management. Psychiatric nursing interventions are guided by the nursing diagnoses. After the patient is released from the hospital, home visits may be needed. Psychotherapy may help manage interpersonal relationships and mood changes. Social services are often needed to obtain disability benefits or services. Use of advanced practice clinicians helps to provide continuity of care (McCann & Baker, 2003).

Priority Care Issues

Patients with SCA are highly susceptible to suicide (Potkin et al., 2003). Living with a persistent psychotic disorder that has a mood component makes suicide a real risk.

NURSING MANAGEMENT: HUMAN RESPONSE TO SCHIZOAFFECTIVE DISORDER

Biologic Domain

Assessment

Assessment of patients with SCA is similar to assessment of those with schizophrenia and affective disorder. A careful history from the patient and family is crucial. The history should contain a description of the full range and duration of symptoms the patient has experienced and those observed by the family; this information is important for predicting outcomes. A patient who has had symptoms for a relatively long period of time has greater difficulty in overcoming effects of the psychosis, which may cause function to deteriorate.

A thorough systems assessment is important to discover any physiologic problems the patient is experiencing, such as sleep pattern disturbances, difficulties with self-care, or poor nutritional habits.

Nursing Diagnoses for the Biologic Domain

Common nursing diagnoses for the biologic domain are Disturbed Thought Process, Disturbed Sensory Perception, and Insomnia. Because of the variety of problems in patients with SCA, almost any nursing diagnosis could be generated. The persistent nature of this disorder lends itself to numerous and varied problems that must all be addressed (see Nursing Care Plan 19.1).

Interventions for the Biologic Domain

Patient Education

Interventions are based on the needs identified in the biopsychosocial assessment (Fig. 19.1). Establishing a regular sleep pattern by setting a routine can help to promote or re-establish normal patterns of rest. Educating the patient about the six food groups in the Food Guide Pyramid and about what constitutes good nutrition can improve nutritional status. Help the patient to notice self-care deficits, especially those caused by lack of motivation. For deficits created by severe mood symptoms, establishing a routine and setting goals can be useful.

Pharmacologic Interventions

An in-depth history of the patient's medication is important in evaluating response to past medications and predicting response to the present regimen.

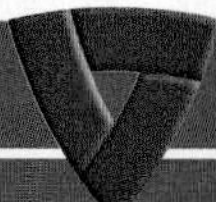

Nursing Care Plan 19.1

Patient With Schizoaffective Disorder

Ms. B is a 28-year-old divorced woman with a 4-year-old daughter. They reside with Ms. B's parents. Ms. B is a hairdresser and tries to work, but she becomes stressed in the workplace, which results in her being fired. She has never applied for disability. Her parents are stressed because of the exacerbations of her illness and caring for her child.

Ms. B has had numerous hospitalizations for aggressive behavior, noncompliance with medications, and receiving medications from various physicians, which results in inappropriate psychiatric management. She is medication seeking and is often prescribed benzodiazepines and diet pills by her primary care physician.

The patient has an ingrained delusional system that makes it hard to introduce reality orientation and feedback. She believes that her ex-husband has sexually abused their child. She has gone to numerous attorneys to try and prosecute the ex-husband to no avail because of the lack of evidence to prove any abuse.

For the last 2 years, Ms. B has believed that a bank guard is in love with her. She is adamant about him protecting her and her child. She states that he watches over them. They have no contact other than speaking to each other when she enters the bank. She has been seeing a man the past 9 months, but states that she really does not care much for him and it is hard for her to move forward in the relationship because she loves the bank guard.

Medications have included antidepressants, neuroleptics (typical and atypical), mood stabilizers, benzodiazepines, sleep medications, and anticonvulsants. She often complains of being depressed and yet is noncompliant with the antidepressant medications when they are prescribed.

Setting: Intensive Care Psychiatric Unit In a General Hospital

Baseline Assessment: Ms. B is admitted to the hospital through the ER. She was hearing voices and was delusional. She has not been taking medications for several months. She is oriented in all spheres and well nourished but unkempt. She is verbalizing delusions about a man at the bank. She cannot sleep well and reportedly goes outdoors at night and yells at a bank guard. Reality feedback increases her agitation. She denies any problems.

Associated Psychiatric Diagnosis		Medications
Axis I:	Schizoaffective disorder	None
Axis II:	Deferred	
Axis III:	None	
Axis: IV:	Social problem (maintaining relationships) Economic problem (no income) Occupation problem (unemployed)	
Axis V:	Current, 28 Potential, 60	

Continued

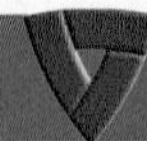

Nursing Care Plan 19.1 *(Continued)*

Nursing Diagnosis 1: Ineffective Individual Coping

Defining Characteristics	Related Factors
Inability to meet role expectations Anxiety Delusions Inability to problem solve	Chronicity of the condition Inadequate psychological resources secondary to delusions Inadequate coping skills Inadequate psychological resources to adapt to residential setting

Outcomes

Initial	Discharge
1. Identify coping pattern 2. Identify stressors 3. Identify personal strengths 4. Accept support through the nursing relationship	5. Manage own behavior 6. Medication compliance 7. Reduction of delusions

Interventions

Interventions	Rationale	Ongoing Assessment
Initiate a nurse–patient relationship to develop trust.	Through the use of the nurse–patient relationship, the patient will be able to maintain compliance with the treatment plan.	Determine whether patient is able to relate to the nurse.
Facilitate the identification of stressors in patient's environment.	To be able to cope with stressors, they need to be identified by the patient.	Assess whether patient is able to identify and verbalize stressors.
Develop coping strategies to manage environmental stressors.	Patient needs to develop realistic strategies to handle environmental stressors.	Determine whether patient-identified strategies are realistic.
Help patient to identify personal strengths.	By identifying personal strengths, patient will increase confidence in using coping strategies.	Assess patient's ability to incorporate coping strategies into her daily routine.
Assist patient to understand the disorder and its management.	By understanding the disorder, patient can develop ways to manage her disorder.	Assess the patient's level of understanding of the disease.
Facilitate emotional support for the family.	Supported family is better equipped to support patient.	Assess family's ability to seek emotional support from the staff.
Teach coping skills	By developing positive coping skills, anxiety and agitation will decrease.	Assess patient's ability to learn the skills to manage stressors.

Evaluation

Outcomes	Revised Outcomes	Interventions
Within the nursing relationship, Ms. B. was able to understand how coping skills can reduce stressors.	Support the patient's ability to recognize stressor and apply coping skills.	Discuss stressors and means of applying coping skills.
Increased insight into what behavior is appropriate has helped the patient to decrease verbalization of delusions.	Provide ongoing support to maintain present level of functioning.	Discuss behavior and provide reality feedback.

Nursing Diagnosis 2: Disturbed Thought Processes

Defining Characteristics	Related Factors
Delusions Impulsivity Medication noncompliance	Ingrained delusions Decreased ability to process secondary to delusions

Continued

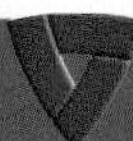

Nursing Care Plan 19.1 *(Continued)*

Outcomes

Initial	Discharge
1. Maintain reality orientation. 2. Communicate clearly with others. 3. Expresses delusional material less frequently.	4. Identify situations that contribute to delusions. 5. Identify how delusions affect life situations. 6. Use coping strategies to deal with delusions. 7. Recognize changes in behavior.

Interventions

Interventions	Rationale	Ongoing Assessment
Promote medication compliance.	Compliance will reduce delusions.	Assess for side effects: heat intolerance, neuroleptic malignant syndrome, renal failure, constipation, dry mouth, increased appetite, salivation, nausea, vomiting, tardive dyskinesia, seizures, somnolence, agitation, insomnia, dizziness.
Teach actions, effects, and side effects of medications.	The more knowledgeable patients are about medication, the more likely they will comply.	Assess ability to understand information.
Support reality testing through helping patient to differentiate thoughts and feelings in relationship to situations.	When comparing thoughts with the situations, patients can develop skills to refute delusions.	Assess for medication compliance.
Monitor verbalization of delusional material.	To determine whether medication is reducing delusional thoughts.	Assess verbalization of delusional material.
Identify stressors that promote delusions.	If patient is able to identify stressors that promote delusions, she can manage the stressors to effectively decrease delusions.	Assess patient's ability to recognize stressors when they occur.
Assist patient in developing skills to deal with delusions (recognizing delusional themes can help the patient in distinguishing between reality- and nonreality-based patterns).	Even though medication can reduce the occurrence of delusions, they may continue in some people with decreased intensity. Cognitive-behavioral skills are important in dealing with these altered thoughts.	Monitor patient's ability to handle delusions.

Evaluation

Outcomes	Revised Outcomes	Interventions
Delusions will be less ingrained.	Continue to practice skills in reality orientation and communication.	Support verbalization of reality-based thoughts.
Patient verbalized action, effect, dosage, and side effects of medications.	Take prescribed medication regularly.	Give positive feedback for understanding of medication.
Medication compliance		Initiate pill counts.

Summary: Ms. B was discharged from the hospital. Verbalization of delusions had not decreased. She was less anxious. She is presently on Abilify 30 mg at bedtime, Effexor XR 75 mg AM, Xanax 0.5 mg AM, and Seroquel 50 mg at bedtime. Mother is helping by filling a weekly medication box. At times Ms B. is questioning her delusions.

Investigate adherence to past treatment to determine the probability of successful intervention. Develop a plan to increase compliance, based on past problems with adherence. For example, use medication boxes and calendars and get help from others in managing the medication. Recognizing medication side effects quickly and intervening promptly to alleviate them will help maintain patient compliance. Helping understand the need for medications is essential.

Mood and psychotic symptoms are equally important and should be evaluated throughout treatment. Atypical antipsychotic agents are generally prescribed because of their efficacy and safe side-effect profile. Clozapine, reported effective for SCA by several authorities, can reduce hospitalizations and risk for suicide (Potkin et al., 2003). A significant portion of patients whose symptoms have resisted other neuroleptic agents experience improvement with clozapine therapy (Volavka et al., 2002). Atypical antipsychotic agents may have **thymoleptic** (mood stabilizing), as well as antipsychotic, effects. Aripiprazole's antidepressant response in SCA may replace polypharmacy, thus reducing drug costs,

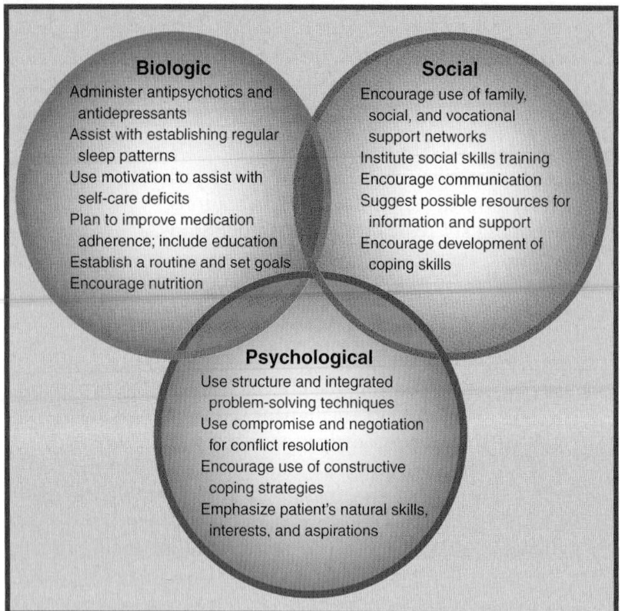

FIGURE 19.1. Biopsychosocial interventions for patients with schizoaffective disorder.

risk of drug interactions, and potential adverse drug effects (Marder et al., 2003). Quetiapine has been found effective (Bech, 2001). Dosage is the same as that used for treating schizophrenia, but lower dosage ranges may also be effective.

• NCLEXNOTE

The medication regimen for patients with schizoaffective disorder will be complex and may include antipsychotics, mood stabilizers, antidepressants, and occasional antianxiety agents.

In many cases, symptoms of depression disappear when psychotic symptoms decrease. If depressive symptoms persist, adjunctive use of an antidepressant agent may be helpful. Successful use of anticonvulsant agents for this disorder has been documented in several clinical trials (Dietrich, Kropp, & Emrich, 2001). Mood stabilizers, which can decrease the frequency and intensity of episodes, may be an alternative adjunctive medication for mood states associated with the bipolar type.

Administering and Monitoring Medications

One of the greatest challenges in pharmacologic interventions is monitoring target symptoms and identifying changes in symptom pattern. Patients can switch from being relatively calm to being very emotional. Whether the patient is overreacting to an environmental event or mood symptoms have changed and the patient requires a medication change can be determined only through careful observation and documentation.

Adherence to medication regimens is critical to a successful outcome. Patients need an opportunity to discuss barriers to compliance.

Managing Side Effects. Monitoring medication side effects in patients with SCA is similar to that in patients with schizophrenia. Extrapyramidal side effects, weight gain, and sedation should be assessed and documented.

Monitoring for Drug Interactions. Avoid using lithium with antipsychotic medications. A few patients taking haloperidol and lithium have experienced an encephalopathic syndrome, followed by irreversible brain damage. Lithium may interact similarly with other antipsychotic agents. It may also prolong the effects of neuromuscular blocking agents. Use of nonsteroidal anti-inflammatory drugs may increase plasma lithium levels. Diuretics and angiotensin-converting enzyme inhibitors should be prescribed cautiously with lithium, which is excreted through the kidney (see Chapter 8 for more information).

Teaching Points 

- Instruct patients to take medications as prescribed.
- Determine whether the patient has sufficient resources to purchase and obtain medications.
- Have the patient write down the prescribed medication and time of administration.
- Explain the target symptom for each medication (e.g., psychosis and mood for atypical antipsychotic agents, mood for antidepressant and mood stabilizer drugs).
- Caution patients about orthostatic hypotension and instruct them to get up slowly from a lying or sitting position. Also advise them to maintain adequate fluid intake.
- Advise patients to contact their case managers or health care providers if they experience dramatic changes in body temperature (neuroleptic malignant syndrome [NMS]), inability to control motor movement (dystonia), or dizziness.
- Advise patients to avoid over-the-counter medications unless a prescriber is consulted.
- Advise patients taking olanzapine and clozapine to monitor body weight and report rapid weight gains.
- Advise patients to report symptoms of diabetes mellitus (frequent urination, excessive thirst, etc.).

Psychological Domain

Assessment

The patient's level of insight into his or her illness may play a role in the course and treatment of SCA. Patients

BOX 19.2

Using Reflection: Overreacting to Stresses

Incident: A patient living in the community told a community health nurse that she refused to let her children go to school because of a terrorist threat in another state.

Reflection: At first the nurse thought that the patient had overslept and had made an excuse for not sending her children to school. Upon further analysis the nurse realized that the patient was overreacting to a stressful situation. Overreaction is one of the characteristics of schizoaffective disorder. The patient was experiencing extreme stress and needed to develop coping strategies for her overreaction to these types of events.

with SCA tend to have better insight than those with schizophrenia (Pini, Cassano, Dell'Osso, & Amador, 2001). Stressors should be evaluated because they may trigger symptoms. Uncovering or exploratory techniques should generally be avoided. Mental status and reality contact may be compromised. Assessment of anxiety level or reactions to stressful situations is important because the combination of these symptoms with psychosis increases the patient's risk for suicide (Box 19.2).

Nursing Diagnoses for Psychological Domain

In SCA, individuals vacillate between mood dysregulation and disturbed thinking. Typical nursing diagnoses for this domain include Hopelessness, Powerlessness, Ineffective Coping, Low Self-esteem, and Impaired Social Interaction (Fig. 19.2).

Interventions for Psychological Domain

Using appropriate interpersonal modalities is important to help the patient, family, and social and vocational support networks cope with the onslaught of acute episodes and recuperative periods. Patients with SCA have fewer awareness deficits than do patients with schizophrenia. Structured, integrated, and problem-solving psychotherapeutic interventions should be used to develop or increase the patient's insight. Psychoeducational interventions can help to decrease symptoms, enhance recognition of early regression, and hone psychosocial skills (see Box 19–3).

Social Domain

Assessment

Social dysfunction is common in patients with diagnoses of SCA. Premorbid adjustment, such as marital status and adolescent social adjustment, may influence patients' level of functioning at the time of diagnosis and their prognoses. Assess for social skill deficits and problems with interpersonal conflicts, particularly in men. Assessment of an adult patient's childhood may give a clue to the patient's current level of social functioning. Assess the patient's use of fantasy and fighting as a means of coping. Patients who report the most severe peer rejection present with the angriest dispositions and display antisocial behaviors.

Nursing Diagnoses for the Social Domain

Because of their mood and thought disturbances, these individuals will have significant problems in the social

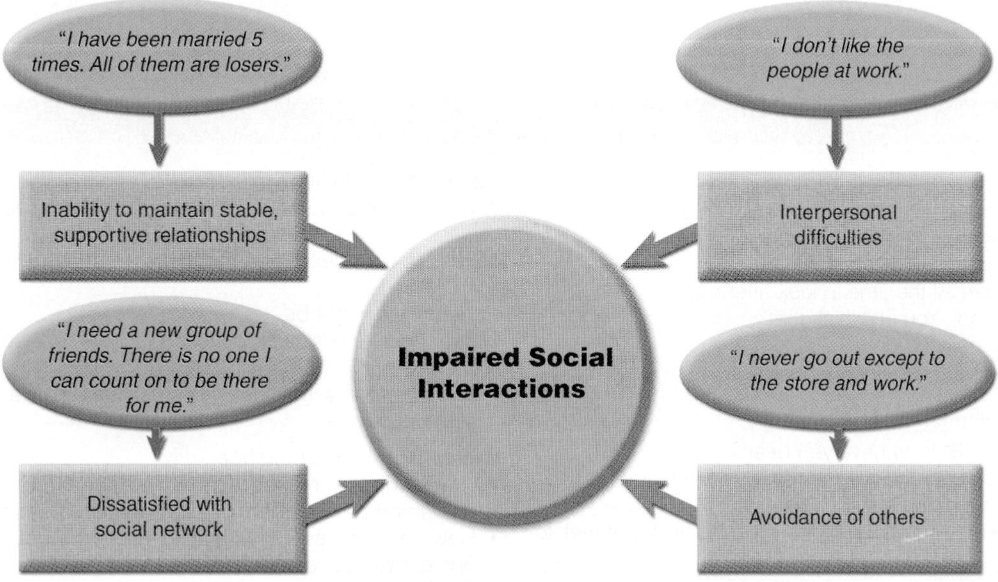

FIGURE 19.2. Nursing diagnosis concept map: Impaired Social interactions.

BOX 19.3

Psychoeducation Checklist: Schizoaffective Disorder

When caring for the patient with schizoaffective disorder, be sure to include the caregiver as appropriate and address the following topic areas in the teaching plan:

- Psychopharmacologic agents (antipsychotic or antidepressants), if used, including drug action, dosage, frequency, and possible adverse effects
- Methods to enhance adherence
- Sleep measures
- Consistent routines
- Goal setting
- Nutrition
- Support networks
- Problem solving
- Positive coping strategies
- Social and vocational skills training

domain. Typical nursing diagnoses include Compromised Family Coping, Impaired Home Maintenance, and Social Isolation.

Interventions for the Social Domain

Social skills training is useful for remediating social deficits and may result in positive social adjustment. Positive results include improved interpersonal competence and decreased symptom severity. Help in identifying feelings and in developing realistic goals, along with supportive therapy, can integrate insight into the disease process. Education focusing on conflict-resolution skills, promoting compromise, negotiation, and expression of negative feelings, can help the patient achieve positive social adjustment. Social skills can be improved through role playing and assertiveness training. Supportive, nurturing, and nonconfrontational interventions help to minimize anxiety and improve understanding (see Box 19.4).

Helping the patient to develop coping skills is essential. Teach communication skills to decrease conflicts and environmental negativity. Memory is linked with development of social skills; psychotic symptoms may interfere with retention of these skills, resulting in slower learning. These patients require long-term, intense social training.

Families are at risk for ineffective coping. Family members face many of the same issues faced by families of patients with schizophrenia and are often puzzled by the patient's emotional overreaction to normal daily stresses. Frequent arguments may lead to verbal and physical abuse.

Evaluation and Treatment Outcomes

Teaching skills to patients with SCA often takes longer than teaching other patients. When evaluating progress related to interventions, be patient if outcomes are not completely met. Psychoeducation results in increased knowledge of the illness and treatment, increased medication compliance, fewer relapses and hospitalizations, briefer inpatient stays, increased social function, decreased family tension, and lighter family burdens (Andres, Pfammatter, Garst, Teschner, & Brenner, 2000). Maintain realistic outcomes and praise small successes to promote positive outcomes (Fig. 19.3).

BOX 19.4

Therapeutic Dialog: Ms. B's "Delusions"

Ineffective Communication

Nurse: Hello, Ms. B, what has been happening?
Patient: The guy from the bank keeps me up all night.
Nurse: That's not possible.
Patient: He's there all the time to look after me.
Nurse: No, he's not. You just think that.
Patient: No, he really is. He is helping me.
Nurse: He does not even know who you are.

Effective Communication

Nurse: Hello, Ms. B. How have you been?
Patient: That guy from the bank is really bothering me.
Nurse: What is he doing?
Patient: He keeps me up all night. I go out in the street to yell at him.
Nurse: Have you actually seen him at night?
Patient: No, but I know he is there.
Nurse: How can he be there when you cannot see him?
Patient: He can't.
Nurse: Does it seem that the thoughts about him come from your mind?
Patient: This might be.
Nurse: Your illness often causes thoughts that are not reality based.
Patient: It seems real but yet so unreal. Those are sort of stupid thoughts.

Critical Thinking Challenge

- How could the nurse's approach in the first scenario have prevented development of a therapeutic relationship?
- How can the second scenario benefit the patient in developing insight into her delusions?
- Discuss the differences between the two approaches.

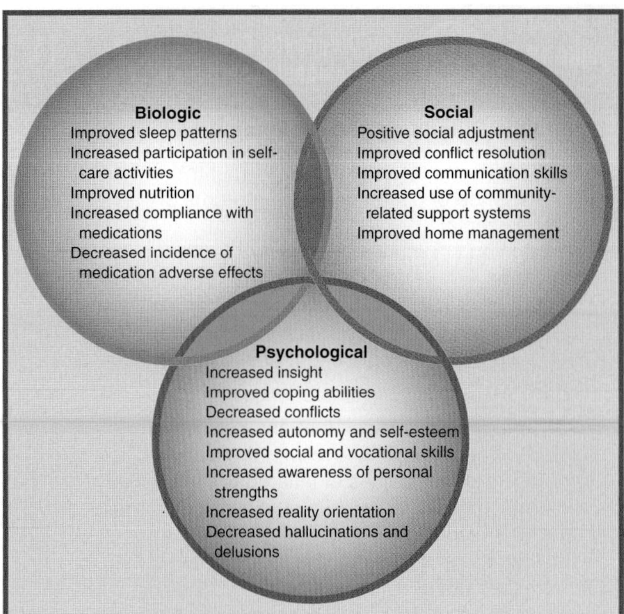

FIGURE 19.3. Biopsychosocial outcomes for patients with SCA.

Continuum of Care

Inpatient-Focused Care

Hospitalization may be required during acute psychotic episodes or when suicidal ideations are present. This structured environment protects the patient from self-harm (i.e., suicidal, assaultive, financial, legal, vocational, or social). During periods of acute psychosis, offering reassurance in a soft, nonthreatening voice, and avoiding confrontational stances, will help the patient begin to trust the staff and nursing care (see Chapter 10). Avoid seclusion and restraint and keep environmental stimulation to a minimum. Use the patient's coping capabilities to reinforce constructive aspects of functioning and enable a return to autonomy.

Emergency! Care

Emergency care is needed during symptom exacerbation. Psychosis, mood disturbance, and medication-related adverse effects account for most emergency situations. During an exacerbation of psychosis, patients may become agitated or aggressive. Assaultive behavior can be managed by using therapeutic techniques (see Chapter 38) and pharmacologic management. If medications are used, benzodiazepines such as lorazepam are usually given. Patients are then evaluated for antipsychotic therapy. Possible medication-related adverse effects include NMS as a reaction to dopamine antagonists or serotonin intoxication, especially if the patient is taking an atypical antipsychotic agent and a selective serotonin reuptake inhibitor (see Chapter 18).

Family Intervention 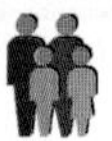

Helping families support the patient in the home or a community placement is an integral part of nursing care. With patient permission, key family members can be included in home visits to learn about symptoms, medications, and side effects. By collaborating with family members, the nurse can strengthen the patient's willingness to follow treatment, monitor symptoms, and continue with rehabilitation and recovery.

Community Treatment

After the patient is released from the hospital, graduated levels of care (i.e., partial hospitalization, day treatment, group home) can help the patient to return to a more normal environment. Programs that foster building and practicing social and vocational skills are appropriate and should also incorporate the patient's natural skills, interests, and aspirations because they are as important as problems and deficits.

Because this illness is episodic, the person with SCA requires close and continued follow-up in the outpatient setting by psychiatrists, nurses, and therapists. These patients require ongoing medication management, supportive and cognitive therapy, and symptom management. If symptoms intensify, hospitalization may be required until they are brought under control.

DELUSIONAL DISORDER

Clinical Course

Delusional disorder is a psychotic disorder characterized by nonbizarre, logical, stable, and well-systematized delusions that occur in the absence of other psychiatric disorders. **Delusions** are false, fixed beliefs unchanged by reasonable arguments. Although delusions are a symptom of many psychotic disorders, in delusional disorder, the delusions are **nonbizarre delusions**, that is, they are characterized by adherence to possible situations that could occur in real life and are plausible in the context of the person's ethnic and cultural background (APA, 2000).

Examples of real-life situations include being followed, poisoned, infected, loved at a distance, or deceived by a spouse or lover. A diagnosis of delusional disorder is based on the presence of one or more nonbizarre delusion for at least 1 month (APA, 2000). Delusions are the primary symptom of this disorder (Box 19.5).

BOX 19.5

Using Reflection: A Missed Opportunity

Incident: A patient in primary care insists that he is being stalked by his former boss who wants the patient's newly developed computer program. He refuses to see any mental health professionals. The nurse focuses on the patient's physical problems and ignores his delusional thoughts.

Reflection: Later, the nurse reflected on the meaning and significance of the patient's beliefs. Could the patient be a victim of stalking? Does the patient have a delusional disorder and need treatment? Does he need further evaluation? Would he hurt anyone? Unfortunately, the nurse will not know the meaning or significance of the statement without further assessment.

The course of delusional disorder is variable. Onset can be acute, or the disorder can occur gradually and become chronic. Patients with this disorder usually live with their delusions for years, rarely receiving psychiatric treatment. They are seldom brought to the attention of health care providers unless their delusion relates to their health (somatic delusion), or they act on the basis of their delusion and violate legal or social rules. Full remissions can be followed by relapses.

Apart from the direct impact of the delusion, psychosocial functioning is not markedly impaired. The person's clarity of thinking and behavior and emotional responses are usually consistent with the delusional focus. In general, behavior is not odd or bizarre. In fact, behavior is remarkably normal, except when the patient focuses on the delusion. At that time, thinking, attitudes, and mood may change abruptly. Personality does not usually change, but the patient is gradually, progressively involved with the delusional concern (APA, 2000).

Diagnostic Criteria

Delusional disorder is characterized by the presence of nonbizarre delusions and includes several subtypes: erotomanic, grandiose, jealous, somatic, mixed, and unspecified (Table 19.2). These subtypes represent the prominent theme of the delusion. A patient who has met criteria A for schizophrenia does not receive a diagnosis of delusional disorder (see Chapter 18 for criteria A). Although hallucinations may be present, they are not prominent (APA, 2000).

If mood episodes occur with this disorder, the total duration of the mood episode is relatively brief compared with the total duration of the delusional period. The delusion is not caused by the direct physiologic effects of substances (i.e., cocaine, amphetamines, marijuana) or a general medical condition (i.e., Alzheimer's disease, systemic lupus erythematosus). Because delusional disorder is uncommon and possesses features that are characteristic of other illnesses, the differential diagnosis has clear-cut logic. It is a diagnosis of exclusion requiring careful evaluation. Distinguishing this disorder from schizophrenia and mood disorders with psychotic features is difficult (APA, 2000).

Table 19.2  **Key Diagnostic Characteristics of Delusional Disorder 297.1** 

Diagnostic Criteria and Target Symptoms

- Nonbizarre delusions of at least 1 month's duration
- No presence of characteristic symptoms of schizophrenia
- Functioning not markedly impaired; behavior not odd or bizarre
- If concurrent with delusions, mood disorders relatively brief in comparison with delusional periods
- Not a direct physiologic effect of substance or medical condition

Erotomanic type: delusions that another person of usually higher status is in love with the person
Grandiose type: delusions of inflated worth, power, knowledge, identity, or special relationship to a deity or famous person
Jealous type: delusions that the individual's sexual partner is unfaithful
Persecutory type: delusions that person or someone close to person is being malevolently treated in some way
Somatic type: delusion that person has some physical defect or general medical condition
Mixed type: delusions characteristic of more than one of the above types; no one theme predominates
Unspecified type: delusion cannot be clearly identified or described

Associated Findings

- Social, marital, or work problems
- Ideas of reference
- Irritable mood
- Marked anger and violent behavior (especially with jealous type)

The prevalence of delusional disorder is about three per 10,000 general population. It is a rare disease even in psychiatric samples (Meloy, 1999). Research data are limited because numbers of recorded case studies and participants are small, and the studies lack systematic description, assessment, and diagnosis.

Delusional disorder may be associated with dysfunction in the frontal-subcortical systems and with temporal dysfunction, particularly on the left side (Fujii, Ahmed, & Takeshita, 1999).

Subtypes

Erotomanic Delusions

The concept of **erotomania** dates from the 17th century. Erotomania rarely appears in the pure or primary form. Secondary erotomania, which occurs with other psychiatric conditions, is more common. Differential diagnosis is important for excluding other significant psychiatric disorders or histologic conditions.

The erotomanic subtype is characterized by the delusional belief that the patient is loved intensely by the "loved object," who is usually married, of a higher socioeconomic status, or otherwise unattainable. The patient believes that the loved object's position in life would be in jeopardy if his or her true feelings were known. In addition, the patient is convinced that he or she is in amorous communication with the loved object. The loved object is often a public figure (e.g., movie star, politician) but may also be a common stranger. The patient believes that the loved object was the first to make advances and fall in love. The patient may entertain some delusional beliefs about a sexual relationship with the loved object, yet the beliefs are unfounded. The delusion, which often idealizes romantic love and spiritual union, rather than sexual attraction (APA, 2000), becomes the central focus of the patient's existence.

The patient may have minimal or no contact with the loved object and often keeps the delusion secret, but efforts to contact the loved object through letters, telephone calls, gifts, visits, surveillance, and stalking are also common. The patient may in many cases transfer his or her delusion to another loved object. There is some evidence that celebrity worship is associated with cognitive deficits (McCutcheon, Ashe, Houran, & Maltby, 2003).

Patients with erotomanic delusional disorder are generally unattractive; are often lower-level employees; lead withdrawn, lonely lives; are single with poor interpersonal relationships; and have limited sexual contacts or are sexually repressed. Clinical patients are mostly women, who do not usually act out their delusions. Forensic patients are mostly men, who tend to be more aggressive and can become violent in pursuit of the loved object, although the loved object may not be the object of the aggression. Men in particular come into contact with the law in their pursuit of the loved object or in a misguided effort to rescue the loved object from some imagined danger. Orders of protection are generally ineffective, and criminal charges of stalking or harassment that lead to incarceration are ineffective as a long-term solution to the problem (Harmon, Rosner, & Owens, 1995; Munro, 1999). The result is repeated arrests and psychiatric examinations, followed by ineffective treatment. Patients are rarely motivated to seek psychiatric treatment. This disorder is difficult to control, contain, or treat. The patient seldom gives up the belief that he or she is loved by the loved object. Separation from the loved object is the only satisfactory means of intervention (APA, 2000). Cognitive rigidity arising from frontal-subcortical dysfunction may contribute to maintaining erotic delusions and result in inability to alter a belief system (Fujii et al., 1999).

Grandiose Delusions

Patients presenting with grandiose delusions are convinced they have a great, unrecognized talent or have made an important discovery. A less common presentation is the delusion of a special relationship with a prominent person (i.e., an adviser to the President) or of actually being a prominent person (i.e., the President). In the latter case, the person with the delusion may regard the actual prominent person as an impostor. Other grandiose delusions may be religious in nature, such as a delusional belief that he or she has a special message from a deity (APA, 2000; Munro, 1999).

Jealous Delusions

The central theme of the jealous subtype is the unfaithfulness or infidelity of a spouse or lover. The belief arises without cause and is based on incorrect inferences justified by "evidence" (i.e., rumpled clothing, spots on sheets) the patient has collected. The patient usually confronts the spouse or lover with a host of such evidence. An associated feature is paranoia. The patient may attempt to intervene in the imagined infidelity by secretly following the spouse or lover or by investigating the imagined lover (APA, 2000; Munro, 1999).

Delusions of jealousy are difficult to treat and may diminish only with separation, divorce, or the death of the spouse or lover. Except in the elderly, such patients generally are male. Jealousy is a powerful, potentially dangerous emotion. Aggression, even violent behavior, may result. Litigious behavior is common, and symptoms with forensic aspects are often seen. Care is essential in determining how to deal with this patient.

Somatic Delusions

Somatic delusions, a mix of psychotic and somatic symptoms, have been described for more than 100 years. The central theme of somatic delusions involves bodily functions or sensations. These patients believe they have physical ailments. Delusions of this nature are fixed, inarguable, and intense, with the patient totally convinced of the physical nature of the somatic complaint. The delusion occurs in the absence of other medical or psychiatric conditions. Medication can cause tactile hallucinations that result directly from the physiologic effects of the medication; when the medication or drug is removed, the symptoms disappear. Somatic delusions are manifested in the following beliefs (APA, 2000):

- A foul odor is coming from the skin, mouth (delusions of halitosis), rectum, or vagina
- Insects have infested the skin (delusional parasitosis)
- Internal parasites have infested the digestive system

- A certain body part is misshapen or ugly (contrary to visible evidence)
- Parts of the body are not functioning (e.g., large intestine, bowels)

The delusion of infestation by insects cannot occur without sensory perceptions, which constitute tactile hallucinations. The patient vividly describes crawling, itching, burning, swarming, and jumping on the skin surface or below the skin. The patient maintains the conviction that he or she is infested with parasites in the absence of objective evidence to the contrary.

Patients with somatic delusions present a dilemma for health care systems because of their excessive use of health care resources. They seek repeated medical consultations with dermatologists, entomologists, infectious disease specialists, and general practitioners. They seek treatment from primary care physicians and refuse psychiatric referral. Even if they seek psychiatric help, these patients typically do not comply with long-term psychiatric intervention. Patients often go through elaborate rituals to cleanse themselves or their surroundings of the perceived pests, collecting hair, scabs, and skin flakes as evidence of an infection. They insist on being given unnecessary medical tests and procedures and are consequently at risk for increased morbidity because of invasive evaluation. Anger and hostility are common among this group, and behavioral characteristics include shame, depression, and avoidance.

The somatic subtype is rare but may be underdiagnosed. Both genders are affected equally, but when onset occurs in late middle age, female patients tend to predominate. Studies of somatic delusions have been marred by methodologic uncertainties, and factors limiting investigation include rarity of the disease, lack of contact with psychiatrists, and noncompliance with the medication regimen. A variant of the somatic subtype is body dysmorphic disorder, which is classified under somatoform disorders in the *Diagnostic and Statistical Manual of Mental Disorders, 4th edition, text revision* (DSM-IV-TR) (see Chapter 23).

Unspecified Delusions

In the mixed subtype, no one delusional theme predominates, and the patient presents with two or more types of delusions. In the unspecified subtype, the delusional beliefs cannot be clearly determined, or the predominant delusion is not described as a specific type. Patients are usually women who experience feelings of depersonalization and derealization and have negative-associated paranoid features. The delusions can be short-lived, recurrent, or persistent. This subtype also includes delusions of **misidentification** (i.e., illusions of doubles), wherein a familiar person is replaced by an impostor. For example, the patient may believe that close family members have assumed the persona of strangers, or that people they know can change into other people at will. This type of delusion occurs rarely and is generally associated with schizophrenia, Alzheimer's disease, or other organic conditions (APA, 2000).

Persecutory delusions, the most common type seen, are not listed as a separate subtype in the DSM-IV-TR, but they are addressed as a subtype of delusional disorder in the text (APA, 2000). The central theme of persecutory delusions is the patient's belief that he or she is being conspired against, cheated, spied on, followed, poisoned, drugged, maliciously maligned, harassed, or obstructed in pursuit of long-term goals. The patient exaggerates small slights, which become the focus of the delusion.

The focus of persecutory delusions is often on some injustice that must be remedied by legal action (querulous paranoia). Patients often seek satisfaction by repeatedly appealing to courts and other government agencies (Harmon et al., 1995; Munro, 1999). These patients are often angry and resentful and may even behave violently toward the people the patient believes are persecuting him or her. The course may be chronic, although the patient's preoccupation with the delusional belief often waxes and wanes. The clarity, logic, and systematic elaboration of this delusional theme leaves a remarkable stamp on this condition (APA, 2000).

Epidemiology and Risk Factors

Delusional disorder is relatively uncommon in clinical settings (APA, 2000). The best estimate of its prevalence in the population is about 0.03%, but precise information is lacking (APA, 2000). Lifetime morbidity is between 0.05% and 0.1% because of the late age of onset.

Few risk factors are associated with delusional disorder. Patients can live with their delusions without psychiatric intervention because their behavior is normal, although if delusions are somatic, patients risk unnecessary medical interventions. Acting on delusions carries a risk for intervention by law enforcement agencies or the legal system. Suicide attempts are neither more nor less common than in the general population (Grunebaum et al., 2001).

Age of Onset

Delusional disorder can begin in adolescence and occurs in middle to later adulthood. Onset occurs at a later age than among patients with schizophrenia. A prevalence of 2% to 4% has been reported in the elderly (APA, 2000).

Gender

Gender does not appear to affect the overall frequency of most delusional disorders (APA, 2000). Patients with erotomanic delusions are generally women; in forensic settings, most people with this disorder are men. Men also tend to experience more jealous delusions, except in the elderly population, in which women outnumber men.

Ethnicity and Culture

A person's ethnic, cultural, and religious background must be considered in evaluating the presence of delusional disorder. The content of delusions varies between cultures and subcultures (APA, 2000).

Family 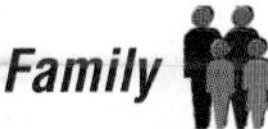

An increased familial risk and familial genetic factors are unknown.

Comorbidity

Mood disorders are frequently found in patients with delusional disorders. Typically mild symptoms of depression such as irritable or dysphoric mood are present. Delusional disorder may also be associated with obsessive-compulsive disorder and paranoid, schizoid, or avoidant personality disorder (APA, 2000).

Etiology

The cause of delusional disorder is unknown. The only major feature of this condition is the formation and persistence of the delusions. Few have investigated possible neurophysiologic and neuropsychological causes of delusional disorder, and theories of causation are contradictory. No psychological or social theories of causation are addressed in the literature.

Biologic Theories

Neuropathologic

In patients with delusional disorder, MRI shows a degree of temporal lobe asymmetry. However, these differences are subtle, so delusional disorder may involve a neurodegenerative component (Ota et al., 2003). The tactile hallucinations of somatic delusions may arise from sensory alterations in the nervous system (Baker, Cook, & Winokur, 1995) or from sensory input that has been misinterpreted because of subtle cortical changes associated with aging.

Genetic and Biochemical

Delusional disorder is probably biologically distinct from other psychotic disorders, yet little or no attention has been paid to genetic factors. Delusions may involve faulty processing of essentially intact perceptions, whereby perceptions become linked with an interpretation that has deep emotional significance but no verifiable basis (Conway et al., 2002; McGuire et al., 2001). Alternately, a complex, malfunctioning dopaminergic system may lead to delusions (Morimoto et al., 2002). This explanation could lead to the argument that a particular delusion depends on the "circuit" that is malfunctioning. Denial of reality has been linked to right posterior cortical dysfunction. Some authors have proposed a combination of biological and early life experiences as etiological components (Bentall, Corcoran, Howard, Blackwood, & Kinderman, 2001). It has been theorized recently that delusions may arise from dysfunction in the entorhinal cortex, which is located in the inner parts of the temporal lobes and serves as a relay between the prefrontal cortex and the hippocampus (Arehart-Treichel, 2004).

Interdisciplinary Treatment

Few if any interdisciplinary treatments are associated with delusional disorder because patients rarely receive attention from health care providers. Pharmacologic intervention is often based on symptoms. For example, patients with somatic delusions are treated for the specific complaints with which they present. Use of benzodiazepines may be common with this disorder because complaints are vague.

Priority Care Issues

By the time a patient with a diagnosis of delusional disorder is seen in a psychiatric setting, he or she has generally had the delusion for a long time. It is deeply ingrained and many times unshakable, even with psychopharmacologic intervention. These patients rarely comply with medication regimens.

Male patients who have the erotomanic subtype are likely to require special care because they are more likely than other patients to act on their delusions (for example, by continued attempts to contact the loved object, or stalking). This group is generally seen in forensic settings.

NURSING MANAGEMENT: HUMAN RESPONSE TO DELUSIONAL DISORDER

Biologic Domain

Assessment

Body systems are assessed to evaluate any physical problems. In people with somatic delusional disorder, assessment may be tedious because of the number and variety of presenting symptoms. Complaints are explored to develop a complete symptom history and to determine whether symptoms have a physical basis or are delusional. Past history of each complaint should be determined because this information may affect outcome. The more recent the onset, the more favorable the prognosis.

• NCLEXNOTE

NCLEXNOTE By definition, delusions are fixed, false beliefs that cannot be changed by reasonable arguments. The nurse should assess the patient's delusion to evaluate its significance to the patient and the patient's safety and the safety of others. The nurse should not dwell on the delusion or try to change it.

Most patients who receive diagnoses of delusional disorder do not experience functional difficulties or impairments. Self-care patterns may be disrupted in patients with the somatic subtype by the elaborate processes used to treat perceived illness (e.g., bathing rituals, creams). Sleep may be disrupted because of the central and overpowering nature of the delusions.

A complete medication history, past and present, is also important to determine the patient's past response and what agents the individual perceives as effective. Examining the patient's records for tests and procedures may help to substantiate the individual's complaints and symptoms.

Nursing Diagnoses for the Biologic Domain

The nursing diagnoses for the biologic domain depend on the type of delusions that are manifested and the response to these symptoms. For example, for a woman with the somatic delusion that insects are crawling on her, Disturbed Sensory Perception (Tactile) would be appropriate. For others who are fearful of poisoning, Imbalanced Nutrition, Less Than Body Requirements, may be a useful diagnosis. Refusal of medication may support a nursing diagnosis of Ineffective Therapeutic Regimen Management.

Interventions for Biologic Domain

Interventions are based on the problems identified during assessment (Fig. 19.4). Each is addressed individually. The nurse helps the patient to establish routines that can resolve problems and promote healthy functioning. A mechanism for managing the patient's medication regimen is developed.

Somatic Interventions

Delusional disorder has a reputation of being chronic and resistant to treatment. Treating somatic disorder is difficult because of the patient's insistence that the problem is not psychiatrically related. Many patients with delusional disorder are seen only by nonpsychiatric specialists, who use expensive and ineffective treatments. Patients with this disorder may adhere poorly to psychiatric pharmacotherapy, which is most likely related to the lack of insight about their illness (Nose, Barbui, & Tansella, 2003). Realistic and modest goals are most sensible. Establishing a therapeutic relationship is fundamental but far from simple.

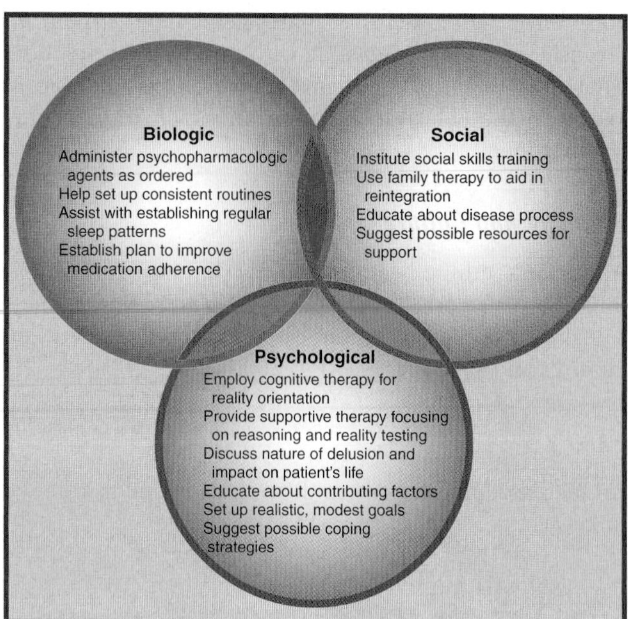

FIGURE 19.4. Biopsychosocial interventions for patients with delusional disorder.

Pharmacologic Interventions

Sparse literature is available about using psychiatric medications in delusional disorder, and the available reports conflict. Antipsychotic agents are useful in improving acute symptoms by decreasing agitation and the intensity of the delusion. They may also be effective in the long term, but little formal information exists to support this theory.

Administering and Monitoring Medications

Compliance in this population is problematic. Patients do not adhere to medication regimens and require monitoring of target symptoms. Look for an opportunity to discuss medications and barriers to compliance.

Managing Side Effects

Management of side effects is similar to that in other disorders that have a delusional component. The nurse assesses for NMS, extrapyramidal side effects, weight gain, and sedation.

Monitoring for Drug Interactions

Interactions are similar to those seen with medications for other disorders. A detailed list of prior and current medications must be elicited from these patients, especially those with somatic delusions, because they may be receiving medications from many different practitioners.

Teaching Points 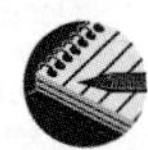

Instruct patients to take medication as prescribed. Determine whether the patient has sufficient resources to purchase and obtain medications, and explain target symptoms for each medication. Caution patients not to take over-the-counter medications without consulting their provider.

Psychological Domain

Assessment

Patients with delusional disorder show few if any psychological deficits, and those that do occur are generally related directly to the delusion. In these patients, average or marginally low intelligence is characteristic. Use of the Minnesota Multiphasic Personality Inventory, a clinical scale that identifies paranoid symptom deviation, may be useful in substantiating the diagnosis.

Mental status is not generally affected. Thinking, orientation, affect, attention, memory, perception, and personality are generally intact. Presenting reality-based evidence in an attempt to change the person's delusion can be helpful in determining whether the belief can be altered with sufficient evidence. If mental status is altered, this fact is generally brought to the health professional's attention by a third party, such as police, family member, neighbor, physician, or attorney. In these cases, the person has usually acted in some manner to draw attention to himself or herself. Talk with the person to grasp the nature of the delusional thinking: theme, impact on the person's life, complexity, systematization, and related features.

Nursing Diagnoses for the Psychological Domain

There are numerous nursing diagnoses that could be generated based upon assessment of the psychological domain. Ineffective Denial, Impaired Verbal Communication, Deficient Knowledge, and Risk for Loneliness are some examples. The nursing diagnoses of Readiness for Enhanced Self-concept, Chronic Low Self-esteem, Anxiety, Fear, and Powerlessness may also be generated.

Interventions for the Psychological Domain

Patients with delusional disorder are treated most effectively in outpatient settings with supportive therapy that allays the person's anxiety. Initiating discussion of the troubling experiences and consequences of the delusion and suggesting a means for coping may be successful. Assisting the person toward a more satisfying general adjustment is desirable (see Box 19.6).

Insight-oriented therapy is not useful because there is no benefit in trying to prove the delusion is not true, arguing the person out of the delusion, or telling the individual that the delusion is imaginary. Cognitive therapy with supportive therapy that focuses on reasoning or reality testing to decrease delusional thinking, or modifying the delusion itself, may be helpful. Educational interventions can aid the patient in understanding how factors such as sensory impairment, social and physical isolation, and stress contribute to the intensity of this disorder.

In certain instances, hospitalization is needed in response to dangerous behavior that could include aggressiveness, poor impulse control, excessive psychological tension, unremitting anger, and threats. Suicide can be a concern, but most patients are not at risk. If hospitalization is required, the person needs to be approached tactfully, and legal assistance may be necessary.

BOX 19.6

Psychoeducation Checklist Delusional Disorder

When caring for the patient with delusional disorder, be sure to include the caregiver, as appropriate, and address the following topic areas in the teaching plan:

- Psychopharmacologic agents (antipsychotic or antidepressants), if used, including drug action, dosage, frequency, and possible adverse effects
- Identification of troubling experiences
- Consequences of delusions
- Realistic goal setting
- Positive coping strategies
- Safety measures
- Social training skills
- Family participation in therapy

Social Domain

Assessment

A common characteristic of individuals with delusional disorder is normal behavior and appearance unless their delusional ideas are being discussed or acted on. The cultural background of the person with delusional disorder has to be evaluated. Ethnic and cultural systems have different beliefs that are accepted within their individual context but not outside their group. Problems can occur in social, occupational, or interpersonal areas. Social function is generally impaired, and social isolation is common among this group. Most are employed, but they generally hold low-level jobs.

Many are married. If the person's family or life partner is supportive, compliance is enhanced, and outcomes are improved. Married women have a better chance for a positive outcome than do unmarried women.

In general, the person's social and marital functioning is more likely to be impaired than their intellectual or occupational functioning.

When social or occupational functioning is poor, difficulties are related to the delusion. Thus, assessing the person's capacity to act in response to the delusion is important. What is the person's level of impulsiveness (i.e., related to behaviors of suicide, homicide, aggression, or violence)? Establishing as complete a picture of the person as possible, including the person's subjective private experiences and concrete psychopathologic symptoms, helps to reduce uncertainty in the assessment process.

Nursing Diagnoses for the Social Domain

Several nursing diagnoses can be generated from the assessment data for the social domain. Ineffective Coping, Interrupted Family Processes, and Ineffective Role Performance are examples.

Interventions for the Social Domain

People with diagnoses of delusional disorder often become socially isolated. The secretiveness of their delusions and the importance the delusions have in their life are central to this phenomenon. Social skills training tailored to the patient's specific deficits can help to improve social adaptation. Family therapy can help the person reintegrate into the family; family education and patient education will enhance understanding of the patient and the disease process. However, group therapy would not be beneficial because the patient lacks insight into the origin of the delusion. Families face many of the same issues as families of patients with other disorders involving delusions, but the stress of dealing with this disorder is not as great. Families are at risk for ineffective coping.

Evaluation and Treatment Outcomes

For patients with delusional disorders, the greater the lack of insight and the poorer the compliance with medication regimens, the more difficult it is to teach the individual. Resistance is typical, and the person is not amenable to interventions. The patient rarely, if ever, develops full insight, and the symptoms related to the original diagnosis are not likely to disappear completely. In evaluating progress, the nurse must remember that outcomes are often not met completely. The nurse should maintain realistic outcomes and praise small successes to promote positive outcomes (Fig. 19.5).

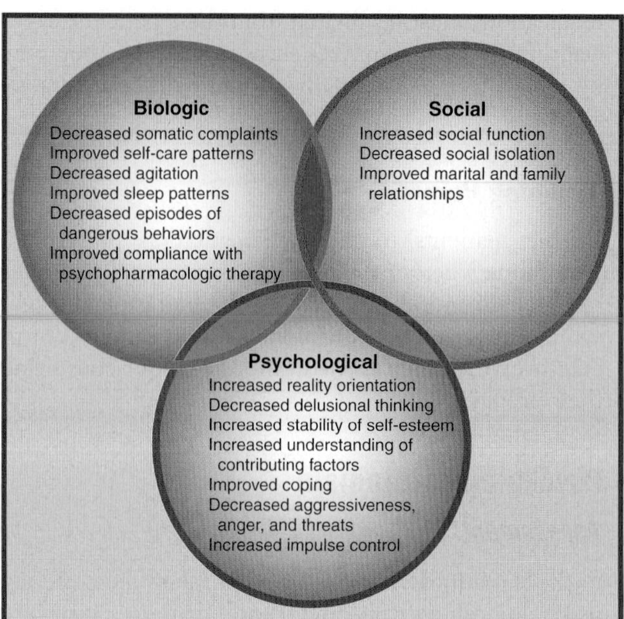

FIGURE 19.5. Biopsychosocial outcomes for patients with delusional disorder.

Continuum of Care

Inpatient-Focused Care

Hospitalization rarely occurs and is usually initiated by the legal or social violations. The hospital environment protects the patient from further legal intervention. Insight-oriented interventions help the patient to understand his or her situation. Avoid confrontational situations; use the patient's coping abilities to reinforce constructive aspects of functioning to enable a return to autonomy.

Emergency! Care

Emergency care is seldom required, unless the patient has had an incident with the law or legal system. The patient may be agitated or aggressive because the delusion, which is perceived as real, has been interrupted.

Family Intervention 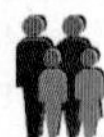

Family therapy may be helpful. By helping the family to develop mechanisms to cope with the patient's delusions, nurses help the family to be more supportive and understanding of the patient.

Community Treatment

Patients with diagnoses of delusional disorder are treated most effectively in an outpatient setting. They should be encouraged to seek psychiatric treatment. Insight-

Table 19.3 Other Psychotic Disorders

Disorder	Definition
Schizophreniform disorder	This disorder is identical to schizophrenia except the total duration of the illness can be less than 6 months (must be at least 1 month) and there may not be impaired social or occupational functioning.
Schizoaffective disorder	This disorder is characterized by an uninterrupted period of illness during which at some time there is a major depressive, manic, or mixed episode along with two of the following symptoms of schizophrenia: delusions, hallucinations, disorganized speech, disorganized or catatonic behavior, or negative symptoms (affective flattening, alogia, or avolition).
Delusional disorder	This disorder is characterized by the presence of nonbizarre delusion and includes several subtypes: erotomanic, grandiose, jealous, somatic, mixed, and unspecified.
Brief psychotic disorder	In this disorder, there is a sudden onset of at least one positive psychotic symptom that lasts at least 1 day but less than 1 month. Eventually, the individual has a full return to normal.
Shared psychotic disorders (*folie à deux*)	In this disorder, one person who is in a close relationship with another person who already has a psychotic disorder with prominent delusions also develops the delusion.
Other psychotic disorders due to substances such as drugs and alcohol	The prominent hallucinations or delusions are judged to be due to the physiologic effects of substances (drugs, alcohol).

American Psychiatric Association. (2000). *Diagnostic and statistical manual of mental disorders* (4th ed., text revision). Washington, DC: Author.

oriented therapy to develop an understanding of the patient's delusion may be helpful. Medications are not often used with delusional disorder, but antipsychotic agents or benzodiazepines are helpful during exacerbations. Other treatments include supportive therapy, development of coping skills, cognitive therapy, and social skills training. Family therapy may be helpful.

OTHER PSYCHOTIC DISORDERS

Other disorders have psychoses as their defining features. The nursing care of patients with these disorders is not discussed specifically, but the generalist psychiatric nurse has the ability to apply care used with other disorders to the disorders presented here (Table 19.3).

Schizophreniform Disorder

The essential features of schizophreniform disorder are identical to those of criteria A for schizophrenia, with the exception of the duration of the illness, which can be less than 6 months (APA, 2000). However, symptoms must be present for at least 1 month to be classified as a schizophreniform disorder (Table 19.4). This diagnosis is also used as provisional if symptoms have lasted more than 1 month but it is uncertain whether the person will recover before the end of the 6-month period. Some research has suggested that this illness may be an early manifestation of schizophrenia (Iancu, Dannon, Ziv, & Lepkifker, 2002).

Altered social or occupational functioning may occur but is not necessary. Most patients experience interruption in one or more areas of daily functioning (APA, 2000).

Brief Psychotic Disorder

In brief psychotic disorder, the length of the episode is at least 1 day but less than 1 month. The onset is sudden and includes at least one of the positive symptoms of criteria A for schizophrenia found in Chapter 18 (see also Table 19.4). Differentiating this illness from bipolar SCA is important (Marneros, Pillmann, Haring, Balzuweit, & Bloink, 2002).

The person generally experiences emotional turmoil or overwhelming confusion and rapid, intense shifts of affect (APA, 2000). Although episodes are brief, impairment can be severe, and supervision may be required to protect the person. Suicide is a risk, especially in younger patients. A predisposition to develop a brief psychotic disorder may include pre-existing personality disorders (APA, 2000). The person's ethnic and cultural background should also be considered in relation to the social or religious context of the symptoms presented. This disorder is uncommon but usually appears in early adulthood (APA, 2000).

Shared Psychotic Disorder

In shared psychotic disorder (*folie à deux*), a person develops a close relationship with another individual ("inducer" or "primary case") who has a psychotic disorder with prominent delusions (APA, 2000; Trabert, 1999) (see Table 19.4). With this disorder, the person believes and shares part or all of the inducer's delusional beliefs. The content of the delusions depends on the inducer, who is the dominant person in the relationship and imposes the delusions on the passive person (APA, 2000). This disorder is somewhat more common in women, and

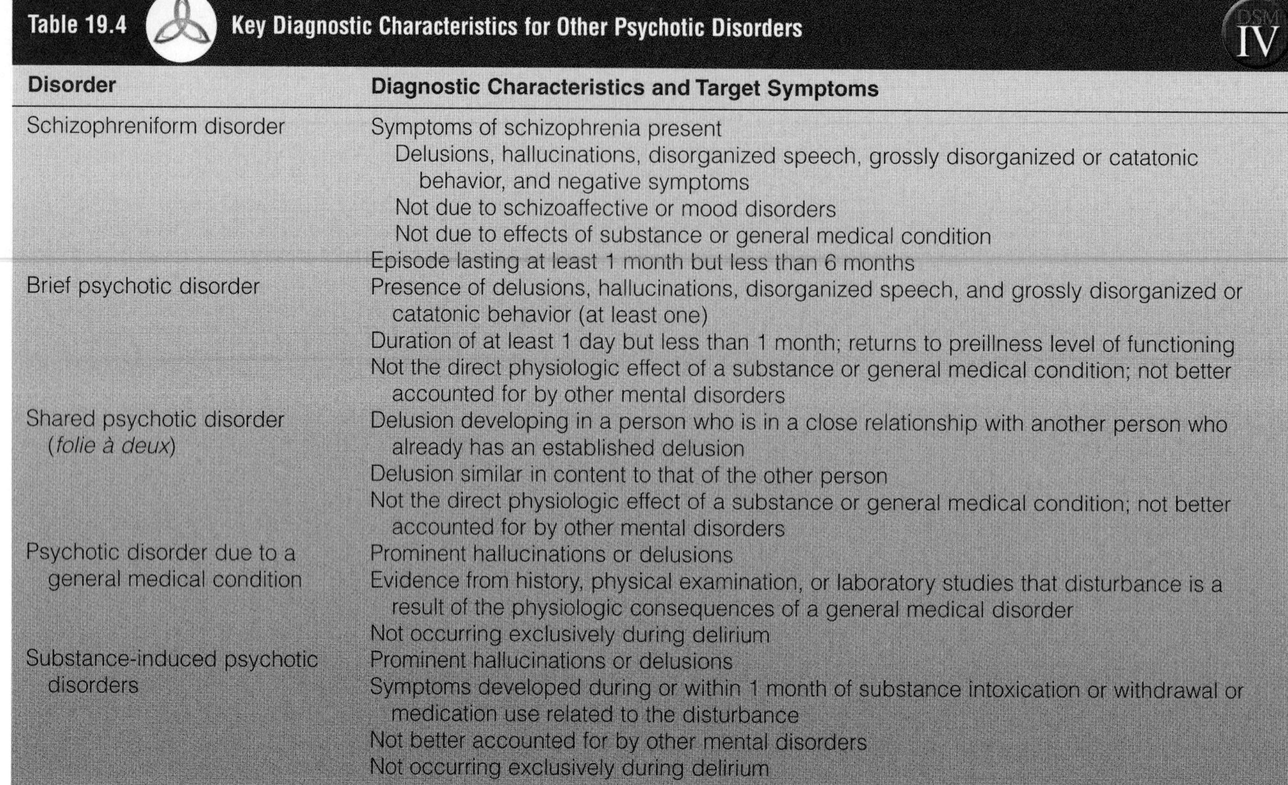

Table 19.4 Key Diagnostic Characteristics for Other Psychotic Disorders DSM IV

Disorder	Diagnostic Characteristics and Target Symptoms
Schizophreniform disorder	Symptoms of schizophrenia present Delusions, hallucinations, disorganized speech, grossly disorganized or catatonic behavior, and negative symptoms Not due to schizoaffective or mood disorders Not due to effects of substance or general medical condition Episode lasting at least 1 month but less than 6 months
Brief psychotic disorder	Presence of delusions, hallucinations, disorganized speech, and grossly disorganized or catatonic behavior (at least one) Duration of at least 1 day but less than 1 month; returns to preillness level of functioning Not the direct physiologic effect of a substance or general medical condition; not better accounted for by other mental disorders
Shared psychotic disorder (*folie à deux*)	Delusion developing in a person who is in a close relationship with another person who already has an established delusion Delusion similar in content to that of the other person Not the direct physiologic effect of a substance or general medical condition; not better accounted for by other mental disorders
Psychotic disorder due to a general medical condition	Prominent hallucinations or delusions Evidence from history, physical examination, or laboratory studies that disturbance is a result of the physiologic consequences of a general medical disorder Not occurring exclusively during delirium
Substance-induced psychotic disorders	Prominent hallucinations or delusions Symptoms developed during or within 1 month of substance intoxication or withdrawal or medication use related to the disturbance Not better accounted for by other mental disorders Not occurring exclusively during delirium

the age of onset is variable. Delusional beliefs are usually shared by people who have lived together for a long time in relative social isolation. However, family members rarely share the same delusional belief. When the relationship is interrupted, the passive person's delusional beliefs decrease or disappear (APA, 2000).

Treatment is sought infrequently (Trabert, 1999). When care is sought, the inducer usually brings the situation to clinical treatment (APA, 2000). If the passive person is removed from the setting, 93% have a favorable course even with no treatment (Trabert). If the inducer receives no intervention, the course is usually chronic.

Psychotic Disorders Attributable to Substance

Patients with a psychotic disorder attributable to a substance present with prominent hallucinations or delusions that are the direct physiologic effects of a substance (e.g., drug abuse, toxin exposure) (APA, 2000) (see Table 19.4). During intoxication, symptoms continue as long as the use of the substance continues. Withdrawal symptoms can occur for as long as 4 weeks. Differential diagnosis is recommended.

SUMMARY OF KEY POINTS

- Schizoaffective disorder has symptoms typical of both schizophrenia and mood disorders but is a separate disorder. Although these patients experience mood problems most of the time, the diagnosis of schizoaffective disorder depends on the presence of positive symptoms (i.e., delusions or hallucinations) without mood symptoms at some time during the uninterrupted period of illness.
- Although controversy and discussion continue about whether schizoaffective disorder is truly a separate disorder, the DSM-IV-TR now identifies it as separate.
- Patients with schizoaffective disorder have fewer awareness deficits and appear to have more insight than do patients with true schizophrenia, a fact that can be used in teaching patients to control symptoms, recognize early regression, and develop psychosocial skills.
- Patients with schizoaffective disorder will likely never be medication free. Intermittent antipsychotic dosing is best for patients who can detect recurring symptoms and institute their own drug therapy.

- Nursing care for patients with schizoaffective disorder is focused on minimizing psychiatric symptoms through promoting medication maintenance and on helping patients maintain optimal levels of functioning. Interventions center on developing social and coping skills through supportive, nurturing, and nonconfrontational approaches. The nurse must be constantly attuned to the mood state of the patient and help the patient learn to solve problems, resolve conflict, and cope with social situations that trigger anxiety.
- Delusional disorder is characterized by stable, well-systematized, and logical nonbizarre delusions that could occur in real life and are plausible in the context of the patient's ethnic and cultural background. These delusions may or may not interfere with an individual's ability to function socially. Patients typically deny any psychiatric basis for their problem and refuse to seek psychiatric care. Patients whose delusions relate to somatic complaints are often seen on medical-surgical units of hospitals. Diagnosis otherwise is often made only when patients act on the basis of their delusions and violate the law or social rules.
- Delusional disorder is further classified as a particular subtype, depending on the nature and content of the patient's delusions, including erotomanic, grandiose, jealous, somatic, mixed, and unspecified.
- Patients with delusional disorder usually do not experience functional difficulties or mental status impairments. Their thinking, orientation, affect, attention, memory, perception, and personality generally remain intact.
- The therapeutic relationship is crucial to the successful treatment of the patient with delusional disorder. Nurses must be aware of the patient's fragile self-esteem and unusual sensitivities and anxieties and try to establish a trusting relationship through a flexible, nonjudgmental approach that promotes empathy, trust, and support while keeping physical and emotional detachment.

CRITICAL THINKING CHALLENGES

1 Mr. J. first received a diagnosis of schizophrenia, but after experiencing extreme mood disturbances, finally received a diagnosis of schizoaffective disorder. During a recent outpatient visit, he confides to a nurse that he just has stress and does not think that he really has any psychiatric problems. Identify assessment areas that should be pursued before the patient leaves his appointment. How would you confront the denial?

2 Ms. S. believed that she had bipolar disorder. At a recent clinic visit, she was told that she most probably had schizoaffective disorder. The patient asked the nurse how a bipolar disorder could turn into schizoaffective disorder. Identify three appropriate responses to her question.

3 A patient with schizoaffective disorder is prescribed an antipsychotic agent (Risperdal) and a mood stabilizer (Depakote). The patient asks you why both medications are needed. Develop the best response for this question. Be thorough.

4 At an interdisciplinary treatment team meeting, the nurse recommends that a woman with schizoaffective disorder attend an anger management group. The rest of the team believes that only a mood stabilizer is needed. Develop the rationale for attending the anger management group in addition to medication supplementation.

5 A patient was prescribed olanzapine (Zyprexa) and an antidepressant (Lexapro) for the treatment of schizoaffective disorder. Since her last monthly visit, she gained 15 pounds. She is considering discontinuing her medication regimen because of the weight gain. Develop a plan to address her weight gain and her intention to discontinue her medication regimen.

6 A. has received a diagnosis of schizoaffective disorder, and B. has received a diagnosis of delusional disorder. How would the symptoms differ? Would there be any similarities? If so, what would they be?

7 Identify and explain each of the subtypes of delusional disorder.

8 An elderly person in a nursing home has a delusion that her husband is having an affair with her sister. Discuss nonpharmacologic nursing interventions that should be implemented with this patient. How would you explain her delusion to her husband? Choose one of the subtypes of delusion and develop a plan for clinical management, focusing on psychiatric nursing care, for a patient experiencing this condition.

9 A patient convincingly informs you that she is having an affair with a famous actor. They both attended the same college about the same time. How would you determine if this patient's belief is a delusion or reality? Is it important that the nurse understand whether the relationship is real? Explain the rationale for your answer.

10 A patient informs a student nurse that he is a member of the Secret Service and that he is undercover. He asks the nurse to keep the secret. The student considers several possible responses, including redirecting the patient to a different topic and confronting him with the reality of his hospitalization. Discuss the best response to this patient's comment.

Misery: 1990. This movie stars James Caan as Paul Sheldon and Kathy Bates as Annie Wilkes. Sheldon is the writer of a popular mystery series who finishes his last novel in a secluded cabin in Colorado. After being rescued in a blizzard by Annie Wilkes, he becomes her prisoner when she prevents him from leaving his cabin. Annie is in love with him but is demanding and possessive. She identifies with the heroine in his latest novel, and is outraged at the conclusion of the novel.

SIGNIFICANCE: Annie demonstrates the thinking patterns associated with delusional disorder.

VIEWING POINTS: Identify the disturbed thinking that Annie demonstrates. Part of Annie's behavior seems normal and other behaviors are illogical. How are they linked?

REFERENCES

American Psychiatric Association (APA). (1980). *Diagnostic and statistical manual of mental disorders* (3rd ed.). Washington, DC: Author.

American Psychiatric Association (APA). (2000). *Diagnostic and statistical manual of mental disorders* (4th ed., text revision). Washington, DC: Author.

Andres, K., Pfammatter, M., Garst, F., Teschner, C., & Brenner, H. D. (2000). Effects of a coping-oriented group therapy for schizophrenia and schizoaffective patients: A pilot study. *Acta Psychiatrica Scandinavica, 101*(4), 318–322.

Arehart-Treichel, J. (2004). Delusions linked to brain region, but why? *Psychiatric News, 39*(19), 21.

Baker, P. B., Cook, B. L., & Winokur, G. (1995). Delusional infestation: The interference of delusions and hallucinations. *Psychiatric Clinics of North America, 18*(2), 345–361.

Bech, P. (2001). The significance of delusions in depressive disorders. *Current Opinions in Psychiatry, 14*(1), 47–49.

Bentall, R. P., Corcoran, R., Howard, R., Blackwood, N., & Kinderman, P. (2001). Persecutory delusions: A review and theoretical integration. *Clinical Psychology Review, 21*(8), 1143–1192.

Conway, C. R., Bollini, A. M., Graham, B. G., Keefe, R. S., Schiffman, S. S., & McEvoy, J. P. (2002). Sensory acuity and reasoning in delusional disorder. *Comprehensive Psychiatry, 43*(3), 175–178.

Crow, T. J., & Harrington, C. A. (1994). Etiopathogenesis and treatment of psychosis. *Annual Review of Medicine, 45*, 219–234.

DeLisi, L. E., Shaw, S. H., Crow, T. J., Shields, G., Smith, A. B., Larach, V. W., et al. (2002). A genome-wide scan for linkage to chromosomal regions in 382 sibling pairs with schizophrenia or schizoaffective disorder. *American Journal of Psychiatry, 159*(5), 803–812.

Dietrich, D. E., Kropp, S., & Emrich, H. M. (2001). Oxcarbazepine in affective and schizoaffective disorders. *Pharmacopsychiatry, 34*(6), 242–250.

Evans, J. D., Heaton, R. K., Paulsen, J. S., McAdams, L. A., Heaton, S. C., & Jeste, D. V. (1999). Schizoaffective disorder: A form of schizophrenia or affective disorder? *Journal of Clinical Psychiatry, 60*(12), 874–882.

Fabisch, K., Fabisch, H., Langs, G., Macheiner, H., Fitz, W., & Honigl, D. (2001). Basic symptoms and their contribution to the differential typology of acute schizophrenic and schizoaffective disorders. *Psychopathology, 34*(1), 15–22.

Fujii, D. E., Ahmed, I., & Takeshita, J. (1999). Neuropsychologic implications in erotomania: Two case studies. *Neuropsychiatry, Neuropsychology and Behavioral Management, 12*(2), 110–116.

Getz, G. E., DelBello, M. P., Fleck, D. E., Zimmerman, M. E., Schwiers, M. L., & Strakowski, S. M. (2002). Neuroanatomic characterization of schizoaffective disorder using MRI: A pilot study. *Schizophrenia Research, 55*(1–2), 55–59.

Gooding, D. C., & Tallent, K. A. (2002). Spatial working memory performance in patients with schizoaffective psychosis versus schizophrenia: A tale of two disorders? *Schizophrenia Research, 15*(3), 209–218.

Grunebaum, M. F., Oquendo, M. A., Harkavy-Friedman, J. M., Ellis, S. P., Li, S., Haas, G. L., Malone, K. M., & Mann. J. J. (2001). Delusions and suicidality. *American Journal of Psychiatry, 158*(5), 742–747.

Harmon, R. B., Rosner, R., & Owens, H. (1995). Obsessional harassment and erotomania in a criminal court population. *Journal of Forensic Science, 41*(2), 188–196.

Huxley, N. A., Rendall, M., & Sederer, L. (2000). Psychosocial treatments in schizophrenia: A review of the past 20 years. *Journal of Nervous and Mental Disease, 188*(4), 187–201.

Iancu, I., Dannon, P. N., Ziv, R., & Lepkifker, E. (2002). A follow-up study of patients with DSM-IV schizophreniform disorder. *Canadian Journal of Psychiatry, 47*(1), 56–60.

Kasanin, J. (1933). The acute schizo-affective psychoses. *American Journal of Psychiatry, 13*, 97–126.

Lewine, R. R., Hudgins, P., Brown, F., Caudle, J., & Risch, S. C. (1995). Differences in qualitative brain morphology findings in schizophrenia, major depression, bipolar disorder, and normal volunteers. *Schizophrenia Research, 15*(3), 253–259.

Maj, M., Pirozzi, R., Formicola, A. M., Bartoli, L., & Bucci, P. (2000). Reliability and validity of the *DSM-IV* diagnostic category of schizoaffective disorder: Preliminary data. *Journal of Affective Disorders, 57*(1–3), 95–98.

Marder, S. R., McQuade, R. D., Stock, E., Kaplita, S., Marcus, R., Safferman, A. Z., et al. (2003). Aripiprazole in the treatment of schizophrenia: Safety and tolerability in short-term, placebo-controlled trials. *Schizophrenia Res, 61*, 123–136.

Marneros, A. (2003). The schizoaffective phenomenon: The state of the art. *Acta Psychiatrica Scandinavica Supplementum, 418*, 29–33.

Marneros, A., Pillmann, F., Haring, A., Balzuweit, S., & Bloink, R. (2002). The relation of 'acute and transient psychotic disorder' (ICD-10 F23) to bipolar schizoaffective disorder. *Journal of Psychiatric Research, 36*(3), 165–171.

Mathews, C. A., Glidden, D., & Hargreaves, W. A. (2002). The effect of diagnostic rates of assigning patients to ethnically focused inpatient psychiatric units. *Psychiatric Services, 53*(7), 823–829.

McCann, T. V., & Baker, H. (2003). Models of mental health nurse–general practitioner liaison: Promoting continuity of care. *Journal of Advanced Nursing, 41*(5), 471–479.

McGuire, L., Junginger, J., Adams, S. G. Jr., Burright, R., & Donovick, P. (2001). Delusions and delusional reasoning. *Journal of Abnormal Psychology, 110*(2), 259–266.

McCutcheon, L. E., Ashe, D. D., Houran, J., & Maltby, J. (2003). A cognitive profile of individuals who tend to worship celebrities. *The Journal of Psychology, 137*(4), 309–322.

Meloy, J. R. (1999). Erotomania, triangulation and homicide. *Journal of Forensic Science, 44*(2), 421–424.

Moller, H. J., Bottlender, R., Gross, A., Hoff, P., Wittmann, J., Wegner, U., & Strauss, A. (2002). The Kraepelinian dichotomy: Preliminary results of a 15-year follow-up study on functional psychoses: Focus on negative symptoms. *Schizophrenia Research, 56*(1–2), 878–894.

Morimoto, K., Miyatake, R., Nakamura, M., Watanabe, T., Hirao, T., & Suwaki, H. (2002). Delusional disorder: Molecular genetic evidence for dopamine psychosis. *Neuropsychopharmacology, 26*(6), 794–801.

Munro, A. (1999). *Delusional disorder.* Cambridge, MA: Cambridge University Press.

Nose, M., Barbui, C., & Tansella, M. (2003), How often do patients with psychosis fail to adhere to treatment programmes? A systematic review. *Psychological Medicine, 33*(7), 1149–1160.

Ota, M., Mizukami, K., Katano, T., Sato, S., Takeda, T., & Asada, T. (2003). A case of delusional disorder, somatic type with remarkable improvement of clinical symptoms and single photon emission computed tomography findings following modified electroconvulsive therapy. *Progress in Neuro-psychopharmacology & Biological Psychiatry, 27*(5), 881–884.

Pini, S., Cassano, G. B., Dell'Osso, L., & Amador, X. F. (2001). Insight into illness in schizophrenia, schizoaffective disorder, and mood disorders with psychotic features. *American Journal of Psychiatry, 158*(1), 122–125.

Potkin, S. G., Alphs, L., Hsu, C., Krishnan, K., Anand, R., Young, F. K., Meltzer, H., & Green, A. (2003). Predicting suicidal risk in schizophrenic and schizoaffective patients in a prospective two-year trial. *Biological Psychiatry, 54*(4), 444–452.

Radomsky, E. D., Haas, G. L., Mann, J. J., & Sweeney, J. A. (1999). Suicidal behavior in patients with schizophrenia and other psychotic disorders. *American Journal of Psychiatry, 156*(10), 1590–1595.

Regenold, W. T., Thapar, R. K., Marano, C., Gavirneni, S., & Kondapavuluru, P. V. (2002). Increased prevalence of type 2 diabetes mellitus among psychiatric inpatients with bipolar I affective and schizoaffective disorders independent of psychotropic drug use. *Journal of Affective Disorders, 70*(1), 19–26.

Reichenberg, A., Weiser, M., Rabinowitz, J., Caspi, A., Schmeidler, J., Mark, M., Kaplan, Z., & Davidson, M. (2002). A population-based cohort study of premorbid intellectual, language, and behavioral functioning in patients with schizophrenia, schizoaffective disorder and nonpsychotic bipolar disorder. *American Journal of Psychiatry, 159*(12), 2027–2035.

Rietschel, M., Krauss, H., Muller, D. J., Schulze, T. G., Knapp, M., Marwinski, K., et al. (2000). Dopamine d3 receptor variant and tardive dyskinesia. *European Archives of Psychiatry and Clinical Neuroscience, 250*(1), 31–35.

Scott, T. F., Price, T. R., George, M. S., Brillman, J., & Rothfus, W. (1993). Midline cerebral malformations and schizophrenia. *Journal of Neuropsychiatry and Clinical Neurosciences, 5*(3), 287–293.

Swoboda, E., Conca, A., Konig, P., Waanders, R., & Hansen, M. (2001). Maintenance electroconvulsive therapy in affective and schizoaffective disorder. *Neuropsychobiology, 43*(1)I, 23–28.

Trabert, W. (1999). Shared psychotic disorder in delusional parasitosis. *Psychopathology, 32*(1), 30–34.

Volavka, J., Czobor, P., Sheitman, B., Lindenmayer, J. P., Citrome, L., McEvoy, J. P., et al. (2002). Clozapine, olanzapine, risperidone, and haloperidol in the treatment of patients with chronic schizophrenia and schizoaffective disorder. *American Journal of Psychiatry, 159*(2), 255–262.

CHAPTER 20

Mood Disorders: Management of Moods and Suicidal Behavior

Barbara Jones Warren, revised from a chapter by Sandra J. Wood and Katharine P. Bailey

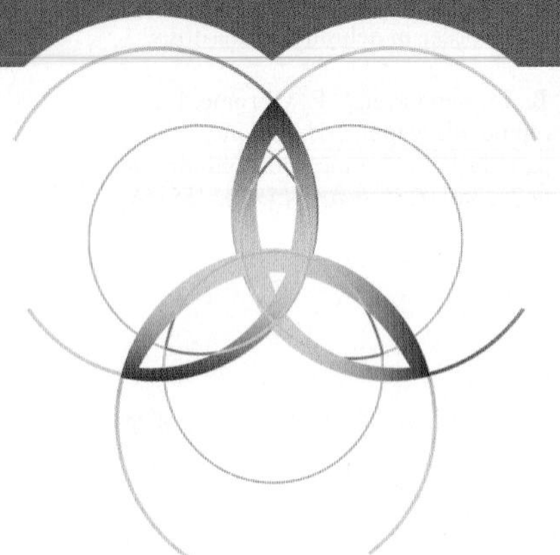

KEY CONCEPTS

- mania
- mood
- mood disorders
- suicidal behavior

LEARNING OBJECTIVES

After studying this chapter, you will be able to:

- Describe the prevalence and incidence of mood disorders and suicide within American society.
- Delineate the clinical symptoms and course of mood disorders and suicidal behavior.
- Analyze the biopsychosocial theories that formulate the education, practice, and research basis in caring for patients who are diagnosed with a mood disorder and who exhibit suicidal behavior.
- Analyze the human responses to mood disorders.
- Discuss the biopsychosocial nursing clinical reasoning processes for patients diagnosed with mood disorders and for those who exhibit suicidal behavior.
- Formulate nursing diagnoses with strategies, interventions, and evaluative approaches that address the cultural needs of persons diagnosed with mood disorders and for those who exhibit suicidal behavior.

KEY TERMS

• affect • bipolar • cyclothymic disorder • depressive episode • dysthymic disorder • euphoria • expansive mood • hypomanic episode • lability of mood • manic episode • mixed episode • rapid cycling • unipolar

Depression is an overwhelming disorder. Well over 17 million people are affected within the United States alone, and it is projected that depression will overtake cardiovascular disease as the major world-wide health concern by the 21st century. The clinical symptoms and course of depressive phenomena is a complex, dynamic biopsychosocial process involving lifespan and cultural aspects. Unless appropriately treated, depression persists over time, having a significant negative effect on life and increasing the risk of suicide. Psychiatric nurses are uniquely positioned to address this pandemic health concern.

The World Health Organization (WHO) predicts that mood disorders will be the number one public health problem in the 21st century. In the United States, mental disorders account for more than 15% of the disease burden for all diseases and a little more than the burden for all types of cancer. Mood disorders are associated with high levels of impairment in occupation, social, and physical functioning and cause as much disability and distress to patients as chronic medical disorders (United States Department of Health and Human Services [U.S. DHHS], 1999). Mood disorders often go undetected and untreated. Studies suggest that more than two-thirds of people with bipolar disorder have their disease misdiagnosed (Hirschfeld, Lewis, & Vornik, 2003). The incidence of misdiagnosis is often greater for persons from culturally and ethnically diverse populations, as their explanation of their symptomatology may be expressed using different terminology than do persons who are not from these populations (U.S. Department of Health and Human Services [U.S. DHHS], 2001). Although health care resources are expended on testing for atypical physical symptom patterns, the opportunity to make use of effective pharmaceutical and psychological treatments often is missed. In addition, because suicide is a significant risk in mood disorders, these disorders have a greater impact on premature mortality. Nurses practicing in any health care setting need to develop competence in assessing patients for the presence of a mood disorder and, if suspected, provide appropriate educational and clinical interventions or referral.

KEY CONCEPT Mood is a pervasive and sustained emotion that colors one's perception of the world and how one functions in it. Normal variations in mood occur as responses to specific life experiences. Normal mood variations, such as sadness, euphoria, and anxiety, are time limited and are not associated with significant functional impairment.

KEY CONCEPT Mood disorders, as defined in the *Diagnostic and Statistical Manual of Mental Disorders*, 4th edition, text revision ([DSM-IV-TR]; American Psychiatric Association [APA], 2000), are recurrent disturbances or alterations in mood that cause psychological distress and behavioral impairment.

KEY CONCEPT Suicidal behavior Suicidal behavior is defined as the occurrence of persistent thought patterns and actions that indicate a person is thinking about, planning, or enacting suicide.

The primary alteration is in mood, rather than in thought or perception. Several terms describe **affect** or outward emotional expression (see Chapter 10) including the following:

- *Blunted*: significantly reduced intensity of emotional expression
- *Flat*: absent or nearly absent affective expression
- *Inappropriate*: discordant affective expression accompanying the content of speech or ideation
- *Labile*: varied, rapid, and abrupt shifts in affective expression
- *Restricted or constricted*: mildly reduced in the range and intensity of emotional expression

Normal range of mood or affect varies considerably both within and between different cultures (this issue is addressed in Ethnic and Cultural Differences).

Primary mood disorders include both depressive disorders (**unipolar**) and manic-depressive (**bipolar**) disorders. The *DSM-IV-TR* has established specific criteria for diagnostic classification of these disorders, including criteria for severity (a change from previous functioning), duration (at least 2 weeks), and clinically significant distress or impairment. Mood episodes are the "building blocks" for the mood disorder diagnoses. The *DSM-IV-TR* describes four categories of mood episodes: major depressive episode, manic episode, mixed episode, and hypomanic episode. This chapter focuses on the depressive disorders and bipolar disorder. The *DSM-IV-TR* categorizes mood disorders as follows:

- *Depressive disorders*: major depressive disorder, single or recurrent; dysthymic disorder; and depressive disorder not otherwise specified (NOS)
- *Bipolar disorders*: bipolar I disorder, bipolar II disorder, cyclothymic disorder, and bipolar disorder NOS
- *Mood disorder* caused by a general medical condition
- *Substance-induced mood disorder*
- *Mood disorder NOS*

DEPRESSIVE DISORDERS

Clinical Course

The primary *DSM-IV-TR* criterion for major depressive disorder is one or more major depressive episodes. In a major **depressive episode**, either a depressed mood or a loss of interest or pleasure in nearly all activities must be present for at least 2 weeks. Four of seven additional symptoms must be present: disruption in sleep, appetite (or weight), concentration, energy; psychomotor agitation or retardation; excessive guilt or feelings of worthlessness; and suicidal ideation (see Table 20.1). Individuals often describe themselves as depressed, sad, hopeless, discouraged, or "down in the dumps." If individuals complain of feeling "blah," having no feelings, or feeling anxious, a depressed mood can sometimes be inferred from their facial expression and demeanor (APA, 2000).

Dysthymic disorder is a milder but more chronic form of major depressive disorder. The *DSM-IV-TR* cri-

Table 20.1  **Key Diagnostic Characteristics for Major Depressive Disorder 296.xx**
Major depressive disorder, single episode 296.2x
Major depressive disorder, recurrent 296.3x

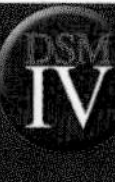

Diagnostic Criteria and Target Symptoms	Associated Findings
• Change from previous level of functioning during a 2-week period Depressed mood Markedly diminished interest or pleasure in all or almost all activities Significant weight loss when not dieting, or weight gain or change in appetite Insomnia or hypersomnia Psychomotor agitation or retardation Fatigue or loss of energy Feelings of worthlessness or excessive or inappropriate guilt Diminished ability to think or concentrate, or indecisiveness Recurrent thoughts of death, recurrent suicidal ideation without a specific plan, or a suicide attempt or specific plan for committing suicide • At least one symptom is depressed mood, or loss of interest or pleasure • Significant distress or impairment of social, occupational, or other important areas of functioning • Not a direct physiologic effect of substance or medical condition • Not better accounted for by bereavement, schizoaffective disorder; not superimposed on schizophrenia, schizophreniform disorder, delusional disorder, or psychotic disorder not otherwise specified	*Associated Behavioral Findings* • Tearfulness, irritability, brooding, obsessive rumination, anxiety, phobias, excessive worry over physical health, and complaints of pain • Possible panic attacks • Difficulty with intimate relationships • Difficulties with sexual functioning • Marital problems • Occupational problems • Substance abuse, such as alcohol • High mortality rate; death by suicide • Increased pain and physical illness • Decreased physical, social, and role functioning • May be preceded by dysthymic disorder

teria for dysthymic disorder are depressed mood for most days for at least 2 years and two or more of the following symptoms: poor appetite or overeating; insomnia or oversleeping; low energy or fatigue; low self-esteem; poor concentration or difficulty making decisions; and feelings of hopelessness. The not otherwise specified (NOS) category includes disorders with depressive features that do not meet strict criteria for major depressive disorder.

Major depressive disorder is commonly a progressive, recurrent illness. With time, episodes tend to occur more frequently, become more severe, and are of a longer duration. About 25% of patients experience a recurrence during the first 6 months after a first episode, and about 50% to 75% have a recurrence within 5 years. The mean age of onset for major depressive disorder is about 40 years; 50% of all patients have an onset between the ages of 20 and 50 years. During a 20-year period, the mean number of episodes is five or six. Symptoms usually develop during a period of days to months. About 50% of patients have significant depressive symptoms before the first identified episode. An untreated episode typically lasts 6 to 13 months, regardless of the age of onset. In one report, only 6% to 14% of depressed suicide victims were adequately treated and only 8% to 17% of all suicide victims were under treatment with prescribed psychiatric medications (Goldsmith, Pellmar, Kleinman, Bunny, 2002).

Depressive Disorders in Special Populations

Children and Adolescents

Depressive disorders in children have manifestations similar to those seen in adults with a few exceptions. In major depressive disorder, children are less likely to experience psychosis, but when they do, auditory hallucinations are more common than delusions. They are more likely to have anxiety symptoms, such as fear of separation, and somatic symptoms, such as stomach aches and headaches. They may have less interaction with their peers and avoid play and recreational activities that they generally have participated in. Mood may be irritable, rather than sad, especially in adolescents. The risk of suicide, which peaks during the mid-adolescent years, is very real in children and adolescents. Mortality from suicide, which increases steadily through the teens, is the third leading cause of death for that age group. Findings from research indicate that deaths due to illegal drug use and automobile accidents may be the outcome of adolescent depression and suicidal ideation (U.S. DHHS, 1999).

Elderly People

Most older patients with symptoms of depression do not meet the full criteria for major depression. However, it is estimated that 8% to 20% of older adults in the community and as many as 37% in primary care settings experience depressive symptoms. Treatment is successful in 60% to 80%, but response to treatment is slower than in younger adults. Depression in elderly people often is associated with chronic illnesses, such as heart disease, stroke, and cancer; symptoms may have a more somatic focus. Depressive symptomatology in this group may be confused with symptoms of dementia or cerebral vascular accidents. Hence, differential diagnosis may be required to ascertain the root and cause of symptoms. Suicide is a very serious risk for the older adult, especially men. People older than age 65 years have the highest suicide rates of any age group. There is a greater likelihood of death in or following a suicide attempt in the elderly. In those 85 years and older, the suicide rate is the highest, at 21 suicides per 100,000 persons (Goldsmith et.al, 2002; U.S. DHHS, 1999).

Epidemiology

In any year, approximately 7% of Americans will experience a mood disorder generally recognized as either depression or mania. This percentage translates into an estimated 11 million people every year. It also appears that the chances of experiencing major depressive disorder are increasing in progressively younger age groups (U.S. DHHS, 1999). Major depressive disorder is twice as common in adolescent and adult women as in adolescent and adult men. Prepubertal boys and girls are equally affected. Major depressive disorders often co-occur with other psychiatric and substance-related disorders. Depression often is associated with a variety of medical conditions, particularly endocrine disorders, cardiovascular disease, neurologic disorders, autoimmune conditions, viral or other infectious diseases, certain cancers, and nutritional deficiencies, or as a direct physiologic effect of a substance (e.g., a drug of abuse, a medication, other somatic treatment for depression, or toxin exposure) (APA, 2000).

FAME AND FORTUNE

Wilbur Wright (1867–1912):
Genius Inventor

Public Persona

Of the Wright brothers, Wilbur and Orville, Wilbur Wright is viewed as the real genius and the one who developed intellectual control over the problem of flight. Although his brother, Orville, had inventive skills and was an ideal counterpart, Wilbur was the one who envisioned things that others could not see. Together, the brothers had the skill to build what they imagined. They once built a wagon that reduced the wheel friction so that it could haul 10 times as much as before. In his early teens, Wilbur invented a machine to fold newspapers, and Orville built a small printing press for a newspaper he started.

Personal Realities

Wilbur Wright suffered with depression that started after an injury he sustained when he was hit in the face with a bat during a game. Complications followed from the medication he received, which affected his heart. He then developed an intestinal disorder, which caused him to abandon his college plans and remain secluded for 4 years. He felt that he could never realize his goal of becoming a clergyman. During his poor health and seclusion, he cared for his mother who was ill with tuberculosis that would eventually cause her death. After his mother died, Wilbur emerged from his depression and he and his brother went into the printing business together. Later, they focused on airplanes and flying.

Source: Crouch, T.D. (1990). *The Bishop's Boys: A Life of Wilbur and Orville Wright.* New York: W.W. Norton & Company.

Ethnic and Cultural Differences

Prevalence rates are unrelated to race. Culture can influence the experience and communication of symptoms of depression. Persons from culturally and ethnically diverse populations may formulate and describe their depressive symptomatology differently than the language proposed for descriptions of these symptoms in the diagnostic criteria of the *DSM-IV-TR* (2000). For example, expressions like "heart-brokenness" (Native American and Middle Eastern), "brain fog" (persons from the West Indies), "zar" and "running amok" may be used in place of such terms as "depressed, sad, hopeless and discouraged" (APA, 2000).

In some cultures, somatic symptoms, rather than sadness or guilt, may predominate (Baker, 2001). For example, language such as "nervous" may be used by persons from Latino and Mediterranean cultures to describe their depressive symptomatology. Individuals from various Asian cultural groups may have complaints of weakness, tiredness, or imbalance. "Problems of the heart" (in Middle Eastern cultures) or of being "heartbroken" (among Hopi Indians) may be the way that persons from these cultural groups express their depressive experiences. Culturally distinctive experiences need to be assessed in order to ascertain any presence of depressive disorder from a "normal" cultural emotional response (APA, 2002).

Risk Factors

Depression is so common that it is sometimes difficult to identify risk factors. The generally agreed-on risk factors include the following:

- Prior episode of depression
- Family history of depressive disorder
- Lack of social support
- Lack of coping abilities

- Presence of life and environmental stressors
- Current substance use and/or abuse
- Medical comorbidity

Etiology

Genetics

Family, twin, and adoption studies demonstrate that genetic influences undoubtedly play a substantial role in the etiology of mood disorders. Major depressive disorder is more common among first-degree biologic relatives of people with this disorder than among the general population. Currently, a major research effort is focusing on developing a more accurate paradigm regarding the contribution of genetic factors to the development of mood disorders (Alda, 2001).

Neurobiologic Hypotheses

Neurobiologic theories of the etiology of depression emerged in the 1950s. These theories posit that major depression is caused by a deficiency or dysregulation in central nervous system (CNS) concentrations of the neurotransmitters norepinephrine, dopamine, and serotonin or in their receptor functions. These hypotheses arose in part from observations that some pharmacologic agents elevated mood, and subsequent studies identified their mechanisms of action. All antidepressants currently available have their therapeutic effects on these neurotransmitters or receptors. Current research focuses on the synthesis, storage, release, and uptake of these neurotransmitters, as well as on postsynaptic events (e.g., second-messenger systems) (Donati & Rasenick, 2003).

Neuroendocrine and Neuropeptide Hypotheses

Major depressive disorder is associated with multiple endocrine alterations, specifically of the hypothalamic–pituitary–adrenal axis, the hypothalamic–pituitary–thyroid axis, the hypothalamic–growth hormone axis, and the hypothalamic–pituitary–gonadal axis. In addition, there is mounting evidence that components of neuroendocrine axes (e.g., neuromodulatory peptides such as corticotropin-releasing factor) may themselves contribute to depressive symptoms. Evidence also suggests that the secretion of these hypothalamic and growth hormones is controlled by many of the neurotransmitters implicated in the pathophysiology of depression (Hanley & Van de Kar, 2003).

Psychoneuroimmunology

Psychoneuroimmunology is a recent area of research into a diverse group of proteins known as *chemical messengers* between immune cells. These messengers, called cytokines, signal the brain and serve as mediators between immune and nerve cells. The brain is capable of influencing immune processes, and conversely, immunologic response can result in changes in brain activity (Kronfol & Remick, 2000). The specific role of these mechanisms in psychiatric disease pathogenesis remains unknown.

Psychological Theories

Psychodynamic Factors

Most psychodynamic theorists acknowledge some debt to Freud's original conceptualization of the psychodynamics of depression, which ascribes etiology to an early lack of love, care, warmth, and protection and resultant anger, guilt, helplessness, and fear regarding the loss of love. The ensuing conflict between wanting to be loved and fear of rejection engenders pathologic self-punitiveness (also conceptualized as aggression turned inward), self-rejection, low self-esteem, and depressive symptoms (see Chapter 6).

Behavioral Factors

The behaviorists hold that depression occurs primarily as the result of a severe reduction in rewarding activities or an increase in unpleasant events in one's life. The resultant depression then leads to further restriction of activity, thereby decreasing the likelihood of experiencing pleasurable activities, which, in turn, intensifies the mood disturbance.

Cognitive Factors

The cognitive approach maintains that irrational beliefs and negative distortions of thought about the self, the environment, and the future engender and perpetuate depressive affects (see Chapter 6).

Developmental Factors

Developmental theorists posit that depression may be the result of loss of a parent through death or separation or lack of emotionally adequate parenting. These factors may delay or prohibit the realization of appropriate developmental milestones.

Social Theories

Family Factors 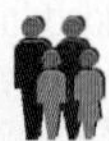

Family theorists ascribe maladaptive patterns in family interactions as contributing to the onset of depression, particularly "ambivalent, abusive, rejecting, or highly dependent family relationships" (APA, 2002, p. 495).

Social Factors

Major depression may follow adverse or traumatic life events, especially those that involve the loss of an important human relationship or role in life. Social isolation, deprivation, and financial deprivation are risk factors (APA, 2002).

Interdisciplinary Treatment of Disorder

Although depressive disorders are the most commonly occurring mental disorders, they are usually treated within the primary care setting, not the psychiatric setting. Individuals with depression enter mental health settings when their symptoms become so severe that hospitalization is needed, usually for suicide attempts, or if they self-refer because of incapacitation. Interdisciplinary treatment of these disorders, which are often lifelong, needs to include a wide array of health professionals in all areas. The specific goals of treatment are:

- Reduce/control symptoms and, if possible, eliminate signs and symptoms of the depressive syndrome.
- Improve occupational and psychosocial function as much as possible.
- Reduce the likelihood of relapse and recurrence.

Priority Care Issues

The overriding concern for people with mood disorders is safety, because these individuals may experience self-destructive thoughts and suicidal ideations. Hence, the assessment of possible suicide risk should be routinely conducted in any person who is incurring depressive symptomatology (see Chapter 17).

Family Response to Disorder 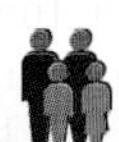

Depression in one member affects the whole family. Spouses, children, parents, siblings, and friends experience frustration, guilt, and anger when the family member is immobilized and cannot function. It is often hard for others to understand the depth of the mood and how disabling it can be. Financial hardship can occur when the family member cannot go to work and spends days in bed. The lack of understanding and difficulty of living with a depressed person can lead to abuse. Women between the ages of 18 and 45 years constitute the majority of those experiencing depression. This incidence may affect women's ability to not only have a productive life and take care of themselves but to also take care of their children or other family members they may have responsibility for. Moreover, research indicates that the incidence of depression may be higher in children whose mothers incur depression (U.S. DHHS, 2001).

NURSING MANAGEMENT: HUMAN RESPONSE TO DEPRESSIVE DISORDER

The diagnosis of major depressive disorder is made when *DSM-IV-TR* criteria are met. An awareness of the risk factors for depression, a comprehensive and culturally competent biopsychosocial assessment, history of illness, and past treatment are key to formulating a treatment plan and to evaluating outcomes (Taylor, 2003; Warren, 2002). Interviewing a family member or close friend about the patient's day-to-day functioning and specific symptoms may be helpful in determining the course of the illness, current symptoms, and level of functioning.

Biologic Domain

Assessment

Because some symptoms of depression are similar to those of some medical problems or side effects of medication therapies, biologic assessment must include a physical systems review and thorough history of medical problems, with special attention to CNS function, endocrine function, anemia, chronic pain, autoimmune illness, diabetes, or menopause. Additional medical history includes surgeries; medical hospitalizations; head injuries; episodes of loss of consciousness; and pregnancies, childbirths, miscarriages, and abortions. A complete list of prescribed and over-the-counter medications should be compiled, including the reason a medication was prescribed or its use discontinued. A physical examination is recommended with baseline vital signs and baseline laboratory tests, including comprehensive blood chemistry panel, complete blood counts, liver function tests, thyroid function tests, urinalysis, and electrocardiograms (Chapter 10). Biologic assessment also includes evaluating the patient for the characteristic neurovegetative symptoms listed below.

• NCLEXNOTE

NCLEXNOTE

In determining severity of depressive symptoms, nursing assessment should explore physical changes in appetite and sleep patterns and decreased energy. And considering the possibility of suicide should always be a priority with patients who are depressed. Assessment and documentation of suicide risk should always be included in patient care.

- *Appetite and weight changes*: In major depression, changes from baseline include decrease or increase in appetite with or without significant weight loss or gain (i.e., a change of more than 5% of body weight in 1 month). Weight loss occurs when not dieting. Older adults with moderate to severe depression need to be assessed for dehydration as well as weight changes.

- *Sleep disturbance*: The most common sleep disturbance associated with major depression is insomnia. *DSM-IV-TR's* definitions of insomnia are divided into three categories: initial insomnia (difficulty falling asleep); middle insomnia (waking up during the night and having difficulty returning to sleep); or terminal insomnia (waking too early and being unable to return to sleep). Less frequently, the sleep disturbance is hypersomnia (prolonged sleep episodes at night or increased daytime sleep). The individual with either insomnia or hypersomnia complains of not feeling rested upon awakening.
- *Decreased energy, tiredness, and fatigue*: Fatigue associated with depression is a subjective experience of feeling tired regardless of how much sleep or physical activity a person has had. Even the smallest tasks require substantial effort.

• NCLEXNOTE

NCLEXNOTE

Remember the three major assessment categories listed above. A question may state several patient symptoms and expect the student to recognize that the patient being described is depressed.

In addition to a physical assessment including weight and appetite, sleep habits, and fatigue factors, an assessment of current medications should be completed. The frequency and dosage of prescribed medication, over-the-counter medication, and use of herbal or culturally related medication treatments should be explored. In depression, the nurse must always assess the lethality of the medication the patient is taking. For example, if a patient has sleeping medications at home, the individual should be further queried about the number of pills in the bottle. Patients also need to be assessed for their use of alcohol, marijuana, and other mood-altering medications, as well as herbal substances because of the potential for drug–drug interactions. For example, patients taking antidepressants that affect serotonin regulation could also be taking St. John's wort (hypericum perforatum) to fight depression. The combined drug and herb could interact to cause serotonin syndrome (altered mental status, autonomic dysfunction, and neuromuscular abnormalities).

Nursing Diagnoses for Biologic Domain

There are several nursing diagnoses that could be formulated based on assessment data, including insomnia, Imbalanced Nutrition, Fatigue, Self-care Deficit, and Nausea. Other diagnoses that should be considered are Disturbed Thought Processes and Sexual Dysfunction.

Interventions for Biologic Domain

Because weeks or months of disturbed sleep patterns and nutritional imbalance only make depression worse, counseling and education should aim to establish normal sleep patterns and healthy nutrition.

Teaching Physical Care 

Encouraging patients to practice positive sleep hygiene and eat well-balanced meals regularly helps the patient move toward remission or recovery. Activity and exercise are also important for improving depressed mood state. Most people find that regular exercise is hard to maintain. People who are depressed may find it impossible. When teaching about exercise, it is important to start with the current level of patient activity and increase slowly. For example, if the patient is spending most of the time in bed, encouraging the patient to get dressed every day and walk for 5 or 10 minutes may be all that patient can tolerate. Gradually, patients should be encouraged to have a regular exercise program and to slowly increase their food intake.

Pharmacologic Interventions

An antidepressant is selected based primarily on an individual patient's target symptoms, genetic responses related to cultural, racial, and ethnic influences and an individual agent's side-effect profile (Warren, in press). Failure to consider these influences may increase the risk of aversive and injurious side effects (Institue of Medicine, 2003; U.S. DHHS, 2001). There are other factors that may influence choice:

- Prior medication response
- Drug interactions and contraindications
- Medication responses in family members
- Concurrent medical and psychiatric disorders
- Patient needs and requirements based on cultural healthcare beliefs and values
- Patient age
- Cost of medication

Medication therapy should be reviewed on a regular basis in order to ascertain whether changes and/or discontinuation of medications might be needed. The treatment and clinical management of psychiatric disorders are divided into the acute phase, continuation phase, maintenance phase, and, when indicated, discontinuation of medication use.

• NCLEXNOTE

Patients may be reluctant to take prescribed antidepressant medications or may self-treat depression based on their cultural beliefs and values (U.S. DHHS, 2001). A culturally competent nursing care and teaching plan needs to address the importance for adherence to a medication regimen and emphasize any potential drug–drug interactions.

- *Acute phase*. The primary goal of therapy for the acute phase is symptom reduction or remission. The objective is to choose the right match of medication and dosage for the patient. Careful monitoring and follow-up are essential during this phase to assess patient response to medications, adjust dosage if necessary, identify and address side effects, and provide patient support and education.
- *Continuation phase*. The goal of this treatment phase is to decrease the risk for relapse (a return of the current episode of depression). If a patient experiences a response to an adequate trial of medication, use of the medication generally is continued at the same dosage for at least 4 to 9 months after the patient returns to a clinically well state.
- *Maintenance phase*. For patients who are at high risk for recurrence (see Risk Factors), the optimal duration of maintenance treatment is unknown but is measured in years, and full-dose therapy is required for effective prophylaxis (Schatzberg, Cole, & DeBattista, 2003).
- *Discontinuation of medication use*. The decision to discontinue active treatment should be based on the same factors considered in the decision to initiate maintenance treatment. These factors include the frequency and severity of past episodes, the persistence of dysthymic symptoms after recovery, the presence of comorbid disorders, and patient preference. Many patients continue taking medications for their lifetime.

Administering Antidepressant Medication Therapy

Antidepressant medications have proved effective in all forms of major depression. To date, controlled trials have shown no single antidepressant drug to have greater efficacy in the treatment of major depressive disorder. Antidepressant medications can be grouped as follows:

- Selective serotonin reuptake inhibitors (SSRIs), which currently include escitalopram oxalate (Lexapro), fluoxetine (Prozac), sertraline (Zoloft), fluvoxamine (Luvox), paroxetine (Paxil), and citalopram (Celexa) (see Box 20.1 for more information); Serotonin norepinephrine reuptake inhibitors (SNRIs), which include venlafaxine (Effexor), nefazodone (Serzone), and duloxetine (Cymbalta);
- Cyclic antidepressants, which include the tricyclic antidepressants (TCAs), and maprotiline (a tetracyclic);
- monoamine oxidase inhibitors (MAOIs), which include phenelzine (Nardil), tranylcypromine (Parnate), and selegiline (Emsam);
- other antidepressants, which include bupropion (Wellbutrin), a norepinephrine dopamine reuptake inhibitor, mirtazapine (Remeron), an α_2 antagonist, and trazadone (Desyrel), a serotonin-2 antagonist/reuptake inhibitor. See Chapter 8 for list of antidepressant medications, usual dosage range, half-life, and therapeutic blood levels. For more information, see Box 20.2.

The first-generation drugs, the TCAs and MAOIs, are being used less often than the second-generation drugs, the SSRIs and atypical antidepressants. Second-generation drugs selectively target the neurotransmitters and receptors thought to be associated with depression and to minimize side effects. The side-effect profiles of the two generations of drugs are significantly different as well (Table 20.2). The efficacy of the MAOIs is well established. Evidence suggests their distinct advantage in treating a specific subtype of depression, so-called atypical depression (characterized by increased appetite, reverse diurnal mood variation, and hypersomnia), depression with panic symptoms, or social phobia (Schatzberg et al., 2003). Given the complexity of their use, MAOIs usually are reserved for patients whose depression fails to respond to other antidepressants or patients who cannot tolerate typical antidepressants.

Monitoring Medications

Patients should be carefully observed when taking antidepressant medications (Box 20.3). In the depths of depression, saving medication for a later suicide attempt is quite common. All of the antidepressants have boxed warnings for suicidality in children and adolescents. During antidepressant treatment, there is ongoing monitoring of vital signs, plasma drug levels as appropriate, liver and thyroid function tests, complete blood counts, and blood chemistry. Responsibilities include ensuring that patients are receiving a therapeutic dosage, helping in the evaluation of compliance, monitoring side effects, and helping to prevent toxicity. (Therapeutic blood levels for antidepressant medications are listed in Chapter 8.) Table 20.3 indicates various pharmacologic and nonpharmacologic interventions for the various side effects of antidepressant

BOX 20.1

Drug Profile: Escitalopram oxalate (Lexapro)

DRUG CLASS: Antidepressant

RECEPTOR AFFINITY: A highly selective serotonin reuptake inhibitor with low affinity for 5HT 1-7 or α- and β- adrenergic, dopamine D1-5, histamine H1-3, muscarinic M1-5, and benzodiazepine receptors or for Na^+, K^+, Cl^-, and Ca^{++} ion channels that have been associated with various anticholinergic, sedative, and cardiovascular side effects.

INDICATIONS: Treatment of major depressive disorder, generalized anxiety disorder.

ROUTES AND DOSAGES: Available as 5-, 10-, and 20-mg oral tablets.

Adults: Initially 10 mg once a day. May increase to 20 mg after a minimum of a week. Trials have not shown greater benefit at the 20-mg dose.

Geriatric: The 10-mg dose is recommended. Adjust dosage related to the drug's longer half-life and the slower liver metabolism of elderly patients.

Renal impairment: No dosage adjustment is necessary for mild to moderate renal impairment.

Children: Safety and efficacy not established in this population.

HALF LIFE (PEAK EFFECT): 27–32 h (4–7 h)

SELECTED ADVERSE REACTIONS: Most common adverse events include insomnia, ejaculation disorder, diarrhea, nausea, fatigue, increased sweating, dry mouth, somnolence, dizziness, and constipation. Most serious adverse events include ejaculation disorder in males; fetal abnormalities and decreased fetal weight in pregnant patients; serotonin syndrome if co-administered with MAOIs, St. John's Wort, or SSRIs, including citalopram (Celexa), of which escitalopram (Lexapro) is the active isomer.

BOXED WARNING: Suicidality in children and adolescents.

WARNINGS: There is potential for intraction with MAOIs. Lexapro should not be used in combination with a MAOI or within 14 days of discoutinuing a MAOI.

SPECIFIC PATIENT/FAMILY EDUCATION:

- Do not take in combination with citalopram (Celexa) or other SSRIs or MAOIs. A 2-week washout period between escitalopram and SSRIs or MAOIs is recommended to avoid serotonin syndrome.
- Families and caregivers should be advised of the need for close observation and communication with the prescriber.
- Notify prescriber if pregnancy is possible or being planned. Do not breast-feed while taking this medication.
- Use caution driving or operating machinery until certain escitalopram does not alter physical abilities or mental alertness.
- Notify prescriber of any OTC medications, herbal supplements, or home remedies being used in combination with escitalopram.
- Ingestion of alcohol in combination with escitalopram is not recommended, although escitalopram does not seem to potentiate mental and motor impairments associated with alcohol.

Source: RX List available at http://www.rxlist.com/cgi/generic/lexapro.htm.

BOX 20.2

Drug Profile: Mirtazapine (Remeron)

DRUG CLASS: Antidepressant

RECEPTOR AFFINITY: Believed to enhance central noradrenergic and serotonergic activity antagonizing central presynaptic α_2-adrenergic receptors. Mechanism of action unknown.

INDICATIONS: Treatment of depression.

ROUTES AND DOSAGE: Available as 15- and 30-mg tablets.

Adults: Initially, 15 mg/d as a single dose preferably in the evening before sleeping. Maximum dosage is 45 mg/d.

Geriatric: Use with caution; reduced dosage may be needed.

Children: Safety and efficacy not established.

HALF-LIFE (PEAK EFFECT): 20–40 h (2 h)

SELECTED ADVERSE REACTIONS: Somnolence, increased appetite, dizziness, weight gain, elevated cholesterol/triglyceride and transaminase levels, malaise, abdominal pain, hypertension, vasodilation, vomiting, anorexia, thirst, myasthenia, arthralgia, hypoesthesia, apathy, depression, vertigo, twitching, agitation, anxiety, amnesia, increased cough, sinusitis, pruritus, rash, urinary tract infection, mania (rare), agranulocytosis (rare).

BOXES WARNING: Suicidality in children and adolescents.

WARNING: Contraindicated in patients with known hypersensitivity. Use with caution in the elderly, patients who are breastfeeding, and those with impaired hepatic function. Avoid concomitant use with alcohol or diazepam, which can cause additive impairment of cognitive and motor skills.

SPECIFIC PATIENT/FAMILY EDUCATION:

- Take the dose once a day in the evening before sleep.
  - Families and caregivers should be advised of the need for dose obervation and communication with the prescriber
- Avoid driving or performing tasks requiring alertness.
- Notify prescriber before taking any OTC or other prescription drugs.
- Avoid alcohol or other CNS depressants.
- Notify prescriber if pregnancy is possible or planned.
- Monitor temperature and report any fever, lethargy, weakness, sore throat, malaise, or other "flu-like" symptoms.
- Maintain medical follow-up, including any appointments for blood counts and liver studies.

Table 20.2 Side Effects of Antidepressant Medications

Generic (Trade) Drug Name	Side Effects: Anticholinergic	Sedation	Orthostatic Hypotension	Gastrointestinal Distress	Weight Gain
Tricyclics: Tertiary Amines					
Amitriptyline (Elavil)	+4	+4	+2	0	+4
Clomipramine (Anafranil)	+3	+3	+2	+1	+4
Doxepin (Sinequan)	+2	+3	+2	0	+3
Imipramine (Tofranil)	+2	+2	+3	+1	+3
Tricyclics: Secondary Amines					
Amoxapine (Asendin)	+3	+2	+1	0	+1
Desipramine (Norpramin)	+1	+1	+1	0	+1
Nortriptyline (Aventyl, Pamelor)	+2	+2	+1	0	+1
SSRIs					
Fluoxetine (Prozac)	0/+1	0/+1	0/+1	+3	0
Sertraline (Zoloft)	0	0/+1	0	+3	0
Paroxetine (Paxil)	0	0/+1	0	+3	0
Fluvoxamine (Luvox)	0/+1	0/+1	0/+1	+3	0
Citalopram (Celexa)	0/+1	0/+1	0/+1	+3	0
Escitalopram (Lexapro)	0/+1	0/+1	0/+1	+3	0
Atypical: Antidepressants					
Venlafaxine (Effexor)	0	0	0	+3	0
Trazodone (Desyrel)	0	+1	+3	+1	+1
Nefazodone (Serzone)	0/+1	+1	+2	+2	0/+1
Bupropion (Wellbutrin)	+2	+2	+1	0	0/+1
Mirtazapine (Remeron)	+3	+4	+3	+3	+2

0 = absent or rare
0/+1 = lowest likelihood
+4 = highest likelihood

medications. See Chapter 8 for diet restrictions for those taking MAOIs. Low doses of selegiline (Emsam), 6 mg/24 hours, do not require diet restriction according to the package insert.

Baseline orthostatic vital signs should be obtained before initiation of any medication, and in the case of medications known to have an impact on vital signs, such as TCAs, MAOIs, or venlafaxine, they should be monitored on a regular basis. If these medications are administered to children or elderly patients, the dosage should be lowered to accommodate the physiologic state of the individual.

Tools for monitoring medication effects are objective observations, vital signs, the patient's subjective reports, and the administration of rating scales over the course of treatment. Responsibilities include ensuring that

BOX 20.3

Guidelines: *Monitoring and Administering Antidepressant Medications*

Nurses should do the following in administering/monitoring antidepressant medications:

- Observe the patient for cheeking or saving medications for a later suicide attempt.
- Monitor vital signs: obtain baseline data, before the initiation of medications (such as orthostatic vital signs and temperature).
- Monitor periodically liver and thyroid function tests, blood chemistry, and complete blood count as appropriate and compare with baseline values.
- Monitor patient symptoms for therapeutic response and report inadequate response to prescriber.
- Monitor patient for side effects and report to the prescriber serious side effects or those that are chronic and problematic for the patient. (Table 20.3 indicates pharmacologic and nonpharmacologic interventions for common side effects.)
- Monitor drug levels as appropriate. (Therapeutic drug levels for antidepressants are listed in Chapter 8.)
- Monitor dietary intake as appropriate, especially with regard to MAOI antidepressants.
- Inquire about patient use of other medications, alcohol, "street" drugs, OTC medications, and/or herbal supplements that might alter the desired effects of prescribed antidepressants.

Table 20.3 Interventions to Relieve Side Effects of Antidepressants

Side Effect	Pharmacologic Intervention	Nonpharmacologic Intervention
Dry mouth, caries, inflammation of the mouth	Bethanechol 10–30 mg tid Pilocarpine drops	Sugarless gum Sugarless lozenges 6–8 cups water per day Toothpaste for dry mouth
Nausea, vomiting	Change medication	Take medication with food Soda crackers, toast, tea
Weight gain	Change medication	Nutritionally balanced diet Daily exercise
Urinary hesitation	Bethanechol 10–30 mg tid	6–8 cups water per day
Constipation	Stool softener	Bulk laxative Daily exercise 6–8 cups water per day Diet rich in fresh fruits, vegetables, and grains
Diarrhea	OTC antidiarrheal	Maintain fluid intake
Orthostatic hypotension		Increase hydration Sit or stand up slowly
Drowsiness	Shift dosing time Lower medication dose Change medication	One caffeinated beverage at strategic time Do not drive when drowsy No alcohol or other recreational drugs Plan for rest time
Fatigue	Lower medication dose Change medication	Daily exercise
Blurred vision	Bethanechol 10–30 mg tid Pilocarpine eyedrops	Temporary use of magnifying lenses until body adjusts to medication
Flushing, sweating	Terazosin 1 mg qd Lower medication dose Change medication	Frequent bathing Lightweight clothing
Tremor	β-blockers Lower medication dose	Reassure patient that tremor may decrease as patient adjusts to medication. Notify caregiver if tremor interferes with daily functioning.

patients are receiving a therapeutic dosage (therapeutic blood levels for antidepressant medications are found in Chapter 8), assessing adherence to the medication regimen, and evaluating compliance.

Individualizing dosages is essential for achieving optimal efficacy. When the newer antidepressants are used, this is usually done by fine-tuning medication dosage based on patient feedback. The TCAs, including imipramine (Tofranil), desipramine (Norpramin), amitriptyline (Elavil), and nortriptyline (Pamelor), have standardized valid plasma levels that can be useful in determining therapeutic dosages, although therapeutic plasma levels may vary from individual to individual. Blood samples should be drawn as close as possible to 12 hours away from the last dose. The newer antidepressants do not have established standardized ranges, and optimal dosing is based on efficacy and tolerability.

Monitoring and Managing Side Effects

First-Generation Antidepressants: TCAs and MAOIs. The most common side effects associated with TCAs are the antihistaminic side effects (sedation and weight gain) and anticholinergic side effects (potentiation of CNS drugs, blurred vision, dry mouth, constipation, urinary retention, sinus tachycardia, and decreased memory).

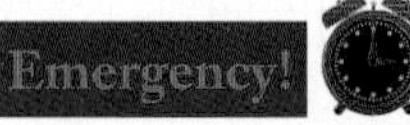

If possible, TCAs should not be prescribed for patients at risk for suicide. Lethal doses of TCAs are only three to five times the therapeutic dose, and more than 1 g of a TCA is often toxic and may be fatal. Death may result from cardiac arrhythmia, hypotension, or uncontrollable seizures.

Serum TCA levels should be evaluated when overdose is suspected. In acute overdose, almost all symptoms develop within 12 hours. Anticholinergic effects are prominent: dry mucous membranes, warm and dry skin, blurred vision, decreased bowel motility, and urinary retention. CNS suppression (ranging from drowsiness to coma) or an agitated delirium may occur. Basic overdose treatment includes induction of emesis, gastric lavage, and cardiorespiratory supportive care. The most common side effects of MAOIs are headache, drowsiness, dry mouth, constipation, blurred vision, and orthostatic hypotension.

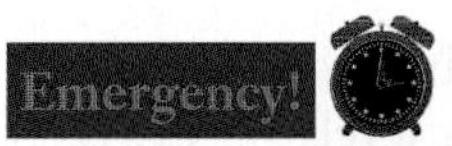

If coadministered with food or other substances containing tyramine (e.g., aged cheese, beer, red wine), MAOIs can trigger a hypertensive crisis that may be life threatening. Symptoms include sudden, severe pounding or explosive headache in the back of the head or temples, racing pulse, flushing, stiff neck, chest pain, nausea and vomiting, and profuse sweating.

MAOIs are more lethal in overdose than are the newer antidepressants and thus should be prescribed with caution if the patient's suicide potential is elevated (see Chapter 8). An MAOI generally is given in divided doses to minimize side effects. These drugs are used cautiously in patients who are suicidal because of their relative lethality compared with the newer antidepressants.

Selected adverse effects of MAOIs include headache, drowsiness, dry mouth and throat, insomnia, nausea, agitation, dizziness, constipation, asthenia, blurred vision, weight loss, and postural hypotension. Although priapism was not reported during clinical trials, the MAOIs are structurally similar to trazodone, which has been associated with priapism (prolonged painful erection).

Second-generation Antidepressants: SSRIs and Other Antidepressants. Serotonin syndrome is a potentially serious side effect caused by drug-induced excess of intrasynaptic serotonin (5-hydroxytryptamine [5-HT]; see Chapter 8). First reported in the 1950s, it was relatively rare until the introduction of the SSRIs. Serotonin syndrome is most often reported in patients taking two or more medications that increase CNS serotonin levels by different mechanisms (Nolan & Scoggin, 2001). The most common drug combinations associated with serotonin syndrome involve the MAOIs, the SSRIs, and the TCAs. Although serotonin syndrome can cause death, it is mild in most patients, who usually recover with supportive care alone. Unlike neuroleptic malignant syndrome, which develops within 3 to 9 days after the introduction of neuroleptic medications (see Chapter 18), serotonin syndrome tends to develop within hours or days after initiating or increasing the dose of serotonergic medication or adding a drug with serotomimetic properties. The symptoms include altered mental status, autonomic dysfunction, and neuromuscular abnormalities. At least three of the following must be present for a diagnosis: mental status changes, agitation, myoclonus, hyperreflexia, fever, shivering, diaphoresis, ataxia, and diarrhea. In patients who also have peripheral vascular disease or atherosclerosis, severe vasospasm and hypertension may occur in the presence of elevated serotonin levels. In addition, in a patient who is a slow metabolizer of SSRIs, higher-than-normal levels of these antidepressants may circulate in the blood. Medications that are not usually considered serotonergic, such as dextromethorphan (Pertussin) and meperidine (Demerol), have been associated with the syndrome (Bernard & Bruera, 2000).

The most important emergency interventions are stopping use of the offending drug, notifying the physician, and providing necessary supportive care (e.g., intravenous fluids, antipyretics, cooling blanket). Severe symptoms have been successfully treated with antiserotonergic agents, such as cyproheptadine (Sorenson, 2002).

Monitoring for Drug Interactions

Although SSRIs and newer atypical antidepressants produce fewer and generally milder side effects, which improves patient tolerability and compliance, there are some side effects to note. Among the most common are

- insomnia and activation
- headaches
- gastrointestinal symptoms
- weight gain

Sexual side effects, primarily diminished interest and performance, are also reported with some SSRIs, particularly sertraline. The most potentially harmful, but preventable, side effect or interaction of SSRIs is serotonin syndrome (Box 20.4).

BOX 20.4

Emergency: Serotonin Syndrome

CAUSE: Excessive intrasynaptic serotonin

HOW IT HAPPENS: Combining medications that increase CNS serotonin levels, such as SSRIs + MAOIs; SSRIs + St. John's wort; or SSRIs + diet pills; dextromethorphan or alcohol, especially red wine; or SSRI + street drugs, such as LSD, MMDA, or Ecstasy.

SYMPTOMS: Mental status changes, agitation, ataxia, myoclonus, hyperreflexia, fever, shivering, diaphoresis, diarrhea

TREATMENT: Assess all medication, supplements, foods, and recreational drugs ingested to determine the offending substances.

Discontinue any substances that may be causative factors. If symptoms are mild, treat supportively on outpatient basis with propranolol and lorazepam and follow-up with prescriber.

If symptoms are moderate to severe, hospitalization may be needed with monitoring of vital signs and treatment with intravenous fluids, antipyretics, and cooling blankets.

FURTHER USE: Assess on a case-by-case basis and minimize risk factors for further medication therapy.

The atypical antidepressant nefazodone (once a more popular medication) has been shown to raise hepatic enzyme levels in some patients, potentially leading to hepatic failure. Trazodone administration has been associated with erectile dysfunction and priapism. Bupropion can cause seizures, particularly in patients at risk for seizures. Bupropion has also been associated with the development of psychosis because it is dopaminergic, and its use should be avoided in patients with schizophrenia. Venlafaxine can cause blood pressure to increase, although this side effect appears to be dose related and can be controlled by lowering the dose (APA, 2002).

Potential drug interactions associated with agents that are metabolized by the cytochrome P-450 systems should be considered when children or elderly patients are treated (see Chapter 7). Five of the most important enzyme systems are 1A2, 2D6, 2C9, 2C19, and 3A4. The 1A2 system is inhibited by the SSRI fluvoxamine. Thus, other drugs that use the 1A2 system will no longer be metabolized as efficiently. For example, if fluvoxamine is given with theophylline, the theophylline dosage must be lowered, or else blood levels of theophylline will rise and cause possible side effects or toxic reactions, such as seizures. Fluvoxamine also affects the metabolism of atypical antipsychotics. On the other hand, smoking and caffeine can induce 1A2 system activity. This means that smokers may need to be given a higher dose of medications that are metabolized by this system (Stahl, 2006).

Fluoxetine (Prozac) and paroxetine (Paxil) are potent inhibitors of 2D6. One of the most significant drug interactions is caused by SSRI inhibition of 2D6 that in turn causes an increase in plasma levels of TCAs. If there is concomitant administration of an SSRI and a TCA, the plasma drug level of TCA should be monitored and probably reduced. In the 3A4 system, some SSRIs (fluoxetine, fluvoxamine, and nefazodone) will raise the levels of alprazolam (Xanax) or triazolam (Halcion) through enzyme inhibition, requiring reduction of dosage of the benzodiazepine. For more information see Table 20.4.

Teaching Points 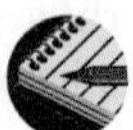

If depression goes untreated or is inadequately treated, episodes can become more frequent, more severe, longer in duration, and can lead to suicide. Patient education involves explaining this pattern and the importance of continuing medication use after the acute phase of treatment to decrease the risk for future episodes. Patient concerns regarding long-term antidepressant therapy need to be assessed and addressed. All teaching points need to be developed and delivered using a culturally competent approach in order to enhance adherence within patients (U.S. DHHS, 2001; Warren, 2002).

Even after the first episode of major depression, medication should be continued for at least 6 months to 1 year after the patient achieves complete remission of symptoms. If the patient experiences a recurrence after tapering the first course of treatment, the regimen should be reinstituted for at least another year, and if the illness reoccurs, medication should be continued indefinitely (Schatzberg et al., 2003).

Table 20.4 Drug–Drug Interactions: Antidepressants

Antidepressant	Other Drug	Effect of Interaction/Treatment
Fluvoxamine	Theophylline	Increased theophylline level: seizures. Tx: Reduce theophylline levels when administering with fluvoxamine.
Fluoxetine, Paroxetine	TCAs Benzodiazepines Phenothiazines	Increased in plasma levels of TCA. Tx: Reduce TCA levels when giving with fluoxetine or paroxetine.
Fluoxetine, Fluvoxamine, Nefazadone	Alprazolam Benzodiazepines	Increased plasma levels of alprazolam. Tx: Reduce dose of alprazolam when administered with benzodiazepines.
Nefazodone	Digoxin Benzodiazepines Antihistamines	Increased levels of digoxin, antihistamines, and benzodiazepines. Tx: Reduce dose of nefazodone when giving with these medications.
Fluvoxamine	Caffeine Nicotine	Lowered levels of fluvoxamine. Tx: Increase dose of fluvoxamine in smokers or patients whose coffee, tea, or caffeinated drink intake is high.
SSRIs	Warfarin	Increased prothrombin time, bleeding. Tx: Monitor closely, decrease dose of warfarin if giving with SSRIs.
SSRIs	Lithium TCAs Barbiturates	Increased CNS effects of SSRIs. Tx: Adjust dosage of SSRI.
SSRIs	Phenytoin	Increased serum levels of phenytoin. Tx: Adjust dosage of phenytoin.

Source: Stahl, 2006.

Teaching Points 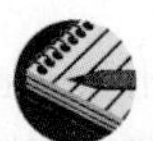

Patients should be advised not to take the herbal substance St. John's wort if they are also taking prescribed antidepressants. St. John's wort also should not be taken if the patient is taking nasal decongestants, hay fever and asthma medications containing monoamines, amino acid supplements containing phenylalanine, or tyrosine. The combination may cause hypertension.

Other Somatic Therapies

Electroconvulsive Therapy Although its therapeutic mechanism of action is unknown, electroconvulsive therapy (ECT) is an effective treatment for severe depression. It is generally reserved for patients whose disorder is refractory or intolerant to initial drug treatments and who are so severely ill that rapid treatment is required (e.g., patients with malnutrition, catatonia, or suicidality).

ECT is contraindicated for patients with increased intracranial pressure. Other high-risk patients include those with recent myocardial infarction, recent cerebrovascular accident, retinal detachment, or pheochromocytoma (tumor on the adrenal cortex or other tumors) and those at risk for complications of anesthesia. Older age has been associated with a favorable response to ECT. Because depression can increase mortality risk for the elderly, in particular, and some elderly patients do not respond well to medication, effective treatment is especially important for this age group (Blazer, Hybels, & Pieper, 2001).

Interventions for the Patient Undergoing ECT The American Nurses Association (2000) defines the role of the nurse in the care of the patient undergoing ECT to include providing educational and emotional support for the patient and family, assessing baseline or pretreatment level of function, preparing the patient for the ECT process, and monitoring and evaluating the patient's response to ECT, sharing it with the ECT team, and modifying treatment as needed (see Chapter 8 for more information). The actual procedure, possible therapeutic mechanisms of action, potential adverse effects, contraindications, and nursing interventions are described in detail in Chapter 8.

Light Therapy (Phototherapy) Light therapy is described in Chapter 8. Given current research, light therapy is an option for well-documented mild to moderate seasonal, nonpsychotic, winter depressive episodes in patients with recurrent major depressive or bipolar II disorders, including children and adolescents (Glod & Baisden, 1999; Zahourek, 2000). There is also evidence that light therapy can modestly improve symptoms in nonseasonal depression, especially when administered during the first week of treatment, in the morning, for those experiencing sleep deprivation (Tuunainen, Kripke, & Endo, 2004).

Psychological Domain

Assessment

The mental status examination is an effective clinical tool to evaluate the psychological aspects of major depression because the focus is on disturbances of mood and affect, thought processes and content, cognition, memory, and attention. The comprehensive mental status examination is described in detail in Chapter 10.

Mood and Affect

The person with depression has a sustained period of feeling depressed, sad, or hopeless and may experience anhedonia (loss of interest or pleasure). The patient may report "not caring anymore" or not feeling any enjoyment in activities that were previously considered pleasurable. In some individuals, this may include decrease in or loss of libido (sexual interest or desire) and sexual function. Depressed mood may be severe enough to provoke thoughts of suicide.

Numerous assessment scales are available for assessing depression. Easily administered self-report questionnaires can be valuable detection tools. These questionnaires cannot be the sole basis for making a diagnosis of major depressive episode, but they are sensitive to depressive symptoms. The following are five commonly used self-report scales:

- General Health Questionnaire (GHQ)
- Center for Epidemiological Studies Depression Scale (CES-D)
- Beck Depression Inventory (BDI)
- Zung Self-Rating Depression Scale (SDS)
- PRIME-MD

Clinician-completed rating scales may be more sensitive to improvement in the course of treatment, assess symptoms in relationship to the *DSM-IV-TR* depressive criteria, and may have a slightly greater specificity than do self-report questionnaires in detecting depression. These include the following:

- Hamilton Rating Scale for Depression (HAM-D)
- Montgomery-Asberg Depression Rating Scale (MADRS)
- National Institute of Mental Health Diagnostic Interview Schedule (DIS)

Thought Content

Depressed individuals often have an unrealistic negative evaluation of their worth or have guilty preoccupations or ruminations about minor past failings. Such individuals often misinterpret neutral or trivial day-to-day events as evidence of personal defects, and they have an exaggerated sense of responsibility for untoward events. As a result they feel hopeless, helpless, worthless, and powerless. The possibility of disorganized thought processes (e.g., tangential or circumstantial thinking) and perceptual disturbances (e.g., hallucinations, delusions) should also be included in the assessment.

Suicidal Behavior

Patients with major depression are at increased risk for suicide. Suicide risk should be assessed initially and throughout the course of treatment. Suicidal ideation includes thoughts that range from a belief that others would be better off if the person were dead or thoughts of death (passive suicidal ideation) to actual specific plans for committing suicide (active suicidal ideation). The frequency, intensity, and lethality of these thoughts can vary and can help to determine the seriousness of intent. The more specific the plan and the more accessible the means, the more serious is the intent. Risk factors that must be carefully considered are the availability and adequacy of social supports, past history of suicidal ideation or behavior, presence of psychosis or substance abuse, and decreased ability to control suicidal impulses.

Cognition and Memory

Many individuals with depression report impaired ability to think, concentrate, or make decisions. They may appear easily distracted or complain of memory difficulties. In older adults with major depression, memory difficulties may be the chief complaint and may be mistaken for early signs of a dementia (pseudodementia) (APA, 2000). When the depression is fully treated, the memory problem often improves or fully resolves.

Nursing Diagnoses for the Psychological Domain

Nursing diagnoses focusing on the psychological domain for the patient with a depressive disorder are numerous. If patient data lead to the diagnosis of Risk for Suicide, the patient should be further assessed for plan, intent, and accessibility of means. Other nursing diagnoses include Hopelessness, Low Self-Esteem, Ineffective Individual Coping, Decisional Conflict, Spiritual Distress, and Dysfunctional Grieving.

Interventions for the Psychological Domain

Although pharmacotherapy is usually the primary treatment method for major depression, patients also can benefit from psychosocial and psychoeducational treatments. The most commonly used therapies are described. For patients with severe or recurrent major depressive disorder, the combination of psychotherapy (including interpersonal therapy, cognitive behavioral therapy, behavior therapy, or brief dynamic therapy) and pharmacotherapy has been found to be superior to treatment with a single modality. Adding a course of cognitive behavioral therapy may be an effective strategy for preventing relapse in patients who have had only a partial response to pharmacotherapy alone (APA, 2000). Clinical practice guidelines suggest that the combination of medication and psychotherapy may be particularly useful in more complex situations (e.g., depression in the context of concurrent, chronic general-medical or other psychiatric disorders, or in patients who fail to experience complete response to either treatment alone). Recent studies suggest that short-term cognitive and interpersonal therapies may be as effective as pharmacotherapy in milder depressions. Psychotherapy in combination with medication may also be used to address collateral issues, such as medication adherence or secondary psychosocial problems (Casacalenda, Perry, & Looper, 2002).

• NCLEXNOTE

NCLEXNOTE A cognitive therapy approach is recommended for helping persons restructure the negative thinking processes related to a person's concept of self, others, and the future. This approach should be included in most nursing care plans for patients with depression.

Therapeutic Relationship

One of the most effective therapeutic tools for treating any psychiatric disorder is the therapeutic alliance, a helpful and trusting relationship between clinician and patient. The alliance is built from a number of activities, including the following:

- Establishment and maintenance of a supportive relationship
- Availability in times of crisis
- Vigilance regarding dangerousness to self and others
- Education about the illness and treatment goals
- Encouragement and feedback concerning progress
- Guidance regarding the patient's interactions with the personal and work environment
- Realistic goal setting and monitoring

Interacting with depressed individuals is challenging because they tend to be withdrawn and have difficulty expressing feelings and engaging in interpersonal interactions. The therapeutic alliance may be enhanced through the use of cognitive therapy as well as the nurse's ability to win the patient's trust through the use of culturally competent strategies in the context of empathy (see Box 20.5).

BOX 20.5

Therapeutic Dialogue: Approaching the Depressed Patient

George Sadder is a 70-year-old retired businessman who has been admitted to a day treatment program because of complaints of stomach pains, insomnia, and hopelessness. He has withdrawn from social activities he previously enjoyed, such as golfing and going out to eat with his wife and friends. This morning he sits in a chair by himself, rather than joining a group activity.

Ineffective Approach

Nurse: "Hi, Mr. Sadder. My name is Sally. How are you feeling today?"

Mr. S: "Lousy, just lousy! I didn't sleep well last night, and my stomach is killing me!"

Nurse: "Oh, that is too bad! Have you had any breakfast?"

Mr. S: "No! Didn't I say that my stomach is killing me?"

Nurse: "Maybe eating breakfast would help your stomach pain."

Mr. S: "You don't know anything about my pain!" (Gets up and walks away.)

Effective Approach

Nurse: "Hi. My name is Sally."

Mr. S: "Hello, Sally. My name is George Sadder."

Nurse: "I'd like to sit down with you, if that is OK."

Mr. S: "If you want, but I am not much of a talker."

Nurse: "That's OK. We can talk or not, whatever you wish."

Mr. S: (Patient winces)

Nurse: "You just winced. Are you in pain?"

Mr. S: "Yes, my stomach has been killing me lately."

Nurse: "What do you usually do to ease the pain?"

Mr. S: "I usually take an antacid with my meals but forgot this morning."

Nurse: "I'll see if I can get some for you now."

Mr. S: "Thanks. When my stomach settles down, maybe we can talk."

Nurse: "That would be fine. I'll check back with you in a few minutes."

Critical Thinking Challenge

- What ineffective techniques did the nurse use in the first scenario and how did they impair communication?
- What effective techniques did the nurse use in the second scenario and how did they facilitate communication?

• NCLEXNOTE

Establishing the patient–nurse relationship with a person who is depressed requires an empathic, quiet approach that is grounded in the nurse's understanding of the cultural needs of the patient.

Cognitive Therapy

Cognitive therapy has been successful in reducing depressive symptoms during the acute phase of major depression (APA, 2002) (see Chapter 11). This therapy uses techniques, such as thought stopping and positive self-talk, to dispel irrational beliefs and distorted attitudes. In one study, remission rates after cognitive therapy were comparable to those after pharmacotherapy (Casacalenda et al., 2002). The use of cognitive therapy in the acute phase of treatment combined with medication has grown in the past few years and now may be considered as first-line treatment for mildly to moderately depressed outpatients.

Behavior Therapy

Behavior therapy has been effective in the acute treatment of patients with mild to moderately severe depression, especially when combined with pharmacotherapy. Therapeutic techniques include activity scheduling, self-control therapy, social skills training, and problem solving. The efficacy of behavior therapy in the continuation and maintenance phase of depression has not been subjected to controlled studies (APA, 2002). Behavior therapy techniques are described in Chapter 10.

Interpersonal Therapy

Interpersonal therapy seeks to recognize, explore, and resolve the interpersonal losses, role confusion and transitions, social isolation, and deficits in social skills that may precipitate depressive states (APA, 2002). It maintains that losses must be mourned and related affects appreciated, that role confusion and transitions must be recognized and resolved, and that social skills deficits must be overcome to acquire social supports. Some evidence in controlled studies suggests that interpersonal therapy is more effective in reducing depressive symptoms with certain populations, such as depressed patients with human immunodeficiency virus infection, and less successful with patients who have personality disorders (APA, 2002) (see Chapter 22).

Family and Marital Therapy 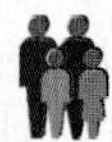

Patients who perceive high family stress are at risk for greater future severity of illness, higher use of health services, and higher health care expense. Marital and family problems are common among patients with mood disorders; comprehensive treatment requires that these problems be assessed and addressed. They may be a consequence of the major depression but may also predispose persons to develop depressive symptoms and/or inhibit recovery and resilience processes. Research suggests that marital and family therapy may reduce depressive symptoms and the risk for relapse in patients with marital and family problems (Thase, 2000). The depressed spouse's depression has marked impact on the marital adjustment of the nondepressed spouse. It is recommended that treatment approaches be designed to help couples be supportive of each other, to adapt, and to cope with the depressive symptoms within the framework of their ongoing marital relations (Mead, 2002). Many family nursing interventions (discussed in detail in Chapter 13) may be used by the psychiatric nurse in providing targeted family-centered care. These include:

- Monitoring patient and family for indicators of stress.
- Teaching stress management techniques.
- Counseling family members on coping skills for their own use.
- Providing necessary knowledge of options and support services.
- Facilitating family routines and rituals.
- Assisting family to resolve feelings of guilt.
- Assisting family with conflict resolution.
- Identifying family strengths and resources with family members.
- Facilitating communication among family members.

Group Therapy

The role of group therapy in treating depression is based on clinical experience, rather than on systematic controlled studies. It may be particularly useful for depression associated with bereavement or chronic medical illness. Individuals may benefit from the example of others who have dealt successfully with similar losses or challenges. Survivors can gain self-esteem as successful role models for new group members. Medication support groups can provide information to the patient and to family members regarding prognosis and medication issues, thereby providing a psychoeducational forum.

Teaching Patients and Families 

Patients with depression and their significant others often incorrectly believe that their illness is their own fault and that they should be able to "pull themselves up by their boot straps and snap out of it." Persons from some cultural groups believe that the symptoms of depression may be a result of someone placing a hex on the affected person because the person has done something evil (Warren, in press). It is vital to be culturally competent to be effective in teaching patients and their families about the treatment modalities for depression.

Patients need to know the full range of suitable treatment options before consenting to participate in treatment. The nurse can provide opportunities for them to question, discuss, and explore their feelings about past, current, and planned use of medications and other treatments (ANA, 2000). Developing strategies to enhance adherence and to raise awareness of early signs of relapse can be important aids to increasing treatment efficacy (see Box 20.6).

BOX 20.6

Psychoeducation Checklist: Major Depressive Disorder

When caring for the patient with a major depressive disorder, be sure to include the following topic areas in the teaching plan:

- Psychopharmacologic agents, including drug action, dosing frequency, and possible adverse effects
- Risk factors for recurrence, signs of recurrence
- Adherence to therapy and treatment program
- Nutrition
- Sleep measures
- Self-care management
- Goal setting and problem solving
- Social interaction skills
- Follow-up appointments
- Community support services

Social Domain

Assessment

Social assessment focuses on the individual's developmental history, family psychiatric history, patterns of relationships, quality of support system, education, work history, and impact of physical or sexual abuse on interpersonal function (see Chapter 10). Including a family member or close friend in the assessment process can be helpful. Changes in patterns of relating (especially social withdrawal) and changes in level of occupational functioning are commonly reported and may represent a significant deterioration from baseline behavior. Increased use of "sick days" may occur. The family's level of support and understanding of the disorder also need to be assessed. For people who are depressed, special attention should be given to the individual's spiritual dimension and religious background (see Box 20.7).

Nursing Diagnoses for the Social Domain

Nursing diagnoses common for the social domain include Ineffective Family Coping, Ineffective Role Performance, Interrupted Family Processes, and Caregiver Role Strain (if the patient is also a caregiver).

BOX 20.7

***Using Reflection:* Assessment of Spiritual Distress**

Incident: A patient expresses extreme guilt over a childhood incident involving a teenage pregnancy that resulted in her child being anonymously adopted. The child is now an adult and is trying to contact her. She tells the nurse that she has committed an unforgivable sin.

Reflection: The nurse listened for several minutes and reflected on the meaning of the patient's statements and observed how distraught the patient appeared. The nurse then asked the patient if she would want to see the hospital chaplain for further clarification. The patient was greatly relieved and requested help from a chaplain.

Interventions for the Social Domain

Individuals experiencing depression have often withdrawn from daily activities, such as engaging in family activities, attending work, and participating in community activities. During hospitalization, patients often withdraw to their rooms and refuse to participate in unit activity. Nurses are challenged to help the patient balance the need for privacy with the need to return to normal social functioning. Depressed patients should never be approached in an overly enthusiastic manner; that approach will irritate them and block communication. On the other hand, patients should be encouraged to set realistic goals to reconnect with their families and communities. Explain to patients that attending social activities, even though they do not feel like it, will promote the recovery process and help patients achieve those goals.

Milieu Therapy

While hospitalized, milieu therapy (see Chapter 10) helps depressed patients maintain socialization skills and continue to interact with others. When depressed, people are often unaware of the environment and withdraw into themselves. On a psychiatric unit, depressed patients should be encouraged to attend and participate in unit activities. These individuals have a decreased energy level and thus may be moving more slowly than others; however, their efforts should be praised.

Safety. In many cases, patients are commonly admitted to the psychiatric hospital because of a suicide attempt. Suicidality should continually be evaluated, and the patient should be protected from self-harm (see Chapter 17). During the depths of depression, patients may not have the energy to complete a suicide. As patients begin to feel better and have increased energy, they may be at a greater risk for suicide. If a previously depressed patient appears to become energized overnight, he or she may have made a decision to commit suicide and thus may be relieved that the decision is finally made. The nurse may misinterpret the mood improvement as a positive move toward recovery; however, this patient may be very intent on suicide. These individuals should be carefully monitored to maintain their safety.

Other Interventions

Nurses are exceptionally well positioned to engage patients and their families in the active process of improving daily functioning, increasing knowledge and skill acquisition, and increasing independent living. Consumer-oriented support groups can help to enhance the self-esteem and the support network of participating patients and their families. Advice, encouragement, and the sense of group camaraderie may make an important contribution to recovery (APA, 2000). Organizations providing support and information include the Depression and Bipolar Support Network (DBSA), National Alliance for the Mentally Ill (NAMI), and the Mental Health Association and Recovery, Inc. (a self-help group).

Interventions for Family Members 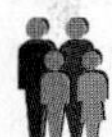

The family needs education and support during and after the treatment of family members. Because major depressive disorder is a recurring disorder, the family needs information about specific antecedents to a family member's depression and what steps to take. For example, one patient may routinely become depressed during the fall of each year, with one of the first symptoms being excessive sleepiness. For another patient, a major loss, such as a child going to college or the death of a pet, may precipitate a depressive episode. Families of elderly patients need to be aware of the possibility of depression and related symptoms, often occurring after the deaths of friends and relatives. Families of children who are depressed often misinterpret depression as behavior problems.

MOVIE viewing GUIDES

Evaluation and Treatment Outcomes

The major goals of treatment are to help the patient to be as independent as possible and to achieve stability, remission, and recovery from major depression. It is often a lifelong struggle for the individual. Ongoing evaluation of the patient's symptoms, functioning, and quality of life should be carefully documented in the patient's record in order to monitor outcomes of treatment.

Continuum of Care

Individuals with depressive disorders may initially present in inpatient and outpatient medical and primary care settings, emergency rooms, and inpatient and outpatient mental health settings. Nurses should be able to recognize depression in these patients and make appropriate interventions or referrals. The continuum of care beyond these settings may include partial hospitalization or day treatment programs; individual, family, or group psychotherapy; home visits, and ethnopsychopharmacotherapy. Although most patients with major depression are treated in outpatient settings, brief hospitalization may be required if the patient is suicidal or psychotic.

Nurses working on inpatient units provide a wide range of direct services, including administering and monitoring medications and target symptoms, conducting psychoeducational groups, and more generally, structuring and maintaining a therapeutic environment. Nurses providing home care have an excellent opportunity to detect undiagnosed depressive disorders and make appropriate referrals.

Nursing practice requires a coordinated, ongoing interaction among patients, families, and providers to deliver comprehensive services. This includes using the complementary skills of both psychiatric and medical care colleagues for forming overall goals, plans, and decisions and for providing continuity of care as needed (ANA, 2000). Collaborative care between the primary care provider and mental health specialist is also key to achieving remission of symptoms and physical well-being, restoring baseline occupational and psychosocial functioning, and reducing the likelihood of relapse or recurrence (Fig. 20.1).

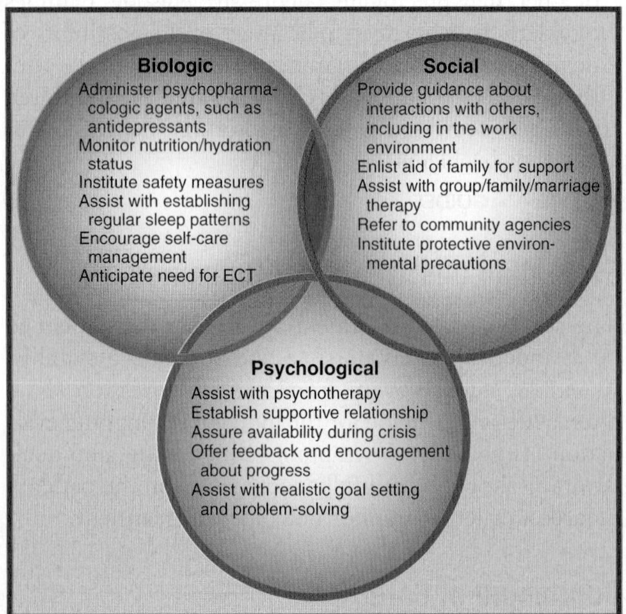

FIGURE 20.1. Biopsychosocial interventions for patients with major depressive disorder (ECT, electroconvulsive therapy).

BIPOLAR DISORDERS (MANIC-DEPRESSIVE DISORDERS)

Diagnostic Criteria

Bipolar disorder is distinguished from depressive disorders by the occurrence of manic or hypomanic (i.e., mildly manic) episodes in addition to depressive episodes. The *DSM-IV-TR* divides bipolar disorders into three major groups: bipolar I (periods of major depressive, manic, or mixed episodes); bipolar II (periods of major depression and hypomania); and **cyclothymic disorder** (periods of hypomanic episodes and depressive episodes that do not meet full criteria for a major depressive episode) (Table 20.5). These are described later. The specifiers describe either the most recent mood episode or the course of recurrent episodes; for example, "bipolar disorder I, most recent episode manic, severe with psychotic features."

KEY CONCEPT Mania is primarily characterized by an abnormally and persistently elevated, expansive, or irritable mood for a duration of at least 1 week (or less, if hospitalized).

A **manic episode** is a distinct period (of at least 1 week, or less, if hospitalized) during which there is an abnormally and persistently elevated, expansive, or irritable mood (APA, 2000). Elevated mood is characterized as **euphoria** (exaggerated feelings of well-being) or elation, during which the person may describe feeling "high," "ecstatic," "on top of the world," or "up in the clouds." **Expansive mood** is characterized by inappropriate lack of restraint in expressing one's feelings and frequently overvaluing one's own importance. Expansive qualities include an unceasing and indiscriminate enthusiasm for interpersonal, sexual, or occupational interactions. Manic episodes can also consist of irritable mood, in which the person is easily annoyed and provoked to anger, particularly when the person's wishes are challenged or thwarted. In addition, manic episodes can consist of alterations between euphoria and irritability (**lability of mood**). To meet full *DSM-IV-TR* criteria, three (or four if the mood is irritable) of seven additional symptoms must be present: inflated self-esteem or grandiosity; decreased need for sleep; being more talkative or having pressured speech; flight of ideas or racing thoughts; distractibility; increase in goal-directed activity or psychomotor agitation; and excessive involvement in pleasurable activities that have a high potential for painful consequences. The disturbance must be severe enough to cause marked impairment in social activities, occupational functioning, and interpersonal relationships or to require hospitalization to prevent self-harm.

During a manic episode, decreased need to sleep is accompanied by increased energy and hyperactivity. The individual often remains awake for long periods at night

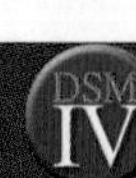

Table 20.5 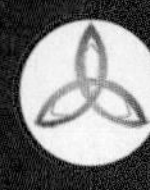

Key Diagnostic Characteristics of Bipolar I Disorder 296.xx
296.0x—Bipolar I, single manic episode
296.40—Bipolar I, most recent episode hypomanic
296.4x—Bipolar I, most recent episode manic
296.6x—Bipolar I, most recent episode mixed
296.5x—Bipolar I, most recent episode depressed
296.7—Bipolar I, most recent episode unspecified

Diagnostic Criteria and Target Symptoms

- Presence of one or more manic episodes or mixed episodes, including one or more major depressive episodes

Manic episode

- Abnormally and persistently elevated, expansive, or irritable mood for at least 1 week
- Persistence of inflated self-esteem and grandiosity
- Decreased need for sleep
- More talkative than usual or pressure to keep talking
- Flight of ideas or racing thoughts
- Distractibility
- Increased goal-directed activity or psychomotor agitation
- Excessive involvement in pleasurable activities with high potential for painful results (such as unrestrained buying sprees, foolish business investments)
- Marked impairment in occupational functioning or in usual social activities or relationships; possible hospitalization to prevent harm; psychotic features

Major depressive episode (symptoms appear nearly every day)

- Depressed mood most of the day
- Markedly diminished interest or pleasure in all or most all activities for most of the day
- Significant weight loss when not dieting; weight gain or increase or decrease in appetite
- Insomnia or hypersomnia
- Psychomotor agitation or retardation
- Fatigue or loss of energy
- Feelings of worthlessness or excessive or inappropriate guilt
- Diminished ability to concentrate or indecisiveness
- Recurrent thoughts of death, suicidal ideation without a specific plan, suicide attempt or specific plan for committing suicide
- Not bereavement
- Clinically significant distress or impairment in social, occupational, or other important areas of functioning

Mixed episode

- Criteria for both manic and major depressive episodes nearly every day for at least 1 week
- Hospitalization to prevent harm; psychotic features

Hypomanic episode

- Distinct period of persistently elevated, expansive, or irritable mood through at least 4 days
- Clearly different from usual nondepressed mood
- Same symptoms as that for manic episode but does not cause impairment in social or occupational functioning or necessitate hospitalization

Associated Findings

Associated Behavioral Findings

Manic episode

- Resistive to efforts for treatment
- Disorganized or bizarre behavior
- Change in dress or appearance
- Possible gambling and antisocial behavior

Major depressive episode

- Tearfulness, irritability
- Obsessive rumination
- Anxiety
- Phobia
- Excessive worry over physical symptoms
- Complaints of pain
- Possible panic attacks
- Difficulty with intimate relationships
- Marital, occupational, or academic problems
- Substance abuse
- Increased use of medical services
- Attempted or complete suicide attempts

Mixed episode

- Similar to those for manic and depressive episodes

Hypomanic episodes

- Sudden onset with rapid escalation within 1–2 d
- Possibly precede or are followed by major depressive episode

Associated Physical Examination Findings

Manic episode

- Mean age of onset for first manic episode after age 21–30 yrs
- Possible child abuse, spouse abuse, or other violent behavior during severe manic episodes
- Associated problems involving school truancy, school failure, occupational failure, divorce, or episodic antisocial behavior

(Continued on following page)

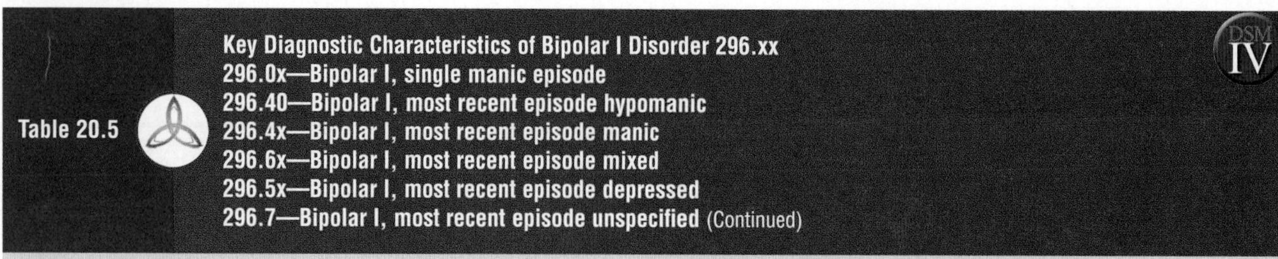

Table 20.5 Key Diagnostic Characteristics of Bipolar I Disorder 296.xx
296.0x—Bipolar I, single manic episode
296.40—Bipolar I, most recent episode hypomanic
296.4x—Bipolar I, most recent episode manic
296.6x—Bipolar I, most recent episode mixed
296.5x—Bipolar I, most recent episode depressed
296.7—Bipolar I, most recent episode unspecified (Continued)

Diagnostic Criteria and Target Symptoms	Associated Findings
• Unequivocal change in function, uncharacteristic of person when asymptomatic • Change observable by others • Not severe enough to cause marked impairment in social or occupational functioning or to require hospitalization; no psychotic features • Episode not better accounted for by other disorders such as schizoaffective disorder and not superimposed on schizophrenia, schizophreniform, delusional, or psychotic disorders • Not a direct physiologic effect of substance or other medical condition	***Associated Laboratory Findings*** ***Manic episodes*** • Polysomnographic abnormalities • Increased cortisol secretion • Absence of dexamethasone nonsuppression • Possible abnormalities with norepinephrine, serotonin, acetylcholine, dopamine, or GABA neurotransmitter ***Major depressive episode*** • Sleep electroencephalogram abnormalities • Possible abnormalities with norepinephrine, serotonin, acetylcholine, dopamine, or GABA neurotransmitter systems

or wakes up several times full of energy. Increased motor activity and agitation, which may be purposeful at first (e.g., cleaning the house), may deteriorate into inappropriate or disorganized actions. The individual may get involved unrealistically in several new endeavors that may entail overspending or sexual encounters or drug or alcohol use, or high-risk activities such as driving too fast or taking up dangerous sports (see Box 20.8). The individual becomes overly talkative, feels pressured to continue talking, and at times is difficult to interrupt. Thoughts become disorganized and skip rapidly among topics that often have little relationship to each other. This decreased logical connection between thoughts is termed *flight of ideas*. Patients with mania have inflated self-esteem, which may range from unusual self-confidence to grandiose delusions. Other psychiatric disorders can have symptoms that mimic a manic episode. Schizophrenia, schizoaffective disorder, anxiety disorders, some personality disorders (borderline personality disorder and histrionic personality disorder), substance abuse involving stimulants, and adolescent conduct disorders should be ruled out when making a diagnosis of mania. The *DSM-IV-TR* criteria for a **mixed episode** are met when the criteria for both a manic episode and a major depressive episode are met and are present for at least 1 week. Individuals who are having a mixed episode usually exhibit high anxiety, agitation, and irritability. The criteria for a **hypomanic episode** are the same as for a manic episode, except that the time criterion is at least 4 days, rather than 1 week, and no marked impairment in social or occupational functioning is present.

The *DSM-IV-TR* criteria for cyclothymic disorder are the presence for at least 2 years of numerous periods with hypomanic symptoms and numerous periods with depressive symptoms that do not meet full criteria for a major depressive episode.

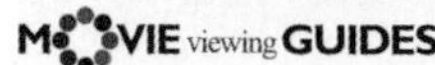

Secondary Mania

Mania can be caused by medical disorders or their treatments or by certain substances of abuse (e.g., certain metabolic abnormalities, neurologic disorders, CNS tumors, and medications) (Strakowski & Sax, 2000).

Rapid Cycling Specifier

Rapid cycling can occur in both bipolar I and bipolar II disorders. In its most severe form, rapid cycling includes

BOX 20.8

Clinical Vignette: The Manic Patient

Mr. Bell was a day trader on the stock market. Initially he was quite successful and, as a result, upgraded his lifestyle with a more expensive car, a larger, more luxurious house, and a boat. When the stock market declined dramatically, Mr. Bell continued to trade, saying that if he could just find the "right" stock he could earn back all of the money he had lost. He spent his days and nights in front of his computer screen, taking little or no time to eat or sleep. He defaulted on his mortgage and car and boat payments and was talking nonstop to his wife. She brought him to the hospital for evaluation

What Do You Think?

- What behavioral symptoms of mania does Mr. Bell exhibit?
- What cognitive symptoms of mania does Mr. Bell exhibit?

continuous cycling between subthreshold mania and depression or hypomania and depression (Suppes et al., 2001). The essential feature of rapid cycling is the occurrence of four or more mood episodes that meet criteria for manic, mixed, hypomanic, or depressive episode during the previous 12 months.

The *DSM-IV-TR* criteria for cyclothymic disorder are at least 2 years of numerous periods with hypomanic symptoms and numerous periods with depressive symptoms that do not meet full criteria for a major depressive episode.

Clinical Course

Bipolar disorder is a chronic, cyclic disorder. There is general agreement that later episodes of illness occur more frequently than earlier episodes, and increased frequency of episodes or more continuous symptoms have been reported in patients who experienced onset at an earlier age and who have a significant family history of illness. Some patients may have unpredictable and variable symptoms of the illness (Suppes et al., 2001). An additional feature of bipolar disorder is rapid cycling. Mixed states have been associated with increased suicidal ideation compared with pure mania (Maser et al., 2002). Bipolar disorder can lead to severe functional impairment as manifested by alienation from family, friends, and coworkers; indebtedness; job loss; divorce; and other problems of living (Rothbaum & Astin, 2000).

Bipolar Disorder In Special Populations

Children and Adolescents

Bipolar disorder in children has been recognized only recently. Although it is not well studied, depression usually appears first. Somewhat different than in adults, the hallmark of childhood bipolar disorder is intense rage. Children may display seemingly unprovoked rage episodes for as long as 2 to 3 hours. The symptoms of bipolar disorder reflect the developmental level of the child. Children younger than 9 years exhibit more irritability and emotional lability; older children exhibit more classic symptoms, such as euphoria and grandiosity. The first contact with the mental health system often occurs when the behavior becomes disruptive, possibly 5 to 10 years after its onset. These children often have other psychiatric disorders, such as attention deficit hyperactivity disorder and conduct disorder (Mohr, 2001) (see Chapter 29).

Elderly People

Geriatric patients with mania demonstrate more neurologic abnormalities and cognitive disturbances (confusion and disorientation) than do younger patients. It generally was believed that the incidence of mania decreases with age because this population was thought to consist of only those individuals who had a diagnosis in younger years and managed to survive into old age. Recently, late-onset bipolar disorder was identified when researchers found evidence of an increased incidence of mania with age, especially in women after age 50 years and in men in the eighth and ninth decades. Late-onset bipolar disorder is more likely related to secondary mania and consequently has a poorer prognosis because of comorbid medical conditions (Kilbourne, 2005).

Epidemiology

Distribution and Age of Onset

Bipolar disorder has a lifetime prevalence of 0.4% to 1.6% in the general adult population (APA, 2000). Most patients with bipolar disorder experience significant symptoms before age 25 years (Suppes et al., 2001). The estimated mean age of onset is between 21 and 30 years. Nearly 20% of patients with bipolar disorder diagnosed demonstrated symptoms before the age of 19 years (Mohr, 2001). Estimates of the prevalence of mania in elderly psychiatric patients are as high as 19%, with prevalence in nursing home patients estimated at about 10% (McDonald, 2000).

Gender, Ethnic, and Cultural Differences

Although no significant gender differences have been found in the incidence of bipolar I and II diagnoses, gender differences have been reported in phenomenology, course, and treatment response. In addition, some data show that female patients with bipolar disorder are at greater risk for depression and rapid cycling than are male patients, whereas male patients are at greater risk for manic episodes (Grunze, Amann, Dittmann, & Walden, 2002; Yildiz & Sachs, 2003). No significant differences have been found based on race or ethnicity (APA, 2000).

Comorbidity

The two most common comorbid conditions are anxiety disorders (most prevalent: panic disorder and social phobia) and substance use (most commonly alcohol and marijuana). Individuals with a comorbid anxiety disorder are more likely to experience a more severe course. A history of substance use further complicates the course of illness and results in less chance for remission and poorer treatment compliance (Sajatovic, Blow, & Ignacio, 2006).

Etiology

Current theories of the etiology of mood disorders are associated with chronic abnormalities of neurotransmission, which are thought to result in compensatory but maladaptive changes in brain regulation. In addition, use of controlled structural and functional imaging studies of patients with mood disorders have generated hypotheses that dysfunction of the CNS is associated with specific structural brain abnormalities and functional CNS alterations (Sheline, 2003).

Chronobiologic Theories

Sleep disturbance is an important aspect of depression and mania. Sleep patterns appear to be regulated by an internal biologic clock center in the hypothalamus. Artificially induced sleep deprivation is known to precipitate mania in some patients with bipolar disorder (Grunze et al., 2002). Because a number of neurotransmitter and hormone levels follow circadian patterns, sleep disruption may lead to biochemical abnormalities that affect mood. Seasonal changes in light exposure also trigger affective episodes in some patients, typically depression in winter and hypomania in the summer in the northern hemisphere (Lewy, Lefler, Emens, & Bauer, 2006).

Sensitization and Kindling Theory

Sensitization (increase in response with repetition of the same dose of drug) and the related phenomenon of kindling (subthreshold stimulation of a neuron generates an action potential; see Chapter 7) refer to animal models. Repeated chemical or electrical stimulation of certain regions of the brain produces stereotypical behavioral responses or seizures. The amount of the chemical or electricity required to evoke the response or seizure decreases with each experience. These phenomena have been used as models to explain why, over time, affective episodes, particularly those seen in patients with bipolar disorder, recur in shorter and shorter cycles and with less relation to environmental precipitants. It is hypothesized that repeated affective episodes might be accompanied by progressive alteration of brain synapses that lower the threshold for future episodes and increase the likelihood of illness. The kindling theory also helps explain the value of using antiseizure medication, such as carbamazepine and valproic acid, for mood stabilization.

FAME AND FORTUNE

Virginia Woolf (1882–1941):
British Novelist

Public Persona

Virginia Woolf, an early feminist and accomplished novelist, came from a long line of writers with a history of mental illness on both sides of the family. Many believe that Virginia Woolf suffered from bipolar disorder. Unfortunately, there was little treatment in her time.

Personal Realities

She experienced mood swings most of her life and had her first mental breakdown at age 13 following her mother's death. She had several more episodes in which she heard voices and once threw herself out of a window. During periods of remission, Woolf was very creative and productive. During her last episode of illness, she committed suicide at the age of 59.

Source: Virginia Woolf, http://www.online-literature.com/virginia_woolf/

Genetic Factors

First-degree biologic relatives of individuals with bipolar I disorder have elevated rates of bipolar I disorder (4% to 24%), bipolar II disorder (1% to 5%), and major depressive disorder (4% to 24%) (APA, 2000). Results from family, adoption, and twin studies indicate that bipolar disorder is highly heritable (McCuffin et al., 2003). Nevertheless, the mode of transmission and its genetic relationship to other mood disorders have not been definitively identified.

Psychological and Social Theories

Most psychological and social theories of mood disorders focus on loss as the cause of depression in genetically vulnerable individuals. Mania is considered to be a biologically rooted condition, but when viewed from a psychological perspective, mania is usually regarded as a condition that arises from an attempt to overcompensate for depressed feelings, rather than a disorder in its own right. It is now generally accepted that environmental conditions contribute to the timing of an episode of illness, rather than cause the illness (Johnson, Andersson-Lundman, Aberg-Wistedt, & Mathe, 2000).

Interdisciplinary Treatment of Disorders

Patients with bipolar disorder have a complex set of issues and likely will be treated by an interdisciplinary team. Nurses, physicians, social workers, psychologists, and activity therapists all have valuable expertise for patients with bipolar disorder. For children with bipolar disorder, school teachers and counselors are included in the team. For elderly patients, the primary care physician becomes part of the team. An important treatment goal is to minimize and prevent either manic or depressive episodes, which tend to accelerate over time. The fewer the episodes, the more likely the person can live a normal, productive life. Another important goal is to help the patient and family to learn about the disorder and manage it throughout a lifetime.

Priority Care Issues

During a manic episode, protection of the patient is a priority. It is during a manic episode that poor judgment and impulsivity result in risk-taking behaviors that can have dire consequences for the patient and family. For example, one patient withdrew all the family money from the bank and gambled it away. Risk for suicide is always a possibility. During a depressive episode, the patient may feel that life is not worth living. During a manic episode, the patient may believe that he or she has supernatural powers, such as the ability to fly. As patients recover from a manic episode, they may be so devastated by the consequences of impulsive behavior and poor judgment during the episode that suicide seems like a reasonable option.

Family Response to Disorder 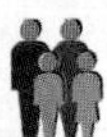

Bipolar disorder can devastate families, who often feel that they are on an emotional merry-go-round, particularly if they have difficulty understanding the mood shifts. A major problem for family members is dealing with the consequences of impulsive behavior during manic episodes, such as excessive debt, assault charges, and sexual infidelities.

NURSING MANAGEMENT: HUMAN RESPONSE TO BIPOLAR DISORDER

The nursing care of patients with bipolar disorder is one of the most interesting yet greatest challenges in psychiatric nursing. In general, the behavior of patients with bipolar disorder is normal between mood episodes. The ideal nursing care occurs during a period of time when the nurse can see the patient in the acute illness phase and in remission. Nursing care of bipolar depression should be approached in a manner similar to that used for major depressive disorder, as described previously.

Biologic Domain

Assessment

With regard to the biologic domain, the assessment emphasis is on evaluating symptoms of mania and, most particularly, changes in sleep patterns. The assessment should follow the guidelines in Chapter 10. In the manic phase of bipolar disorder, the patient may not sleep, resulting in irritability and physical exhaustion. Because eating habits usually change during a manic or depressive episode, the nurse should assess changes in diet and body weight. Because patients with mania may experience malnutrition and fluid imbalance, laboratory studies, such as thyroid function, should be completed. Abnormal thyroid functioning can be responsible for the mood and behavioral disturbances. During a manic phase, patients often become hypersexual and engage in risky sexual practices. Changes in sexual practices should be explored.

Pharmacologic Assessment

When a patient is in a manic state, the previous use of antidepressants should be assessed because a manic episode may be triggered by antidepressant use. In such cases, use of antidepressants should be discontinued. Many times, manic or depressive episodes occur after patients stop taking their mood stabilizer, at which time the reason for stopping the medication should be explored. Patients may stop taking their medications because of side effects or because they no longer believe they have a mental disorder. Special attention should also focus on the use of alcohol and other substances. Usually, a drug screen is ordered to determine current use of substances.

Nursing Diagnoses for Biologic Domain

Among nursing diagnoses in this domain are Insomnia; Sleep Deprivation; Imbalanced Nutrition; Hypothermia, Deficient Fluid Volume; and Noncompliance if patients have stopped taking their medication. If patients are in the depressive phase of illness, the previously discussed diagnoses for depression should be considered.

Interventions for Biologic Domain

Physical Care

In a state of mania, the patient's physical needs are rest, adequate hydration and nutrition, and re-establishment of physical well-being. Self-care has usually deteriorated. For a patient who is unable to sit long enough to eat, snacks and high-energy foods should be provided that can be eaten while moving. Alcohol should be avoided. Sleep hygiene is a priority but may not be realistic until medications take effect. Limiting stimuli can be helpful in decreasing agitation and promoting sleep.

• NCLEXNOTE

NCLEXNOTE Protection of patients with mania is always a priority. Ongoing assessment should focus on irritability, fatigue, and potential for harming self or others.

Teaching Points 

Once the patient's mood stabilizes, the nurse should focus on monitoring changes in physical functioning in sleep or eating behavior and teaching patients to identify antecedents to mood episodes. A regular sleep routine should be maintained if possible. High-risk times for manic episodes, such as changes in work schedule (day to night), should be avoided if possible. Patients should be taught to monitor the amount of their sleep each night and report decreases in sleep of more than 1 hour per night because this may be a precursor to a manic episode.

Intervention With Mood Stabilizers

Pharmacotherapy is essential in bipolar disorder to achieve two goals: rapid control of symptoms and prevention of future episodes or, at least, reduction in their severity and frequency. Pharmacotherapy continues through the various phases of bipolar disorder:

- ***Acute phase.*** The goal of treatment in the acute phase is symptom reduction and stabilization. Therefore, for the first few weeks of treatment, mood stabilizers may need to be combined with antipsychotics or benzodiazepines, particularly if the patient has psychotic symptoms, agitation, or insomnia. If the clinical situation is not an emergency, patients usually start on a low dose and gradually increase the dose until maximum therapeutic benefits are achieved. Once stabilization is achieved, the frequency of serum level monitoring should be every 1 to 2 weeks during the first 2 months and every 3 to 6 months during long-term maintenance. Medications most commonly used for mood stabilization in bipolar disorder are discussed here and in Chapter 8.
- ***Continuation phase.*** The treatment goal in this phase is to prevent relapse of the current episode or cycling into the opposite pole. It lasts about 2 to 9 months after acute symptoms resolve. The usual pharmacologic procedure in this phase is to continue the mood stabilizer while closely monitoring the patient for signs or symptoms of relapse.
- ***Maintenance phase.*** The goal of treating this phase is to sustain remission and to prevent new episodes. The great weight of evidence favors long-term prophylaxis against recurrence after effective treatment of acute episodes. It is recommended that long-term or lifetime prophylaxis with a mood stabilizer be instituted after two manic episodes or after one severe manic episode or if there is a family history of bipolar disorder.
- ***Discontinuation.*** Like the course of major depressive disorder, the course of bipolar disorder typically is recurrent and progressive. Therefore, the same issues and principles regarding the decision to continue or discontinue pharmacotherapy apply.

The mainstays of somatic therapy are the mood-stabilizing drugs. The three agents that show significant efficacy in controlled trials are lithium carbonate (Lithium), divalproex sodium (Depakote), and carbamazepine (Tegretol) (Table 20.6). Both lithium and divalproex sodium have U.S. Food and Drug Administration (FDA) approval for treating acute bipolar I mania, as do most of the atypical antipsychotics.

Lithium Carbonate Lithium is the most widely used mood stabilizer (see Box 20.9). Combined response rates from five studies demonstrate that 70% of patients experienced at least partial improvement with lithium therapy. However, for most patients, lithium is not a fully adequate treatment for all phases of the illness, and particularly during the acute phase, supplemental use of antipsychotics and benzodiazepines is often beneficial. During acute depressive episodes, supplemental use of antidepressants is most often indicated (Keck et al., 2000). Because of its significant side-effect burden (Table 20.7), lithium is poorly tolerated in at least one third of treated patients and has the narrowest gap between therapeutic and toxic concentrations of any routinely prescribed psychotropic agent (Belmaker & Yaroslavsky, 2000). Predictors of poor response to lithium in acute mania include a history of poor response, rapid cycling, dysphoric symptoms, mixed symptoms of depression and mania, psychiatric comorbidity, and medical comorbidity (Alda & Grof, 2000).

Table 20.6 Mood Stabilizing Medications

Generic (Trade) Drug Name	Usual Dosage Range (daily)	Half-life (h)
Lithium (Eskalith, Lithane)	600–1,800 mg	17–36
Divalproex sodium (Depakote)	15–60 mg/kg	6–16
Carbamazepine (Tegretol)	200–1,200 mg	25–65
Olanzapine (Zyprexa)	5–20 mg	21–54
Risperidone (Risperdal)	1–6 mg	20

• NCLEXNOTE

NCLEXNOTE Reviewing blood levels of lithium carbonate and divalproex sodium are ongoing nursing assessments for patients receiving these medications. Side effects of mood stabilizers vary.

Lithium is a salt, and the interaction between lithium levels and sodium levels in the body and the relationship between lithium levels and fluid volume in the body remain crucial issues in its safe, effective use. The higher the sodium levels are in the body, the lower the lithium level will be, and vice versa. Thus, changes in dietary sodium intake can affect lithium blood levels that, in turn, may affect therapeutic results or increase the incidence of side effects. The same applies to fluid volume. If body fluid decreases significantly because of a hot climate, strenuous exercise, vomiting, diarrhea, or drastic reduction in fluid intake, then lithium levels can rise sharply, causing an increase in side effects, progressing to lethal lithium toxicity. Persons from African descent may not therapeutically respond to lithium because they may develop toxic symptoms more rapidly than persons from other cultural groups due to their chemical sensitivity to salt and sodium pump irregular-

BOX 20.9

Drug Profile: Lithium (Eskalith)

DRUG CLASS: Mood stabilizer

RECEPTOR AFFINITY: Alters sodium transport in nerve and muscle cells, increases norepinephrine uptake and serotonin receptor sensitivity, slightly increases intraneuronal stores of catecholamines, delays some second messenger systems. Mechanism of action is unknown.

INDICATIONS: Treatment and prevention of manic episodes in bipolar affective disorder.

ROUTES AND DOSAGE: 150-, 300-, and 600-mg capsules. Lithobid, 300-mg slow-release tablets; Eskalith CR, 450-mg controlled-release tablets; Lithium citrate, 300-mg/5 mL liquid form.

Adult: In acute mania, optimal response is usually 600 mg tid or 900 mg bid. Obtain serum levels twice weekly in acute phase. Maintenance: Use lowest possible dose to alleviate symptoms and maintain serum level of 0.6–1.2 mEq/L. In uncomplicated maintenance obtain serum levels every 2–3 months. Do not rely on serum levels alone. Monitor patient side effects.

Geriatric: Increased risk for toxic effects, use lower doses, monitor frequently.

Children: Safety and efficacy in children younger than 12 y has not been established.

HALF-LIFE (PEAK EFFECT): mean, 24 h (peak serum levels in 1–4 h). Steady state reached in 5–7 d.

SELECT ADVERSE REACTIONS: Weight gain.

WARNING: Avoid use during pregnancy or while breastfeeding. Hepatic or renal impairments increase plasma concentration.

SPECIFIC PATIENT/FAMILY EDUCATION:

- Avoid alcohol or other CNS depressant drugs.
- Notify prescriber if pregnancy is possible or planned. Do not breast-feed while taking this medication.
- Notify prescriber before taking any other prescription, OTC medication, or herbal supplements.
- May impair judgment, thinking, or motor skills; avoid driving or other hazardous tasks.
- Do not abruptly discontinue use.

Table 20.7 Lithium Blood Levels and Associated Side Effects

Plasma Level	Side Effects or Symptoms of Toxicity
<1.5 mEq/L Mild side effects	Metallic taste in mouth Fine hand tremor (resting) Nausea Polyuria Polydipsia Diarrhea or loose stools Muscular weakness or fatigue Weight gain Edema Memory impairments
1.5–2.5 mEq/L Moderate toxicity	Severe diarrhea Dry mouth Nausea and vomiting Mild to moderate ataxia Incoordination Dizziness, sluggishness, giddiness, vertigo Slurred speech Tinnitus Blurred vision Increasing tremor Muscle irritability or twitching Asymmetric deep tendon reflexes Increased muscle tone
>2.5 mEq/L Severe toxicity	Cardiac arrhythmias Blackouts Nystagmus Coarse tremor Fasciculations Visual or tactile hallucinations Oliguria, renal failure Peripheral vascular collapse Confusion Seizures Coma and death

ities (Herrera, Lawson, & Sramek, 1999); anticonvulsant agents may be more appropriate. However, the key is to start the dose low and increase slowly in order to maximize the therapeutic response and avoid overshooting the therapeutic window. See Table 20.8 for lithium interactions with other drugs. See Chapter 8 for further discussion of lithium's possible mechanisms of action, pharmacokinetics, side effects, and toxicity.

Emergency! 

If symptoms of moderate or severe toxicity (e.g., cardiac arrhythmias, blackouts, tremors, seizures) are noted, withhold additional doses of lithium, immediately obtain a blood sample to analyze the lithium level, and push fluids if the patient can take fluids. Contact the physician for further direction about relieving the symptoms. Mild side effects tend to subside or can be managed by nursing measures (see Table 20.9).

Divalproex sodium

Divalproex sodium (Depakote), an anticonvulsant, has a broader spectrum of efficacy and has about equal benefit for patients with pure mania as for those with other forms of bipolar disorder (i.e., mixed mania, rapid cycling, comorbid substance abuse, and secondary mania). Moreover, in one large placebo-controlled study, patients taking divalproex sodium experienced a longer period of stable mood than did patients taking lithium or placebo (Bowden et al., 2000). Whereas divalproex is usually initiated at 250 mg twice a day or lower, in the inpatient setting, it can be initiated in an oral loading dose using 20 to 30 mg/kg body weight (see Box 20.10). This may speed the reduction of manic symptoms and diminish the need for antipsychotics

Table 20.8 Lithium Interactions With Medications and Other Substances

Substance	Effect of Interaction
Angiotensin-converting enzyme inhibitors, such as: • Captopril • Lisinopril • Quinapril	Increases serum lithium; may cause toxicity and impaired kidney function
Acetazolamide	Increases renal excretion of lithium, decreases lithium levels
Alcohol	May increase serum lithium level
Caffeine	Increases lithium excretion, increases lithium tremor
Carbamazepine	Increases neurotoxicity, despite normal serum levels and dosage
Fluoxetine	Increases serum lithium levels
Haloperidol	Increases neurotoxicity, despite normal serum levels and dosage
Loop diuretics, such as furosemide	Increases lithium serum levels, but may be safer than thiazide diuretics; potassium-sparing diuretics (amiloride, spirolac-tone) are safest
Methyldopa	Increases neurotoxicity without increasing serum lithium levels
Nonsteroidal antiinflammatory drugs, such as:	Decreases renal clearance of lithium
• Diclofenac	Increases serum lithium levels by 30%–60% in 3–10 d
• Ibuprofen	Aspirin and sulindac do not appear to have the same effect
• Indomethacin	
• Piroxicam	
Osmotic diuretics, such as: • Urea • Mannitol • Isosorbide	Increases renal excretion of lithium and decreases lithium levels
Sodium chloride	High sodium intake decreases lithium levels; low sodium diets may increase lithium levels and lead to toxicity
Thiazide diuretics, such as: • Chlorothiazide • Hydrochlorothiazide	Promotes sodium and potassium excretion; increases lithium serum levels; may produce cardiotoxicity and neurotoxicity
Tricyclic antidepressants	Increases tremor; potentiates pharmacologic effects of tricyclic antidepressants

early in the course of therapy (Hirschfeld, Baker, Wozniak, Tracy, & Sommerville, 2003). Baseline liver function tests and a complete blood count with platelets should be obtained before starting therapy, and patients with known liver disease should not be given divalproex sodium. There is a boxed warning for hepatotoxicity. Optimal blood levels appear to be in the range of 50 to 150 ng/mL. Levels may be obtained weekly until the patient is stable, and then every 6 months. Divalproex sodium is associated with increased risk for birth defects. Cases of life-threatening pancreatitis have been reported in adults and children receiving valproate, either initially or after several years of use. Some cases were described as hemorrhagic, with a rapid progression from onset to death. If pancreatitis is diagnosed, valproate use should be discontinued.

Carbamazepine

Carbamazepine, an anticonvulsant, also has mood-stabilizing effects. Data from various studies suggest that it may be effective in patients who experience no response to lithium. In addition, patients with secondary mania appear to be more responsive to carbamazepine than to lithium (Strakowski & Sax, 2000). Carbamazepine is metabolized by CYP3A4 and induces CYP1A2 and 3A4. The most common side effects of carbamazepine are dizziness, drowsiness, nausea, and vomiting, which may be avoided with slow incremental dosing. Carbamazepine has a boxed warning for aplastic anemia and agranulocytosis, but frequent clinically unimportant decreases in white blood cell counts occur. Estimates of the rate of severe blood dyscrasias vary from one in 10,000 patients treated to a more recent estimate of one in 125,000 (Schatzberg et al., 2003). Mild, nonprogressive elevations of liver function test results are relatively common. Carbamazepine is associated with increased risk for birth defects.

In patients older than 12 years, carbamazepine is begun at 200 mg once or twice a day. The dosage is increased by no more than 200 mg every 2 to 4 days, to 800 to 1,000 mg a day, or until therapeutic levels or effects are achieved. It is important to monitor for blood dyscrasias and liver damage. Liver function tests and complete blood counts with differential are minimal pretreatment laboratory tests and should be repeated about 1 month after initiating treatment, and at 3 months, 6 months, and yearly. Other yearly tests should include electrolytes, blood urea nitrogen, thy-

Table 20.9 Interventions for Lithium Side Effects

Side Effect	Intervention
Edema of feet or hands	Monitor intake and output, check for possible decreased urinary output. Monitor sodium intake. Patient should elevate legs when sitting or lying. Monitor weight.
Fine hand tremor	Provide support and reassurance, if it does not interfere with daily activities. Tremor worsens with anxiety and intentional movements; minimize stressors. Notify prescriber if it interferes with patient's work and compliance will be an issue. More frequent smaller doses of lithium may also help.
Mild diarrhea	Take lithium with meals. Provide for fluid replacement. Notify prescriber if becomes severe; may need a change in medication preparation or may be early sign of toxicity.
Muscle weakness, fatigue, or memory and concentration difficulties	Provide support and reassurance; this side effect will usually pass after a few weeks of treatment. Short-term memory aids such as lists or reminder calls may be helpful. Notify prescriber if becomes severe or interferes with the patient's desire to continue treatment.
Metallic taste	Suggest sugarless candies or throat lozenges. Encourage frequent oral hygiene.
Nausea or abdominal discomfort	Consider dividing the medication into smaller doses, or give it at more frequent intervals. Give medication with meals.
Polydipsia	Reassure patient that this is a normal mechanism to cope with polyuria.
Polyuria	Monitor intake and output. Provide reassurance and explain nature of side effect. Also explain that this causes no physical damage to kidneys.
Toxicity	Withhold medication. Notify prescriber. Use symptomatic treatments.

roid function tests, urinalysis, and eye examinations. Carbamazepine levels are measured monthly until the patient is on a stable dosage. Studies suggest that blood levels in the range of 8 to 12 ng/mL correspond to therapeutic efficacy. See Table 20.10 for carbamazepine's interactions with other drugs. See Chapter 8 for further discussion of carbamazepine's possible mechanisms of action, pharmacokinetics, side effects, and toxicity.

BOX 20.10

Drug Profile: Divalproex Sodium (Depakote)

Drug Class: Antimania agent

Receptor Affinity: Thought to increase level of inhibitory neurotransmitter, GABA, to brain neurons. Mechanism of action is unknown.

Indications: Mania, epilepsy, migraine.

Routes and Dosage: Available in 125-mg delayed-release capsules, and 125-, 250-, and 500-mg enteric-coated tablets.

Adult Dosage: Dosage depends on symptoms and clinical picture presented; initially, the dosage is low and gradually increased depending on the clinical presentation.

Half-Life (Peak Effect): 6–16 h (1–4 h)

Select Adverse Reactions: Sedation, tremor (may be dose related), nausea, vomiting, indigestion, abdominal cramps, anorexia with weight loss, slight elevations in liver enzymes, hepatic failure, thrombocytopenia, transient increases in hair loss.

Boxed Warning: Hepatotoxicity, teratogenicity, pancreatitis

Warning: Use cautiously during pregnancy and lactation. Contraindicated in patients with hepatic disease or significant hepatic dysfunction. Administer cautiously with salicylates; may increase serum levels and result in toxicity.

Specific Patient/Family Education:

- Take with food if gastrointestinal upset occurs.
- Swallow tablets or capsules whole to prevent local irritation of mouth and throat.
- Notify prescriber before taking any other prescription or OTC medications or herbal supplements.
- Avoid alcohol and sleep-inducing or OTC products.
- Avoid driving or performing activities that require alertness.
- Do not abruptly discontinue use.
- Keep appointments for follow-up, including blood tests to monitor response.

Table 20.10 Selected Medication Interactions With Carbamazepine

Interaction	Drug Interacting With Carbamazepine
Increased carbamazepine levels	Erythromycin Cimetidine Propoxyphene Isoniazid Calcium-channel blockers (Verapamil) Fluoxetine Danazol Diltiazem Nicotinamide
Decreased carbamazepine levels	Phenobarbital Primidone Phenytoin
Drugs whose levels are decreased by carbamazepine	Oral contraceptives Warfarin, oral anticoagulants Doxycycline Theophylline Haloperidol Divalproex sodium Tricyclic antidepressants Acetaminophen—increased metabolism, but also increased risk for hepatotoxicity

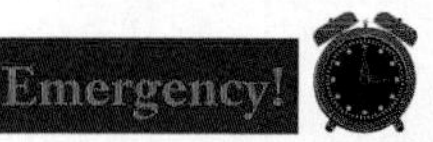

Both valproate and carbamazepine may be lethal if high doses are ingested. Toxic symptoms appear in 1 to 3 hours and include neuromuscular disturbances, dizziness, stupor, agitation, disorientation, nystagmus, urinary retention, nausea and vomiting, tachycardia, hypotension or hypertension, cardiovascular shock, coma, and respiratory depression.

Lamotrigine

Lamotrigine (Lamictal) is recently approved by the FDA for the maintenance treatment of bipolar disorder (www.FDA.gov). It may be particularly effective for rapid cycling and in the depressed phase of bipolar illness. If lamotrigine is given with valproic acid (Depakote), the dose should be reduced. Depakote decreases the clearance of lamotrigine. Lamotrigine does have a "boxed warning" for skin rash. Nurses should be especially vigilant for the appearance of any skin rash. If a rash does appear, it is most likely benign. However, it is not possible to predict whether the rash is benign or serious (Stevens-Johnson syndrome).

Other Anticonvulsants

In small clinical trials, case reports, and anecdotal evidence, newer anticonvulsants also show promise as mood stabilizers. Initial evidence suggests that gabapentin (Neurontin) may be effective for acute mania, mood stabilization, and rapid cycling. Topiramate (Topamax) has been used mostly as add-on therapy in mixed patient samples with refractory mood disorders. A characteristic of topiramate is that it is more associated with weight loss than weight gain. Controlled trials are needed to evaluate further the efficacy of these and other anticonvulsants (Schatzberg et al., 2003).

Intervention With Antidepressants

Acute bipolar depression has received little scientific study in comparison with unipolar depression. Antidepressant drugs may cause either a switch to mania or a mixed state or may induce rapid cycling. Unfortunately, lithium or anticonvulsants are not as effective against depression as they are against mania. However, in a few patients, lithium or anticonvulsants can be used alone with good antidepressant effects. The most common treatment of bipolar depression is an antidepressant combined with a mood stabilizer to "protect" the patient against a manic switch. The antidepressant agents are the same as those used in unipolar illness, although they are sometimes given in lower dosages and for shorter periods of time as a precaution.

Intervention With Antipsychotics

Antipsychotics are prescribed for patients who experience psychosis as a part of bipolar disorder. If patients cannot tolerate mood stabilizers, antipsychotics may be given, instead of antidepressants, to stabilize the moods. Generally, the antipsychotic dosage is lower than what is prescribed for patients with schizophrenia.

Administering and Monitoring Medication

During acute mania, patients may not believe that they have a psychiatric disorder and refuse to take medication. Because their energy is still high, they can be very creative in avoiding medication. Once patients begin to take medications, symptom improvement should be evident. If a patient is very agitated, a benzodiazepine may be given for a short period.

Monitoring and Managing Side Effects

It is unlikely that patients will take only one medication; they may receive several. In some instances, one agent will be used to augment the effects of another, such as supplemental thyroid hormone to boost antidepressant response in depression. Possible side effects for each medication should be listed and cross-referenced. When a side effect appears, the nurse should document the side effect and notify the prescriber so that further evaluation can be made. In some instances, medications should be changed.

Monitoring for Drug Interactions

It is a well-established practice to combine mood stabilizers with antidepressants or antipsychotics. The previously discussed drug interactions should be considered when caring for a person with bipolar disorder. A big challenge is monitoring alcohol, drugs, over-the-counter medications, and herbal supplements. A complete list of all medications should be maintained and evaluated for any potential interaction (see Table 20.4 for specific drug interactions).

Teaching Points 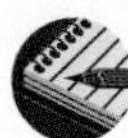

For patients who are taking lithium, it is important to explain that a change in salt intake can affect the therapeutic blood level. If there is a reduction in salt intake, the body will naturally retain lithium to maintain homeostasis. This increase in lithium retention can lead to toxicity. Once stabilized on a lithium dose, salt intake should remain constant. This is fairly easy to do, except during the summer, when excessive perspiration can occur. Patients should increase salt intake during periods of perspiration, increased exercise, and dehydration. Most mood stabilizers and antidepressants can cause weight gain. Patients should be alerted to this potential side effect and should be instructed to monitor any changes in eating, appetite, or weight. Weight reduction techniques may need to be instituted. Patients also should be clearly instructed to check with the nurse or physician before taking any over-the-counter medication, herbal supplements, or any other complementary and alternative treatment approaches (Leininger & McFarland, 2006; Spector, 2004).

Other Somatic Interventions: Electroconvulsive Therapy

ECT may be a treatment alternative for patients with severe mania who exhibit unremitting, frenzied physical activity. Other indications for ECT are acute mania that is unresponsive to antimanic agents or high suicide risk. ECT is safe and effective in patients receiving antipsychotic drugs. Use of valproate or carbamazepine will elevate the seizure threshold, requiring some adjustments in treatment.

Psychological Domain

Assessment

The assessment of the psychological domain should follow the process explained in Chapter 10. Individuals with bipolar disorder can usually participate fully in this part of the assessment.

Mood

By definition, bipolar disorder is a disturbance of mood. If the patient is depressed, using an assessment tool for depression may help determine the severity of depression. If mania predominates, evaluating the quality of the mood (elated, grandiose, irritated, or agitated) becomes important. Usually, mania is determined by clinical observation.

Cognition

In a depressive episode, the individual may not be able to concentrate enough to complete cognitive tasks, such as those called for in the Mini Mental State Exam (MMSE). During the acute phase of a manic or depressive episode, mental status may be abnormal, and in a manic phase, judgment is impaired by extremely rapid, disjointed, and distorted thinking. Moreover, feelings such as grandiosity can interfere with normal executive functioning.

Thought Disturbances

Psychosis commonly occurs in patients with bipolar disorder, especially during acute episodes of mania. Auditory hallucinations and delusional thinking are part of the clinical picture. In children and adolescents, psychosis is not so easily disclosed.

Stress and Coping Factors

Stress and coping are critical assessment areas for a person with bipolar disorder. A stressful event often triggers a manic or depressive episode. In some instances, there are no particular stresses that preceded the episode, but it is important to discuss the possibility. Determining the patient's usual coping skills for stresses lays the groundwork for developing interventional strategies. Negative coping skills, such as substance use or aggression, should be identified because these skills need to be replaced with positive coping skills.

Risk Assessment

Patients with bipolar disorder are at high risk for injury to self and others, with 10% to 15% of patients completing suicide. Child abuse, spouse abuse, or other violent behaviors may occur during severe manic episodes; thus, patients should be assessed for suicidal or homicidal risk (APA, 2000). The risk of relapse and poorer treatment outcomes are associated with obesity. Preventing and treating obesity in patients with bipolar disorder could decrease the morbidity and mortality related to physical illness, enhance psychological well-being, and possibly improve the course of the disorder (Fagiolini, Kupfer, Houck, Novick, & Frank, 2003).

Nursing Diagnoses for the Psychological Domain

Nursing diagnoses associated with the psychological domain of bipolar disorder include Disturbed Sensory

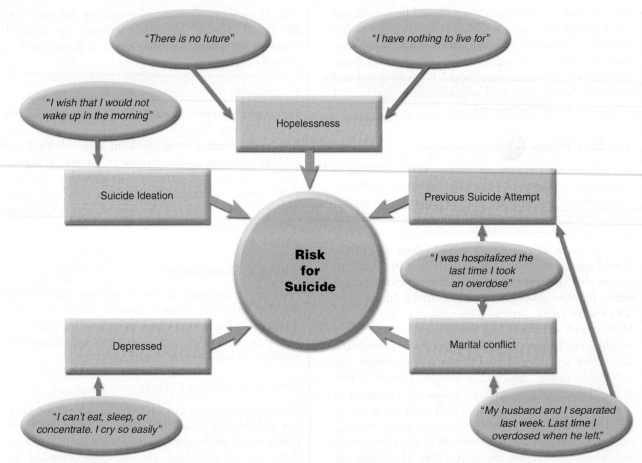

FIGURE 20.2. Nursing diagnosis concept map: risk for Suicide.

Perception; Disturbed Thought Processes; Defensive Coping; Risk for Suicide; Risk for Violence; and Ineffective Coping (see Figure 20.2).

Interventions for the Psychological Domain

Pharmacotherapy is the primary treatment for bipolar disorder but is often unsuccessful unless adjunctive psychosocial interventions are included in the treatment plan. Integration of psychotherapeutic techniques with pharmacotherapy is strongly recommended by clinicians *and* patients (Thase & Sachs, 2000). The most common psychotherapeutic approaches include psychoeducation, individual cognitive-behavioral therapy, individual interpersonal therapy, and adjunctive therapies, such as those for substance use (Rothbaum & Astin, 2000).

Several risk factors associated with bipolar disorders make patients more vulnerable to relapses and resistant to recovery. Among these are high rates of nonadherence to medication therapy, obesity, marital conflict, separation, divorce, unemployment, and underemployment. The goals of psychosocial interventions are to address risk factors and associated features that are difficult to address with pharmacotherapy alone. Particularly important are improving medication adherence, decreasing the number and length of hospitalizations and relapses, enhancing social and occupational functioning, improving quality of life, increasing the patient and family's acceptance of the disorder, and reducing the suicide risk (Rothbaum & Astin, 2000).

Psychoeducation 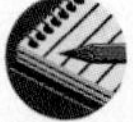

Psychoeducation is designed to provide information on bipolar disorder and successful treatment and recovery and usually focuses on medication adherence. The nurse can provide information about the illness and obstacles to recovery. Helping the patient to recognize warning signs and symptoms of relapse and to cope with residual symptoms and functional impairment are important interventions. Resistance to accepting the illness and to taking medication, the symbolic meaning of medication taking, and worries about the future can be discussed openly. In the interest of improved medication adherence, listening carefully to the patient's concerns about the medication, dosing schedules and dose changes, and side effects are helpful

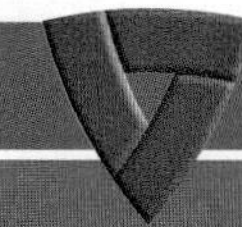

Nursing Care Plan 20.1

The Patient With Bipolar Disorder

JR, a 43-year-old, single woman, lives in a metropolitan city and works for a large travel agency booking corporate business trips. She has a history of alcohol abuse that began when she was in high school. Initially, she relied on alcohol for stress reduction but gradually began abusing it. Her mother, grandfather, and sister all committed suicide within the past several years. JR's father has remarried and moved out of the area. JR has one brother whom she sees occasionally.

Three years ago, JR left her husband after 15 years of an unhappy marriage and moved into a small condominium in a less affluent neighborhood. She began having symptoms of bipolar mixed disorder at that time, when she sold all her clothes, bleached her hair blonde, and began cruising the bars. She would consume excessive amounts of alcohol and often end up spending the night with a stranger. At first her behavior was attributed to her recent divorce. When she began missing work and charging excessively on her credit cards, her friends and two children became concerned and convinced her to seek help for her behavior.

JR received a diagnosis of manic episode, and treatment with lithium carbonate was initiated. Her mood stabilized briefly, but she had two more manic episodes within the next 18 months. Shortly after her last manic episode, she became severely depressed and attempted suicide. TCAs and MAOIs were tried, but she discontinued taking them after a significant weight gain. Once her depression lifted, her mood was stable for several months.

About 2 months ago, JR began missing work again because of depression. She refused to take any antidepressants and just wanted to "wait it out." She often boasted that her one success in life was helping people travel and have a good time. Last week she was told that her position was being eliminated because of a company issue. Now she believes that she is a failure as a wife, as an employee, and as a woman. She became despondent and finally took an overdose to "end it all."

Setting: Intensive Care Psychiatric Unit In A General Hospital

Baseline Assessment: JR is a 43-year-old single woman transferred from ICU after a 3-day hospitalization following a suicide attempt with an overdose of multiple prescriptions and alcohol. She had her first manic episode 3 years before, and subsequently has had symptoms of a mixed bipolar mood disorder most of the time. Medication with lithium carbonate has not protected her from mood swings, and prior trials of TCAs and MAOIs have been unsuccessful. She is currently depressed, with pressured speech, agitation, irritability, sensory overload, inability to sleep, and anorexia.

Associated Psychiatric Diagnosis

Axis I: Bipolar I disorder, most recent episode mixed, severe, without psychotic features
Axis II: Deferred (none apparent in her history and she is currently too ill for personality disorder to be assessed)
Axis III: Hypothyroidism
Axis IV: Social problems (very poor marriage of 15 years, death by suicide of mother, grandfather, one sister)
Axis V: GAF = Current 50
Potential 85

Medications

Lithium carbonate 300 mg tid × 2 years
L-thyroxine 0.1 mg q AM × 1 d
Clonazepam 0.5 mg bid for sleep and agitation
Carbamazepine added on transfer to be titrated up to 400 mg tid

Nursing Diagnosis 1: Risk Suicide

Defining Characteristics

Attempts to inflict life-threatening injury to self
Expresses desire to die
Poor impulse control
Lack of support system

Related Factors

Feelings of helplessness and hopelessness secondary to bipolar disorder
Depression
Loss secondary to finances/job, divorce

Outcomes

Initial

1. Develop a no self-harm contract.
2. Remain free from self-harm.
3. Identify factors that led to suicidal intent and methods for managing suicidal impulses if they return.
4. Accept treatment of depression by trying the SSRI antidepressants.

Discharge

5. Discuss the complexity of bipolar disorder.
6. Identify the antecedents to depression.

Continued

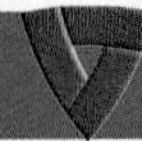

Nursing Care Plan 20.1 *(Continued)*

Interventions

Interventions	Rationale	Ongoing Assessment
Initiate a nurse–patient relationship by demonstrating an acceptance of JR as a worthwhile human being through the use of nonjudgmental statements and behavior.	A sense of worthlessness often underlies suicide ideation. The positive therapeutic relationship can maintain the patient's dignity.	Assess the stages of the relationship and determine whether a therapeutic relationship is actually being formed. Identify indicators of trust.
Initiate suicide precautions per hospital policy.	Safety of the individual is a priority with people who have suicide ideation (see Chapter 36).	Determine intent to harm self—plan and means.
Obtain a no self-harm contract.	A contract can help the patient resist suicide by providing a way of resisting impulses.	Determine patient's ability to commit to a contract.

Evaluation

Outcomes	Revised Outcomes	Interventions
Has not harmed self, denies suicidal thought/intent after realizing that she is still alive.	Absence of suicidal intent will continue.	Discontinue suicide precautions; maintain ongoing assessment for suicidality.
Made a no self-harm contract with nurse, agrees to keep it after discharge.	Maintain a no self-harm contract with outpatient mental health provider.	Support and reinforce this contract.
JR agreed to try to treat her depression by initiating treatment with Prozac.		

Nursing Diagnosis 2: Chronic Low Self-Esteem

Defining Characteristics	Related Factors
Long-standing self-negating verbalizations	Failure to stabilize mood
Expressions of shame and guilt	Unmet dependency needs
Evaluates self as unable to deal with events	Feelings of abandonment secondary to separation from significant other
Frequent lack of success in work and relationships	Feelings of failure secondary to loss of job, relationship problems
Poor body presentation (eye contact, posture, movements)	Unrealistic expectations of self
Nonassertive/passive	

Outcomes

Initial	Discharge
1. Identify positive aspects of self.	3. Verbalize acceptance of personal limitations.
2. Modify excessive and unrealistic expectations of self.	4. Report freedom from most symptoms of depression.
	5. Begin to take verbal and behavioral risks.

Interventions

Interventions	Rationale	Ongoing Assessment
Enhance JR's sense of self by being attentive, validating your interpretation of what is being said or experienced, and helping her verbalize what she is expressing nonverbally.	By showing respect for the patient as a human being who is worth listening to, the nurse can support and help build the patient's sense of self.	Determine whether patient confirms interpretation of situation and if she can verbalize what she is expressing nonverbally.
Assist to reframe and redefine negative statements ("not a failure, but a setback").	Reframing an event positively rather than negatively can help the patient view the situation in an alternative way.	Assess whether the patient can actually view the world in a different way.
Problem solve with patient about how to approach finding another job.	Work is very important to adults. Losing a job can decrease self-esteem. Focusing on the possibility of a future job will provide hope for the patient.	Assess the patient's ability to problem solve. Determine whether she is realistic in her expectations.

Continued

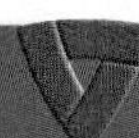

Nursing Care Plan 20.1 *(Continued)*

Interventions

Interventions	Rationale	Ongoing Assessment
Encourage positive physical habits (healthy food and eating patterns, exercise, proper sleep).	A healthy lifestyle promotes well-being, increasing self-esteem.	Determine JR's willingness to consider making lifestyle changes.
Teach patient to validate consensually with others.	Low self-esteem is generated by negative interpretations of the world. Through consensual validation, the patient can determine whether others view situations in the same way.	Assess JR's ability to participate in this process.
Teach esteem-building exercises (self-affirmations, imagery, use of humor, meditation/prayer, relaxation).	There are many different approaches that can be practiced to increase self-esteem.	Assess JR's energy level and ability to focus on learning new skills.
Assist in establishing appropriate personal boundaries.	In an attempt to meet their own needs, people with low self-esteem often violate other people's boundaries and allow others to take advantage of them. Helping patients establish their own boundaries will improve the likelihood of needs being met in an appropriate manner.	Assess JR's ability to understand the concept of boundary violation and its significance.
Provide an opportunity within the therapeutic relationship to express thoughts and feelings. Use open-ended statements and questions. Encourage expression of both positive and negative statements. Use movement, art, and music as means of expression.	The individual with low self-esteem may have difficulty expressing thoughts and feelings. Providing them with several different outlets for expression helps to develop skills for expressing thoughts and feelings.	Monitor thoughts and feelings that are expressed in order to help the patient examine them.
Explore opportunities for positive socialization.	Individuals with low self-esteem may be in social situations that reinforce negative valuation of self. Helping patient identify new positive situations will give other options.	Assess whether the new situations are potentially positive or are a re-creation of other negative situations.
JR began to identify positive aspects of self as she began to modify excessive and unrealistic expectations of self.	Strengthen ability to affirm positive aspects and examine expectations related to work and relationships.	Refer to mental health clinic for cognitive-behavioral psychotherapy with a feminist perspective.
She verbalized that she would probably never work for the company again and that it would never be the same. She verbalized that she would need more assertiveness skills in her relationships.	Identify important aspects of job so that she can begin looking for a job that had those characteristics.	Attend a women's group that focuses on assertiveness skills.
As JR's mood improved, she was able to sleep through the night, and she began eating again—began feeling better about herself.	Maintain a stable mood to promote positive self-concept.	Monitor mood and identify antecedents to depression.

Nursing Diagnosis 3: Ineffective Individual Coping

Defining Characteristics	Related Factors
Verbalization in inability to cope or ask for help	Altered mood (depression) caused by changes secondary to body chemistry (bipolar disorder)
Reported difficulty with life stressors	Altered mood caused by changes secondary to intake of mood-altering substance (alcohol)
Inability to problem solve	Unsatisfactory support system
Alteration in social participation	Sensory overload secondary to excessive activity
Destructive behavior toward self	Inadequate psychological resources to adapt to changes in job status
Frequent illnesses	
Substance abuse	

Continued

Nursing Care Plan 20.1 (Continued)

Outcomes

Initial	Discharge
1. Accept support through the nurse–patient relationship. 2. Identify areas of ineffective coping. 3. Examine the current efforts at coping. 4. Identify areas of strength. 5. Learn new coping skills.	6. Practice new coping skills. 7. Focus on strengths.

Interventions

Interventions	Rationale	Ongoing Assessment
Identify current stresses in JR's life, including her suicide attempt and the bipolar disorder.	When areas of concern are verbalized by the patient, she will be able to focus on one issue at a time. If she identifies the mental disorder as a stressor, she will more likely be able to develop strategies to deal with it.	Determine whether JR is able to identify problem areas realistically. Continue to assess for suicidality.
Identify JR's strengths in dealing with past stressors.	By focusing on past successes, she can identify strengths and build on them in the future.	Assess if JR can identify any previous successes in her life.
Assess current level of depression using Beck's Depression Inventory or a similar one and intervene according to assessed level.	Severely depressed or suicidal individuals need assistance with decision making, grooming and hygiene, and nutrition.	Continue to assess for mood and suicidality.
Assist JR in discussing, selecting, and practicing positive coping skills (jogging, yoga, thought stopping).	New coping skills take a conscious effort to learn and will at first seem strange and unnatural. Practicing these skills will help the patient incorporate them into her coping strategy repertoire.	Assess whether JR follows through on learning new skills.
Educate regarding the use of alcohol and its relationship to depression.	Alcohol is an ineffective coping strategy because it actually exacerbates the depression.	Assess for the patient's willingness to address her drinking problem.
Assist patient in coping with bipolar disorder, beginning with education about it.	A mood disorder is a major stressor in a patient's life. To manage the stress, the patient needs a knowledge base.	Determine JR's knowledge about bipolar disorder.
Administer lithium as ordered (give with food or milk). Reinforce the action, dosage, and side effects. Review laboratory results to determine whether lithium is within therapeutic limits. Assess for toxicity. Recommend a normal diet with normal salt intake; maintenance of adequate fluid intake.	Lithium carbonate is effective in the treatment of bipolar disorder but must be managed. Patient should have a thorough knowledge of the medication and side effects.	Assess for target action, side effects, and toxicity.
Administer carbamazepine as ordered, to be titrated up to 400 mg tid. Observe for presence of hypersensitivity to the drug. Teach about action, dosage, and side effects. Emphasize the possibility of drug interaction with alcohol, some antibiotics, TCAs, and MAOIs.	Carbamazepine can be effective in bipolar disorder. However, it can increase CNS toxicity when given with lithium carbonate.	Assess for target action, side effects, and toxicity.
Administer thyroid supplement as ordered. Review laboratory results of thyroid functioning. Discuss the symptoms of hypothyroidism and how they are similar to depression. Emphasize the importance of taking lithium and L-thyroxine. Explain about the long-term effects of lithium on thyroid functioning.	Hypothyroidism can be a side effect of lithium carbonate and also mimics symptoms of depression.	Determine whether patient understands the relationship between thyroid dysfunction and lithium carbonate.

Continued

Nursing Care Plan 20.1 (Continued)

Evaluation

Outcomes	Revised Outcomes	Interventions
Clonazepam 0.5 mg bid for sleep and agitation.		
JR easily engaged in a therapeutic relationship. She examined the areas in her life where she coped ineffectively.	Establish a therapeutic relationship with a therapist at the mental health clinic.	Refer to mental health clinic.
She identified her strengths and how she coped with stressors and especially her illness in the past. She is willing to try antidepressants again, in hopes of not having the weight gain.	Continue to view illness as a potential stressor that can disrupt life.	Seek advice immediately if there are any problems with medications.
She learned new problem-solving skills and reported that she learned a lot about her medication. She is committed to complying with her medication regimen. She identified new coping skills that she could realistically do. She will focus on strengths.	Continue to practice new coping skills as stressful situations arise.	Discuss with therapist the outcomes of using new coping skills. Attend Alcoholics Anonymous if alcohol is used as a stress reliever.

(see Box 20.11). Health teaching and weight management should be a component of any psychoeducation program. In addition to individual variations in body weight, many of the medications (divalproex sodium, lithium, antidepressants, olanzapine) are associated with weight gain. Monitoring weight and developing individual weight management plans can reduce the risk of relapse and increase the possibility of medication adherence.

Psychotherapy

Long-term psychotherapy may help prevent both mania and depression by reducing the stresses that trigger episodes and increasing the patient's acceptance of the need for medication. Patients should be encouraged to keep their appointments with the therapist, be honest and open, do the assigned homework, and give the therapist feedback on how the treatment is working (Kahn, Ross, Printz, & Sachs, 2000).

BOX 20.11

Psychoeducation Checklist: Bipolar I Disorder

When caring for the patient with a bipolar I disorder, be sure to include the following topic areas in the teaching plan:

- Psychopharmacologic agents, including drug action, dosage, frequency, and possible adverse effects
- Medication regimen adherence
- Strategies to decrease agitation and restlessness
- Safety measures
- Self-care management
- Follow-up laboratory testing
- Support services

Social Domain

Assessment

One of the tragedies of bipolar disorder is its effect on social and occupational functioning. Cultural views of mental illness influence the patient's acceptance of the disorder. During illness episodes, patients often behave in ways that jeopardize their social relationships. Losing a job and going through a divorce are common events. When performing an assessment of social function, the nurse should identify changes resulting from a manic or depressive episode.

Nursing Diagnoses for the Social Domain

Nursing diagnoses for adults can include Ineffective Role Performance; Interrupted Family Processes; Impaired Social Interaction; Impaired Parenting; and Compromised Family Coping. The diagnoses for children and adolescents can include Delayed Growth and Development and Caregiver Role Strain in family coping with a member with a bipolar disorder.

Interventions for the Social Domain

Interventions focusing on the social domain are integral to nursing care for all ages. During mania, patients usually violate others' boundaries. Roommate selection for patients requiring hospital admittance needs to be carefully considered. If possible, a private room is ideal because patients with bipolar disorder tend to irritate others, who quickly tire of the intrusiveness. These patients may miss the cues indicating anger and aggression from others. The nurse should protect the manic patient from self-harm, as well as harm from other patients.

Support groups are helpful for people with this disorder. Participating in groups allows the person to meet others with the same disorder and learn management and preventive strategies. Support groups also are helpful in dealing with the stigma associated with mental illnesses.

Family Interventions 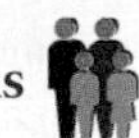

Marital and family interventions are often needed at different periods in the life of a person with bipolar disorder. For the family with a child with this disorder, additional parenting skills are needed to manage the behaviors. The goals of family interventions are to help the family understand and cope with the disorder. Interventions may range from occasional counseling sessions to intensive family therapy.

Family psychoeducation strategies have been shown to be particularly useful in decreasing the risk of relapse and hospitalization. In a study of 53 patients with mania, half were assigned to a 9-month family-focused psychoeducational group and half to individually focused treatment. Those in family-focused treatment were less likely to be rehospitalized (Rea et al., 2003). For more information see Box 20.12.

Evaluation and Treatment Outcomes

Desired treatment outcomes are stabilization of mood and enhanced quality of life. Primary tools for evaluating outcomes are nursing observation and patient self-report (see Nursing Care Plan 20.1 and Interdisciplinary Treatment Plan 20.1).

Continuum of Care

Inpatient Management

Inpatient admission is the treatment setting of choice for patients who are severely psychotic or who are an immediate threat to themselves or others. In acute mania, nursing interventions focus on patient safety because patients are prone to injury due to hyperactivity and often are unaware of injuries they sustain. Distraction may also be effective when a patient is talking or acting inappropriately. Removal to a quieter environment may be necessary if other interventions have not been successful, but the patient should be carefully monitored. Because during acute mania, patients are often impulsive, disinhibited, and interpersonally inappropriate, the nurse should avoid direct confrontations or challenges.

Medication management (Fig. 20.3), including control of side effects and promotion of self-care, are major nursing responsibilities during inpatient hospitalization. Nurses should be familiar with drug–drug interactions (Table 20.4) and with interventions to help control side effects.

Intensive Outpatient Programs

Intensive outpatient programs for several weeks of acute-phase care during a manic or depressive episode are used when hospitalization is not necessary or to prevent or shorten hospitalization. These programs are usually called *partial hospitalization* or *day hospitalization.* Close medication monitoring and milieu therapies that foster restoration of a patient's previous adaptive abilities are the major nursing responsibilities in these settings.

Setting up frequent office visits and crisis telephone calls are additional nursing interventions that can help to shorten or prevent hospitalization during the acute phase of a manic episode. Family sessions or psychoeducation that includes the patient are alternatives. Severely and persistently ill patients may need ongoing intensive treatment, but the frequency of visits can be decreased for patients whose conditions stabilize and who enter the continuation or the maintenance phase of treatment.

BOX 20.12

Research for Best Practice: Help for Families Affected by Bipolar Disorder

Rea, M. M., Tompson, M. C., Miklowitz, D. J., Goldstein, M. J., Hwang, S., & Mintz, J. (2003). Family-focused treatment versus individual treatment for bipolar disorder: results of a randomized clinical trial. Journal of Consulting Clinical Psychology, 71(3), 482–492.

The Question: Is family-focused treatment as effective or more or less effective than individual treatment for bipolar disorder?

Methods: A qualitative study of families' responses to severe mental illness involved 29 participants representing 17 families who were interviewed three times in 2 years. Interviews were analyzed using a comparative technique that described families' responses to these mental illnesses. Living with ambiguity of mental illness was the central concern.

Findings: These families attempted to live normally and sought to control the impact of the illness. The family goals included managing crises, containing and controlling symptoms, and crafting a notion of "normal." The strategies that the families used were being vigilant, setting limits on patients, invoking logic, dealing with sense of loss, seeing patients' strengths, and taking on roles. This study revealed that families were profoundly affected by the social contexts of mental illness.

Implications for Nursing: Families are the informal caregivers and develop their own strategies for dealing with family members with mental illnesses. Including families in psychoeducation programs can facilitate a partnership with the family and allow sharing of successful strategies.

INTERDISCIPLINARY TREATMENT PLAN 20.1

Patient With Bipolar Disorder Community Mental Health Center Treatment Program for JR, a 43-year-old Female

Admission Date:	*Date of This Plan:*	*Type of Plan: Check Appropriate Box*
		☐ Initial ☐ Master ☐ 30 ☐ 60 ☐ 90 ☐ Other

Treatment Team Present:
M. Jones, MD; S. Smith, RNC; T. Thompson, PhD (psychologist); G. Bond, LCSW (social worker); V. Stevens, BA (rehabilitation counselor)

DIAGNOSIS (DSM-IV-TR):

AXIS I: Bipolar I
AXIS II: Deferred
AXIS III: Hypothyroidism
AXIS IV: Social Problems
AXIS V:
Current GAF: 50
Highest Level GAF This Past Year: 85

ASSETS (MEDICAL, PSYCHOLOGICAL, SOCIAL, EDUCATIONAL, VOCATIONAL, RECREATIONAL):

1. Controls illness through medication and monthly visits for brief counseling and stress management.
2. Lives independently in apartment.
3. Works at a library and has good relationships with boss and coworkers.
4. Easily makes friends.

MASTER PROBLEM LIST

				Change	
Prob No.	*Date*	*Problem*	*Code*	*Code*	*Date*
1	1/12/08	Ineffective coping: Does not want to go to work because of intense grief for mother's death.		R	2/12/08
2	1/12/08	Mood disturbance. Patient is very depressed, not eating or sleeping.		R	4/14/08
3	6/12/08	Mood changes with the seasons. Needs monitoring of mood.		T	
4	6/12/08	Interpersonal issues interfering with ability to work at library.		T	

CODE T = Problem must be addressed in treatment.
N = Problem noted and will be monitored.
X = Problem noted, but deferred/inactive/no action necessary.
O = Problem to be addressed in aftercare/continuing care.
I = Problem incorporated into another problem.
R = Resolved.

INDIVIDUAL TREATMENT PLAN PROBLEM SHEET

#1 Problem/Need:	*Date Identified*	*Problem Resolved/Discontinuation Date*
	1/12/08	Ongoing

Cyclic mood changes, usually according to the season. Medication needs to be re-evaluated and adjusted according to mood changes. Stress is often the precipitant to mood changes. Needs updating on information about bipolar disorder.

(Continued on following page)

INTERDISCIPLINARY TREATMENT PLAN 20.1 (Continued)

Patient With Bipolar Disorder Community Mental Health Center Treatment Program for JR, a 43-year-old Female

Objective(s)/Short-Term Goals:	*Target Date*	*Achievement Date*
1. Monitor mood changes. 2. Adjust medications as needed.	Every 3 months	
Treatment Interventions:	*Frequency*	*Person Responsible*
1. Evaluate mood changes.	Every 3 months or as needed.	RN
2. Adjust medications.	Every 3 months or as needed.	MD
3. Medication education.	Weekly class.	RN
4. Stress management techniques.	Weekly class for 6 weeks.	Psychologist
Responsible QMHP	*Patient or Guardian*	*Staff Physician*
Signature Date	Signature Date	Signature Date

Spectrum of Care

In today's health care climate, with efforts to reduce hospitalization, most patients with bipolar disorder are treated as outpatients. Hospitalizations are usually brief, and treatment focuses on restabilization. Patients with mood disorders are likely to need long-term medication regimens and supportive psychotherapy to function in the community. Therefore, medication regimens and additional treatment planning need to be tailored to individual needs. Patients need extended and continued follow-up to monitor medication trials and side effects, reinforce self-care management, and provide continued psychosocial support.

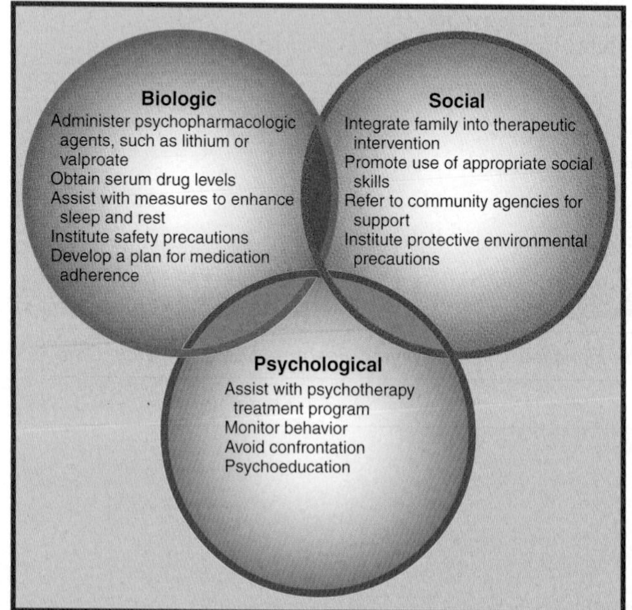

FIGURE 20.3. Biopsychosocial interventions for patients with bipolar I disorder.

Mental Health Promotion

Mental health promotion activities should be the focus during remissions. During this period, patients have an opportunity to learn new coping skills that promote positive mental health. Stress management and relaxation techniques can be practiced for use when needed. A plan for managing emerging symptoms can also be developed during this period.

SUMMARY OF KEY POINTS

- Mood disorders are characterized by persistent or recurring disturbances in mood that cause significant psychological distress and functional impairment. Moods can be broadly categorized as manic or dysphoric (typified by exaggerated feelings of elation or irritability) or depressive or dysthymic (typified by feelings of sadness, hopelessness, loss of interest, and fatigue).
- Primary mood disorders include both depressive disorders (unipolar depression) and manic-depressive disorders (bipolar disorders).
- Genetics undoubtedly plays a role in the etiology of mood disorders. Risk factors include family history of mood disorders, prior mood episodes, lack of social support, stressful life events, substance use, and medical problems, particularly chronic or terminal illnesses.

■ The recommended depression treatment guidelines include antidepressant medication, alone or with psychotherapeutic management or psychotherapy; electroconvulsive therapy for severe depression; or light therapy (phototherapy) for patients with seasonal depressive symptoms.

■ Nurses must be knowledgeable regarding culturally competent strategies related to the use of antidepressant medications, pharmacologic therapeutic effects and associated side effects, toxicity, dosage ranges, and contraindications. Nurses must also be familiar with electroconvulsive therapy protocols and associated interventions. Patient education and the provision of emotional support during the course of treatment are also nursing responsibilities.

■ Many symptoms of depression, such as weight and appetite changes, sleep disturbance, decreased energy, and fatigue, are similar to those of medical illnesses. Assessment includes a thorough medical history and physical examination to detect or rule out medical or psychiatric comorbidity.

■ Biopsychosocial assessment includes assessing mood, speech patterns, thought processes and thought content, suicidal or homicidal thoughts, cognition and memory, and social factors, such as patterns of relationships, quality of support systems, and changes in occupational functioning. Several self-report scales are helpful in evaluating depressive symptoms.

■ Establishing and maintaining a therapeutic nurse–patient relationship is key to successful outcomes. Nursing interventions that foster the therapeutic relationship include being available in times of crisis; providing understanding and education to patients and their families regarding goals of treatment; providing encouragement and feedback concerning the patient's progress; providing guidance in the patient's interpersonal interactions with others and work environment; and helping to set and monitor realistic goals.

■ Psychosocial interventions for mood disorders include self-care management, cognitive therapy, behavior therapy, interpersonal therapy, patient and family education regarding the nature of the disorder and treatment goals, marital and family therapy, and group therapy that includes medication maintenance support groups and other consumer-oriented support groups.

■ Bipolar disorders are characterized by one or more manic episodes or mixed mania (co-occurrence of manic and depressive states) that cause marked impairment in social activities, occupational functioning, and interpersonal relationships and may require hospitalization to prevent self-harm.

■ Manic episodes are periods in which the individual experiences abnormally and persistently elevated, expansive, or irritable mood characterized by inflated self-esteem, decreased need to sleep, excessive energy or hyperactivity, racing thoughts, easy distractibility, and inability to stay focused. Other symptoms can include hypersexuality and impulsivity.

■ Similar to treatment of major depressive disorder, pharmacotherapy is the cornerstone of treatment of bipolar illness, but adjunctive psychosocial interventions are needed as well. Pharmacologic therapy includes treatment with mood stabilizers alone or in combination with antipsychotics or benzodiazepines if psychosis, agitation, or insomnia are present and antidepressants for unremitted depression. Electroconvulsive therapy is a valuable alternative for patients with severe mania that does not respond to other treatment.

■ Recent major advances in bipolar disorder treatment research validate the efficacy of integrated psychosocial and pharmacologic treatment involving family or couples therapies, psychoeducational programs, and individual cognitive-behavioral or interpersonal therapies.

CRITICAL THINKING CHALLENGES

1 Describe how you would do a suicide assessment on a patient in a physician's office who comes in distraught and expressing concerns about her ability to cope with her current situation.

2 Describe how you would approach the patient described in the previous thinking challenge if you determined that she was suicidal.

3 Discuss difficulties in the differential diagnosis of bipolar disorder in the manic phase and other medical and/or psychiatric disorders. List the information you would use to rule out the other diagnosis when dealing with a patient who appears to have mania.

4 Describe how you would approach a patient who is expressing concern that the diagnosis of bipolar disorder will negatively affect his/her social and work relationships.

5 Your depressed patient does not seem inclined to talk about his/her depression. Describe the measures you would take to initiate a therapeutic relationship with him/her.

6 Your patient with mania is experiencing physical hyperactivity that is interfering with his/her sleep and nutrition. Describe the actions you would take to meet the patient's needs for nutrition and rest.

7 Prepare a hypothetical discussion with a patient with potential bipolar disorder concerning the advantages/disadvantages of lithium versus divalproex sodium for treatment of bipolar disorder.

8 Prepare a hypothetical discussion with a depressed patient with potential unipolar disorder concerning the advantages and disadvantages of each of the major classifications of antidepressants.
9 Think about all of the above situations and relate them to persons from culturally and ethnically diverse populations (e.g., African, Latino, or Asian descent; Jewish or Jehovah Witness religions; across the lifespan individuals from children to elderly populations).

About Schmidt. 2002. This movie is about a 67-year-old man, Warren Schmidt, played by Jack Nicholson, who retires from his job as an insurance company executive. He experiences work withdrawal and a lack of direction for his retirement. His wife, Helen, irritates him, and he has no idea what to do to fill his days. While watching television one day he is moved to sponsor a child in Africa with whom he begins a long, one-sided correspondence. When his wife dies unexpectedly, he is initially numb, then sad, and finally angry when he discovers that she had an affair with his best friend many years ago. He is estranged from his only daughter, Jeanie, whose wedding to Randall, a man he feels is beneath her, is imminent. The movie follows Warren as he searches for connection and meaning in his life.

SIGNIFICANCE: Warren Schmidt demonstrates a common phenomenon among the elderly when they retire. He also shows the impact of grief superimposed on initial dysthymia or depression.

VIEWING POINTS: Look for the changes in Schmidt's manifestations of depression in different situations. Note how he experiences the various stages of grieving. What do you think about Schmidt's search for significance and meaning in his life?

Dead Poet's Society. 1989. This film portrays John Keating, played by Robin Williams, as a charismatic English teacher in a conservative, New England prep school for boys in 1959. John brings his love of poetry to the students and encourages them to follow their dreams and talents and make the most of every day. His efforts put him at odds with administration of the school, particularly the headmaster, played by Norman Lloyd, as well as Tom Perry, the father of one of his students, played by Kurtwood Smith. Tom's son, Neil, played by Robert Sean Leonard, chooses to act in a school play despite the objection of his father to any extracurricular activities. When Neil cannot reconcile his love of theater and his father's expectations that he pursue a career in medicine, he kills himself. John Keating blames himself for the death, as does the school administration. He is fired by the administration but has a moment of pride when his students demonstrate their ability to think and act for themselves.

SIGNIFICANCE: This film accurately portrays the sensitivity of adolescents and their longing for worthwhile role models. It also shows adolescent growth and development in a realistic manner. It demonstrates the combination of factors that accompany a decision to commit suicide. We can see how Neil feels caught between his desires and the demands of his father. In the cultural context of the late 1950s, few children or adolescents dared to challenge or defy their parents, especially such a domineering man as Tom Perry.

VIEWING POINTS: Look for the differences in Neil's behavior with his peers and his father or other adults besides Mr. Keating. What, if any, clues do you get that Neil might attempt suicide? What actions by any of the main characters might have prevented his suicide?

Mr. Jones. 1993. This film is about a musician, Mr. Jones, played by Richard Gere, and his psychiatrist. In his manic state, Mr. Jones is a charismatic, charming individual who persuades a contractor to hire him, proceeds to the roof of the building, and prepares to fly off the roof. He withdraws large sums of money from the bank. He knows that he has bipolar disorder but refuses to take his medication because of the side effects. He has episodes of depression during which he becomes suicidal. Once hospitalized, he struggles with trying to find a life on medication.

SIGNIFICANCE: Viewers can gain insight into the impact of mental illness on the promising career of a classical musician. This film illustrates the ways in which interpersonal relationships are affected by a psychiatric disorder. Unfortunately, the unethical romantic relationship between Mr. Jones and his psychiatrist detracts from the quality of the film's content.

VIEWING POINTS: Why does the diagnosis of paranoid schizophrenia not fit Mr. Jones' clinical picture in the admitting room? Identify the antecedents to the manic and depressive episodes. At what point is the physician–patient relationship first compromised? Are there early warning signs that should have alerted the psychiatrist that she was violating professional boundaries?

REFERENCES

Alda, M., & Grof, P. (2000). Genetics and lithium response in bipolar disorders. In J. C. Soares & S. Gershon (Eds.), *Bipolar disorders: Basic mechanisms and therapeutic implications* (pp. 529–543). New York: Marcel Dekker, Inc.

Alda, M. (2001). Genetic factors and treatment of mood disorders. *Bipolar Disorders, 3*(6), 318.

American Nurses Association. (2000). *Scope and standards of psychiatric–mental health clinical nursing practice.* Washington, DC: Author.

American Psychiatric Association (APA). (2000). *Diagnostic and statistical manual of mental disorders* (4th ed., text revision [DSM-IV-TR]). Washington, DC: Author.

American Psychiatric Association (APA). (2002). *Compendium of practice guidelines for the treatment of psychiatric disorders.* Washington, DC: Author.

Baker, F. M. (2001). Diagnosing depression in African Americans. *Community Mental Health Journal, 37*(1), 31–34.

Belmaker, R. H., & Yaroslavsky, Y. (2000). Perspectives for new pharmacological interventions. In J. C. Soares & S. Gershon (Eds.), *Bipolar disorders: Basic mechanisms and therapeutic implications* (pp. 507–527). New York: Marcel Dekker, Inc.

Bernard, S. A., & Bruera, E. (2000). Drug interactions in palliative care. *Journal of Clinical Oncology, 18*(8), 1780–1799.

Blazer, D. G., Hybels, C. F., & Pieper, C. F. (2001). The association of depression and mortality in elderly persons: A case for multiple independent pathways. *Journal of Gerontology: Medical Sciences, 56A*(8), 505–509.

Bowden, C. L., Calabrese, J. R., McElroy S. L., Gyulai, L., Wassef, A., Petty, F., et al. (2000). A randomized placebo-controlled 12 month trial of divalproex and lithium in treatment of out patients with bipolar disorder. *Archives of General Psychiatry, 57*, 481–489.

Bowden, C. L., Calabrese, J. R., Sachs, G., Yatham, L. N., Asghar, S. A., Hompland, M., et al. (2003). A placebo-controlled 18-month trial of lamotrigine and lithium maintenance treatment in recently manic or hypomanic patients with bipolar 1 disorder. *Archives of General Psychiatry, 60*(4), 392–400.

Casacalenda, N., Perry, J. C., & Looper, K. (2002). Remission in major depressive disorder: a comparison of pharmacotherapy, psychotherapy, and control condition. *American Journal of Psychiatry, 159*(8), 1354–1360.

Donati, R. J., & Rasenick, M. M. (2003). G protein signaling and the molecular basis of antidepressant action. *Life Science, 73*(1), 1–17.

Fagiolini, A., Kupfer, D. J., Houck, P. R., Novick, D. M., & Frank, E. (2003). Obesity as a correlate of outcome in patients with bipolar I disorder. *American Journal of Psychiatry, 160*(1), 112–117.

Glod, C. A., & Baisden, N. (1999). Seasonal affective disorder in children and adolescents. *Journal of the American Psychiatric Nurses Association (Psychobiology Perspectives), 5*(1), 29–31.

Goldsmith, S. K., Pellmar, T. C., Kleinman, A. M., & Bunney, W. E., (Eds.), (2002*). Reducing suicide: A national imperative*. Institute of Medicine, Washington, DC: The National Academies Press.

Grunze, H., Amann, B., Dittmann, S., & Walden, J. (2002). Clinical relevance and possibilities of bipolar rapid cycling. *Neuropsychobiology, 45*(Suppl 1), 20–26.

Hanley, N. R., & Van de Kar, L. D. (2003). Serotonin and the neuroendocrine regulation of the hypothalamic-pituitary-adrenal axis in health and disease. *Vitamins and Hormones: Advances in Research and Applications, 66*, 189–225.

Herrar, J. M., Lawson, W. B., Sramek, J. J. (eds.), 1999. Cross cultural psychiatry. New York: John Wiley & Sons.

Hirschfeld, R. M., Baker, J. D., Wozniak, P., Tracy, K., & Sommerville, K. W. (2003). The safety and early efficacy of oral-loaded divalproex versus standard-titration divalproex, lithium, olanzapine, and placebo in the treatment of acute mania associated with bipolar disorder. *Journal of Clinical Psychiatry, 64*(7), 841–846.

Hirschfeld, R. M., Lewis, L., & Vornik, L. A. (2003). Perceptions and impact of bipolar disorder: How far have we really come? Results of the national depressive and manic-depressive association 2000 survey of individuals with bipolar disorders. *Journal of Clinical Psychiatry, 64*(2), 161–174.

Johnson, L., Andersson-Lundman, G., Aberg-Wistedt, A., & Mathe, A. A. (2000). Age of onset in affective disorder: Its correlation with hereditary and psychosocial factors. *Journal of Affective Disorders, 59*(2), 139–148.

Kahn, D. A., Ross, R., Printz, D. J., & Sachs, G. S. (2000). Treatment of bipolar disorder: A guide for patients and families. In G. S. Sachs, D. J. Printz, D. A. Kahn, D. Carpenter, & J. P. Docherty (Eds.), The expert consensus guideline series: Medication treatment of bipolar disorder 2000. *Postgraduate Medicine Special Report*, April 2000, pp. 1–8.

Keck, P. E., Mendlwicz, J., Calabrese, J. R., Fawcett, J., Suppes, T., Vestergaard, P. A., & Carbonell, C. (2000). A review of randomized controlled clinical trials in acute mania. *Journal of Affective Disorders, 59*(Suppl.1), 31–37.

Kilbourne, A.M. (2005). Bipolar disorder in late life: future directions in efficacy and effectiveness research. *Current Psychiatry Reports, 7*(1), 10–7.

Kronfol, Z., & Remick, D. G. (2000). Cytokines and the brain: Implications for clinical psychiatry. *American Journal of Psychiatry, 157*(5), 683–694.

Leininger, M. M., & McFarland, M. R. (2006). *Culture care diversity and universality: A worldwide nursing theory.* Boston: Jones & Barlett Publishers.

Lewy, A. J., Lefler, B. J., Emens, J. S., & Bauer, V. K. (2006). The circadian basis of winter depression. www.pnas.org/cgi/doi/10.1073/pnas.0602425103. Retrieved March 31, 2007.

Maser, J. D., Akiskal, H. S., Schettler, P., Scheftner, W., Mueller, T., Endicott, J., et al. (2002). Can temperament identify affectively ill patients who engage in lethal or near-lethal suicidal behavior? A 14-year prospective study. *Suicide Life Threatening Behavior, 32*(1), 10–32.

McCuffin, P., Rijsdijk, F., Andrew, J., Sham, P., Katz, R., & Cardno, A. (2003). The heritability of bipolar affective disorder and the genetic relationship to unipolar depression. *Archives of General Psychiatry, 60*(5), 497–502.

McDonald, W. M. (2000). Epidemiology, etiology, and treatment of geriatric mania. *Journal of Clinical Psychiatry, 61*(Suppl. 13), 3–11.

Mead, D. E. (2002). Marital distress, co-occurring depression, and marital therapy: Review. *Journal of Marital and Family Therapy, 28*(3), 299–314.

Mohr, W. (2001). Bipolar disorder in children. *Journal of Psychosocial Nursing, 39*(3), 12–23.

National Academy of Sciences, Institute of Medicine (IOM). (2003). *Unequal treatment: Confronting racial and ethnic disparities in health care.* Washington, DC: National Academies Press.

Nolan, S., & Scoggin, J. A. (2001). Serotonin syndrome: Recognition and management. *US Pharmacist, 23*(2). www.uspharmacist.com. Retrieved March 31, 2007.

Rea, M. M., Tompson, M. C., Miklowitz, D. J., Goldstein, M. J., Hwang, S., & Mintz, J. (2003). Family-focused treatment versus individual treatment for bipolar disorder: Results of a randomized clinical trial. *Journal of Consulting Clinical Psychology, 71*(3), 482–492.

Rothbaum, B. O., & Astin, M. C. (2000). Integration of pharmacotherapy and psychotherapy for bipolar disorder. *Journal of Clinical Psychiatry, 61*(Suppl. 9), 68–75.

Sajatovic, M., Blow, F. C., & Ignacio, R. V. (2006). Psychiatric comorbidity in older adults with bipolar disorder. *International Journal of Geriatric Psychiatry, 21*(6), 582–587.

Schatzberg, A. F., Cole, J. O., & DeBattista, C. (2003). *Manual of clinical psychopharmacology* (4th ed.). Washington, DC: American Psychiatric Publishing, Inc.

Sheline, Y. I. (2003). Neuroimaging studies of mood disorder effects on the brain. *Biological Psychiatry, 54*(3), 338–352.

Sorenson, S. (2002). Serotonin syndrome. *Utox Update, 4*(4), 1–2.

Spector, R. (2004). *Cultural diversity in health & illness* (6th ed.). Upper Saddle River, NJ: Prentice-Hall.

Stahl, S. (2006). *Essential psychopharmacology: Neuroscientific basis and practical applications.* Cambridge: Cambridge University Press.

Strakowski, S. M., & Sax, K. W. (2000). Secondary mania: A model of the pathophysiology of bipolar disorder. In J. C. Soares & S. Gershon (Eds.), *Bipolar disorders: Basic mechanisms and therapeutic implications.* New York: Marcel Dekker, Inc.

Suppes, T., Leverich, G. S., Keck, P. E, Nolan, W. A., Denicoff, K. D., Altschuler, L. L., et al. (2001). The Stanley Foundation for bipolar treatment outcome network: Demographics and illness characteristics of the first 261 patients. *Journal of Affective Disorders, 67*(1–3), 45–59.

Taylor, J. S. (2003). Confronting "culture" in medicine's "culture of no culture." *Academic Medicine, 78*(6):555–559,

Thase, M. E. (2000). Modulation of biological factors by psychotherapeutic interventions. In J. C. Soares & S. Gershon (Eds.), *Bipolar disorders: Basic mechanisms and therapeutic implications.* New York: Marcel Dekker, Inc.

Thase, M. E., & Sachs, G. S. (2000). Bipolar depression: Pharmacotherapy and related therapeutic strategies. *Biological Psychiatry, 48*, 558–572.

Tuunainen, A., Kripke, D.F., Endo, T. (2004). Light therapy for non-seasonal depression. The Cochrane Database of Systematic Reviews: Issue 2. Chichester, UK: John Wiley & Sons, Ltd.

United States Department of Health and Human Services (U.S. DHHS). (2001). *Mental health: Culture, race, and ethnicity: A supplement to mental health: A report of the Surgeon General*. Rockville, MD: U.S. DHHS, Substance Abuse and Mental Health Services Administration, Center for Mental Health Services, National Institutes of Health, National Institute of Mental Health. United States Department of Health and Human Services (U.S. DHHS). (1999). *Mental Health: A report of the Surgeon General*. Rockville, MD: U.S. DHHS, Substance Abuse and Mental Health Services Administration, Center for Mental Health Services, National Institutes of Health, National Institute of Mental Health.

Warren, B. J. (in press). Psychosocial bases for understanding human behavior within a cultural context. In C. J. Cornwell (Ed.), *Psychiatric mental health nursing: An evidenced approach to clinical care*. Baltimore, MD: Lippincott.

Warren, B. J. (2002). Interlocking paradigm of cultural competence: A model for psychiatric mental health nursing practice. *Journal of the American Psychiatric Nurses Association, 8*(6), 209–213.

Yildiz, A., & Sachs, G. S. (2003). Do antidepressants induce rapid cycling? A gender-specific association. *Journal of Clinical Psychiatry, 64*(7), 814–818.

Zahourek, R. (2000). Alternative, complementary or integrative approaches to treating depression. *Journal of the American Psychiatric Nurses Association, 6*(3), 77–86.

CHAPTER 21

Anxiety Disorders: Management of Anxiety and Panic

Judith E. Forker

LEARNING OBJECTIVES

After studying this chapter, you will be able to:

- Differentiate normal anxiety responses from those suggestive of an anxiety disorder.
- Discuss the epidemiology, etiology, symptomatology, and treatment of selected anxiety disorders.
- Discuss the neurobiologic underpinnings of the anxiety disorders.
- Discuss biopsychosocial treatment approaches used for patients with anxiety disorders.
- Identify nursing diagnoses used in providing nursing care for patients with anxiety disorders.
- Develop a nursing care plan through the continuum of care for patients with panic disorder.
- Identify biopsychosocial indicators for four levels of anxiety and nursing interventions appropriate for each level.

KEY CONCEPTS

- anxiety
- compulsions
- obsessions
- panic

KEY TERMS

• agoraphobia • anxiolytic • depersonalization • distraction • exposure therapy • flooding • implosive therapy • interoceptive conditioning • panic attacks • panic control treatment • panicogenic • phobia • positive self-talk • systematic desensitization

Anxiety is an uncomfortable feeling of apprehension or dread that occurs in response to internal or external stimuli and can result in physical, emotional, cognitive, and behavioral symptoms. All symptoms of anxiety disorders can be found in healthy individuals given particular circumstances.

Symptoms of anxiety that negatively affect the individual's ability to function in work or interpersonal relationships are considered symptomatic of an anxiety disorder. The anxiety disorders discussed in this chapter include panic disorder, obsessive-compulsive disorder (OCD), generalized anxiety disorder (GAD), phobias, posttraumatic stress disorder (PTSD), and acute stress disorder. Dissociative disorders are not classified as anxiety disorders; however, they are included as part of this chapter because overwhelming anxiety is a cardinal symptom of these disorders.

Panic disorder receives particular attention in this chapter, in part because of the frequency with which people experiencing panic symptoms seek emergency medical care. There is also significant overlap of symptoms and interventions applicable to other anxiety disorders. OCD is highlighted because patients with this disorder often do not seek medical attention and because diagnosing and treating this condition is difficult.

NORMAL VERSUS ABNORMAL ANXIETY RESPONSE

Anxiety is an unavoidable, human condition that takes many forms and serves different purposes. One's response to anxiety can be positive and motivate one to act, or it can produce paralyzing fear, causing inaction. Normal anxiety is described as being of realistic intensity and duration for the situation and is followed by relief behaviors intended to reduce or prevent more anxiety (Peplau, 1989). Normal anxiety response is appropriate to the situation, can be dealt with without repression, and can be used to help the patient identify what underlying problem has caused the anxiety.

During a perceived threat, rising anxiety levels cause physical and emotional changes in all individuals. A normal emotional response to anxiety consists of three parts: physiologic arousal, cognitive processes, and coping strategies. Physiologic arousal, or the fight-or-flight response, is the signal that an individual is facing a threat. Cognitive processes decipher the situation and decide whether the perceived threat should be approached or avoided. Coping strategies are employed to resolve the threat. Table 21.1 summarizes many physical, affective, cognitive, and behavioral symptoms associated with anxiety. The factors that determine whether anxiety is a symptom of a mental disorder are the intensity of anxiety relative to the situation, the trigger for the anxiety, and the particular symptom clusters that manifest the anxiety. Table 21.2 describes the four degrees of anxiety and associated perceptual changes and patterns of behavior.

OVERVIEW OF ANXIETY DISORDERS

Anxiety disorders are the most common of the psychiatric illnesses treated by health care providers. Direct and indirect costs of treating anxiety disorders are in the tens of billions of dollars. It is estimated that more than 19 million people are affected by anxiety disorders (Duque & Neugroschl, 2002). Women seem to experience anxiety disorders more often than do men. At high risk are smokers, individuals younger than 45 years, those separated or divorced, survivors of abuse, and those in low socioeconomic groups (Isensee, Wittchen, Stein, Hofler, & Lieb, 2003; Sheikh, Leskin, & Klein, 2002). Anxiety disorders may also be associated with other mental or physical co-morbidities such as heart disease, respiratory disease, and mood disorders (Goodwin & Pine, 2002; Lavie & Milani, 2004).

Anxiety disorders affect individuals of all ages. Of depressed elderly patients, 35% will have at least one anxiety disorder diagnosis (Lenze et al., 2000). Children and adolescents also experience anxiety disorders. If left untreated, symptoms persist, gradually worsen, and sometimes lead to suicidal ideation and suicide attempts (Sareen et al., 2005). A single patient may concurrently have more than one anxiety disorder or other psychiatric disorders as well.

Anxiety disorders tend to be chronic and persistent illnesses, with full recovery more likely among those who do not have other mental or physical diseases (Rodriquez, Weiseberg, Pagano, Bruce, Spencer, Culepper, & Keller, 2006). In the primary care setting, most patients with anxiety disorders present with a coexisting physical disorder (Bruce et al., 2005).

Special Populations

Prompt identification, diagnosis, and treatment of anxiety disorders may be difficult for special populations such as children and elderly patients. Often, the symptoms suggestive of anxiety disorders may go unnoticed by caregivers or are misdiagnosed because they mimic cardiac or pulmonary pathology, rather than a psychological disturbance.

Children

Anxiety disorders are the psychiatric disorders most frequently treated in children, with the percentage of children affected comparable with that of asthma (Castellanos & Hunter, 2000). Young patients with anxiety disorders often experience separation anxiety disorder and OCD, and the symptoms can be insidious. During these stages in a young person's life, fear of strangers and other signs of anxiety are developmentally appropriate. If left undiagnosed and untreated, the condition typically worsens to the point that the child is unable to carry out his or her responsibilities. Children and adolescents with anxiety disorders have higher rates of suicidal behavior, early parenthood, drug and alcohol dependence, and educational underachievement later in life (Woodward, 2001).

Some evidence suggests a relationship between childhood separation anxiety disorder and atopic disorders (asthma, hives, hay fever, and eczema) and adult-onset panic disorder (Slattery et al., 2002). Research is ongoing to discover predictors of anxiety disorders in adulthood.

Elderly People

Many people subscribe to the myth that elderly people do not experience depression or anxiety disorders because they have little to worry about, but in fact, many elderly people experience depression, substance abuse, or anxiety disorders. This combination of depressive and anxiety symptoms has been shown to decrease social functioning, increase somatic (physical) symptoms, and increase depressive symptoms (Duque & Neugroschl, 2002). Because the elderly population is at risk for suicide, special assessment of anxiety symptoms is essential.

PANIC DISORDER

Panic is an extreme, overwhelming form of anxiety often experienced when an individual is placed in a real or per-

Table 21.1 Symptoms of Anxiety

Physical		
Cardiovascular	*Neuromuscular*	*Gastrointestinal*
Sympathetic	Increased reflexes	Loss of appetite
Palpitations	Startle reaction	Revulsion toward food
Heart racing	Eyelid twitching	Abdominal discomfort
Increased blood pressure	Insomnia	Diarrhea
Parasympathetic	Tremors	*Parasympathetic*
Actual fainting	Rigidity	Abdominal pain
Decreased blood pressure	Spasm	Nausea
Decreased pulse rate	Fidgeting	Heartburn
Respiratory	Pacing	Vomiting
Rapid breathing	Strained face	*Eyes*
Difficulty getting air	Unsteadiness	Dilated pupils
Shortness of breath	Generalized weakness	*Urinary Tract*
Pressure of chest	Wobbly legs	*Parasympathetic*
Shallow breathing	Clumsy motions	Pressure to urinate
Lump in throat	*Skin*	Increased frequency of urination
Choking sensations	Face flushed	
Gasping	Face pale	
Parasympathetic	Localized sweating (palm region)	
Spasm of bronchi	Generalized sweating	
	Hot and cold spells	
	Itching	
Affective	**Cognitive**	**Behavioral**
Edgy	*Sensory-Perceptual*	Inhibited
Impatient	Mind is hazy, cloudy, foggy, dazed	Tonic immobility
Uneasy	Objects seem blurred/distant	Flight
Nervous	Environment seems different/unreal	Avoidance
Tense	Feelings of unreality	Speech dysfluency
Wound-up	Self-consciousness	Impaired coordination
Anxious	Hypervigilance	Restlessness
Fearful	*Thinking Difficulties*	Postural collapse
Apprehensive	Cannot recall important things	Hyperventilation
Scared	Confused	
Frightened	Unable to control thinking	
Alarmed	Difficulty concentrating	
Terrified	Difficulty focusing attention	
Jittery	Distractibility	
Jumpy	Blocking	
	Difficulty reasoning	
	Loss of objectivity and perspective	
	Tunnel vision	
	Conceptual	
	Cognitive distortion	
	Fear of losing control	
	Fear of not being able to cope	
	Fear of physical injury or death	
	Fear of mental disorder	
	Fear of negative evaluations	
	Frightening visual images	
	Repetitive fearful ideation	

Adapted from Beck, A. T., & Emery, C. (1985). *Anxiety disorders and phobias: A cognitive perspective* (pp. 23–27). New York: Basic Books.

ceived life-threatening situation. Panic is normal during periods of threat but abnormal when it is continuously experienced in situations that pose no real physical or psychological threat. Some people experience heightened anxiety because they fear experiencing another panic attack. This type of panic interferes with the individual's ability to function in everyday life and is characteristic of panic disorder.

Table 21.2 Degrees of Anxiety

Degree of Anxiety	Effects on Perceptual Field and on Ability to Focus Attention	Observable Behavior
Mild	Perceptual field widens slightly. Able to observe more than before and to see relations (make connection among data). Learning is possible.	Is aware, alerted, sees, hears, and grasps more than before. Usually able to recognize and name anxiety easily.
Moderate	Perceptual field narrows slightly. Selective inattention: does not notice what goes on peripheral to the immediate focus but can do so if attention is directed there by another observer.	Sees, hears, and grasps less than previously. Can attend to more if directed to do so. Able to sustain attention on a particular focus; selectively inattentive to contents outside the focal area. Usually able to state "I am anxious now."
Severe	Perceptual field is greatly reduced. Tendency toward dissociation: to not notice what is going on outside the current reduced focus of attention; largely unable to do so when another observer suggests it.	Sees, hears, and grasps far less than previously. Attention is focused on a small area of a given event. Inferences drawn may be distorted because of inadequacy of observed data. May be unaware of and unable to name anxiety. Relief behaviors generally used.
Panic (terror, horror, dread, uncanniness, awe)	Perceptual field is reduced to a detail, which is usually "blown up," i.e., elaborated by distortion (exaggeration), or the focus is on scattered details; the speed of the scattering tends to increase. Massive dissociation especially of contents of self-system. Felt as enormous threat to survival. Learning is impossible.	Says, "I'm in a million pieces," "I'm gone." "What is happening to me?" Perplexity, self-absorption. Feelings of unreality. Flights of ideas, or confusion. Fear. Repeats a detail. Many relief behaviors used automatically (without thought). The enormous energy produced by panic must be used and may be mobilized as rage. May pace, run, or fight violently. With dissociation of contents of self-system, there may be very rapid reorganization of the self, usually going along pathologic lines; e.g., a "psychotic break" is usually preceded by panic.

From Pepau, H. (1989). Theoretical constructs: Anxiety, self, and hallucinations. In A. O'Tool, & S. Welt (Eds.). *Interpersonal theory in nursing practice: Selected works of Hildegarde. E. Peplau.* New York: Springer.

KEY CONCEPT Panic is a normal but extreme, overwhelming form of anxiety often experienced when an individual is placed in a real or perceived life threatening situation.

Clinical Course of Panic Disorder

Panic disorder is a lifelong disorder that typically peaks in the teenage years and then again in the 30s. The disorder can surface in childhood or after the fourth decade of life. However, the disorder does not usually manifest after the third decade of life (American Psychiatric Association [APA], 2000). Panic disorder is treatable, but studies have shown that even after years of treatment, many cases remain symptomatic (APA, 2000; Gardos, 2000). In some cases, symptoms may even worsen.

Panic disorder is a chronic condition that has several exacerbations and remissions during the course of the disease. It is characterized by the appearance of disabling attacks of panic that often lead to other symptoms, such as phobias.

Panic Attacks

Panic attacks are sudden, discrete periods of intense fear or discomfort that are accompanied by significant physical and cognitive symptoms. The physical symptoms include palpitations, chest discomfort, rapid pulse, nausea, dizziness, sweating, paresthesias, trembling or shaking, and a feeling of suffocation or shortness of breath. Cognitive symptoms include disorganized thinking, irrational fears, depersonalization, and decreased ability to communicate. Feelings of impending doom or death, fear of going crazy or losing control, and desperation are common.

• NCLEXNOTE

Physical symptoms of panic attack are similar to cardiac emergencies. These symptoms are physically taxing and psychologically frightening to patients. Recognition of the seriousness of panic attacks should be communicated to the patient.

A panic attack usually peaks at 10 minutes but can last as long as 30 minutes, followed by a gradual return to normal functioning. Individuals with panic disorder experience recurrent, unexpected panic attacks followed by persistent concern about experiencing subsequent panic attacks. They fear implications of the attacks, and they have behavioral changes related to the attacks (APA, 2000).

Panic attacks cause fear of death because they mimic symptoms of a heart attack. Individuals often seek emergency medical care because they feel as if they are dying,

BOX 21.1

Clinical Vignette: Panic Disorder

M, a 22-year-old man, has experienced several life changes, including a recent engagement, loss of his father to cancer and heart disease, graduation from college, and entrance to the workforce as a computer engineer in a large inner-city company. Because of his active lifestyle, his sleep habits have been poor. He frequently uses sleeping aids at night and now drinks a full pot of coffee to start each day. He has started smoking to "relieve the stress." While sitting in heavy traffic on the way to work, he suddenly experienced chest tightness, sweating, shortness of breath, feelings of being "trapped," and foreboding that he was going to die. Fearing a heart attack, he went to an emergency room, where his discomfort subsided within a half hour. After several hours of testing, the doctor informed him that his heart was healthy. During the next few weeks, he experienced several episodes of feeling trapped and slight chest discomfort on his drive to work. He fears future "attacks" while sitting in traffic and while in his crowded office cubicle.

What Do You Think?

- What risk factors does M have that might contribute to the development of panic attacks?
- What lifestyle changes do you think would help M reduce stress?

but most will have a negative cardiac workup. People experiencing panic attacks may also believe that the attacks stem from an underlying major medical illness (APA, 2000). Even with sound medical testing and assurance of no underlying disease, these people often remain unconvinced. Panic attacks can occur in individuals first experiencing certain anxiety-provoking medical conditions, such as asthma, or in initial trials of illicit substance use. However, individuals with panic disorder continue to experience panic attacks with or without predisposing conditions (Box 21.1). All panic attacks are either internally or externally driven. Externally driven panic attacks may result, for example, from actually seeing a feared object. An internally driven panic attack results from an uncomfortable, internal feeling. Sensations of being too hot or cramped in a small room might provoke panic attacks. APA (2000) defines these categories.

AGORAPHOBIA AND OTHER PHOBIAS

Panic attacks can lead to the development of **phobias**, or persistent, unrealistic fears of situations, objects, or activities. People with phobias will go to great lengths to avoid the feared objects or situations to deter panic attacks. Box 21.2 presents examples of common phobias.

Agoraphobia, fear of open spaces, commonly co-occurs with panic disorder. Agoraphobia, which may occur after panic attacks, leads to avoidance behaviors. It begins with an intense, irrational fear of being in open spaces, being alone, or being in public places where escape might be difficult or embarrassing. The person fears that if a panic attack occurred, help would not be available, so he or she avoids such situations. Such avoidance interferes with routine functioning and eventually renders the person afraid to leave the safety of home.

BOX 21.2

Common Phobias

Acrophobia (fear of heights)
Agoraphobia (fear of open spaces)
Ailurophobia (fear of cats)
Algophobia (fear of pain)
Arachnophobia (fear of spiders)
Brontophobia (fear of thunder)
Claustrophobia (fear of closed spaces)
Cynophobia (fear of dogs)
Entomophobia (fear of insects)
Hematophobia (fear of blood)
Microphobia (fear of germs)
Nyctophobia (fear of night or dark places)
Ophidiophobia (fear of snakes)
Phonophobia (fear of loud noises)
Photophobia (fear of light)
Pyrophobia (fear of fire)
Topophobia (stage fright)
Xenophobia (fear of strangers)
Zoophobia (fear of animal or animals)

FAME AND FORTUNE

Charles Darwin (1809–1882)

Theory of Evolution

Public Persona

Charles Darwin, credited as the first scientist to gain wide acceptance of the theory of natural selection, might never have published his seminal work, *Origin of the Species,* had it not been for his psychiatric illness. Born in England, Charles Darwin, the grandson of a famous poet, inventor, and physician was expected to accomplish great things. However, his childhood years were troublesome. When he was sent to Cambridge to study medicine, card playing and drinking became his main activities. After meeting a botantist, however, his life changed and he embarked on a 5-year expedition to the Pacific coast of South America.

Personal Realities

Darwin described his sensation of fear, accompanied by troubled beating of the heart, sweat, and trembling of muscles. Thought to have panic disorder, he constantly worried about what he thought he knew until he finally published his ideas on paper. In 1859, *The Origin of Species by Means of Natural Selection* was published. In 1882 he died and was buried in Westminster Abbey.

SOURCE: Darwin, C. (1887). *The life and letters of Charles Darwin.* New York: Appleton & Co.

Some affected individuals continue to face feared situations, but with significant trepidation (i.e., going in public only to pay bills, or to take children to school).

In many cases, agoraphobia develops quickly after a few panic attacks, but the resulting avoidance behaviors do not decrease the severity of the panic attacks (APA, 2000). Other patients can reduce panic attacks by dodging certain instances that precipitate attacks. Many of these individuals may be able to confront a situation if accompanied by someone else; for example, going out in public may be manageable with a friend.

Diagnostic Criteria

Panic disorder is characterized by the onset of panic attacks. Although panic attack does not have a specific DSM code, this disorder affects the person significantly. A person who has a diagnosis of panic attacks has periods of intense fear, at which time at least four physical or psychological symptoms are manifested. These symptoms include palpitations, sweating, shaking, shortness of breath or smothering, sensations of choking, chest pain, nausea or abdominal distress, dizziness, derealization or depersonalization, fear of going crazy, fear of dying, paresthesias, and chills or hot flashes (APA, 2000).

There are two types of panic disorder: with and without agoraphobia. Both types include recurrent and unexpected panic attacks, followed by 1 month or more of consistent concern about having another attack, worrying about the consequences of having another attack, or changing behavior because of fear of the attacks (see Table 21.3).

Epidemiology

Lifetime prevalence estimates of panic disorder without agoraphobia are 3.7% and with agoraphobia is 1.1%. The estimates of isolated panic attacks are 22.7% of the

Table 21.3  **Key Diagnostic Characteristics of Panic Disorder With or Without Agoraphobia** 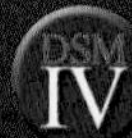

Diagnostic Criteria	Target Symptoms
Panic Disorder Without Agoraphobia Recurrent unexpected panic attacks and 1 month or more (after an attack) of one of the following: • Persistent concern about additional attacks • Worry about the implications of the attack or its consequences • Significant changes in behavior related to the attacks Absence of agoraphobia Not a direct physiologic effect of a substance or medical condition *Panic Disorder With Agoraphobia* Meets criteria for panic disorder, including panic attacks Experiences agoraphobia Not better accounted for any another mental disorder, such as a specific phobia or social phobia (e.g., avoidance limited to social situations because of fear of embarrassment) *Agoraphobia:* Anxiety about being in places or situations from which escape might be difficult (or embarrassing) or in which help may not be available in the event of having an unexpected or situationally predisposed panic attack or panic-like symptoms Fears typically involve characteristic clusters of situations that include being outside the home alone; being in a crowd or standing in a line; being on a bridge; and traveling in a bus, train, or automobile Situations are avoided (e.g., travel is restricted) or endured, with marked distress or anxiety about having a panic attack or panic-like symptoms; or the presence of a companion is required	*Panic Attacks* Discrete period of intense fear or discomfort with four (or more) of the following symptoms that develop abruptly and reach a peak within 10 minutes: • Palpitations, pounding heart, or accelerated heart rate • Sweating • Trembling or shaking • Sensations of shortness of breath or smothering • Feelings of choking • Chest pain or discomfort • Nausea or vomiting • Feeling dizzy, unsteady, lightheaded, or faint • Derealization (feeling of unreality) or depersonalization (being detached from oneself) • Fear of losing control or going crazy • Fear of dying • Paresthesias (numbness or tingling sensations) • Chills or hot flushes Great apprehension about the outcome of routine activities and experiences Loss or disruption of important interpersonal relationships Demoralization Possible major depressive episode *Associated Physical Examination Findings* • Transient tachycardia • Moderate elevation of systolic blood pressure *Associated Laboratory Findings* • Compensated respiratory alkalosis (decreased carbon dioxide, decreased bicarbonate levels, almost normal pH) *Other Targets for Treatment* • Loss or disruption of important interpersonal or occupational activities • Demoralization • Possible major depressive episode

population. It is highly associated with depression, medical conditions including hypertension, and cigarette smoking. Patients experiencing panic disorder with agoraphobia tend to have more coexisting anxiety disorders, anxiety attacks, and anticipatory anxiety than do patients who have panic disorder without agoraphobia (Kessler, Chiu, Jin, Ruscio, Shear, & Walters, 2006).

Evidence suggests gender-related differences in the prevalence of panic disorder. Women appear more likely to experience panic disorder with agoraphobia and more likely to experience panic symptoms after remission (Sheikh, Leskin, & Klein, 2002; Smoller et al., 2003). In the National Comorbidity Survey 1990–1992 (8,098 participants), 3.5% of women experienced panic disorder in their lifetimes, and 2.3% experienced panic disorder in the year preceding the survey. No difference in the prevalence of panic disorders was found between African Americans and Caucasians, but Hispanic people appeared to be affected less commonly (Kessler, 2002).

Etiology

Genetic Theories

There appears to be a substantial familial predisposition to panic disorder with an estimated heritability of 48%. Research findings are establishing associations between the serotonergic and noradrenergic pathways including variants of the serotonin receptor 1A gene, the monoamine oxidase A gene, and the norepinephrine transporter gene (Freitag et al., 2006). More research is needed to analyze this phenomenon.

Neuroanatomic Theories

Certain neurologic abnormalities have also been identified in patients with panic disorder. The most common abnormalities are found in the "fear network" of the brain, i.e., the amygdala, the hippocampus, thalamus, and in the midbrain, pons, medulla, and cerebellum (Sakai et al., 2005).

Biochemical Theories

Identification of neurotransmitter involvement in panic disorder has evolved from neurochemical studies with **panicogenic** substances known to produce panic attacks, such as yohimbine, fenfluramine, norepinephrine, epinephrine, sodium lactate, and carbon dioxide.These substances are often used in studies to stimulate a panic attack.

Serotonin and Norepinephrine

Serotonin and norepinephrine are both implicated in panic disorders. Norepinephrine effects acts on those systems most affected by a panic attack—the cardiovascular, respiratory, and gastrointestinal systems. Serotonergic neurons are distributed in central autonomic and emotional motor control systems regulating anxiety states and anxiety-related physiological and behavioral responses (Abrams, Johnson, Hay-Schmidt, Mikkelsen, Shekhar, & Lowry, 2005). Recent research is beginning to clarify the interaction between norepinephrine and serotonin (Freitag et al., 2006).

Gamma-Aminobutyric Acid

Gamma-aminobutyric acid (GABA) is the most abundant inhibitory neurotransmitter in the brain. GABA receptor stimulation causes several effects, including neurocognitive effects, reduction of anxiety, and sedation. GABA stimulation also results in increased seizure threshold.

Abnormalities in the benzodiazepine–GABA–chloride ion channel complex have been implicated in panic disorder (Goddard, Mason, Appel, Rothmna, Gueorguieva, Behar, & Krystal, 2004).

Hypothalamic–Pituitary–Adrenal Axis

Recent research implicates a role of the HPA axis in panic disorders. A current explanation is that as stress hormones are activated, anxiety increases, which can lead to a panic attack (Graeff, Garcia-Leal, Del-Ben, & Guimaraes, 2005) (see Chapter 14).

Psychoanalytic and Psychodynamic Theories

Psychodynamic theories contribute to the understanding of panic disorders by explaining the importance of the development of anxiety after separation and loss. Patients with panic disorder report greater numbers and severity of recent personal losses at symptom onset than do healthy control subjects. Several studies have examined the prevalence of a history of childhood physical or sexual abuse among patients with panic and other anxiety disorders (Katerndahl, Burge, & Kellog, 2005; Kendler, Hettema, Butera, Gardner, & Prescott, 2003; Safren, Gershuny, Marzol, Otto, & Pollack, 2002).

In a study of the background and personality traits of individuals with panic disorder, several commonalities were found, including being fearful or shy as a child; remembering their parents as angry, critical, or frightening; having feelings of discomfort with aggression; having long-term feelings of low self-esteem; and experiencing a stressful life event associated with frustration and resentment that preceded the initial onset of symptoms (Shear, Cooper, Klerman, Busch, & Shapiro, 1993).

Cognitive-Behavioral Theories

Learning theory underlies most cognitive-behavioral theories of panic disorder. Classic conditioning theory suggests that one learns a fear response by linking an adverse or fear-provoking event, such as a car accident, with a previously neutral event, such as crossing a bridge. One becomes conditioned to associate fear with crossing a bridge. Applying this theory to people with panic disorder has limitations. Phobic avoidance is not always developed secondary to an adverse event.

Further development of this theory led to an understanding of **interoceptive conditioning**, which pairs a somatic discomfort, such as dizziness or palpitations, with an impending panic attack. For example, during a car accident, the individual may experience rapid heartbeat, dizziness, shortness of breath, and panic. Subsequent experiences of dizziness or palpitations, unrelated to an anxiety-provoking situation, incite anxiety and panic. Many cognitive theorists further expound that people with panic disorder may misinterpret mild physical sensations (sweating, dizziness), causing panic as a result of learned fear (catastrophic interpretation). Some researchers hypothesize that individuals with a low sense of control over their environment or with a particular sensitivity to anxiety are vulnerable to misinterpreting normal stress. Controlled exposure to anxiety-provoking situations and cognitive countering techniques has proven successful in reducing the symptoms of panic.

Risk Factors

Family history, substance and stimulant use or abuse, smoking tobacco, and severe stressors are risk factors for panic disorder. Female gender is also a risk factor because females have more panic symptoms than do males. People who have several anxiety symptoms and those who experience separation anxiety during childhood often develop panic disorder later in life (Hayward, Killen, & Kraemer, 2000; Slattery et al., 2002). Early life traumas, history of physical or sexual abuse, socioeconomic or personal disadvantages, and behavioral inhibition by adults have been associated with an increased risk for anxiety disorders in children (Friedman et al., 2002; Katerndahl et al., 2005; Kendler et al., 2003; Woodward, 2001).

Comorbidity

Patients may experience more than one anxiety disorder and depression, eating disorders, substance use or abuse, or schizophrenia (Goldstein, Herrmann, & Shulman, 2006). Although people with panic disorder are thought to have more somatic complaints than the general population, panic disorder correlates with certain medical conditions, including vertigo, cardiac disease, gastrointestinal disorders, and asthma. Patients with mitral valve prolapse, migraine headaches, and hypertension may also have an increased incidence of panic disorder. One might ponder whether these medical conditions result from panic disorder or are discovered more often as a result of increased contacts with health care providers. Whichever the case, people with panic disorder have reported to their health care providers that they feel as if they are in poor physical or psychological health.

Interdisciplinary Treatment of Panic Disorder

Nurses are pivotal in stabilizing the inpatient by providing a safe and therapeutic environment. The nurse also administers medication, monitors its effects, and develops an individual care plan to meet the patient's needs. Advanced practice nurses, licensed clinical social workers, or licensed counselors provide individual psychotherapy sessions as appropriate. Often, a clinical psychologist administers psychological testing and interprets the test results to assist with appropriate diagnosis and to tailor treatment.

Priority Care Issues

People with panic disorder are often depressed and consequently are at high risk for suicide. Adolescents with panic disorder may be at higher risk for suicidal thoughts or attempt suicide more often than other adolescents (Valentiner, Gutierrez, & Blacker, 2002; Sareen et al., 2005). As many as 15% of patients with panic disorder commit suicide; women with both panic disorder and depression or panic disorder and substance abuse are especially at risk (APA, 2000).

Because panic disorder manifests during the childbearing years, the pregnant patient should be assessed carefully for an underlying panic disorder. Although pregnancy may actually protect the mother from developing panic symptoms, postpartum onset of panic disorder requires particular attention. During a time that tremendous effort is spent on family, postpartum onset of panic disorder negatively affects lifestyle and decreases self-esteem in affected women, leading to feelings of overwhelming personal disappointment.

NURSING MANAGEMENT: HUMAN RESPONSE TO PANIC DISORDER

Physiologic symptoms tend to be the impetus for patients to seek medical assistance because the symptoms overlap with other medical and psychiatric illnesses. Often, patients are seen in emergency rooms as they seek treatment for their physical symptoms. Biologic, psychological, and social assessments unveil potential underlying pathology and guide the nurse to an accurate nursing diagnosis.

Biologic Domain

Assessment

Skillful assessment is required to rule out life-threatening causes, including cardiac or neurologic involvement. Once it is determined that the patient does not have other medical problems, the nurse should assess for the characteristic symptoms of panic attack. If the panic attack occurs in the presence of the nurse, direct assessment of the symptoms should be made and documented. Questions to ask the patient might include the following:

- What did you experience preceding and during the panic episode, including physical symptoms, feelings, and thoughts?
- When did you begin to feel that way? How long did it last?
- What is it that caused you to feel and think that way?
- Have you experienced these symptoms in the past? If so, under what circumstances?
- Has anyone in your family ever had similar experiences?
- What do you do when you have these experiences that help you to feel safe?
- Have the feelings and sensations ever gone away on their own?

Substance Use

Assessment for panicogenic substance use, such as sources of caffeine, pseudoephedrine, amphetamines, cocaine, or other stimulants may rule out contributory issues either related or unrelated to panic disorder. Tobacco use can also contribute to the risk for panic symptoms. Many individuals with panic disorder use alcohol or central nervous system (CNS) depressants in an effort to self-medicate anxiety symptoms, and withdrawal from CNS depressants may produce symptoms of panic.

Sleep Patterns

Sleep is often disturbed in patients with panic disorder. In fact, panic attacks can occur during sleep, and the patient may fear sleep for this reason. Nurses should closely assess the impact of sleep disturbance because fatigue may increase anxiety and susceptibility to panic attacks.

Physical Activity

Active participation in a routine exercise program requires assessment. If the patient does not exercise routinely, define the barriers. If exercise is avoided because of chronic muscle tension, poor muscle tone, muscle cramps, general fatigue, exhaustion, or shortness of breath, the symptoms may indicate poor physical health.

Nursing Diagnoses for the Biologic Domain

Appropriate nursing diagnoses for the individual with panic disorder include Anxiety, Risk for Self-Harm, Social Isolation, Powerlessness, and Ineffective Family Coping. Other diagnoses may apply after the nurse has completed a thorough psychiatric nursing assessment and developed an individual services plan (care plan).

Interventions for the Biologic Domain

The course of panic disorder culminates in phobic avoidance as the afflicted person attempts to avoid situations that increase panic. Because identifying and avoiding anxiety-provoking situations is important during therapy, drastically changing lifestyle to avoid situations does not aid recovery. Interventions that focus on the physical aspects of anxiety and panic are particularly helpful in reducing the number and severity of the attacks, giving patients a rapid sense of accomplishment and control.

Breathing Control

Hyperventilation is common. Often, people are unaware that they take rapid, shallow breaths when they become anxious.

Teaching Points 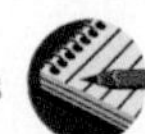

Teaching patients breathing control can be helpful. Focus on the breathing and help them to identify the rate, pattern, and depth. If the breathing is rapid and shallow, reassure the patient that exercise and breathing practice can help change this breathing pattern. Next, assist the patient in practicing abdominal breathing by performing the following exercises:

- Instruct the patient to breathe deeply by inhaling slowly through the nose. Have him or her place a hand on the abdomen just beneath the rib cage.
- Instruct the patient to observe that when one is breathing deeply, the hand on the abdomen will actually rise.
- After the patient understands this process, ask him or her to inhale slowly through the nose counting to five, pause, and then exhale slowly through pursed lips.
- While the patient exhales, direct attention to feeling the muscles relax, focusing on "letting go."
- Have the patient repeat the deep abdominal breathing for 10 breaths, pausing between each inhalation and exhalation. Count slowly. If the patient complains of light-headedness, reassure him or her that this is a normal feeling while deep breathing. Instruct

the patient to stop for 30 seconds, breathe normally, and then start again.

- The patient should stop between each cycle of 10 breaths and monitor normal breathing for 30 seconds.
- This series of 10 slow abdominal breaths, followed by 30 seconds of normal breathing, should be repeated for 3 to 5 minutes.
- Help the patient to establish a time for daily practice of abdominal breathing.

Abdominal breathing may also be used to interrupt an episode of panic as it begins. Once patients have learned to identify their own early signs of panic, they can learn the four-square method of breathing, which helps divert or decrease the severity of the attack. Patients should be instructed as follows:

- Advise the patient to practice during calm periods and to begin by inhaling slowly through the nose, count to four, then hold the breath for a count of four.
- Next, direct the patient to exhale slowly through pursed lips to a count of four and then rest for a count of four (no breath).
- Finally, the patient may take two normal breaths and repeat the sequence.

After patients practice the skill, the nurse should assist patients in identifying the physical cues that will alert them to use this calming technique.

Nutritional Planning

Maintaining regular and balanced eating habits reduces the likelihood of hypoglycemic episodes, lightheadedness, and fatigue.

Teaching Points 

To help teach the patient about healthful eating and ways to minimize physical factors contributing to anxiety, the nurse may:

- Advise the patient to reduce or eliminate substances in the diet that promote anxiety and panic, such as food coloring, monosodium glutamate, and caffeine (withdrawal from which may stimulate panic). Patients need to plan to reduce caffeine consumption and then eliminate it from their diet. Many over-the-counter (OTC) remedies are now used to boost energy or increase mental performance, and some of these contain caffeine. A thorough assessment should be made of all OTC products to assess the potential of anxiety-provoking ingredients.
- Instruct the patient to check each substance consumed and note whether symptoms of anxiety occur and whether the symptoms are relieved by not consuming the product.

Relaxation Techniques

Teaching the patient relaxation techniques is another way to help individuals with panic and anxiety disorders. Some are unaware of the tension in their bodies and first need to learn to monitor their own tension. Isometric exercises and progressive muscle relaxation are helpful methods to learn to differentiate muscle tension from muscle relaxation. This method of relaxation is also helpful when patients have difficulty clearing the mind, focusing, or visualizing a scene, which are often required in other forms of relaxation, such as meditation. Box 21.3 provides one method of progressive muscle relaxation.

Increased Physical Activity

Physical exercise can effectively decrease the occurrence of panic attacks by reducing muscle tension, increasing metabolism, and relieving stress. Exercise programs reduce many of the precipitants of anxiety by improving circulation, digestion, endorphin stimulation, and tissue oxygenation. In addition, exercise lowers cholesterol levels, blood pressure, and weight. After assessing for contraindications to physical exercise, assist the patient in establishing a routine exercise program. Engaging in 10- to 20-minute sessions on treadmills or stationary bicycles two to three times weekly is ideal during winter months. Casual walking or bike riding during seasonal weather promotes health. Help the patient to identify community resources that promote exercise.

Pharmacologic Interventions

Antidepressants (selective serotonin-reuptake inhibitors [SSRIs], serotonin-norepinephrine reuptake inhibitors (SNRIs), tricyclic antidepressants (TCAs), and monoamine oxidase inhibitors (MAOIs) and antianxiety medication (benzodiazepines) have been shown to be effective in panic disorders (see Table 21.4). The use of the TCAs for the treatment of panic disorder is declining significantly and their use will not be discussed in this chapter. The MAOIs are reserved for those who do not respond to the SSRIs or SNRIs. See Chapters 8 and 20 for nursing care for patients taking TCAs and MAOIs.

Selective Serotonin Reuptake Inhibitors (SSRIs)

The SSRIs are recommended as the first drug option in the treatment of panic disorder. They have the best safety profile, and if side effects occur, they tend to be present early in treatment before the therapeutic effect takes place. Hence, SSRIs should be started at low doses and titrated every five to seven days. Antidepressant therapy is recommended for long-term treatment of the disorder and antianxiety as adjunctive treatment (Katon, 2006).

BOX 21.3

Implementing Progressive Muscle Relaxation

Choose a quiet, comfortable location where you will not be disturbed for 20 to 30 minutes. Your position may be lying or sitting, but all parts of your body should be supported, including your head. Wear loose clothing, taking off restrictive items, such as glasses and shoes.

Begin by closing your eyes and clearing your mind. Moving from head to toe, focus on each part or your body and assess the level of tension. Visualize each group of muscles as heavy and relaxed.

Take two or three slow abdominal breaths, pausing briefly between each breath. Imagine the tension flowing from your body.

Each muscle group listed below should be tightened (or tensed isometrically) for 5 to 10 seconds and then abruptly released; visualize this group of muscles as heavy, limp, and relaxed for 15 to 20 seconds before tightening the next group of muscles. There are several methods to tighten each muscle group, and suggestions are provided below. Each muscle group may be tightened two to three times until relaxed. Do not overtighten or strain. You should not experience pain.

- Hands (tighten by making fists)
- Biceps (tighten by drawing forearms up and "making a muscle")
- Triceps (extend forearms straight, locking elbows)
- Face (grimace, tightly shutting mouth and eyes)
- Face (open mouth wide and raise eyebrows)
- Neck (pull head forward to chest and tighten neck muscles)
- Shoulders (raise shoulders toward ears)
- Shoulders (push shoulders back as if touching them together)
- Chest (take a deep breath and hold for 10 seconds)
- Stomach (suck in your abdominal muscles)
- Buttocks (pull buttocks together)
- Thighs (straighten legs and squeeze muscles in thighs and hips)
- Leg calves (pull toes carefully toward you, avoid cramps)
- Feet (curl toes downward and point toes away from your body)

Finally, repeat several deep abdominal breaths and mentally check your body for tension. Rest comfortably for several minutes, breathing normally, and visualize your body as warm and relaxed. Get up slowly when you are finished.

Table 21.4 Medication for Panic Disorder

Medication	Starting Dose mg/day	Therapeutic Dose	Side Effects
Selective serotonin-reuptake inhibitors (SSRIs)			Class effects include nausea, anorexia, tremors, anxiety, sexual dysfunction, jitteriness, insomnia
Fluoxetine (Prozac)	10	20–60	Class effects
Sertraline (Zoloft)	25	50–200	Class effects, loose stools
Paroxetine (Paxil)	10	10–60	Class effects, drowsiness, fatigue, weight
Paroxetine (controlled release) (Paxil CR)	12.5	12.5–25	Class effects
Fluvoxamine (Luvox)	50	50–300	Class effects
Citalopram (Celexa)	10	20–60	Class effects
Escitalopram (Lexapro)	10	10–30	Class effects
Serotonin-norepinephrine reuptake inhibitors (SNRIs)			Class effects: Nausea, sweating, dry mouth, dizziness, insomnia, somnolence, sexual dysfunction, hypertension at dosages >300
Venlafaxine (Extended Release) (Effexor XR)	37.5	75–300	Class effects
Tricyclic Antidepressants (TCAs)			Class effects: sedation, weight gain, dry mouth, urinary hesitancy, constipation, orthostatic hypotension, and slow conduction time through the bundle of His
Imipramine (Tofranil)	10–25	50–300	Class effects
Nortriptyline (Pamelor)	10–25	25–125	Class effects
Desipramine (Norpramin)	10–25	25–300	Class effects
Benzodiazepines			Class effects: sedation, cognitive slowing, physical dependence
Clonazepam (Klonopin)	0.25 3 × daily	0.5–1.5 3 × daily	Class effects
Alprazolam (Xanax)	0.25 3 × daily	0.5–1.5 3 × daily	Class effects
Lorazepam (Ativan)	0.25 3 × daily	0.5–1.5 3 × daily	Class effects

The SSRIs produce anxiolytic effects by increasing the transmission of serotonin by blocking serotonin reuptake at the presynaptic cleft. The initial increase in serotonergic activity with SSRIs may cause temporary increases in panic symptoms and even panic attacks (Brauer, Nowicki, Catalano, & Catalano, 2002). After 4 to 6 weeks of treatment, anxiety subsides, and the antianxiety effect of the medications begins. Increased serotonin activity in the brain is believed to decrease norepinephrine activity. This decrease lessens cardiovascular symptoms of tachycardia and increased blood pressure that are associated with panic attacks (Gorman, Kent, Sullivan, & Coplan, 2000). See Chapter 20 for administration and monitoring side effects.

• NCLEXNOTE

Psychopharmacologic treatment is almost always needed. Antidepressants are the medication of choice. Antianxiety medication is used only for short periods of time.

Serotonin-Norepinephrine Reuptake Inhibitors (SNRIs)

The SNRIs increase levels of both serotonin and norepinephrine by blocking their reuptake presynaptically. Classified as antidepressants, the SNRIs are also used in anxiety disorders. Venlafaxine (Effexor) is the most commonly used SNRI (see Table 21.4). These medications have been shown to reduce severity of panic and anticipatory anxiety. Like the SSRIs, they should not be abruptly discontinued (Katon, 2006).

Benzodiazepine Therapy

High-potency benzodiazepines have produced antipanic effects, and their therapeutic onset is much faster (hours, not weeks) than that of antidepressants (Table 21.4). Therefore, benzodiazepines are tremendously useful in treating intensely distressed patients. Alprazolam (Xanax), lorazepam (Ativan), and clonazepam (Klonopin) are widely used for panic disorder. They are well tolerated but carry the risk for withdrawal symptoms upon discontinuation of use (see Box 21.4). Benzodiazepines are still commonly used for panic disorder even though SSRIs are recommended for first-line treatment of panic disorder (Bruce et al., 2004).

Administering and Monitoring Benzodiazepines

Treatment may include administering benzodiazepines concurrently with antidepressants for the first 4 weeks, then tapering the benzodiazepine to a maintenance dose. This strategy provides rapid symptom relief but avoids the complications of long-term benzodiazepine use. Benzodiazepines with short half-lives do not accumulate in the body, whereas benzodiazepines with half-lives of longer than 24 hours tend to accumulate with chronic treatment, are removed more slowly, and produce less intense symptoms on discontinuation of use (see Chapter 8).

Short-acting benzodiazepines, such as alprazolam, are associated with rebound anxiety, or anxiety that increases after the peak effects of the medication have decreased. Medications with short half-lives (alprazo-

BOX 21.4

Drug Profile: ***Alprazolam (Xanax)***

DRUG CLASS: Antianxiety agent

RECEPTOR AFFINITY: Exact mechanism of action is unknown; believed to increase the effects of γ-aminobutyrate.

INDICATIONS: Management of anxiety disorders, short-term relief of anxiety symptoms or depression-related anxiety, panic attacks with or without agoraphobia. Unlabeled uses for school phobia, premenstrual syndrome, and depression.

ROUTES AND DOSAGES: Available in 0.25-, 0.5-, 1-, and 2-mg scored tablets.

Adults: For anxiety: Initially, 0.25 to 0.5 mg PO tid titrated to a maximum daily dose of 4 mg in divided doses. For panic disorder: Initially, 0.5 mg PO tid increased at 3- to 4-d intervals in increments of no more than 1 mg/d. For school phobia: 2 to 8 mg/d PO. For premenstrual syndrome: 0.25 mg PO tid.

Geriatric patients: Initially, 0.25 mg bid to tid, increased gradually as needed and tolerated.

HALF-LIFE (PEAK EFFECT): 12 to 15 h (1–2 h)

SELECTED ADVERSE REACTIONS: Transient mild drowsiness, initially; sedation, depression, lethargy, apathy, fatigue, light-headedness, disorientation, anger, hostility, restlessness, headache, confusion, crying, constipation, diarrhea, dry mouth, nausea, and possible drug dependence.

WARNINGS: Contraindicated in patients with psychosis, acute narrow angle glaucoma, shock, acute alcoholic intoxication with depressed vital signs, pregnancy, labor and delivery, and breast-feeding. Use cautiously in patients with impaired hepatic or renal function, and severe debilitating conditions. Risk for digitalis toxicity if given concurrently with digoxin. Increased CNS depression if taken with alcohol, other CNS depressants, and propoxyphene (Darvon).

SPECIFIC PATIENT/FAMILY EDUCATION:

- Avoid using alcohol, or sleep-inducing or other OTC drugs.
- Take drug exactly as prescribed and do not stop taking the drug without consulting health care provider.
- Take drug with food if gastrointestinal upset occurs.
- Avoid driving a car or performing tasks that require alertness if drowsiness or dizziness occurs.
- Report any signs and symptoms of adverse reactions.
- Notify health care provider if severe dizziness, weakness, or drowsiness persists; rash or skin lesions, difficulty voiding, palpitations, or swelling of extremities occur.

lam, lorazepam) should be given in three or four doses spaced throughout the day, with a higher dose at bedtime to allay anxiety-related insomnia. Clonazepam, a longer-acting benzodiazepine, requires less frequent dosing and has a lower risk for rebound anxiety.

Because of their depressive CNS effects, benzodiazepines should not be used to treat patients with comorbid sleep apnea. In fact, these drugs may actually decrease the rate and depth of respirations. Exercise caution in elderly patients for these reasons. Discontinuing medication use requires a slow taper during a period of several weeks to avoid rebound anxiety and serious withdrawal symptoms. Benzodiazepines are not indicated in the chronic treatment of patients with substance abuse but can be useful in quickly treating anxiety symptoms until other medications take effect.

Symptoms associated with withdrawal of benzodiazepine therapy are more likely to occur after high doses and long-term therapy. They can also occur after short-term therapy. Withdrawal symptoms manifest in several ways, including psychological (apprehension, irritability, insomnia, and dysphoria), physiological (tremor, palpitations, vertigo, sweating, muscle spasm, seizures), and perceptual (sensory hypersensitivity, depersonalization, feelings of motion, metallic taste).

Monitoring Side Effects The side effects of benzodiazepine medications generally include headache, confusion, dizziness, disorientation, sedation, and visual disturbances. Sedation should be monitored after beginning medication use or increasing the dose. The patient should avoid operating heavy machinery until the sedative effects are known.

Monitoring for Drug Interactions Drugs that interact with benzodiazepines include TCAs and digoxin; interaction may result in increased serum TCA or digoxin levels. Alcohol and other CNS depressants, while used with benzodiazepines, increase CNS depression. Their concomitant use is contraindicated. Histamine-2 blockers (cimetidine) used with benzodiazepines may potentiate sedative effects. Monitor closely for effectiveness in patients who smoke; cigarette smoking may increase the clearance of benzodiazepines.

Teaching Points 

Warn patients to avoid alcohol because of the chance of CNS depression. In addition, warn them not to operate heavy machinery until the sedative effects of the medication are known.

Psychological Domain

Assessment

A complete psychological assessment is necessary to determine patterns of panic attacks, characteristic symptoms in attacks, and the patient's emotional, cognitive, or behavioral responses (see Chap. 10). A comprehensive assessment includes overall mental status, suicidal tendencies and thoughts, cognitive thought patterns, and avoidance behavior patterns. Moreover, a complete psychological evaluation provides the health care professional with a picture of the patient's baseline psychiatric condition. The nurse assesses the behavioral responses of the patient during the interview, noting topics that elicit behaviors suggesting the patient is uncomfortable or nervous (twisting hair, leg movements). The patient's self-concept is assessed, and present and past coping strategies are discussed to determine how the patient handles stress. Finally, a risk assessment is performed to determine the risk for developing psychiatric disorders, the threats to the patient's well-being, and the risk for symptom deterioration (see Chapter 10).

Self-Report Scales

Self-evaluation is difficult in panic disorder. Often the memories of the attack and its triggers are irretrievable. Several tools are available to characterize and rate the patient's state of anxiety. Examples of these symptom and behavioral rating scales are provided in Box 21.5. All of these tools are self-report measures and as such are limited by the individual's self-awareness and openness. However, the Hamilton Rating Scale for Anxiety (HAM-A), provided in Table 21.5, is an example of a scale rated by the clinician (Hamilton, 1959). This 14-item scale reflects both psychological and somatic aspects of anxiety.

Mental Status Examination

During mental status examination, individuals with panic disorder may exhibit anxiety symptoms, including restlessness, irritability, poor concentration, and apprehensive behavior. Disorganized thinking, irrational fears, and decreased ability to communicate often occur during a panic attack. Assess by direct questioning if the patient is experiencing suicidal thoughts, especially if the person is abusing substances or is taking antidepressant medications.

Assessment of Cognitive Thought Patterns

Catastrophic misinterpretations of trivial physical symptoms can trigger panic symptoms. Once identified, these thoughts should serve as a basis for individualizing patient education to counter such false beliefs. Table 21.6 presents a scale to assess catastrophic misinterpretations of the symptoms of panic.

Several studies have found that individuals who feel a sense of control have less severe panic attacks. Individuals who fear loss of control during a panic attack often make the following type of statements:

Table 21.5 Hamilton Rating Scale for Anxiety

Max Hamilton designed this scale to help clinicians gather information about anxiety states. The symptom inventory provides scaled information that classifies anxiety behavior and assists the clinician in targeting behaviors and achieving outcome measures. Provide a rating for each indicator based on the following scale:

0 = None 1 = Mild 2 = Moderate
3 = Severe 4 = Severe, grossly disabling

Item	Symptoms	Rating
Anxious mood	Worries, anticipation of the worst, fearful anticipation, irritability	
Tension	Feelings of tension, fatigability, startle response, moved to tears easily, trembling, feelings of restlessness, inability to relax	
Fear	Of dark, strangers, being left alone, animals, traffic, crowds	
Insomnia	Difficulty in falling asleep, broken sleep, unsatisfying sleep and fatigue on waking, dreams, nightmares, night terrors	
Intellectual (cognitive)	Difficulty concentrating, poor memory	
Depressed mood	Loss of interest, lack of pleasure in hobbies, depression, early waking, diurnal swings	
Somatic (sensory)	Tinnitus, blurring of vision, hot and cold flushes, feelings of weakness, picking sensation	
Somatic (muscular)	Pains and aches, twitching, stiffness, myoclonic jerks, grinding of teeth, unsteady voice, increased muscular tone	
Cardiovascular symptoms	Tachycardia, palpitations, pain in chest, throbbing of vessels, fainting feelings, missing beat	
Respiratory symptoms	Pressure or constriction in chest, choking feelings, sighing, dyspnea	
Gastrointestinal symptoms	Difficulty in swallowing, wind, abdominal pain, burning sensation, abdominal fullness, nausea, vomiting, borborygmi, looseness of bowels, loss of weight, constipation	
Genitourinary symptoms	Frequency of micturition, urgency of micturition, amenorrhea, menorrhagic, development of frigidity, premature ejaculation, loss of libido, impotence	
Autonomic symptoms	Dry mouth, flushing, pallor, tendency to sweat, giddiness, tension headache, raising of hair	
Behavior at interview	Fidgeting, restlessness or pacing, tremor of hands, furrowed brow, strained face, sighing or rapid respiration, facial pallor, swallowing, belching, brisk tendon jerks, dilated pupils, exophthalmos	

From Hamilton, M. (1959). The assessment of anxiety states by rating. *British Journal of Medical Psychology, 32,* 54.

BOX 21.5

Rating Scales for Assessment of Panic Disorder and Anxiety Disorders

Panic Symptoms

Panic-Associated Symptom Scale (PASS)

Argyle, N., Delito, J., Allerup, P., et al. (1991). The Panic-Associated Symptom Scale: Measuring the severity of panic disorder.*Acta Psychiatrica Scandinavica, 83,* 20–26.

Acute Panic Inventory

Dillon, D. J., Gorman, J. M., Liebowitz, M. R., et al. (1987). Measurement of lactate-induced panic and anxiety. *Psychiatry Research, 20,* 97–105.

National Institute of Mental Health Panic Questionnaire (NIMH PQ)

Scupi, B. S., Maser, J. D., & Uhde, T. W. (1992). The National Institute of Mental Health Panic Questionnaire: An instrument for assessing clinical characteristics of panic disorder. *Journal of Nervous and Mental Disease, 180,* 566–572.

Cognitions

Anxiety Sensitivity Index

Reiss, S., Peterson, R. A., & Gursky, D. M. (1986). Anxiety sensitivity, anxiety frequency, and the prediction of fearfulness. *Behaviour Research and Therapy, 24,* 1–8.

Agoraphobia Cognitions Questionnaire

Chambless, D. L., Caputo, G. C., Bright, P., & Gallagher, R. (1984). Assessment of fear in agoraphobics: The Body Sensations Questionnaire and the Agoraphobic Cognitions Questionnaire.*Journal of Consulting and Clinical Psychology, 52,* 1090–1097.

(Continued on following page)

BOX 21.5

Rating Scales for Assessment of Panic Disorder and Anxiety Disorders (Continued)

Body Sensations Questionnaire
Chambless, D. L., Caputo, G. C., Bright, P., & Gallagher, R. (1984). Assessment of fear in agoraphobics: The Body Sensations Questionnaire and the Agoraphobic Cognitions Questionnaire. *Journal of Consulting and Clinical Psychology, 52,* 1090–1097.

Phobias

Mobility Inventory for Agoraphobia
Chambless, D. L., Caputo, G. C., Jasin, S. E., et al. (1985). The mobility inventory for agoraphobia. *Behavior Research and Therapy, 23,* 35–44.

Fear Questionnaire
Marks, I. M., & Matthews, A. M. (1979). Brief standard self-rating for phobic patients. *Behaviour Research and Therapy, 17,* 263–267.

Anxiety

State-Trait Anxiety Inventory (STAI)
Spielberger, C. D., Gorsuch, R. L., & Luchene, R. E. (1976). *Manual for the State-Trait Anxiety Inventory.* Palo Alto, CA: Consulting Psychologists Press.

Penn State Worry Questionnaire (PSWQ)
16 items developed to assess the trait of worry.
Meyer, T., Miller, M., Metzger, R., & Borkovec, T. (1990). Development and validation of the Penn State Worry Questionnaire. *Behaviour Research and Therapy, 28(6),* 487–495.

Beck Anxiety Inventory
21 items rating severity of symptoms on a 4-point scale. Beck, A., Epstein, N., Brown, G., & Steer, R. (1988). An inventory for measuring clinical anxiety: The Beck Anxiety Inventory. *Journal of Consulting and Clinical Psychology, 56,* 893–897.

- "I feel trapped."
- "I'm afraid others will know, or I'll hurt someone."
- "I feel alone. I can't help myself."
- "I'm losing control."

These individuals also tend to show low self-esteem, feelings of helplessness, demoralization, and overwhelming fears of experiencing panic attacks. They may have difficulty with assertiveness or expressing feelings.

Nursing Diagnoses for the Psychological Domain

Anxiety is the primary nursing diagnosis applied to patients with any of these disorders, although many diagnoses address the individual areas regarding one's inability to manage the stress of the disorder (see Figure 21.1). Other diagnoses include Risk for Self-Harm, Social Isolation, Powerlessness, and Ineffective Family Coping. Diagnoses specific to physical panic symptoms such as dizziness, hyperventilation, and so forth are likely. These diagnoses may be applied to all the anxiety disorders covered in this chapter. Outcomes will vary.

Interventions for the Psychological Domain

Because medications treat only the biologic aspects of anxiety, psychological interventions are used to provide the patient with skills to minimize anxiety. The nurse can assist the patient in identifying triggers to anxiety and countering these triggers with individualized psychological measures. Distraction techniques, positive self-talk, panic control treatment, exposure therapy, implosion therapy, and cognitive-behavioral therapy (CBT) can be useful.

Consistent, supportive reassurance should be given to the patient in crisis. Reassure the patient that the panic symptoms are only temporary. After the crisis,

Table 21.6 Panic Attack Cognitions Questionnaire

Rate each of the following thoughts according to the degree to which you believe each thought contributes to your panic attack.

1 = Not at all 3 = Quite a lot
2 = Somewhat 4 = Very much

1. I'm going to die.	1	2	3	4
2. I'm going insane.	1	2	3	4
3. I'm losing control.	1	2	3	4
4. This will never end.	1	2	3	4
5. I'm really scared.	1	2	3	4
6. I'm having a heart attack.	1	2	3	4
7. I'm going to pass out.	1	2	3	4
8. I don't know what people will think.	1	2	3	4
9. I won't be able to get out of here.	1	2	3	4
10. I don't understand what is happening to me.	1	2	3	4
11. People will think I am crazy.	1	2	3	4
12. I'll always be this way.	1	2	3	4
13. I am going to throw up.	1	2	3	4
14. I must have a brain tumor.	1	2	3	4
15. I'll choke to death.	1	2	3	4
16. I'm going to act foolish.	1	2	3	4
17. I'm going blind.	1	2	3	4
18. I'll hurt someone.	1	2	3	4
19. I'm going to have a stroke.	1	2	3	4
20. I'm going to scream.	1	2	3	4
21. I'm going to babble or talk funny.	1	2	3	4
22. I'll be paralyzed by fear.	1	2	3	4
23. Something is physically wrong with me.	1	2	3	4
24. I won't be able to breathe.	1	2	3	4
25. Something terrible will happen.	1	2	3	4
26. I'm going to make a scene.	1	2	3	4

Adapted from Clum, G. A. (1990). Panic attack cognitions questionnaire. *Coping with panic: A drug-free approach to dealing with anxiety attacks.* Pacific Grove, CA: Brooks/Cole.

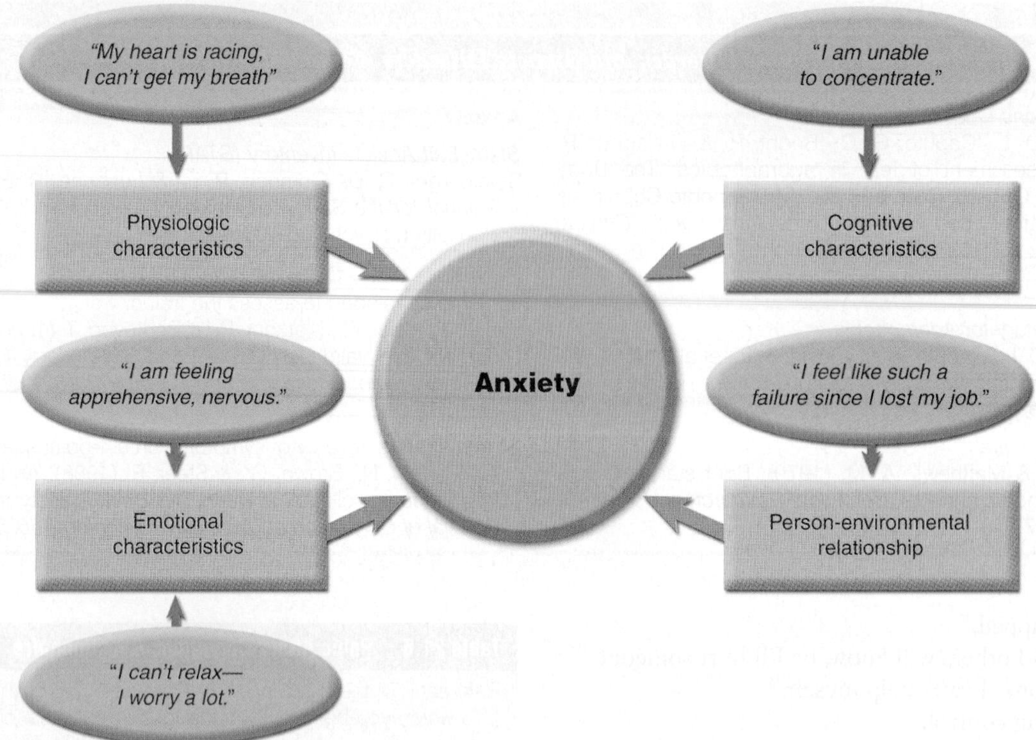

FIGURE 21.1. Nursing diagnosis concept map: anxiety.

the patient should be encouraged to vent his or her feelings. The feedback received from the patient should be used to revise or tailor the care plan.

Peplau devised general guidelines for nursing interventions that might be successful in treating patients with anxiety. These interventions help the patient attend to and react to input other than the subjective experience of anxiety. They are designed to help the patient focus on other stimuli and cope with anxiety in any form (Table 21.7). These general interventions apply to all anxiety disorders and therefore will not be reiterated in subsequent sections. Biopsychosocial interventions are addressed under the pertinent headings in Figure 21.2.

Table 21.7 Nursing Interventions Based On Degrees of Anxiety

Degree of Anxiety	Nursing Interventions
Mild	Assist patient to use energy anxiety provides to encourage learning.
Moderate	Encourage patient to talk: to focus on one experience, to describe it fully, then to formulate the patient's generalizations about that experience.
Severe	Allow relief behaviors to be used but do not ask about them. Encourage the patient to talk: ventilation of random ideas is likely to reduce anxiety to moderate level.
Panic	Stay with the patient. Allow pacing and walk with the patient. No content inputs to the patient's thinking should be made by the nurse. (They burden the patient, who will distort them.) Be direct with the fewest number of words: e.g., "Drink this" (give liquids to replace lost fluids and to relieve dry mouth); "Say what's happening to you," "Talk about yourself," or "Tell what you feel now" (to encourage ventilation and externalization of inner, frightening experience). Pick up on what the patient says, e.g., Pt: "What's happening to me—how did I get here?" N: "Say what you notice." Use short phrases to the point of the patient's comment. Do not touch the patient; patients experiencing panic are very concerned about survival, are experiencing grave threat to self, and usually distort intentions of all invasions of their personal space.

From Peplau, H. (1989). Theoretical constructs: Anxiety, self, and hallucinations. In A. O'Toole & S. Welt (Eds.), *Interpersonal theory in nursing practice: Selected works of Hildegarde E. Peplau.* New York: Springer.

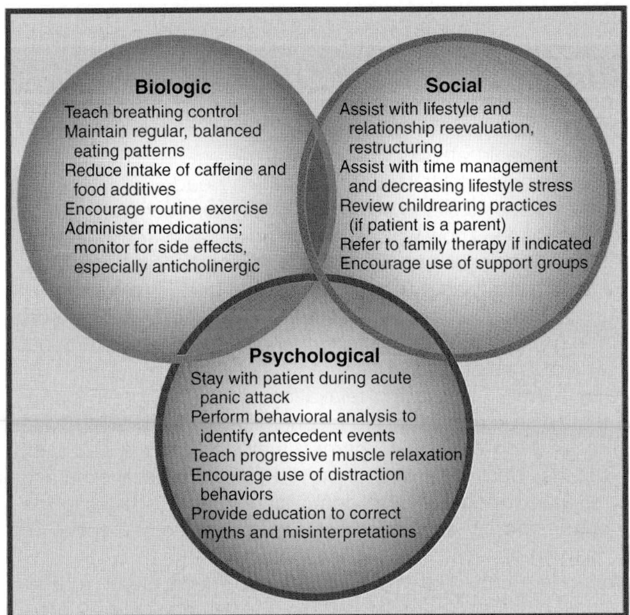

Biologic
Teach breathing control
Maintain regular, balanced eating patterns
Reduce intake of caffeine and food additives
Encourage routine exercise
Administer medications; monitor for side effects, especially anticholinergic
Social
Assist with lifestyle and relationship reevaluation, restructuring
Assist with time management and decreasing lifestyle stress
Review childrearing practices (if patient is a parent)
Refer to family therapy if indicated
Encourage use of support groups
Psychological
Stay with patient during acute panic attack
Perform behavioral analysis to identify antecedent events
Teach progressive muscle relaxation
Encourage use of distraction behaviors
Provide education to correct myths and misinterpretations

FIGURE 21.2. Biopsychosocial interventions for patients with panic disorder.

Distraction

Once patients can identify the early symptoms of panic, they may learn to implement **distraction** behaviors that take the focus off the physical sensations. Some distraction activities include initiating conversation with a nearby person or engaging in physical activity (e.g., walking, gardening, or house cleaning). Performing simple repetitive activities such as snapping a rubber band against the wrist, counting backward from 100 by threes, or counting objects along the roadway might deter an attack.

Positive Self-Talk

During states of increased anxiety and panic, individuals can learn to counter fearful or negative thoughts by using planned and rehearsed positive coping statements, called **positive self-talk**. "This is only anxiety, and it will pass," "I can handle these symptoms," and "I'll get through this" are examples of positive self-talk. These types of positive statements can give the individual a focal point and reduce fear when panic symptoms begin. Handheld cards that carry positive statements can be carried in a purse or wallet so that the person can retrieve them quickly when panic symptoms are felt (see Box 21.6).

Panic Control Treatment

Panic control treatment involves intentional exposure (through exercise) to panic-invoking sensations such as dizziness, hyperventilation, tightness in chest, and sweating. Identified patterns become targets for treatment. Patients are taught to use breathing training and cognitive restructuring to manage their responses and are instructed to practice these techniques between therapy sessions to adapt the skills to other situations.

Exposure Therapy

Exposure therapy is the treatment of choice for agoraphobia. The patient is repeatedly exposed to real or simulated anxiety-provoking situations until he or she becomes desensitized and anxiety subsides.

Systematic Desensitization

Systematic desensitization, another exposure method used to desensitize patients, exposes the patient to a hierarchy of feared situations that the patient has rated from least to most feared. The patient is taught to use muscle relaxation as levels of anxiety increase through multisituational exposure. Planning and implementing exposure therapy requires special training. Because of the multitude of outpatients in treatment for agoraphobia, exposure therapy would be a useful tool for home health psychiatric nurses. Outcomes of home-based exposure treatment are similar to clinic-based treatment outcomes.

Implosive Therapy

Implosive therapy is a provocative technique useful in treating agoraphobia in which the therapist identifies phobic stimuli for the patient and then presents highly anxiety-provoking imagery to the patient, describing the feared scene as dramatically and vividly as possible. **Flooding** is a technique used to desensitize the patient to the fear associated with a particular anxiety-provoking stimulus. Desensitizing is done by presenting feared objects or situations repeatedly without session breaks until the anxiety dissipates. For example, a patient with ophidiophobia might be presented with a real snake repeatedly until his or her anxiety decreases.

Cognitive-Behavioral Therapy

CBT is a highly effective tool for treating panic disorder. It has been considered first-line treatment for panic and other anxiety disorders and is often used in conjunction with medications, including the SSRIs, in treating panic disorder (Kampman, Keijsers, Hoogduin, & Hendriks, 2002). The goals of CBT include helping the patient to manage his or her anxiety and correcting anxiety-provoking thoughts through interventions, including cognitive restructuring, breathing training, and psychoeducation.

Psychoeducation

Psychoeducation programs help to educate patients and families about the symptoms of panic. Individuals

BOX 21.6

Therapeutic Dialogue: Panic Disorder With Agoraphobia

Panic Disorder With Agoraphobia

Mark, a 55-year-old Caucasian man, was admitted 4 days ago to the psychiatric unit with exacerbation of anxiety symptoms and panic attacks during the last 3 weeks. He has a 30-year history of uncontrolled anxiety that is refractory to medications and psychotherapy. On admission, he stated that he feels suicidal at times because he thinks his life is not within his control. He feels embarrassed, angry, and "trapped" by his disorder. During the past 24 hours, Mark is seen crying at times; he also isolates himself in his room. Michelle, Mark's nurse, enters his room to make a supportive contact and to assess his current mental status.

Ineffective Approach

Nurse: Oh... Why are you crying?

Patient: (Looks up, gives a nervous chuckle) Obviously, because I'm upset. I am tired of living this way. I just want to be normal again. I can't even remember what that feels like.

Nurse: You look normal to me. Everyone has bad days. It'll pass.

Patient: I've felt this way longer than you've been alive. I've tried everything and nothing works.

Nurse: You're not the first depressed person that I've taken care of. You just need to go to groups and stay out of your room more. You'll start feeling better.

Patient: (Angrily) Oh, it's just that easy. You have no idea what I'm going through! You don't know me! You're just a kid.

Nurse: I can help you if you help yourself. A group starts in 5 minutes, and I'd like to see you there.

Patient: I'm not going to no damn group! I want to be alone so I can think!

Nurse: (Looks about anxiously) Maybe I should come back after you've calmed down a little.

Effective Approach

Nurse: Mark, I noticed that you are staying in your room more today. What's troubling you?

Patient: (Looks up) I feel like I've lost complete control of my life. I'm so anxious and nothing helps. I'm tired of it.

Nurse: I see. That must be difficult. Can you tell me more about what you are feeling right now?

Patient: I feel like I'm going crazy. I worry all the time about having panic attacks. They make me scared I'm going to die. Sometimes I think I'd be better off dead.

Nurse: (Remains silent, continues to give eye contact)

Patient: Do you know what it's like to be a prisoner to your emotions? I can't even go out of the house sometimes and when I do, it's terrifying. I don't know what to think anymore.

Nurse: Mark, you have lived with this disorder for a long time. You say that the medications do not work to your liking, but what has helped you in the past?

Patient: Well, I learned in relaxation group that panic symptoms are probably caused by chemicals in my brain that are not working correctly. I learned that medications can help, but they don't work well for me. I tried an exposure plan and relaxation techniques to deal with my fears of leaving the house and my chronic anxiety. That did help some, but it's scary to do.

Nurse: It sounds like you have learned much about your illness, one that can be treated, so that you don't always have to feel this way.

Patient: This is easier to say right now when I'm here and can get help if I need it. It's hard to remember this when I'm in the middle of a panic attack and think I'm dying.

Nurse: It's harder when you're alone?

Patient: Much harder! And I'm alone so much of the time.

Nurse: Let's talk about some ways you can manage your panics when you're alone. Tell me some of the techniques you've learned.

Critical Thinking Challenge

- What tone is established by the nurse's opening question in the first scenario?
- Which therapeutic communication techniques did the nurse use in the second scenario to avoid the pitfalls encountered in the first scenario?
- What information was uncovered in the second scenario that was not touched on in the first?
- What predictions can you make about the interpersonal relationship likely to develop between the nurse and the patient in each scenario?

with panic disorder legitimately fear going crazy, losing control, or dying because of their physical symptoms. Attempting to convince a patient that such fears are groundless only heightens anxiety and impedes communication. Information and physical evidence, such as electrocardiogram results and laboratory test results, should be presented in a caring and open manner that demonstrates acceptance and understanding of their situation.

Box 21.7 suggests topics for individual or small-group discussion. It is especially important to cover such topics as the differences between panic attacks and heart attacks, the difference between panic disorder and other psychiatric disorders, and the effectiveness of various treatment methods.

Social Domain

Individuals with anxiety disorders, especially panic disorder and social phobias, often deteriorate socially as the disorder takes its toll on relationships with family and friends. If the disorder becomes severe enough, the person may become completely isolated. Therefore, the social domain must be assessed and treated.

Assessment

Marital and parental functioning can be adversely affected by panic disorder. During the assessment, the nurse should try to grasp the patient's understanding of how panic disorder with or without severe avoidance

BOX 21.7

Psychoeducation Checklist

Panic Disorder

When caring for the patient with panic disorder, be sure to include the following topic areas in the teaching plan:

- Psychopharmacologic agents (anxiolytics or antidepressants) if ordered, including drug action, dosage, frequency, and possible adverse effects
- Breathing control measures
- Nutrition
- Exercise
- Progressive muscle relaxation
- Distraction behaviors
- Exposure therapy
- Time management
- Positive coping strategies

behavior has affected his or her life along with that of the family. Pertinent questions include the following:

- How has the disorder affected your family's social life?
- What limitations related to travel has the disorder placed on you or your family?
- What coping strategies have you used to manage symptoms?
- How has the disorder affected your family members or others?

Cultural Factors

Cultural competence calls for the understanding of cultural knowledge, cultural awareness, cultural assessment skills, and cultural practice. Therefore, cultural differences must be considered in the assessment of panic disorder. Different cultures interpret sensations, feelings, or understandings differently. For example, symptoms of anxiety might be seen as witchcraft or magic (APA, 2000). Several cultures do not have a word to describe "anxiety" or "anxious" and instead may use words or meanings to suggest physical complaints. In addition, showing anxiety may be a sign of weakness in some cultures (Chen, Reich, & Chung, 2002). Many Asian OTC herbal remedies contain substances that may induce panic by increasing the heart rate, basal metabolic rate, blood pressure, and sweating (Chen et al, 2002). Diet pills and ginseng are two examples.

Nursing Diagnoses for the Social Domain

Social Isolation, Impaired Social Interaction, and Risk for Loneliness are usually supported with assessment data. Because the whole family is affected by one member's symptoms, Interrupted Family Processes may also occur.

Interventions for the Social Domain

Individuals with panic disorder, especially those with significant anxiety sensitivity, may need assistance in reevaluating their lifestyle. Time management can be a useful tool. In the workplace or at home, underestimating the time needed to complete a chore or being overly involved in several activities at once increases stress and anxiety. Procrastination, lack of assertiveness, and difficulties with prioritizing or delegating tasks intensify these problems.

Writing a list of chores to be completed and estimating time to complete them provides concrete feedback to the individual. Crossing out each activity as it is completed helps the patient to regain a sense of control and accomplishment. Large tasks should be broken into a series of smaller tasks to minimize stress and maximize sense of achievement. Rest, relaxation, and family time—frequently omitted from the daily schedule—must be included.

Family Response to Disorder 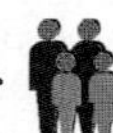

Families afflicted with panic disorder have difficulty with overall communication. Parents with agoraphobia may become critical of their child-rearing abilities, which may cause their children to be overly dependent. Parents with panic disorder may inadvertently cause excessive fears, phobias, or excessive worry in their children. Individuals will need a tremendous amount of support and encouragement from significant others.

Pharmacologic treatment for panic disorder also affects the family in other ways. Medications used to treat panic disorder readily cross the placenta and are excreted in breast milk, potentially barring breastfeeding women from treatment. Pregnancy may actually protect against certain anxiety disorders, but postpartum onset of such disorders is not uncommon. Decisions about taking medications during pregnancy and breast-feeding may lead to guilt, anxiety, and an exacerbation of symptoms.

• NCLEXNOTE

Cognitive therapy techniques give patients with anxiety a sense of control over the recurring threats of panic and obsessions.

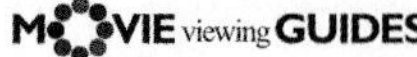

Evaluation and Treatment Outcomes

Patients can be assisted to keep a daily log of the severity of anxiety and the frequency, duration, and severity of panic episodes. This log will be a basic tool for monitoring progress as symptoms decrease. Rating scales may also be helpful to monitor changes in misinterpretations

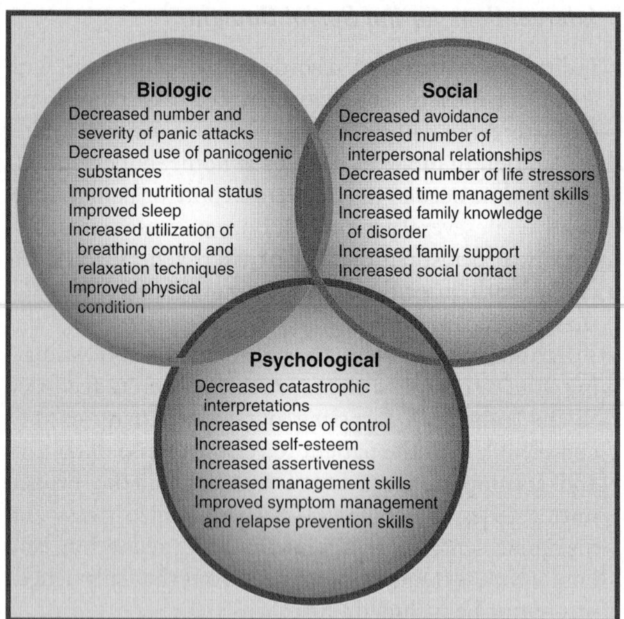

FIGURE 21.3. Biopsychosocial outcomes for patients with panic disorder.

or other symptoms related to panic. Medications alone provide significant short-term improvement for many individuals, but a long-term combination of psychosocial and pharmacologic treatment is usually necessary.

Although many researchers consider panic disorder a chronic, long-term condition, the positive results from outcome studies should be shared with patients to provide encouragement and optimism that patients can learn to manage these symptoms. Outcome studies have demonstrated success with panic control treatment, CBT therapy, exposure therapy, and various medications specific to certain symptoms. Figure 21.3 illustrates a number of examples of biopsychosocial treatment outcomes for individuals with panic disorder.

Continuum of Care

As with any disorder, continuum of patient care across multiple settings is crucial. Patients are treated in the least restrictive environment that will meet their safety needs. As the patient progresses through treatment, the environment of care changes from an emergency or inpatient setting to outpatient clinics or individual therapy sessions.

Inpatient-Focused Care

Inpatient settings provide control for the stabilization of the acute panic symptoms. Medication use often is initiated here because patients who show initial panic symptoms require in-depth assessment to determine the etiology. The patient is formally introduced to the disorder after the diagnosis is made. As crisis stabilization begins, medication management, milieu, and psychotherapies are introduced, and outpatient discharge linkage appointments are set.

Emergency! 

Because individuals with panic disorder are likely to first present for treatment in an emergency room or primary care setting, nurses working in these settings should be involved in early recognition and referral. Consultation with a psychiatrist or mental health professional by the primary care physician can decrease both costs and overall patient symptoms (Katon, Roy-Byrne, Russo, & Cowley, 2002). Unnecessary emergency department visits cause soaring health care costs. Several interventions may be useful in reducing the number of emergency room visits related to panic symptoms. Psychiatric consultation and nursing education can be provided in the emergency department to explore other avenues of treatment. Remembering that the patient experiencing a panic attack is in crisis, nurses can take several measures to help alleviate symptoms, including the following:

- Stay with the patient and maintain a calm demeanor. (Anxiety often produces more anxiety, and a calm presence will help calm the patient.)
- Reassure the patient that you will not leave, that this episode will pass, and that he or she is in a safe place. (The patient often fears dying and cannot see beyond the panic attack.)
- Give clear, concise directions, using short sentences. Do not use medical jargon.
- Walk or pace with the patient to an environment with minimal stimulation. (The patient in panic has excessive energy.)
- Administer PRN anxiolytic medications as ordered and appropriate. (Pharmacotherapy is effective in treating acute panic.)

After the panic attack has resolved, allow the patient to vent his or her feelings. This often helps the patient in clarifying his or her feelings.

Family Interventions 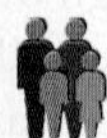

In addition to learning the symptoms of panic disorder, nurses should have information sheets or pamphlets available concerning the disorder and any medications prescribed. Parents, especially single parents, will need assistance in child rearing and may benefit from services designed to provide some respite. Moreover, the entire family will need support in adjusting to the disorder. A referral for family therapy may be indicated. Involving the entire family in the therapy process is imperative. Families experience the symptoms, treatments, clinical setbacks, and recovery from chronic mental illnesses as a unit. Misunderstandings, misconceptions, false information, and stigma of mental illness, singly or collectively, impede recovery efforts.

Community Treatment

Most individuals with panic disorder will be treated on an outpatient basis. Referral lists of community resources and support groups are useful in this setting. Nurses are more directly involved in treatment, conducting psychoeducation groups on relaxation and breathing techniques, symptom management, and anger management. Advanced practice nurses conduct CBT and individual and family psychotherapy. In addition, medication monitoring groups re-emphasize the role of the medications, monitor for side effects, and enhance treatment compliance overall. See Nursing Care Plan 21.1 and the Interdisciplinary Treatment Plan 21.1 that follows it.

OBSESSIVE-COMPULSIVE DISORDER

OCD is a psychiatric disorder characterized by severe obsessions or compulsions that interfere with normal daily routines. Affected patients feel that they have no control over the obsessions and compulsions, which have devastating consequences for patients.

Obsessions are characterized by excessive, unwanted thoughts or impulses that occur repetitively, causing se-

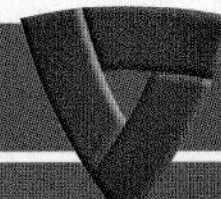

Nursing Care Plan 21.1

The Patient With Panic Disorder

Bill is a 65-year-old African American, unmarried man who began having his first panic attacks after he retired from a post office position 2 years ago. He has been able to live alone until recently, when his daughter became concerned that he was isolating himself and refused to drive to pay bills or to go to the grocery store for food. He admitted to being fearful of leaving because of extreme nervousness and fear of a panic attack. His daughter convinced him to seek help, and he is now in a day treatment program at a local facility. He is able to attend the program most days.

Setting: Day Treatment Program, Adult Psychiatric Services

Baseline Assessment: Bill averages three or four panic attacks per week. His mental status is normal, with no cognitive impairment. MMSE is within normal limits. He is depressed but does not meet criteria for a mood disorder. He misses his job and feels as if part of his identity is lost. Vital signs are normal. He has a known 10-year history of hypertension, with a heart attack at the age of 57 years. He would like to "get rid of the feeling of nervousness" and be able to enjoy life like he did before retirement.

Associated Psychiatric Diagnosis

Axis I: Panic disorder with agoraphobia
Axis II: None
Axis III: History of hypertension
Axis IV: Social problems (unable to leave home)
GAF = Current 60
Potential 90

Medications

Paroxetine CR (Paxil) 12.5 mg every day
Lisinopril (Zestril) 20 mg daily
Lorazepam (Ativan) 1 mg every 6 hours PRN for extreme anxiety

Nursing Diagnosis 1: Anxiety

Defining Characteristics

Trembling, increased pulse
Fearful, irritable, scared, worried
Apprehensive

Related Factors

Impending panic attacks
Panic attacks

Outcomes

Initial

Develop skills to decrease impact of panic attack

Long-term

Carry out normal daily living and social activities outside of the house

Continued

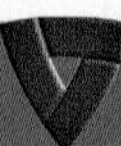

Nursing Care Plan 21.1 (Continued)

Interventions

Interventions	Rationale
Meet daily with Bill to assess if he has had a panic attack within the last 24 hours.	Asking Bill to monitor panic attacks will provide data regarding potential antecedents to attacks.
Using a calm, reassuring approach, encourage verbalization of feelings, perceptions, and fears. Identify periods of time when anxiety level is at its highest.	Discussing the experience of anxiety will help the patient notice when his anxiety increases.
Teach Bill how to perform relaxation techniques.	Having strategies to deal with impending panic attack will decrease the intensity of the experience.
Teach Bill about the actions and side effects of paroxetine. Explain the purposes of the medication. Track the number of PRN medications that are used for anxiety. Also, monitor for use of alcohol and herbal supplements.	Panic attacks are neurobiologic occurrences that respond to medications.

Ongoing Assessment

Determine whether Bill has had a panic attack.
Explore the antecedents and determine whether he was able to practice techniques from education programs.
Observe effectiveness of his technique and changes in anxiety/panic episodes.
Determine whether panic attacks decrease over time and whether there are side effects.
Determine his commitment to living a more normal life.

Evaluation

Outcomes	Revised Outcomes	Interventions
Bill's panic attacks decreased to once a week. Attended day treatment program every day. Able to go to grocery store.	Increase social activity outside of house.	Meet with Bill twice a week to monitor progress. Continue to reinforce the use of strategies in managing anticipatory anxiety.

vere anxiety and distress. Common obsessions include fears of contamination, pathologic doubt, the need for symmetry and completion, thoughts of hurting someone, and thoughts of sexual images (APA, 2000). Compulsions are repetitive actions or behaviors employed in an attempt to neutralize the anxiety felt from the obsession. For example, people with obsessive thoughts of becoming contaminated with dirt may wash their hands repeatedly to prevent contamination.

KEY CONCEPT Obsessions are unwanted, intrusive, and persistent thoughts, impulses, or images that cause anxiety and distress. Obsessions are considered ego-dystonic because they are not under the patient's control and are incongruent with the patient's usual thought patterns

KEY CONCEPT Compulsions are behaviors that are performed repeatedly, in a ritualistic fashion, with the goal of preventing or relieving anxiety and distress caused by obsessions.

Obsessions and compulsions are not necessarily signs of a psychiatric disorder if they are short lived and do not persistently interfere with the person's ability to function. However, obsessions can consume a person's judgment to the degree that most of his or her day is spent performing actions in an attempt to minimize severe anxiety.

Clinical Course

The typical age of onset of OCD is in the early 20s to mid-30s. Although symptoms of OCD often begin in childhood, many patients receive treatment only after the disorder has significantly affected their lives. The astute parent may notice that the child spends great amounts of time on trivial tasks or has falling grades because of poor concentration. Symptom onset of the disorder is gradual, and 15% of afflicted people show progressive decline in social and occupational functioning (APA, 2000). Men are affected more often as children and are most commonly affected by obsessions. Women have a higher incidence of checking and cleaning rituals, with onset typically in the early 20s (Castle & Groves, 2000). This chronic disorder is characterized by episodes of symptom amelioration and exacerbation, and is reported to have a lifetime prevalence of between 1.5% and 3% (Crino, Slade, & Andrews, 2005).

During the course of the disorder, the patient begins to realize that the obsessive thoughts and compulsive actions

INTERDISCIPLINARY TREATMENT PLAN 21.1

The Patient With Panic Disorder

ADULT PSYCHIATRIC CENTER DAY TREATMENT PROGRAM FOR BILL, A 65-YEAR–OLD MALE

Admission Date:	*Date of This Plan:*	*Type of Plan: Check Appropriate Box*				
5/26/08	5/27/08	☐ Initial Master	☐ 30	☐ 60	☐ 90	☐ Other

Treatment Team Present:
Smith, M., MD; S. Jones, RNC; G. Stevens, LCSW (social worker); V. Bond (Music Therapist)

DIAGNOSIS (DSM-IV-TR):

Axis I:	Panic disorder with agoraphobia
Axis II:	None
Axis III:	History of cardiac problems (hypertension)
Axis IV:	Social problems (unable to leave home)
Axis V:	Current GAF: 60
	Highest level GAF this past year: 90

ASSETS (MEDICAL, PSYCHOLOGICAL, SOCIAL, EDUCATIONAL, VOCATIONAL, RECREATIONAL):

1. No physical illness evident
2. Cognitive abilities intact, normal MMSE, wants to get better
3. Family supportive. Daughter is primary support and helps with cleaning and shopping. Able to live alone. Has a few friends. Is able to drive.
4. Now retired. Worked as a postal deliverer for many years. Enjoys card games with friends. Able to maintain his own home.

MASTER PROBLEM LIST

Change Prob. No.	*Date*	*Problem*	*Code*	*Code*	*Date*
1.	5/25/08	Recurring panic attacks interfere with his ability to engage in social activities and maintain independence			
2.					
3.					
4.					
5.					
6.					
7.					
8.					

CODE T = Problem must be addressed in treatment.
N = Problem noted and will be monitored.
X = Problem noted, but deferred/inactive/no action necessary.
O = Problem to be addressed in aftercare/continuing care.
I = Problem incorporated into another problem.
R = Resolved.

INDIVIDUAL TREATMENT PLAN PROBLEM SHEET

#1 Problem/Need:	*Date Identified*	*Problem Resolved/Discontinuation Date*
Recurring panic attacks interfere with his ability to engage in social activities and maintain independence.	5/26/08	

Objective(s)/Short-Term Goals:	*Target Date*	*Achievement Date*
1. Patient reports that he experiences no more than two panic attacks per week (down from 2–3 daily)	6/25/08	
2. Patient begins to go places outside of home.	7/25/08	

(Continued on following page)

INTERDISCIPLINARY TREATMENT PLAN 21.1 (Continued)

Treatment Interventions:	*Frequency*	*Person Responsible*
Attend day treatment program	Daily	RN monitor attendance
Relaxation group	Daily	AT
Panic Disorders Education Group	Daily	SW, RN
Individual counseling for monitoring anxiety and panic attacks	Daily	RN
Medications for anxiety and prevention of panic attacks	Daily	MD/RN
Family support group (patient's family)	Weekly	SW

Describe Patient Participation (and/or family, guardian, other agencies, significant others):

Responsible QMHP		**Patient or Guardian**		**Staff Physician**	
Signature	Date	Signature	Date	Signature	Date

are excessive and unnecessary but continues to have the thoughts and feels compelled to perform the actions.

Comorbidity

Tourette's syndrome has an interesting relationship with OCD. There are similar alterations in brain functioning, and the two disorders often occur together (Johannes et al., 2003; Luo et al., 2004). Other psychiatric disorders co-occur as well. As many as one third of patients with OCD subsequently experience depression because of OCD's effects on their lifestyle (Overbeek, Schruers, Vermetten, & Greiz, 2002). A significant number of older depressed patients have OCD (Fireman, Koran, Levanthal, & Jacobson, 2001). In addition, as many as 60% of people with OCD experience panic attacks. Recent literature suggests that bipolar disorder and cyclothymic disorder may be comorbid with OCD (Kirkby, 2003; Perugi et al., 2002). The lifetime risk for panic disorder, mood disorders, social phobia, specific phobias, disorders of impulse control, and eating disorders is greater in patients with OCD than in the general population (Kaye, Bulik, Thorton, Barbarich, & Masters, 2006).

Because the pressure to perform compulsions resulting from obsessions is untenably stressful, many patients self-medicate to relieve the anxiety produced by obsessive thoughts. About one third will experience substance abuse or dependence in their lifetime. In addition, some patients may abuse benzodiazepines and other anxiolytics, hypnotics, or sedatives.

Personality disorders are also prevalent in OCD, occurring in more than 80% of patients. Most prevalent are cluster C disorders (see Chapter 20). Obsessive-compulsive personality disorder was once thought to predispose an individual to OCD, which thus was the coexisting disorder most commonly diagnosed. However, dependent personality disorder most frequently coexists with OCD and is diagnosed in about half of patients. Also occurring at rates higher than those for the general population are obsessive-compulsive, avoidant, borderline, schizotypal, and paranoid personality disorders. Cluster A personality disorders may predict poorer treatment outcomes.

Diagnostic Criteria

The APA (2000) described five diagnostic criteria for OCD (see Table 21.8).

- Criterion A. The presence of obsessions or compulsions. Obsessions are defined as (1) persistent thoughts, images, or impulses that are intrusive and inappropriate, causing marked anxiety and (2) are not simply excessive fretting over real-life situations; (3) the person tries to ignore or suppress the thoughts, or tries to neutralize them by some other thought or action; and (4) the person understands that the thoughts are a product of his or her own mind. Compulsions are defined as (1) repetitive behaviors that the person feels he or she must perform because of the thoughts or because of rules that must be rigidly followed, and (2) actions performed to reduce stress or to prevent a catastrophe from occurring. The actions and thoughts are not realistically connected and are excessive to the situation.
- Criterion B. At some point in the disorder, the patient recognizes that the thoughts and actions are unreasonable or excessive. This criterion does not apply to children.
- Criterion C. The presence of the thoughts and rituals causes severe disturbance in daily routines, relationships, or occupational function and are time consuming, taking longer than 1 hour a day to complete.
- Criterion D. The thoughts or behaviors are not a result of another Axis 1 disorder.
- Criterion E. The thoughts or behaviors are not a result of the presence of a substance or a medical condition.

Table 21.8  **Key Diagnostic Characteristics of Obsessive-Compulsive Disorder 300.3** 

Diagnostic Criteria and Target Symptoms

- Recurrent obsession or compulsions
  - *Obsessions:* inappropriate and intrusive recurrent and persistent thoughts, impulses, or images causing marked anxiety or distress that are not simply excessive worries
  - Attempts to ignore, suppress, or neutralize obsessions with some other thought or action
  - Recognizes them as a product of his or her own mind
  - *Compulsions:* repetitive behaviors (such as hand-washing, ordering, checking) or mental acts (such as praying, counting) person feels driven to perform in response to obsession or according to rigid rules
  - Acts aimed at preventing or reducing the distress or preventing some dreaded event or situation
  - Compulsions not connected realistically with what they are designed to neutralize or prevent or are clearly excessive
- Recognition by person that obsessions or compulsions are excessive or unrealistic (if not, specify with poor insight)
- Obsessions or compulsions are excessive or unrealistic
- Marked distress that is time-consuming or significantly interfering with normal routine and functioning
- If another psychiatric disorder present, content of obsessions or compulsions not restricted to it
- Not a direct physiologic effect of substance use or medical condition

Associated Behavioral Findings

- Avoidance of situations involving the content of the obsession or compulsion
- Hypochondriacal concerns with frequent physician visits
- Guilt
- Sleep disturbances
- Excessive use of alcohol or sedative, hypnotic, or anxiolytic medications
- Compulsion performance a major life activity; may lead to serious marital, occupational, or social disability

Associated Physical Examination Findings

- Possible dermatologic problems caused by excessive washing with water or caustic cleaning agents

Associated Laboratory Findings

- Increased autonomic activity when confronted with circumstances that trigger obsession

The specifier "With Poor Insight" is added if the patient does not see that the thoughts or behaviors are excessive or unreasonable.

Special Populations

OCD affects people of all ages. Identification, diagnosis, and treatment of OCD is necessary for recovery and optimal functioning.

Children

OCD affects between 1% and 2.3% or more of children and adolescents (APA, 2000). Because children subscribe to myths, superstition, and magical thinking, obsessive and ritualistic behaviors may go unnoticed. Behaviors such as touching every third tree, avoiding cracks in the sidewalk, or consistently verbalizing fears of losing a parent in an accident may have some underlying pathology, but are common behaviors in childhood. Typically, parents notice that a child's grades begin to fall as a result of decreased concentration and great amounts of time spent performing rituals.

Elderly People

OCD typically manifests in childhood and the second decade of life. It can be a lifelong illness, lasting more than 30 years (Mataix-Cols et al., 2002). Predictors of poor outcomes during lifelong treatment include initial symptom onset during childhood, low social functioning, and the presence of both obsessions and compulsions (Castle & Groves, 2000).

Epidemiology

OCD has a 2.5% lifetime prevalence and a 1-year prevalence rate of 0.5% to 2.1% in the adult population. Rates are similar among women and men. First-degree relatives of people with OCD have a higher prevalence rate than the general population. Early onset OCD increases the chances of OCD in relatives and predicts poorer treatment outcomes (Busatto, 2001).

Many obsessive thoughts and compulsive acts are common in OCD. Checking rituals are common in this disorder, and those who perform these rituals are usually considered to be perfectionists. These patients must have objects in a certain order, perform motor activities in a rigid fashion, or arrange things in perfect symmetry. They may take a great deal of time to complete even the simplest task. These individuals tend to experience discontent, rather than anxiety, when things are not symmetrical or perfect. Other patients have magical thinking and perform compulsive rituals to ward off an imagined disaster. They use counting rituals to perform doing-and-undoing rituals (e.g., repeatedly turning on and off the alarm clock) to help them feel that a disaster will not occur. Hoarders feel compelled to check their belongings repeatedly to see that all is accounted for, and they may check the garbage to ensure that nothing of value was discarded.

Some patients have obsessions surrounding aggressive acts of hurting someone or themselves. After hitting a bump in the road, for example, these patients may obsess for hours over whether or not they hit a person. Parents may have recurrent intrusive thoughts that they may hurt their child.

Patients with religious obsessions obsess over the meaning of sins and whether they have followed the letter of the law. They tend to be hypermoral and have the need to confess. They may view their obsessions as a form of religious suffering. These patients are often resistant to treatment. Religious obsessions are most common where severe religious restrictions exist. Diagnosis is not made unless the thoughts or rituals clearly exceed cultural or religious norms, occur at inappropriate times as described by members of the same religion or culture, or interfere with social obligations (APA, 2000).

People with OCD are highly somatic and frequently seek medical treatment for physical symptoms, often just to get reassurance. Acquired immunodeficiency syndrome, cancer, heart attacks, and sexually transmitted diseases are some of the most common obsessional fears.

Etiology

During the 1990s, research evidence from neuroimaging studies, neurochemical studies, and treatment advances substantiated a predominantly neurobiologic basis for OCD. The following sections provide a brief overview of these findings and evidence pointing to genetic vulnerability. Psychological factors are also discussed because of their contributions to the disorder. Because no one explanation accounts for all aspects of OCD, a combination of factors will probably be found to produce the disorder.

Biologic Theories

Genetic, neuropathologic, and biochemical research, reviewed in this section, suggests that OCD has a biologic basis involving several neuroanatomic structures.

Genetic

OCD occurs more often in people who have first-degree relatives with OCD or with Tourette's disorder than it does in the general population. Some studies have also shown an increased prevalence of anxiety and mood disorders in relatives of individuals who have OCD. Twin studies have indicated that OCD occurs more frequently in both siblings of monozygotic twins than of dizygotic twins. Furthermore, Mundo and colleagues (2000) discovered a link between the pathogenesis of OCD and the 5-HT (β_{1D}) receptor gene. This discovery may lead to breakthroughs in pharmacologic treatments of OCD. Overall, genetic linkage to OCD is an area of needed research.

Neuropathologic

Structural neuroimaging studies using computed tomography and magnetic resonance imaging performed to find total-volume differences in brain structure have shown that people with OCD have enlarged basal ganglia (caudate, putamen, and globus pallidus) (Pujol et al., 2004).

Positron emission tomography and single-photon emission computed tomography reveal differences in cerebral glucose metabolism between patients with OCD and control subjects (see Chapter 16). Variation in methods of measurement produces some inconsistencies in the research findings. However, the most replicated results demonstrate increased glucose metabolism in the caudate nuclei (part of the basal ganglia), the orbitofrontal gyri (the gyri directly above the orbit of the eye), and the cingulate gyri (considered to be part of the limbic system). Studies measuring cerebral blood flow and glucose metabolism in patients with OCD during exposure to feared stimuli and during relaxation have further implicated these regions of the brain (Mataix-Cols, Wooderson, Lawrence, Brammer, Speckens, & Phillips, 2004).

Biochemical

Serotonin plays a role in OCD. It has been studied through challenge tests in which serotonin agonists were administered to patients with OCD and control subjects. The most convincing evidence for serotonin's role is that serotonin-specific antidepressants relieve the symptoms of OCD for most patients. A single neurotransmitter is unlikely to be entirely responsible for OCD, but to date, serotonin is the only neurotransmitter to have been implicated. Conventional and novel antipsychotic medications and mood stabilizers have been used in conjunction with serotonin-targeting medications to treat refractory symptoms, indicating that other biochemical processes exist (Foa et al., 2005).

Psychological Theories

Although psychological theories of OCD have not been scientifically tested, the rich literature describing clinical examples and case histories help us to understand the symptoms and behaviors related to OCD. In addition, behavioral treatment of individuals with severe compulsions has resulted in symptom improvement.

Psychodynamic

The psychodynamic theory hypothesizes that OCD symptoms and character traits arise from three unconscious defense mechanisms: isolation (separation of affect from a thought or impulse), undoing (an act performed with the goal of preventing consequences of a thought or impulse), and reaction formation (behavior and consciously stated attitudes that oppose underlying impulses). Classic psychoanalytic theory describes OCD as regression from the oedipal phase to the anal phase of development (see Chapter 7). This regression occurs when the patient becomes anxious about retaliation or loss of love. The anal phase is ambivalent, sadistic, and preoccupied with anger and dirt, thus the frequent occurrence of aggression and cleanliness obsessions.

Behavioral

Behavioral explanations for OCD stem from learning theory. From this viewpoint, obsessions are seen as conditioned stimuli. Through being associated with noxious events, stimuli that are usually considered neutral become anxiety provoking. The individual then engages in activities to escape or avoid the anxiety. Compulsions develop as the individual discovers behaviors that successfully reduce the obsessional anxiety. As the principles of operant conditioning indicate, the more the behaviors decrease the anxiety, the more likely the individual is to continue using them. However, the rituals or behaviors preserve the fear response because the person avoids the initial stimuli and thus never extinguishes the compulsion. Interrupting this cycle is the focus of behavioral therapy in treating an individual with OCD.

Risk Factors

Studies have found a link between infection with β-hemolytic streptococci and OCD (Arnold & Richter, 2001; Kurlan & Kaplan, 2004). High rates of OCD have also been found among individuals who are young, divorced or separated, and unemployed. OCD appears to be less common among African Americans than among non-Hispanic Caucasians.

Interdisciplinary Treatment

Patients with OCD can be difficult to treat because of their symptoms and the pathology of the disease. The obsessions and compulsions consistently interfere with recovery efforts during the treatment course. Staff may have differing opinions about the amount of control the patient has over the behavior, but these differences of opinion must be resolved, and all staff must be consistent in their expectations and acceptance of the patient's behaviors, to keep these patients from becoming frustrated or confused regarding expectations during treatment (Box 21.8).

BOX 21.8

Clinical Vignette: Obsessive-Compulsive Disorder

Robert, a 32-year-old man, is a new patient at a local psychiatric unit. He admitted himself to have his medicines evaluated because his obsessive thoughts and depression have worsened since his recent divorce. While in the hospital, he has quickly become viewed as a "problem patient" because he hoards linens and demands a new bar of soap for each of his five daily showers. He is compelled to open and close his door five times when he leaves or enters his room but does not know why. This behavior has led to arguments with his roommate. In an effort to "help him," the psychiatric technicians locked his bathroom door to prevent him from showering so frequently. He tried to enter his bathroom to shower, and panicked when the technicians refused to allow him to shower, telling him "You can live without it." After receiving PRN medication for extreme anxiety, Robert signed out of the hospital against medical advice because of embarrassment and anger toward the nursing staff.

What Do You Think?

- How could the technicians have handled the situation differently so as to not disrupt Robert's or the unit's clinical care?
- What nursing interventions might be appropriate in providing Robert's care?

Priority Care Issues

As with any patient with a psychiatric disorder, a suicide assessment must be completed. Although patients with OCD do not usually become suicidal as a direct result of anxiety, the disorder greatly distresses the patient, who realizes the pointlessness and absurdity of the behaviors. Often, the patient has tolerated symptoms for quite some time before seeking treatment. The patient may feel a sense of hopelessness and helplessness and may contemplate suicide to end the suffering. An additional risk for suicide is created by the high probability of major depression, which often accompanies OCD. Patients may feel a need to punish themselves for their intrusive thoughts (e.g., religious coupled with sexual obsessions). Some patients have aggressive obsessions, and external limits may have to be imposed for protection of others (see Chapter 34).

NURSING MANAGEMENT: HUMAN RESPONSE TO OBSESSIVE-COMPULSIVE DISORDER

Obsessions create tremendous anxiety, and patients perform compulsions to relieve the anxiety temporarily. If the compensatory ritual is not performed, the person feels increased anxiety and distress. Common compulsions include washing, cleaning, checking, counting, repeating actions, ordering (e.g., insisting that items be stored in a particular manner), confessing (e.g., repeatedly describing past misconduct), and requesting assurances.

Individuals with OCD do not consider their compulsions pleasurable. Often they recognize them as odd and may initially try to resist them. Resistance eventually fails, and patients incorporate repetitive behaviors into daily routines, performing activities in a specific, ritual order. If this sequence is disturbed, the person experiences extreme anxiety until the process can be repeated in the correct sequence (Table 21.8).

The most common obsession is fear of contamination and results in compulsive hand washing. Fear of contamination usually focuses on dirt or germs, but other materials may be feared as well, such as toxic chemicals, poison, radiation, and heavy metals. Patients with contamination obsessions report anxiety as their most common effect, but shame and disgust, linked with embarrassment and guilt, also are experienced.

Patients with OCD may become incapacitated by their symptoms and may spend most of their waking hours locked in a cycle of obsessions and compulsions. They may even become unable to complete a task as simple as walking through a door without performing rituals. Interpersonal relationships suffer, and the patient may actively isolate himself or herself. Patients with OCD may employ dissociation as a defense mechanism.

Depersonalization, a dissociative-type symptom common in OCD, is a nonspecific experience in which the individual loses the sense of personal identity and feels strange or unreal. The repetitive acts or compulsions of OCD are sometimes experienced by the individual as if the body is performing these acts without the person's intention or will. Patients with OCD who have dissociative symptoms tend to have more severe OCD symptoms, are more often depressed, and are more likely to have a coexisting personality disorder.

Biologic Domain

Assessment

Patients with OCD do not have a higher prevalence of physical disease. However, they may complain of multiple physical symptoms. With late-onset OCD (after 35 years of age) and with symptoms that occur with a febrile illness, cerebral pathology should be excluded. Each patient with OCD should be assessed for dermatologic lesions caused by repetitive hand washing, excessive cleaning with caustic agents, or bathing. Osteoarthritic joint damage secondary to cleaning rituals may be observed.

Nursing Diagnoses for the Biologic Domain

Patients with OCD may present with various symptoms, depending on the particular obsession and the compulsions that have evolved to cope with that obsession. As a result, the nursing diagnoses applied to patients with this disorder can run the gamut from the primary diagnosis of Anxiety to other physiologic disturbances of the compulsion, such as Impaired Skin Integrity, which may result from continuous hand washing. Outcomes depend on the nursing diagnoses and treatments selected.

Interventions for the Biologic Domain

Electroconvulsive Therapy

The effect of ECT on decreasing obsessions and compulsions has not been extensively studied. However, it may be helpful in treating symptoms that occur with depression. It also may be used to treat depressive symptoms in patients who have not experienced response to other treatments and who are at risk for suicide. Nursing's role in caring for the patient undergoing ECT is outlined in Chapter 18.

Psychosurgery

Psychosurgery has been used to treat extremely severe OCD that has not responded to prolonged and intensive drug treatment, behavioral therapy, or a combination of the two. Modern stereotactic surgical techniques that produce lesions of the cingulum bundle (a bundle of connective tissue) or anterior limb of the internal capsule (a region near the thalamus and part of the circuit connecting to the cortex) may bring about substantial clinical benefit in some patients without causing significant morbidity (Kim et al., 2003). Other treatment options include radiotherapy and deep brain stimulation in which electrical current is applied through an electrode inserted into the brain (Anderson & Ahmed, 2003).

Maintaining Skin Integrity

For the patient with cleaning or hand-washing compulsions, attention to skin condition is necessary. Encourage the patient to use tepid water when washing and hand cream after washing. Remove harsh, abrasive soaps and replace with moisturizing soaps. Attempt to decrease the frequency of washing by agreeing on a time schedule and time-limited washing.

Psychopharmacologic Treatment

The SSRIs and TCAs are considered to be the most effective treatment agents used for OCD. Clomipramine was the first drug to produce significant advances in treating OCD. Other medications have proved effective, including sertraline, fluoxetine, fluvoxamine, and paroxetine. Other drugs may be used to treat refractory OCD symptoms, including lithium, risperidone (Risperdal), quetiapine (Seroquel), olanzapine (Zyprexa), and haloperidol (Haldol). Neuroleptic augmentation is generally reserved for refractory symptoms.

Administering and Monitoring Medications

Antidepressants used to treat OCD are often given in higher doses than those normally used to treat depression. Aggressive treatment may be indicated to bring the symptoms under control. Thus, medication effects must be closely monitored, including signs of toxicity, to provide safe and adequate care. These medications often take several weeks or months to relieve compulsions, and even longer to decrease obsessions.

Clomipramine pharmacotherapy should begin at 25 mg daily, taken at night, with gradual titration during a period of 2 weeks to 150 mg to 250 mg daily, in divided doses. The maximum dose for children is 200 mg daily. This drug is not approved for children younger than 10 years.

Sertraline and fluvoxamine are indicated for OCD and should be initiated at 50 mg daily (25 mg daily in children). Sertraline can be titrated to a maximum dose of 200 mg daily but incrementally increased no less frequently than once a week. Fluvoxamine can be titrated by 50 mg daily, every 4 to 7 days, to a maximum daily dose of 300 mg. Doses greater than 100 mg should be divided. For children ages 8 to 11 years, start at 25 mg daily and increase by 25 mg every 4 to 7 days to a maximum daily dose of 200 mg. For children older than 11 years, 300 mg is the maximum daily dose.

Paroxetine or fluoxetine should be started at 20 mg daily, usually in the morning. Paroxetine can be titrated by 10 mg per week to a maximum of 60 mg daily. Fluoxetine dosage is titrated according to patient response to a maximum of 80 mg daily. The usual effective dose is 20 to 40 mg daily. Neither paroxetine nor fluoxetine is approved for the treatment of OCD in children.

Monitoring Side Effects

Side effects pose a particular problem for some individuals who are preoccupied with somatic concerns. Unwanted physical symptoms from the medications can become the focus of obsessions. These individuals particularly need frequent reassurance that they are not becoming physically ill and that the side effects are a common response to medication. To ignore or minimize these concerns will only heighten the patient's anxiety and potentially interfere with the desire to continue treatment.

Common side effects of clomipramine include significant sedation, anticholinergic side effects, and an increased risk for seizures. Dizziness, tremulousness, and headache are frequent complaints. Administration at night minimizes complaints of sedation and fatigue. Research is being conducted to compare responses to clomipramine and venlafaxine, a serotonin-norepinephrine reuptake inhibitor (SNRI) in the treatment of OCD. One preliminary study shows that venlafaxine may be as efficacious as clomipramine but with fewer harsh side effects (Albert, Aguglia, Maina, & Bogetto, 2002).

SSRIs all cause sedation, dizziness, somnolence, and headache. In addition, sexual dysfunction is a common complaint in patients being treated with fluvoxamine, sertraline, paroxetine, or fluoxetine. The SSRIs can cause excitability when first started. Monitor patients for insomnia and adjust the dosing time if needed. Weight gain can occur with SSRIs but is relatively rare. Research to curb this effect, possibly with mood stabilizing medications, is ongoing (Van Ameringen, Mancini, Pipe, Campbell, & Oakman, 2002).

Monitoring for Drug Interactions

All antidepressant medications interact with MAOIs, causing hypertensive crises; interaction with tryptophan may cause serotonin syndrome. Therefore, concomitant use should be avoided. Fluoxetine also interacts with thioridazine, TCAs, and lithium. Paroxetine interacts with thioridazine, histamine-2 blockers (cimetidine), phenytoin, digoxin, and warfarin. The use of thioridazine, cisapride, diazepam, and pimozide is contraindicated with fluvoxamine.

Because of the extensive list of drug–drug interactions associated with these medications, a prudent nurse will consult a drug reference handbook before administering medications. Quick recognition of signs and symptoms of interactions or toxic symptoms is imperative for safe care.

Teaching Points

Nurses play an important interdisciplinary role in managing medication for patients with OCD, which includes educating patients and families about medications. Because patients may become discontented with perceived lack of effect, they should be informed that these medications may take several weeks before their effects are felt. All patients should be warned not to abruptly stop taking prescribed medications.

Patients should be instructed to avoid alcohol and not to operate heavy machinery while taking these medications until the sedative effects are known. Instruct patients to inform their providers about any OTC medications they are taking because some will interact with these medications.

Psychological Domain

Assessment

The nurse should assess the type and severity of the patient's obsessions and compulsions. If the assessment occurs in a hospital, remember that some patients with OCD experience a transient decrease in symptoms when admitted to a hospital; therefore, enough time must be allowed for an accurate assessment. If time is unavailable, family members or significant others may provide an important source of information, with the patient's permission.

Most individuals will appear neatly dressed and groomed, cooperative, and eager to answer questions. Orientation and memory are not usually impaired, but patients may be distracted by obsessional thoughts. Individuals with severe symptoms may be preoccupied with fears or with discussing their obsessions, but in most instances, direct questions must be asked to reveal symptoms. For example, the nurse may begin indirectly by asking how long it takes the individual to dress in the morning or leave the house, but usually follow-up questions are needed, such as: Do you find yourself frequently returning to the house to make sure that you have turned off the lights or the stove, even when you know that you have already checked this? Does this happen every day? Are you ever late for work or for important appointments?

Speech will be of normal rate and volume, but often, individuals with an obsessional style of thinking will exhibit circumferential speech. This speech is loaded with irrelevant details but eventually addresses the question. Listening may be frustrating and require considerable patience, but you must remember that such speech is part of the disorder and may be beyond the patient's awareness. Continually interrupting and redirecting them can interfere with establishing a therapeutic relationship, especially in the initial assessment. Redirection should be done in a gentle and noncritical manner to allow the patient to refocus.

Identifying the degree to which the OCD symptoms interfere with the patient's daily functioning is important. Several rating scales can be used to identify symptoms and monitor improvement. Examples of these scales are provided in Box 21.9. Some of these scales are to be used by the nurse; others are self-rating scales. The Yale-Brown Obsessive Compulsive Scale (Y-BOCS) is a popular, clinician-rated 16-item scale that obtains separate subtotals for severity of obsessions and compulsions. The Maudsley Obsessive-Compulsive Inventory is a 30-item, true–false, self-assessment tool that may help the individual to recognize individual symptoms.

BOX 21.9

Rating Scales for Assessing Obsessive-Compulsive Symptoms

Yale-Brown Obsessive Compulsive Scale (Y-BOCS)
Goodman, W., Price, L., Rasmussen, S., et al. (1989). The Yale-Brown Obsessive Compulsive Scale (Y-BOCS): Part I. Development, use and reliability. *Archives of General Psychiatry, 46,* 1006–1011.

The Maudsley Obsessional-Compulsive Inventory (MOC)
Rachman, S., & Hodgson, R. (1980). *Obsessions and Compulsions.* New York: Prentice-Hall.

The Leyton Obsessional Inventory
Cooper, J. (1970). The Leyton Obsessional Inventory. *Psychiatric Medicine, 1,* 48.

Interventions for the Psychological Domain

The nurse's interpersonal skills are crucial to successful intervention with the patient who has OCD. Nurses must control their own anxiety. The nurse should interact with the patient in a calm, nonauthoritarian fashion without exhibiting any disapproval of the patient or the patient's behaviors, while demonstrating empathy about the distress that the disorder has caused (see Box 21.10). This approach is one of the most effective means available for communicating appreciation for the individual, as separate from the illness.

BOX 21.10

Using Reflection: Developing Self-Awareness

Incident: An energetic, excitable nurse told a patient who has OCD to hurry up and get dressed in order to get to the cafeteria for lunch. A few minutes later the patient is found sorting his clothes, making no progress toward getting dressed.

Reflection: The nurse reflected on her interaction with the patient. Although the nurse knew that interacting with a patient with OCD affected the level of anxiety the patient would feel, she was direct, hurried, and too autocratic in her approach to the patient. A calm, nonconfrontational approach would have been better.

Response Prevention

An effective behavioral intervention for patients with OCD who perform rituals is exposure with response prevention. The patient is exposed to situations or objects that are known to induce anxiety but is asked to refrain from performing the ritualistic behaviors. One goal of this procedure is to help the patient understand that resisting the rituals while exposed to the object of anxiety is less stressful and time-consuming than performing the rituals. Another goal is to confound the expectation of distressing outcomes and eventually extinguish the compulsive behaviors. Most patients improve with exposure and response prevention, but few become completely symptom free.

Thought Stopping

Thought stopping is used with patients who have obsessional thoughts. The patient is taught to interrupt obsessional thoughts by saying "Stop!" either aloud or subvocally. This activity interrupts and delays the uncontrollable spiral of obsessional thoughts. Research supporting this technique is scant; however, practitioners have found it useful in multimodal treatment with exposure and response prevention, relaxation, and cognitive restructuring.

Relaxation Techniques

Patients with OCD experience insomnia because of their heightened anxiety levels. Relaxation exercises may be helpful in improving sleep patterns. These exercises do not affect OCD symptoms, but they may be used to decrease anxiety. The nurse may also teach the patient other relaxation measures, such as deep breathing, taking warm baths, meditation, music therapy, or other quiet activities.

Cognitive Restructuring

Cognitive restructuring is a method of teaching the patient to restructure dysfunctional thought processes by defining and testing them (Beck & Emery, 1985). Its goal is to alter the patient's immediate, dysfunctional appraisal of a situation and perception of long-term consequences. The patient is taught to monitor automatic thoughts, then to recognize the connection between thoughts, emotional response, and behaviors. The distorted thoughts are examined and tested by for-or-against evidence presented by the therapist, which helps the patient to realistically assess the likelihood that the feared event will happen if the compulsive behavior is not performed. The patient begins to analyze his or her thoughts as incongruent with reality. For example, even if the alarm clock is not checked 30 times before going to bed, it will still go off in the morning, and the patient will not be disciplined for tardiness at work. Maybe it needs to be checked only once or twice.

Cue Cards

Cue cards are tools used to help the patient restructure thought patterns. They contain statements that are positively oriented and pertain to the patient's specific obsessions and compulsions. Cue cards use information from the patient's symptom hierarchy, an organizational system that breaks down the obsessions and compulsions from least to most anxiety provoking. These cards can help reinforce the belief that the patient is safe and can tolerate the anxiety caused by delaying or controlling compulsive rituals. Examples of cue cards are in Box 21.11.

Psychoeducation

Psychoeducation is a crucial nursing intervention for the patient with OCD. Knowledge is power, and the more the patient knows about his or her disorder, the more control he or she will have over symptoms.

Teaching Points 

The patient should be instructed not only about the biologic components of OCD but also about its treatments and disease course. Treatment is a shared responsibility between the patient and the provider, and the patient should be included in the medication and treatment decision-making processes. If local support groups are available, the patient should be referred to reduce feelings of uniqueness and embarrassment about the disease. Family education is also important, so that the patient will have help in practicing behavioral homework (Box 21.12).

Social Domain

Assessment

Nurses must consider sociocultural factors when evaluating OCD. At times, cultural or religious beliefs may

BOX 21.11

Examples of Cue Card Statements

- It's the OCD, not me.
- These are only OC thoughts; OC thoughts don't mean action; I will not act on the thoughts.
- My anxiety level goes up but will always go down. I never sat with the anxiety long enough to see that it would not harm me.
- Trust myself.
- I did it right the first time.
- Checking the locks again won't keep me safe. I really am safe in the world.

BOX 21.12

Psychoeducation Checklist

Obsessive-Compulsive Disorder

When caring for the patient with OCD, be sure to include the patient's caregiver, if appropriate, and address the following topic areas in the teaching plan:

- Psychopharmacologic agents (SSRIs, MAOIs, lithium, or anxiolytics) if ordered, including drug action, dosage, frequency, and possible adverse effects
- Skin care measures
- Ritualistic behaviors and alternative activities
- Thought stopping
- Relaxation techniques
- Cognitive restructuring
- Community resources

be misunderstood and mistaken for obsessions or compulsions. These beliefs and actions must be evaluated in the context of the individual's culture. If these beliefs are consistent with his or her social or cultural environment, are not harmful to the individual or others, and do not interfere with individual functioning in that environment, they are not considered symptoms of OCD.

Interventions for the Social Domain

- For the hospitalized patient, unit routines must be carefully and clearly explained to decrease fear of the unknown.
- At least initially, do not prevent the patient from engaging in rituals because the patient's anxiety level will increase.
- Recognize the significance of the rituals to the person and empathize with the patient's need to perform them.
- Assist the patient in arranging a schedule of activities that incorporates some private time but also integrates the patient into normal unit activities.

Family Response to Disorder

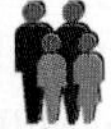

Marital status appears to be affected by OCD. Patients with OCD tend to remain single more often than do people without the disorder. They also have higher rates of celibacy, possibly because they fear being dirty or becoming contaminated. The divorce rate is lower than would be expected, given the stress of living with this disorder, and patients with OCD are able to draw their families gradually into accommodating abnormal behavior. For example, the families of patients with cleaning compulsions may forego normal family and social activities to "help" the patient complete compulsive cleaning of the family home and decrease the anxiety level in the household. Family assessment will reveal the amount of education and support needed and will begin the partnership among the patient, family, and treatment team. Evaluate the family's understanding of the disorder and of proposed treatments. Are they able and willing to help the patient practice cognitive and behavioral techniques? Are they knowledgeable about prescribed medicines? These questions offer a wonderful opportunity for patient and family education.

Family members offer a perspective on the severity of the patient's illness. Family members are experts in the patient's rituals and may observe subtle changes. Evaluate the family's response to changes in the patient's behavior as treatment progresses. You may have to discuss how the family will manage the changes brought about by a decrease in rituals (see Box 21.13). If obsessions and compulsions make it difficult for the individual to leave the home or function at work, financial difficulties may result. These factors should be assessed and appropriate assistance obtained through social services when necessary.

MOVIE viewing GUIDES

BOX 21.13

Research for Best Practice

Stengler-Wenzke, K., Trosbach, J., Dietrich, S., & Angermeyer, M. C.. (2004). Coping strategies used by the relatives of people with obsessive-compulsive disorder. Journal of Advanced Nursing, 48(1):35–42.

THE QUESTION A number of investigations have described coping strategies of relatives of patients with schizophrenia and other psychiatric disorders. But there have been no studies reported in the literature focusing on family coping strategies and OCD. Yet OCD is known to be a disease which negatively affects the quality of life of both the patient and the family.

METHODS Narrative interviews were conducted with family members of patients with OCD to explore their experience of burden and the coping strategies they had developed in response. Interviews were analyzed using a grounded theory approach.

FINDINGS Family members described experiencing different burdens and a variety of methods in attempts to cope with their relatives with OCD. Some families focused on patients' resources, seeking ways to support the patient, while others described assisting in rituals or actively opposing the patient's symptoms.

IMPLICATIONS FOR NURSING Findings from this study highlight the importance of evaluating the family's understanding of OCD, their experience of burden, and their styles of coping and support as they interact with their relative with OCD. Nurses can engage the family in a partnership to support the treatment plan, and teach positive coping strategies that will lessen the burden and anxiety of responding to their relative with OCD. Parents and spouses can be included in the teaching plan, with a focus on such topics as:

Biologic and psychological treatment approaches;
Medication management;
Strategies for social support;
Health-promoting responses to ritualistic behaviors.

Evaluation and Treatment Outcomes

Several methods can be used to measure the response to treatment, including nursing care: changes in Y-BOCS scores or other rating scales, remission of presenting symptoms, and the ability to complete activities of daily living. The patient should be able to participate in social or group activities with a degree of comfort and without self-harming or aggressive intent. He or she should also be able to demonstrate common knowledge of OCD by describing its symptoms, biologic basis, and treatments.

Continuum of Care

The symptoms of OCD can become debilitating. The symptoms wax and wane throughout treatment. As the focus of treatment shifts from inpatient to outpatient environments, patients must be assessed continually to ensure favorable patient outcomes through early intervention should symptoms resurface.

Inpatient-Focused Care

In an inpatient setting, the presence of a patient with severe OCD may present a nursing management challenge. These patients require a significant amount of staff time. They may monopolize bathrooms or showers or have disruptive rituals involving eating. Nurses play an integral role in treating the patient with OCD. The nurse should help the patient perform activities of daily living to ensure that they are completed. Monitoring medication effects, teaching psychoeducation groups, ensuring adequate caloric intake, and providing individual patient counseling are additional inpatient interventions.

Emergency!

Individuals with OCD frequently use medical services long before they seek psychiatric treatment. Therefore, early recognition of symptoms and referral are important concerns for nurses working in primary care and other medical settings. Once individuals are referred, most psychiatric treatment of OCD occurs on an outpatient basis. Although only individuals with severely debilitating symptoms or self-harming thoughts and actions are hospitalized, patients may experience intense anxiety symptoms to the point of panic. In such an emergency, benzodiazepines and other anxiolytics can be used.

Family Interventions 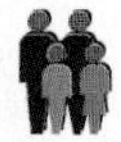

The families of patients with OCD will need to be educated about the etiology of the disorder. Understanding the biologic basis of the disorder should decrease some of the stigma and embarrassment they may feel about the bizarre nature of the patient's obsessions and compulsions. Education about both biologic and psychological treatment approaches should be provided.

Family assistance in monitoring symptom remission and medication side effects is invaluable. Family members can also assist the patient with behavioral and cognitive interventions.

When caring for the patient with OCD, be sure to include the patient's caregiver, if appropriate, and address the following topic areas in the teaching plan:

- Medications, including drug action, dosage, frequency, and possible adverse effects
- Skin care measures
- Ritualistic behaviors and alternative activities
- Thought stopping
- Relaxation techniques
- Cognitive restructuring
- Community resources

Community Treatment

Partial hospitalization programs and day treatment programs care for most patients with OCD. They allow patients to maintain significant independence while beginning medications and behavioral therapies. During inpatient treatment, the multidisciplinary treatment team should discuss the intensity of the required outpatient treatment. Some patients require outpatient treatment daily when symptoms are increased. Maintenance outpatient therapy may be scheduled weekly or twice weekly for several weeks until the symptoms are well controlled. Community agency visits are recommended to monitor medication.

GENERALIZED ANXIETY DISORDER

Generalized anxiety disorder (GAD) is characterized by excessive worry and anxiety (apprehensive expectation). It affects about 4% of the population, and is twice as common in women than men (Rabatin & Keltz, 2002). Individuals with this disorder experience excessive worry and anxiety almost daily for at least months. The anxiety does not usually pertain to a specific situation; rather, it concerns a number of real-life activities or events. Ultimately, the excessive worry and anxiety cause great distress and interfere with the patient's daily personal or social life.

Clinical Course

The onset of GAD is insidious. Many patients complain of being chronic worriers. GAD affects individuals of all ages. About half the individuals presenting for treatment report onset in childhood or adolescence, although onset after 20 years of age is also common. Adults with GAD often worry about matters such as their job, household finances, health of family members, or simple matters, such as household chores or being late for appointments. The intensity of the worry fluctuates, and stress tends to intensify the worry and anxiety symptoms (APA, 2000).

Patients with GAD may exhibit mild depressive symptoms, such as dysphoria. They are also highly somatic, with complaints of multiple clusters of physical symptoms, including muscle aches, soreness, and gastrointestinal ailments (APA, 2000). In addition to physical complaints, patients with GAD often experience poor sleep habits, irritability, trembling, twitching, poor concentration, and an exaggerated startle response. People with this disorder often present in a primary care setting, with a chief complaint of somatic symptoms (Rollman et al., 2005). Yet this highly prevalent disorder is rarely diagnosed and treated in the community (Stein et al., & Roy-Byrne, 2004).

Generally speaking, patients with GAD feel frustrated, disgusted with life, demoralized, and hopeless. They may state that they cannot remember a time that they did not feel anxious. They experience a sense of ill-being and uneasiness and a fear of imminent disaster. Over time, they may recognize that their chronic tension and anxiety is unreasonable.

Comorbidity

Patients with GAD often have other psychiatric disorders. Roughly three quarters of patients with GAD have at least one additional current or lifetime psychiatric diagnosis. The most common comorbid disorders are major depressive disorder, social phobia, specific phobia, panic disorder, and dysthymia. Lenze et al. (2000) found that 27.5% of depressed elderly patients have a comorbid anxiety disorder; Beekman et al. (2000) found that 30.3% of patients with GAD also had major depressive disorder.

Alcoholism is a significant problem associated with GAD. Patients with GAD may use alcohol, anxiolytics, or barbiturates to relieve anxiety symptoms, but this self-medication potentially leads to dependency.

Diagnostic Criteria

The APA (2000) describes several diagnostic features of GAD: excessive worry and anxiety about several issues that occurs more days than not for a period of at least 6 months (Criterion A). The patient has little or no control over the worry (Criterion B). The anxiety and worry are accompanied by at least three of the following symptoms for at least 6 months: sleep disturbance, becoming easily fatigued, restlessness, poor concentration, irritability, and muscle tension (Criterion C). The worry and anxiety focuses are not limited to the qualities of another psychiatric diagnosis, including panic disorder, social phobia, OCD, separation anxiety disorder, anorexia nervosa, somatization disorder, or hypochondriasis and do not exclusively occur with PTSD (Criterion D). The worry and anxiety cause significant impairment in social, occupational, or another significant area of functioning (Criterion E). Finally, the disturbance is not substance induced or caused by a general medical condition and does not occur exclusively with a mood, psychotic, or pervasive developmental disorder (Criterion F) (see Table 21.9).

Table 21.9 Key Diagnostic Characteristics of General Anxiety Disorder

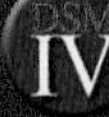

Diagnostic Criteria and Target Symptoms	Associated Findings
• Excessive anxiety and worry (apprehensive expectation) occurring for more days than not for at least 6 months involving a number of events or activities Restlessness or feeling keyed up or on edge Being easily fatigued Difficulty concentrating or mind going blank Irritability Muscle tension Sleep disturbance • Difficulty controlling the worry • Focus of anxiety and worry not confined to another psychiatric disorder • Clinically significant distress or impairment of functioning resulting from anxiety, worry, or physical symptoms • Not a direct physiologic effect of a substance or medical condition • Does not occur exclusively during a mood disorder, psychotic disorder, or pervasive developmental disorder	*Associated Behavioral Findings* • Possible depressive symptoms *Associated Physical Examination Findings* • Muscle tension with twitching, trembling, feeling shaky, and muscle aches and soreness • Clammy cold hands, dry mouth, sweating, nausea or diarrhea, "lump in the throat"

Special Populations

GAD may be overdiagnosed in children because symptoms overlap with those of other psychiatric disorders (APA, 2000). In addition, children have to meet only one of the additional symptoms outlined in Criterion C (rather than three, as adults do). Children with GAD manifest their symptoms through worry about their performance in school or sports and often excel in these areas (Castellanos & Hunter, 2000). Somatic complaints in children with GAD are heightened. Children may also worry about trivial issues, such as what clothes to wear or about physical appearance or social interactions. Children with the disorder tend to be perfectionistic and conforming, seeking frequent approval from parents or authority figures.

Elderly people also experience GAD, although anxiety in old age has not received much attention. Nonetheless, many elderly patients in depression and anxiety studies meet the criteria for GAD or have significant anxiety symptoms (Beekman et al., 2000; Lenze et al., 2000; Wang, Berglund, & Kessler, 2000). Elderly patients with GAD have been treated with benzodiazepines, which are known to produce memory and motor impairment.

Epidemiology

Because comorbid psychiatric diagnoses are common, assessing the true prevalence of this disorder is difficult. However, GAD is common, affecting nearly 4% of the population at any given time. The lifetime prevalence rate is nearly 5%. Of those presenting at anxiety disorder clinics, 25% have GAD and a primary or comorbid diagnosis (APA, 2000). In clinical settings, women and men are fairly equally distributed. In wider studies, roughly 66% of patients with GAD are female (APA, 2000).

Etiology

Biologic theories of causation for GAD have not been extensively studied. GAD may not be a true disease in itself, but rather a phase of other psychiatric disorders. Nonetheless, the fact that GAD has consistent symptoms, which can be controlled with medication, have led investigators to consider several biologic possibilities.

Neurochemical Theories

Symptoms suggesting activation of the sympathetic nervous system are common in GAD, and studies have found evidence of norepinephrine system dysregulation. Venlafaxine, a serotonin-norepinephrine reuptake inhibitor (SNRI), is approved for the treatment of GAD. Medications that act on serotonin, such as the SSRIs, are also effective in treating anxiety. This fact has led investigators to explore whether serotonin dysfunction is related to GAD. Although more research is needed to understand the underlying pathophysiology, serotonin and the GABA–benzodiazepine receptor complex appear to be involved. However, although the effects of benzodiazepines in reducing the symptoms of anxiety have been well documented, little research has been done to clarify the function of GABA and the benzodiazepine receptors in GAD (Mathew et al., 2004).

Genetic Theories

Few studies have examined genetic and familial factors in the etiology of GAD. One study of twins revealed that GAD is a moderately inheritable disorder. Individuals with GAD may have a genetic vulnerability that predisposes them to anxiety sensitivity. Biologic foundations involved in the development of anxiety disorders might be the same ones responsible for depression (APA, 2000; Hettema, & Prescott, & Kendler, 2004; Wade, Bulik, Prescott, & Kendler, 2004). The family environment might also play an important role because one may become anxious through learned behavior.

Psychological Theories

Cognitive-behavioral theory regarding the etiology of GAD proposes that the disorder results from inaccurate assessment of perceived environmental dangers. These inaccuracies result from selective focus on negative details, distorted information processing, and an overly pessimistic view of one's coping ability. Psychoanalytic theory postulates that anxiety represents unresolved unconscious conflicts. Sources of anxiety change in different developmental stages and include such conflicts as fear of separation or fear of loss of love.

Sociologic Theories

Although there are no specific sociocultural theories related to the development of GAD, a high-stress lifestyle and multiple stressful life events may be contributors. Kindling results from overstimulation or repeated stimulation of nerve cells by environmental stressors. Individuals with GAD are hypersensitive to stress and anxiety-provoking events.

Risk Factors

Unresolved conflicts, cognitive misinterpretations, and life stressors are examples of potential contributors to the development of the disorder. Patients may have a genetic predisposition to anxiety sensitivity. Behavioral inhibition, characterized by shyness, fear, or becoming withdrawn in unfamiliar situations, may be a risk factor for GAD and other anxiety disorders (Castellanos & Hunter, 2000).

NURSING MANAGEMENT: HUMAN RESPONSE TO GENERALIZED ANXIETY DISORDER

Nursing assessment and intervention for individuals with GAD include many of the same biopsychosocial considerations that apply to panic disorder. Assessment of the patient's anxiety symptoms should include the following questions; answers are used to tailor individual approaches:

- How do you experience anxiety symptoms?
- Are your symptoms primarily physical, psychological, or both?
- Are you aware when you are becoming anxious?
- Are you aware that anxiety induces the physical symptoms?
- What coping mechanisms do you routinely use to deal with anxiety?
- What life stressors add to these symptoms? What changes can you make to reduce these stressors?

Biologic Domain

Assessment

Diet and Nutrition

Some ordinary food stimulants, such as caffeine, are known to induce anxiety symptoms, and patients with GAD may be hypersensitive to them. Many OTC medications can alter mood and may increase anxiety symptoms. A concrete step that patients with GAD can take to reduce anxiety is to eliminate caffeine from their diets. Nurses can help patients achieve a caffeine-free state through education and dietary management, while assisting with pain relief for the headache that often accompanies caffeine withdrawal. Additional substances that can provoke anxiety are diet pills, amphetamines, ginseng, and ma huang (Chen, Reich, & Chung, 2002).

Sleep Patterns

Sleep disturbance is a common symptom for individuals with GAD, so the patient's sleep pattern should be assessed closely. Alcohol should be avoided because it disturbs the sleep cycle. Help the patient with measures that promote sleep, such as eating the last meal of the day in the early evening, avoiding fluids after 8:00 PM, and taking a warm bath before bedtime.

Interventions for Biologic Domain

The physical symptoms of anxiety and the neurotransmitter systems involved suggest that several medications can be effective in treating GAD. Benzodiazepines are most commonly used, but antidepressants (paroxetine, imipramine, and venlafaxine), buspirone, and β-blockers have all proved effective.

Administering and Monitoring Medications

Although widely used in patients with GAD, benzodiazepine treatment remains somewhat controversial. If the patient self-medicates, benzodiazepines may complicate treatment because of their addictive qualities. However, many people with GAD are reluctant to take prescribed medications, and most do not seek treatment until their level of suffering is substantial. Benzodiazepines offer quick relief from anxiety symptoms until the antidepressant therapeutic effects are felt, which may take a few weeks. Hydroxyzine shows promise for treating GAD and may provide an alternative to benzodiazepines (Llorca et al., 2002).

Buspirone. Buspirone (BuSpar) is an anxiolytic that acts by inhibiting spontaneous firing of serotonergic neurons in the dorsal raphe and by antagonism of 5-HT1a receptors in the dorsal raphe, hippocampus, and parts of the frontal cortex. Buspirone does not interact with benzodiazepine receptors and may increase brain noradrenergic and dopaminergic activity (see Chapter 9 for additional information). Buspirone must be taken for 3 to 4 weeks before its anxiolytic effects are felt. This delay may be difficult for patients to tolerate, particularly if they have used benzodiazepines in the past and are familiar with their rapid onset of action. Although buspirone effectively treats anxiety symptoms, patients may discontinue the treatment because of the lag in therapeutic effect.

Antidepressants. Venlafaxine, paroxetine, and imipramine have proven effective in treating GAD. They have serotonergic and noradrenergic effects, which are believed to reduce anxiety symptoms (Flynn & Chen, 2003).

Monitoring Side Effects

TCAs (imipramine) and benzodiazepines cause significant side effects and drug interactions that require ongoing monitoring. (See the discussions of these medications in the section on treatment of panic disorder.)

Buspirone side effects include dizziness, insomnia, drowsiness, and nervousness. Dry mouth, blurred vision, and abdominal distress can occur but are uncommon.

Venlafaxine has a relatively benign side-effect profile. Anticholinergic effects, including dry mouth and constipation, are common. This drug also causes dizziness, nervousness, and insomnia. Transient hypertension occurs in some patients; therefore, blood pressure should be monitored. Gastrointestinal effects (nausea and vomiting) can occur as well.

Monitoring for Drug Interactions

Venlafaxine and buspirone both interact with MAOIs, and neither should be initiated within 14 days of treatment of each other. Although buspirone does not increase alcohol-induced impairment, it is prudent to avoid use of alcohol because it depresses the CNS.

Teaching Points 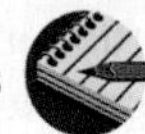

Teaching points for venlafaxine and buspirone include informing the patient that the anxiolytic effects of the medication will not be felt for several weeks. Warn patients against operating heavy machinery until they know the effects of the medication. If benzodiazepine therapy is being tapered and buspirone therapy started, instructions to the patient should include a warning not to discontinue use of the benzodiazepine suddenly because of the risks of withdrawal, including rebound anxiety and seizures.

Psychological and Social Domains

Psychological and social assessment and intervention strategies for GAD are similar to those for panic disorder; refer to the section on panic disorder.

Cognitive and behavioral therapies, effective treatments for GAD, are generally underused. Outcome studies indicate that cognitive treatment achieves significant reductions in the severity of somatic and anxiety symptoms, with many patients regaining normal function. Combining relaxation, supportive, and cognitive therapies may potentiate therapeutic effects.

Evaluation and Treatment Outcomes

Nursing diagnoses that apply to GAD are the same as for panic disorder, including Anxiety; Powerlessness; Sleep Pattern; Low Self-Esteem; and Disturbed, Ineffective Family Coping. Interventions are individualized and are focused on the patient and the family in controlling or coping with the anxiety. Interventions for panic disorder apply to controlling the symptoms of GAD.

Treatment outcomes for patients with GAD include reducing the frequency and intensity of anxiety and controlling the factors that stimulate or provoke this uncomfortable state. Specifically, evaluation can focus on the individual's ability and skills in using techniques that control anxiety, such as relaxation, positive self-talk, and stress management. Reducing personal and environmental stress; eliminating certain foods and drinks, such as caffeine, in the diet; and developing strategies to deal with stressful family situations are outcome successes.

Continuum of Care

Like patients with panic disorder, patients with GAD often seek treatment in emergency rooms or from medical internists because of the physical symptoms associated with the illness. Only about one third of patients with GAD seek psychiatric treatment (APA, 2000), and many patients do not seek any treatment. Many patients with GAD who do seek treatment consult internists, cardiologists, or neurologists for their physiologic symptoms. Nurses in these settings must be aware of the disorder and able to provide necessary assessment and intervention. Nurses in home health settings have an excellent opportunity to identify symptoms of undiagnosed GAD and make appropriate referrals.

Inpatient and outpatient management of GAD is similar to the treatments detailed in the section on panic disorder. Because anxiety produces more anxiety, a calm, reassuring, and nonjudgmental approach is necessary. Whether treatment is home or clinic based, both the patient and the provider must actively participate in monitoring and managing environmental stress levels. Patients need a relaxing and unstimulating environment. Reducing noise and lowering lights induces relaxation; methods such as breathing control exercises, progressive muscle relaxation, and other interventions discussed previously in this chapter may also be helpful (see Box 21.14).

Specific Phobia

Specific phobia (formally simple phobia) is a disorder marked by persistent fear of clearly discernible, circumscribed objects or situations, which often leads to avoidance behaviors. The lifetime prevalence rates range from 7% to 11%, and the disorder generally affects women twice as much as men. It has a bimodal distribution, peaking in childhood and then again in the 20s. The

BOX 21.14

Psychoeducation Checklist

Generalized Anxiety Disorder

When caring for the patient with generalized anxiety disorder, be sure to include the following topic areas in the teaching plan:

- Psychopharmacologic agents (benzodiazepines, antidepressants, nonbenzodiazepine anxiolytics, and/or β-blockers) if ordered, including drug action, dosage, frequency, and possible adverse effects
- Breathing control
- Nutrition and diet restriction
- Sleep measures
- Progressive muscle relaxation
- Time management
- Positive coping strategies

focus of the fear in specific phobia may result from the anticipation of being harmed by the phobic object. For example, dogs are feared because of the chance of being bitten or automobiles are feared because of the potential of crashing. The focus of fear may likewise be associated with concerns about losing control, panicking, or fainting on exposure to the phobic object.

Anxiety is usually felt immediately on exposure to the phobic object, and the level of anxiety is usually related to both the proximity of the object and the degree to which escape is possible. For example, anxiety heightens as a cat approaches a person who fears cats, and lessens when the cat moves away. At times, the level of anxiety escalates to a full panic attack, particularly when the person must remain in a situation from which escape is deemed to be impossible. Fear of specific objects is fairly common, and the diagnosis of specific phobia is not made unless the fear significantly interferes with functioning or causes marked distress. Assessment differentiates simple phobia from other diagnoses with overlapping symptoms. Box 21.2 lists a number of specific phobias. Among adult patients who are seen in clinical settings, the most to least common phobias are situational phobias, natural environment phobias, blood–injection–injury phobia, and animal phobias. The most common phobias among community samples are of heights, mice, spiders, and insects (APA, 2000).

Blood-injection-injury type phobia merits special consideration because the phobia surrounds medical treatments. The physiologic processes that are exhibited during phobic exposure include a strong vasovagal response, which significantly increases blood pressure and pulse, followed by deceleration of the pulse and lowering of blood pressure in the patient. Monitor closely when giving required injections or medical treatments.

About 75% of patients with blood–injection–injury phobia report fainting on exposure. Factors that may predispose individuals to specific phobias may include traumatic events, unexpected panic attacks in the presence of the phobic object or situation, observation of others experiencing a trauma, or repeated exposure to information warning of dangers, such as parents repeatedly warning young children that dogs bite.

Phobic content must be evaluated from an ethnic or cultural background. In many cultures, fears of spirits or magic are common. They should be considered part of a disorder only if the fear is excessive in the context of the culture, causes the individual significant distress, or impairs the ability to function.

Psychotropic drugs have not been effective in the treatment of specific phobia. Anxiolytics may give short-term relief of phobic anxiety, but there is no evidence that they affect the course of the disorder. The treatment of choice for specific phobia is exposure therapy. Patients who are highly motivated can experience success with treatment (Newman, Erickson, Przeworski, & Dzus, 2003).

Social Phobia

Social phobia (social anxiety disorder) involves a persistent fear of social or performance situations in which embarrassment may occur. Exposure to a feared social or performance situation nearly always provokes immediate anxiety and may trigger panic attacks. People with social phobias fear that others will scrutinize their behavior and judge them negatively. They often do not speak up in crowds out of fear of embarrassment. They will go to great lengths to avoid feared situations. If avoidance is not possible, they will suffer through the situation with visible anxiety.

People with social phobia appear to be highly sensitive to disapproval or criticism, tend to evaluate themselves negatively, and have poor self-esteem and a distorted view of personal strengths and weaknesses. They may magnify personal flaws and underrate any talents. They often believe others would act with more assertiveness in a given social situation. Men and women with social phobia tend to have difficulties with dating and with sexual relationships (Bodinger et al., 2002). Children tend to underachieve in school because of test-taking anxiety. This is an important area that should be assessed in all patients.

Generalized social phobia is diagnosed when the individual experiences fears related to most social situations, including public performances and social interactions. These individuals are likely to demonstrate deficiencies in social skills, and their phobias interfere with their ability to function. Generalized social phobia may be linked to low dopamine receptor binding, as suggested by recent research (Schneier et al., 2000).

People with social phobias fear and avoid only one or two social situations. Classic examples of such situations are eating, writing, or speaking in public or using public bathrooms. The most common fears for individuals with social phobia are public speaking, fear of meeting strangers, eating in public, writing in public, using public restrooms, and being stared at or being the center of attention.

Pharmacotherapy is a relatively new area of research in treating social phobia. SSRIs are used to treat social phobia because they significantly reduce social anxiety and phobic avoidance (Stein, Fyer, Davidson, Pollack, & Wiita, 1999). Paroxetine has proven effective for long-term treatment (Stein, Versiani, Hair, & Kumar, 2002). Benzodiazepines are also used to reduce anxiety caused by phobias. Providing referrals for appropriate psychiatric treatment is a critical nursing intervention.

Posttraumatic Stress Disorder

PTSD affects roughly 8% of the general population, and women are more likely than men to be affected. PTSD is defined by characteristic symptoms that develop after a traumatic event involving a personal experience of threatened death, injury, or threat to physical integrity. It may also include witnessing such an event happening to another person or learning that a family member or close friend has experienced such an event. Examples of traumatic events are violent personal assault, military combat, natural disasters, terrorist attack, being taken hostage, incarceration as a prisoner of war, torture, automobile accident, or being diagnosed with a life-threatening illness.

Patients with PTSD re-experience the event through distressing images, thoughts, or perceptions and may have recurrent nightmares. In addition, the patient may experience flashbacks and exhibit extreme stress on exposure to an event or image that resembles the traumatic event (e.g., fireworks may bring back memories of war). Patients may avoid discussing the event altogether or avoid people and places that remind them of the traumatic event. Patients may experience difficulty sleeping, irritability, poor concentration, exaggerated startle response, or hypervigilance (APA, 2000).

Risk factors for PTSD include a prior diagnosis of acute stress disorder (Brewin, Andrews, Rose, & Kirk, 1999). Pre-existing personality; extent, duration, and intensity of trauma involved; environmental issues; high levels of anxiety; low self-esteem, and existing personality difficulties may increase the likelihood of PTSD developing.

Sertraline is approved for treating PTSD. Treatment begins at 25 mg daily and is titrated to a maximum of 200 mg/d. Minipress, an antihypertensive agent, has been found to decrease recurrent nightmares in patients with PTSD (Raskind et al., 2002). This is an area for future research.

Acute Stress Disorder

Acute stress disorder involves the development of anxiety, dissociation, and other symptoms after a recent exposure to a traumatic stressor. Stressors include those specified for PTSD. Within 4 weeks of the traumatic event and lasting for at least 2 days, the patient continually re-experiences the event, avoids situations that remind him or her of the event, and has increased anxiety and excitation that negatively affect his or her lifestyle. The patient must have three dissociative symptoms, including numbing, detachment, a reduction of awareness to one's surroundings, derealization, depersonalization, or dissociative amnesia (APA, 2000). After 1 month, the diagnosis is changed to PTSD if symptoms persist.

Dissociative Disorders

Dissociative disorders are thought to be responses to extreme external or internal events or stressors. Prevalence is higher among people who experience childhood physical or sexual abuse than among others. The onset of these disorders may be sudden or occur gradually, and the course of each may be long-term or transient.

Dissociation, or a splitting from self, may occur as a form of coping with severe anxiety. The essential feature of the five disorders in this class involves a failure to integrate identity, memory, and consciousness. This class of disorders includes dissociative amnesia, the inability to recall important, yet stressful information; dissociative fugue, unexpected travel away from home with the inability to recall one's past and confusion about personal identity or the assumption of a new identity; depersonalization disorder, the feeling of being detached from one's mental processes; dissociative identity disorder, formerly multiple personality disorder (see Chapter 35); and dissociative disorder not otherwise specified. See Table 21.10 for diagnostic criteria and assessment findings. Persons with dissociative disorders may also have comorbid substance abuse, mood disorders, personality disorders (Cluster B), or PTSD. Treatment options include the use of antidepressants to treat underlying mood and anxiety. Psychotherapy options include hypnotherapy, cognitive-behavioral therapy, and psychoanalytic psychotherapy to discover the triggers that lead to heightened anxiety and dissociation.

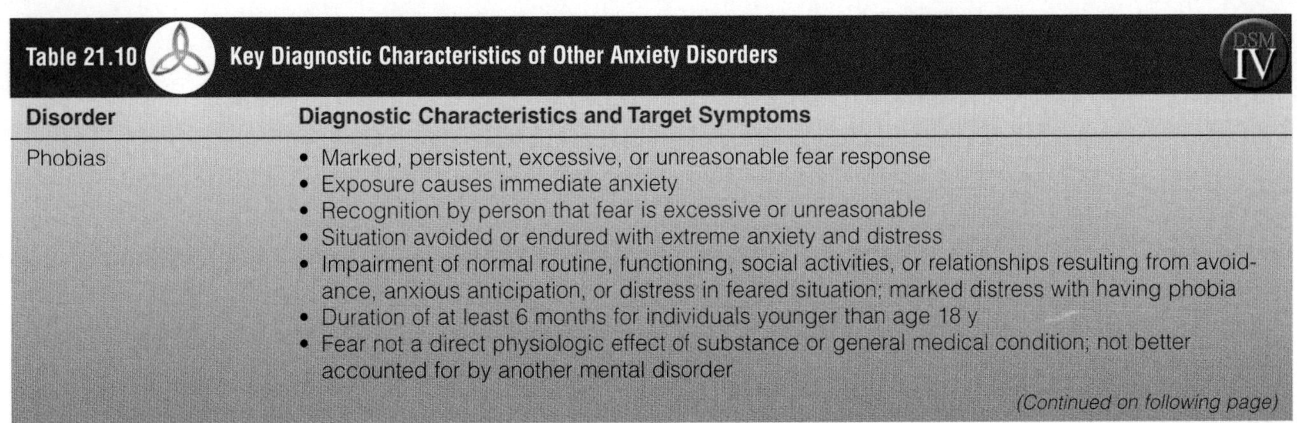

Table 21.10 Key Diagnostic Characteristics of Other Anxiety Disorders DSM IV

Disorder	Diagnostic Characteristics and Target Symptoms
Phobias	• Marked, persistent, excessive, or unreasonable fear response • Exposure causes immediate anxiety • Recognition by person that fear is excessive or unreasonable • Situation avoided or endured with extreme anxiety and distress • Impairment of normal routine, functioning, social activities, or relationships resulting from avoidance, anxious anticipation, or distress in feared situation; marked distress with having phobia • Duration of at least 6 months for individuals younger than age 18 y • Fear not a direct physiologic effect of substance or general medical condition; not better accounted for by another mental disorder

(Continued on following page)

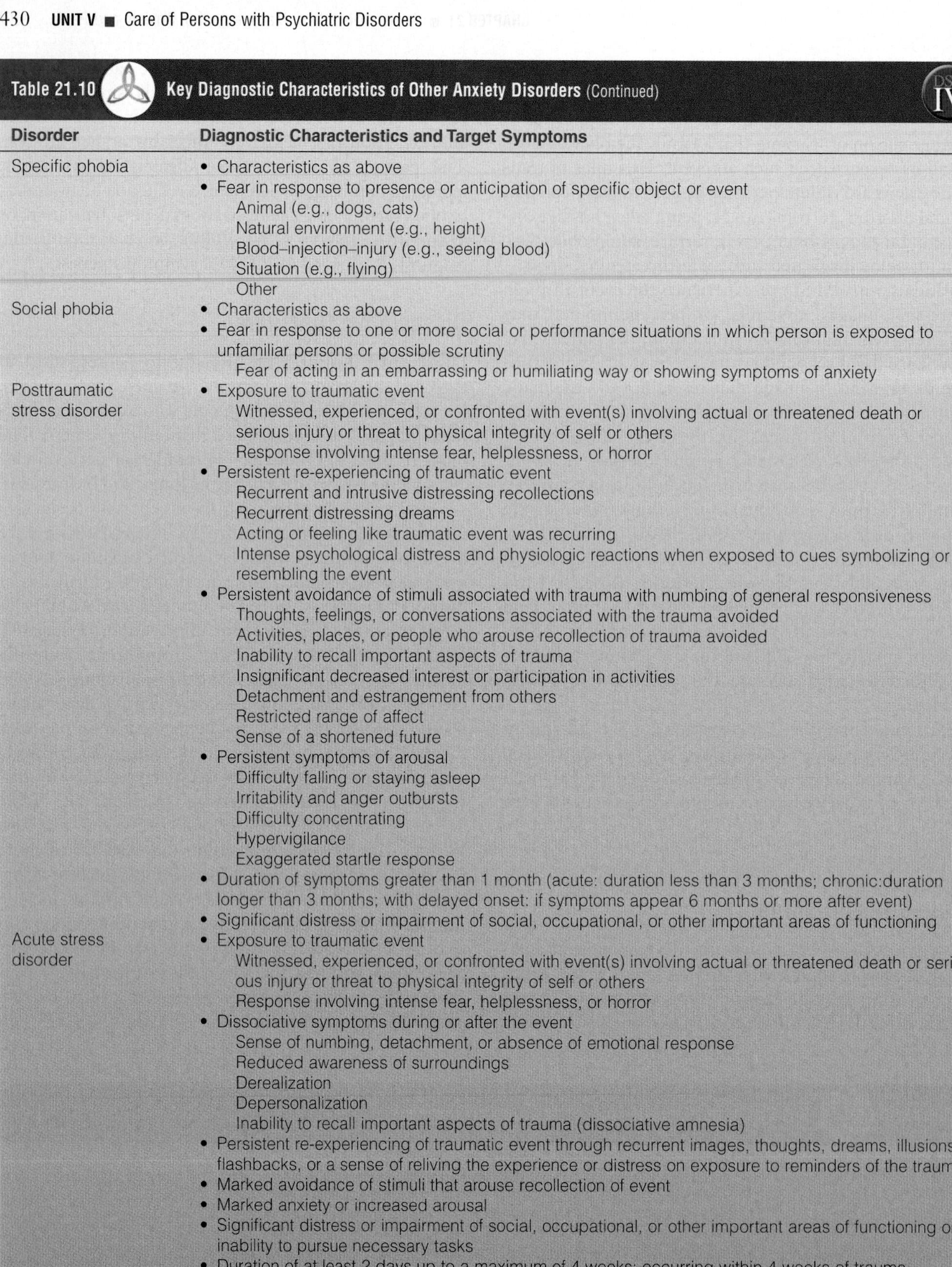

Table 21.10 Key Diagnostic Characteristics of Other Anxiety Disorders (Continued) DSM IV

Disorder	Diagnostic Characteristics and Target Symptoms
Specific phobia	• Characteristics as above • Fear in response to presence or anticipation of specific object or event Animal (e.g., dogs, cats) Natural environment (e.g., height) Blood–injection–injury (e.g., seeing blood) Situation (e.g., flying) Other
Social phobia	• Characteristics as above • Fear in response to one or more social or performance situations in which person is exposed to unfamiliar persons or possible scrutiny Fear of acting in an embarrassing or humiliating way or showing symptoms of anxiety
Posttraumatic stress disorder	• Exposure to traumatic event Witnessed, experienced, or confronted with event(s) involving actual or threatened death or serious injury or threat to physical integrity of self or others Response involving intense fear, helplessness, or horror • Persistent re-experiencing of traumatic event Recurrent and intrusive distressing recollections Recurrent distressing dreams Acting or feeling like traumatic event was recurring Intense psychological distress and physiologic reactions when exposed to cues symbolizing or resembling the event • Persistent avoidance of stimuli associated with trauma with numbing of general responsiveness Thoughts, feelings, or conversations associated with the trauma avoided Activities, places, or people who arouse recollection of trauma avoided Inability to recall important aspects of trauma Insignificant decreased interest or participation in activities Detachment and estrangement from others Restricted range of affect Sense of a shortened future • Persistent symptoms of arousal Difficulty falling or staying asleep Irritability and anger outbursts Difficulty concentrating Hypervigilance Exaggerated startle response • Duration of symptoms greater than 1 month (acute: duration less than 3 months; chronic:duration longer than 3 months; with delayed onset: if symptoms appear 6 months or more after event) • Significant distress or impairment of social, occupational, or other important areas of functioning
Acute stress disorder	• Exposure to traumatic event Witnessed, experienced, or confronted with event(s) involving actual or threatened death or serious injury or threat to physical integrity of self or others Response involving intense fear, helplessness, or horror • Dissociative symptoms during or after the event Sense of numbing, detachment, or absence of emotional response Reduced awareness of surroundings Derealization Depersonalization Inability to recall important aspects of trauma (dissociative amnesia) • Persistent re-experiencing of traumatic event through recurrent images, thoughts, dreams, illusions, flashbacks, or a sense of reliving the experience or distress on exposure to reminders of the trauma • Marked avoidance of stimuli that arouse recollection of event • Marked anxiety or increased arousal • Significant distress or impairment of social, occupational, or other important areas of functioning or inability to pursue necessary tasks • Duration of at least 2 days up to a maximum of 4 weeks; occurring within 4 weeks of trauma • Not a direct physiologic effect of a substance or general medical condition; not better accounted for by other mental disorder
Dissociative identity disorder	• Two or more distinct identities or personality states—each with own pattern of perceiving, relating to, and thinking about the environment and the self • Control of person's behavior by at least two of the identities • Inability to recall important personal information; too extensive to be due to forgetfulness • Not a direct physiologic effect of a substance or general medical condition

SUMMARY OF KEY POINTS

- Anxiety-related disorders are the most common of all psychiatric disorders and comprise a wide range of disorders, including panic disorder, OCD, GAD, phobias, acute stress disorder, PTSD, and dissociative disorder.
- The anxiety disorders share the common symptom of recurring anxiety but differ in symptom profiles. Panic attacks occur in many of the disorders.
- Those experiencing anxiety disorders have a high level of physical and emotional illness and often experience dual diagnoses with other anxiety disorders, substance abuse, or depression. These disorders often render individuals unable to function effectively at home or at a job.
- Patients with panic disorder are often seen in a number of health care settings, frequently in hospital emergency rooms or clinics, presenting with a confusing array of physical and emotional symptoms. Skillful assessment is required to eliminate possible life-threatening causes.
- Current research points to a combination of biologic and psychosocial factors that cause persistent anxiety. The initial stage of panic attack seems to be biologically generated by neural activity in the brain stem. There is also biologic evidence that anticipatory anxiety is linked to the kindling phenomenon occurring in the limbic system, which lowers one's biologic threshold for response to stressors. The last stage of phobic avoidance is a learned phenomenon that involves considerable cognitive activity, occurring in the prefrontal cortex. Other research demonstrates that there are also personality traits that predispose individuals to anxiety disorders, including low self-esteem, external locus of control, some negative family influences, and some traumatic or stressful precipitating event. These biologic and psychosocial components combine to yield a true biopsychosocial theory of causation.
- Treatment approaches for all anxiety-related disorders are somewhat similar, including pharmacotherapy, psychological treatments, or often a combination of both.
- Nurses at the generalist level use interventions from each of the dimensions—biologic, psychological, and social. Approaching these patients with knowledge of the disorder, understanding, and calm is crucial. Nurses can be instrumental in crisis intervention, medication management, and psychoeducation.
- Psychoeducation is crucial in the management of anxiety disorders and includes methods to help patients control and cope with the anxiety reactions (i.e., control of breathing, stress reduction, and relaxation techniques), education regarding medication side effects and management, and education of family members to understand these disorders.
- OCD is a rather rare disorder but is often difficult to diagnose because patients do not often seek help. It is characterized by unwanted, intrusive, and persistent thoughts (i.e., fear of germ contamination) that cause so much anxiety and distress that the individual feels compelled to perform ritualistic, repetitive actions (excessive hand washing and cleaning) to reduce the agonizing anxiety.

CRITICAL THINKING CHALLENGES

1. How does patient culture affect the assessment of anxiety?
2. How might one differentiate shyness from social anxiety disorder?
3. How might the etiology of depression and anxiety be similar, as antidepressant medications are used to treat both?
4. What are some of the barriers in assessing pathologic anxiety in children? Are anxiety disorders underdiagnosed or overdiagnosed in children? Explain.
5. What role might parents, aside from genetics, play in contributing to the development of anxiety disorders in their offspring?
6. What are the risks and benefits of treating anxiety disorders with benzodiazepine medications in persons with substance abuse?
7. Pregnancy appears to protect against the development of some anxiety disorders, and postpartum onset of anxiety disorders is not uncommon. What biopsychosocial dynamics may be involved?

Dirty Filthy Love: 2004. Mark Furness (played by Michael Sheen) is an architect whose marriage and career is threatened by his OCD and Tourette's syndrome. The story is about his divorce, his best friend's matchmaking efforts, and a woman who introduces him to therapy, a healthy relationship, and unconditional love.

VIEWING POINTS: Differentiate Mark's response to his Tourette's and OCD. Which disorder is ultimately more problematic?

If Mark were your patient, what medication would you expect to be prescribed? Identify teaching needs related to medication and the obsessions and compulsions.

Explain the dynamics of the relationship of Mark and Charlotte. Can you identify Charlotte's mental disorder?

As Good As It Gets: 1997. Novelist Melvin Udall, played by Jack Nicholson, lives in his own world of obsessive-compulsive behavior patterns, avoiding cracks in sidewalks and rigidly adhering to a regimen of daily breakfasts in the café, where single mom Carol Connelly, played by Helen Hunt, works. Udall's world is changed when he unwillingly becomes a sitter for his next-door neighbor's dog. A friendship leading to a romance develops between Udall and Connelly.

VIEWING POINTS: Identify the behaviors that indicate that Udall has an anxiety disorder. Observe feelings that are generated in you by Udall's behavior. How are Udall's friends able to tolerate his behavior?

REFERENCES

Abrams, J. K., Johnson, P. L., Hay-Schmidt, A., Mikkelsen, J. D., Shekhar, A., & Lowry, C.A. (2005). Serotonergic systems associated with arousal and vigilance behaviors following administration of anxiogenic drugs. *Neuroscience, 133*(4), 983–997.

Albert, U., Aguglia, E., Maina, G., & Bogetto, F. (2002). Venlafaxine versus clomipramine in the treatment of obsessive-compulsive disorder: A preliminary single-blind, 12 week, controlled study. *Journal of Clinical Psychiatry, 63*(11),1004–1009.

Anderson, D., & Ahmed, A. (2003). Treatment of patients with intractable obsessive-compulsive disorder with anterior capsular stimulation. *Journal of Neurosurgery, 98*(5), 1104–1109.

American Psychiatric Association (APA). (2000). *Diagnostic and statistical manual of mental disorders* (4th ed., text revision). Washington, DC: Author.

Arnold, P., & Richter, M. (2001). Is obsessive-compulsive disorder an autoimmune disease? *Canadian Medical Association Journal, 165*(10), 1353–1358.

Beck, A., & Emery, G. (1985). *Anxiety disorders and phobias: A cognitive perspective.* New York: Basic Books.

Beekman, A., de Beurs, E., Von Balkom, A., et al. 2000. Anxiety and depression in later life: Co-occurrence and communality of risk factors. *American Journal of Psychiatry, 157*, 1.

Bodinger, L., Hermesh, H., Aizenberg, D., Valevski, A., Marom, S., Shiloh, R., et al. (2002). Sexual function and behavior in social phobia. *Journal of Clinical Psychiatry, 63(10)*, 874–879.

Brauer, H., Nowicki, P., Catalano, G., & Catalano, M. (2002). Panic attacks associated with citalopram. *Southern Medical Journal, 95*(9), 1088–1089.

Brewin, C., Andrews, B., Rose, S., & Kirk, M. (1999). Acute stress disorder and posttraumatic stress disorder in victims of violent crime. *American Journal of Psychiatry, 156*(3), 360–366.

Bruce, S., Vasile, R., Goisman, R., Salzman, C., Spencer, M., Machan, J., & Keller, M. (2003). Are benzodiazepines still the medication of choice for patients with panic disorder with or without agoraphobia? *American Journal of Psychiatry, 160*(8), 1432–1438.

Bruce, S., Yonkers, K., Otto, M, Eisen, J., Weisberg, R., Pagano, M., et al. (2005). Influence of psychiatric comorbidity on recovery and recurrence in generalized anxiety disorder, social phobia, and panic disorder: a 12-year prospective study. *American Journal of Psychiatry, 162(6)*, 1179–1187.

Busatto, G. (2001). Regional cerebral blood flow abnormalities in early-onset obsessive-compulsive disorder: An exploratory SPECT study. *Journal of the American Academy of Child and Adolescent Psychiatry, 40*(3), 347–354.

Castellanos, D., & Hunter, T. (2000). Anxiety disorders in children and adolescents. *Southern Medical Journal, 92*(10), 946–954.

Castle, D. & Groves, G. (2000). The internal and external boundaries of obsessive-compulsive disorder. *Australian and New Zealand Journal of Psychiatry 34*(2), 249–255.

Chen, J-P., Reich, L., & Chung, H. (2002). Anxiety disorders. *Western Journal of Medicine, 176*(4), 249–253.

Clum, G. A. (1990). Panic Attack Cognitions Questionnaire. *Coping with panic: A drug-free approach to dealing with anxiety attacks.* Pacific Grove, CA: Brooks/Cole.

Cooper, J. (1970). The Leyton Obsessional Inventory. *Psychiatric Medicine, 1*, 48.

Crino, R., Slade, T., & Andrews, G. (2005). The changing prevalence and severity of obsessive-compulsive disorder criteria from DSM-III to DSM-IV. *American Journal of Psychiatry, 162*(5), 876–882.

Dugue, M., & Neugroschl, J. (2002). Anxiety disorders. Helping patients regain stability and calm. *Geriatrics, 57*(8), 27–31.

Fireman, B., Koran, L., Leventhal, J., & Jacobson, A. (2001). The prevalence of clinically recognized obsessive-compulsive disorder in a large health maintenance organization. *American Journal of Psychiatry, 158* (11), 1904–1910.

Flynn, C. & Chen, Y. (2003). Antidepressants for generalized anxiety disorder. *American Family Physician, 68*(9), 1757–1758.

Foa, E., Liebowitz, M., Kozak, M., Davies, S., Campeas, R., Franklin, M., Juppert, J., Kjernisted, K., Rowan, V., Schmidt, A., Simpson, H., & Tu, X. (2005). Randomized, placebo controlled exposure and ritual prevention, clomipramine, and their combination in the treatment of obsessive-compulsive disorder. *American Journal of Psychiatry, 162(1)*, 15–161.

Freitag, C.M., Domschke, D., Rothe, D., Lee, Y.J., Hohoff, C., Gutknecht, L., et al. (2006)., Interaction of serotonergic and noradrenergic gene variants in panic disorder. *Psychiatric Genetics, 16*(2), 59–65.

Friedman, S., Smith, L., Fogel, D., Paradis, C., Viswanathan, R., Ackerman, R., Trappler, B. (2002). The incidence and influence of early traumatic life events in patients with panic disorder: A comparison with other psychiatric outpatients. *Journal of Anxiety Disorders, 16*(3), 259–272.

Gardos, G. (2000). Long-term treatment of panic disorder with agoraphobia in private practice. *Journal of Psychiatric Practice, 6*, 140–146.

Goddard, A., Mason, G., Appel, M., Rothman, D., Gueorguieva, R., Behar, K., & Krystal, J. (2004). Impaired GABA neuronal response to acute benzodiazepine administration in panic disorder. *American Journal of Psychiatry, 161*(12), 2186–2193.

Goldstein, B., Herrmann, N., & Shulman, K. (2006). Comorbidity in bipolar disorder among the elderly: results from an epidemiological community sample. *American Journal of Psychiatry, 163*(2), 319–321.

Goodman, W., Price, L., Rasmussen, S., Mazure, C., Fleischmann, R. L., Hill, C. L., et al. (1989). The Yale-Brown Obsessive Compulsive Scale (Y-BOCS): Part 1. Development, use and reliability. *Archives of General Psychiatry, 46*, 1006–1011.

Goodwin, R., & Pine, D. (2002). Respiratory disease and panic attacks among adults in the United States. *Chest, 122*(2), 645–650.

Gorman, J., Kent, J., Sullivan, G., & Coplan, J. (2000). Neuroanatomical hypothesis of panic disorder, revised. *American Journal of Psychiatry, 157*(4), 493–505.

Graeff, F. G., Garcia-Leal, D., Del-Ben, C. M., & Guimaraes, F. S. (2005). Does the panic attack activate the hypothalamic-pituitary-adrenal axis? *Anais da Academia Brasiliera de Ciencias*, 77(3), 477–491.

Hamilton, M. (1959). The assessment of anxiety states by rating. *British Journal of Medical Psychology, 32*, 54.

Hayward, C., Killen, J., & Kraemer, H. (2000). Predictors of panic attacks in adolescents. *Journal of the American Academy of Child and Adolescent Psychiatry, 39*(2), 207–214.

Hettema, J., Prescott, C., & Kendler, K. (2004). Genetic and environmental sources of covariation between generalized anxiety disorder and neuroticism. *American Journal of Psychiatry, 161*(9), 1581–1587.

Isensee, B., Wittchen, H., Stein, M., Hofler, M., & Lieb, R. (2003). *Archives of General Psychiatry, 60*(7), 692–700.

Johanness, S., Wies inga, B. N., Noges, W., Roda, D., Muller-Vahl, K., R., Emnish, H. M., Dengles, R., Munte, R. F. & Wietrich, D. (2003). Tourette syndrome and obsessive-compulsive disorder: Event-related brain potentials show similar mechanism of frontal inhibition but dissimilar target evaluation process. *Behavior Neurology 14*(1–2); 9–17.

Kampman, M., Keijsers, G., Hoogduin, C., & Hendriks, G. (2002). A randomized, double-blind, placebo-controlled study of the effects of adjunctive paroxetine in panic disorder patients unsuccessfully treated with cognitive-behavioral therapy alone. *Journal of Clinical Psychiatry, 63*(9), 772–777.

Katerndahl, D., Burge, S., & Kellog, N. (2005). Predictors of development of adult psychopathology in female victims of childhood sexual abuse. *Journal of Nervous and Mental Diseases, 193*(4), 258–264.

Katon, W.J., (2006). Panic disorder. *The New England Journal of Medicine, 354*(22), 2360–2367.

Katon, W., Roy-Byrne, P., Russo, J., & Cowley, D. (2002). Cost-effectiveness and cost offset of a collaborative care intervention for primary care patients with panic disorder. *Archives of General Psychiatry, 59*(12), 1098–1104.

Kaye, W. H., Bulik, C., Thorton, L., Barbarich, N., & Masters, K. (2004). Comorbidity of anxiety disorders with anorexia and bulimia nervosa. *American Journal of Psychiatry, 161*(12), 2215–2221.

Kendler, K., Hettema, J., Butera, F., Gardner, C., & Prescott, C. (2003). Life event dimensions of loss, humiliation, entrapment, and danger in the prediction of onsets of major depression and generalized anxiety. *Archives of General Psychiatry, 60*(8), 789–796.

Kessler, R. C. (2002). *National Comorbidity Survey, 1990–1992.* (Computer file). Conducted by University of Michigan, Survey Research Center (2nd ed.) ICPSR. Ann Arbor, MI: Inter-University Consortium for Political and Social Research (producer and distributor).

Kessler, R., Chiu, W., Jin, R., Ruscio, A., Shear, K., & Walters, E. (2006). The epidemiology of panic attacks, panic disorder, and agoraphobia in the National Comorbidity Survey Replication. *Archives of General Psychiatry, 63*(4), 415–424.

Kim, C. H., Chang, J. W., Koo, M. S., Kim, J. W., Suh, H. S., Park, I. H., & Lee, H. S. (2003). Anterior cingulotomy for refractory obsessivecompulsive disorder. *Acta Psychiatrica Scandinavica, 107* (4), 241–243.

Kirkby, K. (2003). Obsessive-compulsive disorder: Towards better understanding and outcomes. *Current Opinion in Psychiatry, 16*(1), 49–55.

Kurlan, R., & Kaplan, E. (2004). The pediatric autoimmune neuropsychiatric disorders associated with streptococcal infection (PANDAS) etiology for tics and obsessive-compulsive symptoms: hypothesis or entity? Practical considerations for the clinician. *Pediatrics, 113*(4), 907–911.

Lavie, C. J., & Milani, R. V. (2004). Prevalence of anxiety in coronary patients with improvement following cardiac rehabilitation and exercise training. *American Journal of Cardiology, 93*(3), 336–339.

Lenze, E., Mulsant, B., Shear, M., Schulberg, H. C., Dew, M. A., Begley, A. E., et al. (2000). Comorbid anxiety disorders in depressed elderly patients. *American Journal of Psychiatry, 157*(5), 722–728.

Llorca, P., Spadone, C., Sol, O., Danniau, A., Bougerol, T., Corruble, E., et al. (2002). Efficacy and safety of hydroxyzine in the treatment of generalized anxiety disorder: A 3 month double-blind study. *Journal of Clinical Psychiatry, 63*(11), 1020–1027.

Luo, F., Leckman, J., Katsovich, L., Findley, D., Grantz, H., Tucker, D., et al. (2004). Prospective longitudinal study of children with tic disorders and/or obsessive-compulsive disorder: relationship of symptom exacerbations to newly acquired streptococcal infections. *Pediatrics, 113*(6), e578–e585.

Mataix-Cols, D., Rauch, S. L., Baer, L., Eisen, J. L., Shera, D. M., Goodman, W. K., et al. (2002). Symptom stability in adult obsessive-compulsive disorder: data from a naturalistic two-year follow-up study. *American Journal of Psychiatry, 159*(2), 263–268.

Mataix-Cols, D., Wooderson, S., Lawrence, N., Brammer, M. J., Speckens, A., & Phillips, M. L. (2004). Distinct neural correlates of washing, checking, and hoarding symptom dimensions in obsessive-compulsive disorder. *Archives of General Psychiatry, 61*(6), 564–576.

Mathew, S. J., Mao, X., Coplan, J. D., Smith, E. L., Sackeim, H. A., Gorman, J. M., & Shungu, D. C. (2004). Dorsolateral prefrontal cortical pathology in generalized anxiety disorder: a proton magnetic resonance spectroscopic imaging study. *American Journal of Psychiatry, 161*(6), 1119–1121.

Mundo, E., Ritcher, M., Sam, F., Macciardi, F., & Kennedy, J. L. (2000). Is the 5-HT (1D beta) receptor gene implicated in the pathogenesis of obsessive compulsive disorder? *American Journal of Psychiatry, 157*(7), 1160–1161.

Newman, M., Erickson, T., Przeworski, A., & Dzus, E. (2003). Self-help and minimal contact therapies for anxiety disorders: Is human contact necessary for therapeutic efficacy? *Journal of Clinical Psychology, 59*(3), 251–274.

Overbeek, T., Schruers, K., Vermetten, E., & Greiz, E. (2002). Comorbidity of obsessive-compulsive disorder and depression: Prevalence, symptom severity, and treatment effect. *Journal of Clinical Psychiatry, 63*(12), 1106–1112.

Peplau, H. (1989). Theoretic constructs: Anxiety, self, and hallucinations. In A. O'Toole & S. Welt (Eds.), *Interpersonal theory in nursing practice: Selected works of Hildegarde E. Peplau.* New York: Springer.

Perugi, G., Toni, C., Frare, F., Travierso, M., Hantouche, E., & Akiskal, H. (2002). Obsessive-compulsive-bipolar comorbidity: A systematic exploration of clinical features and treatment outcome. *Journal of Clinical Psychiatry, 63*(12), 1129–1134.

Pujol, J., Soriano-Mas, C., Alonso, P., Cardoner, N., Menchon, J. M., Deus, J., & Vallejo, J. (2004). Mapping structural brain alterations in obsessive-compulsive disorder. *Archives of General Psychiatry, 61*(7), 720–730.

Rabatin, J., & Keltz, L. B. (2002). Generalized anxiety and panic disorders. *Western Journal of Medicine, 173*(3), 164–168.

Rachman, S., & Hodgson, R. (1980). *Obsessions and compulsions.* New York: Prentice-Hall.

Rapaport, M. H., Wolkow, R., Rubin, A., Hackett, E., Pollack, M., & Ota, K. U. (2001). Sertraline treatment of panic disorder: Results of a long-term study. *Acta Psychiatrica Scandinavica, 104*(4), 289–298.

Raskind, M., Thompson, C., Petrie, E., Dobie, D. J., Rein, R. J., Hoff, D. J., et al. (2002). Prazosin reduces nightmares in combat veterans with posttraumatic stress disorder. *Journal of Clinical Psychiatry, 63*(7), 565–568.

Rodriguez, B. F., Weisberg, R. B., Pagano, M. E., Bruce, S. E., Spencer, M. A., Culpepper, L., & Keller, M. B. (2006). Characteristics and predictors of full and partial recovery from generalized anxiety disorder in primary care patients. *Journal of Nervous and Mental Diseases, 194*(2), 9–97.

Rollman, B. L., Belnap, B. H., Mazumdar, S., Houck, P. R., Zhu, F., & Gardner, W., et al. (2005). A randomized trial to improve the quality of treatment for panic and generalized anxiety disorders in primary care. *Archives of General Psychiatry, 62*(12), 1332–1341.

Roy-Byrne, P. P., Clary, C. M., Miceli, R. J., Colucci, S. V., Xu, Y., Grundzinski, A. N. (2001). The effect of selective serotonin reuptake inhibitor treatment of panic disorder on emergency room and laboratory resource utilization. *Journal of Clinical Psychiatry, 62*(9), 678–682.

Safren, S. A., Gershuny, B. S., Marzol, P., Otto, M. W., & Pollack, M. H. (2002). History of childhood abuse in panic disorder, social phobia, and generalized anxiety disorder. *Journal of Nervous and Mental Disorders, 190*(7), 453–456.

Sakai, Y., Kumano, H., Nishikawa, M., Kakano, Y., Kaiya, H., Imabayashi, E., et al. (2005). Cerebral glucose metabolism associated with a fear network in panic disorder. *Neuroreport. 16*(9), 927–931.

Sareen, J., Cox, B. J., Afifi, T. O., de Graff, R., Asmundson, G. J., ten Have, M., & Stein, M. B. (2005). Anxiety disorders and risk for suicidal ideation and suicide attempts: a population-based longitudinal study of adults. *Archives of General Psychiatry, 62*(11), 1249–1257.

Schneier, F., Liebowitz, M., Abi-Dargham, A., Zea-Ponce, Y., Lin, S. H., Laruelle, M., et al. (2000). Low dopamine D2 receptor binding potential in social phobia. *American Journal of Psychiatry, 157*(3), 457–459.

Shear, M. K., Cooper, A. M., Klerman, G. L., Busch, F. N., & Shapiro, T. (1993). A psychodynamic model of panic disorder. *American Journal of Psychiatry, 150,* 859–866.

Sheikh, J. I., Leskin, G. A., & Klein, D. F. (2002). Gender differences in panic disorder: Findings from the National Comorbidity Survey. *American Journal of Psychiatry, 159*(8), 1438.

Smoller, J. W., Pollack, M. H., Wassertheil-Smoller, S., Barton, B., Hendrix, S. L., Jackson, R. D., et al. (2003). Prevalence and correlates of panic attacks in postmenopausal women: results from an ancillary study to the Women's Health Initiative. *Archives of Internal Medicine, 163*(17), 2041–2050.

Slattery, M., Klein, D., Mannuzza, S., Moulton, J. L. 3rd, Pine, D.S., Klein, R. G., et al. (2002). Relationship between separation anxiety disorder, parental panic disorder, and atopic disorders in children: a controlled high-risk study (Statistical data included). *Journal of the American Academy of Child and Adolescent Psychiatry, 41*(8), 947–954.

Stein, M. B., Fyer, A. J., Davidson, J. R., Pollack, M. J., & Wiita, B. (1999). Fluvoxamine treatment of social phobia (social anxiety disorder): A double-blind, placebo-controlled trial. *American Journal of Psychiatry, 156*(5), 756–760.

Stein, D., Versiani, M., Hair, T., & Kumar, R. (2002). Efficacy of paroxetine for relapse prevention in social anxiety disorder: A 24-week study. *Archives in General Psychiatry, 59* (12), 1111–1118.

Stein, M. B., Sherbourne, C. D., Craske, M. G., Means-Christensen, A., Bystritsky, A., Katon, W., et al. (2004). Quality of care for primary care patients with anxiety disorders. *American Journal of Psychiatry, 161*(12), 2230–2237.

Stengler-Wenzke, K., Trosbach, J., Dietrich, S., & Angermeyer, M. C. (2004). Coping strategies used by the relatives of people with obsessive-compulsive disorder. *Journal of Advanced Nursing, 48*(1), 35–42.

Valentiner, D., Gutierrez, P., & Blacker, D. (2002). Anxiety measures and their relationship to adolescent suicidal ideation and behavior. *Journal of Anxiety Disorders, 16*(1), 11–32.

Van Ameringen, M., Mancini, C., Pipe, B., Campbell, M., & Oakman, J. (2002). Topiramate treatment for SSRI-induced weight gain in anxiety disorders. *Journal of Clinical Psychiatry, 63*(11), 981–984.

Wade, T.D., Bulik, C. M., Prescott, C. A., & Kendler, K. S. (2004). Sex influences on shared risk factors for bulimia nervosa and other psychiatric disorders. *Archives of General Psychiatry, 61*(3), 251–256.

Wang, P., Berglund, P., & Kessler, R. (2000). Recent care of common mental disorders in the United States: Prevalence and conformance with evidenced-based recommendations. *Journal of General Internal Medicine, 15*, 284–292.

Woodward, L. (2001). Life course outcomes of young people with anxiety disorders in adolescence. *Journal of the American Academy of Child and Adolescent Psychiatry, 40*(9), 1086–1093.

CHAPTER 22

Personality and Impulse Disorders: Meaning of Behavior

Barbara J. Limandri, Mary Ann Boyd, Ann Bland, and Beverly Hart

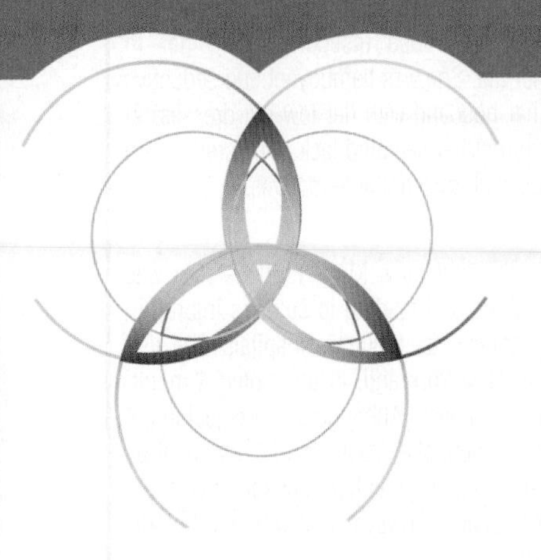

KEY CONCEPTS

- personality
- personality disorder
- personality traits

LEARNING OBJECTIVES

After studying this chapter, you will be able to:

- Identify the common features of personality disorders.
- Distinguish between the concepts of personality and personality disorder.
- Analyze the prevailing biologic, psychological, and social theories explaining the development of personality disorders.
- Discuss the epidemiology of each personality disorder.
- Distinguish among the three clusters of personality disorders.
- Formulate nursing diagnoses and plan interventions for patients with specific personality disorders.
- Compare the psychoanalytic explanation of the borderline personality disorder with biosocial theory.
- Apply the nursing process to individuals with a diagnosis of borderline personality disorder.
- Analyze special concerns within the nurse–patient relationship common to treating those with personality disorders.
- Compare and contrast the impulse-control disorders.

KEY TERMS

• affective instability • attachment • cognitive schema • communication triad • dialectical behavior therapy (DBT) • dichotomous thinking • dissociation • emotional dysregulation • emotional vulnerability • emotions • identity diffusion • impulsivity • inhibited grieving • invalidating environment • kleptomania • parasuicidal behavior • projective identification • psychopath • pyromania • self-identity • separation-individuation • skills groups • sociopath • temperament • thought stopping • trichotillomania

The concept of personality seems deceivingly simple but is very complex. Historically, the term *personality* was derived from the Greek *persona*, the theatrical mask used by dramatic players. Originally, the term had the connotation of a projected pretense or allusion. With time, the connotation changed from being an external surface representation to the internal traits of the individual.

KEY CONCEPT Personality is a complex pattern of characteristics, largely outside of the person's awareness, that comprise the individual's distinctive pattern of perceiving, feeling, thinking, coping, and behaving. The personality emerges from a complicated interaction of biologic dispositions, psychological experiences, and environmental situations.

Today, personality is conceptualized as a complex pattern of psychological characteristics that are not easily altered and that are largely outside of the person's awareness. These characteristics or traits include the individual's specific style of perceiving, thinking, and feeling about self, others, and the environment. These styles or traits are similar across many different social or personal situations and are expressed in almost every facet of functioning. Intrinsic and pervasive, they emerge from a complicated interaction of biologic dispositions, psychological experiences, and environmental situations that ultimately comprise the individual's distinctive personality (Millon, Grossman, Millon, Meagher, & Ramnath, 2004).

PERSONALITY DISORDERS

No sharp division exists between normal and abnormal personality functioning. Instead, personalities are viewed on a continuum from normal at one end to abnormal at the other. Many of the same processes involved in the development of a "normal" personality are responsible for the development of a personality disorder.

KEY CONCEPT A **personality disorder** is an enduring pattern of inner experience and behavior that deviates markedly from the expectations of the individual's culture, is pervasive and inflexible, has an onset in adolescence or early adulthood, is stable with time, and leads to distress or impairment (American Psychiatric Association [APA], 2000, p. 685).

Personality disorders are classified as Axis II diagnoses, separate from the other mental disorders presented thus far, which are classified under Axis I (APA, 2000). Axis II classification was intended to focus attention on behavior patterns that might be overlooked in the light of the more pronounced disorders of Axis I. Frequently, an Axis II diagnosis coexists with an Axis I diagnosis. For example, a person who has a dependent personality disorder might also have symptoms of generalized anxiety disorder when faced with demands to function autonomously. Ten personality disorders are recognized as psychiatric diagnoses and are organized into three clusters based on the dimensions of *odd-eccentric*, *dramatic-emotional*, and *anxious-fearful* behaviors or symptoms.

Cluster A consists of the disorders that most broadly characterize odd and eccentric misfit disorders, including paranoid personality disorder, schizoid personality disorder, and schizotypal personality disorder. People with cluster B disorders show great **impulsivity** (acting without considering the consequences of the act or alternate actions) and emotionality; these disorders consist of antisocial personality disorder (APD), borderline personality disorder (BPD), histrionic personality disorder, and narcissistic personality disorder. Dramatic and erratic behavior best characterizes people with cluster B disorders. Cluster C disorders feature a predominant sense of anxiety and fearfulness and include avoidant personality disorder, dependent personality disorder, and obsessive-compulsive personality disorder.

BPD is highlighted in this chapter because it is severely incapacitating and difficult to treat. APD is also emphasized. Symptoms associated with both of these disorders often provoke negative reactions on the part of the clinician, which interferes with the clinician's ability to provide effective care. Impulse-control disorders are summarized at the end of the chapter. These disorders commonly coexist with other mental disorders.

MOVIE viewing GUIDES

FAME AND FORTUNE

Mary Todd Lincoln (1818–1882)

First Lady

Public Persona

Mary Todd Lincoln, the wife of President Abraham Lincoln, was a complicated and contradictory woman whose insecurities led her to overindulge in many areas of her life. She was flamboyant and seductive in her dress, often surprising her husband with her low-cut dresses. At times, she caused public criticism of her seeming lack of discretion and extension of friendship to people with questionable motives.

Personal Realities

While living in Washington as the first lady, Mary Todd Lincoln was involved in charitable works, visiting and reading to soldiers injured in the Civil War and raising money for events at military hospitals. She also made frequent shopping trips to New York and, in one noted 4-month period, collected about 400 pairs of gloves. Although she was jealous of her husband's attention to other women, she caused public comment by her unorthodox friendships with men as well as her unchaperoned trips. She was highly devoted to her husband, however, and was psychologically immobilized after his death.

Source: www.mrlincolnswhitehouse.org

Personality Disorder Versus Personality Traits

To receive a diagnosis of a personality disorder, an individual must demonstrate the criteria behaviors persistently and to such an extent that they impair the ability to function socially and occupationally. In some people, the underlying feelings and behaviors may be intermittent and interfere interpersonally without impairment.

Instead of having a personality disorder, the individual is said to have traits of the disorder, which also can be noted on Axis II without a formal diagnosis. Changing lifelong personality patterns is difficult and requires much understanding and support.

> **KEY CONCEPT Personality traits** are prominent aspects of personality that are exhibited in a wide range of important social and personal contexts (APA, 2000, p. 770).

Common Features and Diagnostic Criteria

The personality disorder diagnosis is based on abnormal, inflexible behavior patterns of long duration, traced to adolescence or early adulthood that deviate from acceptable cultural norms. These behaviors are pervasive across a broad range of personal and social situations, cause significant distress or impairment to social or occupational functioning, and deviate markedly from expectations of the individual's culture. For immigrants who may be having difficulty learning new acceptable social and cultural behavior patterns and adjusting to a new culture, the diagnosis of a personality disorder may be delayed beyond this difficult adjustment period.

Maladaptive Cognitive Schema

Cognitive schema are patterns of thoughts that determine how a person interprets events. Each person's cognitive schema screen, code, and evaluate incoming stimuli. In personality disorders, maladaptive cognitive schema cause misinterpretation of other people's actions or reactions and of events that result in dysfunctional ways of responding. For example, if a person thinks that no one can be trusted, an innocent, friendly gesture can be interpreted as a suspicious behavior, provoking a hostile response, instead of a reciprocal friendly greeting.

Affectivity and Emotional Instability

Emotions are psychophysiologic reactions that define a person's mood and can be categorized as negative (anger, fright, anxiety, guilt, shame, sadness, envy, jealousy, and disgust), positive (happiness, pride, relief, and love), and neutral (hope, compassion, empathy, sympathy, and contentment). Emotions can affect the ability to learn and function by interfering with accessing and storing information in memory. Negative, intense emotions interfere with memory storage of related events (Hurlemann, Hawellek, Maier, Dolan, 2007).

Impaired Self-identity and Interpersonal Functioning

Self-identity, central to the normal development of one's personality, is formed through an integration of social and occupational roles and affiliations, self-attributed personality traits, attitudes about gender roles, beliefs about sexuality and intimacy, long-term goals, political ideology, and religious beliefs. Without an adequately formed identity, an individual's goal-directed behavior is impaired, and interpersonal relationships are disrupted. Each individual's abilities, limitations, and goals are shaped by one's identity. In personality disorders, self-identity is often disturbed or absent.

Impulsivity and Destructive Behavior

People with personality disorders often come to the attention of the mental health clinician because their impulsive behavior results in negative consequences to others or themselves. They seem unable to consider the consequences of their actions before acting on their impulses. For example, an individual may feel rage toward another and lack skills to resist the impulse to attack that person physically, even though this action may be punished.

CLUSTER A DISORDERS: ODD-ECCENTRIC

Paranoid Personality Disorder: Suspicious Pattern

Personality patterns of a person with paranoid personality disorder are mistrust of others and the desire to avoid relationships in which the individual is not in control or loses power. These individuals are suspicious, guarded, and hostile. They are consistently mistrustful of others' motives, even relatives and close friends. Actions of others are often misinterpreted as deception, deprecation, and betrayal, especially regarding fidelity or trustworthiness of a spouse or friend (Millon et al., 2004). Minor innocuous incidents are often misinterpreted as having sinister or hidden meaning, and suspicions are magnified into major distortions of reality. People with paranoid personalities are unforgiving and hold grudges; their typical emotional responses are anger and hostility. They distance themselves from others and are outwardly argumentative and abrasive; internally, they feel powerlessness, fearful, and vulnerable. Other hallmark features of paranoid personality disorder are persistent ideas of self-importance and the tendency to be rigid and controlled. Blind to their own unattractive behaviors and characteristics, they often attribute these traits to others. Their outward demeanor often seems cold, sullen, and humorless. They want to appear controlled and objective, yet often they react emotionally, displaying signs of nervousness, anger, envy, and jealousy. Orderly by nature, they are hypervigilant to any environmental changes that may loosen their control on the world. Because people with this disorder are extremely sensitive about appearing "strange" or "bizarre," they will not seek mental health care until they decompensate into a psychosis (Table 22.1).

Epidemiology

The prevalence of paranoid personality disorder is reported to be 0.5% to 2.5% in the general population (APA, 2000) but could be even higher. In data derived from the 2001–2002 National Epidemiologic Survey on Alcohol and related conditions, paranoid personality disorder was reported to be the second highest personality disorder (4.41%; N = 43,093) in this study (Grant et al., 2004). In inpatient settings, 10% to 30% of patients have this disorder, and in outpatient settings, 2% to 10% have the disorder (APA, 2000). Axis I disorders, such as generalized anxiety disorder, mood disorders, and schizophrenia, can coexist with paranoid personality disorder, but minor Axis I symptoms usually are not seen. Other Axis II disorders can also coexist, such as narcissistic, avoidant, and obsessive-compulsive personality disorders (Millon et al., 2004).

Table 22.1  **Summary of Diagnostic Characteristics of Cluster A Disorders** 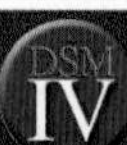

Disorder	*Diagnostic Criteria and Target Symptoms*
Paranoid Personality Disorder 301.0	• Pervasive distrust and suspiciousness of others interpreted as malevolent (often with little or no justification or evidence to support it) Assumption of exploitation, harm, or deception; feelings that others are plotting against him or her with possible sudden attacks (associated with feelings of deep or irreversible injury) at any time for no reason Preoccupation with doubts of loyalty or untrustworthiness of friends and associates; deviation from doubts viewed as support for assumptions Reluctance to confide in others or become close in fear that information will be used against him or her Interpretation of hidden meanings into remarks or events, believing them to be demeaning and threatening Holding of grudges with unwillingness to forgive; minor intrusions arouse major hostility, persisting for long periods of time Quick to react and counterattack to perceived insults—possible pathologic jealousy with recurrent suspiciousness about fidelity of spouse or sexual partner • Not occurring exclusively during course of another psychiatric disorder; not a direct physiologic effect of a general medical condition
Schizoid Personality Disorder 301.20	• Pervasive pattern of detachment from social relating • Restricted range for emotional expression Lacking desire for intimacy Indifference to opportunities for close relationships Little satisfaction from being part of family or social group Preference for alone time rather than being with others; choosing solitary activities or hobbies Little if any interest in having sexual experiences with others Reduced pleasure from sensory, bodily, or interpersonal experiences No close friends or relatives Indifference to approval or criticism from others Emotional coldness, detachment, or flattened affectivity • Not occurring exclusively during course of another psychiatric disorder; not a direct physiologic effect of a general medical condition
Schizotypal Personality Disorder 301.22	• Pervasive pattern of social and interpersonal deficits evidenced by acute discomfort; reduced capacity for close relationships; cognitive and perceptual distortions; and eccentric behavior Ideas of reference Odd beliefs or magical thinking influencing behavior, such as superstitions, and preoccupation with paranormal phenomena, special powers Perceptual alterations Odd thinking and speech Suspiciousness or paranoid ideation Stiff, inappropriate, or constricted interactions Odd or eccentric behavior or appearance Few close friends or confidants (other than first-degree relative) Anxiety in social situations, especially unfamiliar ones; no decrease in anxiety with increasing familiarity • Not occurring exclusively during course of another psychiatric disorder

Etiology

The etiologic factors of paranoid personality disorder are unclear, but there may be a genetic predisposition for an irregular maturation. An underlying excess in limbic and sympathetic system reactivity or a neurochemical acceleration of synaptic transmission may exist. These dysfunctions can give rise to the hypersensitivity, cognitive autism, and social isolation that characterize these patients. As children, these individuals tend to be active and intrusive, difficult to manage, hyperactive, irritable, and have frequent temper outbursts.

Nursing Management

Nurses most likely see these patients for other health problems but will formulate nursing diagnoses based on the patient's underlying suspiciousness. Assessment of these individuals will reveal disturbed or illogical thoughts that demonstrate misinterpretation of environmental stimuli. For example, a man was convinced that his wife was having an affair with the neighbor because his wife and the neighbor left their homes for work at the same time each morning. Although the man's beliefs were illogical, he never once considered that he was wrong. He frequently followed them but never caught them together. He continued to believe they were having an affair. The nursing diagnosis of Disturbed Thought Processes is usually supported by the assessment data.

Because of their inability to develop relationships, these patients are often socially isolated and lack social support systems. Yet, the nursing diagnosis of Social Isolation is not appropriate for the person with paranoid personality disorder because the person does not meet the defining characteristics of feelings of aloneness, rejection, desire for contact with people, and insecurity in social situations.

Nursing interventions based on the establishment of a nurse–patient relationship are difficult to implement because of the patient's mistrust. If a trusting relationship is established, the nurse helps the patient identify problematic areas, such as getting along with others or keeping a job. Through therapeutic techniques such as acceptance, confrontation, and reflection, the nurse and patient examine a problematic area to gain another view of the situation. Changing thought patterns takes time. Patient outcomes are evaluated in terms of small changes in thinking and behavior.

Schizoid Personality Disorder: Asocial Pattern

People with schizoid personality disorder are expressively impassive and interpersonally unengaged (Millon et al., 2004). They tend to be unable to experience the joyful and pleasurable aspects of life. They are introverted and reclusive, and clinically appear distant, aloof, apathetic, and emotionally detached. They have difficulties making friends, seem uninterested in social activities, and appear to gain little satisfaction in personal relationships. In fact, they appear to be incapable of forming social relationships. Interests are directed at objects, things, and abstractions. As children, they engage primarily in solitary activities, such as stamp collecting, computer games, electronic equipment, or academic pursuits such as mathematics or engineering. In addition, there seems to be a cognitive deficit characterized by obscure thought processes, particularly about social matters. Communication with others is confused and lacks focus. These individuals reveal minimum introspection and self-awareness, and interpersonal experiences are described in a very mechanical way (see Table 22.1).

Epidemiology

Schizoid personality disorder is rarely diagnosed in clinical settings. It is estimated that the prevalence of schizoid disorder is 3.13% (Grant et al., 2004). The most prevalent comorbid disorder is avoidant personality disorder, which occurs in 5% of the cases. Dependent and obsessive-compulsive disorders may coexist with schizoid personality disorder (Torgersen, Kringlen, & Cramer, 2001).

Etiology

The etiologic processes are speculative. There may be defects in either the limbic or reticular regions of the brain that may result in the development of the schizoid pattern (Millon et al., 2004). The defects of this personality may stem from an adrenergic–cholinergic imbalance in which the parasympathetic division of the autonomic nervous system is functionally dominant. Excesses or deficiencies in acetylcholine and norepinephrine may result in the proliferation and scattering of neural impulses that may be responsible for the cognitive "slippage" or affective deficits.

Nursing Management

Impaired Social Interactions and Chronic Low Self-esteem are typical diagnoses of patients with schizoid personality disorder. Major treatment goals are to enhance the experience of pleasure, prevent social isolation, and increase emotional responsiveness to others. Because these individuals often lack customary social skills, social skills training is useful in enhancing their ability to relate in interpersonal situations. The primary focus is to increase the patient's ability to feel pleasure. The nurse balances interventions between encouraging enough social activity that prevents the individual from retreating to a fantasy world and too much social activity that becomes intolerable.

The nurse may find working with these individuals unrewarding and become frustrated, feel helpless, or feel bored during the interactions. It is difficult to establish a therapeutic relationship with these individuals because they tend to shy away from interactions. Evaluation of outcomes should be in terms of increasing the patient's feelings of satisfaction with solitary activities.

Schizotypal Personality Disorder: Eccentric Pattern

Persons with the schizotypal personality disorder are characterized by a pattern of social and interpersonal deficits. They are void of any close friends other than first-degree relatives. They have odd beliefs about their world that are inconsistent with their cultural norms. Ideas of reference (incorrect interpretations of events as having special, personal meaning) are often present, as are unusual perceptual delusions and odd, circumstantial, and metaphorical thinking and speech. Their mood is constricted or inappropriate, and they have excessive social anxieties of a paranoid character that do not diminish with familiarity. Their appearance and behavior are characterized as odd, eccentric, or peculiar. They usually exhibit an avoidant behavior pattern (see Table 22.1).

If these individuals do become psychotic, they seem totally disoriented and confused. Many will exhibit posturing, grimacing, inappropriate giggling, and peculiar mannerisms. Speech tends to ramble. Fantasy, hallucinations, and bizarre, fragmented delusions may be present. Regressive acts such as soiling and wetting the bed may occur. These individuals may consume food in an infantile or ravenous manner. Symptoms mirror but fall short of features that would justify the diagnosis of schizophrenia. The person's tendency is to remain socially isolated, dependent on family members or institutions. These patients avoid social interaction that can keep them functional, and well-intentioned relatives or institutional staff will protect them, reinforcing their dependency. People with this disorder are particularly prone to experiencing disorganized schizophrenia.

Epidemiology

The prevalence of schizotypal personality disorder is estimated to range from 0.6% to 5.1%, with a median rate of about 3% of the nonclinical population. In a clinical sample of psychiatric patients, the prevalence ranged from 2.0% to 64%, with a median prevalence of 17.5% (Torgersen et al., 2001). When studying four personality disorders (borderline, schizotypal, avoidant, and obsessive-compulsive), schizotypal personality disorder rates were found to be higher among African Americans when compared with Caucasians (Chavira et al., 2003). This wide variation in prevalence and ethnicity rates may reflect the controversy surrounding the classification of schizotypal disorder as a separate personality disorder, instead of a component of schizophrenia.

Etiology

The etiology of schizotypal personality disorder is unknown. The neurobiological explanation integrates phenomenological, genetic, and cognitive abnormalities. Frontal lobe volume may be preserved in schizotypal personality disorder while temporal volume reductions appear to be common in both disorders. Individuals with schizotypal personality disorder may be spared from psychosis and severe social and cognitive deterioration of chronic schizophrenia by the genetic or environmental factors that promote greater frontal capacity and reduced striatal dopaminergic reactivity (Siever & Davis, 2004). Additional research is needed to determine whether this disorder is a milder form of schizophrenia.

Nursing Management

Depending on the amount of decompensation (deterioration of functioning and exacerbation of symptoms), the assessment of a patient with a schizotypal personality disorder can generate a range of nursing diagnoses. If a person has severe symptoms, such as delusional thinking or perceptual disturbances, the nursing diagnoses are similar to those for a person with schizophrenia (see Chapter 18). If symptoms are mild, the typical nursing diagnoses include Social Isolation, Ineffective Coping, Low Self-esteem, and Impaired Social Interactions.

People with schizotypal personality disorder need help in increasing their sense of self-worth and recognizing their positive attributes. They can benefit from interventions such as social skills training and environmental management that increases their psychosocial functioning. Their odd, eccentric thoughts and behaviors alienate them from others. Reinforcing socially appropriate dress and behavior can improve their overall appearance and ability to relate in the environment. Because they have a hard time generalizing from one situation to another, attention to cognitive skills is important (Waldeck & Miller, 2000).

Continuum of Care

People with cluster A personality disorders are rarely seen in mental health clinics because they seldom admit to mental health problems. They can improve their quality of life through psychotherapy, but their suspiciousness, lack of trust, or impaired social interactions make it difficult to establish a therapeutic relationship. They do not usually seek treatment unless more serious symptoms appear, such as depression or anxiety. Medications are not generally used unless there is coexisting anxiety or depression. Even patients with schizotypal personality disorder have a relatively stable course. Few actually experience schizophrenia or another psychotic disorder (APA, 2000). They too seek health care for other problems, and come to the attention of mental health professionals when their odd behavior interferes with their daily activities. At these times, brief interventions are needed, such as self-care assistance, reality orientation, and role enhancement (Dochterman & Bulechek, 2004).

Nursing care is often provided in a home or clinic setting, with the personality disorder being secondary to the purpose of the care. This means that nurses are focusing on other aspects of patient care and may miss the underlying psychiatric disorder. A psychiatric nursing consult may be needed for these patients to help identify the disorder.

CLUSTER B DISORDERS: DRAMATIC-EMOTIONAL

Borderline Personality Disorder: Unstable Pattern

Clinical Course of Disorder

In 1938, the term *borderline* was first used to refer to a group of disorders that did not quite fit the definition of either neurosis or psychosis (Stern, 1938). The term evolved from the psychoanalytic conceptualization of the disorder as a dysfunctional personality structure. In 1980, BPD was formally recognized as a distinct disorder in the *DSM-III*. In the *DSM-IV-TR*, BPD is defined as "a pervasive pattern of instability of interpersonal relationships, self-image, and affects, and marked impulsivity that begins by early adulthood and is present in a variety of contexts" (APA, 2000, p. 706). Table 22.2 outlines the diagnostic characteristics of BPD.

People with BPD have problems in regulating their moods, developing a sense of self, maintaining interpersonal relationships, maintaining reality-based cognitive processes, and avoiding impulsive or destructive behavior. They appear more competent than they actually are and often set unrealistically high expectations for themselves. When these expectations are not met, they experience intense shame, self-hate, and self-directed anger. Their lives are like soap operas—one crisis after another. Some of the crises are caused by the individual's dysfunctional lifestyle or inadequate social milieu, but many are caused by fate—the death of a spouse or a diagnosis of an illness. They react emotionally with minimal coping skills. The intensity of their dysregulation often frightens themselves and others. Friends, family members, and coworkers limit their contact with the person, which furthers their sense of aloneness, abandonment, and self-hatred. It also diminishes opportunities for learning self-corrective measures.

Remissions from the acute symptoms (self-injurious behaviors and suicide attempts or threats) are fairly common and recurrences are quite rare. Other chronic symptoms such as feelings of intense anger and profound abandonment concerns are more long term problems, but recent research supports that the prognosis for BPD is better than previously recognized (Becker, McGlashan, & Grilo, 2006).

Table 22.2  **Key Diagnostic Characteristics of Borderline Personality Disorder 301.83** 

Diagnostic Criteria and Target Symptoms	*Associated Findings*
• Pervasive pattern of unstable interpersonal relationships, self-image, and affects Frantic efforts to avoid real or imagined abandonment Pattern of unstable and intense interpersonal relationships (alternating between extremes of idealization and devaluation) Identity disturbance (markedly and persistently unstable self-image or sense of self) Impulsivity in at least two areas that are potentially self-damaging (spending, sex, substance abuse, reckless driving, or binge eating) Recurrent suicidal behavior, gestures, or threats; or self-mutilating behavior Affective instability due to a marked reactivity of mood (intense episodes lasting a few hours and only rarely more than a few days) Chronic feelings of emptiness Inappropriate, intense anger or difficulty controlling anger Transient, stress-related paranoid ideation or severe dissociative symptoms • Beginning by early adulthood and presenting in a variety of contexts	***Associated Behavioral Findings*** • Pattern of undermining self at the moment a goal is to be realized • Possible psychotic-like symptoms during times of stress • Recurrent job losses, interrupted education, and broken marriages • History of physical and sexual abuse, neglect, hostile conflict, and early parental loss or separation

Affective Instability

Affective instability (rapid and extreme shift in mood) is a core characteristic of BPD and is evidenced by erratic emotional responses to situations and intense sensitivity to criticism or perceived slights. For example, a person may greet a casual acquaintance with intense affection, yet later, be aloof with the same acquaintance. Friends describe individuals with BPD as moody, irresponsible, or intense. These individuals fail to recognize their own emotional responses, thoughts, beliefs, and behaviors. Persons with BPD also have difficulty recognizing negative facial affects of others and experiencing negative emotions, particularly sadness, anger, and disgust (Bland, Williams, Scharer, & Manning, 2004). Clinically, when a stressful situation is encountered, these individuals react with shifts in emotions. They seem to have limited ability to develop emotional buffers to stressful situations. Regulating anger, anxiety, sadness, and disgust is particularly problematic (Bland et al., 2004).

Identity Disturbances

Identity diffusion occurs when a person lacks aspects of personal identity or when personal identity is poorly developed (Erikson, 1968). Four factors of identity are most commonly disturbed: role absorption (narrowly defining self within a single role), painful incoherence (distressed sense of internal disharmony), inconsistency (lack of coherence in thoughts, feelings, and actions), and lack of commitment (Wilkinson-Ryan & Westen, 2000). Other factors of the personality identity (religious ideology, moral value systems, sexual attitudes) appear to be less important in identity diffusion. Clinically, these patients appear to have no sense of their own identity and direction; this becomes a source of great distress to these patients and is often manifested by chronic feelings of emptiness and boredom. It is not unusual for people with BPD to direct their actions in accord with the wishes of other people. For example, one woman with BPD describes herself: "I am a singer because my mother wanted me to be. I live in the city because my manager thought that I should. I become whatever anyone tells me to be. Whenever someone recommends a song, I wonder why I didn't think of that. My boyfriend tells me what to wear."

Unstable Interpersonal Relationships

People with BPD have an extreme fear of abandonment as well as a history of unstable, insecure attachments (Millon et al., 2004). Most never experienced a consistently secure, nurturing relationship and are constantly seeking reassurance and validation. In an attempt to meet their interpersonal needs, they idealize others and establish intense relationships that violate others' interpersonal boundaries, which leads to rejection. When these relationships do not live up to their expectations, they devalue the person. Continually disappointed in relationships, these individuals, who already are intensely emotional and have a poor sense of self, feel estranged from others and inadequate in the face of perceived social standards. Intense shame and self-hate follow. These feelings often result in self-injurious behaviors, such as cutting the wrist, self-burnings, or head banging.

In social situations, people with BPD use elaborate strategies to structure interactions. That is, they restrict their relationships to ones in which they feel in control. They distance themselves from groups when feeling anxious (which is most of the time) and rarely use their social support system. Even if they are married or have a supportive extended family, they are reluctant to share their feelings. They do not want to burden anyone; they fear rejection and also assume that people are tired of hearing them repeat the same issues (Millon et al., 2004).

Cognitive Dysfunctions

The thinking of people with BPD is dichotomous. Cognitively, they evaluate experiences, people, and objects in terms of mutually exclusive categories (e.g., good or bad, success or failure, trustworthy or deceitful), which informs extreme interpretations of events that would normally be viewed as including both positive and negative aspects. There are also times when their thinking becomes disorganized. Irrelevant, bizarre notions and vague or scattered thought connections are sometimes present, as well as delusions and hallucinations.

Another cognitive dysfunction common in BPD is **dissociation**, or times when thinking, feeling, or behaviors occur outside a person's awareness (Friedel, 2004). Dissociation can be conceptualized on a continuum from minor dissociations of daily life, such as daydreaming, to a breakdown in the integrated functions of consciousness, memory, perception of self or the environment, and sensory-motor behavior. For example, in driving familiar roads, people often get lost in their thoughts or dissociate and suddenly do not remember what happened during that part of the trip. Environmental stimuli are ignored, and there are changes in the perception of reality. The individual is physically present but mentally in another place. Dissociation serves a useful purpose; in the case of driving a familiar road, dissociation alleviates the boredom of driving. It is also a coping strategy for avoiding disturbing events. In dissociating, the person does not have to be aware of or remember traumatic events. There is a strong correlation between dissociation and self-injurious behavior (Zanarini, Ruser, Frankenburg, & Hennen, 2000).

Dysfunctional Behaviors

Impaired Problem Solving. In BPD, there is often failure to engage in active problem solving. Instead, problem solving is attempted by soliciting help from others in a helpless, hopeless manner. Suggestions are rarely taken.

Impulsivity. Impulsivity is also characteristic of people with BPD. Because impulse-driven people have difficulty delaying gratification or thinking through the consequences before acting on their feelings, their actions are often unpredictable. Essentially, they act in the moment and clean up the mess afterward. Gambling, spending money irresponsibly, binge eating, engaging in unsafe sex, and abusing substances are typical of these individuals. They can also be physically or verbally aggressive. Job losses, interrupted education, and unsuccessful relationships are common.

Self-injurious Behaviors. The turmoil and unsuccessful interpersonal relationships and social experiences associated with BPD may lead the person to undermine himself or herself when a goal is about to be reached. The most serious consequences are a suicide attempt or **parasuicidal behavior** (deliberate self-injury with an intent to harm oneself). The prevalence of self-injurious behavior is estimated to be present in half of the patients with BPD (Chapman, Specht, & Cellucci, 2005). Self-injurious behavior can be compulsive (e.g., hair pulling), episodic or repetitive (cutting wrists, arms, or other body parts) and is more likely to occur when the individual with BPD is depressed; has highly unstable interpersonal relationships, especially problems with intimacy and sociability; and is paranoid, hypervigilant (alert, watchful), and resentful. All self-injurious behavior should be considered potentially life threatening and taken seriously.

Borderline Personality Disorder in Special Populations

Many children and adolescents show symptoms similar to those of BPD, such as moodiness, self-destruction, impulsiveness, lack of temper control, and rejection sensitivity. If a family member has BPD, the adolescent should be carefully assessed for this disorder. Because symptoms of BPD begin in adolescence, it makes sense that some of the children and adolescents would meet the criteria for BPD, even though it is not diagnosed before young adulthood. More likely, there are personality traits, such as impulsivity and mood instability, in many adolescents that should be recognized and treated whether or not BPD actually develops.

Epidemiology

The estimated prevalence of BPD in the general population ranges from 0.4% to 2.0%, with a median rate of 1.6%. In clinical populations, BPD is one of the most frequently diagnosed personality disorders (Zimmerman, Rothschild, and Chelminski, 2005). More than three fourths (77%) of the patients with diagnoses of BPD are young women (mean age, mid-20s) (Friedel, 2004). One explanation for this is that it is more socially acceptable for women than men to seek help from the health care system. Another reason is that childhood sexual abuse, which more commonly affects girls, is one of the strongest risk factors for BPD. Gender bias in diagnosing may have a role.

Ample clinical reports show the coexistence of personality disorders with Axis I disorders (mood, substance abuse, eating, dissociative, and anxiety disorders) and other personality disorders (Zimmerman et al., 2005).

Risk Factors

Various studies show that physical and sexual abuse appear to be significant risk factors for BPD (Bandelow et al., 2005). Other studies cite parental loss and separation (Levy, Meehan, Weber, Reynoso, & Clarkin, 2005). Clearly, more studies are needed to identify risk factors for the development of BPD.

Etiology

Evidence supports a biopsychosocial etiology. Recent studies demonstrate differences in brain functioning between those with and without BPD, but also provide evidence that psychological and social factors contribute to the development of the disorder. The following discussion highlights the leading explanations for BPD.

Biologic Theories

There is now clear evidence of central nervous system dysfunction in BPD including possible structural changes (De la Fuente et al., 2006). Magnetic resonance imaging studies of 21 female patients with both BPD and PTSD, compared with a matched healthy control sample, showed that women with BPD had a 16% smaller amygdala than did the healthy control subjects (Driessen et al., 2000).

Biologic abnormalities are associated with three BPD characteristics: affective instability; transient psychotic episodes; and impulsive, aggressive, and suicidal behavior (Pally, 2002). Associated brain dysfunction occurs in the limbic system and frontal lobe and increases the behaviors of impulsiveness, parasuicide, and mood disturbance. A decrease in serotonin activity and an increase in α_2-noradrenergic receptor sites may be related to the irritability and impulsiveness common in people with this disorder (Goodman, New, & Siever, 2004).

It has also been hypothesized that an increase in dopamine may be responsible for transient psychotic states. These dysfunctions could be caused by a number of events, including trauma, epilepsy, and attention-deficit hyperactivity disorder (ADHD). People with BPD manifest psychotic-like symptoms, including paranoid thinking, dissociation, depersonalization, and derealization. These symptoms seem to be associated with intense anxiety. There is some evidence that these symptoms are associated with excessive dopaminergic activity (Friedel, 2004a).

Psychological Theories

Psychoanalytic Theories. The psychoanalytic views of BPD focus on two important psychoanalytic concepts: separation-individuation and projective identification. A person with BPD has not achieved the normal and healthy developmental stage of **separation-individuation**, during which a child develops a sense of self, a permanent sense of significant others (object constancy), and integration of seeing both bad and good components of self (Jørgensen, 2006). Those with BPD lack the ability to separate from the primary caregiver and develop a separate and distinct personality or self-identity. Psychoanalytic theory suggests that these separation difficulties occur because the primary caregivers' behaviors have been inconsistent or insensitive to the needs of the child. The child develops ambivalent feelings regarding interpersonal relationships and therefore has no basis for establishing trusting and secure relationships in the future. Children experience feelings of intense fear and anger in separating themselves from others. This problem continues into adulthood, and they continue to experience difficulties in maintaining personal boundaries and in interpersonal interactions and relationships. Often, these patients falsely attribute to others their own unacceptable feelings, impulses, or thoughts, termed **projective identification**. Projective identification is believed to play an important role in the development of BPD and is a defense mechanism by which people with BPD protect their fragile self-image. For example, when overwhelmed by anxiety or anger at being disregarded by another, they defend against the intensity of these feelings by unconsciously blaming others for what happens to them. They project their feelings onto a significant other with the unconscious hope that the other knows how to deal with it. Projective identification becomes a defensive way of interacting with the world, which leads to more rejection.

Maladaptive Cognitive Processes. Cognitive schemas are important in understanding BPD (and antisocial personality disorder as well). Individuals with personality disorders develop dysfunctional beliefs and maladaptive schemas leading them to misinterpret environmental stimuli continuously, which in turn leads to rigid and inflexible behavior patterns in response to new situations and people (Butler, Brown, Beck, & Grisham, 2002; Lobbestael, Arntz, & Sieswerda, 2005). Because those with BPD have been conditioned to anticipate rejection and disappointment in the past, they become entrenched in a pattern of fear and anxiety regarding encountering new people or situations. They have fears that disaster is going to strike any minute. Early in life, patients with BPD and other personality disorders develop maladaptive schemas or dysfunctional ways of interpreting people and events. Table 22.3 explains 15 major maladaptive schemas at work in those with personality disorders. The work of cognitive therapists is to challenge these distortions in thinking patterns and replace them with realistic ones.

Social Theories: Biosocial Theories

This biosocial viewpoint proposed by Marsha Linehan and colleagues sees BPD as a multifaceted problem, a combination of a person's innate **emotional vulnerability** and his or her inability to control that emotion in social interactions (**emotional dysregulation**) and the environment (Linehan, 1993) (Box 22.1). The emotional dysregulation and aggressive impulsivity entail both social learning and biologic regulation. Much of the neurobiologic research is directed at neurotransmitter functions involving serotonin, norepinephrine, dopamine, acetylcholine, GABA, and vasopressin (Joyce et al., 2006; Gollan, Lee, & Coccaro, 2005). In fact, restoring balance in these systems permits more consistent neural firing between the limbic system and the frontal and prefrontal cortex. When these pathways are functional, the person has greater capacity to think about his or her emotions and modulate behavior more responsibly.

According to the biosocial approach, the ability to control emotion is in part learned from private experiences and encounters with the social environment. BPD is believed to develop when emotionally vulnerable individuals interact with an **invalidating environment**, a social situation that negates private emotional responses and communication. When core emotional responses and communications are continuously dismissed, trivialized, devalued, punished, and discredited (invalidated) by respected or valued persons, the vulnerable individual becomes unsure about their feelings (Fig. 22.1). A minor example of invalidating environment or response follows: The parents of Emily, a 4-year-old girl, tell her that the family is going to grandmother's house for a family meal. The child responds, "I am not going to Gramma's. I hate Stevie (cousin)." The parents reply, "You don't hate Stevie. He is a wonderful child. He is your cousin, and only a spoiled, selfish little girl would say such a thing." The parents have devalued Emily's feelings and discredited her comments, thereby invalidating her feelings and sense of personal worth.

The most severe form of invalidation occurs in situations of child sexual abuse. Often, the abusing adult has told the child that this is a "special secret" between them. The child experiences feelings of fear, pain, and sadness,

Table 22.3 Maladaptive Schemes

Domain	Schemes with Definitions
I. Disconnection & rejection	1. *Abandonment/instability* Important people will not be there 2. *Mistrust/abuse* Other people will use patient for own selfish end 3. *Emotional deprivation* Emotional connection will not be fulfilled 4. *Defectiveness/scheme* One is flawed, bad, or worthless 5. *Social isolation/alienation* Being different from or not fitting in
II. Impaired autonomy & performance	1. *Dependence/incompetence* Belief that one is unable to function on one's own 2. *Vulnerability to harm and illness* Fear that disaster is about to strike 3. *Enmeshment/undeveloped self* Excessive emotional involvement at expense of normal social development 4. *Failure* Belief that one has failed
III. Impaired limits	1. *Entitlement/grandiosity* Belief that one is superior to others entitled to special rights 2. *Insufficient self-control/self-discipline* Difficulty or refusal to exercise sufficient self-control
IV. Other directedness	1. *Subjugation* Excessive surrendering of control to others because of feeling coerced 2. *Self-sacrifice* Excessive focus on voluntarily meeting the needs of others at the expense of one's own gratification 3. *Approval-seeking/recognition-seeking* Excessive emphasis on gaining approval, recognition, or attention
V. Overvigilance & inhibition	1. *Negativity/pessimism* Lifelong focus on negative aspects of life 2. *Emotional inhibition* Excessive inhibition of spontaneous action, feeling, or communication 3. *Unrelenting standard/hypercriticalness* Belief one must meet very high standard, perfectionistic, rigid 4. *Punitiveness* Belief people should be harshly punished

Young, J. E. (2003). *Cognitive therapy for personality disorders: A schema-focused approach.* Sarasota, FL: Professional Resource Press.

BOX 22.1

Behavioral Patterns in Borderline Personality Disorder

1. *Emotional vulnerability.* Person experiences a pattern of pervasive difficulties in regulating negative emotions, including high sensitivity to negative emotional stimuli, high emotional intensity, and slow return to emotional baseline.
2. *Self-invalidation.* Person fails to recognize one's own emotional responses, thoughts, beliefs, and behaviors and sets unrealistically high standards and expectations for self. May include intense shame, self-hate, and self-directed anger. Person has no personal awareness and tends to blame social environment for unrealistic expectations and demands.
3. *Unrelenting crises.* Person experiences pattern of frequent, stressful, negative environmental events, disruptions, and roadblocks—some caused by the individual's dysfunctional lifestyle, others by an inadequate social milieu, and many by fate or chance.
4. *Inhibited grieving.* Person tries to inhibit and over-control negative emotional responses, especially those associated with grief and loss, including sadness, anger, guilt, shame, anxiety, and panic.
5. *Active passivity.* Person fails to engage actively in solving of own life problems but will actively seek problem solving from others in the environment; learned helplessness, hopelessness.
6. *Apparent competence.* Tendency for the individual to appear deceptively more competent than he or she actually is; usually due to failure of competencies to generalize across expected moods, situations, and time, and failure to display adequate nonverbal cues of emotional distress.

Linehan, M. (1993). *Cognitive-behavioral treatment of borderline personality disorder* (p. 10). New York: Guilford Press.

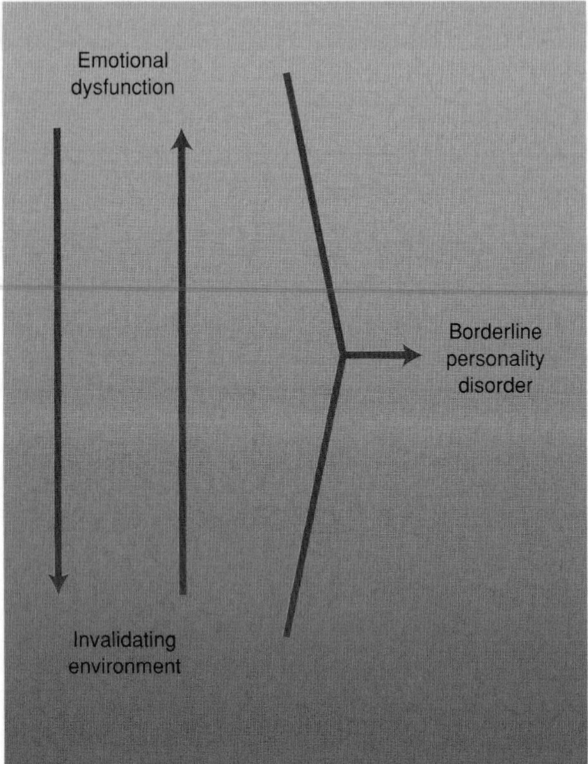

FIGURE 22.1. Biosocial theory of borderline personality disorder. (Courtesy of Marsha M. Linehan, Ph.D., Department of Psychology, Box 351525, University of Washington, Seattle, WA 98195. © 1993 by Marsha M. Linehan.)

yet this trusted adult continuously dismisses the child's true feelings and tells the child what he or she should feel.

Interdisciplinary Treatment

BPD is a very complex disorder that requires the whole mental health care team. Several types of medications are usually needed including mood stabilizers, antidepressants, and anxiolytics; careful medication monitoring is necessary. Psychotherapy is needed to help the individual manage the dysfunctional moods, impulsive behavior, and self-injurious behaviors. Specially trained therapists who are comfortable with the many demands of these patients are needed. These therapists represent a variety of mental health disciplines, including psychology, social work, and advanced practice nursing. This is a lifelong disorder requiring ongoing treatment as the individual copes with multiple interpersonal crises.

Dialectical Behavior Therapy

Dialectical behavior therapy (DBT) combines cognitive and behavior therapy strategies. Clinicians partner with patients and focus on the many interconnected behaviors (e.g., parasuicidal and substance abuse). Patients learn to understand their disorder by actively participating in establishing treatment goals, collecting data about their own behavior, identifying treatment targets, and working with the therapists in changing the problematic behaviors. When used on an inpatient basis, DBT requires total staff commitment and reinforcement and has shown significant improvement in depression, anxiety, and dissociation symptoms and a highly significant decrease in parasuicidal behavior (Linehan et al., 2006). Staff must maintain a positive approach and assume a skills coach role with patients. DBT is more often incorporated into a long-term partial hospitalization and outpatient treatment approach because the greatest effectiveness occurs when skills are reinforced over time and practiced in a variety of daily living settings.

Core interventions include problem solving, exposure techniques (gradual exposure to cues that set off aversive emotions), skill training, contingency management (reinforcement of positive behavior), and cognitive modification. **Skills groups** are an integral part of DBT and are taught in group settings in which patients practice emotional regulation, interpersonal effectiveness, distress tolerance, core mindfulness, and self-management skills.

Emotion regulation skills are taught to manage intense, labile moods and involve helping the patient label and analyze the context of the emotion and develop strategies to reduce emotional vulnerability. Teaching individuals to observe and describe emotions without judging them or blocking them helps patients experience emotions without stimulating secondary feelings that cause more distress. For example, describing the emotion of anger without judging it as being "bad" can eliminate feelings of guilt that lead to self-injury.

Interpersonal effectiveness skills include the development of assertiveness and problem-solving skills within an interpersonal context. *Mindfulness skills* are the psychological and behavioral versions of meditation skills usually taught in Eastern spiritual practice and are used to help the person improve observation, description, and participation skills by learning to focus the mind and awareness on the current moment's activity.

Distress tolerance skills involve helping the individual tolerate and accept distress as a part of normal life. *Self-management skills* focus on helping patients learn how to control, manage, or change behavior, thoughts, or emotional responses to events (Linehan, 1993; van den Bosch, Verheul, Schippers, & van den Brink, 2002).

Family Response to Disorder 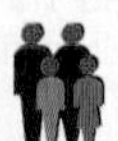

Individuals with BPD are typically part of a chaotic family system, but they usually add to the chaos. Their family often feels captive to these patients. Family members are afraid to disagree with them or refuse to meet their multiple needs, fearing that self-destructive behavior will follow. During the course of the disorder, family members often get "burned out" and withdraw from the patient, only adding to the patient's fear of abandonment.

NURSING MANAGEMENT: HUMAN RESPONSE TO BPD

Persons with BPD may enter the mental health system early (young adulthood or before), because of their chaotic lifestyle. There are unstable moods, problems with interpersonal relationships, low self-esteem, and self-identity issues. Thinking and behavior are dysregulated (see Box 22.2). There are problems in daily living—maintaining intimate relationships, keeping a job, and living within the law (Box 22.3).

They drop in and out of treatment as it suits their mood and usually do not remain with one clinician for long-term treatment. They do not receive consistent treatment and usually seek help from health care workers because of consequences of their numerous life crises, medical conditions, other psychiatric disorders (e.g., depression), or for physical treatment of self-injury. Thus, other problems usually may need attention before the patient's underlying personality disorder can be addressed. Sometimes, the nurse will not know that the person has BPD. However, during an assessment, it becomes clear that these individuals let things bother them more than do others or have an inflexible view of the world. They also seem to have great difficulty changing behavior, no matter the consequences. Because they see the world differently from

BOX 22.2

Response Patterns of Persons With Borderline Personality Disorder

Affective (mood) dysregulation
Mood lability
Problems with anger
Interpersonal dysregulation
Chaotic relationships
Fears of abandonment
Self-dysregulation
Identity disturbance or difficulties with sense of self
Sense of emptiness
Behavioral dysregulation
Parasuicidal behavior or threats
Impulsive behavior
Cognitive dysregulation
Dissociative responses
Paranoid ideation

Courtesy of M. Linehan, Department of Psychology, Box 351525, University of Washington, Seattle, WA 98195-1525, 1993.

BOX 22.3

Clinical Vignette: Borderline Personality Disorder

JS is a 22-year-old single woman who was recently fired from her job as a data entry clerk. She is living with her mother and stepfather, who brought her to the emergency room after finding her crouched in a fetal position in the bathroom, her wrists bleeding. She seemed to be in a daze. This is her first psychiatric admission, although her mother and stepfather have suspected that she has "needed help" for a long time. In high school, she received brief treatment for a potential eating disorder. She remains very thin but is able to eat at least one meal per day. During periods of stress, she will go for days without eating. Joanne is the second of three children. Her parents divorced when she was 3 years old. She has not seen her father since he left. Although she has pleasant memories of her father, her mother has told her that he beat Joanne and her sisters when he was drinking. When Joanne was 6 years old, her older sister died following an automobile accident. Joanne was in the car but was uninjured. As a child, Joanne was seen as a potential singing star. Her natural musical talent attracted her teachers' support, which encouraged her to develop her talent. She received singing lessons and entered state-wide competitions in high school. Although she enjoyed the attention, she was never really comfortable in the limelight and felt "guilty" about having a talent that she sometimes resented. She was able to make friends but found that she was unable to keep them. They described her as "too intense" and emotional. She had one boyfriend in high school, but she was very uncomfortable with any physical closeness. After ending the relationship with the boyfriend, she concentrated on dieting to have a "perfect body." When her dieting attracted her parents' attention, she vowed to eat just enough to keep them "off her back about it." She spent much of her leisure time with her grandmother. She attended college briefly but was unable to concentrate. It was during college and after her grandmother's death that Joanne began cutting her wrists during periods of stress. It seemed to calm her.

After leaving college, Joanne returned home. She had several jobs and short-lived friendships. She was usually fired from her job because of "moodiness," and it would take her several months before she would again find another. She would spend days in her room listening to music. Her recent episode followed being fired from work and spending 3 days in her bedroom.

What Do You Think?

- How would you describe Joanne's mood?
- Are Joanne's losses (father, sister) really severe enough to affect her ability to relate to others now? Do the losses seem to relate to the self-injury?
- What behaviors indicate that there are problems with self-esteem and self-identity?

the average person, they have difficulty in successfully relating to other people and living a satisfying life.

Biologic Domain

Biologic Assessment

People with BPD are usually able to maintain personal hygiene and physical functioning. Because of the comorbidity of BPD and eating disorders and substance abuse, a nutritional assessment may be needed. The assessment should also include the use of caffeinated beverages, such as coffee, tea, soda, and alcohol. With patients who engage in binging or purging, assessment should include examining the teeth for pitting and discoloration, as well as the hands and fingers for redness and calluses caused by inducing vomiting. The patient should be queried about physiologic responses of emotion. Sleep patterns also should be assessed because sleep alterations may suggest coexisting depression or mania.

Physical Indicators of Self-injurious Behaviors. Patients with BPD should be assessed for self-injurious behavior or suicide attempts. It is important to ask the patient about specific self-abusive behaviors, such as cutting, scratching, or swallowing. The patient may wear long sleeves to hide injury on the arms. Specifically asking about thoughts of hurting oneself when experiencing a major upset provides an opportunity for prevention and for coaching the patient toward alternative self-soothing measures.

Pharmacologic Assessment. Patients with BPD may be taking several medications. For example, one patient may be taking a small dose of an antipsychotic and a mood stabilizer. Another may be taking a selective serotonin reuptake inhibitor (SSRI). Initially, patients may be reluctant to disclose all of the medications they are taking because, for many, there has been a period of trial and error. They are fearful of having medication taken away from them. Development of rapport with special attention to a nonjudgmental approach is especially important when eliciting current medication practices. The effectiveness of the medication in relieving the target symptom needs to be determined. Use of alcohol and street drugs should be carefully assessed to determine drug interactions.

Nursing Diagnoses for the Biologic Domain

Nursing diagnoses focusing on the biologic domain include Insomnia, Imbalanced Nutrition, Self-mutilation or Risk for Self-mutilation, and Ineffective Therapeutic Regimen Management.

Interventions for the Biologic Domain

The interventions for the biologic domain may address a whole spectrum of problems. Usually, the patients are managing hydration, self-care, and pain well. This section focuses on those areas most likely to be problematic.

Sleep Enhancement. Facilitation of regular sleep–wake cycles may be needed because of disturbed sleep patterns. Conservative approaches should be exhausted before recommending medication. Establishing a regular bedtime routine, monitoring bedtime snacks and drinks, and avoiding foods and drinks that interfere with sleep should be tried. If relaxation exercises are used, they should be adapted to the tolerance of the individual. Moderate exercises (e.g., brisk walking) 3 to 4 hours before bedtime activates both serotonin and endorphins, thereby enhancing calmness and a sense of well-being before bedtime. For patients who have difficulty falling asleep and experience interrupted sleep, it helps to establish some basic sleeping routines. The bedroom should be reserved for only two activities: sleeping and sex. Therefore, the patient should remove the television, computer, and exercise equipment from the bedroom. If the patient is not asleep within 15 minutes, he or she should get out of bed and go to another room to read, watch television, or listen to soft music. The patient should return to bed when sleepy. If the patient is not asleep in 15 minutes, the same process should be repeated.

Special consideration must be made for patients who have been physically and sexually abused and who may be unable to put themselves in a vulnerable position (such as lying down in a room with other people or closing their eyes). These patients may need additional safeguards to help them sleep, such as a night light or repositioning of furniture to afford easy exit.

Nutritional Balance. The nutritional status of the person with BPD can quickly become a priority, particularly if the patient has coexisting eating disorders or substance abuse. Eating is often a response to stress, and patients can quickly become overweight. This is especially a problem when the patient has also been taking medications that promote weight gain, such as antipsychotics, antidepressants, or mood stabilizers. Helping the patient to learn the basics of nutrition, make reasonable choices, and develop other coping strategies are useful interventions. If patients are engaging in purging or severe dieting practices, teaching the patient about the dangers of both of these practices is important (see Chapter 24). Referral to an eating disorders specialist may be needed.

Prevention and Treatment of Self-injury. Patients with BPD are usually admitted to the inpatient setting because of threats of self-injury. Observing for antecedents of self-injurious behavior and intervening before an episode is an important safety intervention. Patients can learn to identify situations leading to self-destructive behavior and develop preventive strategies. Because patients with BPD are impulsive and may respond to stress by harming themselves, observation of the patient's interactions and assessment of the mood, level of distress, and agitation are important indicators of impending self-injury.

Remembering that self-injury is an effort to self-soothe by activating endogenous endorphins, the nurse can assist the patient to find more productive and enduring ways to find comfort. Linehan (1993) suggests using the Five Senses Exercise:

- Vision (e.g., go outside and look at the stars or flowers or autumn leaves)
- Hearing (e.g., listen to beautiful or invigorating music or the sounds of nature)
- Smell (e.g., light a scented candle, boil a cinnamon stick in water)
- Taste (e.g., drink a soothing, warm, nonalcoholic beverage)
- Touch (e.g., take a hot bubble bath, pet your dog or cat, get a massage)

Pharmacologic Interventions. Less medication is better for people with BPD. Patients should take medications only for target symptoms for a short time (e.g., an antidepressant for a bout with depression) because they may be taking many medications, particularly if they have a comorbid disorder, such as a mood disorder or substance abuse. Pharmacotherapy is used to control emotional dysregulation, impulsive aggression, cognitive disturbances, and anxiety as an adjunct to psychotherapy (Morana & Camara, 2006).

Controlling Emotional Dysregulation. Target symptoms of emotional dysregulation include instability of mood, marked shifts from or to depression, stress-related and transient mood crashes, rejection sensitivity, and inappropriate and intense outbursts of anger. Because decreased central serotonin neurotransmission has been implicated in the emotional dysregulation and impulsive-aggressive behaviors, the antidepressants are frequently used (Binks et al., 2006).

Reducing Impulsivity. Impulsivity, anger outbursts, and mood lability may be treated effectively with the newer GABA-ergic anticonvulsants such as lamotrigine (Lamictal), gabapentin (Neurontin), and topiramate (Topamax) (Nickel et al., 2005). These appear to act by regulating neural firing in the mesolimbic area. Carbamazepine (Tegretol) and lithium have also been used, but these have a less favorable side effect profile. Divalproex is a frequently used drug for impulsivity and aggression (Hollander, Swann, Coccaro, Jiang, & Smith, 2005).

Managing Transient Psychotic Episodes. Antipsychotic medications may be useful when the patient demonstrates thought disorganization, misinterpretation of reality, and high levels of emotional instability. Low doses of antipsychotics are most often used off label (Binks et al., 2006).

Decreasing Anxiety. If a patient is experiencing anxiety, a nonbenzodiazepine such as buspirone (BuSpar) may be used (Box 22.4). Buspirone appears to be an ideal antianxiety drug. Unlike the benzodiazepines, it does not have the sedation, ataxia, tolerance, and withdrawal effects and does not lead to abuse. However, buspirone takes longer to act than do the benzodiazepines. If a patient has been taking benzodiazepines for years, buspirone may not lead to much improvement. When switching from a benzodiazepine to buspirone, the withdrawal symptoms may be unpleasant (or even dangerous), and buspirone will not have any effect on the distress. Because buspirone is a serotonin (5-HT1A) agonist, its use with an SSRI enhances the benefits of both drugs to reduce anxiety and depression symptoms (Stahl, 2000), but exposes the patient to serotonin syndrome risk.

More often, people with BPD find buspirone ineffective if their type of anxiety is intense and accompanied by agitation and aggression. In these instances, SSRIs may be prescribed at higher doses than those used for depression (Best, Williams, & Coccaro, 2002; Gurvits, Koenigsberg, & Siever, 2000).

Monitoring and Administering Medications. In inpatient settings, it is relatively easy to control medications; in other settings, patients must be aware that it is their responsibility to take their medication and monitor the number and type of drugs being taken. Patients who rely on medication to help them deal with stress or those who are periodically suicidal are at high risk for abuse of medications. Patients who have unusual side effects are also at high risk for noncompliance. The nurse determines whether the patient is actually taking medication, whether the medication is being taken as prescribed, the effect on target symptoms, and the use of any over-the-counter drugs, such as antihistamines or sleeping pills.

However, the patient cannot rely just on the medication. Assuming responsibility for taking the medication regularly, understanding the effects of the medication,

BOX 22.4

Drug Profile: Buspirone (Buspar)

DRUG CLASS: Antianxiety agent

RECEPTOR AFFINITY: Binds to serotonin receptors and acts as an agonist to 5-HT_{1B}. Clinical significance unclear. Exact mechanism of action unknown.

INDICATIONS: Management of anxiety disorders or short-term relief of symptoms of anxiety.

ROUTES AND DOSAGE: Available in 5- and 10-mg tablets.

Adults: Initially, 15 mg/d (5 mg tid). Increased by 5 mg/d at intervals of 2–3 d to achieve optimal therapeutic response. Not to exceed 60 mg/d.

Children: Safety and efficacy under 18 years of age not established.

HALF-LIFE (PEAK EFFECT): 3–11 h (40–90 min).

SELECT ADVERSE REACTIONS: Dizziness, headache, nervousness, insomnia, light-headedness, nausea, dry mouth, vomiting, gastric distress, diarrhea, tachycardia, and palpitations.

WARNING: Contraindicated in patients with hypersensitivity to buspirone, marked liver or renal impairment, and during lactation. Alcohol and other CNS depressants can cause increased sedation. Decreased effects seen if given with fluoxetine. Should not be given with MAOIs.

SPECIFIC PATIENT/FAMILY EDUCATION:

- Take drug exactly as prescribed; may take with foods or meals if gastrointestinal upset occurs.
- Avoid alcohol and other CNS depressants.
- Notify prescriber before taking any over-the-counter or prescription medications.
- Avoid driving or performing hazardous activities that require alertness and concentration.
- Use ice chips or sugarless candies to alleviate dry mouth.
- Notify prescriber of any abnormal involuntary movements of facial or neck muscles, abnormal posture, or yellowing of skin or eyes.
- Continue medical follow-up and do not abruptly discontinue use.

and augmenting the medication with other strategies is the most effective approach. The nurse helps the patient assume this responsibility and provides guidance that supports self-efficacy and competence. It is also important for the nurse to emphasize that the medications provide the physiologic balance, but it is the patient's effort and skills that provide the social and behavioral balance. By stressing this, the patient does not overinvest in the medication and feels more confident of her or his own skills.

Side-Effect Monitoring and Management. Patients with BPD appear to be sensitive to many of the medications, and the dose may need to be adjusted based on the side effects they experience. Listen carefully to the patient's description of the side effects. Any unusual side effects should be accurately documented and reported to the prescriber.

Teaching Points 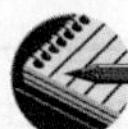

Patients should be educated about the medications and their interactions with other drugs and substances. Interventions include teaching patients about the medication and how and where it acts in the brain and body, helping establish a routine for taking prescribed medication, reporting side effects, and facilitating the development of positive coping strategies to deal with daily stresses, rather than relying on medications. Eliciting the patient's partnership in care improves adherence and thereby outcomes.

Psychological Domain

Psychological Assessment

People with BPD have usually experienced significant losses in their lives that shape their view of the world. They experience **inhibited grieving**, "a pattern of repetitive, significant trauma and loss, together with an inability to fully experience and personally integrate or resolve these events" (Linehan, 1993, p. 89). They have unresolved grief that can last for years and avoid situations that evoke those feelings of separation and loss. During the assessment, the nurse can identify the losses (real or perceived) and explore the patient's experience during these losses, paying particular attention to whether the patient has reached resolution. History of physical or sexual abuse and early separation from significant caregivers may provide important clues to the severity of the disturbances.

Mood fluctuations are common and can be assessed by any number of the depression and anxiety screening scales, or by asking the following questions:

- What things or events bother you and make you feel happy, sad, angry?
- Do these things or events trouble you more than they trouble other people?
- Do friends and family tell you that you are moody?
- Do you get angry easily?
- Do you have trouble with your temper?
- Do you think you were born with these feelings or did something happen to make you feel this way?

Appearance and activity level generally reflect the person's mood and psychomotor activity. Many of those with BPD have been physically or sexually abused and thus should be assessed for depression. A disheveled appearance can reflect depression or an agitated state. When feeling good, these patients can be very engaging; they tend to be dramatic in their style of dress and attract attention, such as by wearing an unusual hairstyle or heavy makeup. Because physical appearance reflects identity, patients may experiment with their appearance and seek affirmation and acceptance from others. Body piercing, tattoos, and other adornments provide a mechanism to define self.

Impulsivity. Impulsivity can be identified by asking the patient if he or she does things impulsively or spur of the moment. Have there been times when you were hurt by your actions or were sorry later that you acted in the way you did? Direct questions about gambling, choices in sexual partners, sexual activities, fights, arguments, arrests, and alcohol drinking habits can also help in identifying areas of impulsive behavior.

From a neurophysiologic perspective, impulsively acting before thinking seems to be mediated by rapid nerve firing in the mesolimbic area. This activates psychomotor responses prior to pathways reaching the prefrontal cortex (Best et al., 2002). Teaching the patient strategies to slow down automatic responses (e.g., deep breathing, counting to 10) buys time to think before acting.

Cognitive Disturbances. The mental status examination of those with BPD usually reveals normal thought processes that are not disorganized or confused, except during periods of stress. Those with BPD usually exhibit **dichotomous thinking**, or a tendency to view things as absolute, either black or white, good or bad, with no perception of compromise. Dichotomous thinking can be assessed by asking patients how they view other people. Evidence of dichotomous thinking is indicated with responses of "good" or "bad," "wonderful" or "terrible."

Dissociation and Transient Psychotic Episodes. There may be periods of dissociation and transient psychotic episodes. Dissociation can be assessed by asking if there is ever a time when the patient does not remember events or has the feeling of being separate from his or her body. Some patients refer to this as "spacing out." By asking specific information about how often, how long, and when dissociation first was used, the nurse can get an idea of how important dissociation is as a coping skill. It is important to ask the person what is happening in the environment when dissociation occurs. Frequent dissociation indicates a highly habitual coping mechanism that will be difficult to change. Because transient psychotic states occur, it is also important to elicit data regarding the presence of hallucinations or delusions, their frequency and circumstances.

Risk Assessment: Suicide or Self-injury. It is critical that patients with BPD be assessed for suicidal and self-damaging behavior, including alcohol and drug abuse. (Suicide assessment is discussed in Chapter 17.) An assessment should include direct questions, asking if the patient thinks about or engages in self-injurious behaviors. If so, the nurse should continue to explore the behaviors: what is done, how it is done, its frequency, and the circumstances surrounding the self-injurious behavior. It is helpful to explain briefly to the patient that sometimes people cut, scratch, or pick at themselves as a way of bringing some relief and comfort. Although the behavior brings temporary relief, it also places the person at risk for infection. Approaching the assessment in this way conveys a sense of understanding and is more likely to invite the patient to disclose honestly.

Nursing Diagnoses for the Psychological Domain

One of the first diagnoses to consider is Risk for Self-mutilation because protection of the patient from self-injury is always a priority. If cognitive changes are present (dissociation and transient psychosis), two other diagnoses may be appropriate: Disturbed Thought Process and Ineffective Coping. The Disturbed Thought Process diagnosis is used if dissociative and psychotic episodes actually interfere with daily living. For example, a secretary could not complete processing letters because she was unable to differentiate whether the voices on the dictating machine were being transmitted by the machine or her hallucinations. The nurse helped her learn to differentiate the hallucinations from dictation. The patient learned to take her headset off, take a deep breath, and listen to her external environment. When she recognized "the voice" as her partner criticizing her, she was able to use her cognitive reframing strategies to refocus on reality.

If the individual copes with stressful situations by dissociating or hallucinating, the diagnosis Ineffective Coping is used. The outcome in this instance would be the substitution of positive coping skills for the dissociations or hallucinations.

Other nursing diagnoses that are typically supported by assessment data include Personal Identity Disturbance, Anxiety, Grieving, Chronic Low Self-esteem, Powerlessness, Post-trauma Response, Defensive Coping, and Spiritual Distress. The identification of outcomes depends on the nursing diagnoses (Fig. 22.2).

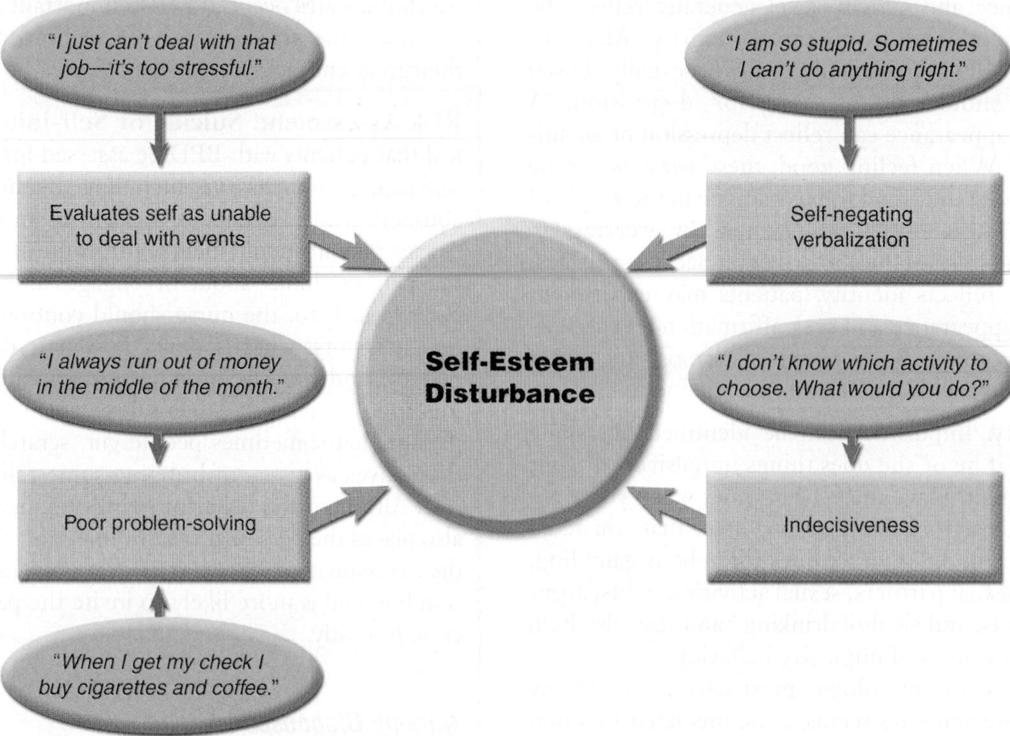

FIGURE 22.2. Nursing diagnosis concept map: chronic low self-esteem.

Interventions for the Psychological Domain

The challenge of working with people with BPD is engaging the patient in a therapeutic relationship that will survive its emotional ups and downs. The patient needs to understand that the nurse is there to coach her or him to develop self-modulation skills. A relationship based on mutual respect and consistency is crucial for helping the patient with those skills. Self-awareness skills are needed by the nurse along with access to clinical supervision by an advanced practice psychiatric–mental health nurse such as a clinical nurse specialist or psychiatric–mental health nurse practitioner (Bland & Rossen, 2005; Bland, Tudor, & Whitehouse; in press). Because patients with BPD are frequently hospitalized, even nurses in acute care settings have an opportunity to develop a long-term relationship (Fig. 22.3).

Generalist psychiatric–mental health nurses do not function as the patient's primary therapists, but they do need to establish a therapeutic relationship that strengthens the patient's coping skills and self-esteem, and supports individual psychotherapy. The therapeutic relationship helps the patient to experience a model of healthy interaction with consistency, limit setting, caring, and respect for others (both self-respect and respect for the patient). Patients who have low self-esteem need help in recognizing genuine respect from others and reciprocating with respect for others. In the therapeutic relationship, the nurse models self-respect by observing personal limits, being assertive, and clearly communicating expectations. (Box 22.5).

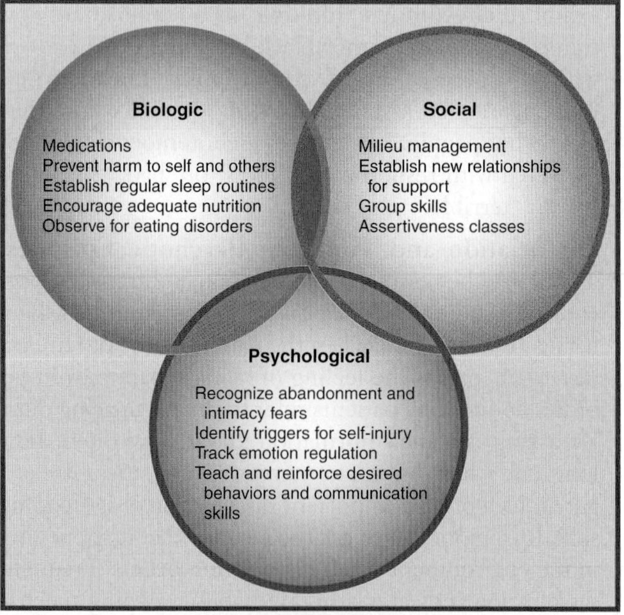

FIGURE 22.3. Biopsychosocial interventions for patients with borderline personality disorder.

BOX 22.5

Research for Best Practice

Hoch, J. S., O'Reilly, R. L., & Carscadden, J. (2006). Relationship management therapy for patients with borderline personality disorder. Psychiatric Services, 57(2), 179–181.

THE QUESTION: Will relationship management therapy reduce the use of seclusion and restraint for patients with hospitalized borderline personality disorder?

METHODS: A retrospective pre-post analysis of 27 adult patients admitted to an inpatient relationship management program was conducted based on the premise that individuals with borderline personality disorder are responsible, competent adults who can choose their own treatment, limited only by the availability of resources and by professional standards of practice. This type of therapy prepares patients for other approaches, such as DBT. All patients with the exception of two had data available for at least 1 year before they enrolled.

FINDINGS: There were no differences in the mean number of hours in seclusion in the year before enrollment compared with the year during enrollment (12 vs 9 hours). Statistical differences were seen in the mean number of hours in restraints before and during the program (33 vs 1 hour).

IMPLICATIONS FOR NURSING: Providing patients with choices of treatment may reduce the behaviors leading to self-harm. Although restraints are rarely used in the United States, this study has potential for shaping a positive treatment experience for patients who are high risk for suicide and self-harm.

Abandonment and Intimacy Fears. A key to helping patients with BPD is recognizing their fears of both abandonment and intimacy. Informing the patient of the length of the relationship as much as possible allows the patient to engage in and prepare for termination with the least pain of abandonment. If the patient's hospitalization is time limited, the nurse overtly acknowledges the limit and reminds the patient with each contact how many sessions remain (see Box 22.6).

In day-treatment and outpatient settings, the duration of treatment may be indeterminate, but the nurse may not be available that entire time. The termination process cannot be casual; this would stimulate abandonment fears. However, some patients end prematurely when the nurse informs them of the impending end as a way to leave before being rejected. Anticipating premature closure, the nurse explores with the patient anticipated feelings, including the wish to run away. After careful planning, the nurse anticipates, in advance, the patient's feelings, discusses how to cope with them, reviews the progress the patient has made, and summarizes what the patient has learned from the relationship that can be generalized to future encounters.

Establishing Personal Boundaries and Limitations. Personal boundaries are highly context specific; for example, stroking the hair of a stranger on the bus would be inappropriate, but stroking the hair and face of one's intimate partner while sitting together would

BOX 22.6

Therapeutic Dialogue: Borderline Personality Disorder

Ineffective Approach

Patient: Hey, you know what? You are my favorite nurse. That night nurse sure doesn't understand me the way you do.
Nurse: Oh, I'm glad you are comfortable with me. Which night nurse?
Patient: You know, Sue.
Nurse: Did you have problems with her?
Patient: She is terrible. She sleeps all night or she is on the telephone.
Nurse: Oh, that doesn't sound very professional to me. Anything else?
Patient: Yeah, she said that you didn't know what you were doing. She said that you couldn't nurse your way out of a paper bag (smiling).
Nurse: She did, did she. (Getting angry.) She should talk.
Patient: Well, I gotta go to group. Where will you be? I feel so much better if I know where you are. I don't know how I can possibly be discharged tomorrow.

Effective Approach

Patient: Hey, you know what? You are my favorite nurse. That night nurse sure doesn't understand me the way you do.
Nurse: I really like you, Sara. Tomorrow you will be discharged, and I'm glad that you will be able to return home. (Nurse avoided responding to "favorite nurse" statement. Redirected interaction to impending discharge.)
Patient: That night nurse slept all night.
Nurse: What was your night like? (Redirecting the interaction to Sara's experience.)
Patient: It was terrible. Couldn't sleep all night. I'm not sure that I'm ready to go home.
Nurse: Oh, so you are not quite sure about discharge? (Reflection.)
Patient: I get so, so lonely. Then, I want to hurt myself.
Nurse: Lonely feelings have started that chain of events that led to cutting, haven't they? (Validation.)
Patient: Yes, I'm very scared. I haven't cut myself for 1 week now.
Nurse: Do you have a plan for dealing with your lonely feelings when they occur?
Patient: I'm supposed to start thinking about something that is pleasant—like spring flowers in the meadow.
Nurse: Does that work for you?
Patient: Yes, sometimes.

Critical Thinking Challenge

- How did the nurse in the first scenario get sidetracked?
- How was the nurse in the second scenario able to keep the patient focused on herself and her impending discharge?

be appropriate. Our personal physical space needs (boundaries) are distinct from behavioral and emotional limits we have. These concepts apply both to the patient and the nurse. Furthermore, limits may be temporary (e.g., "I can't talk with you right now, but after the change of shift, I can be available for 30 minutes").

Testing limits is a natural way of identifying where the boundaries are and how strong they are. Therefore, it is necessary to state clearly the enduring limits (e.g., the written rules or contract) and the consequences of violating them. The limits must then be consistently maintained. Clarifying limits requires making explicit what is usually implicit. Despite the clinical setting (e.g., hospital, day-treatment setting, outpatient clinic), the nurse must clearly state the day, time, and duration of each contact with the patient and remain consistent in those expectations. This may mean having a standing appointment in day treatment or the mental health clinic or noting the time during each shift the nurse will talk individually with the hospitalized patient. The nurse should refrain from offering personal information, which is frequently confusing to the person with BPD. At times, the person may present in a somewhat arrogant and entitled way. It is important for the nurse to recognize such a presentation as reflective of internal confusion and dissonance. Responding in a very neutral manner avoids confrontation and a power struggle, which might also unwittingly reinforce the patient's internal sense of inferiority.

Some additional strategies for establishing the boundaries of the relationship include the following:

- Documenting in the patient chart the agreed-on appointment expectations
- Sharing the treatment plan with the patient
- Confronting violations of the agreement in a nonpunitive way
- Discussing the purpose of limits in the therapeutic relationship and applicability to other relationships.

When patients violate boundaries, it is important to respond right away but without taking the behavior personally. For example, if a patient is flirtatious, simply say something like, "X, I feel uncomfortable with your overly friendly behavior. It seems out of place since we have a professional relationship. That would be more fitting for an intimate relationship that we will never have."

Management of Dissociative States. The desired outcome for someone who dissociates is to reduce or eliminate the dissociative experiences. The natural tendency is to want to "fix it." Unfortunately, there are limited medications for dissociation, but because the SSRIs, dopamine antagonists, and serotonin-dopamine antagonists affect other target symptoms, the dissociative experiences decrease. Because dissociation occurs during periods of stress, the best approach is to help the patient develop other strategies to deal with stress.

The nurse can teach the patient how to identify when he or she is dissociating and then to use some grounding strategies in the moment. Basic to grounding is planting both feet firmly on the floor or ground, then taking a deep abdominal breath to the count of 4, holding it to the count of 4, exhaling to the count of 4, and then holding it to the count of 4. This is called the four-square method of breathing. The benefit of this approach is to bring about a deep, slow breath that activates the calming mechanisms of the parasympathetic system.

After the grounding exercise, the patient uses one or more senses to make contact with the environment, such as touching the fabric of a nearby chair or listening to the traffic noise. As the patient improves in self-esteem and ability to relate to others, the frequency of dissociation should decrease.

Behavioral Interventions. The goal of behavioral interventions is to replace dysfunctional behaviors with positive ones, using the behavioral models discussed in Chapters 6 and 11. The nurse has an important role in helping patients control emotions and behaviors by acknowledging and validating desired behaviors and ignoring or confronting undesired behaviors. Patients often test the nurse for a response, and nurses must decide how to respond to particular behaviors. This can be tricky because even negative responses can be viewed as positive reinforcement for the patient. In some instances, if the behavior is irritating but not harmful or demeaning, it is best to ignore rather than focus on it. However, grossly inappropriate and disrespectful behaviors require confrontation. If a patient throws a glass of water on an assistant because she is angry at the treatment team for refusing to increase her hospital privileges, an appropriate intervention would include confronting the patient with her behavior and issuing the consequences, such as losing her privileges and apologizing to the assistant.

However, this incident can be used to help the patient understand why such behavior is inappropriate and how it can be changed. The nurse should explore with the patient what happened, what events led up to the behavior, what were the consequences, and what feelings were aroused. Advanced practice nurses or other therapists will explore the origins of the patient's behaviors and responses, but the generalist nurse needs to help the patient explore ways to change behaviors involved in the current situation. The laboriousness of this analytical process may be a sufficient incentive for the patient to abandon the dysfunctional behavior.

Emotional Regulation. A major goal of cognitive therapeutic interventions is emotional regulation—recognizing and controlling the expression of feelings. Patients often fail even to recognize their feelings; instead, they respond quickly without thinking about the consequences. Remember, the time needed for taking action is shorter than the time needed for thinking before acting. Pausing makes up for the momentary lag between the limbic and autonomic response and the prefrontal response.

The nurse can help the patient identify feelings and gain control over expressions such as anger, disappointment, or frustration. The goal is for patients to tolerate their feelings without feeling compelled to act out those feelings on another person or on themselves.

A helpful technique for managing feelings is known as the **communication triad**. The triad provides a specific syntax and order for patients to identify and express their feelings and seek relief. The "sentence" consists of three parts:

- An "I" statement to identify the prevailing feeling
- A nonjudgmental statement of the emotional trigger
- What the patient would like differently or what would restore comfort to the situation

The nurse must emphasize with patients that they begin with the "I" statement and the identification of feelings, although many want to begin with the condition. If the patient begins with the condition, the statement becomes accusatory and likely to evoke defensiveness (e.g., "When you interrupt me, I get mad."). Beginning with "I" allows the patient to identify and express the feeling first and take full ownership. For example, the patient who is angry with another patient in the group might say, "Joe, I feel angry ("I" statement with ownership of feeling) when you interrupt me (the trigger or conditions of the emotion), and I would like you to apologize and try not to do that with me (what the patient wants and the remedy)." This simple skill is easy to teach, is easy to reinforce and to encourage others to reinforce, and is a surprisingly effective way of moderating the emotional tone.

Another element of emotional regulation is learning to delay gratification. When the patient wants something that is not immediately available, the nurse can teach patients to distract themselves, find alternate ways of meeting the need, and think about what would happen if they have to wait to meet the need.

The practice of **thought stopping** might also help the patient to control the inappropriate expression of feelings. In thought stopping, the person identifies what feelings and thoughts exist together. For example, when the person is ruminating about a perceived hurt, the individual might say "Stop that" (referring to the ruminative thought) and engage in a distracting activity. Three activities associated with thought stopping are effective:

- Taking a quick deep breath when the behavior is noted (this also stimulates relaxation)
- Visualizing a stop sign or saying "stop" when possible (this allows the person to hear externally and internally)
- Deliberately replacing the undesired behavior with a positive alternative (e.g., instead of ruminating about an angry situation, think about a neutral or positive self-affirmation). The sequencing and combining of the steps puts the person back in control.

Challenging Dysfunctional Thinking. The nurse can often challenge the patient's dysfunctional ways of thinking and challenge the person to think about the event in a different way. When a patient engages in catastrophic thinking, the nurse can challenge by asking, "What is the worst that could happen?" and "How likely would that be to occur?" Or, in dichotomous thinking, when the patient fixates on one extreme perception or alternates between the extremes only, the nurse can ask the patient to think about any examples of exceptions to the extreme. The point of the challenge is not to debate or argue with the patient, but to provide different perspectives to consider. Encouraging patients to keep journals of real interactions to process with the nurse or therapist is another effective way of testing the reality of their thinking and anticipations, affording more choices and flexibility (Box 22.7).

In problem solving, the nurse might encourage the patient to debate both sides of the problem and then search for common ground. Practicing communication and negotiation skills through role playing helps the

BOX 22.7

Challenging Dysfunctional Thinking

Ms. S had worked for the same company for 20 years with a good job record. Following an accident, she made some minor mistakes in her work that she quickly corrected. She informed her company nurse that her work was "really slipping" and that she was fearful of her coworkers' disapproval and getting fired from her job. The nurse asked her to keep a journal of coworkers' comments for the next week. At the next visit, the following dialogue occurred:

Nurse: I noticed that you received several compliments on your work. Even a close friend of your boss expressed appreciation for your work.

Ms. S: It was a light week at work. I really don't believe they meant what they said.

Nurse: I can see how you can believe that one or two comments are not genuine, but how do you account for four and five good reports on your work?

Ms. S: Well, I don't know.

Nurse: It looks like your beliefs are not supported by your journal entries. Now, what makes you think that your boss wants to fire you after 20 years of service?

BOX 22.8

Thought Distortions and Corrective Statements

Thought Distortion	Corrective Statement
Catastrophizing	
"This is the most awful thing that has ever happened to me"	"This is a sad thing, but not the most awful."
"If I fail this course, my life is over."	"If you fail the course, you can take the course again. You can change your major."
Dichotomizing	
"No one ever listens to me."	"Your husband listened to you last night when you told him . . ."
"I never get what I want."	"You didn't get the promotion this year, but you did get a merit raise."
"I can't understand why everyone is so kind at first, then always dumps me when I need them the most."	"It is hard to remember those kind things and times when your friends have stayed with you when you needed them."
Self-Attribution Errors	
"If I had just found the right thing to say, she wouldn't have left me."	"There is not a single right thing to say; and she left you because she chose to."
"If I had not made him mad, he wouldn't have hit me."	"He has a lot of choices in how to respond, and he chose hitting. You are responsible for your feelings and actions."

patient make mistakes and correct them without harm to her or his self-esteem. The nurse also encourages patients to use these skills in their everyday lives and report back on the results, asking patients how they feel applying the skills and how doing so affects their self-perceptions. Success, even partial success, builds a sense of competence and self-esteem (Box 22.8).

Management of Transient Psychotic Episodes. During psychotic episodes with auditory hallucinations, the patient should be protected from harming self or others. In an inpatient setting, the patient should be monitored closely and a determination made as to whether the voices are telling the patient to engage in self-harm (command hallucinations). The patient may be observed more closely and begin taking antipsychotic medication. In the community setting, the nurse should help the patient develop a plan for managing the voices. For example, if the voices return, the patient contacts the clinic and returns for evaluation. There may be a friend or relative who should be contacted or a case manager who can help the patient get the necessary protection if it is needed. In some instances, hearing the voices is a prelude to self-injury. Another person can help the patient resist the voices. Once other aspects of the disorder are managed, the episodes of psychosis decrease or disappear.

Teaching and practicing distress tolerance skills help the patient have power over the voices and control intense emotions. When not experiencing hallucinations, the patient can practice deep abdominal breathing, which calms the autonomic nervous system. Using brainstorming techniques, the patient identifies early internal cues of rising distress while the nurse writes them on an index card for the patient to refer to later. Next, the nurse teaches some skills for tolerating painful feelings or events. To help the patient remember, suggest the mnemonic "A wise mind ACCEPTS" with the following actions:

- Activities to distract from stress
- Contributing to others, such as volunteering or visiting a sick neighbor
- Comparing yourself to people less fortunate than you
- Emotions that are opposite what you are experiencing
- Pushing away from the situation for a while
- Thoughts other than those you are currently experiencing
- Sensations that are intense, such as holding ice in your hand (Linehan, 1993, pp. 165–166).

Patient Education 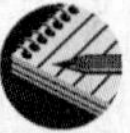

Patient education within the context of a therapeutic relationship is one of the most important, empowering interventions for the generalist psychiatric–mental health nurse to use. Teaching patients skills to resist parasuicidal urges, improve emotional regulation, enhance interpersonal relationships, tolerate stress, and enhance overall quality of life provides the foundation for long-term behavioral changes. These skills can be taught in any treatment setting as a part of the overall facility program (see Box 22.9). If nurses are practicing in a facility where DBT is the treatment model, they can be trained in DBT and can serve as group skills leaders.

BOX 22.9

Psychoeducation Checklist: Borderline Personality Disorder

When caring for the patient with borderline personality disorder, be sure to include the following topic areas in the teaching plan:

- Management of medication, if used, including drug action, dosage, frequency, and possible adverse effects
- Regular sleep routines
- Nutrition
- Safety measures
- Functional versus dysfunctional behaviors
- Cognitive strategies (distraction, communication skills, thought-stopping)
- Structure and limit setting
- Social relationships
- Community resources

Social Domain

Social Assessment

Some individuals with BPD can function very well except during periods when symptoms erupt. They hold jobs, are active in communities, and can perform well. During periods of stress, symptoms often appear. On the other hand, some individuals with severe BPD function poorly; they are always in a crisis, which they have often created.

Social Support Systems. Identification of social supports, such as family, friends, and religious organizations, is the purpose in assessing resources. Knowing how the patient obtains social support is important in understanding the quality of interpersonal relationships. For example, some patients consider their "best friends" nurses, physicians, and other health care personnel. Because this is a false friendship (i.e., not reciprocal), it inevitably leads to frustration and disappointment. However, helping the patient find ways to meet other people and encouraging the patient's efforts are more realistic.

Interpersonal Skills. Assessment of the person's ability to relate to others is important because interpersonal problems are linked to dissociation and self-injurious behavior. Information about friendships, frequency of contact, and intimate relationships will provide data about the person's ability to relate to others. Patients with BPD often are sexually active and may have numerous sexual partners. Their need for closeness clouds their judgment about sexual partners, and it is not unusual to find these patients in abusive, destructive relationships with people with antisocial personality disorder. During assessment, nurses should use their own self-awareness skills to examine their personal response to the patient. How the nurse responds to the patient can often be a clue to how others perceive and respond to this person. For example, if the nurse feels irritated or impatient during the interview, that is a sign that others respond to this person in the same way; on the other hand, if the nurse feels empathy or closeness, chances are this patient can evoke these same feelings in others.

Self-esteem and Coping Skills. Coping with stressful situations is one of the major problems of people with BPD. Assessment of their coping skills and their ability to deal with stressful situations is important. Because the patient's self-esteem is usually very low, assessment of self-esteem can be done with a self-esteem assessment tool or by interviewing the patient and analyzing the assessment data for evidence of personal self-worth and confidence. Self-esteem is highly related to identifying with health care workers. Patients with BPD perceive their families and friends as being weary of their numerous crises and their seeming unwillingness to break the vicious self-destructive cycle. Feeling rejected by their natural support system, these individuals create one within the health system. During periods of crisis or affective instability, especially during the late evening, early morning, or on weekends, they call or visit various psychiatric units asking to speak to specific personnel who formerly cared for them. They even know different nurses' scheduled days off and make the rounds to several hospitals and clinics. Sometimes they bring gifts to nurses or call them at home. Because their newly created social support system cannot provide the support that is needed, the patient continues to feel rejected. One of the goals of the treatment is to help the individual establish a natural support network.

Family Assessment 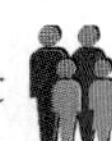

Family members may or may not be involved with the patient. These individuals are often estranged from their families. In other instances, they are dependent on them, which is also a source of stress. Childhood abuse is common in these families, and the perpetrator may be a family member. Ideally, family members are interviewed for their perspectives on the patient's problem. Assessment of any mental disorder in the patient's family and of the current level of functioning is useful in understanding the patient and identifying potential resources for support.

Nursing Diagnoses for the Social Domain

Defensive Coping, Chronic Low Self-esteem, and impaired Social Interaction are nursing diagnoses that address the social problems faced by patients with BPD.

Interventions for the Social Domain

Environmental management becomes critical in caring for a patient with BPD. Because the unit can be structured to represent a microcosm of the patient's community, patients have an opportunity to identify relationship problems, boundary violations, and stressful situations. When these situations occur, the nurse can help the patient cope by finding alternative explanations for the situation and practicing new skills. Individual sessions help the patient to try out some skills, such as putting feelings into words without actions. Role playing may help patients experience different degrees of effectively relating feelings without the burden of hurting someone they care about. Day treatment and group settings are excellent places for patients to learn more effective feeling management and to practice these techniques with each other. The group helps members develop empathy and diffuses attachment to any one person or therapist.

Building Social Skills and Self-esteem. In the hospital, the nurse can use groups to discuss feelings and ways to cope with them. Women with BPD benefit from assertiveness classes and women's health issues classes. Many of the women are involved in abusive relationships and lack the ability to resolve these relationships because of their extreme anxiety regarding separating from those they love and their extreme need to feel connected. These women verbalize desires to leave, but they do not have the strength and self-confidence needed to leave. Exposing them to a different style of interaction as well as validation from other people increases their self-esteem and ability to separate from negative influences.

Exploring Social Supports. Dependency on family members is a problem for many people with BPD. In some families a patient's positive progress may be met with negative responses, and patients in these situations need help in maintaining a separate identity while staying connected to family members for social support. Family support groups sometimes help. Usually, the nurse helps the patient explore new relationships that can provide additional social contacts.

Teaching Effective Ways to Communicate 

An important area of patient education is teaching communication skills. Patients lack interpersonal skill in relating because they often had inadequate modeling and few opportunities to practice. The goals of relationship skill development are to identify problematic behavior that interferes with relationships and to use appropriate behaviors in improving relationships. The starting point is with communication. The nurse teaches the patient basic communication approaches, such as making "I" statements, paraphrasing what the other party says before responding, checking the accuracy of perceptions with others, compromising and seeking common ground, listening actively, and offering and accepting reactions. Besides modeling the behaviors, the nurse guides patients in practicing a variety of communication approaches for common situations. When role playing, the nurse needs to discuss not only what the skills are and how to perform them, but also the feelings patients have before, during, and after the role play.

In day treatment and outpatient settings, the nurse can give the patient homework, such as keeping a journal, applying role-playing skills to actual situations, and observing behaviors in others. In the hospital, the patient can experience the same process, and the nurse is available to offer immediate feedback. Whatever the setting, or even the specific problems addressed, the nurse must keep in mind and remind the patient that change occurs slowly. Thus, working on the problems occurs gradually, with severity of symptoms as the guide to deciding how fast and how much change to expect.

Evaluation and Outcomes

Evaluation and outcomes vary depending on the severity of the disorder, the presence of comorbid disorders, and the availability of resources. For a patient with severe symptoms or continual self-injury, keeping the patient safe and alive may be a realistic outcome. Helping the patient resist parasuicidal urges may take years. In contrast, individuals who rarely need hospitalization and have adequate resources can expect to recover from the self-destructive impulses and learn positive interaction skills that promote a quality lifestyle. Most patients fall somewhere in between, with periods of symptom exacerbation and remission. In these patients, increasing the symptom-free time may be the best indicator of outcomes.

Continuum of Care

Treatment of BPD involves long-term therapy. Hospitalization is sometimes necessary during acute episodes involving parasuicidal behavior, but once this behavior is controlled, patients are discharged. It is important for these individuals to continue with treatment in the outpatient or day treatment setting. They often appear more competent and in control than they are, and nurses must not be deceived by these outward appearances. They need continued follow-up and long-term therapy, including individual therapy, psychoeducation, and positive role models (see **Nursing Care Plan 22.1**).

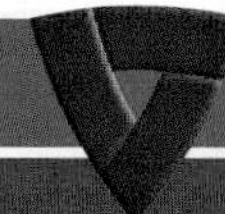

Nursing Care Plan 22.1

Patient With Borderline Personality Disorder

YJ, a 28-year-old, single woman, was brought to the emergency department of a hospital by police officers after finding her in a Burger Chef with superficial self-inflicted lacerations on both forearms. She pleaded with the police not to take her to the hospital. The police report noted that she fluctuated between intense crying and pleading to fighting physically and using foul language. By the time she arrived in the emergency department, however, she was calm, cooperative, pleasant, and charming. When asked why she cut herself, YJ reported she wasn't sure but added that her therapist was leaving today for a 4-week trip to Europe. YJ specifically asked the staff not to call her therapist because "she will be angry with me."

After the emergency physician examined YJ, the advanced practice mental health nurse assessed her developmental and psychiatric history and a summary of recent events, before she reached a provisional diagnosis of borderline personality disorder with a primary nursing diagnosis of risk for self-mutilation related to abandonment anticipation. YJ had several previous self-destructive episodes with minor injuries, only one requiring sutures, and two hospitalizations. She lives with her boyfriend, who is currently on a business trip, and works part time at a bookstore. Her invalid mother lives with her younger sister. There are no other relatives. YJ's father died traumatically in an automobile accident when she was 3 years old. YJ was in the car when it crashed; she received minor injuries.

Because YJ refused to agree not to harm herself, the nurse admitted YJ to the psychiatric unit with suicide precautions. Once on the unit, YJ was assessed by a staff nurse as having a basically normal mental status examination except that her mood was very tearful at times but charming and joking at other times. She said, "Don't mind me, I cry at the drop of a hat sometimes." Toward the middle of the interview she said, "I feel safer here than I ever felt before. It must be you. Are you sure you're just a staff nurse?" YJ agreed to a contract for safety just for today, but added, "Are you going to be my nurse tomorrow? I feel safest with you." When the nurse had completed her assessment, she showed YJ around the unit. As the nurse left her in the day room, YJ said, "My therapist doesn't understand me very well. I don't care if she is going out of town. After 4 years, she hasn't helped. If I had you as a therapist, I wouldn't be here now."

Setting: Inpatient Psychiatric Unit in a General Hospital

Baseline Assessment: YJ, a 28-year-old woman, came into the emergency department with superficial self-inflicted wounds on both forearms. There was a marked discrepancy in her behavior at the scene of the incident reported by emergency medical technicians from her presentation in the emergency department and now on the inpatient unit. She was admitted this time because she refused to agree not to harm herself further if released. She is angry and sad that her therapist is leaving for 4 weeks for a vacation and doesn't know how she will cope while the therapist is gone. She fears the therapist will not return.

Psychiatric Diagnosis	Medications
Axis I: Adjustment disorder with depressed mood Axis II: Borderline personality disorder Axis III: Superficial wounds to both forearms Axis IV: Social support (inadequate social support) Axis V: GAF current = 60; GAF past year = 75	Sertraline (Zoloft) 150 mg qd for anxiety and depression

Nursing Diagnosis 1: Self-Mutilation

Defining Characteristics	Related Factors
Cuts and scratches on body Self-inflicted wounds	Fears of abandonment secondary to therapist's vacation Inability to handle stress

Outcomes

Initial	Discharge
1. Remain safe and not harm herself. 2. Identify feelings before and after cutting herself. 3. Agree not to harm herself over the next 24 h. 4. Identify ways of dealing with self-harming impulses if they return.	5. Verbalize alternate thinking with more realistic base. 6. Identify community resources to provide structure and support while therapist is gone.

Continued

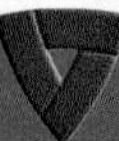

Nursing Care Plan 22.1 *(Continued)*

Interventions

Interventions	Rationale	Ongoing Assessment
Monitor patient for changes in mood or behavior that might lead to self-injurious behavior.	Close observation establishes safety and protection of patient from self-harm and impulsive behaviors.	Document according to facility policy. Continue to observe for mood and behavior changes.
Discuss with patient need for close observation and rationale to keep her safe.	Explanation to patient for purpose of nursing interventions helps her cooperate with the nursing activity.	Assess her response to increasing level of observation.
Administer medication as prescribed and evaluate medication effectiveness in reducing depression, anxiety, and cognitive disorganization.	Allows for adjustment of medication dosage based on target behaviors and outcomes.	Observe for side effects.
After 6–8 h, present written agreement to not harm herself.	Permits patient time to return to more thoughtful ways of responding rather than her previous reactive response. Also permits her to save face and avoid embarrassment of a losing power struggle if presented much earlier.	Observe for her willingness to agree to not harm herself.
Communicate information about patient's risk to other nursing staff.	The close observation should be continued throughout all shifts until patient agrees to resist self-harm urges.	Review documentation of close observation for all shifts.

Evaluation

Outcomes	Revised Outcomes	Interventions
Remained safe without further harming self. Identified fears of abandonment before cutting herself and relief of anxiety afterward. She identified friends to call when fears return and hotlines to use if necessary.	Use hotlines or call friends if fears to harm self return.	Give patient hotline number and ask her to record friends' numbers in an accessible place.
Agreed to not harm herself over the next 3 d.	Does not harm self for 3 d.	Remind her to call someone if urges return.
Enrolled in a day hospital program for 4 wk.	Attend day hospital program.	Follow-up on enrollment.

Nursing Diagnosis 2: Risk for Loneliness

Defining Characteristics	Related Factors
Social isolation	Fear of abandonment secondary to therapist's impending vacation

Outcomes

Initial	Discharge
1. Discuss being lonely. 2. Identify previous ways of coping with loneliness.	3. Identify strategies to deal with loneliness while therapist is away.

Interventions

Interventions	Rationale	Ongoing Assessment
Develop a therapeutic relationship.	People with BPD are able to examine loneliness within the structure of a therapeutic relationship.	Assess her ability to relate and nurse's response to the relationship.

Nursing Care Plan 22.1

Interventions

Interventions	Rationale	Ongoing Assessment
Discuss past experience with therapist being gone with emphasis on how she was able to survive it.	She has survived therapist's absences before. By identifying the strategies she used, she can build on those strengths.	Assess her ability to assume any responsibility for "living through it." This will become a strength.
Acknowledge that it is normal to feel angry when the therapist is gone, but there are other strategies that may help the patient deal with the loneliness besides cutting.	Acknowledging feelings is important. Helping patient focus on the possibility of other strategies for dealing with the anger helps her regain a sense of control over her behavior.	Assess whether she is willing to acknowledge that there are other behavioral strategies of handling anger.
Begin immediate disposition planning with focus on day hospitalization or day treatment for skills training and management of loneliness.	While patient is in hospital, she is out of stressful environment in which she can learn more effective behaviors and use the therapy. Moving out of the hospital and back into outpatient therapy decreases possibility of regression and lost learning (Linehan, 1993).	Assess her willingness to learn new skills within a day treatment setting.
Teach her about stress management techniques. Assign her to anger management group while she is in the hospital.	Learning about ways of dealing with feelings and stressful situations helps the patient with BPD choose positive strategies rather than self-destructive ones.	Monitor whether she actually attends the groups. She should be encouraged to attend.

Evaluation

Outcomes	Revised Outcomes	Interventions
YJ was able to verbalize her anger about her therapist leaving and fears of abandonment. The last two times her therapist went on vacation, the patient became self injurious and was hospitalized for 2 wk.	None	
YJ was willing to be discharged the next day if she could attend day treatment while her therapist was gone.	Identify other strategies of dealing with therapist vacations besides cutting.	Attend stress management, communication, and self-comforting classes.

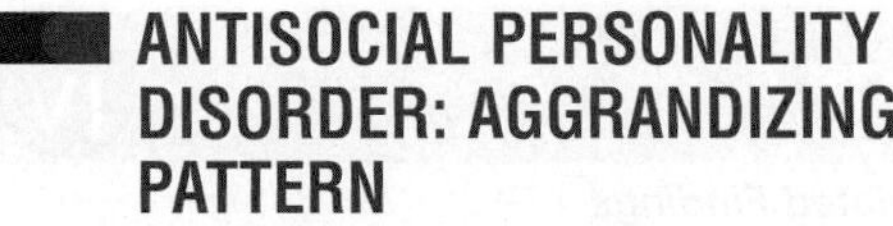

ANTISOCIAL PERSONALITY DISORDER: AGGRANDIZING PATTERN

Clinical Course of Disorder

In the *DSM-IV*, antisocial personality disorder (APD) is defined as "a pervasive pattern of disregard for, and violation of, the rights of others that begins in childhood or early adolescence and continues into adulthood" (APA, 2000, p. 701). The terms **psychopath** or **sociopath** are often used by the general public to refer to persons with an antisocial personality disorder. These individuals are behaviorally impulsive and interpersonally irresponsible. They fail to adapt to the ethical and social standards of the community. They act hastily and spontaneously, are shortsighted, and fail to plan ahead or consider alternatives. They lack a sense of personal obligation to fulfill social and financial responsibilities, including those involved with being a spouse, a parent, an employee, a friend, or member of the community. Disdainful of traditional values, they fail to conform to social norms and values. They enjoy a sense of freedom and relish being unencumbered and unconfined by people, places, or responsibilities. They can be interpersonally engaging, which is often mistaken for a genuine sense of concern for other people. In reality, they lack empathy, are unable to express human compassion, and tend to be insensitive, callous, and contemptuous of others. Easily irritated, they often become aggressive, disregarding the safety of themselves or others. They lack remorse for transgressions. No matter what the consequences, they are rarely able to delay gratification (APA, 2000).

These individuals have faith only in themselves and are secure only when they are independent from those whom they fear will harm or humiliate them. Their need for independence is based on their mistrust of others, rather than an inherent belief in their own self-worth. They are driven by a need to prove their superiority and see themselves as the center of the universe. Some of these individuals openly and flagrantly violate laws, ending up in jail. But most people with APD never come in conflict with the law and, instead, find a niche in society, such as in business, the military, or politics that rewards their competitive, tough behavior (Millon et al., 2004; see Table 22.4). This disorder has a chronic course, but the antisocial behaviors tend to diminish later in life, particularly after the age of 40 years (APA, 2000).

Epidemiology and Risk Factors

The prevalence of antisocial personality disorder in national prevalence studies is 3.6% of the population. This disorder occurs more frequently in men, who are at greater risk for APD than women (Grant et al., 2004).

Age of Onset

To be diagnosed with APD, the individual must have exhibited one or more childhood behavioral characteristics of conduct disorder and ADHD, such as aggression to people or animals, destruction of property, deceitfulness or theft, or serious violation of rules (Box 22.10).

Cultural and Ethnic Differences

People with APD or psychopathic personalities are found in many cultures, including industrialized and nonindustrialized societies. In an analysis of the Inuit of Northwest Alaska, individuals who break the rules when they are known are called *kunlangeta*, meaning "his mind knows what to do but he does not do it" (Murphy, 1976, p. 1026). This term is used for someone who repeatedly lies, cheats, and steals. He is described as someone who does not go hunting and, when the other men are out of the village, takes sexual advantage of the women. In another culture in rural southwest Nigeria, the Yorubas use the word *arankan* to mean a "person who always goes his own way regardless of others, who is uncooperative, full of malice and bullheaded" (Murphy, p. 1026). In both cultures, the healers and shamans do not consider these people treatable.

In the United States, there are prevalence differences found among some of the cultural groups. In the 2001–2002 National Epidemiologic Survey on Alcohol and Related Conditions ($N = 43{,}093$), the odds of antisocial personality disorder were greater among Native Americans and lower among Asians compared with Caucasians (Grant et al., 2004).

Comorbidity

Antisocial personality disorder is associated with several other psychiatric disorders, including mood, anxiety, and other personality disorders. APD is strongly associated with alcohol and drug abuse (Rhee et al., 2006; Goldstein et al., 2006). To be diagnosed with APD as an adult (after the age of 18), the criteria for childhood or adolescence conduct disorder must be met (before the age of 18) (APA, 2000). Conduct disorder in childhood compared with adolescence is associated with greater risk of social phobia, generalized anxiety disorder, drug dependence, and paranoid, schizoid, and avoidant personality disorders (Goldstein et al., 2006).

Table 22.4 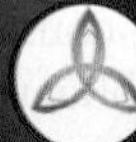 **Key Diagnostic Characteristics of Antisocial Personality Disorder 301.7** 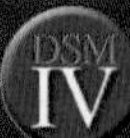

Diagnostic Criteria and Target Symptoms	Associated Findings
• Pervasive pattern of disregard for and violation of the rights of others Failure to conform to social norms with respect to lawful behaviors (repeatedly performing acts that are grounds for arrest) Deceitfulness (repeated lying, use of aliases, or conning others for personal profit or pleasure) Impulsivity or failure to plan ahead Irritability and aggressiveness (repeated physical fights or assaults) Reckless disregard for safety of self or others Consistent irresponsibility (repeated failure to sustain consistent work behavior or honor financial obligations) Lack of remorse (being indifferent to or rationalizing having hurt, mistreated, or stolen from another) • Occurring since 15 years of age • At least 18 years of age • Evidence of conduct disorder with onset before 15 years of age • Not exclusive during the course of schizophrenia or manic episode	***Associated Behavioral Findings*** • Lacking empathy • Callous, cynical, and contemptuous of the feelings, rights, and suffering of others • Inflated and arrogant self-appraisal • Excessively opinionated, self-assured, or cocky • Glib, superficial charm; impressive verbal ability • Irresponsible and exploitative in sexual relationships; history of multiple sexual partners and lack of a sustained monogamous relationship • Possible dysphoria, including complaints of tension; inability to tolerate boredom, and depressed mood.

BOX 22.10

Clinical Vignette: Antisocial Personality Disorder: Male Versus Female

Stasia (female) and Jackson (male) are fraternal twins, 22 years old, who received diagnoses of antisocial personality disorder. The following are their clinical profiles.

Jackson

Jackson is currently in the county jail for the third time. Although his juvenile records begin at age 9 and include misdemeanors and class B felonies, his burglary conviction is his first adult crime. His school teachers thought Jackson was very bright but that he had significant difficulty with peers and authority figures. He fought regularly, was described as a bully, and seemed always to be scamming. At age 16, Jackson dropped out of school and joined a gang.

Jackson's juvenile probation officer explained that Jackson came from a very violent family and neighborhood and described the situation by saying, "If gangs hadn't gotten him, his father would have." His lawyer described him as "a likeable guy, but I wouldn't turn my back on him."

The jail nurse described Jackson as "a real charmer, but nothing is ever his fault." Oddly, he is the only person in the jail with an adequate supply of cigarettes and CDs. "We get along fine. I don't understand why guards have such difficulty with him." Sometimes, the guards send Jackson to the dispensary for injuries, and Jackson plaintively explains to the nurse, "Those guards beat me up again, I don't know why."

Stasia

Stasia was recently hospitalized for the sixth time when one of her male friends beat her. She has been working as a prostitute for 5 years. Her physical examination noted not only multiple bruises but also tattoos that cover 50% of her body. In addition, she has piercings of her tongue, ears, brow, lips, and nipples. She is emotionally volatile, manipulative, and angry. Stasia has many acquaintances and sexual partners, but none are truly intimate. She has periods when she uses drugs regularly.

Stasia and Jackson's mother was jailed when the twins were 18 months old and didn't return until they were 6 years old. They were raised mostly by their paternal grandmother, who hated their mother and reminded Stasia frequently of how much she looked like her mother. Their father, when present, was violent toward Jackson and sexually abused Stasia.

What Do You Think?

- How might gender influence the development of symptoms?
- How might culture influence early recognition of problems and provision of early intervention to prevent future serious mental disorders?
- What are some possible outcomes in this situation?
- How does this case demonstrate the interaction between socialization, biology, and culture?

Etiology

Biologic Theories

The biochemical basis of antisocial disorder is not clearly understood. However, some curious biologic markers have been identified. Gotz and colleagues (1999) found significantly higher antisocial behavior in adolescent and adult men with the XYY sex chromosome abnormality than in control subjects. Serotonin deficiency and low dopamine levels have also been implicated in APD, especially related to impulsive aggression (Goodman et al., 2004). Researchers consistently find dysregulation in catecholamines with changed activity of the dopaminergic pathways in the frontal cortex (Soderstrom, Blennow, Sjodin, & Forsman, 2003). The limbic-prefrontal cortex (Veit et al., 2002) and dorsolateral prefrontal cortex (Dolan & Park, 2002) are specifically implicated, accounting for poor judgment, emotional distance, aggression, and impulsivity (Kiehl et al., 2001).

Psychological Theories

Learning, social behavior, empathy, emotional awareness, and regulation are all directly influenced by the nature of the relationship between the caregiver and child. One of the leading explanations of APD is that these individuals had unsatisfactory attachments in early relationships that led to antisocial behavior in later life. Normal relationships begin with **attachment** that can be defined as

> Behavior that results in a person attaining or retaining proximity to some other differentiated and preferred individual. During the course of healthy development, attachment behavior leads to the development of affectional bonds or attachments, initially between child and parent and later between adult and adult. The forms of behavior and the bonds to which they lead are present and active throughout the life cycle (Bowlby, 1980, p. 39).

An attachment relationship between the child and caregiver depends on the response of both parties. The sense of security in any relationship depends on the quality of the responsiveness experienced with the attachment figure (Smallbone & Dadds, 2000). If the parental figures are overanxious or avoidant, the child does not develop a sense of security with others and instead experiences self as an island (Reti et al., 2002). Secure attachments facilitate a balance between connection to another and the ability to go out into the world autonomously. In a secure attachment, a child feels safe, loved, and valued, but also develops the self-confidence to interact with the rest of the world. Experiences in successive relationships interact with prior experiences to determine an individual's trust in others.

Insecure attachments are formed as a result of faulty interaction between the caregiver and the child and are expressed in relationships as ambivalence, avoidance, or disorganization (Ainsworth, 1989). In APD, a failure to make or sustain stable attachments in early childhood can lead to avoidance of future attachments. Studies have found several childhood situations to be risk factors for developing dysfunctional attachments, such as parental abandonment or neglect, loss of parent or primary caregiver, and physical or sexual abuse. However, evidence supports the theory that ability to foster secure emotional attachments may be a learned parenting skill and that parents who lacked secure attachment relationships in their own childhood may lack the ability to form secure attachment relationships with their own children.

Children are born with a particular **temperament**, a recognizable and distinctive way of behavior that is evident during the first few months of life. Some infants are more relaxed or calm and sleep a lot, whereas others are extremely alert, startled by the slightest noise, cry more, and sleep less. Scientists believe temperament is neurobiologically determined, and many believe that it is central to understanding personality disorders. Children seem to be born with certain temperaments that remain fairly stable throughout development.

Temperament consists of the interaction of two behavioral dimensions—activity and adaptability. Activity patterns in individuals vary along a spectrum, from active or intense children, whose actions display decisiveness and vigor as they continuously relate to their environment, to passive children, who are more cautious and slow to relate to their environment (a wait-and-see pattern of behavior). Adaptability includes a spectrum, with the extreme at one end being the child who is regular in biologic functions such as eating or sleeping, has a positive approach to new stimuli, and maintains a high degree of flexibility in response to changing conditions. At the other end of the adaptability dimension are children who display irregularity in biologic functions, withdrawal reactions to new stimuli, and minimal flexibility in response to change.

Some studies indicate that extreme temperaments make one vulnerable to antisocial behavior patterns. A difficult temperament is characterized by withdrawal from novel stimuli, low adaptability, and intense emotional reactions. Four key behaviors are present in a difficult temperament: aggression, inattention, hyperactivity, and impulsivity. There is a strong relationship between difficult temperament and problem behaviors such as those of ADHD, oppositional behavior, and conduct disorder (Cukrowicz, Taylor, Schatschneider, Iacono, 2006).

Hyperactivity alone is not related to the development of antisocial personality in adults, whereas hyperactivity occurring with aggression and the other behaviors listed is related to APD (Barry et al., 2000; Giancola, 2000; Schubiner et al., 2000). Temperament and problem behaviors are generally consistent throughout a lifetime.

Social Theories

In many cases, individuals with APD come from chaotic families in which alcoholism and violence are the norm. Individuals who have been victims of abuse or neglect, live in a foster home, or had several primary caregivers are more likely to experience antisocial behaviors, especially aggression (Johnson, Cohen, Chen, Kasen, & Brook, 2006; Andrews, Foster, Capaldi, & Hop, 2000). However, it is difficult to separate the influence of social factors on the development of the disorder because the symptoms of APD are social manifestations—unemployment, divorces and separations, and violence.

Interdisciplinary Treatment of Disorder

People with APD rarely seek mental health care because of the disorder itself, but rather for treatment of depression, substance abuse, or uncontrolled anger or for forensic evaluation (Millon et al., 2004). Patients who are admitted through the courts with an Axis I diagnosis often have a comorbid diagnosis of APD. Treatment is difficult and involves helping the patient alter his or her cognitive schema. The overall treatment goals are to develop a nurturing sense of attachment and empathy for other people and situations and to live within the norms of society.

Priority Care Issues

Although they can be interpersonally charming, these patients can become verbally and physically abusive if their expectations are not met. Protection of other patients and staff from manipulative and sometimes abusive behavior is a priority.

Family Response to Disorder 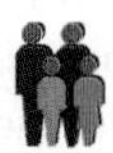

If there are family members, they have probably been abused, mistreated, or intimidated by these patients. For example, one patient sold his mother's possessions while she was at work. Another would abuse his wife after drinking. However, family members may be fiercely loyal to the patient and blame themselves for his or her shortcomings (see Box 22.11).

NURSING MANAGEMENT: HUMAN RESPONSE TO APD

Biologic Domain

Biologic Assessment

Antisocial personality disorder does not significantly impair the biologic dimension unless there are coexisting substance abuse or other Axis I disorders. Because

BOX 22.11

Using Reflection: Who is responsible?

Incident:
An adult patient with APD told the nurse that he had been arrested because his parents and wife would not pay his parking tickets. He further explained that his former boss was responsible for a shortage of funds that caused the patient to be fired. The nurse empathized with the patient and wondered how so many bad things could happen to one person. When family members arrived, they expressed sincere regret for not paying the parking tickets. His wife wondered what she had done wrong.

Reflection:
Upon reflection, the nurse realized that the patient was not assuming responsibility for his own actions. The patient was blaming others for his poor judgment.

substance abuse is a major problem with this population, the physical effects of chronic use of addictive substances must be considered.

Nursing Diagnoses for the Biologic Domain

A common nursing diagnosis in APD is Dysfunctional Family Processes, Alcoholism.

Interventions for Biologic Domain

In instances in which there are coexisting disorders, the personality disorder may actually interfere with interventions aimed at improving physical functioning. For example, a patient with schizophrenia and APD may not develop enough trust within a relationship to examine his or her delusional thoughts or other aspects of dysfunction, such as alcohol or drug abuse.

Psychological Domain

Psychological Assessment

Many patients with APD are committed to health care agencies by the court system. Assessment generally involves using basic psychological assessment tools to evaluate aberrant behaviors.

Nursing Diagnoses for the Psychological Domain

Because so many patients with APD have dysfunctional thinking patterns, a common nursing diagnosis is Disturbed Thought Processes and Risk for Other Directed Violence.

Interventions for the Psychological Domain

Therapeutic relationships are difficult to establish because these individuals do not attach to others and are often unable to use the relationship to change behavior. After the first few meetings with these patients, the nurse may feel that the relationship has a good start, but in reality, a superficial alliance is usually formed. Additional sessions reveal the lack of patient commitment to the relationship. These patients begin to revisit topics discussed in sessions or lose interest in trying to work on problems. By using self-awareness skills and accessing supervision regularly, the nurse can identify blocks in the development of a therapeutic relationship (or lack of) and his or her response to the relationship. The goal of the therapeutic relationship is to identify dysfunctional thinking patterns and develop new problem-solving behaviors.

Self-responsibility facilitation (encouraging a patient to assume more responsibility for personal behavior) is useful with patients with APD (Dochterman & Bulechek, 2004). The nursing activities that are particularly helpful include holding the patient responsible for his or her behavior, monitoring the extent that self-responsibility is assumed, and discussing the consequences of not dealing with responsibilities. The nurse needs to refrain from arguing or bargaining about the unit rules, such as time for meals, use of the television room, and smoking. Instead, positive feedback is given to the patient for accepting additional responsibility or changing behavior.

Self-awareness enhancement (exploring and understanding personal thoughts, feelings, motivation, and behaviors) is another nursing intervention that is important in helping these individuals develop a sense of understanding about relating peacefully to the rest of the world (Dochterman & Bulechek, 2004). Encouraging patients to recognize and discuss thoughts and feelings helps the nurse understand how the patient views the world. The nurse can then use many of the same communication techniques discussed in the section on BPD.

Teaching Points 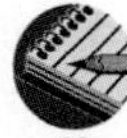

Patient education efforts have to be creative and thought provoking. In teaching a person with APD, a direct approach is best, but the nurse must avoid "lecturing," which the patient will resent. In teaching the patient about positive health care practices, impulse control, and anger management, the best approach is to engage the patient in a discussion about the issue and then direct the topic to the major teaching points. These patients often take great delight in arguing or showing how the rules of life do not apply to them. A sense of humor is important, as are clear teaching goals and avoiding being sidetracked (see Box 22.12).

BOX 22.12

Psychoeducation Checklist: Antisocial Personality Disorder

When caring for the patient with antisocial personality disorder, be sure to include the following topic areas in the teaching plan:

- Positive health care practices, including substance abuse control
- Effective communication and interaction skills
- Impulse control
- Anger management
- Group experience to help develop self-awareness and impact of behavior on others
- Analyzing an issue from the other person's viewpoint
- Maintenance of employment
- Interpersonal relationships and social interactions

Social Domain

Social Assessment

The nursing assessment usually focuses on other problems in addition to the response to the personality disorder. In fact, eliciting data may be difficult because of the basic mistrust individuals with APD have toward authority figures. Patients may not give an accurate history or may embellish aspects to project themselves in a more positive light. Often, they deny any criminal activity, even if they are admitted in police custody. Key areas of assessment are determining the quality of relationships, impulsivity, and the extent of aggression. These individuals do not assume responsibility for their own actions and often blame others for their misfortune. Their disregard for others is manifested in their interactions. For example, one patient with human immunodeficiency virus was engaging in unprotected sex with several different women because he wanted to "have fun as long as I can." He was completely unconcerned about the possibility of transmitting the virus. These individuals often make good first impressions. Self-awareness is especially important for the nurse because of the initial charming quality of many of these individuals. Once these patients realize that the nurse cannot be used or manipulated, they lose interest in the nurse and revert to their normal, egocentric behaviors.

Nursing Diagnoses for the Social Domain

Nursing diagnoses for patients with APD are related to their interpersonal detachment, lack of awareness of others, avoidance of feelings, impulsiveness, and discrepancy between their perception of themselves and others' perception of them. Typical diagnoses are Ineffective Role Performance (unemployment), Ineffective Individual Coping, Impaired Communication, Impaired Social Interactions, Low Self-esteem, and Risk for Violence. Outcomes should be short term and relevant to a specific problem. For example, if a patient has been chronically unemployed, a reasonable short-term outcome would be to set up job interviews, rather than obtain a job.

Interventions for the Social Domain

These patients have a long-standing history of difficulty in interpersonal relationships. In an inpatient unit, interventions can be more intense and focus on helping the patient develop positive interaction skills and experience a consistent environment. For example, the focus of nursing interventions may be the patient's continual disregard of the rights of others. On one unit, a patient continually placed orders for pizzas in the name of another patient who had limited intelligence and was genuinely afraid of the person with APD. The victimized patient always paid for the pizza and gave it to the other patient. When the nursing staff realized what was happening, they confronted the patient with APD about the behavior and revoked his unit privileges.

Group interventions are more effective than individual modalities because other patients and staff can validate or challenge the patient's view of a situation (Messina, Wish, & Nemes, 1999). Problem-solving groups that focus on identifying a problem and developing a variety of alternative solutions are particularly helpful because patient self-responsibility is reinforced when patients remind each other of the better alternatives. Patients are likely to confront each other with dysfunctional schemas or thinking patterns. Teaching patients with APD the same communication techniques as those with BPD will also encourage self-responsibility. These patients often attend groups that focus on the development of empathy.

Milieu interventions, such as providing a structured environment with rules that are consistently applied to patients who are responsible for their own behavior, are important. While living in close proximity to others, the individual with APD will demonstrate dysfunctional social patterns that can be identified and targeted for correction. For example, these patients often violate ward rules, such as no smoking or limitations on the number of visitors, and may bring contraband, such as illegal drugs, to the unit.

Aggressive behavior is often a problem for these individuals and their family members. Like patients with BPD, people with APD tend to be impulsive. Instead of self-injury, these individuals are more likely to strike out at those who are perceived to be interfering with their immediate gratification. Anger control assistance (helping to express anger in an adaptive, nonviolent manner) becomes a priority intervention. Because the expression of anger and aggression develops during a lifetime, these individuals can benefit from anger management techniques.

Social support for these individuals is often minimal, just as it is for individuals with BPD, but the reasons are different. These individuals have often taken advantage of friends and relatives who, in turn, no longer trust them. Helping the patient build a new support system once new skills are learned is usually the only option. For these individuals to develop friends and re-engage family members, they must learn to interact in new ways, develop empathy, and risk an attachment. For many, this never truly becomes a reality.

Family Patterns

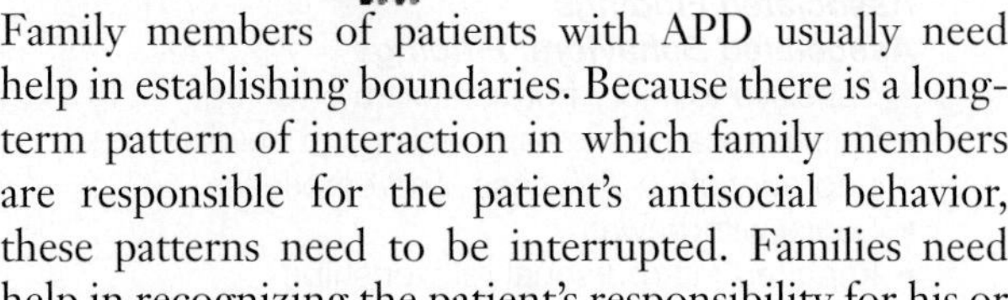

Family members of patients with APD usually need help in establishing boundaries. Because there is a long-term pattern of interaction in which family members are responsible for the patient's antisocial behavior, these patterns need to be interrupted. Families need help in recognizing the patient's responsibility for his or her actions.

Evaluation and Outcomes

The outcomes of interventions for patients with APD need to be evaluated in terms of management of specific problems, such as maintaining employment or developing a meaningful interpersonal relationship. The nurse will most likely see these patients for other health care problems, so that adherence to treatment recommendations and development of health care practices (e.g., reduce smoking and alcohol consumption) can also be factored into the evaluation of outcomes.

Continuum of Care

People with APD rarely seek mental health care (Millon, et al. 2004). Nurses will most likely see these patients in medical–surgical settings for comorbid conditions. Consistency in interventions is necessary in treating the patient throughout the continuum of care.

Histrionic Personality Disorder: Gregarious Pattern

"Attention seeking" and "emotional" describe people with histrionic personality disorders. These individuals are lively and dramatic and draw attention to themselves by their enthusiasm, dress, and apparent openness. They are the "life of the party" and, on the surface, seem interested in others. Their insatiable need for attention and approval quickly becomes obvious. These needs are inflexible and persistent, even after others attempt to meet them. They are moody and often experience a sense of helplessness when others are disinterested in them. They are sexually seductive in their attempts to gain attention and often are uncomfortable within a single relationship. They are highly suggestible and have a tendency to change opinions often. Their appearance is provocative and their speech dramatic. They express strong opinions without supporting facts. Loyalty and fidelity are lacking (APA, 2000) (Table 22.5).

Gender influences the manifestations of this disorder. Women dress seductively, may express dependency on selected men, and may "play" a submissive role. Men may dress in a very masculine manner and seek attention by bragging about athletic skills or successes in the job. Individuals with this disorder have difficulty achieving any true intimacy in interpersonal relationships. They seem to possess an innate sensitivity to the moods and thoughts of those they wish to please. This hyperalertness enables them to maneuver quickly to gain their attention. Then, they attempt to control relationships by their seductiveness at one level but become extremely dependent on their friends at another level. Their demand for constant attention quickly alienates their friends. They become depressed when they are not the center of attention.

Epidemiology

The prevalence of histrionic personality disorder is estimated at 1.8% of the general population (Grant et al., 2004). In mental health settings, the prevalence rate is reported to be 10% to 15% (APA, 2000). There are no gender differences. There is a greater risk of occurrence of this disorder among African Americans than Caucasians. Low-income groups and less educated persons are also at higher risk for occurrence of histrionic personality disorder. Widowed/separated/divorced or never married are at greater risk than married. This disorder co-occurs with borderline, dependent, and antisocial personality disorders. It also exists with anxiety disorders, substance abuse, and mood disorders (Millon et al., 2004).

Etiology

There is a need for research in determining the etiologic factors of histrionic personality disorder. Some speculate that this disorder has a biologic component and that heredity may play a role, but that the biologic influence is less than in some of the previously discussed personality disorders. In infancy and early childhood, these individuals are extremely alert and emotionally responsive. The tendencies for sensory alertness may be traced to responses of the limbic and reticular systems. They

Table 22.5  **Key Diagnostic Characteristics of Histrionic and Narcissistic Personality Disorders 301.50** 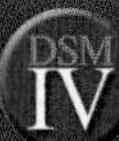

Diagnostic Criteria and Target Symptoms for Histrionic Disorders	Associated Findings
• Pervasive and excessive emotionality and attention-seeking behavior Feelings of being uncomfortable and unappreciated when not the center of attention (lively and dramatic in drawing attention to self) Inappropriately sexually seductive or provocative Shallow and rapidly shifting emotional expression Use of physical appearance to draw attention to self Impressionistic and vague style of speech Exaggerated expression of emotion, theatricality, and self-dramatization Highly suggestible Viewing of relationships as more intimate than they really are	***Associated Behavioral Findings*** • Difficulty achieving emotional intimacy in romantic and sexual relationships • Use of emotional manipulation and seductiveness coupled with marked dependency • Impaired relationships with same-sex friends • Constant demanding of attention, leading to alienation of friends • Craving novelty, excitement, and stimulation; easily bored with routines • Difficulty in situations involving delayed gratification • Increased risk for suicidal gestures and threats for attention
Diagnostic Criteria and Target Symptoms for Narcissistic Disorders	***Associated Findings***
• Pervasive pattern of grandiosity; need for admiration; lack of empathy Grandiose sense of self-importance Preoccupation with fantasies of unlimited success, power or vigilance, beauty, or ideal love Belief of own superiority, specialness, and uniqueness; association with individuals of higher or special status Need for excessive admiration and constant attention Sense of entitlement (unreasonable expectation of highly favorable treatment) Exploitation and taking advantage of others Lack of empathy; difficulty recognizing desires, experiences, and feelings of others Envious of others; feeling that others are envious of him or her Arrogant, haughty behavior or attitudes	***Associated Behavioral Findings*** • Sensitive to injury from criticism or defeat • Criticism causes inward feelings of humiliation, degradation, hollowness, and emptiness • Social withdrawal • Impaired interpersonal relationships • Impaired performance because of intolerance to criticism • Unwilling to take risk in competitive situation when defeat is possible

demonstrate a high degree of dependence on others and a type of dissociation in which they have reduced awareness of their behavior in relation to others (Millon et al., 2004). It is believed these highly alert and responsive infants seek more gratification from external stimulation during their first few months of life. Depending on the responsiveness of caregivers to them, they develop behavior patterns in response to their caregivers. It is believed that these children experience brief, highly charged, and irregular reinforcement from multiple caregivers (parents, siblings, grandparents, foster parents) who are unable to provide consistent experiences.

Parental behavior and role modeling are also believed to contribute to the development of histrionic personality disorder. Many of the women with this disorder reported that they are just like their mother, who is emotionally labile, bored with the routines of home life, flirtatious with men, and clever in dealing with people. It is believed that through role modeling, these children learn and mimic the behaviors observed in caregivers or adults (Millon et al., 2004).

Nursing Management

The ultimate treatment goal for patients with histrionic personality disorder is to correct the tendency to fulfill all their needs by focusing on others to the exclusion of themselves. When these individuals seek mental health care, they have usually experienced a period of social disapproval or deprivation. Their hope is that the mental health providers will help fulfill their needs. Specific goals are needed to protect the person from becoming dependent on a mental health system. In the nursing assessment, the nurse focuses on the quality of the individual's interpersonal relationships. It is common that the person is dissatisfied with his or her partner, and sexual relations may be nonexistent.

During the assessment, the patient will make statements that indicate low self-esteem. Because these individuals believe that they are incapable of handling life's demands and have been waiting for a truly competent person to take care of them, they have not developed a positive self-concept or adequate problem-solving abilities.

Nursing diagnoses that are usually generated include Chronic Low Self-esteem, Ineffective Individual Coping, and Ineffective Sexual Patterns. Outcomes focus on helping the patient develop autonomy, a positive self-concept, and mature problem-solving skills.

A variety of interventions support the outcomes. A nurse–patient relationship that allows the patient to explore positive personality characteristics and develop independent decision-making skills forms the basis of the interventions. Reinforcing personal strengths, conveying confidence in the patient's ability to handle situations, and examining negative perceptions of self can be done within the therapeutic relationship. Encouraging the patient to act autonomously can also improve the individual's sense of self-worth (Dochterman & Bulechek, 2004). Attending assertiveness groups can help increase the individual's self-confidence and improve self-esteem.

Narcissistic Personality Disorder: Egotistic Pattern

People with a narcissistic personality disorder are grandiose, have an inexhaustible need for admiration, and lack empathy. Beginning in childhood, these individuals believe that they are superior, special, or unique and that others should recognize them in this way (APA, 2000). They are often preoccupied with fantasies of unlimited success, power, beauty, or ideal love. They overvalue their personal worth, direct their affections toward themselves, and expect others to hold them in high esteem. They define the world through their own self-centered view. People with narcissistic personality disorder are benignly arrogant and feel themselves above the conventions of their cultural group. They believe they are entitled to be served and that it is their inalienable right to receive special considerations. These individuals are often successful in their jobs but may alienate their significant others, who grow tired of their narcissism (see Table 22.5). Clinically, those with narcissistic personality disorder show overlapping characteristics of BPD.

Epidemiology

The prevalence of narcissistic personality disorder in the general population is estimated to be less than 1%. In the mental health clinical population, the prevalence ranges from 2% to 16% (APA, 2000). In nonclinical samples, the prevalence rate ranges from 0.0% to 0.4% (Lyons, 1995). Narcissistic personality disorder is found in professions that are unusually respected such as law, medicine, and science or those associated with celebrity status. It seems to occur more frequently in men than in women (Millon et al., 2004). It also commonly occurs in only children and among first-born boys in cultural groups in which males have special privileges. This disorder can coexist with other Axis II disorders, such as antisocial, histrionic, and paranoid disorders and Axis I disorders of mood, anxiety, and substance abuse.

Etiology

There is little evidence of any biologic factors that contribute to the development of this disorder. One notion about its development is that it is the result of parents' overvaluation and overindulgence of a child. These children are overly pampered and indulged, with every whim catered to. They learn to view themselves as special beings and to expect special treatment and subservience from others. They do not learn how to cooperate, share, or consider others' desires and interests. An alternate explanation is that the child never truly separated emotionally from his or her primary caregiver and therefore cannot envision functioning independently.

Nursing Management

The nurse usually encounters narcissists in medical settings and in psychiatric settings with a coexisting psychiatric disorder. They are difficult patients who are often snobbish, condescending, and patronizing in their attitudes. It is unlikely that these individuals are motivated to develop sensitivity to others and socially cooperative attitudes and behaviors. Nurses need to use their self-awareness skills in interacting with these patients. The nursing process focuses on the coexisting responses to other health care problems.

Continuum of Care

Patients with histrionic and narcissistic personality disorders do not seek mental health care unless they have a coexisting medical or mental disorder. They are likely to be treated within the community for most of their lives, with the exception of short hospitalizations for nonpsychiatric problems.

CLUSTER C DISORDERS: ANXIOUS-FEARFUL

Avoidant Personality Disorder: Withdrawn Pattern

Avoidant personality disorder is characterized by avoiding social situations in which there is interpersonal contact with others. This avoidance is purposeful and deliberate because of fears of criticism and feelings of inadequacy. These individuals are extremely sensitive to negative comments and disapproval. They engage in interpersonal relationships only when they receive unconditional approval. The behavior becomes problematic when they restrict their social activities and work opportunities because of their extreme fear of rejection. They appear timid, shy, and hesitant. In childhood, they are shy, but instead of growing out of the shyness, it becomes worse in adulthood. They distance themselves from activities that involve personal contact with others. They perceive themselves as socially inept, inadequate, and inferior, which in turn justifies their isolation and rejection by others. They rely on fantasy for gratification of needs, confidence, and conflict resolution. These individuals withdraw into their fantasies as a means of dealing with frustration and anger. They also have underlying feelings of tension, sadness, and anger that vacillate between desire for affection, fear of rebuff, embarrassment, and numbness of feeling (APA, 2000; Millon et al., 2004) (Table 22.6).

Epidemiology

The prevalence of avoidant personality disorder is 2.36% (Grant, 2004). Avoidant personality disorder has been reported in about 10% of outpatients in mental health clinics. The problem with examining the epidemiology of avoidant personality disorder is its potential overlap with the Axis I disorder, generalized social phobia. Several studies found that a significant portion of the patients with diagnoses of social phobia also met criteria for avoidant personality disorder (Ralevski et al., 2005; Shea et al., 2004). More research is needed to clarify the relationship between personality and anxiety disorders.

Etiology

Experts speculate that individuals with avoidant personality disorder experience aversive stimuli more intensely and more frequently than do others because they may possess an overabundance of neurons in the aversive center of the limbic system (Millon et al., 2004). A general biologic vulnerability may be inherited and interact with environmental factors. Research indicates that those with avoidant personality disorder demonstrate significantly less curiosity and novelty seeking than do healthy control subjects (Taylor, Laposa, & Alden, 2004).

Nursing Management

Assessment of these individuals reveals a lack of social contacts, a fear of being criticized, and evidence of

Table 22.6 Key Diagnostic Characteristics of Cluster C Disorders DSM IV

Disorder	Diagnostic Criteria and Target Symptoms
Avoidant Personality Disorder 301.82	• Pervasive pattern of social inhibition with feelings of inadequacy and hypersensitivity to negative evaluation Avoidance of activities involving significant personal contact because of fear of criticism, disapproval, or rejection Lack of willingness for involvement unless certainty of being liked Restraint within intimate relationships for fear of shame or ridicule Preoccupation with criticism or rejection in social situations Inhibition in new interpersonal situations Viewing self as socially inept, personally unappealing, or inferior Unusual reluctance to take personal risks or engage in new activities
Dependent Personality Disorder 301.6	• Pervasive and excessive need for being taken care of, resulting in submission and clinging with fears of separation Advice and reassurance needed from others for decision making Responsibility for major areas of life assumed by others Difficulty expressing disagreement with others for fear of loss of support or approval Difficulty initiating things by self Excessive methods used to obtain support and nurturance from others Uncomfortable and helpless when alone Urgent seeking of another relationship if previous one ends Unrealistic preoccupation with fears of having to take care of self
Obsessive-Compulsive Personality Disorder 301.4	• Pervasive pattern of preoccupation with orderliness, perfectionism, mental and interpersonal control at the expense of flexibility, openness, and efficiency Major point of activity lost because of preoccupation Task completion interfered with because of perfectionism Excessive devotion to work and productivity, excluding friends and leisure Overly conscientious, scrupulous, and inflexible about morality, ethics, or values Difficulty discarding worn-out or worthless objects Reluctance to delegate tasks or work with others Miserly spending attitude Rigidity and stubbornness

chronic low self-esteem. The nursing diagnoses Chronic Low Self-esteem, Social Isolation, and Ineffective Coping can be used. The establishment of a therapeutic relationship is necessary to be able to help these individuals meet their treatment outcomes. The development of the nurse–patient relationship is a slow process and requires an extreme amount of patience on the part of the nurse. These individuals may not have had positive interpersonal relationships and need time to be able to trust that the nurse will not criticize and demean them. Interventions should focus on refraining from any negative criticism, assisting the patient to identify positive responses from others, exploring previous achievements of success, and exploring reasons for self-criticism. The patient's social dimension should be examined for activities that increase self-esteem and interventions focused on increasing these self-esteem–enhancing activities. Social skills training may help reduce symptoms.

Dependent Personality Disorder: Submissive Pattern

People with dependent personality disorder cling to others in a desperate attempt to keep them close. Their need to be taken care of is so great that it leads to doing anything to maintain the closeness, including total submission and disregard for self.

Decision making is difficult or nil. They adapt their behavior to please those to whom they are attached. They lean on others to guide their lives. They ingratiate themselves to others and denigrate themselves and their accomplishments. Their self-esteem is determined by others. Behaviorally, they withdraw from adult responsibilities by acting helpless and seeking nurturance from others. In interpersonal relationships, they need excessive advice and reassurance. They are compliant, conciliatory, and placating. They rarely disagree with others and are easily persuaded. Friends describe them as gullible. They are warm, tender, and noncompetitive. They timidly avoid social tension and interpersonal conflicts (APA, 2000) (see Table 22.6). Dependent personality disorder is associated with suicide and alcoholism (Echeburua, de Medina, & Aizpiri, 2005; Loas et al., 2005).

Epidemiology

According to the *DSM-IV-TR*, dependent personality disorder is one of the most frequently reported disorders in mental health clinics (APA, 2000), but a recent study estimates the prevalence at 0.49% (Grant et al., 2004). The diagnosis is made more frequently in women than in men. This gender difference may represent a sex bias by clinicians because when standardized instruments are used, men and women receive diagnoses at equal rates. The risk of dependent personality disorder is greater for the least educated, widowed/divorced/separated and never married women (Grant).

Etiology

It is likely that there is a biologic predisposition to develop the dependency attachments of this disorder. However, no research studies support a biologic hypothesis. Dependent personality disorder most often is explained as a result of parents' genuine affection, extreme attachment, and overprotection. Children then learn to rely on others to meet basic needs and do not learn the necessary skills for autonomous behavior.

Nursing Management

Nurses can determine the extent of dependency by assessment of self-worth, interpersonal relationships, and social behavior. They should determine whether there is currently someone on whom the person relies (parent, spouse) or if there has been a separation from a significant relationship by death or divorce.

Nursing diagnoses that are usually generated from the assessment data are Ineffective Individual Coping, Low Self-esteem, Impaired Social Interaction, and Impaired Home Maintenance Management. Home management skills may be a problem if the patient does not have the useful skills and now has to make decisions related to finances, shopping, cooking, and cleaning. The challenge of caring for these patients is to help them recognize their dependent patterns, motivate them to want to change, and teach them adult skills that have not been developed, such as balancing a checkbook, planning a weekly menu, and paying bills. Occasionally, if a patient is extremely fatigued, lethargic, or anxious, and the disorder interferes with efforts at developing more independence, antidepressants or antianxiety agents may be used.

These patients readily engage in a nurse–patient relationship and initially will look to the nurse to make all decisions. The nurse can support patients to make their own decisions by resisting the urge to tell them what to do. Ideally, these patients are in individual psychotherapy and working toward long-term personality changes. The nurse can encourage patients to stay in therapy and to practice the new skills that are being learned. Assertiveness training is helpful.

OBSESSIVE-COMPULSIVE PERSONALITY DISORDER: CONFORMING PATTERN

Obsessive-compulsive disorder (OCD) stands out in Axis II because it bears close resemblance to obsessive-compulsive anxiety disorder (Axis I). A distinguishing difference is that those with the anxiety disorder tend to use obsessive thoughts and compulsions when anxious but less so when anxiety decreases. With OCD, the person does not demonstrate obsessions and compulsions as much as an overall rigidity, perfectionism, and control. Individuals with this disorder attempt to maintain control by careful attention to rules, trivial details, procedures, and lists (APA, 2000). These people are not fun. They may be completely devoted to work, which typically has a rigid character, such as maintaining financial records or tracking inventory. They are uncomfortable with unstructured leisure time, especially vacations. Leisure activities are likely to be formalized (season tickets to sports, organized tour groups). Hobbies are approached seriously.

Behaviorally, individuals with OCD are perfectionists, maintaining a regulated, highly structured, strictly organized life. A need to control others and situations is common in personal and in work life. They are prone to repetition and have difficulty making decisions and completing tasks because they become so involved in the details. They can be overly conscientious about morality and ethics and value polite, formal, and correct interpersonal relationships. They also tend to be rigid, stubborn, and indecisive and are unable to accept new ideas and customs. Their mood is tense and joyless. Warm feelings are restrained, and they tightly control the expression of emotions (APA, 2000) (see Table 22.6).

Epidemiology

The prevalence of obsessive-compulsive personality disorder is 1% in the general population and 3% to 10% in individuals receiving treatment in mental health clinics (APA, 2000). However, the prevalence rates could be even higher today. In data derived from the National Epidemiologic Survey on Alcohol and Related Conditions ($N = 43{,}093$), obsessive-compulsive personality disorder (7.88%) was found to be the most prevalent personality disorder of 7 of the 10 *DSM-IV* personality disorders in the general population (Grant et al., 2004). This disorder is associated with higher education, employment, and marriage. Subjects with the disorder had a higher income than did those without the disorder.

Etiology

As with some of the other personality disorders, there is little evidence for a biologic formulation. The basis of the compulsive patterns that characterize obsessive-compulsive personality disorder is parental overcontrol and overprotection that is consistently restrictive and sets distinct limits on the child's behavior. Parents teach these children a deep sense of responsibility to others and to feel guilty when these responsibilities are not met. Play is viewed as shameful, sinful, and irresponsible, leading to dire consequences. They are encouraged to resist the natural inclinations toward play and impulse gratification, and parents try to impose guilt on the child to control behavior.

Nursing Management

These individuals seek mental health care when they have attacks of anxiety, spells of immobilization, sexual impotence, and excessive fatigue. To change the compulsive pattern, psychotherapy is needed. There may be short-term pharmacologic intervention with an antidepressant or anxiolytic as an adjunct.

The nursing assessment focuses on the patient's physical symptoms (sleep, eating, sexual), interpersonal relationships, and social problems. Typical nursing diagnoses include Anxiety, Risk for Loneliness, Decisional Conflict, Sexual Dysfunction, Insomnia, and Impaired Social Interactions. People with OCD realize that they can improve their quality of life, but they will find it extremely anxiety provoking to make the necessary changes. A supportive nurse–patient relationship based on acceptance of the patient's need for order and rigidity will help the person have enough confidence to try new behaviors. Examining the patient's belief that underlies the dysfunctional behaviors can set the stage for challenging the childhood thinking. Because the compulsive pattern was established in childhood, it will take a long time to modify the behavior (see Box 22.13).

Continuum of Care

Long-term therapy is ideal for patients with avoidant personality disorder because it takes time to make the changes. Mental health nurses may see these individuals for other health problems. Encouraging the patient to continue with therapy and contacting the therapist when necessary are important in maintaining continuity of care. These patients are hospitalized only for a coexisting disorder.

BOX 22.13

Using Reflection: Developing Self-Awareness

Incident: An energetic, excitable nurse told a patient who has OCD to hurry up and get dressed in order to get to the cafeteria for lunch. A few minutes later she found the patient sorting his clothes, making no progress toward getting dressed.

Reflection: The nurse reflected on her interaction with the patient. Even though the nurse knew that interacting with a patient with OCD affected the level of anxiety the patient would feel, she was direct, hurried, and was too autocratic in her approach to the patient. She realized that a calm, non-confrontational approach would have been better.

People with dependent and obsessive-compulsive personality disorders are treated primarily in the community. If there is a coexisting disorder or the person experiences periods of depression, hospitalization may be useful for a short period of time.

IMPULSE-CONTROL DISORDERS

This group of mental disorders has this essential feature: irresistible impulsivity. These disorders are not part of other disorders but often coexist with them. The following impulse-control disorders have been identified by the *DSM-IV*:

- Intermittent explosive disorder
- Kleptomania
- Pyromania
- Pathologic gambling
- Trichotillomania

These disorders are characterized by an inability to resist an impulse or temptation to complete an activity that is considered harmful to self or others, an increase in tension before the individual commits the act, and excitement or gratification at the time the act is committed. The release of tension is perceived as pleasurable, but remorse and regret usually follow the act. There are other disorders that have been proposed for inclusion based up possible similarities such as compulsive buying and compulsive Internet use (Grant & Potenza, 2006) (Table 22.7).

Intermittent Explosive Disorder

Episodes of aggressiveness that result in assault or destruction of property characterize people with intermittent explosive disorder. The severity of aggressiveness is out of proportion to the provocation. The episodes can have serious psychosocial consequences, including job loss, interpersonal relationship problems, school expulsion, divorce, automobile accidents, or jail. This diagnosis is given only after all other disorders with aggressive components (delirium, dementia, head injury, BPD, APD, substance abuse) have been excluded. Little is known about this disorder, but it is a more common condition than previously thought. Twelve-month prevalence estimates are 3.9% of the population with a mean of 43 lifetime attacks. Mean age at onset is 14 years of age. It is more common in men than in women and less than 30% ever receive treatment for their anger (Kessler et al., 2006).

The treatment of this disorder is multifaceted. Psychopharmacologic agents are sometimes used as an adjunct to psychotherapeutic, behavioral, and social interventions. Serotonergic antidepressants and GABA-ergic mood stabilizers have been used. Anxiolytics are used for obsessive patients who experience tension states and explosive outbursts. Medication alone is insufficient and anger management should be included in the treatment plan.

Kleptomania

In **kleptomania**, individuals cannot resist the urge to steal, and they independently steal items that they could easily afford. These items are not particularly useful or wanted. The underlying issue is the act of stealing. The term *kleptomania* was first used in 1838 to describe the behavior of several kings who stole worthless objects (Goldman, 1992). These individuals experience an increase in tension and then pleasure and relief at the time of the theft. It is a rare condition that occurs in fewer than 5% of shoplifters (APA, 2000). Because it is considered a "secret" disorder, there is little information about this, but it is believed to last for years, despite numerous convictions for shoplifting. It appears that kleptomania often has its onset during adolescence (Grant & Kim, 2005) (see Table 22.7).

Some shoplifting appears to be related to anxiety and stress, in that it serves to relieve symptoms. In a few instances, brain damage has been associated with kleptomania. Depression is the most common symptom identified in a compulsive shoplifter.

Kleptomania is difficult to detect and treat. There are few accounts of treatment. It appears that behavior therapy is frequently used. Antidepressant medication that helps relieve the depression has been successful in some cases. More investigation is needed (Schatzberg, 2000).

Pyromania

Irresistible impulses to start fires characterize **pyromania**. These individuals are aroused before setting a fire and are fascinated with fires. They are attracted to fires, often becoming regular "fire watchers" or even firefighters. These arsonists, people who intentionally set fires or make an effort at fire setting, are not motivated by aggression, anger, suicidal ideation, or political ideology. They may make advanced preparation for the fire. Little is known about this disorder because only a small number of deliberate firestarters are apprehended and of those individuals, only a few undergo a psychiatric evaluation (Brett, 2003). Most fire setting is not done by people with this disorder. This disorder occurs infrequently, mostly in men (APA, 2000) (see Table 22.7).

Early research demonstrated low serotonin and norepinephrine levels associated with arson (Virkkunen et al., 1994). Little is known about treatment, and as with the other impulse-control disorders, no one approach is uniformly effective. Historically, firestarters generally pos-

Table 22.7 Summary of Diagnostic Characteristics for Impulse-Control Disorders DSM IV

Disorder	Diagnostic Criteria and Target Symptoms
Kleptomania 312.32	• Recurrent failure to resist impulse to steal object that is not needed • Increased tension before theft • Pleasure, gratification, or relief at time of theft • Theft not related to anger or vengeance; not in response to delusion or hallucination • Not better accounted for by another psychiatric disorder
Pyromania 312.23	• Multiple episodes of deliberate and purposeful fire setting • Tension or affective arousal before act • Fascination with, interest in, curiosity about, or attraction to fires Regular fire watchers False alarm setters Pleasure with institution, equipment, and personnel associated with fires • Pleasure gratification or tension relief with fire starting, watching its effects or participating in aftermath • Not done for monetary gain; expression of ideology, anger, or vengeance; concealing criminal activity; improving living conditions; or as a response to hallucination or delusion • Not better accounted for by another psychiatric disorder
Pathologic gambling 312.31	• Persistent and recurrent maladaptive gambling behavior • Disruption of personal, family, or vocational pursuits Preoccupation with gambling Increased amounts of money needed to achieve excitement Unsuccessful efforts to stop, cut back, or control Restlessness and irritability with attempts to control or cut back Means of escape from problems or mood Chasing of losses; attempts to get even Lying to family and others to conceal involvement Commission of illegal acts to finance behavior Significant relationships, job, or opportunities jeopardized or lost Reliance on others for relief of poor financial situation • Not better accounted for by manic episode
Trichotillomania 312.39	• Recurrent pulling of one's hair with subsequent hair loss Brief episodes throughout day or sustained periods of hours Increased during stress and relaxation periods • Increased tension immediately before act and with attempts to resist urge • Gratification, pleasure, or relief with act • Not better accounted for by another psychiatric disorder; not the effect of a general medical condition
Intermittent explosive episode 312.34	• Significant distress and impairment of functioning • Discrete episodes of failing to resist aggressive impulses resulting in serious assaultive acts or property destruction • Degree of aggressiveness grossly out of proportion to provocation or stressor • Not better accounted for by another psychiatric disorder; not a direct physiologic effect of a substance or general medical condition

sess poor interpersonal skills, exhibit low-self esteem, battle depression, and have difficulty managing anger (Brett, 2003). Education, parenting training, behavior contracting with token reinforcement, problem-solving skills training, and relaxation exercises may all be used in the management of the patient's responses. One study found that specifically with boys who set fires, fire safety education and cognitive behavioral therapy proved to be successful intervention approaches with firestarting children and their families (Kolko, Herschell, & Scharf, 2006).

Pathologic Gambling

Social gambling becomes pathologic when it becomes recurrent and disrupts personal, family, or vocational pursuits. These individuals are preoccupied with gambling and experience an aroused, euphoric state during the actual betting. The action of seeking an aroused state is often more important to the pathologic gambler than the desire for money itself (Schmitz, 2005). They are drawn to the games and begin making bigger and bigger bets. Characteristically, they relentlessly chase their losses in an attempt to win them back. They are unable to control their gaming and may lie to family, friends, and employers to hide their gambling. These individuals are highly competitive, energetic, restless, and easily bored. The prevalence is estimated at 1% to 3% of the population (APA, 2000); another study found a 1% to 3% lifetime prevalence (Grant & Kim, 2003). In addition, these individuals may use the thrill of gambling as a way of escaping or lifting a depressed mood (Schmitz, 2005). Of those individuals in treatment for pathologic gambling, 20% have reported attempting suicide (see Table 22.7).

This disorder is conceptualized as similar to alcohol and other substances of dependence (Hall et al., 2000). When substances are used in conjunction with gambling, they cause a deterioration in play and accelerate the progression of the gambling disorder. Other comorbid disorders include depression, ADHD, Tourette's syndrome, and personality disorders (Schmitz, 2005). The disorder has four phases: winning, losing, desperation, and hopelessness. Pathologic gambling can be treated by psychotherapists experienced in this disorder; for many, Gamblers Anonymous is sufficient.

Compulsive gamblers feel omnipotent in their ability to win back what was lost. This omnipotence serves as self-deception that leads to denial. Care of these patients involves confronting their omnipotent beliefs. These individuals quickly irritate staff by their self-assurance and overbearing attitude. Staff education about the disorder is important. Family involvement is also crucial. Families often have been dealing with the patient in a dysfunctional manner. Relapse prevention involves learning about specific cues that trigger the gambling behavior.

With the rise in pathologic gambling and its social consequences, there have been greater efforts to identify supportive pharmacotherapy. Because the underlying mechanisms are anxiety and impulsivity, first-line drugs are SSRIs. These have been moderately effective (Hollander et al., 2000), especially when combined with cognitive-behavioral approaches (Oakley-Browne, Adams, & Mobberly, 2000).

Trichotillomania

Trichotillomania is chronic, self-destructive hair pulling that results in noticeable hair loss, usually in the crown, occipital, or parietal areas, although sometimes of the eyebrows and eyelashes. The patient has an increase in tension immediately before pulling out the hair or when attempting to resist the behavior. After the hair is pulled, the person feels a sense of relief. Some would classify this disorder as one of self-mutilation. It becomes a problem when there is a significant distress or impairment in other areas of function. A hair-pulling session can last several hours, and the individual may ritualistically eat the hairs or discard them. Hair ingestion may result in the development of a hair ball, which can lead to anorexia, stomach pain, anemia, obstruction, and peritonitis. Other medical complications include infection at the hair-pulling site. Hair pulling is done alone, and usually patients deny it. Instead of pain, these persons experience pleasure and tension release (APA, 2000; Woods et al., 2006) (see Table 22.7).

The onset of trichotillomania occurs among children before the age of 5 years and in adolescence. For the young child, distraction or redirection may successfully eliminate the behavior. The behavior in adolescents may begin a chronic course that may last well into adulthood. This disorder is poorly understood. Its prevalence is estimated at 2% to 4% of the population. The cause is unknown (APA, 2000). Initially, it was believed that medications would be helpful in treatment, but evidence does not support these expectations. Cognitive behavior therapy has been shown to be effective in some studies (Woods et al., 2006). More research is needed.

The assessment includes a review of current problems, developmental history (especially school conflicts, learning difficulties), family history, social history, identification of support systems, previous psychiatric treatment, and health history. The cultural context in which the trichotillomania occurs must be taken into consideration because in some cultures, this behavior is viewed as socially acceptable (Kress, Kelly, & McCormick, 2004). Hair-pulling history and pattern is also solicited to determine the duration and severity of the disorder. The typical nursing diagnoses include Self-mutilation, Low Self-esteem, Hopelessness, Impaired Skin Integrity, and Ineffective Denial. Within the therapeutic relationship, a cognitive behavioral approach can be used to help the patient identify when hair pulling occurs, the precipitating events, and the details of the episode. Individuals with trichotillomania report that anxiety, loneliness, anger, fatigue, guilt, frustration, and boredom can all trigger one's hair pulling behaviors (Kress, Kelly, & McCormick, 2004). Current research also showed that persons with chronic hair pulling typically avoid social activities and events. In addition, the economic impact of trichotillomania can be significant in relation to lost work or school days (Wetterneck, Woods, Norberg, & Begotka, 2006). Teaching about the disorder will help patients understand that they are not alone and that others have also suffered with this problem. The goal of treatment is to help the patient learn to substitute positive behaviors for the hair-pulling behavior through self-monitoring of events that precipitate the episodes.

Continuum of Care

Impulse-control disorders require long-term treatment, usually in an outpatient setting. Group therapy is often a facet of treatment because patients can talk in a community where people share common experiences. Hospitalization is rare, except when there are comorbid psychiatric or medical disorders.

SUMMARY OF KEY POINTS

- A personality is a complex pattern of characteristics, largely outside of the person's awareness, that comprise the individual's distinctive pattern of perceiving, feeling, thinking, coping, and behaving. The personality emerges from a complicated interaction of biologic dispositions, psychological experiences, and environmental situations.
- Personality disorder is an enduring pattern of inner experience and behavior that deviates markedly from the expectations of the individual's culture, is pervasive and inflexible, has an onset in adolescence or early adulthood, is stable over time, and leads to distress or impairment.
- In the *DSM-IV*, personality disorders are on Axis II and are organized around three clusters or dimensions: cluster A, odd-eccentric disorders; cluster B, dramatic-emotional disorders; and cluster C, anxious-fearful disorders. Any of the personality disorders can coexist with Axis I disorders.
- People with cluster A personality disorders whose odd, eccentric behaviors often alienate them from others can benefit from interventions such as social skills training, environmental management, and cognitive skill building. Changing patterns of thinking and behaving are difficult and take time; thus, patient outcomes must be evaluated in terms of small changes in thinking and behavior.
- In cluster A, paranoid personality disorder is characterized by a suspicious pattern, schizoid personality disorder by an asocial pattern, and schizotypal personality disorder by an eccentric pattern.
- People with borderline personality disorder (cluster B) have difficulties regulating emotion and have extreme fears of abandonment, leading to dysfunctional relationships; they often engage in self-injury.
- Antisocial personality disorder (cluster B), often synonymous with psychopath or sociopath, includes people who have no regard for and refuse to conform to social rules.
- Patients with cluster B personality disorders often have difficulties with emotional regulation or being able to recognize and control the expression of their feelings, such as anger, disappointment, and frustration. The nurse can help these patients identify feelings and gain control over their feelings and actions by teaching communication skills and techniques, thought-stopping techniques, distraction, or problem-solving techniques.
- Cluster C personality disorders are characterized by anxieties and fears and include avoidant, dependent, and obsessive-compulsive disorders. The obsessive-compulsive personality disorder differs from the obsessive-compulsive anxiety disorder because the individual demonstrates an overall rigidity, perfectionism, and need for control.
- For many patients with personality disorders, maintaining a therapeutic nurse–patient relationship can be one of the most helpful interventions. Through this therapeutic relationship, the patient experiences a model of healthy interaction, establishing trust, consistency, caring, boundaries, and limitations that help to build the patient's self-esteem and respect for self and others. In some personality disorders, nurses will find it more difficult to engage the patient in a true therapeutic relationship because of the patient's avoidance of interpersonal and emotional attachment (i.e., antisocial personality disorder or paranoid personality disorder).
- Patients with personality disorders are rarely treated in an inpatient facility, except during periods of destructive behavior or self-injury. Treatment is delivered in the community and over time. Continuity of care is important in helping the individual change lifelong personality patterns.
- Although not classified as personality disorders, the impulse-control disorders share one of the primary characteristics of impulsivity, which leads to inappropriate social behaviors that are considered harmful to self or others and that give the patient excitement or gratification at the time the act is committed.

CRITICAL THINKING CHALLENGES

1 Define the concepts *personality* and *personality disorder*. When does a normal personality become a personality disorder?

2 Karen, a 36-year-old woman receiving inpatient care, was admitted for depression; she also has a diagnosis of borderline personality disorder. After a telephone argument with her husband, she approaches the nurse's station with her wrist dripping with blood from cutting. What nursing diagnosis best fits this behavior? What interventions should the nurse use with the patient once the self-injury is treated?

3 A 22-year-old man with borderline personality disorder is being discharged from the mental health unit after a severe suicide attempt. As his primary psychiatric nurse, you have been able to establish a thera

peutic relationship with him but are now terminating the relationship. He asks you to meet with him "for just a few sessions" after his discharge because his therapist will be on vacation. What are the issues underlying this request? What should you do? Explain and justify.

4 Compare the psychoanalytic explanation of the development of borderline personality disorder with Linehan's biosocial theory.
5 Compare the characteristics, epidemiology, and etiologic theories of antisocial and borderline personality disorders.
6 Discuss the differences between histrionic and borderline personality disorders.
7 Compare and contrast antisocial and narcissistic personality disorders.
8 Define and summarize the three personality disorders of cluster A. Compare the following among the three disorders:
   a Defining characteristics
   b Epidemiology
   c Biologic, psychological, and social theories
   d Key nursing assessment data
   e Nursing diagnoses and outcomes
   f Specific issues related to a therapeutic relationship
   g Interventions
9 Define and summarize the three personality disorders of cluster C. Compare the following among the three disorders:
   a Defining characteristics
   b Epidemiology
   c Biologic, psychological, and social theories
   d Key nursing assessment data
   e Nursing diagnoses and outcomes
   f Specific issues related to a therapeutic relationship
   g Interventions
10 Define and summarize the impulse-control disorders. Compare the following among the three disorders:
   a Defining characteristics
   b Epidemiology
   c Biologic, psychological, and social theories
   d Key nursing assessment data
   e Nursing diagnoses and outcomes
   f Interventions

Fatal Attraction: 1987. This award-winning film portrays the relationship between a married attorney, Dan Gallagher (played by Michael Douglas), and Alex Forest, a single woman (played by Glenn Close). Their one-night affair turns into a nightmare for the attorney and his family as Alex becomes increasingly possessive and aggressive, demonstrating behaviors characteristic of borderline personality disorder: anger, impulsivity, emotional lability, fear of rejection and abandonment, vacillation between adulation and disgust, and self-mutilation.

VIEWING POINTS: Identify the behaviors of Alex that are characteristics of borderline personality disorder. Identify the feelings that are generated by the movie. With which characters do you identify? For which characters do you feel sympathy? If Alex had lived and been admitted to your hospital, what would be your first priority?

REFERENCES

Ainsworth, M. (1989). Attachments beyond infancy. *American Psychologist, 44*(4), 709–716.

American Psychiatric Association. (2000). *Diagnostic and statistical manual of mental disorders* (4th ed., text revision). Washington, DC: Author.

Andrews, J. A., Foster, S. L., Capaldi, D., & Hop, H. (2000). Adolescent and family predictors of physical aggression, communication, and satisfaction in young adult couples: A prospective analysis. *Journal of Consulting Clinical Psychology, 68*(2), 195–208.

Becker, D. F., McGlashan, T. H., & Grilo, C. M. (2006). Exploratory factor analysis of borderline personality disorder criteria in hospitalized adolescents. *Comprehensive Psychiatry, 47*(2), 99–105.

Bandelow, B., Krause, J., Wedekind, D., Broocks, A., Hajak, G. & Ruther, E. (2005). Early traumatic life events, parental attitudes, family history, and birth risk factors in patients with borderline personality disorder and healthy controls. *Psychiatry Research, 134*(2), 169–179.

Barry, C. T., Frick, P. J., DeShazo, T. M., McCoy, M. G., Ellis, M., & Loney, B. R. (2000). The importance of callous-unemotional traits for extending the concept of psychopathy to children. *Journal of Abnormal Psychology, 109*(2), 335–340.

Best, M., Williams, J. M., & Coccaro, E. F. (2002). Evidence for a dysfunctional prefrontal circuit in patients with an impulsive aggressive disorder. *Processes of the National Academy of Science, 11*(12), 8448–8853.

Binks, C.A., Fenton, M., McCarthy, L., Lee, T., Adams, C.E., Duggan, C. (2006). Pharmacological interventions for people with borderline personality disorder. *Cochrane Database of Systematic Reviews,* Jan 25;(1): CD005653.

Bland, A. R., & Rossen, E. (2005). Clinical supervision of nurses working with patients with borderline personality disorder. *Issues in Mental Health Nursing, 26*(5), 507–517.

Bland, A. R., Williams, C. A., Scharer, K., & Manning, S. (2004). Emotion processing in borderline personality disorders. *Issues in Mental Health Nursing, 25*(7), 655–672.

Bland, A. R., Tudor, G., & Whitehouse, D. M. (in press). Nursing care of inpatients with borderline personality disorder: A literature review. *Perspectives in Psychiatric Care.*

Bowlby, J. (1980). *Loss: Sadness and depression.* New York: Basic Books.

Brett, A. (2003). Kindling theory in arson: How dangerous are firesetters? *Australian and New Zealand Journal of Psychiatry, 38*(6), 419–425.

Butler, A. C., Brown, G. K., Beck, A. T., & Grisham, J. R. (2002). Assessment of dysfunctional beliefs in borderline personality disorder. *Behavioral Research and Therapy, 40*(10), 1231–1240.

Chapman, A. L., Specht, J. W., & Cellucci, T. (2005). Borderline personality disorder and deliberate self-harm: does experiential avoidance play a role? *Suicide & Life-threatening Behavior 35*(4), 388–99.

Chavira, D. A., Grilo, C. M., Shea, T., Yen, S., Gunderson, J.G., et al. (2003). Ethnicity and four personality disorders. *Comprehensive Psychiatry, 44*(5), 483–491.

Cukrowicz, K. C., Taylor, J., Schatschneider, C., & Iacono, W. G. (2006). Personality differences in children and adolescents with attention-deficit/hyperactivity disorder, conduct disorder, and controls. *Journal of Child Psychology and Psychiatry, 47*(2), 151–159.

De la Fuente, J. M., Bobes, J., Vizuete, C., Bascaran, M.T., Morlan, I., & Mendlewicz, J. (2006). Neurologic soft signs in borderline personality disorder. *Journal of Clinical Psychiatry, 67*(4), 541–546.

Dolan, M., & Park, I. (2002). The neuropsychology of antisocial personality disorder. *Psychological Medicine, 32*(3), 417–427.

Driessen, M., Herrmann, J., Stahl, K., Zwaan, M., Meier, S., Hill, A., et al. (2000). Magnetic resonance imaging volumes of the hippocampus and the amygdala in women with borderline personality disorder and early traumatization. *Archives of General Psychiatry, 57*(12), 1115–1122.

Echeburua, E., de Medina, R.B., & Aizpiri, J. (2005). Alcoholism and personality disorders: an exploratory study. *Alcohol & Alcoholism, 40*(4), 323–326.

Erikson, E. (1968). *Identity: Youth and crisis.* New York: Norton.

Friedel, R. O. (2004). *Borderline personality disorder demystified: An essential guide for understanding and living with BPD.* Marlowe & Company: New York.

Friedel, R. O. (2004a). Dopamine dysfunction in borderline personality disorder: A hypothesis. *Neuropsychopharmacology, 29*(6), 1020–1039.

Giancola, P. R. (2000). Temperament and antisocial behavior in preadolescent boys with or without a family history of a substance use disorder. *Psychological Addictive Behaviors, 14*(1), 56–68.

Goldman, M. (1992). Kleptomania: An overview. *Psychiatric Annals, 22*(2), 68–71.

Gollan, J. K., Lee, R., & Coccaro, E. F. (2005). Developmental psychopathology and neurobiology of aggression. *Development & Psychopathology, 17*(4), 1151–1171.

Goodman, M., New, A., & Siever, L. (2004). Trauma, genes, and the neurobiology of personality disorders. *Annals of the New York Academy of Sciences, 1032*, 104–116.

Gotz, M. J., Johnstone, E. C., & Ratcliffe, S. G. (1999). Criminality and antisocial behaviour in unselected men with sex chromosome abnormalities. *Psychological Medicine, 29*(4), 953–962.

Grant, B. F., Hasin, D. S., Stinson, F. D., Dawson, D. A., Chou, S. P., Ruan, W. J., & Pickering, R. P. (2004). Prevalence, correlates, and disability of personality disorders in the United States: Results from the National epidemiologic survey on alcohol and related conditions. *Journal of Clinical Psychiatry, 65*(7), 948–995.

Grant, J. E., & Kim, S. W. (2003). Comorbidity of impulse control disorders in pathological gamblers. *Acta Psychiatrica Scandinavica, 108*(3), 203–207.

Grant, J. E., & Kim, S. W. (2005). Quality of life in kleptomania and pathological gambling. *Comprehensive Psychiatry, 46*(1), 34–37.

Grant, J. E., & Potenza, M. N. (2006). Compulsive aspects of impulse-control disorders. *Psychiatric Clinics of North America, 29(2)*, 539–551.

Goldstein, R. B., Grant, B. F., Ruan, J., Smith, S. M., & Saha, T. D. (2006). Antisocial personality disorder with childhood-vs-adolescence-onset conduct disorder. *The Journal of Nervous and Mental Disease, 194*(9), 667–675.

Gurvits, I. G., Koenigsberg, H. W., & Siever, I. J. (2000). Neurotransmitter dysfunction in patients with borderline personality disorder. *Psychiatric Clinics of North America, 23*(1), 27–40.

Hall, G. W., Carriero, N. J., Takushi, R. Y., Montoya, I. D., Preston, K. L., & Gorelick, D. A. (2000). Pathological gambling among cocaine-dependent outpatients. *American Journal of Psychiatry, 157*(7), 1127–1133.

Hollander, E., DeCaria, C. M., Finkell, J. N., Begaz, R., Wong, C. M., & Carwight, C. (2000). A randomized double-blind fluvoxamine/placebo crossover trial in pathologic gambling. *Biological Psychiatry, 47*(9), 813–817.

Hollander, E., Swann, A. C., Coccaro, E. F., Jiang, P., Smith, T. B. (2005). Impact of trait impulsivity and state aggression on divalproex versus placebo response in borderline personality disorder. *American Journal of Psychiatry, 162*(3), 621–624.

Hurlemann, R., Hawellek, B., Maier, W., Dolan, R. J. (2007). Enhanced emotion-induced amnesia in borderline personality disorder. *Psychological Medicine, 16*; 1–11

Johnson, J. G., Cohen, P., Chen, H., Kasen, S., & Brook, J. S. (2006). Parenting behaviors associated with risk for offspring personality disorder during adulthood. *Archives of General Psychiatry, 63*(5), 579–587.

Jørgensen, C.R. (2006). Disturbed sense of identity in borderline personality. *Journal of Personality Disorders, 20*(6), 618–644.

Joyce, P. R., McHugh, P. C., McKenzie, J. M., Sullivan, P. F., Mulder, R. T., Luty, S. E., et al. (2006). A dopamine transporter polymorphism is a risk factor for borderline personality disorder in depressed patients. *Psychological Medicine, 36(6)*, 807–813.

Kessler, R. C., Coccaro, E. F., Fava, M., Jaeger, S., Jin, R., Walters, E. (2006). The prevalence and correlates of DSM-IV intermittent explosive disorder in the National Comorbidity Survey Replication. *Archives of General Psychiatry, 63*(6), 669–678.

Kiehl, K. A., Smith, A. M., Hare, R. D., Mendrek, A., Forster, B. B., Brink, J., & Liddle, P. F. (2001). Limbic abnormalities in affective processing by criminal psychopaths as revealed by functional magnetic resonance imaging. *Biological Psychiatry, 50*(9), 677–684.

Kolko, D. J., Herschell, A. D., & Scharf, D. M. (2006). Education and treatment of boys who set fires: Specificity, moderators and predictors of recidivism. *Journal of Emotional and Behavioral Disorders, 14*(4), 227–239.

Kress, V. E. W., Kelly, B. L., & McCormick, L. J. (2004). Trichotillomania: Assessment, diagnosis, and treatment. *Journal of Counseling & Development, 1*(82), 185–190.

Linehan, M. (1993). *Cognitive-behavioral treatment of borderline personality disorder.* New York: Guilford Press.

Levy, K. N., Meehan, K. B., Weber, M., Reynoso, J., & Clarkin, J. F. (2005). Attachment and borderline personality disorder: implications for psychotherapy. *Psychopathology, 38*(2), 64–74.

Linehan, M. M., Comtois, K. A, Murray, A. M., Brown, M. Z., Gallop, R. J., Heard, H. L., et al. (2006). Two-year randomized controlled trial and follow-up of dialectical behavior therapy vs therapy by experts for suicidal behaviors and borderline personality disorder. *Archives of General Psychiatry, 63*(7), 57–66.

Loas, F., Guilbaud, O., Perez-Diaz, F., Verrier, A., Stephan, P., Lang, F., et al. (2005). Dependency and suicidality in addictive disorders. *Psychiatry Research, 137*(12), 103–111.

Lobbestael, J., Arntz, A., & Sieswerda, S. (2005). Schema modes and childhood abuse in borderline and antisocial personality disorders. *Journal of Behavior Therapy and Experimental Psychiatry 36*(3), 240–253.

Lyons, M. (1995). Epidemiology of personality disorders. In M. Tsuang, M. Tohen, & G. Zahner (Eds.), *Textbook in psychiatric epidemiology.* New York: Wiley-Liss.

Dochterman, J. M., & Bulechek, G. (2004). *Iowa Intervention Report. Nursing interventions classification* (NIC) (4th ed.). St. Louis: Mosby–Year Book.

Messina, N. P., Wish, E. D., & Nemes, S. (1999). Therapeutic community treatment for substance abusers with antisocial personality disorder. *Journal of Substance Abuse Treatment, 17*(1–2), 121–128.

Millon, T., Grossman, S., Millon, C., Meagher, S., & Ramnath, R. (2004). Personality disorders in modern life(2nd ed.). John Wiley & Sons, Inc.: Hoboken, NJ.

Morana, H. C., & Camara, F. P. (2006). International guidelines for the management of borderline personality disorder. *Current Opinion in Psychiatry, 19*(5), 539–543.

Murphy, J. (1976). Psychiatric labeling in cross-cultural perspective: Similar kinds of disturbed behavior appear to be labeled abnormal in diverse cultures. *Science, 191*(4231), 1019–1028.

Nickel, M. K., Nickel, C., Kaplan, P., Lahmann, C., Muhlbacher, M., Tritt, K., et al. (2005). Treatment of aggression with topiramate in male borderline patients: a double-blind, placebo-controlled study. *Biological Psychiatry, 57*(5), 495–499.

Oakley-Browne, M. A., Adams, P., & Mobberly, P. M. (2000). Interventions for pathological gambling. *Cochrane Database of Systematic Reviews*, (2), CD001521.

Pally, R. (2002), The neurobiology of borderline personality disorder: the synergy of "nature and nurture." *Journal of Psychiatric Practice, 8*(3), 133–142.

Ralevski, E., Sanislow, C. A., Grilo, C. M., Skodol, A. E., Gunderson, J.G., Shea, M.T., et al. (2005). Avoidant personality disorder and social phobia: distinct enough to be separate disorders? *Acta Psychiatrica Scandinavica, 112*(3), 208–214.

Reti, I. M., Samuels, J. F., Eaton, W. W., Bienvenu, O. J. III, Costa, P. T. Jr., & Nestadt, G. (2002). Adult antisocial personality traits are associated with experiences of low parental care and maternal overprotection. *Acta Psychiatrica Scandinavia, 106*(2), 126–133.

Rhee, S. H., Hewitt, J. K., Young, S. E., Corley, R. P., Crowley, T. J., Neale, M. C., & Stallings, M. C. (2006). *Drug & Alcohol Dependence, 84*(1), 85–92.

Schatzberg, A. F. (2000). New indications of antidepressants. *Journal of Clinical Psychiatry, 61*(Suppl 11), 9–17.

Schmitz, J. M. (2005). The interface between impulse-control disorders and addictions: Are pleasure pathway responses shared neurobiological substrates? *Sexual Addiction & Compulsivity, 12*, 149–168.

Schubiner, H., Tzelepis, A., Milberger, S., Lockhart, N., Kruger, M., Kelley, B. J., & Schoener, E. P. (2000). Prevalence of attention-deficit/hyperactivity disorder and conduct disorder among substance abusers. *Journal of Clinical Psychiatry, 61*(4), 244–251.

Shea, M., Stout, R. L., Yen, S., Pagano, M. E., Skodol, A.E., Morey, L.C., et al. (2004). Associations in the course of personality disorders and Axis I disorders over time. *Journal of Abnormal Psychology, 113*(4), 499–508.

Siever, L. J., & Davis, K. L. (2004). The pathophysiology of schizophrenia disorders: Perspectives from the spectrum. *American Journal of Psychiatry, 161*(3), 398–413.

Smallbone, S. W., & Dadds, M. R. (2000). Attachment and coercive sexual behavior. *Sex Abuse, 12*(1), 3–15.

Soderstrom, H., Blennow, K., Sjodin, A. K., & Forsman, A. (2003). New evidence for an association between the CSF HVA: 5-HIAA ratio and psychopathic traits. *Journal of Neurology, Neurosurgery & Psychiatry, 74*(7), 918–921.

Stahl, S. (2000). *Essential psychopharmacology* (2nd ed.). Cambridge: Cambridge University Press.

Stern, A. (1938). A psychoanalytic investigation and therapy in the borderline group of neuroses. *Psychoanalytic Quarterly*, 7, 467–489.

Taylor, C. T., Laposa, J. M., & Alden, L. E. (2004). Is avoidant personality disorder more than just social avoidance? *Journal of Personality Disorders, 18*(6), 571–594.

Torgersen, S., Kringlen, E., & Cramer, V. (2001). The prevalence of personality disorders in a community sample. *Archives of General Psychiatry, 58*(6), 590–596.

van den Bosch, L. M., Verheul, R., Schippers, G. M., & van den Brink, W. (2002). Dialectical behavior therapy of borderline patients with and without substance use problems. Implementation and long-term effects. *Addictive Behaviors, 27*(6), 911–923.

Veit, R., Flor, H., Erb, M., Hermann, C., Lotze, M., Grodd, W., & Birbaumer, N. (2002). Brain circuits in emotional learning in antisocial behavior and social phobia in humans. *Neuroscience Letters, 328*(3), 233–236.

Virkkunen, M., Rawlings, R., Tokola, R., Poland, R. E., Guidotti, A., Nemeroff, C., et al. (1994). CSF biochemistries, glucose metabolism, and diurnal activity rhythms in alcoholic, violent offenders, fire setters, and healthy volunteers. *Archives of General Psychiatry*, 51(1), 20–27.

Waldeck, T. L., & Miller, L. S. (2000). Social skills deficits in schizotypal personality disorder. *Psychiatry Research, 93*(3), 237–246.

Wetterneck, C. T., Woods, D. W., Norberg, M. M., & Begotka, A. M. (2006). The social and economic impact of trichotillomania *Behavioral Interventions* 21, 97–109.

Wilkinson-Ryan, T., & Westen, D. (2000). Identity disturbance in borderline personality disorder: An empirical investigation. *American Journal of Psychiatry, 157*(4), 528–541.

Woods, D. W., Flessner, C., Franklin, M. E., Wetterneck, M.S., Walther, M. R., Anderson, E. R., & Cardona, D. (2006). Understanding and treating trichotillomania: What we know and what we don't know. *Psychiatric Clinics of North America, 29*, 487–501.

Zanarini, M. C., Ruser, T., Frankenburg, F. R., & Hennen, J. (2000). The dissociative experiences of borderline patients. *Comprehensive Psychiatry, 41*(3), 223–227.

Zweig-Frank, H., Paris, J., & Guzder, J. (1994). Psychological risk factors for dissociation and self-mutilation in female patients with borderline personality disorder. *Canadian Journal of Psychiatry, 39*(5), 259–264.

Zimmerman, M., Rothschild, L., & Chelminski, I. (2005). The prevalence of DSM-IV personality disorders in psychiatric outpatients. *American Journal of Psychiatry, 162*(10), 1911–1918.

CHAPTER 23

Somatoform and Related Disorders

Mary Ann Boyd and Victoria Soltis-Jarrett

LEARNING OBJECTIVES

After studying this chapter, you will be able to:

- Explain the concept of somatization and its occurrence in people with mental health problems.
- Discuss the epidemiologic factors related to somatic problems.
- Compare the etiologic theories of somatization disorder from a biopsychosocial perspective.
- Contrast the major differences between somatoform and factitious disorders.
- Discuss human responses to somatization disorder.
- Apply the elements of nursing management to a patient with somatization disorder.

KEY CONCEPT

- somatization

KEY TERMS

• alexithymia • factitious disorders • malingering • pseudologia fantastica • psychosomatic • somatization disorder • somatoform disorders

The connection between the "mind" and "body" has been hypothesized and described for centuries. The term **psychosomatic** originates from psychosomatic medicine and has been traditionally used to describe, explain, and predict the psychological origins of illness and disease. Unfortunately, this notion promotes the assumption that certain diseases are purely "psychological" in nature, thus carrying the meaning that the individual's symptoms are not real or valid. For example, it was once believed that asthma suffers were behaviorally "acting out" their anger, fear, or emotional pain and were seeking attention rather than suffering from an alteration in their respiratory status. This narrow and biased assumption has been challenged in nursing because it has limited the opportunity for the nurse to complete a holistic nursing assessment and plan of care for a patient who is suffering from physical symptoms that are deemed "medically unfounded" (Soltis-Jarrett, 2005). Physical symptoms that are medically unfounded are defined as signs and symptoms for which there is insufficient medical and pathophysiological evidence to explain the individual's level of suffering and complaint. While the individual's signs and symptoms may be unfounded in medicine, nurses have been challenged to find ways of assessing and managing these individuals using an approach to care that is grounded in nursing. Somatization is a concept used in nursing because it focuses on the individual's experience and expression of unexplained physical symptoms This notion acknowledges and respects the individual's expression of their health and illness rather than to label their signs and symptoms as "all in their head" or imaginary (Soltis-Jarrett, 2005). Individuals who present with somatization communicate their symptoms and suffering through bodily sensations, functional changes, and somatic metaphors. This chapter explores the concept of somatization and explains the care of patients whose psychiatric disorder has as its primary characteristic the experience, expression, and manifestation of unexplained physical symptoms.

KEY CONCEPT Somatization is the term used to describe the experience and expression of unexplained physical symptoms through bodily sensations, functional changes, and/or somatic descriptions

Although somatization is common in many psychiatric disorders, including depression, anxiety, and psychosis, it is the primary symptom of somatoform and factitious disorders. Somatoform disorders are a group of psychiatric disorders characterized by bodily signs and symptoms. Therefore, a **somatoform disorder** is one in which the patient experiences and expresses suffering through their reported physical signs and symptoms. A **factitious disorder** is one in which the patient deliberately produces signs of medical or mental disorder and misrepresents their histories or bodily symptoms (American Psychiatric Association [APA], 2000). The major difference between the two diagnostic categories is that in the somatoform disorders, the physical symptoms are not intentionally produced by the patient. The somatoform disorders are clustered into six different clinical syndromes:

1. Somatization disorder
2. Undifferentiated somatoform disorder
3. Conversion disorder
4. Pain disorder
5. Hypochondriasis
6. Body dysmorphic disorder

The factitious disorders include factitious disorder and factitious disorder not specified. This chapter presents the nursing care of persons experiencing a somatoform disorder and factitious disorder. Somatization disorder is explained in detail to illustrate one example of somatoform disorders.

SOMATIZATION

Anyone who feels the pain of a sore throat or the ache of influenza has a somatic symptom (from *soma*, meaning body), but it is not considered to be somatization unless the physical symptoms are unfounded and include bodily sensations, functional changes, or somatic descriptions. There may or may not be an identifiable physiologic cause for the medical problems, and this "lack of cause" engenders great distress for patients as they often repeatedly seek health care professionals for help, diagnosis, and treatment of their physical symptoms. Some practitioners believe that individuals who experience somatization have physical sensations that are amplified, while others have suggested that people who somatize view their personal problems in physical terms, rather than in psychosocial terms. For example, a woman quits her job complaining of chronic fatigue, rather than recognizing that she is emotionally stressed from the constant harassment of a coworker. These practitioners believe that individuals with somatization internalize their stress or cope with life problems and stressors by expressing anxiety, stress, and frustration through their own physical symptoms. Although there are several definitions of somatization, there is no known etiology or cause of this disorder in medicine. Therefore, there is an assumption that there is no cure or treatment for those who suffer from somatoform disorders. However, this is not the case in nursing, as nurses need to recognize that somatization is the patient's expression and experience of their health and illness and not an imaginary or "made up" set of physical symptoms. Therefore nursing needs to be focused on *care* rather than *cure*.

Cultural Differences in Somatization

Because norms, values, and expectations about health and illness are culturally based, physical sensations are experienced and expressed according to culturally defined expectations. In cultures in which the expression of physical discomfort is more acceptable than psychological distress, the disruption of routine body cycles, such as digestive or menstrual cycles, sleep, physical balance, and orientation, are commonly the focus of patient concern, instead of problems in interpersonal relationships, economic crises, death of a spouse, adjustment to marriage, and inability to become pregnant.

Gender and Somatization

Somatic experience appears to be different in men than in women. One group of researchers showed that women were more likely to be diversified somatizers, who have frequent, brief sickness with a variety of complaints. Men were more likely to be asthenic somatizers, with fewer diverse complaints but more chronically disabled by fatigue, weakness, or common minor illnesses (Cloninger, Martin, Guze, & Clayton, 1986; Cloninger, von Knorring, Sigvardsson, & Bohman, 1986).

SOMATIZATION DISORDER

Somatization disorder is defined as multiple physical symptoms that are inadequately explained on the basis of physical and laboratory examinations. The disorder can change with time and can vary from person to person (APA, 2000).

Somatization disorder is further defined as "a polysymptomatic disorder that begins before age 30 years, extends over a period of several years, and is characterized by a combination of pain, gastrointestinal, sexual, and psychoneurological symptoms" (APA, 2000).

Clinical Course

In somatization disorder, patients have recurring, multiple, and clinically significant somatic problems that involve several body systems. Other somatoform disorders are characterized by only one set of complaints, such as conversion disorder (see later discussion) or pain disorder. Physical problems in somatization disorder cut across all body systems, such as gastrointestinal (nausea, vomiting, diarrhea), neurologic (headache, backache), or musculoskeletal (aching legs). The physical illness may last 6 to 9 months. These individuals perceive themselves as being "sicker than the sick" and report all aspects of their health as poor. They are often disabled and cannot work. These individuals typically visit a health care provider at least once annually. They quickly become frustrated with their primary health care providers, who do not seem to appreciate the seriousness of their symptoms and who are unable to verify a particular problem that accounts for their extreme discomfort. Consequently, they "provider-shop," moving from one to another until they find one who will give them new medication, hospitalize them, or perform surgery. Characteristically, these individuals undergo multiple surgeries. People with somatization disorder evoke negative subjective responses in health care providers, who usually wish that the patient would go to someone else.

• NCLEXNOTE

NCLEXNOTE Patients with somatoform disorders will seek health care from multiple providers but will avoid mental health specialists.

Because a psychiatric diagnosis of somatization disorder is made only after numerous unexplained physical problems, psychiatric–mental health nurses do not usually care for these individuals early in the disorder. Instead, nurses in primary care and medical–surgical settings are more likely to encounter these patients.

Diagnostic Criteria

The diagnosis is made when there is a pattern of multiple, recurring, "significant" somatic complaints. Table 23.1 lists the key diagnostic criteria and target symptoms. A significant complaint is one that received medical treatment or for which the symptoms cause impairment in social, occupational, or other areas of functioning (APA, 2000).

Table 23.1  **Key Diagnostic Characteristics of Somatization Disorder 300.81** 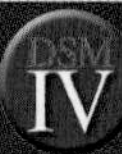

Diagnostic Criteria and Target Symptoms	Associated Findings
• History of many physical complaints beginning before age 30 and occurring over a period of several years • Complaints requiring treatment or causing significant impairment in social, occupational, or other important area of functioning History of pain related to at least four different sites or functions, such as head, abdomen, back, joints, extremities, chest, rectum, during menstruation, during sexual intercourse, or during urination History of at least two gastrointestinal symptoms, such as nausea, bloating, vomiting (other than during pregnancy), diarrhea, or intolerance of several different foods History of at least one sexual or reproductive symptom, such as sexual indifference, erectile or ejaculatory dysfunction, irregular menses, excessive menstrual bleeding, vomiting throughout pregnancy History of one pseudoneurologic symptom or deficit suggesting a neurologic condition not limited to pain, such as conversion symptoms (impaired coordination or balance, paralysis or localized weakness, difficulty swallowing or lump in throat, aphonia, urinary retention, hallucinations, loss of touch or pain sensation, double vision, blindness, deafness, seizures; dissociative symptoms, for example, amnesia, or loss of consciousness other than fainting) • Symptoms cannot be explained by a known general medical condition or direct effects of a substance Symptoms unexplainable or excessive When a general medical condition exists, the physical complaints or resulting impairments are in excess of what would be expected from the history, physical examination, or laboratory findings • Symptoms are not intentionally produced or feigned	***Associated Behavioral Findings*** • Colorful, exaggerated complaints lacking specific factual information • Inconsistent historians • Treatment sought from several physicians with numerous medical examinations, diagnostic procedures, surgeries, and hospitalizations • Anxiety and depressed mood • Impulsive with antisocial behavior, suicide threats and attempts, and marital discord ***Associated Physical Findings*** • Absence of objective findings to fully explain subjective complaints • Possible diagnosis of functional disorders, such as irritable bowel syndrome

Somatization Disorder in Special Populations

Evidence suggests that this disorder occurs in all populations and cultures. The type and frequency of somatic symptoms may differ across cultures.

Children

Although many children experience unexplained medical symptoms, somatization disorder is not usually diagnosed until adolescence. However, children who are diagnosed with somatization disorder have been found to be experiencing anxiety and trauma that are related to their presentation of physical symptoms (Diseth 2005; Muris & Meesters, 2004). Adolescents diagnosed with somatization disorder may initially present with menstrual difficulties, pelvic, and/or abdominal pain. More research is needed to identify risk factors and treatment outcomes (Lieb, Pfister, Mastaler, & Wittchen, 2000).

Elderly People

Somatization disorder is a lifelong trait and can persist into old age, affecting the elderly; however, there is little research specific to this population. Subjective non–well-being (the reporting of never feeling good), rather than objective health measures, may be an indicator of somatization (Schneider et al., 2003) and useful to consider when assessing medically unexplained physical symptoms in the elderly. One of the challenges in nursing is to differentiate the somatic symptoms of this disorder from other medical problems that should be diagnosed and treated. In the elderly, somatic symptoms can represent many things, such as depression, anxiety, chronic insomnia, or bereavement (Drayer, et al., 2005; Sheehan & Banerjee, 1999). Recognizing the complexity of physical manifestations and assessing the patterns of symptoms are important.

Epidemiology

The estimated prevalence of somatization disorder ranges from 0.2% to 2% of the general population (APA, 2000; Grabe et al., 2003). Because these individuals perceive themselves as medically sick and may never see a mental health provider, these estimates may underrepresent the true prevalence. Some estimates are as high as 11% of the population. Thus, in many people, somatization disorder is unrecognized, undiagnosed, and mismanaged in primary care settings (Yates, 2002).

Age of Onset

Somatization disorder, by definition, occurs before the age of 30 years, usually with the first symptom presentation during adolescence. The individual may not receive a diagnosis before the age of 30 years, but one unexplained somatic symptom must be present before this age. This disorder typically has its onset in childhood or adolescence and is remarkably stable, lasting many years into adulthood and into late life (Lieb et al., 2002; Mullick, 2002).

Getting older does not increase the likelihood of receiving a diagnosis of somatization disorder; epidemiologic data indicate that the prevalence of somatization among people younger than 45 years is similar to the rate among those older than 45 years. However, patients who begin to have symptoms after 30 years are not likely to have enough symptoms to meet the criteria in the *Diagnostic and Statistical Manual of Mental Disorders*, 4th ed., text revision (*DSM-IV-TR;* APA, 2000) for somatization disorder and are more likely to have a diagnosable medical problem (Gureje, Simon, Usutn, & Goldberg, 1997).

Gender, Ethnic, and Cultural Differences

Epidemiologic studies have reported that somatization disorder occurs primarily in women, particularly those in lower socioeconomic status and high emotional distress (Ladwig, Marten-Mittag, Erazo, & Gundel, 2001). The prevalence in men in the United States is less than 0.2%. Reports of greater prevalence among men from other countries, such as Greece and Puerto Rico, suggest that cultural factors contribute to the appearance of the disorder. However, the debate regarding the differences in gender expression and increased reporting of somatic symptoms by women in the medical literature has implied that the question at hand may need further exploration into the origins and expression of somatization.

Comorbidity

Somatization disorder frequently coexists with other psychiatric disorders, most commonly depression and anxiety. Others include panic disorder, mania, social phobia, obsessive-compulsive disorder (OCD), psychotic disorders, and personality disorders (Garyfallos et al., 1999). Nurses rarely see patients who have only somatization disorder.

Ultimately, numerous unexplained medical problems also coexist with this disorder because many patients have received medical and surgical treatments, often unnecessary, and are plagued with side effects. A disproportionately high number of women who eventually receive diagnoses of somatization disorder have been treated for irritable bowel syndrome, polycystic ovary disease, and chronic pain. It is estimated that as many as 94% of people with irritable bowel syndrome have psychiatric disorders, especially major depression, anxiety, and somatization disorder (Whitehead, Palsson, & Jones, 2002). Many also have had non–cancer-related hysterectomies. Even after the patient is treated by mental health providers and develops some understanding of the disorder, the physical problems do not disappear.

Etiology

The cause of somatization disorder is unknown. The following are theories regarding the development of the disorder.

Biologic Theories

Neuropathologic Theory

The neuropathology of somatization disorder is unknown. Evidence suggests that there is a decreased activity in certain brain areas, such as the caudate nuclei, left putamen, and right precentral gyrus in somatization disorder (Garcia-Campayo, Sanz-Carrillo, Baringo, & Ceballos, 2001; Hakala et al., 2002). These findings indicate that a hypometabolism may be associated with somatization disorder.

Genetic

Although somatization disorder has been shown to run in families, the exact transmission mechanism is unclear. Strong evidence suggests an increased risk for somatization disorder in first-degree relatives, indicating a familial or genetic effect (APA, 2000). Because many women with somatization disorder live in chaotic families, environmental influence could explain the high prevalence in first-degree relatives. Males in these families show high risk for antisocial personality disorder and substance abuse.

Biochemical Changes

Research is as yet insufficient to identify specific biochemical changes. However, because these patients experience other psychiatric problems, such as depression or panic, clearly many neurobiological changes occur. Women with this disorder often have numerous menstrual problems and often undergo hysterectomies. Because of these symptoms, studies are needed to determine the involvement of the hypothalamic–pituitary–gonadal axis, which regulates estrogen and testosterone secretion.

Psychological Theories

Somatization has been explained as a form of social or emotional communication, meaning the bodily symptoms express an emotion that cannot be verbalized. The adolescent who experiences severe abdominal pain after her parents' argument or the wife who receives nurturing from her husband only when she has back pain are two examples. From this perspective, somatization may be a way of maintaining relationships. Following this line of reasoning, as an individual's physical problems become a way of controlling relationships, so somatization becomes a learned behavior pattern. With time, physical symptoms develop automatically in response to perceived threats. Finally, somatization disorder develops when somatizing becomes a way of life.

Social Theories

Somatization disorders occur everywhere, but the symptoms may vary from culture to culture. In addition, the conceptualization of somatization disorder is primarily Western, although studies in Japan have identified and discussed the notion of somatization as a moral issue rather than a medical problem. Somatization is a more socially acceptable way to express behavior in lieu of being diagnosed as depressed because in Japan, mental illness is perceived as a character flaw (Young, 2003). In many non-Western societies, where the mind–body distinction is not made and symptoms have different meanings and explanations, these physical manifestations are not labeled as a psychiatric disorder (Box 23.1). In Latin American countries, depression is more likely described in somatic symptoms, such as headaches, gastrointestinal disturbances, or complaints of "nerves," rather than sadness or guilt (Jorge, 2003).

BOX 23.1

Somatization in Chinese Culture

In Chinese tradition, the health of the individual reflects a balance between positive and negative forces within the body. Five elements at work in nature and in the body control conditions (fire, water, wood, earth, metal); five viscera (liver, heart, spleen, kidneys, lungs); five emotions (anger, joy, worry, sorrow, fear); and five climatic conditions (wind, heat, humidity, dryness, cold). All illness is explained by imbalances among these elements. Because emotion is related to the circulation of vital air within the body, anger is believed to result from an adverse current of vital air to the liver. Emotional outbursts are seen as results of imbalances among the natural elements, rather than the results of behavior of the person.

The stigma of mental illness in the Chinese culture is so great that it can have an adverse effect on a family for many generations. If problems can be attributed to natural causes, the individual and family are less responsible, and stigma is minimized. The Chinese have a culturally acceptable term for symptoms of mental distress—the closest translation of which would be *neurasthenia*—which comprises somatic complaints of headaches, insomnia, dizziness, aches and pains, poor memory, anxiety, weakness, and loss of energy.

Risk Factors

This disorder tends to run in families, and children of mothers with multiple unexplained somatic complaints are more likely to have somatic problems. Adults are at higher risk for unexplained medical symptoms if they experienced unexplained symptoms as children or if their parents were in poor health when the patient was about 15 years old (Hotopf, Mayou, Wadsworth, & Wessely, 1999). Recent data have confirmed a strong association between sexual trauma exposure and somatic symptoms, illness attitudes, and healthcare utilization in women (Stein et al., 2004) as well as a theoretical relationship between childhood sexual abuse and somatization (Hulme, 2004). Individuals with depression and anxiety are also especially likely to experience somatization (Gureje & Simon, 1999).

Interdisciplinary Treatment

The care of patients with somatization disorders involves three approaches:

- Providing long-term general management of the chronic condition;
- Conservatively treating symptoms of comorbid psychiatric and physical problems;
- Providing care in special settings, including group treatment (Huibers, Beurskens, Bleijenberg, & van Schayck, 2003).

The cornerstone of management is trust and to be believed. Women in one research study reported that it was important for the health care provider to believe their symptoms rather than to doubt or disregard their symptoms (Soltis-Jarrett, 2005). Ideally, the patient should see only one health care provider at regularly scheduled visits. During each primary care visit, the provider should conduct a partial physical examination of the organ system in which the patient has complaints. Physical symptoms are treated conservatively using the least intrusive approach. In the mental health setting, the use of cognitive-behavior therapy (CBT) is promising. In a review of 31 clinical trials, patients treated with CBT improved more than did control subjects in 71% of the studies. Benefits were observed whether or not psychological distress was ameliorated (Kroenke & Swindle, 2000).

NURSING MANAGEMENT: HUMAN RESPONSE TO SOMATIZATION DISORDER

Somatization is the primary response to this disorder. The defining characteristics, depicted in the biopsychosocial model (Fig. 23.1), are so well integrated that

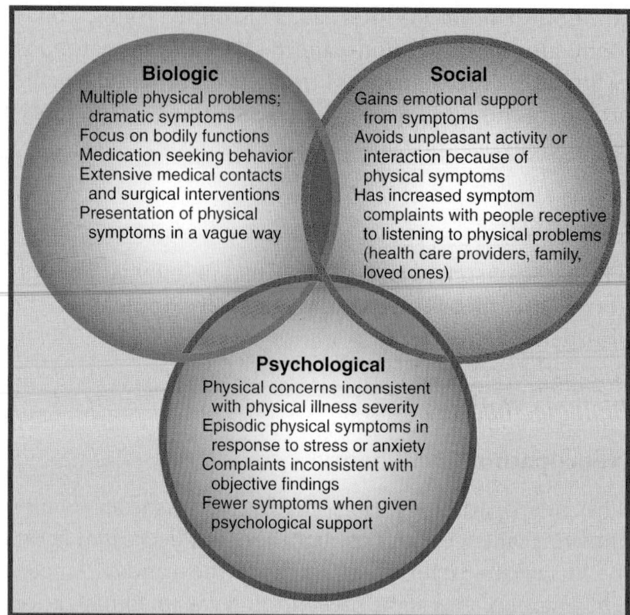

FIGURE 23.1. Biopsychosocial characteristics of patients with somatization disorder.

separating the psychological and social dimensions is difficult. The most common characteristics follow:

- Reporting the same symptoms repeatedly;
- Receiving support from the environment that otherwise might not be forthcoming (such as gaining a spouse's attention because of severe back pain);
- Expressing concern about the physical problems inconsistent with the severity of the illness (being "sicker than the sick").

Biologic Domain

During the assessment interview, allow enough time for the patient to explain all medical problems; a hurried assessment interview blocks communication.

Assessment

Past medical treatment has been ineffective because it did not address the underlying psychiatric disorder. However, psychiatric–mental health nurses typically see these patients for problems related to the coexisting psychiatric disorder, such as depression, not because of the somatization disorder. While taking the patient's history, the nurse will discover that the individual has had multiple surgeries or medical problems and realize that somatization disorder is a strong possibility. If the patient has not already received a diagnosis of somatization disorder, the nurse should screen for it by determining the presence of the most commonly reported problems associated with this disorder, which include

BOX 23.2

Health Attitude Survey

On a scale of 1 to 5, please indicate the extent to which you agree (5) or disagree (1).

Dissatisfaction With Care

1. I have been satisfied with the medical care I have received. (R)
2. Doctors have done the best they could to diagnose and treat my health problems. (R)
3. Doctors have taken my health problems seriously.
4. My health problems have been thoroughly evaluated. (R)
5. Doctors do not seem to know much about the health problems I have had.
6. My health problems have been completely explained. (R)
7. Doctors seem to think I am exaggerating my health problems.
8. My response to treatment has not been satisfactory.
9. My response to treatment is usually excellent. (R)

Frustration With Ill Health

10. I am tired of feeling sick and would like to get to the bottom of my health problems.
11. I have felt ill for quite a while now.
12. I am going to keep searching for an answer to my health problems.
13. I do not think there is anything seriously wrong with my body. (R)

High Utilization of Care

14. I have seen many different doctors over the years.
15. I have taken a lot of medicine recently.
16. I do not go to the doctor often. (R)
17. I have had relatively good health over the years.

Excessive Health Worry

18. I sometimes worry too much about my health.
19. I often fear the worst when I develop symptoms.
20. I have trouble getting my mind off my health.

Psychological Distress

21. Sometimes I feel depressed and cannot seem to shake it off.
22. I have sought help for emotional or stress-related problems.
23. It is easy to relax and stay calm. (R)
24. I believe the stress I am under may be affecting my health.

Discordant Communication of Distress

25. Some people think that I am capable of more work than I feel able to do.
26. Some people think that I have been sick just to gain attention.
27. It is difficult for me to find the right words for my feelings.

(R) indicates items reversed for scoring purposes. Scoring—The higher the score, the more likely somatization is a problem. Noyes, R. Jr., Langbehn, D., Happel, R., Sieren, L., & Muller, B. (1999). Health Attitude Survey: A scale for assessing somatizing patients. *Psychosomatics, 40*(6), 470–478.

dysmenorrhea, lump in throat, vomiting, shortness of breath, burning in sex organs, painful extremities, and amnesia. If the patient has these symptoms, he or she should be seen by a mental health provider qualified to make the diagnosis. Box 23.2 presents the Health Attitude Survey, which can be used as a screening test for somatization.

Review of Systems

Although these patients' symptoms have usually received considerable attention from the medical community, a careful review of systems is important because the appearance of physical problems is usually related to psychosocial problems. Even as the nurse continues to see the patient for mental health problems, an ongoing awareness of biologic symptoms is important, particularly because these symptoms are de-emphasized in the overall management.

Pain is the most common problem in people with this disorder. Because the pain is usually related to symptoms of all the major body systems, it is unlikely that a somatic intervention such as an analgesic will be effective on a long-term basis. The nurse must remember that although there is no medical explanation for the pain, the patient's pain is real and has serious psychosocial implications. A careful assessment should include the following questions:

- What is the pain like?
- What is the extent of the pain?
- What helps the pain get better?
- When is the pain at its worst?
- What has worked in the past to relieve the pain?

Physical Functioning

The actual physical functioning of these individuals is often marginal. They usually have problems with sleep, fatigue, activity, and sexual functioning. Assessment of these areas will generate data to be used in establishing a nursing diagnosis. The amount and quality of sleep are important, as are the times when the individual sleeps. For example, an individual may sleep a total of 6 hours each diurnal cycle, but only from 2:00 to 6:00 AM, plus an afternoon nap.

Fatigue is a constant problem, and a variety of physical problems interfere with normal activity. These patients report overwhelming lack of energy, which makes maintaining usual routines or accomplishing

BOX 23.3

Clinical Vignette: Somatization Disorder and Stress

Ms. J, age 42 years, has been coming to the mental health clinic for 2 years for her nerves. She has seen only the physician for medication, but now has been referred to the nurse's new stress management group because she is experiencing side effects to all the medications that have been tried. The psychiatrist has diagnosed somatization disorder and wants her to learn to manage her "nerves" without medication.

At the first meeting with the nurse, Ms. J was preoccupied with chest pain and bloating that had lasted for the last 6 months. Her chest pain is constant and sharp at times. The pain does not prevent her from going to her job as a waitress but does interfere with meal preparation at night for her family and her ability to have sexual intercourse. She has numerous other physical problems, including allergies to certain perfumes, dysmenorrhea, ovarian polycystic disease (ovarian cysts), chronic urinary tract infections, and rashes. She is constantly fatigued and has frequent leg cramps. She states that she is too tired to fix dinner for her family. On days off from work, she takes a nap in the afternoon, sleeping until evening. She is unable to fall asleep at night.

She believes that she will soon have to have her gallbladder removed because of occasional referred pain to her back and nausea that occurs a couple hours after eating. She is not enthusiastic about a stress management group and does not believe that it will help her problems. However, she has agreed to consider it as long as the psychiatrist will continue prescribing diazepam (Valium).

What Do You Think?

How would you prioritize Ms. J's physical symptoms?
What are some possible explanations for Ms. J's fatigue?

daily tasks impossible. Fatigue is accompanied by the inability to concentrate on simple functions, leading to decreased performance and disinterest in surroundings. Patients tend to be lethargic and listless and often have little energy (Box 23.3).

Female patients with this disorder usually have had multiple gynecologic problems. The reason is not known, but symptoms of dysmenorrhea, painful intercourse, and pain in the "sex organs" suggests involvement of the hypothalamic–pituitary–gonadal axis. Physiologic indicators, such as those produced by laboratory tests, are not available. However, a careful assessment of the patient's menstrual history, gynecologic problems, and sexual functioning is important. It is also important to assess if there is a past or current history of abuse, whether it is sexual, physical, and/or emotional. The physical manifestations of somatization disorder often lead to altered sexual behavior.

Pharmacologic Assessment

A psychopharmacologic assessment of these patients is challenging. Patients with somatization disorder frequently provider-shop, perhaps seeing seven or eight different providers within a year. Because they often receive medications from each provider, they are usually taking a large number of drugs. They tend to protect their sources and may not be truthful in identifying the actual number of medications they are ingesting. A pharmacologic assessment is needed not only because of the number of medications but also because these individuals frequently have unusual side effects or they report that they are "sensitive" to medications. Because of their somatic sensitivity, they often overreact to medication.

These patients spend much of their life trying to find out what is wrong with them. When one provider after another can find little if any explanation for their symptoms, many become anxious. To alleviate their anxiety, they either self-medicate with over-the-counter medications and substances of abuse (e.g., alcohol, marijuana) or find a provider who prescribes an anxiolytic. Because the anxiety of their disorder cannot be treated within a few weeks with an anxiolytic, they become dependent on medication that should not have been prescribed in the first place.

Although anxiolytics have a place in therapeutics, they are not recommended for long-term use and only complicate the treatment of somatoform disorders. These medications should also be avoided because of their addictive qualities. Unfortunately, by the time these individuals see a mental health provider they have already begun taking an anxiolytic for anxiety, usually a benzodiazepine. Many times, they only agree to see a mental health provider because the last provider would no longer prescribe an anxiolytic without a psychiatric evaluation.

Nursing Diagnoses for the Biologic Domain

Because somatization disorder is a chronic illness, patients could have almost any one of the nursing diagnoses at some time in their life. At least one nursing diagnosis likely will be related to the individual's physical state. Fatigue, Pain, and Insomnia are usually supported by the assessment data. The challenge in devising outcomes for these problems is to avoid focusing on the biologic aspects and instead help the patient overcome the fatigue, pain, or sleep problem through biopsychosocial approaches.

Interventions for the Biologic Domain

Nursing interventions that focus on the biologic dimension become especially important because medical treatment must be conservative, and aggressive pharmacologic treatment must be avoided. Each time a nurse sees the patient, time spent on the physical complaints should be respected and believed within a limited time frame. Several biologic interventions, including pain management, activity enhancement, nutrition regulation, relaxation, and pharmacologic interventions, may be useful in caring for patients with somatization disorder.

Pain Management

In pain management, a single approach rarely works. Pain is a primary issue. After a careful assessment of the pain, the nurse should develop nonpharmacologic strategies to reduce it. If gastrointestinal pain is frequent, eating and bowel habits should be explored and modified. For back pain, exercises and consultation from a physical therapist may be useful. Headaches are a challenge. Self-monitoring and tracking them engages the patient in the therapeutic process and helps to identify psychosocial triggers.

Activity Enhancement

Helping the patient establish a daily routine may alleviate some of the difficulty with sleeping, but doing so may be difficult because most of these patients do not work. Encouraging the patient to get up in the morning and go to bed at night at specific times can help the patient to establish a routine. These patients should engage in regular exercise to improve their overall physical state, but they often have numerous reasons why they cannot. This is where the nurse's patience is tested; the nurse ultimately needs to remember that the patient's symptoms are an expression of their suffering.

Nutrition Regulation

Patients with somatization disorder often have gastrointestinal problems and may have special nutritional needs. The nurse discusses with the patient the nutritional value of foods. Because these individuals often take medications that promote weight gain, weight control strategies may be discussed. For overweight individuals, suggest healthy, low-calorie food choices. Teach patients about balancing dietary intake with activity levels to increase their awareness of food choices.

Relaxation

Patients taking anxiety-relieving medication can be taught relaxation techniques to alleviate stress. It will be a challenge to help these patients really use these strategies. The nurse should consider a variety of techniques, including simple relaxation techniques, distraction, and guided imagery (see Chapter 10).

Psychopharmacologic Interventions

No medication is specifically recommended for somatization disorder. Psychiatric symptoms of comorbid disorders, such as depression and anxiety, are treated pharmacologically as appropriate. Usually, the patients who are depressed and/or anxious are taking an antidepressant to treat their symptoms. Depressed mood alone is not an indication for initiation of antidepressant treatment. If depressed mood persists and insomnia, decreased appetite, decreased libido, and anhedonia are also present, aggressive psychopharmacologic management is indicated (Fallon et al., 2003). A wide variety of drugs are available, including the selective serotonin reuptake inhibitors (SSRIs), serotonin/norepinephrine reuptake inhibitors (SNRIs), tricyclic antidepressants (TCAs), and the monoamine oxidase inhibitors (MAOIs) (see Chapter 20). Recently, the use of dual-acting antidepressants (SNRIs) has been shown to be useful in the treatment of the physical symptoms associated with depression. Clinical evidence currently indicates that dual-acting agents such as venlafaxine (Effexor) and duloxetine (Cymbalta) may be beneficial in controlling pain over agents that increase either serotonin (e.g., SSRIs) or norepinephrine (e.g., Wellbutrin) alone. These dual-acting agents are also better tolerated than tricyclic antidepressants and monoamine oxidase inhibitors, therefore minimizing the potential for side effects which can add to the somatic symptoms spectrum (Wise, Arnold, & Maletic, 2005). Seek evidence that the symptoms of anxiety and/or depression have gone into remission for at least 1 year (or more) before discontinuing use of the medication (see Box 23.4).

Phenelzine (Nardil) is one of the MAOIs that has been effective in treating not just depression, but also the chronic pain and headaches common in people with somatization disorder. Food–drug interactions are the most serious side effects of MAOIs. While taking these agents, patients should avoid foods high in tyramine and also certain medications for colds and coughs (see Chapter 8).

Anxiety is treated pharmacologically, similar to depression. The first line of treatment for all anxiety disorders is with a selective serotonin reuptake inhibitor (SSRI). Doses are usually higher than prescribed for depression in order to relieve and manage the symptoms of the anxiety disorders including panic, social phobia, generalized anxiety, OCD, and posttraumatic stress disorder (PTSD). Nonpharmacologic approaches such as biofeedback or relaxation are also

BOX 23.4

Drug Profile: ***phenelzine (Nardil)***

DRUG CLASS: Monoamine oxidase inhibitor

RECEPTOR AFFINITY: Inhibits MAO, an enzyme responsible for breaking down biogenic amines, such as epinephrine, norepinephrine, and serotonin, allowing them to accumulate in neuronal storage sites throughout the central and peripheral nervous systems.

INDICATIONS: Treatment of depression characterized as "atypical, nonendogenous," or "neurotic" or nonresponsive to other antidepressant therapy or in situations in which other antidepressant therapy is contraindicated.

ROUTE AND DOSAGE: Available as 15-mg tablets.

Adults: Initially, 15 mg PO tid, increasing to at least 60 mg/d at a fairly rapid pace consistent with patient tolerance. Therapy at 60 mg/d may be necessary for at least 4 weeks before response occurs. After maximum benefit achieved, dosage reduced gradually over several weeks. Maintenance dose may be 15 mg/d or every other day.

Geriatric: Adjust dosage accordingly because patients over 60 years of age are more prone to develop adverse effects.

Pediatric: Not recommended for children under 16 years of age.

HALF-LIFE (PEAK EFEECTS): Unknown (48–96 h).

SELECTED ADVERSE REACTIONS: Dizziness, vertigo, headache, overactivity, hyperreflexia, tremors, muscle twitching, mania, hypomania, jitteriness, confusion, memory impairment, insomnia, weakness, fatigue, overstimulation, restlessness, increased anxiety, agitation, blurred vision, sweating, constipation, diarrhea, nausea, abdominal pain, edema, dry mouth, anorexia, weight changes, hypertensive crisis, orthostatic hypotension, and disturbed cardiac rate and rhythm.

BOXED WARNING: Suicidality in children and adolescents.

WARNINGS: Contraindicated in patients with pheochromocytoma, congestive heart failure, hepatic dysfunction, severe renal impairment, cardiovascular disease, history of headache, and myelography within previous 24 h or scheduled within next 48 h. Use cautiously in patients with seizure disorders, hyperthyroidism, pregnancy, lactation, and those scheduled for elective surgery. Possible hypertensive crisis, coma, and severe convulsions may occur if administered with tricyclic antidepressants; possible hypertensive crisis when taken with foods containing tyramine. Increased risk for adverse interaction is possible when given with meperidine. Additive hypoglycemic effect can occur when taken with insulin and oral sulfonylureas.

SPECIFIC PATIENT/FAMILY EDUCATION:

- Take drug exactly as prescribed; do not stop taking abruptly or without consulting your health care provider.
  - Families and caregivers of patients should be advised to observe for the emergence of anxiety, agitation, panic attacks, insomnia, irritability, hostility, aggressiveness, impulsivity, akathisia (psychomotor restlessness), hypomania, mania, other unusual changes in behavior, worsening of depression, and suicidal ideation. Such symptoms should be reported to the patient's prescriber or health professional, especially if they are severe, abrupt in onset, or were not part of the patient's presenting symptoms.
- Avoid consuming any foods containing tyramine while taking this drug and for 2 weeks afterward.
- Avoid alcohol, sleep-inducing drugs, over-the-counter drugs such as cold and hay fever remedies and appetite suppressants—all of which may cause serious or life-threatening problems.
- Report any signs and symptoms of adverse reactions.
- Maintain appointments for follow-up blood tests.
- Report any complaints of unusual or severe headache or yellowing of eyes or skin.
- Avoid driving a car or performing any activities that require alertness.
- Change position slowly when going from a lying to sitting or standing position to minimize dizziness or weakness.

quite useful in conjunction with pharmacologic treatment. Benzodiazepines may be used initially in the treatment of anxiety but should be slowly decreased and discontinued because of the psychological and physiological dependence associated with these medications. Buspirone (BuSpar), a nonbenzodiazepine, does not lead to tolerance or withdrawal and may be useful for relief of anxiety. If panic disorder is present, it should be treated aggressively.

Monitoring and Administering Medications

In somatization disorder, patients are usually treated in the community and self-medicated. The nurse should carefully question patients about self-administered medicine and determine which medicines they are currently taking (including over-the-counter and herbal supplements). The nurse should listen carefully to determine effects the patient attributes to the medication. This information should be documented and reported to the rest of the team. The patient should be encouraged to continue taking only prescribed medication and to seek approval before taking any additional over-the-counter or prescribed medications.

Monitoring and Managing Side Effects

These individuals often have atypical reactions to their medications. Side effects should be assessed, but the patient should be encouraged to compare the benefits of the medication with any problems related to side effects. Nurses should also encourage the patients to give the medications enough time to be effective as many medications require up to 6 weeks before the patient has a response and/or the relief of their symptoms.

Monitoring Drug Interactions

In working with patients with somatization disorder, the nurse must always be on the lookout for drug–drug interactions. Medications these patients take for physical problems could interact with psychiatric medications. Patients may be taking alternative medicines, such as herbal supplements, but they usually willingly disclose their experiments (Garcia-Campayo & Sanz-Carrillo, 2000). The patient should be encouraged to use the same pharmacy for filling all prescriptions so that possible reactions can be checked and monitored.

Psychological Domain

The mental status of individuals with somatization disorder can be within normal limits, although most patients report frustration, depression, and hopelessness about their situation. What is most noticeable is their intense focus on their body and the physical symptoms that are causing them distress and disability. Generally, cognition is not impaired. However, these individuals seem preoccupied with the signs and symptoms of their illnesses and may even keep a record of their experiences. Living with illness, diseases, and suffering truly becomes a way of life.

Some individuals with somatization disorder have intense emotional reactions to life stressors and have lead or are leading traumatic or chaotic lives. These patients usually have had a series of personal crises beginning at an early age. Examples include severe sexual and physical abuse and psychological trauma. Typically, a new symptom or medical problem develops during times of emotional stress as well as during anniversaries of losses or traumas that occurred in the patient's lifetime. It is critical that the nurse consider the link between the physical assessment data and the patient's psychological and social history. A thorough history of major psychological events should be compared with the chronology of physical problems. Special attention should be paid to any history of sexual abuse or trauma in the patient's younger years. Early sexual abuse also may prevent the individual from being able to perform sexually or to have chronic abdominal pain or discomfort during sexual relations.

The individual's mood is usually labile, often shifting from extremely excited or anxious to being depressed and hopeless. Response to physical symptoms is usually magnified, such as interpreting a simple cold as pneumonia or a brief chest pain as a heart attack. Family members may not believe the physical symptoms are real and may view them as attention-getting behavior because symptoms often improve when the patient receives attention. For example, a woman who has been in bed for 3 weeks with severe back pain may suddenly feel much better once her children visit her.

There is emerging evidence that some people with somatic symptoms have alexithymia. Research has focused on the construct of **alexithymia** and also whether there are illness patterns for people who have difficulty identifying and expressing their emotion (Duddu, Issac, & Chaturvedi, 2006; Kojima, Senda, Nagaya, Tokudome, & Furukawa, 2003; Porcelli et al., 2003, Waller & Scheidt, 2006).

• NCLEXNOTE

NCLEXNOTE

Encourage and allow patients with somatoform disorder to discuss their physical problems before focusing on psychosocial issues.

Nursing Diagnoses for the Psychological Domain

Nursing diagnoses that target responses to somatization disorder typical of the psychological domain include the following: Anxiety, Ineffective Sexuality Patterns, Impaired Social Interactions, Ineffective Coping, and Ineffective Therapeutic Regimen Management (see Figure 23.2).

Interventions for the Psychological Domain

The choice of psychological intervention depends on the specific problem the patient is experiencing. The most important and ongoing intervention is the maintenance of a therapeutic relationship.

Development of a Therapeutic Relationship

The most difficult aspect of nursing care is developing a sound, positive nurse–patient relationship, yet this relationship is crucial. Without it, the nurse is just one more provider who fails to meet the patient's expectations. Developing this relationship requires time and patience. Therapeutic communication techniques should be used to refocus the patient on psychosocial problems related to the physical manifestations (see Box 23.5).

During periods when symptoms of other psychiatric disorders surface, additional interventions are needed. For example, if depression occurs, additional supportive or cognitive approaches may be needed.

Counseling

Counseling, with a focus on problem solving, is needed from time to time. These patients have chaotic lives

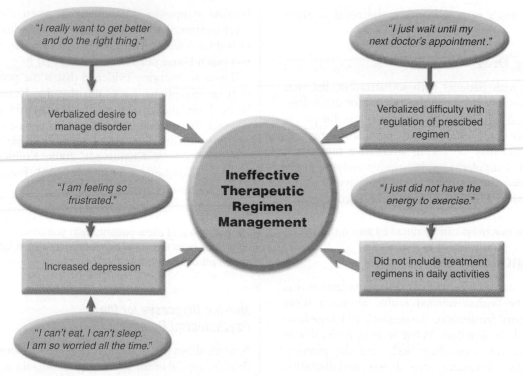

FIGURE 23.2. Nursing Diagnosis Concept Map: Ineffective Therapeutic Regimen Management.

and need support through the multitude of crises. Although they may appear fascinating and at times self-assured, they can easily irritate others because of their constant complaints. The consequences of their impaired social interaction with others must be examined within a counseling framework. It will become evident to the nurse that the patient's problem-solving and decision-making skills could be improved.

BOX 23.5

Therapeutic Dialogue: Establishing a Relationship

Ineffective Approach

Nurse: Good morning, Ms. C.
Patient: I'm in so much pain. Take that breakfast away.
Nurse: You don't want your breakfast?
Patient: Can't you see? I hurt! When I hurt, I can't eat!
Nurse: If you don't eat now, you probably won't be able to have anything until lunch.
Patient: Who cares. I have no intention of being here at lunchtime. I don't belong here.
Nurse: Ms. C, I don't think that your doctor would have admitted you unless there is a problem. I would like to talk to you about why you are here.
Patient: Nurse, I'm just here. It's none of your business.
Nurse: Oh.
Patient: Please leave me alone.
Nurse: Sure, I will see you later.

Effective Approach

Nurse: Good morning, Ms. C.
Patient: I'm in so much pain. Take that breakfast away.
Nurse: (Silently removes tray. Pulls up chair and sits down.)
Patient: My back hurts.
Nurse: Oh, when did the back pain start?
Patient: Last night. It's this bed. I couldn't get comfortable.
Nurse: These beds can be pretty uncomfortable.
Patient: My back pain is shooting down my leg.
Nurse: Does anything help it?
Patient: Sometimes if I straighten out my leg it helps.
Nurse: Can I help you straighten out your leg?
Patient: Oh, it's OK. The pain is going away. What did you say your name is?
Nurse: I'm Susan Miller, your nurse while you are here.
Patient: I won't be here long. I don't belong in a psychiatric unit.
Nurse: While you are here, I would like to spend time with you.
Patient: OK, but you understand, I do not have any psychiatric problems.
Nurse: We can talk about whatever you want. But, since you want to get out of here, we might want to focus on what it will take to get you ready for discharge.

Critical Thinking Challenge

- What communication mistakes did the nurse in the first scenario make?
- What communication strategies helped the patient feel comfortable with the nurse in the second scenario? How is the first scenario different from the second?

BOX 23.6

Psychoeducation Checklist: Somatization Disorder

When caring for the patient with somatization disorder, be sure to include the following topic areas in the teaching plan:

- Psychopharmacologic agents (anxiolytics) if ordered, including drug, action, dosage, frequency, and possible adverse effects.
- Nonpharmacologic pain relief measures
- Exercise
- Nutrition
- Social interaction
- Appropriate health care practices
- Problem-solving
- Relaxation and anxiety-reduction techniques
- Sexual functioning

Identifying stresses and strengthening positive coping responses helps the patient deal with a chaotic lifestyle.

Patient Education: Health

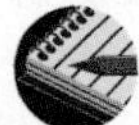

Health teaching is useful throughout the nurse–patient relationship. These patients have many questions about illnesses, symptoms, and treatments. Emphasize positive health care practices and minimize the effects of serious illness. Because of problems in managing medications and treatment, the therapeutic regimen needs constant monitoring, resulting in ample opportunities for teaching. One area that might require special health teaching is impaired sexuality. Because of their long history of physical problems related to the reproductive tract, these patients may have difficulty carrying out normal sexual activity, such as intercourse, reaching orgasm, and so forth. Basic teaching about normal sexual function is often needed (see Box 23.6).

Social Domain

People with this disorder spend excessive time seeking medical care and treating their multiple illnesses. Most are unemployed. Because they believe themselves to be very sick, they also believe that they are disabled and cannot work. Because their symptoms are often inconsistent with any identifiable medical diagnosis, these individuals are rarely satisfied with health care providers, who can find nothing wrong. However, their social network often consists of a series of providers, rather than peers. Identifying a support network requires sorting out the health care providers from family and friends.

Assessment

Family members can also become weary of the individual's constant complaints of physical problems. These individuals sometimes live in chaotic families with multiple problems. In assessing the family structure, other members with psychiatric disorders must be identified. Women may be married to abusive men who have antisocial personality disorders; alcoholism is common. Identifying the positive and negative relationships within the family is important.

Somatization disorder is particularly problematic because it disrupts the family's social life. Changes in routine or major life events often precipitate the appearance of a symptom. For example, a patient may be planning a vacation with the family, but at the last minute decides she cannot go because her back pain has returned and she will not be able to sit in the car. These family disruptions are common.

Nursing Diagnoses for the Social Domain

Some of the nursing diagnoses related to the social domain that are typical of people with somatization disorder include the following: Risk for Caregiver Role Strain, Ineffective Community Coping, Disabled Family Coping, and Social Isolation.

Interventions for the Social Domain

Patients with somatic disorders are usually isolated from their families and communities. Strengthening social relationships and activities often becomes the focus of the nursing care. The nurse should help the patient identify individuals with whom contact is desired, ask for a commitment to contact them, and encourage them to reinitiate a relationship. The nurse should counsel the patient about talking too much about their symptoms with these individuals and emphasize that medical information should be shared with the nurse. The nurse must also ensure that the patient knows when the next appointment is scheduled.

Group Interventions

Although these patients may not be candidates for insight group psychotherapy, they do benefit from cognitive-behavioral groups that focus on developing coping skills for everyday life (Lidbeck, 2003). Because most of the patients are women, participation in groups that address feminist issues should be encouraged to strengthen their assertiveness skills and improve their generally low self-esteem (Figure 23.3).

When leading a group that has members with this disorder, redirection can keep the group from giving too much attention to a person's illness. However, these individuals need reassurance and support while in a group. They may verbalize that they do not fit in or belong in the group. In reality, they are feeling insecure and threatened in the situation. The group leader

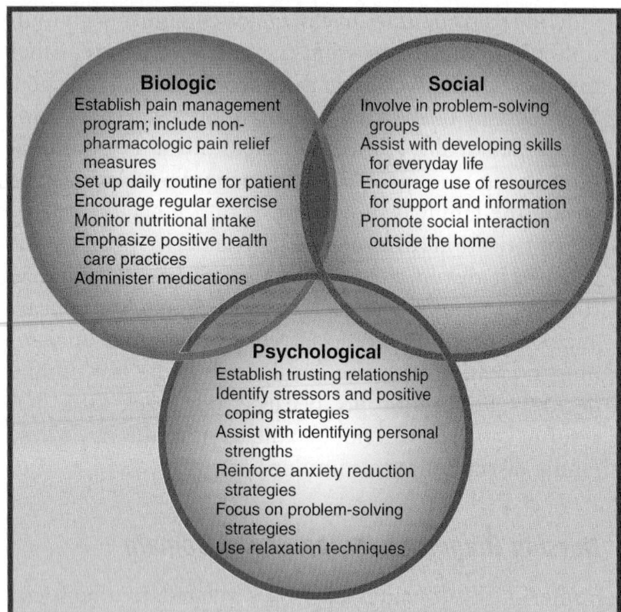

FIGURE 23.3. Biopsychosocial interventions for patients with somatization disorder.

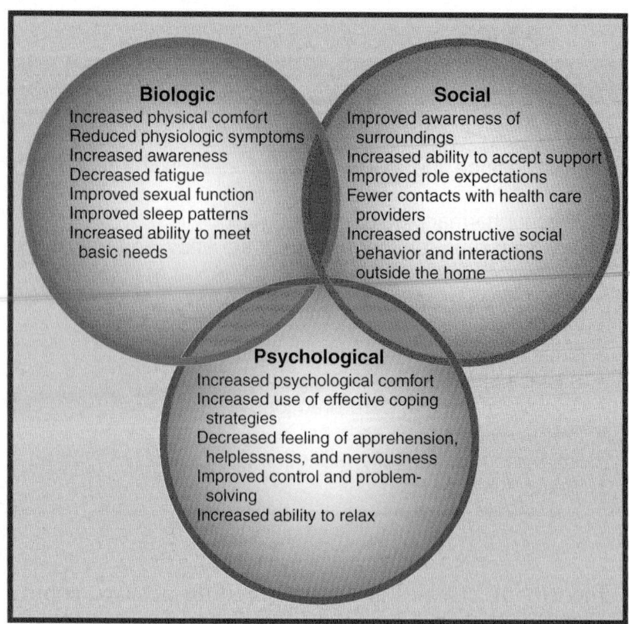

FIGURE 23.4. Biopsychosocial outcomes for patients with somatization disorder.

needs to show patience and understanding in order to engage the individual effectively in meaningful group interaction.

Family Interventions The results of a family assessment often reveal that families of these individuals need education about the disorder, helpful strategies for dealing with the multiple complaints of the patient, and, usually, help in developing more effective communication patterns. Because of the chaotic nature of some of the families and the lack of healthy problem solving, physical, sexual, and psychological abuse may be evident. The nurse should be particularly sensitive to any evidence of current physical or sexual abuse (see Chapter 39).

Evaluation and Treatment Outcomes

The outcomes for patients with somatization disorder should be realistic. Because this is a lifelong disorder, small successes should be expected. Specific outcomes should be identified, such as gradually increasing social contact. Over time, there should be a gradual reduction in the number of health care providers the individual contacts and a slight improvement in the ability to cope with stresses (Figure 23.4).

Continuum of Care

Inpatient Care

Ideally, these individuals will spend minimal time in the hospital. Inpatient stays occur when their comorbid disorders become symptomatic. While an inpatient, the patient should be the responsibility of one primary nurse who provides or oversees all of the nursing care. The inpatient nurse must establish a relationship with the patient (and family) and teach other nursing staff members about this disorder.

Emergency Care

The emergencies these individuals experience may be physical (e.g., chest pain, back pain, gastrointestinal symptoms) or stress responses related to a psychosocial crisis. Occasionally, these individuals become suicidal and require an intensive level of care. Generally speaking, nonpharmacologic interventions should be tried first, with very conservative use of antianxiety medications. All attempts should be made to retrieve records from other facilities.

Community Treatment

These patients can spend a lifetime in the health care system and still have little continuity of care. Switching from provider to provider is detrimental to their long-term care. Most are outpatients. When they are hospitalized, it is usually for evaluation of medical problems. When their comorbid psychiatric disorders, such as depression, become symptomatic, these patients may also be hospitalized for a short time. See Nursing Care Plan 23.1.

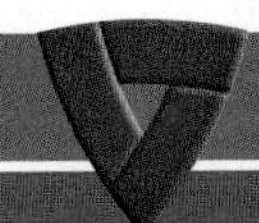

Nursing Care Plan 23.1

Nursing Care Plan for a Patient With Somatization Disorder

SC is a 48-year-old woman who is making her weekly visit to her primary care physician for unexplained multiple somatic problems. This week, her concern is reoccurring abdominal pain that fits no symptom pattern. Upon physical examination, a cause for her abdominal pain could not be found. She is requesting a refill of alprazolam (Xanax) which is the only medication that relieves her pain. She is in the process of applying for disability income because of being completely disabled by neck and shoulder pain. The physician and office staff avoid her whenever possible. The physician will not refill the prescription until SC is evaluated by the consulting mental health team that provides weekly evaluations and services.

Setting: Primary Care Office

Baseline Assessment: 48-year-old Caucasian, obese woman who appears very angry. She resents being forced to see a psychiatric clinician for the only medication that works. She denies any psychiatric problems or emotional distress. SC is wearing a short, black top and slacks that are too tight. Her hair is in curlers and she says that it is too much trouble to comb her hair. Her mental status is normal, but she admits to being slightly depressed and takes the alprazolam for her nerves. She says she has nothing to live for, but denies any thoughts of suicide. She is dependent on her children for everything and feels very guilty about it. She spends most of her waking hours going to various doctors and taking combinations of medications to relieve her pains. She has no friends or nonfamily social contacts because they would not be able to stand her.

Associated Psychiatric Diagnosis

Axis I R/O depression; Somatization disorder
Axis II R/O histrionic personality disorder
Axis III S/P hysterectomy
S/P gastric bypass
S/P carpel tunnel release
Chronic shoulder, neck pain, vertigo
Axis IV Social problems (father died 6 months ago, divorced 9 months)
Economic problems (small pension)
Occupational problems (potential disability)
GAF = Current, 60
Potential, 75

Medications

Premarin, 0.625 mg every day
Alprazolam (Xanax), 25 mg tid
Ranitidine HCL (Zantac), 150 mg with meals
Simethicone, 125 mg qid with meals
Calcium carbonate, 1,200 mg every day
Multiple vitamin, every day
Zolpidem tartrate (Ambien), 10 mg at bedtime PRN
Ibuprofen, 600 mg q4h PRN pain
Maalox, PRN
Preparation H suppositories

Nursing Diagnosis 1: Chronic Low Self-Esteem

Defining Characteristics

Self-negating verbalizations (long-standing)
Hesitant to try new things
Expresses guilt
Evaluates self as being unable to deal with events

Related Factors

Feeling unimportant to family
Feeling rejected by husband
Constant physical problems interfering with normal social activities

Outcomes

Initial	Long-term
Identify need to increase self-esteem	Participate in individual or group therapy for esteem building

Interventions

Interventions	Rationale	Ongoing Assessment
Establish rapport with patient	Individuals with low self-esteem are reluctant to discuss true feelings	Self-exam feelings provoked by patient (discuss with supervisor if interfering with care). Determine if patient is beginning to engage in a relationship.

Continued

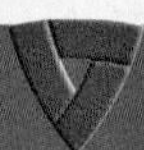

Nursing Care Plan 23.1 (Continued)

Interventions	Rationale	Ongoing Assessment
Encourage patient to spend time dressing and grooming appropriately.	Confidence and self-esteem improve when a person looks well-groomed.	Monitor response to suggestions.
Encourage patient to discuss various somatic problems, but allow some time to discuss psychological and interpersonal issues.	Patients with somatization disorder need time to express their physical problems. It helps them feel valued. The best way to build a relationship is to acknowledge physical symptoms.	Monitor time that patient spends explaining physical symptoms.
Explore opportunities for SC to meet other people with similar, nonmedical interests.	Focusing SC on meeting others will improve the possibilities of increasing contacts.	Observe willingness to identify other interests besides physical problems.

Evaluation

Outcomes	Revised Outcomes	Interventions
SC admitted to having low self-esteem, but was very reluctant to consider meeting new people.	Focus on building self-esteem.	Identify activities that will enhance personal self-esteem.

Nursing Diagnosis 2: Ineffective Therapeutic Regimen Management

Defining Characteristics	Related Factors
Choices of daily living ineffective for meeting health care goal. Verbalizes difficulty with prescribed regimens.	Inappropriate use of benzodiazepines for nerves.

Outcomes

Initial	Long-term
Honestly discuss the use of medications.	Use nonpharmacologic means for stress reduction, especially antianxiety medications.

Interventions

Interventions	Rationale	Ongoing Assessment
Clarify the frequency and purpose of taking alprazolam.	Unsupervised polypharmacy is very common with these patients. Further clarification is usually needed.	Carefully track self-report of medication use; determine if patient is disclosing the use of all medications.
Educate patient about the effects of combining medications, emphasizing negative effects.	Education about combining medication is the beginning of helping patient become effective in medication regimen.	Observe patient's ability and willingness to consider negative effects.
Recommend that patient gradually reduce number of medications and problem-solve other means of managing physical symptoms.	Giving patients clear directions about managing health care regimens needs to be followed up with specific strategies to change behavior.	Evaluate patient's ability to problem solve.

Evaluation

Outcomes	Revised Outcomes	Interventions
Patient disclosed use of medications, but was unwilling to consider changing ineffective use of medication.	Identify next step if primary care physician does not refill prescription.	Discuss the possibility of not being able to obtain alprazolam. Refer patient to mental health clinic for further evaluation.

Mental Health Promotion

Patients with somatization disorder should focus on "staying healthy," instead of focusing on their illness. For these individuals, approaching the topic of health promotion usually has to be within the context of preventing further problems. Setting aside time for themselves and identifying activities that meet their psychological and spiritual needs, such as going to church or synagogue, are important in maintaining a healthy balance.

OTHER SOMATOFORM DISORDERS

The other somatoform disorders have many symptoms that are similar to those of somatization disorder and can be equally as debilitating. The following discussion summarizes the other somatoform disorders and highlights the primary focus of nursing management.

Undifferentiated Somatoform Disorder

Patients who have unexplained physical problems for at least 6 months have diagnoses of undifferentiated somatoform disorder. This disorder is different from somatization disorder in that these patients do not have multiple, unexplained physical problems before 30 years of age; instead, they may have just one. Fatigue, loss of appetite, and gastrointestinal or genitourinary problems are the most common complaints. This disorder is most frequently seen in women of lower socioeconomic status. The course of the disorder is unpredictable, and often another mental or physical disorder is diagnosed. For this disorder, nursing care is similar to that for somatization disorder.

In many other parts of the world, the term *neurasthenia* is used to describe a syndrome of chronic fatigue and weaknesses. In the United States, these individuals receive a diagnosis of undifferentiated somatoform disorder if the condition has lasted for 6 months.

Conversion Disorder

Conversion disorder is a psychiatric condition in which emotional distress or unconscious conflict are expressed through physical symptoms. Patients with conversion disorder can present with pseudoneurologic symptoms including impaired coordination or balance, paralysis, aphonia (inability to produce sound), difficulty swallowing or a sensation of a lump in the throat, and urinary retention. They also may have loss of touch, vision problems, blindness, deafness, and hallucinations. In some instances, they may have seizures (APA, 2000). The patient's symptoms do not follow a neurological course, but rather follow their own perceived conceptualization of the problem. If only the pseudoneurologic symptoms are present, the patient receives a diagnosis of conversion disorder. The nurse must understand that the physical sensation is real for the patient. There is evidence of a relationship between childhood trauma (such as sexual abuse) and conversion disorder (Roelofs, Keijsers, Hoogduin, Naring, & Moene, 2002). In approaching this patient, the nurse treats the conversion symptom as a real symptom that may have distressing psychological aspects. The nurse intervenes by acknowledging the symptom and helps the patient deal with it. As trust develops within the nurse–patient relationship, the nurse can help the patient develop problem-solving approaches to everyday problems.

Pain Disorder

In pain disorder, pain severe enough for the patient to seek medical attention interferes with social and occupational functioning. The onset of the pain is often associated with psychological factors, such as a traumatic or humiliating experience. However, the pain can also be attributed to the onset or worsening of comorbid symptoms of depression and/or anxiety. Because of the pain, the individual often cannot return to work or school. Unemployment, disability, and family problems frequently follow. Pain disorder is believed to be an everyday phenomena and relatively common (Hiller, Rief, & Brahler, 2006). From 10% to 15% of adults in the United States within a given year are disabled by back pain (APA, 2000). Pain disorder may occur at any age. Women experience headaches and musculoskeletal pain more often than do men. Acute pain tends to resolve within a short time; chronic pain may persist for many years. Pain medication should be prescribed conservatively. If mood disorders are also present, mood stabilizers not only treat the depression but also may treat the pain (Maurer, Volz, & Sauer, 1999). Nursing care focuses on helping patients identify strategies to relieve pain and to examine stressors in their lives.

Hypochondriasis

The difference between hypochondriasis and the other somatoform disorders is that patients with hypochondriasis are preoccupied with their fears about developing a serious illness based on their misinterpretation of body sensations. In hypochondriasis, the fear of having an illness continues despite medical reassurance and interferes with the psychosocial functioning. These individuals spend time and money on repeated examinations looking for feared illnesses. For example, an occasional cough or the appearance of a small sore results in the person making an appointment with an oncologist. Hypochondriasis sometimes appears if the patient had a serious childhood illness or if a family member has a serious illness. The prevalence of hypochondriasis in general medical practice is estimated to be between 2% and 7% (APA, 2000). These patients are most likely seen in medical–surgical settings, unless they have a coexisting psychiatric disorder.

Several interventions have been effective in reducing patients' fears of experiencing serious illnesses. CBT, stress management, and group interventions lead to a decrease in intensity and increase in control of symptoms (Fava, Grandi, Rafanelli, Fabbri, & Cazzaro, 2000; Walker, Vincent, Furer, Cox, & Kjemisted, 1999). Whether the positive outcomes result from the intervention itself, or from the symptom validation and increased attention given to the patient, is unknown. Other interventions include the use of SSRIs, which have been successful at decreasing the ruminations and anxiety associated with the patient's fears of experiencing serious illness (Fallon et al., 2003). However, based on these studies, nursing management should include listening to the patient's report of symptoms and fears, validating it by acknowledging that the fears may be real, asking the patient to monitor symptoms in a journal, and encouraging the patient to bring the journal to the next visit. By actually seeing the symptom pattern, the nurse can continue to educate the patient and assess for significant symptoms. The outcome of this approach should be a decrease in fears and better control of the symptoms.

Body Dysmorphic Disorder

Patients with body dysmorphic disorder (BDD) focus on real (but slight) or imagined defects in appearance, such as a large nose, thinning hair, or small genitals. Preoccupation with the defect causes significant distress and interferes with their ability to function socially. They feel so self-conscious that they avoid work or public situations. Some fear that their "ugly" body part will malfunction. This disorder occurs equally in men and women, but few epidemiologic data are available. In anxiety disorders and depression, BDD is estimated to occur in 5% to 40% of patients (APA, 2000). BDD may be present in 25% of patients with anorexia nervosa (Rabe-Jablonska & Tomasz, 2000). In patients receiving dermatology care and cosmetic surgery, the estimate is 6% to 15% (Phillips, Dufresne, Wilkel, & Vittorio, 2000; Uzun et al., 2003).

BDD usually begins in adolescence and continues throughout adulthood. These individuals are not usually seen in psychiatric settings unless they have a coexisting psychiatric disorder or a family member insists on psychiatric attention. BDD is an extremely debilitating disorder and can significantly impair an individual's quality of life (Box 23.7). The obvious nursing diagnosis is Disturbed Body Image. While developing a therapeutic relationship, the nurse should respect these patients' preoccupations and avoid challenging their beliefs. However, the nurse should also assess the extent of preoccupation with the body part. If the patient is actually disfigured, the preoccupation may take on a phobic quality (Newell, 1999). If so, referral to a mental health specialist should be considered. The generalist nurse can help the patient

FAME AND FORTUNE

Leo Tolstoy (1828–1910)
Russian Novelist

Public Persona

Count Leo Tolstoy was one of the giants of 19th century literature. He was raised in wealth and privilege in Czarist Russia. Among the most famous works authored by Tolstoy are the novels *War and Peace* and *Anna Karenina.* Experts believe that his fiction portrays his own inner character. For example, in *War and Peace,* Pierre Bezuhov reflects the life of the author.

Personal Realities

In *Confessions,* Tolstoy describes his depressions, hypochondriasis, and alcoholism.

BOX 23.7

Clinical Vignette: ***Body Dysmorphic Disorder***

K, a 16-year-old girl, for about 6 months has believed that her pubic bone is becoming increasingly dislocated and prominent. She believes that everyone stares at and talks about it. She does not remember a particular event related to the appearance of the symptom, but is absolutely convinced that she can be helped only by a surgical correction of her pubic bone.

She was treated recently for anorexia nervosa with marginal success. Although her weight is nearly normal, she continues to be preoccupied with the looks of her body. She spends almost the entire day in her bedroom, wearing excessively large pajamas, and she refuses to leave the house. Once or twice a day, she lowers herself to the ground and measures, with her fingers, the distance between her pelvic girdle and the ground in order to check the position of the pubic bone.

In desperation, her parents called the clinic for help. The family was referred to a home health agency and a psychiatric home health nurse who arranged for an assessment visit.

What Do You Think?

- How should the nurse approach K? Should an assessment begin immediately?
- From the vignette, identify nursing diagnoses, outcomes, and interventions.

Adapted from Sobanski, E., & Schmidt, M. H. (2000). "Everybody looks at my pubic bone"—a case report of an adolescent patient with body dysmorphic disorder. Acta Psychiatrica Scandinavica, *101,* 80–82.

by developing interventions for other nursing diagnoses that may be present, such as Social Isolation, Low Self-Esteem, and Ineffective Coping. These patients will often be treated with an antidepressant, and in particular an SSRI which targets the underlying anxiety associated with their preoccupation of their perceived disfiguration of their body or body part (Phillips & Najjar, 2003).

FACTITIOUS DISORDERS

The other type of psychiatric disorders characterized by somatization is factitious disorders; patients with these disorders intentionally cause an illness or injury to receive the attention of health care workers. These individuals are motivated solely by the desire to become a patient and develop a dependent relationship with a health care provider. There are two classes of factitious disorders: factitious disorder and factitious disorder, not otherwise specified.

Factitious Disorder

Although feigned illnesses have been described for centuries, it was not until 1951 that the term *Münchausen's syndrome* was used to describe the most severe form of this disorder, which was characterized by fabricating a physical illness, having recurrent hospitalizations, and going from one provider to another (Asher, 1951). Today, this disorder is called factitious disorder and is differentiated from **malingering,** in which the individual who intentionally produces illness symptoms is motivated by another specific self-serving goal, such as being classified as disabled or avoiding work.

Unlike people with borderline personality disorder, who typically injure themselves overtly and readily admit to self-harm, patients with factitious disorder injure themselves covertly. The illnesses are produced in such a manner that the health care provider is tricked into believing that a true physical or psychiatric disorder is present. The *DSM-IV-TR* identifies three subtypes of factitious disorder: (1) one that has predominantly psychological symptoms, (2) one that has predominately physical symptoms (Münchausen's syndrome), and (3) one that has a combination of physical and psychological manifestations, with neither one predominating (APA, 2000).

The self-produced physical symptoms appear as medical illnesses and cut across all body systems. They include seizure disorders, wound-healing disorders, the abscess processes (introduction of infectious material below the skin surface), and feigned fever (rubbing the thermometer). In one study of 42 children and adolescents who falsify chronic illness, most patients were female, and the most commonly reported falsified or induced conditions were fevers, ketoacidosis, purpura, and infections (Libow, 2000).

These patients are extremely creative in simulating illnesses, and they tell fascinating, but false, stories of personal triumph. These tales are referred to as **pseudologia fantastica** and are a core symptom of the disorder. Pseudologia fantastica are stories that are not entirely improbable and often contain a matrix of truth and falsehood. These patients falsify blood, urine, and other samples by contaminating them with protein or fecal material. They self-inject anticoagulants to receive diagnoses of "bleeding of undetermined origin" or ingest thyroid hormones to produce thyrotoxicosis. They also inflict injury on themselves by inserting objects or feces into body orifices, such as the urinary tract, open wounds, or even intravenous tubing. They produce their own surgical scars, especially abdominal, and when treated surgically, they delay wound healing through scratching, rubbing, or manipulating the wound and introducing bacteria into the wound. These patients put themselves in life-threatening situations through actions such as ingesting allergens known to produce an anaphylactic reaction.

Patients who manifest primarily psychological symptoms produce psychotic symptoms such as hallucinations and delusions, cognitive deficits such as memory loss, dissociative symptoms such as amnesia, and conversion symptoms such as pseudoblindness or pseudoparalysis. These individuals often become psychotic, depressed, or suicidal after an unconfirmed tragedy. When questioned about details, they become defensive and uncooperative. Sometimes, these individuals have a combination of both physical and psychiatric symptoms.

Epidemiology

The prevalence of this disorder is unknown because diagnosing it and obtaining reliable data are difficult. Prevalence was reported to be high when researchers were actually looking for the disorder in specific populations. Within large general hospitals, factitious disorders are diagnosed in about 1% of patients with whom mental health professionals consult. The age range of patients with the disorder is between 19 and 64 years. The median age of onset is the early 20s. Once thought to occur predominantly in men, this disorder is now reported predominantly in women. No genetic pattern has been identified, but it does seem to run in families. Many of these people have comorbid psychiatric disorders, such as mood disorders, personality disorders, and substance-related disorders.

Etiology

The etiology of factitious disorders is believed to have a psychodynamic basis. The theory is that these individuals, who were often abused as children, received nurturance only during times of illness; thus, they try to recreate illness or injury in a desperate attempt to receive love and attention. During the actual self-injury, the individual is reported to be in a trancelike, dissociative state. Many patients report having an intimate relationship with a health care provider, either as a child or as an adult, and then experiencing rejection when the relationship ended. The self-injury and subsequent attention is an attempt by the individual to re-enact those experiences and gain control over the situation and the other person. Often, the patients exhibit aggression after being discovered, allowing them to express revenge on their perceived tormenter (Feldman 2004).

These patients are usually discovered in medical–surgical settings. They are hostile and distance themselves from others. Their network is void of friends and family and usually consists only of health care providers, who change at regular intervals. In factitious disorder, the patients fabricate a detailed and exaggerated medical history. When the interventions do not work and the fabrication is discovered, the health care team feels manipulated and angry. When the patient is confronted with the evidence, he or she becomes enraged and often leaves that health care system, only to enter another. Eventually, the person is referred for mental health treatment. The course of the disorder usually consists of intermittent episodes (APA, 2000).

NURSING MANAGEMENT: HUMAN RESPONSE TO FACTITIOUS DISORDER

The overall goal of treatment is for the patient to replace the dysfunctional, attention-seeking behaviors with positive behaviors. To begin treatment, the patient must acknowledge the deception, but confrontation does not appear to lead to acknowledgment (Krahn, Li, & O'Connor, 2003). The mental health team has to accept and value the patient as a human being who needs help. The pattern of self-injury is well established and meets overwhelming psychological needs, so giving up the behaviors is difficult. The treatment is long-term psychotherapy. The generalist psychiatric–mental health nurse will most likely care for the patient during or after periods of feigned illnesses. More is known about the treatment of individuals with factitious physical disorders than of those with psychological disorders.

Assessment

A nursing assessment should focus on obtaining a history of medical and psychological illnesses. Physical disabilities should be identified. Early childhood experiences, particularly instances of abuse, neglect, or abandonment, should be identified to understand the underlying psychological dynamics of the individual and the role of self-injury. Family relationships become strained as the members become aware of the self-inflicted nature of this disorder. Family assessment is important.

Nursing Diagnoses

The nursing diagnoses could include almost any diagnosis: Risk for Trauma, Risk for Self-Mutilation, Ineffective Individual Coping, or Low Self-Esteem.

Desired outcomes include decreased self-injurious behavior and increased positive coping behaviors. Any nursing intervention must be implemented within the context of a strong nurse–patient relationship (Moffatt, 2000).

Nursing Interventions

Nurses must continually examine their own feelings about these patients. The fabrications and deceits provoke anger and a sense of betrayal in the nurse. To be effective with these patients, the nurse must be aware of these feelings and resolve them by developing a better understanding of the underlying psychodynamic issues (Box 23.8). Confronting the patient has been reported effective if the patient feels supported and accepted and if there is clear communication among the patient, the mental health care team, and family members. All care should be centralized within one facility, and the patient should see providers regularly, even when not in active crisis. Offering the patient a face-saving way of giving up the factitious disorder is often crucial. The

BOX 23.8

Using Reflection: Ethical Dilemma

Incident: Walking into a patient's room, the nurse observes a patient purposefully tearing open her sutures. The nurse yells at her to stop and asks her why she is doing that. The patient screams at her to get out and leave her alone. The nurse is upset and tries to understand what she just witnessed. She kept asking "how could she do that when she just went through a major surgery to repair her problem?"

Reflection: Upon reflecting, the nurse realized that her own values were in conflict and that she was very angry with the patient for purposefully traumatizing herself. She then focused on trying to understand the patient's need to carry out such painful self-abuse. She resolved to discuss the behavior with the patient using a nonjudgmental approach in order to help her develop new ways of dealing with the underlying need for self-mutilation.

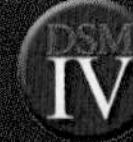

Table 23.2 Key Diagnostic Characteristics of Factitious Disorder
300.16 With predominantly psychological signs and symptoms
300.19 With predominantly physical signs and symptoms
300.19 With combined psychological and physical signs and symptoms

Diagnostic Criteria and Target Symptoms	Associated Findings
• Intentionally producing psychological or physical signs and symptoms Subjective complaints, such as pain in absence of pain Self-inflicted conditions Exaggeration or exacerbation of pre-existing medical conditions Any combination or variation • Motivated by need to assume sick role • Absence of external incentives for behavior	***Associated Behavioral Findings*** • Very dramatic, but vague, inconsistent history • Pathologic lying about history to intrigue listener • Extensive knowledge of medical terminology and hospital routines • Repeated hospitalizations in numerous hospitals, in many locations • Complaints of pain and requests for analgesics common • Eagerly undergo extensive workups with invasive procedures and operations • Deny allegations that symptoms are factitious once revealed, usually followed by rapid discharge against medical advice (With predominantly psychological signs and symptoms) • Claims of depression, suicidal ideation, auditory and visual hallucinations, recent and remote memory loss, and dissociative symptoms • Extremely suggestible • Negativistic and uncooperative when questioned ***Associated Physical Examination*** • Severe right lower quadrant pain with nausea and vomiting, massive hemoptysis, generalized rashes and abscesses, fever of unknown origin, bleeding secondary to ingestion of anticoagulants, and "lupus-like" syndromes • Symptoms limited to person's knowledge, sophistication, and imagination

treatment goal is recovery, not confession. Behavioral techniques that shape new behaviors help the patient move forward toward a new life.

The goal is for care to be given within the context of one system. A team that knows the patient, agrees on a treatment approach, and follows through is crucial to the patient's eventual recovery. For this to happen, the medical, psychiatric, inpatient, and outpatient teams need to communicate with each other on a regular basis. Family members must also be aware of the need for consistent treatment.

Factitious Disorder, Not Otherwise Specified

The diagnosis "factitious disorder, not otherwise specified" is reserved for people who do not quite meet all the diagnostic criteria of factitious disorder (Table 23.2). Within the category of factitious disorder, not otherwise specified, the *DSM-IV-TR* (APA, 2000) includes a rare, but dramatic disorder, factitious disorder by proxy, or Münchausen's by proxy, which involves another person, usually the mother, who inflicts injuries on her child to gain the attention of the health care provider through her child's injuries. These actions include inducing seizures, poisoning, or smothering. This most severe form of child abuse is usually identified in the emergency room. The mother rarely admits injuring the child and thus is not amenable to treatment; the child is removed from the mother's care. This form of child abuse is distinguished from other forms by routine, unwitting involvement of health care workers, who subject the child to physical harm and emotional distress through tests, procedures, and medication trials. Some researchers suspect that children who are abused in this way may later experience factitious disorder (Libow, 2000).

SUMMARY OF KEY POINTS

■ Somatization is psychological stress that is manifested in physical symptoms and is the chief characteristic of somatoform disorders and factitious disorders. The difference between these two types of disorders is that in somatoform disorders, the individuals experience unexplained physical symptoms but do not self-inflict injuries, whereas in factitious disorders, individuals self-inflict injuries to gain medical attention.

- Somatization is affected by sociocultural and gender factors. It occurs more frequently in women than men; in those less educated; those living in urban areas; those who are older, separated, widowed, or divorced; and in Mexican American women more than in non-Hispanic women. It also has been strongly associated with individuals who have been sexually abused as children.
- The somatoform disorders are clustered into six different clinical syndromes: (1) somatization disorder, (2) undifferentiated somatoform disorder, (3) conversion disorder, (4) pain disorder, (5) hypochondriasis, and (6) body dysmorphic disorder. The person with somatization disorder suffers multiple physical problems and symptoms, in contrast to those with other clinical subtypes, in which one major symptom recurs.
- Somatization disorder, the most complex of the somatoform disorders, is a chronic relapsing condition characterized by multiple physical symptoms of unknown origin that develop during times of emotional distress.
- Factitious disorders include two subtypes: (1) factitious disorder and (2) factitious disorder, not otherwise specified. In factitious disorder, physical or psychological symptoms (or both) are fabricated to assume the sick role. Factitious disorder, not otherwise specified includes factitious disorder by proxy, the intentional production of symptoms in others, usually children.
- Identifying and diagnosing somatoform and factitious disorders is very complex because patients with the disorders refuse to accept any psychiatric basis to their problems and often go for years moving from one health care provider to another to receive medical attention and avoid psychiatric assessment.
- These patients are often seen on the medical–surgical units of hospitals and go years without receiving a correct diagnosis. In most cases, they finally receive mental health treatment because of comorbid conditions, such as depression, anxiety, and panic disorder.
- The development of the nurse–patient relationship is crucial to assessing these patients and identifying appropriate nursing diagnoses and interventions. Because these patients deny any psychiatric basis to their problem and continue to focus on their symptoms as being medically based, the nurse must take a flexible, relaxed, and nonjudgmental approach that acknowledges the symptoms but focuses on new ways of coping with stress and avoiding recurrence of symptoms.
- Health teaching is important in helping the individual develop positive lifestyle changes in place of somatization responses. Identifying personal strengths and supporting the development of positive skills improve self-esteem and personal confidence. Teaching the use of biofeedback and relaxation provides the patient with positive coping skills.

CRITICAL THINKING CHALLENGES

1. A depressed young white woman is admitted to a psychiatric unit in a state of agitation. She reports extreme abdominal pain. Her admitting provider tells you that she has a classic case of somatization disorder and to de-emphasize her physical symptoms. Under no circumstances is she to have any pain medication. Conceptualize the assessment process and how you would approach this patient.
2. Compare and contrast somatoform disorders with factitious disorders.
3. Develop a continuum of "self-injury" for patients with borderline personality disorder, somatization disorder, factitious disorder, and factitious disorder by proxy.
4. Develop a teaching plan for an individual who has a long history of somatization disorder but who recently received a diagnosis of breast cancer. How will the patient be able to differentiate the physical symptoms of somatization disorder from those associated with the treatment of her breast cancer?
5. A Chinese American patient was admitted for panic attacks and numerous somatic problems, ranging from dysmenorrhea to painful joints. Results of all medical examinations have been negative. She truly believes that her panic attacks are caused by a weak heart. What approaches should the nurse use in providing culturally sensitive nursing care?
6. A person with depression is started on a regimen of Nardil, 15 mg tid. She believes that she is allergic to most foods but insists on having wine in the evenings because it helps digest her food. Develop a teaching plan that provides the knowledge that she needs to prevent a hypertensive crisis caused by excessive tyramine but that is sensitive to the patient's food preferences.

Freud: 1962. This is an account of Sigmund Freud's life and the development of his early psychiatric theories and treatment. The film focuses on his struggle for acceptance in the Viennese medical community, rather than on the development of his actual theories. However, conversion disorder is depicted in his patients throughout this movie.

SIGNIFICANCE: Somatoform disorders are rarely clearly depicted in films. This movie has examples of people with somatoform disorders.

VIEWING POINTS: Identify the symptoms of somatoform disorder.

REFERENCES

American Psychiatric Association. (2000). *Diagnostic and statistical manual of mental disorders* (4th ed., text revision). Washington, DC: Author.

Asher, R. (1951). Münchausen's syndrome. *Lancet, 1,* 339–341.

Cloninger, C., Martin, R., Guze, S., & Clayton, P. (1986). A prospective follow-up and family study of somatization in men and women. *American Journal of Psychiatry, 143*(7), 873–878.

Cloninger, C., von Knorring, A., Sigvardsson, S., & Bohman, M. (1986). Symptom patterns and causes of somatization in men. II. Genetic and environmental independence from somatization in women. *Genetic Epidemiology, 3*(3), 171–185.

Diseth, T. H. (2005). Dissociation in children and adolescents as reaction to trauma: an overview of conceptual issues and neurobiological factors. *Nordic Journal of Psychiatry, 59(2),* 79–91.

Drayer, R. A., Mulsant, B. H., Lenze, E. J., Rollman, B. L., Dew, M. A., Kelleher, K., et al. (2005). Somatic symptoms of depression in elderly patients with medical comorbidities. *International Journal of Geriatric Psychiatry, (20),* 973–982.

Duddu, V., Issac, M. K., & Chaturvedi, S. K. (2006). Somatization, somatosensory amplification, attribution styles and illness behavior: a review. *International Review of Psychiatry, 18*(1), 25–33.

Fallon, B. A., Qureshi, A. I., Schneier, F. R., Sanchez-Lacay, A., Vermes, D., et al. (2003). An open trial of fluvoxamine for hypochondriasis. *Psychosomatics, 44*(4), 298–303.

Fava, G., Grandi, S., Rafanelli, C., Fabbri, S., & Cazzaro, M. (2000). Explanatory therapy in hypochondriasis. *Journal of Clinical Psychiatry, 61*(4), 317–322.

Feldman, M. D. (2004). Playing sick? Untangling the web of Munchausen syndrome, Munchausen by proxy, malingering factitious disorders. New York: Brunner Rutledge.

Garcia-Campayo, J., & Sanz-Carrillo, C. (2000). The use of alternative medicines by somatoform disorder patients in Spain. *British Journal of General Practice, 50*(455), 487–488.

Garcia-Campayo, J., Sanz-Carrillo, C., Baringo, T., & Ceballos, C. (2001). A SPECT scan in somatization disorder patients: An exploratory study of eleven cases. *The Australian and New Zealand Journal of Psychiatry, 35*(3), 359–363.

Garyfallos, G., Adamopoulou, A., Karastergiou, A., Voikli, M., Ikonomidis, N., Donias, S., et al. (1999). Somatoform disorders: Comorbidity with other *DSM-III-R* psychiatric diagnoses in Greece. *Comprehensive Psychiatry, 40*(4), 299–307.

Grabe, H. J., Meyer, C., Hapke, U., Rumpf, H. J., Freyberger, H. J., Dilling, H., & John, U. (2003). Specific somatoform disorder in the general population. *Psychosomatics, 44*(4), 304–311.

Gureje, O., Simon, G. E., Ustun, T. B., Goldberg, D. P. (1997). Somatization in cross-cultural perspective: A World Health Organization study in primary care. *American Journal of Psychiatry,154*(7), 989–995.

Gureje, O., & Simon, G. E. (1999). The natural history of somatization in primary care. *Psychological Medicine, 29*(3), 669–676.

Hakala, M., Karlsson, H., Ruotsalainen, U., Koponen, S., Bergman, J., Stenman, H., et al. (2002). Severe somatization in women is associated with altered cerebral glucose metabolism. *Psychological Medicine, 32*(8), 1379–1385.

Hiller, W., Rief, W., Brahler, E. (2006). Somatization in the population: from mildly bodily misperceptions to disabling symptoms. *Social Psychiatry and Psychiatric Epidemiology,* in press.

Hotopf, M., Mayou, R., Wadsworth, M., & Wessely, S. (1999). Childhood risk factors for adults with medically unexplained symptoms: Results from a national birth cohort study. *American Journal of Psychiatry, 156*(11), 1796–1800.

Huibers, M. J., Beurskens, A. J., Bleijenberg, G., & van Schayck, C. P. (2003). The effectiveness of psychosocial interventions delivered by general practitioners. *Cochrane Database of Systematic Reviews;(2:, CD3494.*

Hulme, P. A. (2004). Theoretical perspectives on the health problems of adults who experienced childhood sexual abuse. *Issues in Mental Health Nursing, 25,* 339–361.

Jorge, J. R. (2003). Depression in Brazil and other Latin American countries. *Seishin Shinkeigaku Zasshi, 105*(1), 9–16.

Kojima, M., Senda, Y., Nagaya, T., Tokudome, S., & Furukawa, T. A. (2003). Alexithymia, depression and social support among Japanese workers. *Psychotherapy and Psychosomatics, 72*(6), 307–314.

Krahn, L. E., Li, H., & O'Connor, M. K. (2003). Patients who strive to be ill: Factitious disorder with physical symptoms. *American Journal of Psychiatry, 160*(6), 1163–1168.

Kroenke, K., & Swindle, R. (2000). Cognitive-behavioral therapy for somatization and symptom syndromes: A critical review of controlled clinical trials. *Psychotherapy Psychosomatics, 69*(4), 205–215.

Ladwig, K. H., Marten-Mittag, B., Erazo, N., & Gundel, H. (2001). Identifying somatization disorder in a population-based health examination survey: Psychosocial burden and gender differences. *Psychosomatics, 42*(6), 511–518.

Libow, J. A. (2000). Child and adolescent illness falsification. *Pediatrics, 105*(2), 336–342.

Lidbeck, M. (2003). Group therapy for somatization disorders in primary care: Maintenance of treatment goals of short cognitive-behavioural treatment one-and-a half-year follow-up. *Acta Psychiatrica Scandinavica, 107*(5), 449–456.

Lieb, R., Pfister, H., Mastaler, M., & Wittchen, H. U. (2000). Somatoform syndromes and disorders in a representative population sample of adolescents and young adults: Prevalence, comorbidity and impairments. *Acta Psychiatrica Scandinavica, 101*(3), 194–208.

Lieb, R., Zimmermann, P., Friis, R. H., Hofler, M., Tholen, S., & Wittchen, H. U. (2002). The natural course of DSM-IV somatoform disorders and syndromes among adolescents and young adults: A prospective-longitudinal community study. *European Psychiatry, 17*(6), 321–331.

Maurer, I., Volz, H. P., & Sauer, H. (1999). Gabapentin leads to remission of somatoform pain disorder with major depression. *Pharmacopsychiatry, 32*(6), 255–257.

Moffatt, C. (2000). Self-inflicted wounding: Identification, assessment and management. *British Journal of Community Nursing, 5*(1), 34–40.

Mullick, M. S. (2002). Somatoform disorders in children and adolescents. *Bangladesh Medical Research Council Bulletin, 28*(3), 112–122.

Muris, P., Meesters, C. (2004). Children's somatization symptoms: correlations with trait anxiety, anxiety sensitivity, and learning experiences. *Psychological Reports, 94*(3 pt 2), 1269–1275.

Newell, R. J. (1999). Altered body image: A fear-avoidance model of psychosocial difficulties following disfigurement. *Journal of Advanced Nursing, 30*(5), 1230–1238.

Noyes, R. Jr., Langbehn, D., Happel, R., Sieren, L., & Muller, B. (1999). Health Attitude Survey: A scale for assessing somatizing patients. *Psychosomatics, 40*(6), 470–478.

Phillips, K. A., Dufresne, R. J., Wilkel, C. S., & Vittorio, C. C. (2000). Rate of body dysmorphic disorder in dermatology patients. *Journal of American Academy of Dermatology, 42*(3), 436–441.

Phillips, K. A., & Najjar, F. (2003). An open-label study of citalopram in body dysmorphic disorder. *Journal of Clinical Psychiatry, 64*(6), 715–720.

Porcelli, P., Bagby, R. M., Taylor, G. J., DeCarne, M., Leandro, G., & Todarello, O. (2003). Alexithymia as predictor of treatment outcome in patients with functional gastrointestinal disorders. *Psychosomatic Medicine, 65*(5), 911–918.

Rabe-Jablonska, J. J., & Tomasz, M. (2000). The links between body dysmorphic disorder and eating disorders. *European Psychiatry, 15*(5), 302–305.

Roelofs, K.., Keijsers, G. P., Hoogduin, K. A., Naring, G. W., & Moene, F. C. (2002). Childhood abuse in patients with conversion disorders. *American Journal of Psychiatry, 159*(11), 1908–1913.

Schneider, G., Wachter, M., Driesch, G., Kruse, A., Nehen, H. G., & Heuft, G. (2003). Subjective body complaint as an indicator of somatization in elderly patients. *Psychosomatics, 44*(2), 91–99.

Sheehan, B., and Banerjee, S. (1999). Review: Somatization in the elderly. *International Journal of Psychiatry, 14,* 1044–1049.

Sobanski, E., & Schmidt, M. H. (2000). 'Everybody looks at my pubic bone'—A case report of an adolescent patient with body dysmorphic disorder. *Acta Psychiatrica Scandinavica, 101,* 80–82.

Soltis-Jarrett, V. (2005). Assessing and managing medically unexplained physical symptoms in women: Providing "H.O.P.I.," An innovative protocol and treatment program. Poster Presentation. International Psychiatric-Mental Health Nurses Association, Denver, Colorado, April 7, 2006.

Stein, M. B., Lang, A. J., Laffaye, C., Satz, L. E., Lenox, R. J., & Dresselhaus, T. R. (2004). Relationship of sexual assault history to somatic symptoms and health anxiety in women. *General Hospital Psychiatry, 26*(3), 178–183.

Uzun, O., Basoglu, C., Akar, A., Cansever, A., Ozsahin, A., Cetil, M., & Ebrinc, S. (2003). Body dysmorphic disorder in patients with acne. *Comprehensive Psychiatry, 44*(5), 415–419.

Walker, J., Vincent, N., Furer, P., Cox, B., & Kjemisted, K. (1999). Treatment preference in hypochondriasis. *Journal of Behavior Therapy & Experimental Psychiatry, 30*(4), 251–258.

Waller, E., & Scheidt, C. E. (2006). Somatoform disorders as disorders of affect regulation: a development perspective. *International Review of Psychiatry 18*(1), 13–24.

Whitehead, W. E., Palsson, O., & Jones, K. R. (2002). Systematic review of the comorbidity of irritable bowel syndrome with other disorders: What are the causes and implications? *Gastroenterology, 122*(4), 1140–1156.

Wise, T. N., Arnold, L. M., & Maletic, V. (2005). Management of painful physical symptoms associated with depression and mood disorders. *CNS Spectrum, 10*(12, Suppl 19), 1–13.

Yates, W. R. (2002). Somatoform disorders. Retrieved on June 10, 2003, from www.emedicing. com/MED/topic3527.htm.

Young, J. (2003). Mind-body concepts and mental illness: a study of Japanese values. *Seishin Shinkeigaku Zasshi, 105*(8), 1016–1025.

CHAPTER 24

Eating Disorders

Jane H. White

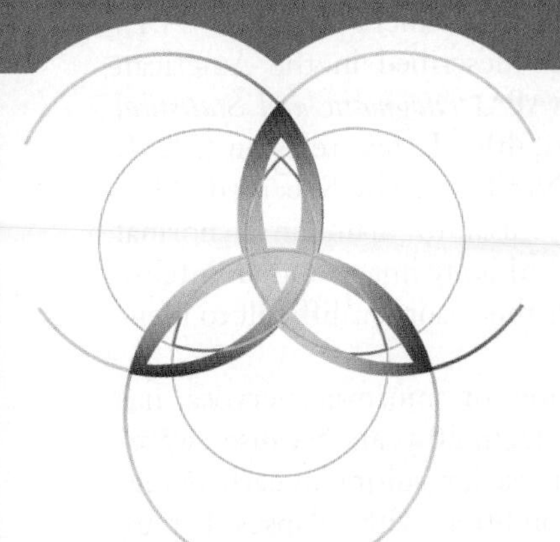

KEY CONCEPTS

- body dissatisfaction
- body image distortion
- dietary restraint
- drive for thinness
- enmeshment
- interoceptive awareness
- sexuality fears

LEARNING OBJECTIVES

After studying this chapter, you will be able to:

- Distinguish the signs and symptoms of anorexia nervosa from those of bulimia nervosa.
- Describe two etiologic theories of both anorexia nervosa and bulimia nervosa.
- Explain the importance of body image, body dissatisfaction, and gender identity in developmental theories that explain etiology of eating disorders.
- Describe the neurobiology and neurochemistry in both anorexia nervosa and bulimia nervosa.
- Explain the impact of sociocultural norms on the development of eating disorders.
- Describe the risk factors and protective factors associated with the development of eating disorders.
- Formulate the nursing diagnoses for individuals with eating disorders.
- Describe the nursing interventions for individuals with anorexia nervosa and bulimia nervosa.
- Differentiate binge eating disorder from bulimia nervosa.
- Analyze special concerns within the nurse–patient relationship for the nursing care of individuals with eating disorders.
- Identify strategies for prevention and early detection of eating disorders.

KEY TERMS

• anorexia nervosa • binge eating • binge eating disorder •body image • bulimia nervosa • cue elimination • self-monitoring

Only since the 1970s have eating disorders received national attention, primarily because several high-profile personalities and athletes with these disorders have received front-page news coverage. Since the 1960s, the increased incidence of anorexia nervosa and bulimia nervosa has prompted mental health professionals to address their causes and devise effective treatments. Moreover, there has been a concomitant increase in research studies addressing this intense obsession with being thin and the dissatisfaction with one's body that underlie these potentially life-threatening disorders. Thus, mental health professionals are crucial to prevention, early diagnosis, and treatment of both anorexia nervosa and bulimia nervosa.

This chapter focuses on anorexia nervosa and bulimia nervosa. In addition, binge eating disorder (BED), a newly identified eating disorder in its infancy relative to research, is briefly considered in this chapter. Symptoms of these disorders, such as dieting, binge eating, and preoccupation with weight and shape, overlap significantly. Experts view these symptoms along a continuum of normal to pathologic eating behaviors (White, 2000a) (Fig. 24.1), an approach that helps to identify subclinical or subthreshold cases. Many individuals with anorexia ner-

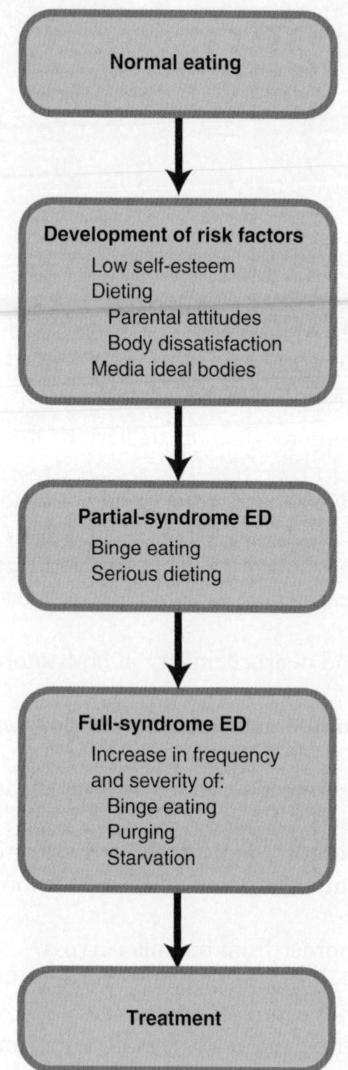

FIGURE 24.1. Progression of Symptoms Leading to an Eating Disorder (ED).

vosa have bulimic symptoms, and many with bulimia nervosa have anorexic symptoms. For this reason, types of anorexia, such as the purging type, and types of bulimia, such as the restricting type, are differentiated based on the predominant symptom the individual uses to restrict food and weight gain. These disorders differ in definition, clinical course, etiologies, and interventions and will be considered separately in this chapter. However, because their risk factors and prevention strategies are similar, they will be discussed together, when considering these two topics.

ANOREXIA NERVOSA

Clinical Course

The onset of **anorexia nervosa** is usually in early adolescence. Onset can be slow, in that serious dieting may be present long before an emaciated body—the result of starvation—is noticed. This discovery often prompts diagnosis. Because the incidence of subclinical or partial-syndrome cases, in which the symptoms are not severe enough to use an anorexia nervosa diagnosis, is higher than that of anorexia nervosa, many young women may not receive early treatment for their symptoms, or in some cases, they receive no treatment (see Fig. 24.1). Partial-syndrome cases are described in the American Psychiatric Association's (APA) *Diagnostic and Statistical Manual of Mental Disorders*, 4th ed., text revision (*DSM-IV-TR*), Eating Disorder Not Otherwise Specified (APA, 2000). The individual's refusal to maintain a normal weight because of a distorted body image and an intense fear of becoming fat makes this disorder difficult to identify and treat.

The long-term outcome of anorexia nervosa has improved during the past 15 to 20 years because awareness of the disease has increased, resulting in early detection. It can be a chronic condition, with relapses that are usually characterized by significant weight loss. However, unlike most mental illnesses, eating disorders are curable (Anderson, 2001). Reporting conclusive outcomes for anorexia nervosa is difficult because of the variety of definitions used to determine recovery. Although patients considered to have recovered have restored normal weight, menses, and eating behaviors, some continue to have distorted body images and be preoccupied with weight and food, many develop bulimia nervosa, and many continue to have symptoms of other psychiatric illnesses. Conclusions from a review of 119 outcome studies revealed that, on average, less than half of patients recovered (Steinhausen, 2002). In these and other studies, about 10% to 25% of patients go on to experience bulimia nervosa (White, 2000b). A poor outcome has been related to an initial lower minimum weight, the presence of purging (vomiting), and a later age of onset.

FAME AND FORTUNE

Karen Carpenter (1950–1983):
An American Musician

Public Persona

Karen Carpenter and her brother were the #1 best-selling American recording artists and performing musicians of the 1970s. In the United States alone, the Carpenters had eight gold albums, five platinum albums, and 10 gold single recordings—all proof of significant professional success.

Personal Realities

In everyday life, however, Karen Carpenter battled with anorexia nervosa for 7 years—starving herself, using laxatives, drinking water, taking dozens of thyroid pills, and purging. Just as she was beginning to overcome the disorder, she died of complications at the age of 32.

Diagnostic Criteria

The diagnostic criteria for anorexia nervosa have been refined in each edition of the *Diagnostic and Statistical Manual for Mental Disorders* (APA, 2000). Research on core symptoms has resulted in very specific criteria (Table 24.1). Originally, the central feature of the disorder was thought to be a distorted body image (Bruch, 1973). Although body image distortion remains an important criterion, recent investigators have highlighted a drive for thinness, perfectionism, and a fear of becoming fat as most essential to diagnosis (Wiederman & Pryor, 2000). Recent refinements to diagnostic criteria have included weight loss of 25 pounds and absence of menses for at least 3 consecutive months or periods (APA, 2000). Box 24.1 lists the common psychological characteristics of eating disorders.

BOX 24.1

Psychological Characteristics Related to Eating Disorders

Anorexia Nervosa	Anorexia Nervosa and Bulimia Nervosa
Decreased interoceptive awareness	Difficulty expressing anger
Sexuality conflict/fears	Low self-esteem
Maturity fears	Body dissatisfaction
Ritualistic behaviors	Powerlessness
	Ineffectiveness
Bulimia Nervosa	Perfectionism
Impulsivity	Dietary restraint
Boundary problems	Obsessiveness
Limit-setting difficulties	Compulsiveness
	Nonassertiveness
	Cognitive distortions

Table 24.1  **Key Diagnostic Characteristics for Anorexia Nervosa** 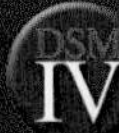

Diagnostic Criteria	Target Symptoms and Associated Findings
• Refusal to maintain body weight at or above a minimally normal weight for age and height • Intense fear of gaining weight or becoming fat, even though underweight • Disturbance in way person experiences body shape or weight • Undue influence of body weight or shape on self-evaluation or denial of seriousness of current low body weight • Absence of at least three consecutive menstrual cycles (in postmenarchal females) • Restricting type: not regularly engaged in binge eating or purging behavior (such as self-induced vomiting or misuse of laxatives, diuretics, or enemas) • Binge eating and purging type: regularly engaging in binge eating or purging behavior	• Depressive symptoms such as depressed mood, social withdrawal, irritability, insomnia, and diminished interest in sex • Obsessive-compulsive features related and unrelated to food • Preoccupation with thought of food • Concerns about eating in public • Feelings of ineffectiveness • Strong need to control one's environment • Inflexible thinking • Limited social spontaneity and overly restrained initiative and emotional expression ***Associated Physical Examination Findings*** • Complaints of constipation, abdominal pain • Cold intolerance • Lethargy and excess energy • Emaciation • Significant hypotension, hypothermia, and skin dryness • Bradycardia and possible peripheral edema • Hypertrophy of salivary glands, particularly the parotid gland • Dental enamel erosion related to induced vomiting • Scars or calluses on dorsum of hand from contact with teeth for inducing vomiting ***Associated Laboratory Findings*** • Leukopenia and mild anemia • Elevated blood urea nitrogen • Hypercholesterolemia • Elevated liver function studies • Electrolyte imbalances, metabolic alkalosis, or metabolic acidosis • Low normal serum thyroxine levels; decreased serum-triiodothyronine levels • Low serum estrogen levels • Sinus bradycardia • Metabolic encephalopathy • Significantly reduced resting energy expenditure • Increased ventricular/brain ratio secondary to starvation

Anorexia nervosa is further categorized into two major types: restricting and purging. We now understand more clearly that many of the clinical features associated with anorexia nervosa may result from malnutrition or semistarvation. For example, classic research on volunteers who have been semistarved and observations of prisoners of war and conscientious objectors has demonstrated that these states are characterized by symptoms of food preoccupation, binge eating, depression, obsession, and apathy. Drastic measures to resist overeating persist long after the semistarvation experience, even when food is plentiful. Table 24.2 presents the medical complications, signs, and symptoms of eating disorders that result from starving or binge eating and purging. Many somatic systems are compromised in individuals with eating disorders.

KEY CONCEPT Body image distortion occurs when the individual perceives his or her body disparately from how the world or society views it.

For adolescents, body image is important because it has a complex psychological impact on overall self-concept and is a crucial factor in determining how adolescents interact with others and think society will respond to them. For most individuals, body image is consistent with how others view them. However, those with anorexia nervosa have a body image severely distorted from reality. Because of this distortion, they see themselves as obese and undesirable, even when they are emaciated. They are unable to accept objective reality and the perceptions of the outside world. Perceptions, attitudes, and behaviors are all part of this disturbance. **Body image** refers to a mental picture of one's own body. Body image disturbance occurs when there is extreme discrepancy between one's own mental picture of his or her body and the perception of the outside world.

Because of this distortion, individuals with anorexia nervosa have an intense drive for thinness. They see themselves as fat, fear becoming fatter, and are "driven" to work toward "undoing" this fear.

KEY CONCEPT Drive for thinness is an intense physical and emotional process that overrides all physiologic body cues.

The individual with anorexia nervosa ignores body cues, such as hunger and weakness, and concentrates all efforts on controlling food intake. The entire mental focus of the young patient with anorexia nervosa narrows to only one goal: weight loss. Typical thought patterns are: "If I gain a pound, I'll keep gaining." This all-or-

Table 24.2 Complications of Eating Disorders

Body System	Symptoms
From Starvation to Weight Loss	
Musculoskeletal	Loss of muscle mass, loss of fat (emaciation) Osteoporosis
Metabolic	Hypothyroidism (symptoms include lack of energy, weakness, intolerance to cold, and bradycardia) Hypoglycemia, decreased insulin sensitivity
Cardiac	Bradycardia, hypotension, loss of cardiac muscle, small heart, cardiac arrhythmias including atrial and ventricular premature contractions, prolonged QT interval, ventricular tachycardia, sudden death
Gastrointestinal	Delayed gastric emptying, bloating, constipation, abdominal pain, gas, diarrhea
Reproductive	Amenorrhea, low levels of luteinizing hormone and follicle-stimulating hormone, irregular periods
Dermatologic	Dry, cracking skin and brittle nails due to dehydration, lanugo (fine baby-like hair over body), edema, acrocyanosis (bluish hands and feet); hair thinning
Hematologic	Leukopenia, anemia, thrombocytopenia, hypercholesterolemia, hypercarotenemia
Neuropsychiatric	Abnormal taste sensation (possible zinc deficiency) Apathetic depression, mild organic mental symptoms, sleep disturbances, fatigue
Related to Purging (Vomiting and Laxative Abuse)	
Metabolic	Electrolyte abnormalities, particularly hypokalemia, hypochloremic alkalosis; hypomagnesemia; increased blood urea nitrogen
Gastrointestinal	Salivary gland and pancreatic inflammation and enlargement with increase in serum amylase; esophageal and gastric erosion (esophagitis) rupture; dysfunctional bowel with haustral dilation; superior mesenteric artery syndrome
Dental	Erosion of dental enamel (perimyolysis), particularly frontal teeth with decreased decay
Neuropsychiatric	Seizures (related to large fluid shifts and electrolyte disturbances), mild neuropathies, fatigue, weakness, mild organic mental symptoms
Cardiac	Ipecac cardiomyopathy arrhythmias

nothing thinking keeps these patients on rigid regimens for weight loss.

The behavior of patients with anorexia nervosa becomes organized around food-related activities, such as preparing food, counting calories, and reading cookbooks. Much behavior concerning what, when, and how they eat is ritualistic. Food combinations and the order in which foods may be eaten, and under which circumstances, can seem bizarre. One patient, for example, would eat only cantaloupe, carrying it with her to all meals outside of her home, and consuming it only if it were cut in smaller than bite-sized pieces and only if she could use chopsticks, which she also carried with her.

Feelings of inadequacy and a fear of maturity are also characteristic of the individual with anorexia nervosa. Weight loss becomes a way for these individuals to experience some sense of control and combat feelings of inadequacy and ineffectiveness. Every lost pound is viewed as a success, and weight loss often confers a feeling of virtuousness. Because these individuals feel inadequate, they fear emotional maturation and the unknown challenges the next developmental stages will bring. For some, remaining physically small is believed to symbolize remaining childlike. Perfectionism has today become a more significantly researched issue in individuals who develop anorexia nervosa and is especially predictive of the development of this disorder in athletes (Ferrand & Brunet, 2004; Hinton & Kubas, 2005). Patients with anorexia nervosa also have difficulty defining feelings because they are confused about or unsure of emotions and visceral cues, such as hunger. This uncertainty is called a lack of interoceptive awareness.

KEY CONCEPT Interoceptive awareness is a term used to describe the sensory response to emotional and visceral cues, such as hunger.

Patients with anorexia nervosa are confused about sensations; therefore, their responses to cues are inaccurate and inappropriate. Often they cannot name feelings they are experiencing, such as anxiety. This profound lack of interoceptive awareness is thought to be partially responsible for developing and maintaining this disorder and some instances of bulimia nervosa.

In addition, patients with anorexia nervosa avoid conflict and have difficulty expressing negative emotions, especially anger (Geller, Cockell, & Goldner, 2000). They have an overwhelming sense of guilt. Whereas anger and conflict avoidance are also common in the families of people with this disorder, a sense of guilt is usually not found in the parents (Berghold & Lock, 2002).

Because of the ritualistic behaviors, all-encompassing focus on food and weight, and feelings of inadequacy that accompany anorexia nervosa, social contacts are gradually reduced, and the patient becomes isolated. With more severe weight loss comes other symptoms, such as apathy, depression, and even mistrust of others.

Epidemiology

In this country, the lifetime prevalence of anorexia nervosa is reported to be from 0.5% to 1%. Anorexia nervosa is less common than bulimia nervosa. A similar prevalence is found in most Westernized countries; the disorder is also more prevalent within U.S. ethnic minorities and those in other countries than previously recognized. Cultural change itself, such as moving to a society such as the United States, may be associated with increased vulnerability to eating disorders, especially when values about physical aesthetics are involved. Ethnic groups of women who are not vulnerable to developing eating disorders have not internalized a thin body as ideal, common in adolescents raised in the United States, and are not dissatisfied with their bodies (Warren et al., 2005). The incidence (new cases) for anorexia nervosa have remained the same during the past decade despite prevention and early intervention efforts, leading some to speculate on the biologic/genetic predisposition for the development of anorexia nervosa (Currin, Schmidt, Treasure & Jick, 2005).

Age of Onset

The age of onset is typically between 14 and 16 years. Some experts have reported an even earlier age of onset. Adolescents are vulnerable because of stressors associated with their development, especially concerns about body image, autonomy, and peer pressure, and their susceptibility to such influences as the media, which extols an ideal body type. An important predictor of anorexia nervosa is early onset menses, as early as 10 or 11 years of age.

Gender Differences

Females are 10 times more likely than males to develop anorexia nervosa. This disparity has been attributed to society's influence on females to achieve an ideal body type. Box 24.2 highlights some of the findings about eating disorders in males.

Ethnic and Cultural Differences

In the United States, eating disorders are slightly more common among Hispanic and Caucasian populations and less common among African Americans and Asians (Bisaga et al., 2005, Streigel-Moore et al., 2003). In the past 15 to 20 years, the incidence among various ethnic groups has increased. Contextual variables that may influence eating disorders in women of color are level of acculturation, socioeconomic status, peer social-

BOX 24.2

Boys and Men With Eating Disorders

Eating disorders in boys and men are becoming more prevalent. Men are more likely to have a later onset than women, and at around age 20.5 years. Boys and men are also more likely to be involved in an occupation or sport in which weight control influences performance, such as wrestling or sports in which low body fat would be advantageous (Baum, 2006).

Men with anorexia nervosa of the restricting type were found to have lower testosterone levels. In studies comparing men and women on psychological characteristics, men had lower drive for thinness and body dissatisfaction scores, but higher perfectionism scores (Joiner, Katz, & Heatherton, 2000).

In another investigation, predictors of binge eating were different for men compared with women. Anger and depression preceded binges in men, whereas dieting failure was the most significant predictor of a binge in women (Costanzo et al., 1999). Men and women did not differ with regard to comorbid conditions, such as depression and substance abuse, but had less reported sexual abuse than did women with eating disorders. In one study, men had prevalence ratios similar to those of women when partial syndrome cases were considered (Woodside et al., 2001). This supports the idea that eating disorders may go undiagnosed in males, and seem much higher in women than they actually are.

ization, family structure, and immigration status (Kuba & Harris, 2001).

Familial Predisposition 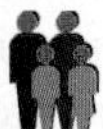

First-degree relatives of people with anorexia nervosa have higher rates of this disorder. Rates of partial syndrome or subthreshold cases among female family members of individuals with anorexia nervosa are even higher (Strober, Pataki, Freeman, & DeAntonio, 2000). Female relatives also have high rates of depression, leading researchers to hypothesize a shared genetic factor may influence development of both disorders. Twin studies have also demonstrated a shared transmission of eating disorders and anxiety disorders; however, the nature of this shared diathesis remains unknown (Keel, Klump, et al., 2005).

Comorbidity

Depression is common in individuals with anorexia nervosa, and these individuals are at risk to attempt suicide (Franko et al., 2004). However, anxiety disorders such as obsessive-compulsive disorder (OCD), phobias, and panic disorder are even more strongly associated with anorexia nervosa (Kaye et al., 2004). In many individuals with anorexia nervosa, OCD symptoms predate the anorexia nervosa diagnosis by about 5 years, leading many researchers to consider OCD a causative or risk factor for anorexia nervosa (Anderluh et al., 2003; Milos et al., 2002). These comorbid conditions often resolve when anorexia nervosa has been treated successfully. In other cases, symptoms of a premorbid condition, such as OCD, remain even though an individual has recovered from anorexia nervosa. This finding has influenced many experts to believe that many of the characteristics of anorexia nervosa, such as perfectionism and making sure that everything is symmetrical or that objects are placed the same distance from each other and the like (symmetry-seeking) are trait, rather than state, characteristics and may actually influence the development of the disorder.

Etiology

Some of the risk factors and the etiologic factors for eating disorders overlap. For example, dieting is a risk factor for the development of anorexia nervosa, but it is also a biologic etiologic factor, and in its most serious form—starving—it is also a symptom. This overlap of risk factors, causes, and symptoms must be kept in mind. Viewing them along a continuum from less to more severe helps with this conceptualization (see Fig. 24.1). Most experts agree that anorexia nervosa (as well as bulimia nervosa) is multidimensional and multidetermined. Figure 24.2 depicts the biopsychosocial etiologic factors for anorexia nervosa.

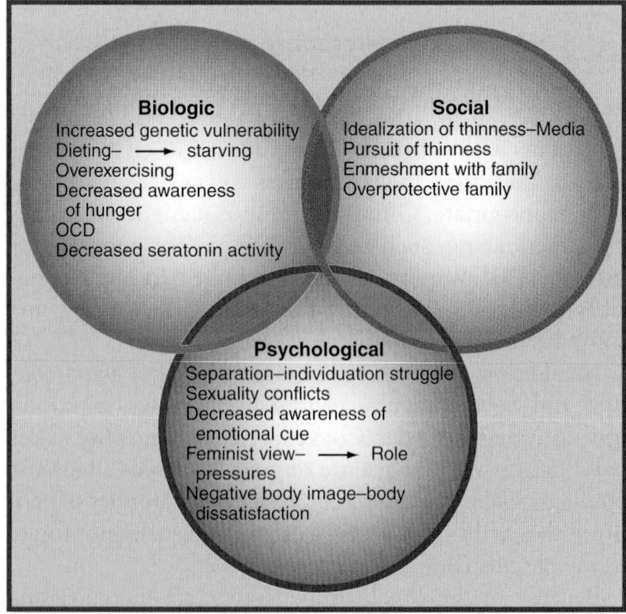

FIGURE 24.2. Biopsychosocial etiologies for patients with anorexia nervosa.

Biologic Theories

Over the past three decades, most of what was researched about the etiology of anorexia nervosa has been focused on psychological factors. However, recently studies using brain imaging have resulted in important information that may refocus the etiology of anorexia nervosa. Studies that have been undertaken show brain gray and white matter volume loss during the ill state of anorexia nervosa and that this remits with recovery. However, studies have also shown that some disturbances, such as neuroreceptor dynamics, regional blood flow, and cerebral glucose metabolism, are activated in the presence of food and body image distortions, shedding some light on the etiology of these features. The fact that these biologic disturbances persist after recovery from anorexia nervosa supports the hypothesis that brain changes are actually traits that may create a vulnerability to the development of eating disorders (Frank et al., 2004). The biopsychosocial model of this interaction best explains the etiology (see Fig. 24.2).

Neuropathologic Theories

Studies have implicated cingulate, frontal, temporal, and parietal regions in anorexia nervosa. Challenges, such as providing the stimulus of food or body images, have been shown to activate some of these regions (see above), raising the possibility of further explanation for the development of body image distortions from other than a cultural or psychological perspective. In a study in which women with eating disorders and those without were presented shapes of women's bodies (underweight, overweight, and normal), those with eating disorders rated the body shapes in all three weight categories as more aversive than did the normal group, and their ratings correlated positively with activity in the right medial apical prefrontal cortex (Uher et al., 2005).

Genetic Theories

Genetic research on eating disorders is in its infancy. Beginning evidence suggests that a specific gene influences anorexia nervosa. However, the existence of comorbid conditions makes it difficult to determine the influence of genetics on anorexia nervosa. Separating genetic influences from environmental influences when twins share a similar family environment is difficult, but investigators reviewing data from twin studies recently demonstrated that the concordance rate for monozygotic twins is higher (44%) than for dizygotic twins (12.5%). Thus, a genetic factor may be involved in the etiology of anorexia nervosa (Bulik et al., 2003).

However, as noted earlier in this chapter, other studies have highlighted a shared genetic transmission of eating disorders and anxiety disorders (Keel et al., 2005). Again, this leads to a conclusion that there may be a shared familial predisposition to the development of an eating disorder.

Biochemical Theories

Studies of neuroendocrine, neuropeptide, vasopressin, oxytocin, and neurotransmitter functioning in patients with eating disorders indicate that these systems may be related to maintaining anorexia nervosa. Endogenous opioids may contribute to denial of hunger in patients with the disorder. Some studies have shown weight gain after patients received opiate antagonists. Thyroid function is also decreased in patients with this disorder. Studies demonstrated that reduced 5-HT (1A) (serotonin pathways) is evident during the illness and the recovery in anorexia nervosa (Frank et al., 2004; Kaye et al., 2005). There is therefore beginning evidence regarding one biologic theory of causation. However, some of the difficulty in drawing definitive conclusions stems from the many comorbid conditions, such as depression and OCD, associated with a diagnosis of anorexia nervosa, which some researchers view as having a shared etiology or risk factor because of a similar serotonergic pathway. Earlier research had theorized that these neurotransmitter and neuroendocrine abnormalities, such as blunted serotonergic function in low-weight patients, were state related and tended to normalize after symptom remission and weight gain (Bailer & Kaye, 2003). Further supporting this relationship to weight loss, a recent study of women with both anorexia nervosa and bulimia nervosa demonstrated a significantly reduced brain-derived neurotrophic factor (BDNF) when compared to healthy women. All of these individuals were malnourished; the reduction of BDNF reduction may represent an adaptive change to counteract the decreased caloric ingestion of women with anorexia nervosa or bulimia nervosa (Monteleone et al., 2005). Thus, currently, until more definitive research is done, these neurochemical neurotransmitter changes should be viewed as indicating a vulnerability in some individuals, who under certain psychological and environmental conditions, such as cultural pressures, starve themselves. Further studies will need to sort out the comorbid brain chemistry findings to establish a firm neurotransmitter etiology for eating disorders.

Psychological Theories

To date, the most widely accepted psychological theory of anorexia nervosa is psychoanalytic. In this theory, key tasks of separation-individuation and autonomy are interrupted. Struggles around identity and role, body image formation, and sexuality fears predominate as a result of developmental arrests.

Because anorexia nervosa is usually diagnosed between 14 and 18 years of age, developmental struggles of adolescence have long been an acceptable theory of causation (Bruch, 1973). Two key conflicts for this age group are autonomy and separation-individuation.

During early adolescence, when individuals begin to establish their independence and autonomy, some girls may feel inadequate or ineffective. They may grow up in families in which they have not had an opportunity to "try out" independence. Thus, dieting and weight control are viewed as a means to defend against these feelings. In later adolescence, when separation-individuation is a developmental task, similar conflicts arise when the adolescent is ill prepared for this stage and feels inadequate and ineffective in going forward emotionally.

Gender identity has been hypothesized to explain the significant difference between the numbers of girls and boys who experience anorexia nervosa and bulimia nervosa. Studies have shown that girls and boys do not differ dramatically in self-esteem until just before adolescence. At the time self-doubt increases in girls, pubertal weight gain can also occur, resulting in a more rounded shape. Thus, normal occurrences can add to confusion about one's identity. Other researchers believe that confusion and self-doubt are aided by conflicting messages that young women receive from society about their roles in life. Young girls may interpret expectations about how they should look, what roles they should perform, and what they should achieve in society as pressures to achieve "all." Young women who aspire to their interpretation of these expectations often try to please others to avoid conflicts around perceived expectations. Feminists have focused on this role pressure as one part of an explanation for the significant increase in eating disorders and for the greater prevalence in females. Box 24.3 outlines some feminist assumptions regarding role, feminism, and the development of eating disorders.

BOX 24.3

Feminist Ideology and Eating Disorders

Since the 1970s, proponents of the feminist cultural model of eating disorders have advanced a position to explain the higher prevalence of these disorders in women. Feminists believe there is a struggle women have today similar to ones they believe women have had in history. They believe that during the Victorian era, "hysteria," a well-known emotional illness, developed as a result of oppression when women were not allowed to express their feelings and opinions and were "silenced" by a male-dominated society. Feminist scholars claim that women today are socialized to avoid self-expression in the face of conflict, seek attachment through putting others first, judge self by external standards, and present an outward compliant self while the inner self grows angry. They believe that the development of an eating disorder is a reaction against these expectations and norms of society (Gutwill, 1994).

Feminists have taken issue with what they call the biomedical model of explanation for the development of eating disorders, seeing it as limiting and patriarchal. It is the recovery of society that must take place to decrease the prevalence of eating disorders. Feminists believe that this will occur only when women are emancipated, given a voice, and socialized differently. They call for more research in which women are coresearchers as well as "subjects," helping to provide the investigators with their own stories and perspectives.

KEY CONCEPT Sexuality fears are often underlying issues for patients with anorexia nervosa. Starvation is viewed as a response to these fears.

In girls, anorexia nervosa usually develops during adolescence, when dating begins. Girls usually experience dating as more stressful than boys do because intimacy is more important to girls. Thus, they tend to attribute the failure of a relationship to an inadequacy in themselves (Streigel-Moore, 1993). During the past several years, girls have become involved sexually at increasingly younger ages. Although they are often ill prepared, they can experience a great deal of pressure from peers to do so. Parents may be unprepared to address sexual activity with daughters at younger ages than expected. If parents are not available to help with decisions, anxiety about them can increase. Bruch (1973) has described self-starvation as the adolescent girl's response to her fear of adult sexuality. Sexual anxieties may promote binge eating as well.

Social Theories

More than with any other psychiatric condition, society plays a significant role in the development of eating disorders. Theories about social norms and expectations explain some of the causes of eating disorders (Brumberg, 1988). The media, the fashion industry, and peer pressure are significant social influences. Magazines and television shows depict young girls and adolescents, with thin and often emaciated bodies, as glamorous. Girls diet because they want to be like these models both in character and appearance. Two of the most common adolescent dieting methods—restricting calories and taking diet pills—have been shown to be influenced by women's beauty and fashion magazines (Thomsen, Weber, & Brown, 2002). A significant study from the 1990s showed that for young girls, dolls such as Barbie negatively influenced their views of normal body types (Brownell & Napolitano, 1995) (see Box 24.4). In addition, many types of media discuss dieting and exercise as ways to achieve success, popularity, power, and the like. Comparing one's own body to the bodies of models produces significant body dissatisfaction, a key characteristic associated with

BOX 24.4

Research for Best Practice: ***Barbie® and Ken®***

Brownell, K., & Napolitano, M. A. (1995). Distorting reality for children: Body size proportions for Barbie and Ken dolls. International Journal of Eating Disorders, 18, 295–298.

The Question: A great deal of research has focused on ideal body types and how these affect American women such as Miss America contestants. This study was designed to examine body proportions in popular dolls, Barbie® and Ken®, to determine the extent to which they vary from the proportions of young, healthy adults.

Methods: Hip, waist, chest, neck length and circumference measurements were taken on men and women, aged 22 to 32 years of normal weight and average height. The same measurements were made on Barbie and Ken dolls, and a ratio of the measurements of the real subjects to doll figures was calculated. The ratio was then applied to estimate changes needed for the subjects to have the same proportional measurements as the dolls.

Findings: The researchers found that for the female subject to attain Barbie's proportions, there would have to be an increase in 24 inches in height, 5 inches in the chest, and 2 to 3 inches in neck length and a decrease of 6 inches in the waist and 0.2 inches in the neck circumference. For the male subject to attain Ken's proportions, he would require increases in height by 20 inches, waist by 10 inches, chest by 11 inches, and neck length by 0.85 inches. The neck circumference for the male would need to increase 7.9 inches.

The results of this study provide more evidence that individuals are exposed to highly unrealistic models for shape and weight. Although Barbie and Ken dolls are not meant to show ideal proportions, the discrepancies are obvious. Healthy, normal-weight children use such models as standards for comparison, leading logically to an outcome of body dissatisfaction.

Implications for Nursing: The findings from this study can be used to assist parents in choosing appropriate models for dolls for children. This research also provides a basis for helping women with eating disorders understand how subtle environmental cues influence the formulation of their ideal body types at an early age.

dieting, low self-esteem, and development of an eating disorder.

KEY CONCEPT In body dissatisfaction, the body becomes overvalued as a way of determining one's worth. Particularly for women with bulimia nervosa, body dissatisfaction has been related to low self-esteem, depression, dieting, bingeing, and purging.

Once the body is considered all-important, the individual begins to compare her body with others, such as those of celebrities. Images from television and fashion magazines are particularly powerful for young girls and adolescents struggling with the tasks of identity and body image formation (Andrist, 2003). Body dissatisfaction resulting from this comparison, in which one's own body is perceived to fall short of an ideal, may be dissatisfaction about one's weight, shape, size, or even a certain body part. Even in the absence of overweight, most adolescents surveyed in numerous studies were dissatisfied with their bodies. Many adolescents act to overcome this dissatisfaction through dieting and overexercising. In a recent study, college women correlated figures that they viewed as overweight with unhappiness and those in the study with eating disorder symptoms had a higher correlation of these two study variables (Viken et al., 2005). In those who have other risk factors and are thus more vulnerable, eating disorder symptoms may develop.

Teasing abut weight has also been linked to the development of eating disorders, especially bulimia. In a recent study of overweight and nonoverweight children 10 to 14 years of age, teasing for the overweight group was associated with bulimic behaviors. For the total group, teasing resulted in higher weight concerns, more loneliness, poorer self-perception of one's physical appearance, higher preference for sedentary/isolative activities, and lower preference for active/social activities (Hayden-Wade et al., 2005).

Family Responses 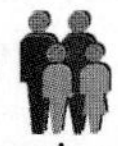

The family of the patient with anorexia has classically been labeled as overprotective, enmeshed, being unable to resolve conflicts, and being rigid regarding boundaries.

KEY CONCEPT Enmeshment refers to an extreme form of intensity in family interactions.

Changes between two family members reverberate through the whole family system. Direct communication is blocked, and one member relays communication from another to a third. In an enmeshed family, the individual gets lost in the system. The boundaries that define individual autonomy are weak. This excessive togetherness intrudes on privacy (Minuchin, Rossman, & Baker, 1978).

Overprotectiveness is defined as a high degree of concern for one another. The parents' overprotectiveness retards the child's development of autonomy and competence (Minuchin et al., 1978). *Rigidity* refers to families who are heavily committed to maintain the status quo and find change difficult. Conflict is avoided, and a strong ethical code or religious orientation is usually the rationale. Today, more is known to amplify this original understanding of the family's impact on the development of anorexia nervosa (see Box 24.5). In summary, no one etiologic factor is predominant in the development of

BOX 24.5

Research for Best Practice: Mothers and Daughters and Weight Concerns

Ogden, J., & Steward, J. (2000). The role of the mother–daughter relationship in explaining weight concern. International Journal of Eating Disorders, 28(11), 78–83.

The Question: The literature highlights two different possible roles for the mother–daughter relationship and how these roles influence the development of weight concerns measured by dietary restraint and body dissatisfaction. The first role is simply the mother's own modeling of her concerns about her weight; the second model influencing weight concerns that was tested is the actual interaction between mothers and daughters.

Methods: Interaction was defined as how autonomous the mother was perceived to be by the daughter, and vice versa, how enmeshed they were emotionally, and the overall view of the mother's role. This study compared the two models of explanation and found no support for the first model, mothers simply being concerned about their own weight and dieting.

Findings: The results showed that high body dissatisfaction and dietary restraint for the daughters were related to the mother's own belief as well as the daughter's view of the mother's low autonomy. When both believed in factors that related to high enmeshment and unclear boundaries, more restraint and body dissatisfaction were found. This study lends support to a complex picture of risk factors in the families of girls who experience eating disorders. Whereas parental attitudes about weight shape and size have been shown to be important influences on body dissatisfaction for girls, modeling autonomy, clear boundaries, and valuing differentiation of family members (nonenmeshment) are also important family functions and tasks.

Implications for Nursing: Assessment of parents and the family before providing psychoeducation should include questions related to whether boundaries are clear and whether members are autonomous or enmeshed.

anorexia nervosa. Biopsychosocial factors converge to contribute to its development.

Risk Factors

Risk factors for developing eating disorders are well known. Similar factors put women at risk for both anorexia nervosa and bulimia nervosa. Risk factors are often classified in the same way as the etiologic categories: biologic, psychological, sociocultural, and family (Fig. 24.3).

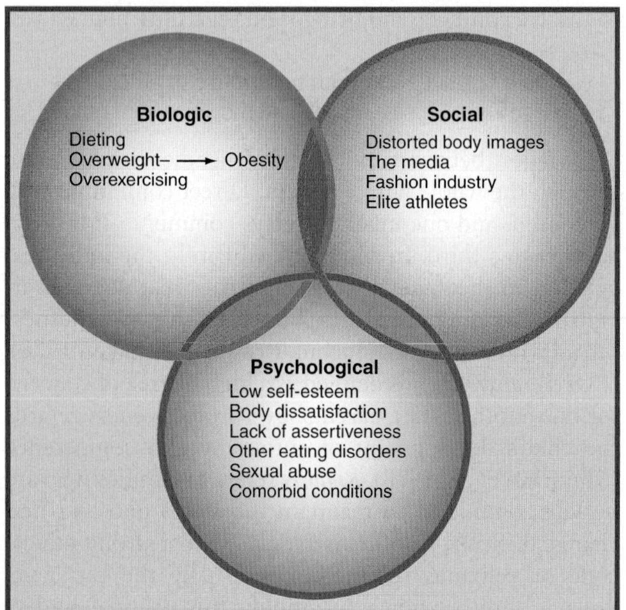

FIGURE 24.3. Biopsychosocial risk factors for anorexia and bulimia nervosa.

Biologic

Dieting despite weight loss or an increase in basal metabolic rate (BMR) are the most significant biologic risk factors studied. Overexercising is also a risk factor. Girls begin to diet at an early age because of body dissatisfaction, a need for control, or a prepubertal weight increase, making both actual weight gain and the fear of weight gain risk factors. In one recent study of nontreatment–seeking overweight children ages 6 to 13, almost 30% of those interviewed and administered the Children's Eating Disorder Examination reported that being overweight preceded dieting and loss of control over eating (Tanofsky-Kraff et al., 2005). Restricting food can lead to starvation, in the case of anorexia nervosa, or to binge eating and purging. A recent large study of high school students (n = 15,349) found that 26% of female students and 10% of males reported abnormal eating and weight control practices in "the last month." Correlates in this study were having an underweight BMI, exercising to control weight, and dieting to control weight as well as weight perception and dissatisfaction. Recently, studies on twins demonstrated evidence that features of perfectionism, a core symptom in anorexia nervosa, may be genetically determined (Tozzi et al., 2004) and thus labeled as a risk factor for its development.

Psychological

Results of numerous studies have shown that low self-esteem, body dissatisfaction, and feelings of ineffectiveness also put individuals at risk for an eating disorder. Much of the recent research on these factors has demonstrated that resilience or protective factors, such as academic achievement, family connectedness, emotional well-being, and positive self-esteem, can mediate these risk factors and prevent development of an eating disorder (Croll, Neumark-Sztainer, Story, & Ireland, 2002). Perfectionism has been highlighted as a significant personality symptom risk factor in eating disorders and studies are underway demonstrating this to be a trait rather than state symptom.

Sociocultural

The media, the fashion industry, and society's focus on the ideal body type are risk factors for eating disorders. In addition, peer pressure and attitudes influence eating behaviors. Some adolescents have reported that dieting, binge eating, and purging were learned behaviors, resulting from peer pressure and a need to conform. Peers and friends, as well as peers in the larger school system, influence unhealthy weight control behaviors among adolescent girls (Eisenberg et al., 2005). In addition, recent research has highlighted another factor that may help to prevent the development of an eating disorder in women who are at risk: women at high risk for developing eating disorders, when exposed to attractive average weight media models, were less likely to endorse thinness and restricting than those high-risk women exposed to thin models (Fister & Smith, 2004).

Athletes are at greater risk for developing eating disorders; perfectionism has been demonstrated to influence this development. The greatest risk factor for disordered eating attitudes for females in a study of swimmers, runners, and soccer players was perfectionism (Hopkinson & Lock, 2004). The female athlete "triad" (symptoms of disordered eating, menstrual dysfunction, and low BMI) has been studied extensively nationally and internationally. In a recent study, both elite (leanness sports such as running and gymnastics) and nonelite athletes (nonleanness sports such as soccer) experienced triad symptoms (Torstveit & Sundgot-Borgen, 2005). Perfectionism is also related to ballet dancers, who are thus at risk. Dancers who exhibit high levels of perfectionism and, perhaps consequently, place themselves in highly competitive environments have been shown to exhibit a significantly increased risk for disordered eating when compared with dancers who are less perfectionistic (Thomas, Keel & Heatherton, 2005). Ballet dancers are also at high risk because of the need to maintain a particular appearance (see Box 24.6).

Family 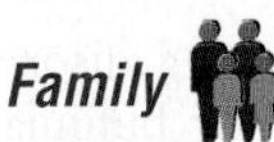

The family, often unwittingly, can transmit unrealistic attitudes about weight, shape, and size. Adolescents are particularly sensitive to comments about their bodies because this is the stage for body image formation. Parental attitudes about weight have been found to influence body dissatisfaction and dieting; parental comments

BOX 24.6

***Research for Best Practice:* Girls and Athletics**

Smolak, L., Murnen, S. K. & Ruble, A. (2000). Female athletes and eating problems: A meta analysis. International Journal of Eating Disorders, 27(4), 371–380.

The Question: Many investigations have highlighted that there are certain groups at risk for eating disorders, such as ballet dancers and gymnasts. Some of these investigations have found conflicting results on which groups are at risk. This is because factors such as the type of sport (e.g., gymnastics), whether the athlete is an elite one, and whether the sport requires a lean look for competition, were considered in only some studies.

Methods: Researchers conducted a comprehensive review and analysis of all of the studies on athletics, dance, and eating disorders symptoms from 1975 to 1999.

Findings: Ballet dancers are one of the most at-risk groups. Contrary to previous assumptions, especially by the popular press, running, swimming, and gymnastics were not as risky as ballet dancing. Although elite versus high school athletes were more at risk than nonathletes, this was not true for elite runners, swimmers, or gymnasts.

Findings from this study are important because healthy athletic competition, which increases confidence, at the middle school and high school level has been shown to be a protective factor in preventing risk factors such as body dissatisfaction from developing into an eating disorder. However, there is a growing body of research on the female athlete triad (amenorrhea, osteoporosis, and disordered eating) especially because of the dramatic increase in women participating in organized sports during the last 30 years. This triad is associated with an imbalance between energy intake and energy expenditure (Golden, 2002). Therefore, the benefits of athletic achievement as a protective factor must be weighed against medical morbidity.

Implications for Nursing: Assessing high-risk groups such as ballet dancers and athletes for the development of eating disorders is important in working in the community and for school health nurses. Nurses can teach parents and adolescents about the value of healthy athletic competition as a protective factor and as a means of intervening in obesity may or may not outweigh potential risks. An accurate assessment of each young woman is important before assuming athletics are "protective."

about weight or shape, or even parents' worrying about their own weight, can influence adolescents in much the same way as the media does. Children of mothers with eating disorders are at risk for developing such disorders, but the degree of risk depends on environmental factors and specific difficulties, such as the child's temperament. In investigations on attitudes, parents of girls with eating disorders were found to have often teased their daughters about their weight, and mothers had overestimated their daughters' weight, but not their sons' (Schwartz, Phares, Tantleff-Dunn, & Thompson, 1999). See Box 24.5 for further information about the role of mother–daughter relationships and body dissatisfaction (Patel, Wheatcroft, Park, & Stein, 2002). Maladaptive paternal behavior, such as low affection, communication, and time spent with a child, has recently been associated with high rates of eating disorders (Johnson, Cohen, Kasen, & Brook, 2002).

Concurrent Disorders

Comorbidity is related to the etiology of eating disorders. Anorexia nervosa puts women at risk for bulimia nervosa. An estimated 25% to 30% of women with anorexia nervosa go on to experience binge eating and purging (White, 2000b). One explanation for this relationship is an incomplete recovery that eventually turns to purging when restricting food intake is no longer effective.

Sexual Abuse

There have been conflicting findings from investigations when the relationship of eating disorders to sexual abuse has been studied. Childhood sexual abuse has often been suggested as a risk factor for eating disorders. Many investigations have supported the notion that, although childhood sexual abuse has occurred in a larger percentage of women with bulimia nervosa than in the general population, this percentage may not be larger than the percentage of women with other psychiatric disorders who have experienced such abuse (Perkins & Luster, 1999). Women with eating disorders who report sexual abuse typically also have comorbid conditions, such as borderline personality disorder and substance abuse disorder (Casper & Lyubomorisky, 1997). Childhood sexual abuse has been viewed as increasing the risk for the development of substance abuse and eating disorder symptoms (Bulik, Prescott, & Kendler, 2001). In a more recent study of girls and boys in the ninth and twelfth grades who reported sexual abuse, there was a significant association between abuse and unhealthy eating behaviors, as well as other symptoms such as a lower self-esteem. Those reporting multiple victimizations had the highest ratio of disordered eating behaviors (Ackard & Neumark-Sztainer, 2003). Although it is unclear how other symptomatology interacts with eating disorder symptoms following abuse, assessing a concurrent history of sexual abuse, and other factors, such as the development of depression must be considered to clarify the nature of this relationship.

Interdisciplinary Treatment

Treatment for the patient with anorexia nervosa focuses on initiating nutritional rehabilitation, resolving conflicts around body image disturbance, increasing effective coping, addressing the underlying conflicts related to maturity fears and role conflict, and assisting the family with healthy functioning and communication. Several methods are used to accomplish these goals during the stages of illness and recovery.

When selecting the type of treatment (i.e., inpatient or outpatient) for anorexia nervosa and bulimia nervosa, clinicians rely on criteria that have been developed to assist them. Typically, the medical complications presented in Table 24.2 influence the decision to hospitalize an individual with an eating disorder. Suicidality is another reason for hospitalization. The criteria for hospital admission are outlined in Table 24.3.

In most instances, a patient with anorexia nervosa must be hospitalized to restore weight. Patients are admitted to a specialized eating disorder unit or program, or to a

Table 24.3 Criteria for Hospitalization of Patients With Eating Disorders

Medical	Psychiatric
• Weight loss, <75% below ideal • Heart rate, <40 beats/min; children <20 beats/min • Temperature, <36°C • Blood pressure, <90/60 mm Hg; children, <80/50 mm Hg • Glucose, <60 mg/dL • Serum potassium, <3 mEq/L • Severe dehydration • Electrolyte imbalance	• Risk for suicide • Severe depression • Failure to comply with treatment • Inadequate response to treatment at another level of care (outpatient)

Adapted from Yoel, J., & Workgroup in Eating Disorders. (2000). Practice guidelines for the treatment of patients with eating disorders. *American Journal of Psychiatry, 157*(1), 1–35.

general psychiatric unit. Because these individuals are often intelligent and engaging and (with the exception of their emaciated state) appear nonimpaired, the severity of the patient's disorder and distress may be underestimated. Particularly in a busy unit where other patients' symptoms of mental illness may be more overt, the needs of patients with eating disorders are at risk for being secondary to those of others because they may be erroneously perceived as less sick (Wolfe & Gimby, 2003). Thus, it is important to remember the high rates of mortality and medical complications among individuals with eating disorders. If the patient's somatic systems are seriously compromised, a medical unit might be the choice for this initial intensive refeeding phase. In most psychiatric units, all members of the team participate in a weight-gain protocol. Dietitians plan this weight-increasing program; physicians, nurses, psychologists, and social workers monitor the refeeding process and its effects on the patient and establish the intensive therapies that must be instituted after the refeeding phase.

The patient's systems must be monitored closely because at the time of admission most patients are severely malnourished (see Table 24.2). Patients usually are placed on a privilege-earning program in which privileges, such as having visitors and receiving passes to go outside the hospital, are earned based on weight gain (see Chapter 10 for a discussion of these programs).

The hospital course goes smoothly at first because the patient with anorexia nervosa resists losing weight. After an acceptable weight (at least 85% of ideal) is established, the patient is discharged to a partial hospitalization program or an intensive outpatient program. The intensive therapies needed to help patients with their underlying issues (e.g., body distortion and maturity fears) and to help families with communication and enmeshment usually begin after refeeding because concentration is usually impaired in the severely undernourished patient with anorexia. Family therapy typically begins while the patient is still hospitalized. Art therapy and psychodrama have been demonstrated to be more effective than traditional group therapy for adolescents with eating disorders, especially during the acute phases of the disease, when the concentration required for verbal therapy may be impaired (Diamond-Raab & Orrell-Valente, 2002).

Pharmacologic Interventions

Research demonstrates that selective serotonin reuptake inhibitors (SSRIs) are not effective for individuals, especially adolescents, who are in the acute phase of this disorder or hospitalized, as initially believed. When compared with individuals not treated with SSRIs, there was no difference between those with anorexia receiving SSRIs and those not receiving these medications either on symptom reduction, including anxiety symptoms, or hospital readmissions (Holtkamp et al., 2005). This lack of efficacy has been hypothesized to be patients' low body weights causing low protein stores as protein is needed for SSRI metabolism. Other experts claim that the symptoms of anorexia nervosa, such as body distortion, hyperkinesis, and apathy, are primarily the result of starvation, which causes changes in brain chemistry. Thus, restoring weight influences symptom remission more significantly than does psychopharmacology. Of course, comorbid conditions such as depression should be treated with appropriate antidepressant medication (see Chapter 20). Some clinical experts who work with these patients have found that the SSRIs can be effective later, during outpatient treatment and after weight restoration. However, in contrast, some researchers have claimed that there is insufficient evidence to support the effectiveness of SSRIs in adolescent anorexia nervosa (Holtkamp et al., 2005). Target symptoms in only some individuals who demonstrate obsessiveness, ritualistic behaviors, and perfectionism will remit with these medications. SSRIs must be used with caution, and the patient's weight must be constantly monitored because, during the initiation phase, some of the SSRIs may cause weight loss.

Priority Care Issues

Mortality is high among patients with anorexia nervosa; the crude rate has been determined to be between 7% and 10%, and therefore higher than for females without anorexia nervosa in the general population (Birmingham et al., 2005). Factors that correlate with death are illness of long duration, bingeing and purging, and comorbid illnesses (Herzog et al., 2000). Substance abuse, particularly severe alcohol use, has been found to predict mortality in patients with anorexia nervosa (Keel et al., 2003; Korndorfer et al., 2003).

NURSING MANAGEMENT: HUMAN RESPONSE TO ANOREXIA NERVOSA DISORDER

Therapeutic Relationship

Establishing a therapeutic relationship with individuals with anorexia nervosa may be difficult initially because they are suspicious and mistrustful. They often express fear of adults, especially health care professionals, whom they believe want to "make them fat." By the time they are hospitalized, mistrust can almost reach a state of paranoia. Because of their low body weight and starvation, they are often impatient and irritable. A firm, accepting, and patient approach is important in working with these individuals. Providing a rationale for all

BOX 24.7

Therapeutic Dialogue: The Patient With an Eating Disorder

Ineffective Approach

Nurse: You haven't eaten your lunch yet.
Patient: I can't. I'm already fat.
Nurse: Look at you, you're skin and bones.
Patient: I'll eat when I go out this afternoon on pass.
Nurse: You can't go on pass. You have to start realizing that you are sick. Because you can't take care of yourself, we are in charge.
Patient: You're trying to control me.
Nurse: We are trying to be responsible.
Patient: I won't eat!
Nurse: We have set up punishments for not eating.
Patient: Then I won't go out! At least I won't get fatter.

Effective Approach

Nurse: You haven't eaten your lunch.
Patient: I can't. I'm already fat.
Nurse: Seeing yourself as fat is part of your eating disorder. We are here to help you.
Patient: I'll eat when I go out on pass.
Nurse: We wrote your behavioral plan together, and you know you will not be able to go out because your pass is dependent on eating both breakfast and lunch. Here!
Patient: You're trying to control me.
Nurse: We are worried about you. That's why we set up this plan. How can I help you now with this meal?
Patient: What if I eat half?
Nurse: No, you must eat all of it. Why don't I sit here while you eat? Eating is scary for you. We can talk about other choices you have on the unit; tonight, you can choose the movie or board games.
Patient: Okay, at least I have some choices.

Critical Thinking Challenge

- What effect did the first interaction have on the patient's behavior? Why?
- In the second interaction, what theories and interventions regarding eating disorders did the nurse use in her approach to the patient?

interventions helps build trust, as does a consistently nonreactive approach. Power struggles over eating are common, and remaining nonreactive is a challenge. During such power struggles, the nurse should always think about his or her own feelings of frustration and need for control (see Box 24.7).

Biologic Domain

Assessment

A thorough evaluation of body systems is important because many systems can be compromised by starvation. A careful history from both the patient with anorexia nervosa and the family, including the length and duration of symptoms, such as fasting, avoiding meals, and overexercising, is necessary to assess altered nutrition. Nursing management involves various biopsychosocial assessment and interventions (see Nursing Care Plan 24.1).

Patients with longer duration of these maladaptive behaviors typically have more difficult and prolonged recovery periods.

• NCLEXNOTE

Eating disorders are serious psychiatric disorders that threaten life. Careful assessment and referral for treatment are important nursing interventions.

The patient's weight is determined using the BMI and a scale. Currently, criteria for discharge require patients to be at least 85% of ideal weight according to height and weight tables. BMI, thought to reflect weight most accurately because exact height is used, is calculated by dividing weight in kilograms squared by height in meters. An acceptable BMI is between about 19 and 25.

Nursing Diagnoses for the Biologic Domain

A primary nursing diagnosis is Imbalanced Nutrition: Less Than Body Requirements.

Interventions for the Biologic Domain

Refeeding, the most important intervention during the hospital or initial stage of treatment (Fig. 24.4), is also the most challenging. The nurse will encounter resistance to weight gain and refusal to eat and must monitor and record all intake carefully as part of the weight gain protocol.

The refeeding protocol typically starts with 1,500 calories a day and is increased slowly until the patient is consuming about 3,500 calories a day in several meals. The usual plan for patients with very low weights is a weight gain of between 1 to 2 pounds a week.

Weight-increasing protocols usually take the form of a behavioral plan, using positive reinforcements (i.e., excursion passes) and negative reinforcements (i.e., returning to bed rest) to encourage weight gain. Help patients to understand that these actions are not punitive. When all staff members agree on a clear protocol for behaviors related to eating and weight gain, reactivity of the staff to the patient is greatly reduced. These

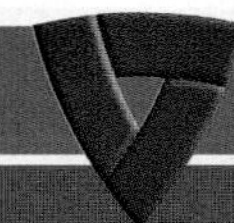

Nursing Care Plan 24.1

The Patient With Anorexia Nervosa

JS is a 16-year-old girl who appears much younger. She is 5′5″ and weighs 92 pounds. She has been treated unsuccessfully in an outpatient clinic and now is being admitted to stabilize her weight. She does not believe that she is too thin and resents being forced to be hospitalized. Hospitalization precipitated by being asked to leave gymnastics team because of low body weight.

Setting: Inpatient Psychiatric Unit

Baseline assessment: JS appears frail, pale, and dressed in oversized clothes. She is tearful, states that she is depressed and angry, and that she has no friends. Physical examination results: bradycardia pulse = 58, hypotension, 88/60, constipation, amenorrhea, dry skin patches, and cold intolerance. Hypokalemia (K+ = 3.5); leukopenia (WBCs <5,000). Dehydration, temperature elevation, 99°F, elevated BUN, abnormal thyroid functioning.

Associated Psychiatric Diagnosis

Axis I: Anorexia nervosa
Binge-eating/purging type
Axis II: None
Axis III: None
Axis IV: Social support (social withdrawal)
GAF = Current 55
Potential 75

Medications

Fluoxetine (Prozac), 20 mg in AM

Nursing Diagnosis 1: Imbalanced Nutrition: Less Than Body Requirements

Defining Characteristics

Unable to increase food intake
Weight more than 20% below ideal weight

Related Factors

Believes she cannot eat most foods
Purges by vomiting "occasionally"
Exercises 6–8 h daily
Sleep pattern disturbed by exercise

Outcomes

Initial

Maintains daily intake of 1,200 calories
Eliminates exercising while in hospital
Ceases purging for 1 week

Long-term

Gains 1–3 pounds
Develops strategies to maintain weight.

Interventions

Interventions	Rationale	Ongoing Assessment
Allow patient to verbalize feelings such as anxiety related to food and weight gain—develop a therapeutic relationship.	Through a relationship and examining her feelings, she may be more likely to cooperate with nutritional regimen.	Determine anxiety level when discussing food and weight gain.
Monitor meals and snacks, record amount eaten.	Severe anorexia is life threatening. Aggressive interventions are needed to ensure adequate intake.	Monitor intake. Assess JS's ability to complete meals on time and without supplements.
Do not substitute other foods for food on patient tray. Limit caffeine intake to 1 cup coffee (soda) daily.	People with anorexia usually "play games" with food. By prohibiting substitution, a more positive approach is encouraged. Caffeine is an appetite suppressant and has a diuretic effect.	Determine how willing JS is to follow nutritional regimen.
Monitor 1 h after meals for purging. Weigh daily in hospital gown after patient has voided. Monitor vital signs daily, electrolytes.	Physical signs of impending complications include evidence of purging, decreasing body weight, hypotension, hyperthermia, and hypokalemia.	Monitor vital signs, weight, and electrolytes, especially potassium.

Continued

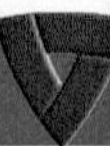

Nursing Care Plan 24.1 *(Continued)*

Evaluation

Outcomes	Revised Outcomes	Interventions
JS gains 5 pounds at the end of $1^1/_2$ weeks. Has been cooperative with meal regimen. She has begun to acknowledge the seriousness of her illness and the life-threatening aspects of severe dieting and purging.	Ceases binge–purge episodes for 1 week. Continues to increase her weight (1–3 pounds/week). Establish and maintain regular, adequate nutritional eating habits	Daily weights while on unsupervised meals. Praise her for her successes. Arrange or discharge to outpatient clinic. Participation in relapse-prevention classes.

Nursing Diagnosis 2: Disturbed Body Image

Defining Characteristics	Related Factors
Verbalizes that she is too fat Perceives herself as unattractive Hides body in large, baggy clothing	Inaccurate perceptions of physical appearance secondary to anorexia nervosa Believes that one can never be too rich or too thin Equates physical fitness and attractiveness with thinness

Outcomes

Initial	Long-term
Verbalizes feelings related to changing body shape and weight. Identifies beliefs about controlling body size.	Acknowledges negative consequences of too little fat on body. Identifies positive aspects of her body and its ability to function.

Interventions

Interventions	Rationale	Ongoing Assessment
Explore JS's beliefs and feelings about body. Maintain a nonjudgmental approach.	To help patient gain a more positive body image, an understanding of her own views is important.	Monitor for statements that identify perceptions of her body. Is her view *distorted* or *dissatisfied*?
Assist patient in identifying positive physical characteristics.	In anorexia, the body is viewed negatively. By focusing on parts of the body that are positive, such as eyes or hands, the patient can begin to experience a positive image of her body.	Observe for patient's reaction to her body. Which areas are viewed positively? Observe for negative statements related to body size and self-esteem.
Clarify patient's views about an ideal body.	Many societal cues idealize an unrealistically thin female body.	Monitor for statements indicating external pressures to lose weight, experiences of teasing about body changes, or evidence of sexual abuse from others.
Provide education related to normal growth of women's bodies, role of fat in protection of body.	Providing education will help in reinforcing a broader view of the importance of a healthy body.	Assess patient's willingness to learn information.

Evaluation

Outcomes	Revised Outcomes	Interventions
JS revealed that she believes that she is too fat but does have positive physical traits—eyes. She believes that those who are overweight have lost control of their lives. She knows some models who are 6' and weigh barely 100 lbs.	Accept alternative beliefs related to her own body.	Gradually, focus on other positive physical aspects of JS's body. Discuss grooming that encourages a more attractive look. Challenge her beliefs about body weights of models.
Willing to read information about normal body functioning.	Accept a new view of body functioning as a complex phenomenon.	Discuss the biologic aspect of the development of body weight. Emphasize multiple factors determine body weight.

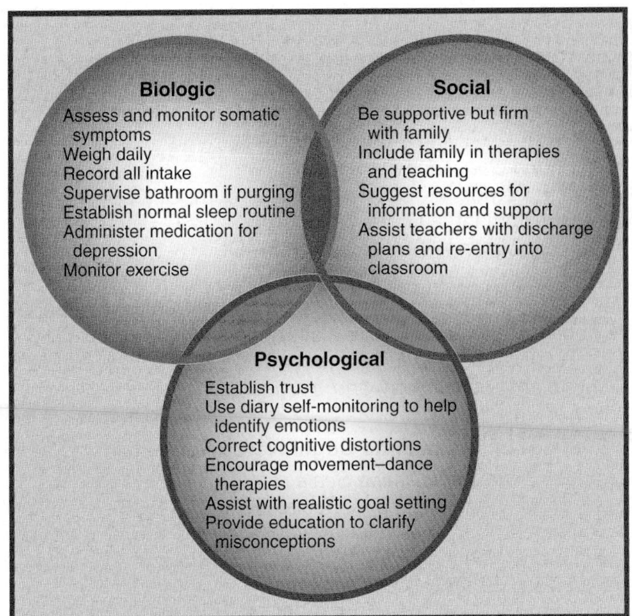

Biologic
Assess and monitor somatic symptoms
Weigh daily
Record all intake
Supervise bathroom if purging
Establish normal sleep routine
Administer medication for depression
Monitor exercise
Social
Be supportive but firm with family
Include family in therapies and teaching
Suggest resources for information and support
Assist teachers with discharge plans and re-entry into classroom
Psychological
Establish trust
Use diary self-monitoring to help identify emotions
Correct cognitive distortions
Encourage movement–dance therapies
Assist with realistic goal setting
Provide education to clarify misconceptions

FIGURE 24.4. Biopsychosocial interventions for patients with anorexia nervosa.

protocols provide ready-made, consistent responses to food-refusal behaviors and should be carried out in a caring and supportive context. On rare occasions when the patient is unable to recognize or accept her illness (denial), nasogastric tube feedings may be necessary.

Menses history also must be explored. Most patients with anorexia nervosa have reached menarche but have experienced amenorrhea for some months because of starvation. A return to regular menses signifies substantial body fat restoration. Sleep disturbance is also common, and these individuals are viewed as hyperkinetic. They sleep little, but usually awake in an energized state. A structured, healthy sleep routine must be established immediately to conserve energy and calorie expenditure because of low weight. To further conserve energy, patients are often relegated to bed rest until a certain amount of weight is regained. Exercise is generally not permitted during refeeding and only with caution after this phase. Inpatients must be closely supervised because they are often found exercising in their rooms, running in place and doing calisthenics.

Psychological Domain

Assessment

The psychological symptoms that patients with anorexia experience are listed in Box 24.1. The classic symptoms of body distortion—fear of weight gain, unrealistic expectations and thinking, and ritualistic behaviors—are easily noted during a clinical interview. Often, people with anorexia nervosa avoid conflict and have difficulty expressing negative emotions, such as anger. Other conflicts, such as sexuality fears and feelings of ineffectiveness, may underlie this disorder. These symptoms may not be apparent during a clinical interview; however, a variety of instruments is available to clinicians and researchers for determining their presence and severity. Box 24.8 lists well-known instruments used to assess psychological symptoms associated with eating disorders. The Eating Attitudes Test is frequently used in community and clinical samples (Box 24.9). There is also a child version of this test, the CHEAT. The results of these paper-and-pencil tests can help identify the most significant symptoms for an individual patient and indicate a focus for interventions, especially therapy.

Nursing Diagnosis for the Psychological Domain

Two common nursing diagnoses in anorexia nervosa are Anxiety and Disturbed Body Image. See Figure 24.5.

Interventions for the Psychological Domain

For interoceptive awareness problems (inability to experience visceral cues and emotions), the nurse can encourage patients to keep a journal. Most patients use a somatic complaint such as "I feel bloated" or "I'm fat" to replace a negative emotion such as guilt or anger. Although refeeding following a state of starvation may cause bloating in some cases, bloating often is imagined and part of body image distortion. Help patients to identify these feelings by having them write a description of the "fat feeling" and list possible underlying emotions and troublesome situations next to this description.

Understanding Feelings

Identifying feelings, such as anxiety and fear, and especially negative emotions, such as anger, is the first step in helping patients to decrease conflict avoidance and develop effective strategies for coping with these feelings.

Do not attempt to change distorted body image by merely pointing out that the patient is actually too thin. This symptom is often the last to resolve itself, and some individuals may take years to see their bodies realistically. However, although this symptom is difficult to abate, patients can continue to fear becoming fat but not be driven to act on the distortion by starving. The fear of becoming fat eventually lessens with time.

The nurse can help individuals with cognitive distortions and unrealistic assumptions to restructure the way they view the world, especially relative to food, eating, weight, and shape. Faulty ways of viewing these situa-

BOX 24.8

Assessment Instruments

1. Tests for Disordered Eating (Symptoms)

Compulsive Eating Scale
Dunn, P. K., & Ondercin, P. (1981). Personality variables related to compulsive eating in college women. *Journal of Clinical Psychology, 31,* 43–49.

Eating Attitudes Test
Garner, D. M., & Garfinkel, P. E. (1979). The Eating Attitudes Test: An index of the symptoms of anorexia nervosa. *Psychosomatic Medicine, 10,* 647–656.

Children's Eating Attitude Test (CHEAT)
Maloney, M., McGuire, J., & Daniels, S. R. (1988). Reliability testing of a children's version of the Eating Attitude Test. *Journal of the American Academy of Child and Adolescent Psychiatry, 27,* 541–543.

Eating Disorder Examination-Questionnaire (EDE-O)
Carolyn Black, Rutgers University Eating Disorders Clinic, 41C Gordon Road, Piscataway, NJ 08854.

Eating Disorder Inventory-2 (EDI-2) and EDI-2 Symptom Checklist (EDI-2-SC).
Psychological Assessment Resources, P.O. Box 998, Odessa, FL 33556 (800-331-8378).

Eating Habits Questionnaire (Restraint Scale)
Herman, C. P., & Mack, D. (1975). Restrained and unrestrained eating. *Journal of Personality, 43,* 647–660.

Yale-Brown-Cornell Eating Disorder Scale (YBC-EDS)
Mazure, C. M., Halmi, K. A., Sunday, S. R., Romano, S. J., & Einhorn, A. M. (1994). Yale-Brown-Cornell Eating Disorder Scale: Development, use, reliability, and validity. *Journal of Psychiatric Research, 28,* 425–445.

2. Tests of Body Dissatisfaction/Body Image

Body Shape Questionnaire (BSQ)
Cooper, P., Taylor, M., Cooper, Z., & Fairburn, C. (1987). The development and validation of the BSQ. *International Journal of Eating Disorders, 6,* 485–494.

Color-a-Person Test
Wooley, S. C., & Kearney-Cooke, A. (1986). Intensive treatment of bulimia and body image disturbance. In K. D. Brownell & J. P. Foreyt (Eds.), *Handbook of eating disorders: Physiology, psychology and treatment of obesity, anorexia, and bulimia* (pp. 476–502). New York: Basic Books.

3. Tests of Emotional and Cognitive Components

Cognitive Behavioral Dieting Scale
Martz, D. M., Sturgis, E. T., & Gustafson, S. B. (1996). Development and preliminary validation of the Cognitive Behavioral Dieting Scale. *International Journal of Eating Disorders, 19,* 297–309.

Emotional Eating Scale
Arrow, B., Kenardy, J., & Agras, W. S. (1995). The emotional eating scale: The development of a measure to assess coping with negative affect by eating. *Internationl Journal of Eating Disorders, 18,* 79–90.

4. Risk Factors Identification

The McKnight Risk Factor Survey
Shisslak, C. M., Renger, R., Sharpe, T., et al. (1999). Development and evaluation of the McKnight Risk Factor Survey for assessing potential risk and protective factors for disordered eating in preadolescent and adolescent girls. *International Journal of Eating Disorders,* 25, 195–214. (versions available for younger and older children).

tions result in ineffective coping. Table 24.4 lists some distortions commonly experienced by individuals with eating disorders and some typical restructuring responses or statements that challenge the distortion, which the nurse can present as more realistic ways of perceiving situations. Other therapies, such as movement and dance therapy, can help the patient experience pleasure from his or her body, although dance should be used cautiously during refeeding because of energy-expenditure concerns. Imagery and relaxation are often used to overcome distortions and to decrease anxiety stemming from a distorted body image. While in the hospital, patients usually are evaluated for discharge to partial hospitalization or to intensive outpatient therapy, depending on the resources available, the extent of family support, and comorbidity. In both instances, the patient and family will participate in a combination of individual and family therapy.

Interpersonal Therapy

Interpersonal therapy (IPT) is a type of treatment that focuses on uncovering and resolving the developmental and psychological issues underlying the disorder. Role transitions, control, and ineffective feelings typically are the focus (McIntosh et al., 2000). Cognitive therapy may also be incorporated to continue to address and change distortions about food and interactions with others.

Family therapy is usually initiated in the hospital and continued more intensively after discharge. The section on Etiology: Family discusses some of the family symptoms, such as enmeshment, which are the focus of the therapy.

Patient Education 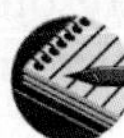

When weight is restored and concentration is improved, patients with anorexia nervosa can benefit from psychoeducation. Although these individuals have a wealth of knowledge about food and calories, they also have misinformation that needs clarifying. For example, they are often unclear about the role of "fats" in a healthy diet and try to be as "fat free" as possible. A thorough assessment of their knowledge is important because they seem to be "walking calorie books" with little information on the role of all of the nutrients and the importance of including them in a healthy diet.

BOX 24.9
Eating Attitudes Test

Please place an (x) under the column that applies best to each of the numbered statements. All of the results will be strictly confidential. Most of the questions relate to food or eating, although other types of questions have been included. Please answer each question carefully. Thank you.

	Always	Very Often	Often	Sometimes	Rarely	Never
1. Like eating with other people	—	—	—	—	—	×
2. Prepare foods for others but do not eat what I cook	×	—	—	—	—	—
3. Become anxious before eating	×	—	—	—	—	—
4. Am terrified about being overweight	×	—	—	—	—	—
5. Avoid eating when I am hungry	×	—	—	—	—	—
6. Find myself preoccupied with food	×	—	—	—	—	—
7. Have gone on eating binges in which I feel that I may not be able to stop	×	—	—	—	—	—
8. Cut my food into small pieces	×	—	—	—	—	—
9. Am aware of the calorie content of foods that I eat	×	—	—	—	—	—
10. Particularly avoid foods with a high carbohydrate content (e.g., bread, potatoes, rice)	×	—	—	—	—	—
11. Feel bloated after meals	×	—	—	—	—	—
12. Feel that others would prefer I ate more	×	—	—	—	—	—
13. Vomit after I have eaten	×	—	—	—	—	—
14. Feel extremely guilty after eating	×	—	—	—	—	—
15. Am preoccupied with a desire to be thinner	×	—	—	—	—	—
16. Exercise strenuously to burn off calories	×	—	—	—	—	—
17. Weigh myself several times a day	×	—	—	—	—	—
18. Like my clothes to fit tightly	—	—	—	—	—	×
19. Enjoy eating meat	—	—	—	—	—	×
20. Wake up early in the morning	×	—	—	—	—	—
21. Eat the same foods day after day	×	—	—	—	—	—
22. Think about burning up calories when I exercise	×	—	—	—	—	—
23. Have regular menstrual periods	—	—	—	—	—	×
24. Am aware that other people think I am too thin	×	—	—	—	—	—
25. Am preoccupied with the thought of having fat on my body	×	—	—	—	—	—
26. Take longer than others to eat	×	—	—	—	—	—
27. Enjoy eating at restaurants	—	—	—	—	—	×
28. Take laxatives	×	—	—	—	—	—
29. Avoid foods with sugar in them	×	—	—	—	—	—
30. Eat diet foods	×	—	—	—	—	—
31. Feel that food controls my life	×	—	—	—	—	—
32. Display self-control around food	×	—	—	—	—	—
33. Feel that others pressure me to eat	×	—	—	—	—	—
34. Give too much time and thought to food	×	—	—	—	—	—
35. Suffer from constipation	—	×	—	—	—	—
36. Feel uncomfortable after eating sweets	×	—	—	—	—	—
37. Engage in dieting behavior	×	—	—	—	—	—
38. Like my stomach to be empty	×	—	—	—	—	—
39. Enjoy trying new rich foods	—	—	—	—	—	×
40. Have the impulse to vomit after meals	×	—	—	—	—	—

Scoring: The patient is given the questionnaire without the X's, just blank. 3 points are assigned to endorsements that coincide with the X's; the adjacent alternatives are weighted as 2 points and 1 point, respectively. A total score of more than 30 indicates significant concerns with eating behavior.

• NCLEXNOTE

Setting realistic eating goals is one of the most helpful interventions for patients with eating disorders. Because individuals with anorexia nervosa are often perfectionistic, they often set unrealistic goals.

Teaching Points 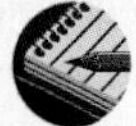

One of the most helpful skills the nurse can teach is to set realistic goals around food and also around other activities or tasks. Because of perfectionism, patients with anorexia often set unrealistic goals and end up

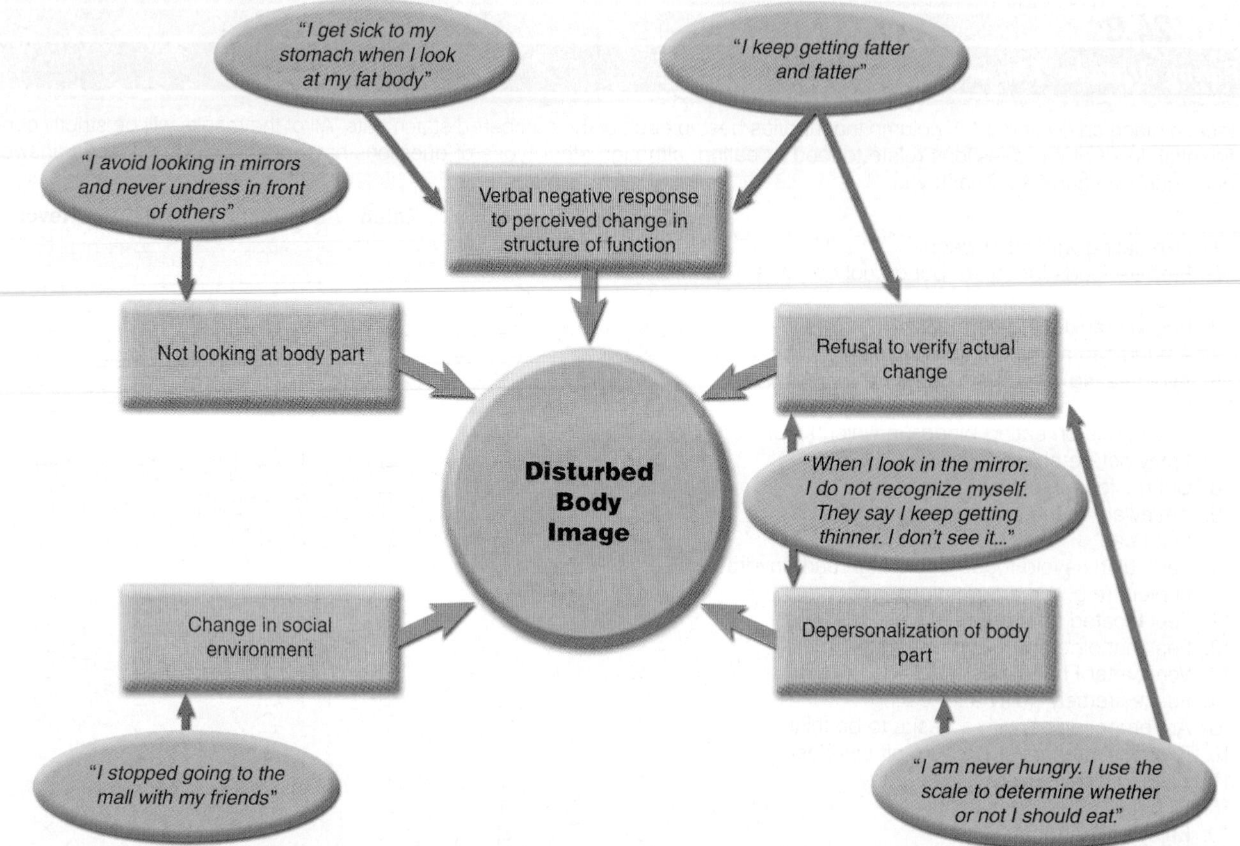

FIGURE 24.5. Nursing Diagnosis Concept Maps: Disturbed Body Image.

frustrated. The nurse can help them establish smaller, more realistic, attainable goals (see Box 24.10).

Families and friends are eager to help the patient with anorexia but often need direction. Box 24.11 provides a list of strategies that may assist them.

Social Domain

Nursing Diagnosis for the Social Domain

Ineffective Coping is a predominant nursing diagnosis with regard to the social domain.

Table 24.4 Congnitive Distortions Typical of Patients With Eating Disorders,With Restructuring Statements

Distortion	Clarification or Restructuring
Dichotomous or all-or-nothing thinking "I've gained 2 pounds, so I'll be up by 100 pounds soon."	"You have never gained 100 pounds, but I understand that gaining 2 pounds is scary."
Magnification "I binged last night, so I can't go out with anyone."	"Feeling bad and guilty about a binge are difficult feelings, but you are in treatment and you have been monitoring and changing your eating."
Selective abstraction "I can only be happy 10 pounds lighter."	"When you were 10 pounds lighter, you were hospitalized. You can choose to be happy about many things in your life."
Overgeneralization "I didn't eat anything yesterday and did okay, so I don't think not eating for a week or two will harm me."	"Any starvation harms the body, whether or not outward signs were apparent to you. The more you starve, the more problems your body will encounter."
Catastrophizing "I purged last night for the first time in 4 months—I'll never recover."	"Recovery includes up and downs, and it is expected you will still have some mild but infrequent symptoms."

BOX 24.10

Psychoeducation Checklist: Anorexia Nervosa

When caring for the patient with anorexia nervosa, be sure to include the following topic areas in the teaching plan:

- Psychopharmacologic agents, if used, including drug, action, dosage, frequency, and possible adverse effects
- Nutrition and eating patterns
- Effect of restrictive eating or dieting
- Weight monitoring
- Safety and comfort measures
- Avoidance of triggers
- Self-monitoring techniques
- Trust
- Realistic goal setting
- Resources

Interventions for the Social Domain

Younger patients with anorexia nervosa may have lost some school time because of hospitalization. Integrating back into a school and classroom setting is difficult for most. Shame and guilt about having an eating disorder and being hospitalized must be addressed. Because these patients typically have isolated themselves before hospitalization and treatment, renewing friendships and relationships with peers may provoke anxiety. Involving school nurses and teachers in the re-entry process may help.

Denial, guilt, and subsequent greater overprotectiveness are common reactions of the family, especially when hospitalization has been necessary. Family therapy is important if the patient still lives at home. Skilled therapists are able to help family members with their feelings, increase effective communication, decrease protectiveness, and resolve guilt. Often, siblings become resentful of the patient with an eating disorder because of the significant amount of attention they get from the parents. Having siblings attend family sessions to discuss these feelings and the effect the illness has had on them is helpful.

BOX 24.11

What Family and Friends Can Do to Help Those With Eating Disorders

- Tell the person you are concerned, you care, and you would like to help. Suggest that the person seek professional help from a physician or therapist.
- If the person refuses to seek professional help, encourage reaching out to an adult, such as a teacher, school nurse, or counselor.
- Do not discuss weight, the number of calories being consumed, or particular eating habits. Do try to talk about things other than food, weight, counting calories, and exercise.
- Avoid making comments about a person's appearance. Concern about weight loss may be interpreted as a compliment; comments regarding weight gain may be felt as criticism.
- It will not help to become involved in a power struggle. You cannot force the person to eat.
- You can offer support. Ultimately, however, the responsibility and the decision to accept help and to change rest with the person.
- Read and educate yourself regarding these disorders.

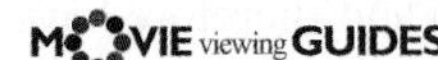

Evaluation And Treatment Outcomes

Several factors influence the outcome of treatment for anorexia nervosa. Particularly long duration of symptoms and low weight when treatment begins predict poor outcomes, whereas family support and involvement generally improve outcomes. Comorbid conditions and their severity will also influence recovery. Although patients are discharged from the hospital when their weight has reached 85% of what is considered ideal, restoration of healthy eating and changes in maladaptive thinking may not have yet occurred. Individuals often continue to restrict foods. Therefore, without intensive outpatient treatment, including nutritional counseling and support, they are unlikely to recover fully. Distorted thinking and eating patterns can set the stage for a relapse and later for the possible development of bulimia nervosa. Many of the instruments used to assess eating disorder symptoms can be used throughout the patient's treatment to evaluate attitudes and thinking processes that continue to prevent full recovery (see Box 24.8).

Continuum of Care

Hospitalization

Hospitalization is required based on criteria noted in Table 24.3. Anorexia nervosa in its acute stage is unlikely to be manageable in outpatient settings.

Emergency Care 

Emergency care is not usually needed for individuals with anorexia nervosa. Family members and peers usually notice the weight loss and emaciation before patients' systems are compromised to the degree that they require emergency treatment. If systems are compromised enough to warrant emergency treatment, patients usually are admitted immediately for inpatient care.

Family Assessment and Intervention 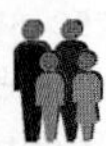

The family of the person with anorexia will need extensive treatment and follow-up. The therapist, psychologist, advanced practice nurse, or social worker meets regularly, at least once a week, with the individual and the family. This method has been demonstrated to be more effective than family therapy without the patient or individual therapy alone (Robin et al., 1999). The family therapy focuses on such issues as separation-individuation, autonomy, ineffective communication, and practical issues, such as how parents can effectively monitor food intake. Many family theorists believe that eating disorders develop because of family dysfunction and therefore have some unrealized meaning for each family. For example, the patient may be attempting to keep a splitting, divorcing, or estranged family together with her illness. In other instances, parents may be trying to prevent a daughter from separating and individuating because they are emotionally unprepared for this process. The development of an eating disorder may be a reaction to these situations. The therapy helps to uncover these meanings and to improve effective parenting.

Outpatient Treatment

After refeeding, treatment of anorexia nervosa takes place on an outpatient basis and involves individual and family therapy, nutrition counseling to reinforce healthy eating patterns and attitudes, and physician visits to monitor weight and evaluate somatic recovery. Support groups, often suggested, should not be substituted for therapy. In fact, some self-directed support groups that lack professional leadership can actually delay or prevent needed professional treatment. However, after full recovery, support groups are useful in maintaining recovery.

Prevention

Eating disorders are among the most preventable mental disorders. Instruments such as the McKnight Risk Factor Survey (Shisslak et al., 1999), which measure the presence and degree of risk factors, can be used to plan prevention or treatment after early detection (see Box 24.8). National eating disorder awareness and advocacy groups work toward educating the general public, those at risk, and those who work with groups at risk, such as teachers and coaches. They also monitor the media and work to remove unhealthy advertisements and articles that appear in magazines appealing to young girls. A list of on-line resources and some programs and their purposes are found in the Web Links section of thePoint.

Prevention and early detection strategies for parents and schoolteachers are often the focus of school nurses and mental health nurses who work in the community. Some of these strategies appear in Table 24.5 and are based on the research on risk factors and protective factors. These protective factors, such as confidence and healthy competition in athletics, have been shown to prevent the development of an eating disorder for individuals who were at risk (Taylor et al., 1998). Dieting, being overweight, and body dissatisfaction are examples of risk factors underlying the development of eating disorders that can be reversed with early identification and intervention.

Table 24.5 Prevention Strategies for Parents and Children

Parents	Children
Education	***Education***
Real vs. ideal weight	Peer pressure regarding eating, weight
Influence of attitudes, behaviors, teasing	Menses, puberty, normal weight gain
Ways to increase self-esteem	Strategies for obesity
Role of media: TV, magazines	Ways to develop or improve self-esteem
Signs and symptoms	Body image traps: media, retail clothing
Interventions for obesity	Adapting and coping with problems
Boys at risk also	Reporting friends with signs of eating disorders
Observe for rituals	**Screening** for risk factors
Supervision of eating and exercise	**Assessment** for treatment
	Follow-up: monitor for relapse

BULIMIA NERVOSA

Bulimia nervosa is a relatively newly identified disorder: until about 25 years ago, it was thought to be a type of anorexia nervosa. However, findings from extensive investigations have identified its characteristics as a separate entity. It is more prevalent than anorexia nervosa. Individuals with bulimia nervosa are usually older at onset than are those with anorexia nervosa. The disorder generally is not as life threatening as anorexia nervosa. The usual treatment is outpatient therapy. Outcomes are better for bulimia nervosa than for anorexia nervosa, and mortality rates are lower.

Clinical Course

There are few outward signs associated with bulimia nervosa. Individuals binge and purge in secret and are typically of normal weight; therefore, it does not come to the attention of parents and peers as readily as does anorexia nervosa. Treatment consequently can be delayed for years as individuals attempt on their own to get their eating under control. Patients usually initiate their own treatment when control of their eating becomes impossible. Once treatment is undertaken and completed, patients typically recover completely, except in cases in which personality disorders and comorbid serious depression are also present.

Patients with bulimia nervosa present as overwhelmed and overly committed individuals, "social butterflies" who have difficulty with setting limits and establishing appropriate boundaries. They have an enormous number of rules regarding food and food restriction, and they feel shame, guilt, and disgust about their binge eating and purging. They may also be impulsive in other areas of their lives, such as spending.

Diagnostic Criteria

The key characteristics for the diagnosis of bulimia nervosa appear in Table 24.6 (also see Box 24.1). There are two types of bulimia nervosa: purging type and restricting type. Patients with the restricting type are similar to those with anorexia nervosa. However, in bulimia, restricting is followed by binge eating, which is then followed by another period of restricting. In the purging type, binge eating is followed by purging. The difference between purging in the patient with anorexia and purging in the patient with bulimia is the severe weight loss and amenorrhea that accompanies anorexia nervosa. Bulimia nervosa involves engaging in recurrent episodes of binge eating and compensatory purging in the form of vomiting or using laxatives, diuretics, or emetics, or in nonpurging compensatory behaviors, such as fasting or overexercising in order to avoid weight gain. These episodes must occur at least twice a week for a period of at least 3 months in order to meet the *DSM-IV-TR* criteria (APA, 2000). People with this disorder may binge and purge as many as several times a day.

Binge eating is defined as rapid, episodic, impulsive, and uncontrollable ingestion of a large amount of food during a short period of time, usually 1 to 2 hours. Eating is followed by feelings of guilt, remorse, and often self-contempt, leading to purging. To assuage the out-of-control feeling, severe dieting is instituted, and these restrictions, referred to as *dietary restraint*, precipitate the next binge. The restrictions are viewed as "rules," such as no sweets, no fats, and so forth. Each binge seems to influence stricter and stricter rules about what cannot be consumed, leading to more frequent binge eating. This cycle has prompted clinicians to focus treatment primarily on interventions related to dietary restraint. When dietary restraint is resolved, binge eating is decreased, and generally the purging that follows binge eating also is decreased.

KEY CONCEPT Dietary restraint has been described by researchers in the field of eating disorders as a way to explain the relationship between dieting and binge eating (Polivy & Herman, 1993).

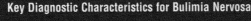

Table 24.6  **Key Diagnostic Characteristics for Bulimia Nervosa** 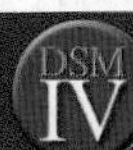

Diagnostic Criteria	Target Symptoms and Associated Findings
• Recurrent episodes of binge eating • Characterized by both of the following: eating in a discrete period of time an amount larger than most people would eat during a similar period of time and under similar circumstances; sense of lack of control over eating during the episode • Recurrent inappropriate compensatory behavior to prevent weight gain, such as self-induced vomiting, misuse of laxatives, diuretics, enemas, or other medications; fasting; or excessive exercise • Binge eating and inappropriate compensatory behaviors occurring on average at least twice a week for 3 months • Self-evaluation unduly influenced by body shape and weight • Not occurring exclusively during episodes of anorexia nervosa • *Purging type:* regular engagement in self-induced vomiting or misuse of diuretics, laxatives, or enemas • *Nonpurging type:* use of other inappropriate compensatory behaviors, such as fasting or excessive exercise without regular engagement in self-induced vomiting, or misuse of laxatives, diuretics, or enemas	• Usually within normal weight range, possible overweight or underweight • Restriction of total calorie consumption between binges, selecting low-calorie foods while avoiding foods perceived to be fattening or likely to trigger a binge • Increased frequency of depressive symptoms and anxiety symptoms • Possible substance abuse or dependence involving alcohol or stimulants ***Associated Physical Examination Findings*** • Loss of dental enamel • Chipped, ragged, or moth-eaten teeth appearance • Increased incidence of dental caries • Scars on dorsum of hand from manually inducing vomiting • Cardiac and skeletal myopathies from use of syrup of ipecac for vomiting • Menstrual irregularities • Dependence on laxatives • Esophageal tears ***Associated Laboratory Findings*** • Fluid and electrolyte abnormalities • Metabolic alkalosis (from vomiting) or metabolic acidosis (from diarrhea) • Mildly elevated serum amylase levels

Dieters' deprivation, or restraint, whether real or imagined, contributes to overeating and bingeing. Deprivation may operate in a straightforward fashion by instigating a drive toward repletion. Another possibility is that deprivation alters one's perceptual reactivation to attractive food cues, making them more irresistible. Attempted deprivation may make dieters more prone to feel distress over their dietary "failures," especially if dieting has become a way to overcome body dissatisfaction and to compensate for distress through binge eating. Whether the eating is influenced by the attraction of forbidden foods or by internal needs to assuage failure, there is significant evidence that restraining one's intake is a precondition for bouts of overeating.

A number of studies have uncovered a group of individuals who binge in the same way as those with bulimia nervosa but who do not purge or compensate for binges through other behaviors. This disorder is now classified in a temporary way in the *DSM-IV-TR* as binge eating disorder (BED). These individuals also differ in that most of them are also obese. Box 24.12 describes BED and the current understanding about this disorder. Because this is a newly recognized disorder, until additional research clarifies its symptoms, etiology, and treatment, it is now described in the Appendix of the *DSM-IV-TR* (APA, 2000). Clinicians classify BED as an "eating disorder not otherwise specified" until it has been researched further for inclusion as a separate diagnosis in the *DSM-IV-TR*. Its etiology is believed to be similar to that of bulimia nervosa. The treatment of binge eating disorder is still in the investigative stages, and most experts use interventions similar to those used for bulimia nervosa.

BOX 24.12

Binge Eating Disorder

Binge eating disorder (BED), although still in the research stage to refine its characteristics for inclusion in the *DSM-IV-TR* (APA, 2000) as a separate entity, is estimated to affect 3% to 4% of the population. The criteria for BED consist of binge eating, which includes both the ingestion of a large amount of food in a short period of time and a sense of loss of control during the binge; distress regarding the binge; eating until uncomfortably full; and feelings of guilt or depression following the binge. Purging does not occur with BED, and this differentiates it from bulimia nervosa. In addition, investigators have shown that individuals with BED have lower dietary restraint and are higher in weight, even though many are not obese, than those with bulimia nervosa. It has been estimated that 10% to 30% of obese individuals have BED. Some women with bulimia nervosa have reported that they binged without purging for several years before developing bulimia nervosa at as young as age 10 years (Bulik et al., 1998).

Cognitive-behavior therapy has not been as effective for BED as it is for bulimia nervosa. Investigations have shown that sertraline has been effective in reducing binges. Topiramate, used for epilepsy, has been studied for use for BED and was found to decrease binge eating and appetite. Some weight loss was also a result of treatment with this medication. More studies are needed to confirm its effectiveness (Shapira, Goldsmith, & McElroy, 2000).

Bulimia Nervosa in Special Populations

Bulimia nervosa occurs in all age groups. It is not as common in children as in adolescents and adults; children appear more likely to have binge eating disorder (BED) (APA, 2000). This finding has only recently been reported, and more data are needed to substantiate this theory.

Epidemiology

Lifetime prevalence of bulimia nervosa is reported to be from 3% to 8%, depending on whether clinical or community populations are sampled. Stricter criteria are used when clinical groups are studied, making the prevalence rate lower. The occurrence is more common than that of anorexia nervosa (APA, 2000). The incidence of BN has been decreasing over the past decade; this decrease is not attributable to changes in service utilization, thereby suggesting a change in sociocultural factors is involved in its development (Keel, Heatherton & 2005).

Age of Onset

Typically, the age of onset is between 18 and 24 years. The incidence of bulimia nervosa is increasing among women between 25 and 45 years but has been relatively stable in the typical age group (Pawluck & Gorey, 1998).

Gender Differences

As with anorexia nervosa, females are 10 times more likely than males to experience bulimia nervosa. Box 24.2 highlights differences in males with eating disorders.

Ethnic and Cultural Differences

Bulimia nervosa is related to culture in the same way as anorexia nervosa. In Western cultures and those becoming westernized in their norms, the focus on achieving a thin body ideal underlies the dieting and dietary restraint that sets up the trajectory toward a diagnosable eating disorder. Hispanic and white women have higher rates than do Asian and African American women. The difference as noted earlier in the chapter has much to do with how women from specific cultural backgrounds internalize the thin ideal.

Comorbidity

The most common comorbid conditions are substance abuse and dependence, depression, and OCD. In one study, women continued having OCD after remission of their bulimic symptoms, underlining the notion that some comorbid conditions may occur before the eating disorder, are trait-related features, and may actually have a role in precipitating the disorder (von Ranson, Kaye, Weltzin, Rao, & Matsunaga, 1999).

Cluster B, Axis II disorders, such as borderline personality disorder, are also found frequently in these individuals (Matsunaga et al., 2000), and many women with bulimia nervosa have had anorexia nervosa previously.

Etiology

Some of the predisposing or risk factors for anorexia nervosa and bulimia nervosa overlap with theories of causality (see Fig. 24.3). For example, dieting puts an individual at risk for the development of bulimia nervosa. The dieting can turn into dietary restraint, a symptom that leads to binge eating and purging. However, not all individuals who diet experience bulimia nervosa. The interplay of other risk factors (e.g., body dissatisfaction and separation individuation issues) most likely explains the development of this disorder.

Biologic Theories

Some progress has been made in understanding the biologic causes of bulimia nervosa. Dieting, one of the most important causative factors, occurs in this country in girls as young as 8 years of age (Hill & Pallin, 1998). Dieting is believed to affect serotonergic regulation. As in anorexia nervosa, overexercising has also contributed to some of the symptoms of bulimia nervosa, especially in individuals with the restricting type of this disorder. In one recent study, women with restricting food behaviors influenced the development of eating-related thoughts when they were compared with nonrestraining women (O'Connell et al., 2005)

Neuropathologic

The changes noted in the brain by MRI are the result of eating dysregulation, rather than the cause. As with anorexia nervosa, these changes often disappear when symptoms such as dietary restraint, binge eating, and purging remit.

Genetic and Familial Predispositions 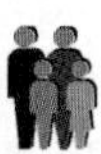

A specific gene responsible for bulimia nervosa has not been conclusively identified. Recently, twin studies have been reviewed to determine the role genetics might play in the development of bulimia nervosa. Whereas it has been widely recognized that environment also plays a role, in several twin studies, genetic influences outweighed environmental ones (Bulik et al., 2000). In one twin study, researchers demonstrated that there was a significant linkage on chromosome 10p in families of individuals with bulimia nervoxa (Bulik et al., 2003). Findings continue to be treated with caution because sorting out environmental and genetic influences is difficult when twins live in the same environment.

Biochemical

The most frequently studied biochemical theory in bulimia nervosa relates to lowered brain serotonin neurotransmission. People with bulimia nervosa are believed to have altered modulation of central serotonin neuronal systems (Kaye et al., 2000).

Studies have typically looked to tryptophan, an amino acid and serotonin precursor, to explain this mechanism. Findings from several studies have demonstrated that women with bulimia nervosa experience symptoms of depressed mood, a desire to binge, and an increase in weight and shape concerns when tryptophan is depleted (Bell, Hood & Nutt, 2005). To further advance these findings, in another study, women who had recovered from bulimia nervosa (i.e., symptoms had remitted) were examined after ingestion of a formula to deplete tryptophan. They returned to symptoms of a desire to binge, preoccupation with shape, and depressed mood (Wolfe et al., 2000). Chronic depletion of plasma tryptophan is thought to be one of the major mechanisms whereby persistent dieting can lead to the development of eating disorders in vulnerable individuals.

Psychological and Social Theories

Psychological factors in the etiology of bulimia nervosa have been studied extensively, and most experts believe that these factors converge with environmental or sociocultural factors within individuals with a biologic predisposition, causing symptoms to develop. As with anorexia nervosa, psychoanalytic developmental theories that explain separation-individuation are important in causality. Because the age of onset for bulimia nervosa is late adolescence, going away to college, for example, may represent the first physical separation for some adolescents, who are unprepared for the emotional separation. In addition, an inability to set limits and develop healthy boundaries leads to a sense of being overwhelmed and "drained." In most instances, women with bulimia nervosa are not assertive and have difficulty saying no, fearing that they will not be liked. Overwhelming feelings often lead to binge eating, either to avoid or to distract oneself from feelings such as resentment, or binge eating can serve to assuage emptiness, or to fill up a "drained" self with food.

Cognitive Theory

Many experts view cognitive theory as influential in eating disorder symptoms. It explains the distorted thinking present in people with bulimia nervosa. This explanation is similar for depression, in which a particular thought pattern is learned (see Chapter 11 for an explanation of cognitive theory). Many experts view bulimia nervosa as a disorder of thinking, in that distortions are the basis of behaviors such as binge eating and purging. Psychological triggering mechanism models explain that cues such as stress, negative emotions, and even environmental cues (e.g., the presence of attractive food) play a role in etiology. However, today these cognitive and triggering theories are viewed as an explanation for maintaining the binge eating once it has been established, rather than an explanation of causality.

The same sociocultural factors that underlie anorexia nervosa play a significant role in the development of bulimia nervosa.

Family 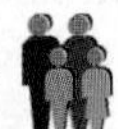

The families of individuals who experience bulimia nervosa are reported to be chaotic, with few rules and unclear boundaries. Often, there is an overly close or enmeshed relationship between the daughter and mother. Daughters may relate that their mother is their "best friend." The boundaries are blurred in that the mother may interact with the daughter as a confidante, and this unhealthy relating further impedes the separation-individuation process. The daughters often feel guilty about separation and responsible for their mother's happiness and emotional well-being (see Box 24.5). Some research on families of individuals with bulimia nervosa has found them to be unempathic and unavailable.

In summary, as with anorexia nervosa, theories of causation do not individually explain the development of bulimia nervosa. Rather, the convergence of many of these factors at a vulnerable stage of individual development best explains causality.

Risk Factors

The risk or predisposing factors for bulimia nervosa are similar to those for anorexia nervosa (see Fig. 24.3). Society's influences, such as the media and peer pressure, underlie the desire to achieve an ideal thin body type. Comparing oneself to these ideal body types leads to body dissatisfaction. These factors influence behaviors such as dietary restraint and overexercising. Dietary restraint leads to binge eating, and purging ensues because of a fear of becoming fat.

Interdisciplinary Treatment

Individuals with bulimia nervosa benefit from a comprehensive multifaceted treatment approach. The goals for treatment for individuals with bulimia nervosa focus on stabilizing and then normalizing eating, which means stopping the binge–purge cycles; restructuring dysfunctional thought patterns and attitudes, especially about eating, weight, and shape; teaching healthy boundary setting; and resolving conflicts about separation-individuation. Treatment usually takes place in an outpatient setting, except when the patient is suicidal or when past outpatient treatment has failed (Table 24.3).

In addition to intensive psychotherapy, usually cognitive-behavioral therapy (CBT) or IPT and pharmacologic interventions are also necessary. The SSRIs demonstrated effectiveness in treating binge eating and purging, even without comorbid depression. Nutrition counseling is an important part of outpatient treatment to stabilize and normalize eating. Some mental health professionals, psychologists, advanced practice psychiatric nurses, and social workers specialize in treating eating disorders, often working with nutritionists who also have expertise in working with this population. Group psychotherapy and support groups are also used. Family therapy is not usually a part of the treatment because many people with bulimia nervosa live on college campuses away from home or are older and on their own. Usually, treatment becomes less intensive as symptoms remit. Therapy focuses on psychological issues, such as boundary setting and separation-individuation conflicts and on changing problematic behaviors and dysfunctional thinking using CBT.

• NCLEXNOTE

NCLEXNOTE

Therapeutic relationships and cognitive interventions are a priority in the nursing care of patients with eating disorders.

Priority Care Issues

Because of the comorbid conditions of depression and borderline personality disorder, some individuals with bulimia nervosa may become suicidal. They are also often at risk for self-mutilation. Because they display high levels of impulsivity, shoplifting, and overspending, financial and legal difficulties have been associated with bulimia nervosa.

NURSING MANAGEMENT: HUMAN RESPONSE TO BULIMIA NERVOSA DISORDER

The primary nursing diagnoses for patients with bulimia nervosa are Imbalanced Nutrition: Less Than Body Requirements, Powerlessness, Anxiety, and Ineffective Coping. Establishing a therapeutic relationship precedes biopsychosocial assessment and interventions.

Therapeutic Relationship

Individuals with bulimia nervosa experience a great deal of shame and guilt. They also often have an intense need to please and be liked and may approach the nurse–patient relationship in a superficial manner. They are too ashamed to discuss their symptoms but do not want to disappoint others, so they may discuss more social or unrelated issues in an attempt to engage the nurse (Box 24.13). A nonjudgmental, accepting approach, stressing the importance of the relationship and outlining its purpose, are important at the outset. Explaining the nature of the relationship and the goals of therapy will help clarify the boundaries.

Biologic Domain

Despite that most individuals with bulimia nervosa maintain normal weights, the physical ramifications of this disorder may be similar to those of anorexia nervosa. Hypokalemia can contribute to muscle weakness and fatigability, as well as to the development of cardiac arrhythmias, palpitations, and cardiac conduction defects. Patients who purge risk fluid and electrolyte abnormalities that can further compromise cardiac status. Neuropsychiatric disturbances, such as poor concentration and attention, and sleep disturbances are common.

BOX 24.13

***Using Reflection:* Understanding the "Need to Please"**

Incident: A nurse became very angry upon discovering that her patient with bulimia had been reporting to the nurse that she was no longer purging. The nurse had worked closely with the patient who disclosed many other psychological issues. The nurse felt that the patient had manipulated her.

Reflection: Upon reflection, the nurse began to see the situation differently. The patient was very connected to the nurse who had made it clear that purging was unacceptable. Fearful of rejection, the patient did not want to disappoint the nurse and focused on other issues.

Assessment

The nurse should assess current eating patterns, determine the number of times a day the individual binges and purges, and note dietary restraint practices. Sleep patterns and exercise habits are also important.

Nursing Diagnoses for the Biologic Domain

Imbalanced Nutrition: Less Than Body Requirements and Disturbed Sleep Pattern are typical nursing diagnoses for the biologic domain.

Interventions for the Biologic Domain

If the patient is admitted to the hospital, meals and all food intake must be strictly monitored to normalize eating. Bathroom visits should also be supervised to prevent purging. Outpatients are asked to record their intake, binges, and purges to form a foundation for changing behaviors with CBT. Because individuals with bulimia nervosa have chaotic lifestyles and are often overcommitted, sleep may be a low priority. Sleep-deprived individuals may assume that food would be helpful, and they begin to eat, triggering a binge. To encourage regular sleep patterns, patients should go to bed and rise at about the same time every day.

Pharmacologic Interventions

Whereas pharmacologic intervention is effective for symptom remission in bulimia nervosa, experts agree that the combination of CBT and medication has had the best results (Wilson et al., 1999). Fluoxetine (Prozac) has been the most studied for bulimia nervosa in clinical trials (see Box 24.14). Effective doses are usually 60 mg per day, a higher dosage than that used to treat depression. Sertraline (Zoloft) has also been used effectively. These medications, prescribed for binge eating and purging, are effective, decreasing both binge eating and purging episodes, even when depression is not present (Milano et al., 2005; Goldstein, Wilson, Arscroft, & Al-Banna, 1999). The most important concern in using these medications is decreased appetite and weight loss during the first few weeks of administration. Weight should be monitored, especially during this period.

Monitoring and Administration of Medication

The intake of medication must be monitored for possible purging after administration. The effect of the medication will depend on whether it has had time to absorb.

Teaching Points 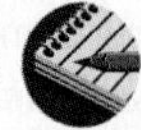

Patients should be instructed to take medication as prescribed. SSRIs must be taken in the morning because

BOX 24.14

Drug Profile: Fluoxetine Hydrochloride (Prozac)

DRUG CLASS: Selective serotonin reuptake inhibitor

RECEPTOR AFFINITY: Inhibits central nervous system neuronal uptake of serotonin with little effect on norepinephrine; thought to antagonize muscarinic, histaminergic, and α-adrenergic receptors.

INDICATIONS: Treatment of depressive disorders, obsessive compulsive disorder, bulimia nervosa, and panic disorder.

ROUTES AND DOSAGE: Available in 10- and 20-mg capsules and 20 mg/5 mL oral solution

Adults: 20 mg/d in the morning, not to exceed 80 mg/d. Full antidepressant effect may not be seen for up to 4 weeks. If no improvement, dosage is increased after several weeks. Dosages >20 mg/d are administered twice daily. For eating disorders: typically 40 mg to 60 mg/d recommended.

Geriatric: Administer at lower or less-frequent doses; monitor responses to guide dosage.

Children: Safety and efficacy have not been established.

HALF-LIFE (PEAK EFFECT): 2 to 3 d (6–8 h)

SELECTED ADVERSE REACTIONS: Headache, nervousness, insomnia, drowsiness, anxiety, tremors, dizziness, lightheadedness, nausea, vomiting, diarrhea, dry mouth, anorexia, dyspepsia, constipation, taste changes, upper respiratory infections, pharyngitis, painful menstruation, sexual dysfunction, urinary frequency, sweating, rash, pruritus, weight loss, asthenia, and fever

BOXED WARNING: Suicidality in children and adolescents

WARNINGS: Avoid use in pregnancy and while breast-feeding. Use with caution in patients with impaired hepatic or renal function and diabetes mellitus. Possible risk for toxicity if taken with tricyclic antidepressants.

SPECIAL PATIENT AND FAMILY EDUCATION:

- Be aware that drug may take up to 4 weeks to get full antidepressant effect.
- Take drug in the morning or divided doses, if necessary.
- Families and caregivers of pediatric patients being treated with antidepressants should monitor patient for agitation, irritation, unusual changes in behavior
- Report any adverse reactions.
- Avoid driving a car or performing hazardous activities because the drug may cause drowsiness or dizziness.
- Eat small, frequent meals to help with complaints of nausea and vomiting.

they can cause insomnia. Patients should be informed that any weight loss they initially experience is temporary and is usually regained after a few weeks, when the medication dosage has stabilized.

Psychosocial Domain

Assessment

For the individual with bulimia nervosa, psychological assessment focuses on cognitive distortions—cues or stimuli that lead to dysfunctional behavior affecting symptom development—and knowledge deficits. The psychological characteristics typical of patients with bulimia nervosa are presented in Box 24.1.

Individuals with bulimia nervosa display a significant number of cognitive distortions, examples of which are found in Table 24.4. These thought patterns form the basis for "rules" and lead the way to destructive eating patterns. During routine history taking, patients relate many of these erroneous assumptions. Situations that produce feelings of being overwhelmed and powerless need to be explored, as does the patient's ability to set boundaries, control impulsivity, and maintain quality relationships. These underlying issues precipitate binge eating. Body dissatisfaction should be openly explored. Several assessment tools are available to gauge such characteristics as body dissatisfaction and impulsivity (see Box 24.8). Mood is an important area for evaluation because many people with bulimia nervosa also have depression. Symptoms of depression, especially the vegetative signs, should be thoroughly explored (see Chapter 20).

Nursing Diagnoses for the Psychosocial Domain

Deficient Knowledge, Disturbed Thought Processes, and Powerlessness are among the common diagnoses for the social domain.

Interventions for the Psychosocial Domain

Both CBT and IPT have been used for individuals with bulimia nervosa. The combination of CBT and pharmacologic interventions is best for producing an initial decrease in symptoms (Leung, Waller, & Thomas, 2000; Mitchell, Peterson, Meyers, & Wunderlich, 2001).

Behavioral therapy alone has not been as effective as CBT. IPT has had positive outcomes but may take longer to change binge eating and purging symptoms. Although binge eating may persist, little work can be done on underlying interpersonal issues, such as boundary setting, because the patient is intent on feeling out of control with eating. Therefore, cognitive therapy is begun first, to address the distorted thinking processes influencing dietary restraint, binge eating, and purging. Decreasing these symptoms will eliminate the out-of-control feelings.

CBT is usually conducted in a group, with one or two sessions a week. A series of sessions is instituted to change dysfunctional thinking, rigid rules about eating, and impulsive behaviors. The cognitive interventions focus on distorted or dysfunctional thought patterns.

Behavioral Techniques

The behavioral techniques, such as **cue elimination** and response prevention, require self-monitoring to individualize the therapy. **Self-monitoring** is accomplished using a diary, in which the patient records binges and purges and precipitating emotions and environmental cues. Emotional and environmental cues are identified, and alternative responses are suggested, tried, and reinforced. When a cue or stimulus leads to a dysfunctional or unhealthy response, the response can be eliminated, or an alternate, healthier response to the cue can be substituted, tried, and then reinforced. Figure 24.6 gives two examples of behavioral interventions. In example 1, for the patient with anorexia nervosa, the response is modified or altered to a healthier one; in example 2, for the patient with bulimia nervosa, the cue is changed to produce a different, healthier response. Other techniques, such as postponing binges and purges through distraction, a technique to interrupt the cycle, are also effective.

Psychoeducation

In addition to cognitive and behavioral techniques, educational strategies are also incorporated into CBT during weekly sessions.

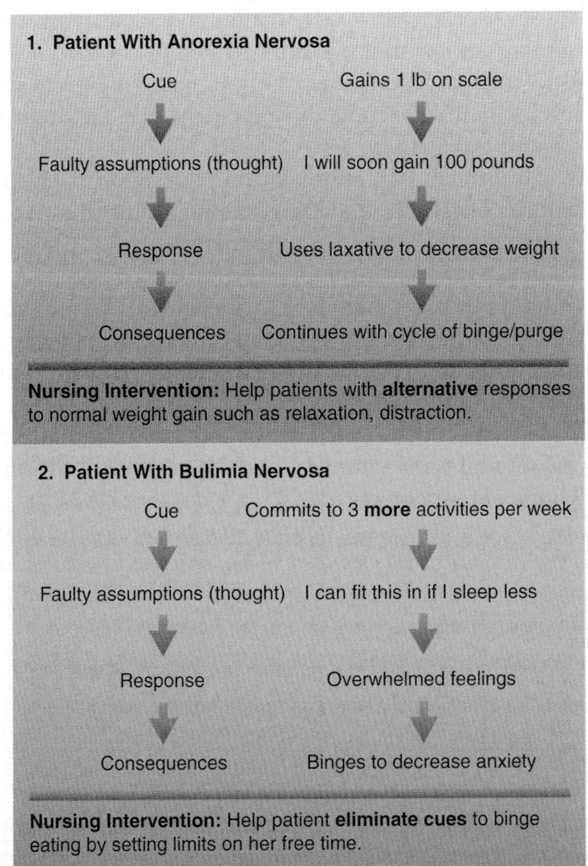

FIGURE 24.6. Examples of the relationship of cues, thoughts, responses and behavioral interventions.

Teaching Points

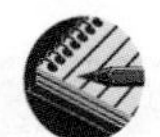

For individuals with bulimia nervosa, psychoeducation focuses on setting boundaries and healthy limits, developing assertiveness, learning nutritional concepts related to healthy eating, and clarifying misconceptions about food. Although earlier studies demonstrated that women with eating disorders have an above average knowledge of nutrition, further work has demonstrated that those with subclinical eating disorders do not have an above average knowledge of nutrition, making this component of treatment essential (Breen & Espelage, 2004). Rules that result from dichotomous thinking also must be addressed because of their role in dietary restraint and resulting binge eating.

Group Therapy

Group therapy is cost-effective and increases learning more effectively than does individual treatment because patients learn from each other as well as from the nurse, therapist, or leader. Some experts have recommended 12-step programs for treating bulimia nervosa. However, many clinicians who work in this specialty have noted that these programs, with their strict rules, can be counterproductive for patients with bulimia nervosa, who already have rigid rules and are "abstinent" in many ways that lead to binge eating. Broad parameters regarding food choices (e.g., all foods allowed in moderation) in combination with knowledge about healthy eating should be encouraged instead.

After symptoms subside, patients can concentrate on interpersonal issues in therapy, such as a fused relationship with their mother, or feelings of inadequacy and low self-esteem, which often underlie their lack of assertiveness.

The nurse can assist patients to understand the binge–purge cycle and the role of rigid rules in contributing to this cycle. The value of eating meals regularly to ward off hunger and reduce the possibility of a binge is also important. Patients who abuse laxatives must be taught that, although these drugs produce water-weight loss, they are ineffective for true, lasting weight loss. Patients also need information about potassium depletion, electrolyte imbalances, dehydration, and the medical consequences of binge eating and purging. Other topics for psychoeducation are included in Box 24.15.

Evaluation and Treatment Outcomes

Patients with bulimia nervosa have better recovery outcomes than do those with anorexia nervosa. Outcomes have improved since the early 1990s, partially because of earlier detection, research on what treatments are most effective, and neuropharmacologic research and advances. Experts in the field of eating disorders report a 69% to

BOX 24.15

Psychoeducation Checklist: Bulimia Nervosa

When caring for the patient with bulimia nervosa, be sure to include the following topic areas in the teaching plan:

- Psychopharmacologic agents, if used, including drug, action, dosage, frequency, and possible adverse effects
- Binge–purge cycle and effects on body
- Nutrition and eating patterns
- Hydration
- Avoidance of cues
- Cognitive distortions
- Limit setting
- Appropriate boundary setting
- Assertiveness
- Resources
- Self-monitoring and behavioral interventions
- Realistic goal setting

70% recovery rate with CBT and medication (Keel et al., 1999). Other studies comparing various methods (such as supportive therapy) have also demonstrated that CBT produces the best results (Wilson et al., 1999). Because CBT requires a specialist's care, current treatment research is exploring the use of self-help models, including manuals that can be combined with psychopharmacology (Mitchell et al., 2001). Frequency of binge eating and purging and severity of dietary restraint at initial treatment, depression, and borderline personality disorder predict a poor outcome after treatment (Bulik et al., 1998; Keel et al., 1999). Good outcome has been associated with a shorter duration of illness; receiving treatment within the first few years of illness is associated with an 80% recovery rate (Reas, Williamson, Martin, & Zucker, 2000).

Continuum of Care

Although patients with bulimia nervosa are less likely than those with anorexia nervosa to require hospitalization, those with extreme dehydration and electrolyte imbalance, depression and suicidality, or symptoms that have not remitted with outpatient treatment need hospitalization.

However, most treatment takes place in outpatient settings. After treatment, referrals to recovery groups and support groups are important to prevent relapse. Rarely do patients with bulimia nervosa require emergency care.

Prevention

As with anorexia nervosa, preventing bulimia nervosa requires effort on the part of teachers, school nurses, parents, and society as a whole. Because many of the risk factors are seen early in children attending elementary school, educating school nurses and teachers is an important focus for psychiatric–mental health nurses working in the community. Protective factors that mediate between risk factors and the development of an eating disorder must be emphasized and developed. Table 24.5 covers important prevention strategies for parents and their children or adolescents.

Society has begun to engage in an effort to help young girls. The federal government has developed a website called "girl power" devoted to self-confidence in such areas as body image.

SUMMARY OF KEY POINTS

- Anorexia nervosa and bulimia nervosa have some common symptoms but are classified as discrete disorders in the *DSM-IV-TR*.
- Eating disorders are best viewed along a continuum that includes subclinical or partial-syndrome disorders; because these disorders occur more frequently than full syndromes, they are often overlooked but, once identified, can be prevented from worsening.
- Similar factors predispose individuals to the development of anorexia nervosa and bulimia nervosa, and these factors represent a biopsychosocial model of risk. These disorders are preventable, and identifying risk factors assists with prevention strategies.
- Etiologic factors contribute in combination to the development of eating disorders; no one factor provides an explanation.
- Treatment of anorexia nervosa almost always includes hospitalization for refeeding; bulimia nervosa is treated primarily on an outpatient basis.
- For patients with bulimia nervosa, CBT improves symptoms sooner than does interpersonal therapy, and CBT is most effective when combined with medication. For patients with anorexia, family therapy plus individual interpersonal therapy is the most effective.
- Pharmacotherapy can be effective for bulimia nervosa but not for anorexia nervosa, especially during acute malnourishment.
- The outcomes for bulimia nervosa are better than those for anorexia nervosa. The type and severity of comorbid conditions and the length of the illness influence outcomes.

CRITICAL THINKING CHALLENGES

1 Discuss the potential difficulties and risks in attempting to treat a patient with anorexia nervosa in an outpatient setting.

2 A patient in the clinic is seen for bulimia nervosa and is prescribed fluoxetine. She reports great success immediately and attributes this to weight lost. What are your concerns and interventions?
3 Parents are often in need of support and suggestions for how to help prevent eating disorders. Develop a teaching program and include the topics and rationale for suggestions chosen.
4 Identify the important nursing management components of a refeeding program for a hospitalized patient with anorexia nervosa.
5 Bulimia nervosa is often described as a closet disorder with secretive binge eating and purging. Identify the signs and symptoms of each system involved for someone with this disorder.
6 Positive outcomes for the recovery of bulimia nervosa and anorexia nervosa are dependent on many factors. Identify the factors that promote positive outcomes and those related to poorer outcomes and prognosis.

REFERENCES

Ackard, D.M. & Neumark-Sztainer, D. (2003). Multiple sexual victimizations among adolescent boys and girls: prevalence and associations with eating behaviors and psychological health. *Journal of Child Sexual Abuse, 12*(1), 17–37.

American Psychiatric Association (APA). (2000). *Diagnostic and statistical manual of mental disorders* (4th ed., text revision). Washington, DC: Author.

Anderson, A. (2001). Progress in eating disorder research. *American Journal of Psychiatry, 158*, 515–517.

Andrist, L. (2003). Media images, body dissatisfaction, and disordered eating in adolescent women. *The American Journal of Maternal/Child Nursing, 28*(2), 119–123.

Anderluh. M.B., Tchanturia, K., Rabe-Hesketh, S., & Treasure, J. (2003). childhood obsessive-compulsive personality traits in adult women with eating disorders; defining a broader eating disorder phenotype. *American Journal of Psychiatry.* 160(2). 242–247.

Arrow, B., Kenardy, J., & Agras, W. S. (1995). The Emotional Eating Scale: The development of a measure to assess coping with negative affect by eating. *International Journal of Eating Disorders, 18*, 79–90.

Baum, A. (2006) eating disorders in the male athlete. Sports Medicine 36, (1), 1–6.

Bailer, U. F., & Kaye, W. H. (2003). A review of neuropeptide and neuroendocrine dysregulation in anorexia and bulimia nervosa. *Current Drug Targets CNS Neuronal Disorders, 2*(1), 53–59.

Berghold, K. M., & Lock, J. (2002). Assessing guilt in adolescents with anorexia nervosa. *American Journal of Psychotherapy, 56*(3), 378–390.

Bell C.J., Hood, S.D., Nutt. D.J. (2005). Acute tryptophan depletion: Clinical effects and implications. *Australia & New Zealand Journal of Psychiatry*, 39(7), 565–574.

Birmingham, C.L., Su, J., Hlyansky, J.A., Goldner, E.M. & Gao, M. (2005). The mortality rate from anorexia nervosa. *International Journal of Eating Disorders, 38*(2), 143–146.

Bisaga, K. Whitaker, A., Davies, M. Chuang, S, Feldman, J & Walsh, B.T. (2005). Eating disorder and depressive symptoms in urban high school girls from different ethnic backgrounds. *Journal of Developmental and Behavioral Pediatrics, 26*(4), 257–266.

Breen, H.B. & Espelage, D.L> (2004). Nutrition expertise in eating disorders. *Eating and Weight Disorders, 9*(2), 120–125

Brownell, K., & Napolitano, M. A. (1995). Distorting reality for children: Body size proportions of Barbie and Ken dolls. *International Journal of Eating Disorders, 18*, 295–298.

Bruch, H. (1973). *Eating disorders: Obesity, anorexia nervosa and the person within*. New York: Basic Books.

Brumberg, J. (1988). *Fasting girls: The emergence of anorexia nervosa as a modern disease*. Cambridge: Harvard University Press.

Bulik, C. M., Sullivan, P. F., Joyce, P. M., Carter, F. A., & McIntosh, V. V. (1998). Prediction of one-year outcome in bulimia nervosa. *Comprehensive Psychiatry, 39*(4), 206–254.

Bulik, C. M., Sullivan, P., Wade, T., & Kendler, K. (2000). Twin studies of eating disorders: A review. *International Journal of Eating Disorders, 27*, 1–20.

Bulik, C.M., Prescott, C.A., Kendler, K.S. (2001). Features of childhood sexual abuse and the development of psychiatric and substance abuse disorders. *British Journal of Psychiatry, 179*, 444–449.

Bulik, C.M., Devlin, B., Bacanu, S.A., Thornton, L., Kump, K.L., Fichter, M.M., Halmi. K.A., Kaplan, A.S., Strober, M., Woodside, D.B., Bergen, A.W., Ganjei, J.K., Crow, S., Mitchell, J., Rotondo, A., Mauri, M., Cassano, G., Keel, P., Berretini, W.H., & Kaye, WH. (2003). Significant linkage on chromosome 10p in families with bulimia nervosa. *American Journal of Human Genetics*, 72(1), 200–207.

Casper, R. C., & Lyubomorisky, S. (1997). Individual psychopathology relative to reports of unwanted sexual experiences as predictors of a bulimic eating pattern. *International Journal of Eating Disorders, 21*, 229–236.

Cooper, P., Taylor, M., Cooper, Z., & Fairburn, C. (1987). The development and validation of the BSQ. *International Journal of Eating Disorders, 6*, 485–494.

Costanzo, P. R., Musante, G. J., Friedman, K. E., Kern, L. S., & Tomlinson, K. (1999). The gender specificity of emotional, situational, and behavioral indicators of binge eating in a diet-seeking obese population. *International Journal of Eating Disorders, 26*(2), 205–210.

Croll, J., Neumark-Sztainer, D., Story, M., & Ireland, M. (2002). Prevalence and risk and protective factors related to disordered eating behaviors among adolescents: Relationship to gender and ethnicity. *Journal of Adolescent Health, 13*(2), 166–175.

Currin, L., Schmidt, U., Treasure, J. & Jick, H. (2005). Time trends in eating disorder incidence. *British Journal of Psychiatry*, 186, 132–135.

Diamond-Raab, L., & Orrell-Valente, J. K. (2002). Art therapy, psychodrama and verbal therapy. An integrative model of group therapy in the treatment of adolescents with anorexia nervosa and bulimia nervosa. *Child and Adolescent Psychiatric Clinics of North America, 11*(2), 343–364.

Dunn, P. K., & Ondercin, P. (1981). Personality variables related to compulsive eating in college women. *Journal of Clinical Psychology, 31*, 43–49.

Eisenberg., M.E., Neumark-Sztainer , D., Story, M., & Perry, C. (2005). The role of social norms and friends' influences on unhealthy weight-control among adolescent girls. *Social Science and Medicine, 60*(6), 1165–1173.

Ferrand, C. & Brunet, E. (2004). Perfectionism and risk for disordered eating among young French male cyclists of high performance. *Perception and Motor Skills* 99(3), 959–967.

Fister, S.M. & Smith, G.T. (2004). Media effects on expectancies: exposure to realistic female imahes as a protective factor. *Psychology of Addictive Behaviors, 18*(4), 394–397.

Frank, G.K., Bailer, U.F., Henry S. Wagner,A. & Kaye W.H. (2004). Neuroimaging studies in eating disorders. *Central Nervous System, 9*(7), 539–548.

Franko, D.L., Keel, P.K., Dorer, D.L. Blais, M.A., Delinsky, S.S., Eddy, K.T., Charat, V., Renn, R, & Herzog, D.B. (2005). What predicts suicide attempts in women with eating disorders? *Psychological Medicine, 34*(5), 843–853.

Garner, D. M., & Garfinkel, P. E. (1979). The Eating Attitudes Text: An index of the symptoms of anorexia nervosa. *Psychosomatic Medicine, 10*, 647–656.

Geller, J., Cockell, S., & Goldner, E. (2000). Inhibited expression of negative emotions and interpersonal orientation in anorexia nervosa. *International Journal of Eating Disorders, 28*, 8–19.

Goldstein, D. J., Wilson, M. G., Arscroft, R. C., & Al-Banna, M. (1999). Effectiveness of fluoxetine therapy in bulimia nervosa regardless of comorbid depression. *International Journal of Eating Disorders, 25*, 19–28.

Gutwill, S. (1994). Women's eating problems: Social context and the internalization of culture. In C. Bloom, A. Gitter, S. Gutwill, et al. (Eds.), *Eating problems: A feminist psychoanalytic treatment model* (pp. 1–27). New York: Basic Books.

Golden, N.H. (2002). A review of the female athlete triad (amenorrhea, osteoporosis and disordered eating). *International Journal of Adolescent Mental Health*, 14(1), 9–17.

Hayden-Wade, H.A., Stein, R.I.,, Ghaderi, A., Saelens, B.E., Zabinski, M.E., and Wilfley, D.E. Prevalence characteristics and correlates of teasing experiences among overweight children vs. non-overweight peers. *Obestity Research*, 13(8), 1381–1392.

Herman, C. P., & Mack, D. (1975). Restrained and unrestrained eating. *Journal of Personality, 43*, 647–660.

Herzog, D. B., Greenwood, D. N., Dorer, D. J., Flores, A. T., Ekeblad, E. R., Richards, A., et al. (2000). Mortality in eating disorders: A descriptive study. *International Journal of Eating Disorders, 28*(1), 20–26.

Hill, A., & Pallin, V. (1998). Dieting awareness and low self-worth: Related issues in 8-year-old girls. *International Journal of Eating Disorders, 24*, 405–413.

Hinton, P.S. & Kubas, K.L. (2005). Psychosocial correlates of disordered eating in female collegiate athlete: validation of the ATHLETE questionnaire *Journal of American College Health*, 54(3), 149–156.

Holtkamp, K., Konrad, K., Kaiser, N., Ploenes, Y., Heussen, N. Grzella, I. & Herpetz-Dahlmann, B. (2005). A retrospective study of SSRI treatment in adolescent anorexia nervosa: insufficient evidence for efficacy. *Journal of Psychiatric Research*, 39(3), 303–310.

Hopkinson, R.A/ & Lock, J. (2004). Athletics, perfectionism, and disordered eating. *Eating and Weight Disordered* 9(2), 99–106.

Johnson, J. G., Cohen, P., Kasen, S., & Brook, J. S. (2002). Childhood adversities associated with risk for eating disorders or weight problems during adolescence or early adulthood. *American Journal of Psychiatry, 159*, 394–400.

Joiner, T. E., Katz, J., & Heatherton, T. F. (2000). Personality factors differentiate late adolescent females and males with chronic bulimic symptoms. *International Journal of Eating Disorders, 27*, 191–197.

Kaye, W. H., Frank, G.K., Bailer, U.F., Henry, S.E. et al (2005). Serotonin alterations in anorexia and bulimia nervosa: new insights from imaging studies. *Physiology & Behavior*, 85 91), 73–81.

Kaye, W. H., Gendall, K. A., Fernstrom, M. H., Fernstrom, J. D., McConaha, C. W., & Weltzin, T. E. (2000). Effects of acute tryptophan depletion on mood in bulimia nervosa. *Biological Psychiatry, 47*(2), 151–157.

Kaye, W. H., Klump, K.L., Frank, G. K., & Strober, M. (2000). Anorexia and bulimia. *Annual Review of Medicine*, 51, 299–313.

Keel, P. K., Dorer, D. J., Eddy, K. T., Franco, D., Charatan, D. L., & Herzog, D. B. (2003). Predictors of mortality in eating disorders. *Archives of General Psychiatry, 60*, 179–183.

Keel, P.K., Healtherton, T.F., Dorer, D.J., Joiner, T.E., & Zalta, A.K. (2006). Point prevalence of bulimia nervosa in 1982, 1992, and 2002. *Psychological Medicine*, 36(1), 119–127.

Keel, P.K., Klump, K.L., Miller, K.B., McGue, M. & Iacono, W.G. (2005). Shared transmission of eating disorders and anxiety disorders. *International Journal of Eating Disorders*, 38(2), 99–105.

Keel, P. K., Mitchell, J. E., Miller, K. B., Davis, T. L., & Crow, S. J. (1999). Long-term outcome of bulimia nervosa. *Archives of General Psychiatry, 56*, 63–69.

Korndorfer, S. R., Lucas, A. R., Suman, V. J., Crowson, C. S., Krahn, L. E., & Melton, L. J. III (2003). Long-term survival of patients with anorexia nervosa: A population based study in Rochester, MN. *Mayo Clinic Proceedings, 78*(3), 278–284.

Kuba, S. A., & Harris, D. J. (2001). Eating disturbances in women of color: An exploratory study of contextual factors in the development of disordered eating in Mexican-American women. *Health Care for Women International, 22*(3), 281–298.

Leung, N., Waller, G., & Thomas, G. (2000). Outcome of group cognitive-behavioral therapy for bulimia nervosa: The role of core beliefs. *Behaviour Research and Therapy, 38*(2), 145–156.

Mazure, C. M., Halmi, K., Sunday, S. R., Romano, S. J., & Einhorn, A. M. (1994). Yale-Brown-Cornell Eating Disorder Scale: Development, use, reliability, and validity. *Journal of Psychiatric Research*, 28, 425–445.

Maloney, M., McGuire, J., & Daniels, S. R. (1988). Reliability testing of a children's version of the Eating Attitude Test. *Journal of the American Academy of Child and Adolescent Psychiatry, 27*, 541–543.

Martz, D. M., Sturgis, E. T., & Gustafson, S. B. (1996). Development and preliminary validation of the Cognitive Behavioral Dieting Scale. *International Journal of Eating Disorders, 19*, 297–309.

Matsunaga, H., Kaye, W. H., McConaha, C., Plotnikov, K., Pollice, C., & Rao, R. (2000). Personality disorders among subjects recovered from eating disorders. *International Journal of Eating Disorders, 27*, 353–357.

McIntosh, V. V., Bulik, C. M., McKenzie, J. M., et al. (2000). Interpersonal psychotherapy for anorexia nervosa. *International Journal of Eating Disorders*, 27, 125–139.

Milos, G., Spindler, A., Ruggiero, G., Klaghofer, R., Schnyder, V. (2002). Comorbidity of obsessive-compulsive disorders and duration of eating disorders. *International Journal of Eating Disorders, 36*(3), 284–289.

Mazure, C. M., Halmi, K. A., Sunday, S. R., Romano, S. J., & Einhorn, A. M. (1994). Yale-Brown-Cornell Eating Disorder Scale: Development, use, reliability, and validity. *Journal of Psychiatric Research, 28*, 425–445.

McIntosh, V. V., Bulik, C. M., McKenzie, J. M., Luty, S. E., & Jordan, J. (2000). Interpersonal psychotherapy for anorexia nervosa. *International Journal of Eating Disorders, 27*, 125–139.

Minuchin, S., Rossman, B. L., & Baker, L. (1978). *Psychosomatic families*. Cambridge: Harvard University Press.

Mitchell, J. E., Peterson, C. B., Meyers, T., & Wunderlich, S. (2001). Combining pharmacotherapy in the treatment of patients with eating disorders. *Psychiatric Clinics of North America, 24*(2), 315–323.

Milano, W., Siano, C., Putrella, C., Caoasso, A. (2005). Treatment of bulimia nervosa with fluvoxamine: a randomized control trial. *Advanced Therapeutics* 22(3), 278–283.

Monteleone, P.Fabrazzo, M., Martiadis, V., Serritella, C., Pannuto, M. & Maj, M. (2005). Circulatig brain-derived neurotrophic factor is decreased in women with AN and BN but not in women with binge- eating disorder: relationships to comorbid depression, psychpathology, and hormonal variables. *Psychological Medicine*, 35 (6), 897–905.

O'Connell, C., Larkin, K., Mizes, J.S. Fremouw, W. (2005). The impact of caloric preloading on attempts at food and eating-related suppression in restrained and unrestrained eaters. *International Journal of Eating Disorders, 38(1), 42–48.*

Ogden, J., & Steward, J. (2000). The role of the mother–daughter relationship in explaining weight concern. *International Journal of Eating Disorders, 28*(11), 78–83.

Patel, P., Wheatcroft, R., Park, R. J., & Stein, A. (2002). The children of mothers with eating disorders. *Clinical Child and Family Psychological Review, 5*(1), 1–19.

Pawluck, D. E., & Gorey, K. M. (1998). Secular trends in the incidence of anorexia nervosa: Integrative review of population based studies. *International Journal of Eating Disorders, 23*, 347–352.

Perkins, D. F., & Luster, T. (1999). The relationship between sexual abuse and purging: Findings from a community wide survey of female adolescents. *Child Abuse and Neglect, 23*, 371–382.

Polivy, J., & Herman, C. P. (1993). Etiology of binge eating: Psychological mechanisms. In C. G. Fairburn & G. T. Wilson (Eds.), *Binge eating: Nature, assessment and treatment* (pp. 173–205). New York: Guilford.

Reas, D. L., Williamson, D. A., Martin, C. K., & Zucker, N. L. (2000). Duration of illness predicts outcome for bulimia nervosa: A long term follow up study. *International Journal of Eating Disorders, 27*, 428–434.

Robin, A. L., Siegel, P. T., Moye, A. W., Gilroy, M., Dennis, A. B., & Sikand, A. (1999). A controlled comparison of family versus individual therapy for adolescents with anorexia nervosa. *Journal of the American Academy of Child and Adolescent Psychiatry, 38*(12), 1482–1489.

Schwartz, D., Phares, V., Tantleff-Dunn, S., & Thompson, J. K. (1999). Body image, psychological functioning, and parental feedback regarding physical appearance. *International Journal of Eating Disorders, 18*, 339–344.

Shapira, N. A., Goldsmith, T. D., & McElroy, S. L. (2000). Treatment of binge eating disorder with topiramate: A clinical case series. *Journal of Clinical Psychiatry, 61*(5), 368–372.

Shisslak, C., Renger, R., Sharpe, T., Crago, M., McKnight, K. M, Gray, N., et al. (1999). Development and evaluation of the McKnight Risk Factor Survey for assessing potential risk and protective factors for disordered eating in preadolescent and adolescent girls. *International Journal of Eating Disorders, 25*, 195–214.

Smolak, L., Murnen, S. K., & Ruble, A. (2000). Female athletes and eating problems: A meta analysis. *International Journal of Eating Disorders*, 27(4), 371–380.

Steinhausen, H. C. (2002). The outcome of anorexia nervosa in the 20th century. *The American Journal of Psychiatry, 159*, 1284–1293.

Streigel-Moore, R. (1993). Etiology of binge eating: A developmental perspective. In C. G. Fairburn & G. T. Wilson (Eds.), *Binge eating, nature, assessment and treatment* (pp. 144–172). New York: Guilford.

Strober, M., Pataki, C., Freeman, R., & DeAntonio, M. (1999). No effect of adjunctive fluoxetine on eating behavior or weight phobia during the inpatient treatment of anorexia nervosa: An historical case controlled study. *Journal of Child and Adolescent Psychopharmacology, 9*(3), 195–201.

Streigel-Moore R.H., Dohm, FA., Kraemer, H.C., Taylor, C.B., Daniel, S., Crawford, P.B., & Schreiber, G.B.(2003). Eating disorders in black and white women. *American Journal of Psychiatry, 160*(7), 1326–31.

Strober, M., Freeman, R., Lampert, C., et al. (2000). Controlled family study of anorexia nervosa and bulimia nervosa: Evidence of shared liability and transmission of partial syndromes.

Taylor, C. B., Sharpe, T., Shisslak, C., Bryson, S., Estes, L. S., Gray, N., et al. (1998). Factors associated with weight loss in adolescent girls. *International Journal of Eating Disorders, 24*, 31–42.

Tanofsky-Kraff, M., Faden, D., Yanovski, S.Z., Wilfley, D.E. & Yanovski, J.A. (2005). The perceived onset of dieting and loss of control eating behaviors in overweight children. *International Journal of Eating Disorders, 38*(2), 112–122.

Thomsen, S. R., Weber, M. M., & Brown, L. B. (2002). The relationship between reading beauty and fashion magazines and the use of pathogenic dieting methods among adolescent females. *Adolescence, 37*(145), 1–18.

Thomas, J.J., Keel, P.K. & Heatherton, T.F. (2005). Disordered eating attitudes and behaviors in ballet students: examination of environmental and individual risk factors. *International Journal of Eating Disorders, 38*(3), 263–268.

Tortsveit, M.K. & Sundgot-Borgen, J. (2005). The female athlete traid exists in both elite athletes and controls. *Medicine, Science, Sports & Exercise*, 37(9), 1449–1459.

Tozzi, F., Aggen, S.H., Neale, B.M., Anderson, C.B., Mazzeo, S.E., Neale, M.C., & Bulik, C.M. (2004). The structure of perfectionism: a twin study *Journal of Behavior & Genetics*, 34(5), 483–494.

Uher, R. et al. (12 authors)(2005). Functional neuroanatomy of body shape perception in health and eating-disordered women. *Biological Psychiatry, 58*(12), 990–997.

von Ranson, K. M., Kaye, W. H., Weltzin, T. E., Rao, R., & Matsunaga, H. (1999). Obsessive-compulsive disorder symptoms before and after recovery from bulimia nervosa. *American Journal of Psychiatry, 156*(11), 1703–1708.

Viken, R.J. Treat, T.A. Bloom, S.L. & McFall, R.M. (2005). Illosory correlation of body types and unhappiness: covariation bias and its relationships to eating disorder symptoms. *International Journal of Eating Disorders, 38*(1), 65–72.

Warren, C.S., Gleaves, D.H., Cepeda-Benito, A., Fernandez Mdel, c., Rodriguez-Ruiz, S. (2005). Ethnicity as a protective factor against internalization of a thin ideal and body dissatisfaction. *International Journal of Eating Disorders, 37*(3), 241–249.

White, J. H. (2000a). Eating disorders in elementary and middle school children: Risk factors, early detection and prevention. *The Journal of School Nursing, 16*(2), 26–35.

White, J. H. (2000b). Symptom development in bulimia nervosa: A comparison of women with and without a history of anorexia nervosa. *Archives of Psychiatric Nursing, 14*(2), 81–92.

Wiederman, M., & Pryor, T. (2000). Body dissatisfaction, bulimia, and depression among women: The mediating role of drive for thinness. *International Journal of Eating Disorders, 27*, 90–95.

Wilson, G. T., Loeb, K. L., Walsh, B. T., Labouvie, E., Petkova, E., Liu, X., & Waternaux, C. (1999). Psychological versus pharmacological treatments of bulimia nervosa: Predictors and processes of change. *Journal of Consulting and Clinical Psychology, 67*(4), 451–459.

Wolfe, B. E., & Gimby, L. B. (2003). Caring for the hospitalized patient with an eating disorder. *The Nursing Clinics of North America, 38*, 75–99.

Wolfe, B. E., Metzger, E. D., Levine, J. M., Finkelstein, D. M., Cooper, T. B., & Jimerson, D. C. (2000). Serotonin function following remission from bulimia nervosa. *Neuropsychopharmacology, 22*(3), 257–263.

Wooley, S. C., & Kearney-Cooke, A. (1986). Intensive treatment of bulimia and body image disturbance. In K. D. Brownell & J. P. Foreyt (Eds.), *Handbook of eating disorders: Physiology, psychology and treatment of obesity, anorexia, and bulimia* (pp. 476–502). New York: Basic Books.

Woodside, D. B., Garfinkel, P. E., Lin, E., Goering, P., Kaplan, A. S., Goldbloom, D. S., & Kennedy, S. H. (2001). Comparison of men with full or partial eating disorders, men without eating disorders, and women with eating disorders in the community. *American Journal of Psychiatry, 158*, 570–574.

Yoel, J., & Workgroup in Eating Disorders. (2000). Practice guidelines for the treatment of patients with eating disorders. *American Journal of Psychiatry, 157*(1), 1–35.

CHAPTER 25

Substance-Related Disorders

Barbara G. Faltz, Harvey "Skip" Davis, and Richard V. Wing

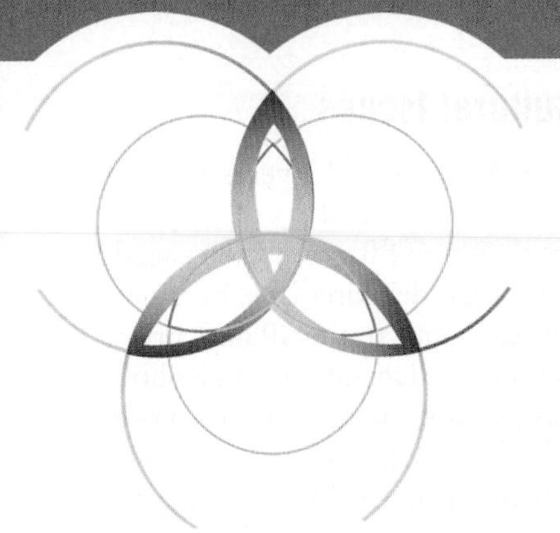

LEARNING OBJECTIVES

After studying this chapter, you will be able to:

- Describe the actions, effects, and withdrawal symptoms of alcohol, marijuana, stimulants, sedatives, hallucinogens, opiates, dissociative anesthetics, and inhalants
- Discuss the evidence that serves as a basis of care and treatment of persons with substance abuse disorders.
- Formulate nursing diagnoses based on a biopsychosocial assessment of people with substance use disorders.
- Compare intervention approaches to substance use disorders.
- Implement treatment interventions for patients with substance-related disorders.

KEY CONCEPTS

- Addiction
- denial
- motivation

KEY TERMS

• abuse • alcohol withdrawal syndrome • Alcoholics Anonymous • anhedonia • brief intervention • codependence • confabulation • confrontation • countertransference • craving • delirium tremens • dependence • detoxification • hallucinogen • harm reduction • inhalants • Korsakoff's psychosis • methadone maintenance • opiates • peer assistance programs • relapse • substance-related disorders • tolerance • use • Wernicke's syndrome • withdrawal

Ancient and modern history chronicles the negative impact of alcohol and drug dependence on various cultures and civilizations. The human use and abuse of alcohol and other drugs has been around since the beginning of history; so too have the subsequent social and emotional problems that accompany substance dependence. Alcohol, tobacco, and other drug problems have reached epidemic proportions in the United States, with incidence rising in younger age groups, particularly among adolescents and young adults. The risk of exposure to illegal drugs is now a threat to children, adolescents, and young adults in almost every local neighborhood, community, and school. Healthy People 2010 has identified substance dependence as a major health issue (U.S. Department of Health and Human Services [DHHS], 2000).

Specific health concerns include: (1) the risk for spread of human immunodeficiency virus (HIV) infection, hepatitis B and C, tuberculosis, and other communicable diseases among alcohol and other drug users; (2) premature deaths or traumatic injuries caused by drug overdoses or other unsafe activities or practices engaged in while under the influence of alcohol or drugs (e.g., motor vehicle accidents); and (3) domestic violence. The medical and social implications of these health problems are profound for a new generation of children who are now at risk for the serious medical, developmental, learning, and psychological problems associated with exposure to drugs and alcohol.

This chapter reviews addiction, types of substance use, biologic and psychological effects, current theories of substance use disorders, and interventions available for treatment.

KEY CONCEPT Addiction is a condition of continued use of substances despite adverse consequences.

The role of the nurse is discussed in assessment and planning interventions to help meet the needs of patients and family members who seek treatment. Professional issues regarding chemical dependency within the nursing profession are also examined.

SUBSTANCE USE

Definitions and Terms

The following terms are used to describe behavior patterns regarding substance use:

- **Use** is when a person drinks alcohol or swallows, smokes, sniffs, or injects a mind-altering substance.
- **Abuse** is when a person uses alcohol or drugs for the purpose of intoxication or, in the case of prescription drugs, for purposes beyond their intended use.
- **Dependence** refers to physiological dependence as evidenced by tolerance and withdrawal or impairment in social and occupational functioning resulting from the pathological and repeated use of substances.
- **Withdrawal** is the adverse physical and psychological symptoms that occur when a person ceases using a substance.
- **Detoxification** is the process of safely and effectively withdrawing a person from an addictive substance, usually under medical supervision.
- **Relapse** is the recurrence of alcohol- or drug-dependent behavior in an individual who has previously achieved and maintained abstinence for a significant time beyond the period of detoxification.

Diagnostic Criteria

The American Psychiatric Association's (APA, 2000) *Diagnostic and Statistical Manual of Mental Disorders*, 4th ed., text revision (*DSM-IV-TR*) classifies **substance-related disorders** as disorders related to taking a drug of abuse, including alcohol, amphetamines, cannabis (marijuana), cocaine, hallucinogens, inhalants, nicotine, opioids, phencyclidine, sedatives-hypnotics, anxiolytics, caffeine, or other unknown substances. These disorders are further categorized as those related to the abuse of a substance, those related to dependence on a substance, or those induced by intoxication or withdrawal. The *DSM-IV-TR* outlines diagnostic criteria for both substance abuse and dependence (Table 25.1).

Epidemiology and Cultural Issues

About half (50.3%) of Americans over 12 years or 121 million people report being current drinkers of alcohol. In a national survey, more than one fifth of persons aged 12 or older participated in binge drinking (five or more drinks on one occasion) at least once in the 30 days prior to the survey. Fifteen million are dependent on alcohol; 16% of the population has alcoholism and 80% or more of the alcohol consumed in the United States is consumed by people with alcoholism (NIDA, 2005a). In 2004, rates of binge drinking and heavy alcohol use were highest among young adults ages 18 to 25 years (Substance Abuse and Mental Health Services Administration [SAMHSA], 2005).

In 2004, an estimated 14 million Americans (6.3% of the population 12 years of age and older) were current illicit drug users. Marijuana, the most commonly used illicit drug, was used by 76.4% (14.6 million) of current illicit drug users; however, marijuana use is declining in the adolescent population after peak use in the late 1990s (SAMHSA, 2005).

The current estimate is that there are 3.6 million cocaine users (National Institute on Drug Abuse [NIDA], 2005). Studies indicate that the number of students who have ever used hallucinogens or dissociative anesthetics is reflecting a downward trend for LSD (lysergic acid diethylamide) and a slight increase in the use of PCP (phencyclidine), whereas the use of other hallucinogens and dissociatives appears to have leveled (NIDA, 2005a; 2005b).

In 2002, 13,000 youth between the ages of 12 and 17 had used heroin at least once in the past year, compared with 12,000 in 2003. Among the general population age 12 and older, 404,000 had used annually in 2002, compared with 314,000 in 2003 (Wu, et al. 2003). The Drug Abuse Warning Network (DAWN) lists heroin among the four most frequently mentioned drugs reported in drug-related death cases in 2002 (SAMHSA, 2002). Nationwide, treatment of heroin-related problems in emergency departments has increased 35% since 1995.

Recently, a substantial new epidemic of heroin abuse has been developing in the United States and spreading to middle-class users. The proportion of people inhaling or smoking heroin and the number of people seeking treatment has continued to increase (NIDA,

Table 25.1  DSM-IV Substance-Related Disorders 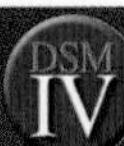

Substance Disorder	Diagnostic Criteria
Substance Dependence	
Alcohol dependence Amphetamine dependence Cannabis dependence Cocaine dependence Hallucinogen dependence Inhalant dependence Nicotine dependence Opioid dependence Phencyclidine dependence Sedative, hypnotic, or anxiolytic dependence Polysubstance dependence	Maladaptive pattern of substance use leading to clinically significant impairment or distress • Impairment manifested by three or more of the following: tolerance (need for markedly increased amounts of the substance to reach intoxication or desired effect), withdrawal, substance often taken in large amounts or over a longer period than was intended, persistent desire or unsuccessful efforts to cut down or control use, much time spent in activities necessary to obtain the substance or use it, reduction or cessation of important social, occupational, or recreational activities, use continued despite knowledge of having persistent or recurrent physical or psychological problem likely to have been caused or exacerbated by the substance
Substance Abuse	
Alcohol abuse Amphetamine abuse Cannabis abuse Cocaine abuse Hallucinogen abuse Inhalant abuse Opioid abuse Phencyclidine abuse Sedative, hypnotic, or anxiolytic abuse	• Maladaptive pattern of substance use leading to clinically significant impairment or distress • Impairment manifested by three or more of the following occurring within a 12-month period: Recurrent use, resulting in failure to fulfill major role obligations at work, school, or home Recurrent use in situations that are physically hazardous Recurrent substance-related legal problems Continued use despite feeling persistent or recurrent effects of the substance
Substance Intoxication	
Alcohol intoxication Alcohol intoxication delirium Amphetamine intoxication Amphetamine intoxication delirium Caffeine intoxication Cannabis intoxication Cannabis intoxication delirium Cocaine intoxication Cocaine intoxication delirium Hallucinogen intoxication Hallucinogen intoxication delirium Opioid intoxication Opioid intoxication delirium Inhalant intoxication Inhalant intoxication delirium Phencyclidine intoxication, delirium Sedative, hypnotic, or anxiolytic intoxication	• Symptoms never met criteria for substance dependence • Reversible substance-specific syndrome due to recent ingestion or exposure to a substance • Clinically significant maladaptive behavioral or psychological changes due to effect of substance on central nervous system, developing during or shortly after use of substance • Symptoms not due to general medical condition, nor better accounted for by another mental disorder
Substance Withdrawal	
Alcohol withdrawal, delirium Amphetamine withdrawal Cocaine withdrawal Opioid withdrawal Sedative, hypnotic, or anxiolytic withdrawal, delirium	• Development of substance-specific syndrome due to cessation or reduction in substance use, previously heavy and prolonged • Syndrome causing significant distress or impairment in social, occupational, or other important areas of functioning

2005b). In 2004, the number of new nonmedical users of oxycodone was 615,000, with an average age at first use of 24.5 years. Estimates of oxycodone initiation show a steady increase in the number of initiates from 1995, the year this drug was first available, through 2003 (SAMHSA, 2005).

African Americans

Alcohol is the drug most widely used by African American youth. Although African American youth use both licit and illicit substances at lower rates than do Caucasians, they have experienced more associated health and legal problems than have other ethnic groups (SAMHSA, 2005). Frequent heavy drinking in Caucasians aged 18 to 29 drops as they age, but rates of heavy drinking and alcohol problems remain high in the same age group of African Americans who were exposed to more alcohol advertising in magazines and television programs than their Caucasian counterparts (Hanson, 2003).

Latino Americans

The prevalence of drug use is alarmingly high among Mexican American and Puerto Rican adolescent boys, who have a much higher use of marijuana than the Cuban American or other Latin American students (SAMHSA, 2005). Of the Latino Americans, Mexican American men report the most frequent, heavy drinking and alcohol-related problems. Cuban Americans report the lowest percentages of problems. For women, fewer intergroup differences exist than for men (Delva, 2005).

Asians and Pacific Islanders

As a general pattern, Asian and Pacific Islanders have a lower prevalence rate of substance dependence than any other group, but the rate is increasing particularly among the Native Hawaiian/Pacific Islanders. Alcohol use is also increasing significantly among Asian Americans, who constitute one of the fastest growing U.S. minority populations (SAMHSA, 2005). Several cultural patterns and attitudes have been suggested as influencing factors:

1. Public drunkenness is viewed as unacceptable and disgraceful behavior.
2. Drinking is viewed as primarily a male activity, and many Asian women do not drink.
3. Seeking professional help is viewed as a sign of character weakness, particularly in Asian men.
4. Asian flushing syndrome, a physiologic reaction that occurs in 47% to 85% of Asian Americans, resulting in a red cutaneous flush or rash that appears on the face and body and particularly the ears after drinking alcohol, may serve as deterrent to drinking excessively.

The Asian flushing syndrome has been associated with the lack of the liver enzyme acetaldehyde dehydrogenase, which results in an initial rapid rate of alcohol metabolism and sudden buildup of acetaldehyde, a toxic byproduct of alcohol metabolism (Collins & McNair, 2002).

Native Americans

Studies indicate that alcohol and other drug use prevalence rates are highest among members of Native American groups (OAS/SAMHSA, 2003). Alcohol dependence is a leading cause of morbidity and mortality in Native Americans. Recent studies suggest that marijuana, alcohol, tobacco, and stimulant dependence have a genetic influence. In a Southwest California Native American community, there appears to be several chromosomal regions linked to alcohol dependence (Ehlers et al., 2004; Wilhelmsen & Ehlers, 2005). These results add support to a long-held belief that some Native Americans were genetically predisposed to alcoholism.

Gender Differences

Changes in women's roles during the past century are most likely responsible for the narrowing of the gender gap in substance use. Worldwide, men consume more alcohol and abuse drugs more than women (Holmila & Raitasalo, 2005). In the United States, higher prevalence of abuse disorders is related to early age of initiation of behavior, not necessarily gender. Gender differences are being studied according to type of substance, ethnicity, and biological predisposition. Generally, men abuse cocaine and heroin more than women, who are more likely to abuse prescription drugs. Drug and alcohol use patterns in women vary with age, education, marital status, employment, race and ethnicity, and the alcohol or drug usage of spouse or significant other (Collins & McNair, 2002; Holdcraft & Iacono, 2004; Zilberman, Tavares, & el-Guebaly, 2003; Green, Perrin, & Polen, 2004)

Comorbidity

Many substance-dependent people have comorbid mental disorders. Some disorders are in part a byproduct of long-term substance dependence; others predispose the individual to alcohol or drug abuse. Whatever the reason, nurses should be aware that substance-dependent patients often have anxiety disorders, phobias, or obsessive-compulsive and affective disorders, such as major depression and dysthymia (Fu et al., 2002). Other coexisting mental disorders include attention deficit hyperactivity disorder (Winstanley, Eagle & Robbins, 2006; Kalbag & Levin, 2005) and personality disorders (Marmorstein

& Iacono (2005). These are discussed in detail in Chapters 22 and 28.

Alcohol- and drug-dependent individuals are at high risk for death caused by drug overdose but are also at increased risk for death from other causes, including homicide, suicide, and opportunistic infections, such as HIV, secondary to drug injection. Earlier studies have well documented the connection between alcohol dependence and increased risk for diabetes mellitus, gastrointestinal problems, hypertension, liver disease, and stroke (Hendriks & van Tol, 2005).

Etiology

The disease model of substance abuse is a biopsychosocial one. It encompasses the body, the mind, and society's influences in studying the disease and formulating treatment (Amodia, Cano, & Eliason, 2005). Recent biologic studies in humans and animals have confirmed a genetic predisposition underpinning drinking behaviors and significant genetic differences in self-administration for several other drugs, yet no precise genetic marker has been established. Recent evidence from genetics, neurochemistry, and pharmacology has revealed the essential biologic component of alcoholism—that it is a chronic and progressive disease that must be treated. This disease is influenced not just by the biologic components but also by the individual's temperament and feelings about self (psychological components) and environmental factors, such as parental and family relationships and peer pressure (social components). To understand and treat substance-dependent people, nurses must understand and treat all facets of this illness (see Figure 25.1).

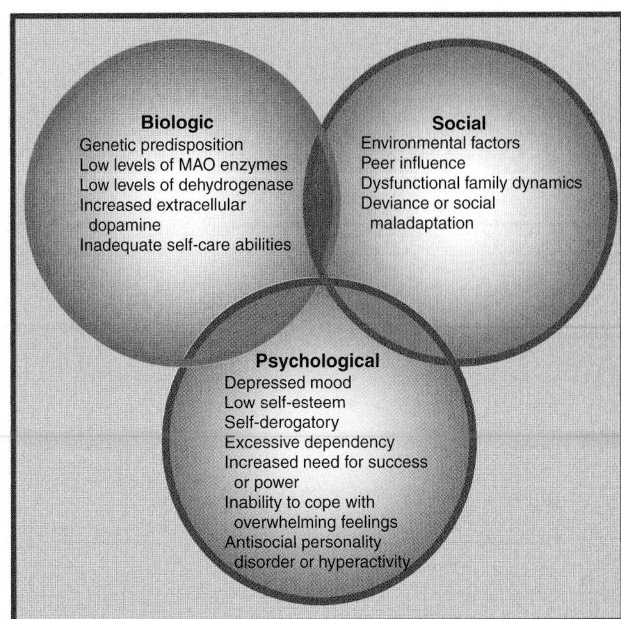

FIGURE 25.1. Biopsychosocial etiologies for patients with substance abuse.

ALCOHOL

Alcohol (or ethanol) is a sedative anesthetic found in various proportions in liquor, wine, and beer. Alcohol produces a sedative effect by depressing the central nervous system (CNS). This effect causes the individual to experience relaxed inhibitions, heightened emotions, mood swings that can range from bouts of gaiety to angry outbursts, and cognitive impairments such as reduced concentration or attention span, and impaired judgment and memory. Depending on the amount of alcohol ingested, the effects can range from feelings of mild sedation and relaxation, to confusion and serious impairment of motor functions and speech, to severe intoxication that can result in coma, respiratory failure, and death. See Table 25.2 for a summary of the effects of abused substances.

The intensity of CNS impairments depends on how much alcohol is consumed in a given period of time and how rapidly the body metabolizes it. Intoxication is determined by the level of alcohol in the blood, called **blood alcohol level** (BAL). The body can metabolize 1 oz of liquor, a 5-oz glass of wine, or a 12-oz can of beer per hour without intoxication. Table 25.3 shows normal physiologic responses at various blood alcohol levels. Excessive or long-term abuse of alcohol can adversely affect all body systems, and the effects can be serious and permanent. Box 25.1 lists the major physical complications of alcohol abuse in the major organ systems.

Years of alcohol abuse can cause cerebellar degeneration from increased levels of acetaldehyde, a toxic byproduct of alcohol metabolism, and can result in impaired coordination, a broad-based unsteady gait, and fine tremors. Sedative-hypnotic long-term effects include disturbances in rapid eye movement (REM) sleep and chronic sleep disorders. Although certain alcohol-related cognitive impairment is reversible with abstinence, long-term alcohol abuse can cause specific neurologic complications that lead to organic brain disorders, known as alcohol-induced amnestic disorders (discussed later). People who abuse alcohol can exhibit various patterns of use. Some engage in heavy drinking on a regular or daily basis; others may abstain from drinking during the week and engage in heavy drinking on the weekends; still others can experience longer periods of sobriety interspersed with bouts of binge drinking (several days of intoxication).

Thus, all patients should be screened not only for alcohol use disorders, but also for drinking patterns or behaviors that may place them at increased risk for experiencing adverse health effects or alcoholism. Risky (binge) drinkers who have not yet become alcohol dependent often can be treated successfully within a primary care set-

Table 25.2 Summary of Effects of Abused Substances, Overdose, Withdrawal Syndromes, and Prolonged Use

Substance	Route	Effects (E) and Overdose (O)	Withdrawal Syndrome	Prolonged Use
Alcohol	Oral	E: Sedation, decreased inhibitions, relaxation, decreased coordination, slurred speech, nausea O: Respiratory depression, cardiac arrest	Tremors; seizures, increased temperature, pulse, and blood pressure; delirium tremens	Affects all systems of the body. Can lead to other dependencies.
Stimulants (amphetamines, cocaine)	Oral, IV, inhalation, smoking	E: Euphoria, initial CNS stimulation then depression, wakefulness, decreased appetite, insomnia, paranoia, aggressiveness, dilated pupils, tremors O: Cardiac arrhythmias/arrest, increased or lowered blood pressure, respiratory depression, chest pain, vomiting, seizures, psychosis, confusion, seizures, dyskinesias, dystonias, coma	Depression: psychomotor retardation at first, then agitation; fatigue then insomnia; severe dysphoria and anxiety; cravings, vivid, unpleasant dreams; increased appetite. Amphetamine withdrawal is not as pronounced as cocaine withdrawal.	Is often alternated with depressants. Weight loss and resulting malnutrition and increased susceptibility to infectious diseases. May produce schizophrenia-like syndrome with paranoid ideation, thought disturbance, hallucinations, and stereotyped movements
Cannabis (marijuana, hashish, THC)	Smoking, oral	E: Euphoria or dysphoria, relaxation and drowsiness, heightened perception of color and sound, poor coordination, spatial perception and time distortion, unusual body sensations (weightlessness, tingling, etc.), dry mouth, dysarthria, and food cravings O: Increased heart rate, reddened eyes, dysphoria, lability, disorientation		Can decrease motivation and cause cognitive deficits (inability to concentrate, memory impairment).
Hallucinogens (LSD, MDMA)	Oral	E: Euphoria or dysphoria, altered body image, distorted or sharpened visual and auditory perception, depersonalization, bizarre behavior, confusion, incoordination, impaired judgment and memory, signs of sympathetic and parasympathetic stimulation, palpitations (blurred vision, dilated pupils, sweating) O: Paranoia, ideas of reference, fear of losing one's mind, depersonalization, derealization, illusions, hallucinations, synesthesia, self-destructive/aggressive behavior, tremors		"Flashbacks" or HPPD may occur after termination of use.
Phencyclidine (PCP)	Oral, inhalation, smoking	E: Feeling superhuman, decreased awareness of and detachment from the environment, stimulation of the respiratory and cardiovascular system, ataxia, dysarthria, decreased pain perception O: Hallucinations, paranoia, psychosis, aggression, adrenergic crisis (cardiac failure, CVA, malignant hyperthermia, status epilepticus, severe muscle contractions)		"Flashbacks," HPPD, organic brain syndromes with recurrent psychotic behavior, which can last up to 6 months after not using the drug, numerous psychiatric hospitalizations and police arrests.
Opiates (heroin, codeine)	Oral, injection, smoking	E: Euphoria, sedation, reduced libido, memory and concentration difficulties, analgesia, constipation, constricted pupils O: Respiratory depression, stupor, coma	Abdominal cramps, rhinorrhea, watery eyes, dilated pupils, yawning, "goose flesh," diaphoresis, nausea, diarrhea, anorexia, insomnia, fever (see Table 25–5)	Can lead to criminal behavior to get money for drugs, risk for infection-related to needle use (e.g., HIV, endocarditis, hepatitis).

Substance	Route	Effects (E) and Overdose (O)	Withdrawal Syndrome	Prolonged Use
Sedatives, hypnotics, anxiolytics	Oral, injection	E: Euphoria, sedation, reduced libido, emotional lability, impaired judgment O: Respiratory depression, cardiac arrest	Anxiety rebound and agitation, hypertension, tachycardia, sweating, hyperpyrexia, sensory excitement, motor excitation, insomnia, possible tonic-clonic convulsions, nightmares, delirium, depersonalization, hallucinations	Often alternated with stimulants, use with alcohol enhances chance of overdose, risk for infection related to needle use.
Inhalants (glue, lighter fluid)	Inhalation	E: Euphoria, giddiness, excitation O: CNS depression: ataxia, nystagmus, dysarthria, coma and convulsions	Similar to alcohol but milder, with anxiety, tremors, hallucinations, and sleep disturbance as the primary symptoms	Long-term use can lead to liver and renal failure, blood dyscrasias, damage to the lungs. CNS damage (OBS, peripheral neuropathies, cerebral and optic atrophy, parkinsonism).
Nicotine	Smoking	E: Stimulation, enhanced performance and alertness, and appetite suppression O: Anxiety	Mood changes (craving, anxiety) and physiologic changes (poor concentration, sleep disturbances, headaches, gastric distress, and increased appetite)	Increased chance for cardiac disease and lung disease.
Caffeine	Oral	E: Stimulation, increased mental acuity, inexhaustability O: Restlessness, nervousness, excitement, insomnia, flushing, diuresis, gastrointestinal distress, muscle twitching, rambling flow of thought and speech, tachycardia or cardiac arrhythmia, agitation	Headache, drowsiness, fatigue, craving, impaired psychomotor performance, difficulty concentrating, yawning, nausea	Physical consequences are under investigation.

CNS, central nervous system; CVA, cerebrovascular accident; GI, gastrointestinal; HIV, human immunodeficiency virus; HPPD, hallucinogen persisting perceptual disorder; OBS, organic brain syndrome.

Table 25.3 Behavior and Blood Alcohol Levels

Number of Drinks	Blood Alcohol Levels (mg%)	Behavior
1–2	0.05	Impaired judgment, giddiness, mood changes
5–6	0.10	Difficulty driving and coordinating movements
10–12	0.20	Motor functions severely impaired, resulting in ataxia. There is emotional lability.
15–20	0.30	Stupor, disorientation, and confusion
20–24	0.40	Coma
25	0.50	Respiratory failure, death

ting (Ballesteros, Gonzalez-Pinto, Querajeta, & Cerino, 2004).

Biologic Responses to Alcohol

Alcohol makes the neuronal membranes more permeable to potassium (K^+) and chloride (Cl^-) and closes sodium (Na^+) and calcium (Ca^{++}) channels. This increased permeability depresses the CNS, and adrenergic activity raises blood pressure and heart rate. Alcohol is metabolized in the liver as a carbohydrate into carbon dioxide and water. The breakdown process (oxidation) of the compound ethanol (CH_3CH_2OH) is ethanol → acetaldehyde + water → acetic acid → carbon dioxide + water. Acetaldehyde is toxic and is usually broken down by acetaldehyde dehydrogenase. Rapid alcohol intake can cause an accumulation of acetaldehyde, which then combines with the neurotransmitters dopamine and serotonin to produce tetrahydroisoquinolines and β-carbolines. Physical dependence on alcohol becomes a problem when central nervous system cells require alcohol to function normally.

People who have abused alcohol for long periods of time often experience alcohol **tolerance**, a phenomenon producing a more rapid metabolism of alcohol and decreased response to sedating, motor, and anxiolytic effects. These individuals may demonstrate higher blood alcohol levels than normal (listed in Table 25.3) before they experience symptoms of intoxication. The locus ceruleus, a brain structure that normally inhibits the action of ethanol, is believed to be instrumental in the development of alcohol tolerance.

BOX 25.1

Medical Complications of Alcohol Dependence

- **Cardiovascular System:** Cardiomyopathy, congestive heart failure, hypertension
- **Respiratory System:** Increased rate of pneumonia and other respiratory infections
- **Hematologic System:** Anemias, leukemia, hematomas
- **Nervous System:** Withdrawal symptoms, irritability, depression, anxiety disorders, sleep disorders, phobias, paranoid feelings, diminished brain size and functioning, organic brain disorders, blackouts, cerebellar degeneration, neuropathies, palsies, gait disturbances, visual problems
- **Digestive System** and **Nutritional Deficiencies:** Liver diseases (fatty liver, alcoholic hepatitis, cirrhosis), pancreatitis, ulcers, other inflammations of the gastrointestinal (GI) tract, ulcers and GI bleeds, esophageal varices, cancers of the upper GI tract, pellagra, alcohol amnestic disorder, dermatitis, stomatitis, cheilosis, scurvy
- **Endocrine and Metabolic:** Increased incidence of diabetes, hyperlipidemia, hyperuricemia, and gout
- **Immune System:** Impaired immune functioning, higher incidence of infectious diseases, including tuberculosis and other bacterial infections
- **Integumentary System:** Skin lesions, increased incidence of infection, burns, and other traumatic injury
- **Musculoskeletal System:** Increased incidence of traumatic injury, myopathy
- **Genitourinary System:** Hypogonadism, increased secondary female sexual characteristics in men (hypoandrogenization and hyperestrogenization), impotence in males, electrolyte imbalances due to excess urinary secretion of potassium and magnesium

Alcohol Withdrawal Syndrome

Alcohol withdrawal syndrome, which occurs after alcohol consumption is reduced or when abstaining from alcohol after prolonged use, causes changes in vital signs, diaphoresis, and gastrointestinal and CNS adverse effects. The severity of withdrawal symptoms ranges from mild to severe, depending on the length and amount of alcohol use. Symptoms include increased heart rate and blood pressure, diaphoresis, mild anxiety, restlessness, and hand tremors (Table 25.4). In patients with alcoholism or in chronic drinkers, the alcohol withdrawal syndrome usually begins within 12 hours after abrupt discontinuation or attempt to decrease consumption. Only 5% of individuals with alcohol dependence ever experience severe complications of withdrawal, such as **delirium tremens** or grand mal (tonic–clonic) seizures.

• NCLEXNOTE

NCLEXNOTE Alcohol abuse continues to require nursing assessment and interventions in all settings. Patients who abuse alcohol for long periods of time are at high risk for delirium tremens. Observing for signs of seizure activity is a priority nursing intervention.

Alcohol-Induced Amnestic Disorders

Alcohol is directly toxic to the brain, causing atrophy of the frontal cortex and eventually chronic brain syndrome. Patients with alcohol-induced amnestic disorders

Table 25.4 Alcohol Withdrawal Syndrome

	Stage I: Mild	Stage II: Moderate	Stage III: Severe
Vital signs	Heart rate elevated, temperature elevated, normal or slightly elevated systolic blood pressure	Heart rate 100–120 bpm; elevated systolic blood pressure and temperature	Heart rate, 120–140 bpm; elevated systolic and diastolic blood pressures; elevated temperature
Diaphoresis	Slightly	Usually obvious	Marked
Central nervous system	Oriented, no confusion, no hallucinations	Intermittent confusion; transient visual and auditory hallucinations and illusions, mostly at night	Marked disorientation, confusion, disturbing visual and auditory hallucinations, misidentification of objects, delusions related to the hallucinations, delirium tremens, disturbances in consciousness
	Mild anxiety and restlessness	Painful anxiety and motor restlessness	Agitation, extreme restlessness, and panic states
	Restless sleep	Insomnia and nightmares	Unable to sleep
	Hand tremors, "shakes," no convulsions	Visible tremulousness, rare convulsions	Gross uncontrollable tremors, convulsions common
Gastrointestinal system	Impaired appetite, nausea	Anorexia, nausea and vomiting	Rejecting all fluid and food

usually have a history of many years of heavy alcohol use and are generally older than 40 years. Symptom onset can be gradual or develop over many years. Impairment can be severe, and once the disorder is established, it can persist indefinitely.

Wernicke's syndrome is caused by thiamine deficiency and is not exclusive to alcoholism. Wernicke's encephalopathy presents with oculomotor dysfunctions (bilateral abducens nerve palsy), ataxia, and confusion. Encephalopathy often evolves when thiamine deficiency is chronic and untreated. **Korsakoff's psychosis**, also known as alcohol amnestic disorder, is characterized by both retrograde and anterograde amnesia with sparing of intellectual function. **Confabulation,** telling a plausible, but imagined scenario that fills in memory gaps, is a key feature and used to compensate for memory loss. As many as half of patients with Korsakoff's psychosis do not experience significant improvement even if alcohol is no longer used (Miller & Hester, 2003).

Pharmacologic Treatment of Alcohol Withdrawal

Several medications can help an individual overcome the symptoms of alcohol withdrawal: benzodiazepines; long-acting CNS depressants, which produce sedation and reduce anxiety symptoms; and antipsychotic medications. Antianxiety and sedating drugs, such as benzodiazepines, are useful when substituted for the shorter-acting drug alcohol.

Benzodiazepines usually are administered when there are elevations in heart rate, blood pressure, and temperature and on the presence of tremors. Patients can be given 5 to 10 mg of diazepam (Valium) every 2 to 4 hours, or 25 to 100 mg of chlordiazepoxide hydrochloride (Librium) every 4 hours. Medication given early in the course of withdrawal and in sufficient dosages can prevent the development of delirium tremens. Should withdrawal delirium occur, higher doses are used, with careful monitoring of the patient to prevent overdose. These drugs are also extremely effective during withdrawal as anticonvulsants because they act more rapidly than does phenytoin (Dilantin), which can take 7 to 10 days to reach therapeutic levels. Seizures, if they occur, usually do so within the first 48 hours of withdrawal.

Disulfiram (Antabuse) is not a treatment or cure for alcoholism, but it can be used as adjunct therapy to help deter some individuals from drinking while using other treatment modalities to teach new coping skills to alter abuse behaviors (see Box 25.2). Disulfiram plus even small amounts of alcohol produces adverse effects. In severe reactions, there may be respiratory depression, cardiovascular collapse, arrhythmias, myocardial infarction, acute congestive heart failure, unconsciousness, convulsions, and death.

Naltrexone was originally used as a treatment for heroin abuse, but it is now approved for treatment of alcohol dependence. Naltrexone is formulated in a once-daily dose in pill form and a monthly injection. The precise mechanism of action for naltrexone's effect is unknown; however, reports from successfully treated patients suggest three kinds of effects: (1) can reduce **craving** (the urge or desire to drink); (2) can help maintain abstinence, and (3) can interfere with the tendency to want to drink more if a recovering patient slips and has a drink. Naltrexone may be particularly useful in patients who continue to drink heavily (Leavitt, 2002; McCaul, Wand, Eissenberg, Rohde, & Cheskin, 2000). (See Box 25.3.)

BOX 25.2

Drug Profile: *Disulfiram (Antabuse)*

DRUG CLASS: Antialcoholic agent, enzyme inhibitor

RECEPTOR AFFINITY: Inhibits the enzyme aldehyde dehydrogenase, blocking oxidation of alcohol and allowing acetaldehyde to accumulate to concentrations 5 to 10 times higher than normal in the blood during alcohol metabolism. Believed to inhibit norepinephrine synthesis.

INDICATIONS: Management of selected patients with chronic alcohol use who want to remain in a state of enforced sobriety.

ROUTE AND DOSAGE: Available in 250- and 500-mg tablets

Adults: Initially, a maximum dose of 500 mg/d PO in a single dose for 1–2 weeks. Maintenance dosage of 125 to 500 mg/d PO not to exceed 500 mg/d, continued until patient is fully recovered socially, and a basis for permanent self-control is established.

HALF-LIFE (PEAK EFFECT): Unclear (12 h)

SELECTED ADVERSE REACTIONS: Drowsiness, fatigue, headache, metallic or garlic-like aftertaste. If taken with alcohol: flushing, throbbing in head and neck, throbbing headaches, respiratory difficulty, nausea, copious vomiting, sweating, thirst, chest pain, palpitations, dyspnea, hyperventilation, tachycardia, hypotension, syncope, weakness, vertigo, blurred vision, confusion; severe reactions may include arrhythmias, cardiovascular collapse, acute congestive heart failure, and unconsciousness.

WARNINGS: Never administer to an intoxicated patient or without the patient's knowledge. Do not administer until patient has abstained from alcohol for at least 12 hours. Contraindicated in patients with severe myocardial disease, coronary occlusion, or psychoses, or in patients receiving current or recent treatment with metronidazole, paraldehyde, alcohol, or alcohol-containing preparations. Use cautiously in patients with diabetes mellitus, hypothyroidism, epilepsy, cerebral damage, chronic and acute nephritis, hepatic cirrhosis or dysfunction.

POSSIBLE DRUG INTERACTIONS: Concomitant administration of phenytoin, diazepam, or chlordiazepoxide may cause increased serum levels and risk for drug toxicity. Increased prothrombin time caused by disulfiram may lead to a need to adjust dosage of oral anticoagulants.

SPECIFIC PATIENT/FAMILY EDUCATION

- Take the drug daily; take it at bedtime if it makes you dizzy or tired. Crush or mix tablets with liquid if necessary.
- Do not take any form of alcohol (such as beer, wine, liquor, vinegars, cough mixtures, sauces, aftershave lotions, liniments, or cologne); doing so may cause a severe unpleasant reaction.
- Wear or carry medical identification with you at all times to alert any medical emergency personnel that you are taking this drug.
- Keep appointments for follow-up blood tests.
- Avoid driving or performing tasks that require alertness if drowsiness, fatigue, or blurred vision occur.
- Know that the metallic aftertaste is transient and will disappear after use of the drug is discontinued.

BOX 25.3

Drug Profile: *Naltrexone (Trexan)*

DRUG CLASS: Narcotic antagonist

RECEPTOR AFFINITY: Binds to opiate receptors in the CNS and competitively inhibits the action of opioid drugs, including those with mixed narcotic agonist–antagonist properties.

INDICATIONS: Adjunctive treatment of alcohol or narcotic dependence as part of a comprehensive treatment program.

ROUTE AND DOSAGE: Available in 50-mg tablets

Adults: For alcoholism: 50 mg/d PO; for narcotic dependence: initial dose of 25 mg PO; if no signs or symptoms seen, complete dose with 25 mg. Usual maintenance dose is 50 mg/d PO.

Children: Safety has not been established for use in children younger than 18 y.

HALF-LIFE (PEAK EFFECT): 3.9–12.9 h (60 min)

SELECTED ADVERSE REACTIONS: Difficulty sleeping, anxiety, nervousness, headache, low energy, abdominal pain/cramps, nausea, vomiting, delayed ejaculations, decreased potency, skin rash, chills, increased thirst, joint and muscle pain

WARNINGS: Contraindicated in pregnancy and patients allergic to narcotic antagonists. Use cautiously in narcotic addiction because may produce withdrawal symptoms. Do not administer unless patient has been opioid free for 7–10 d. Also, use cautiously in patients with acute hepatitis, liver failure, depression, suicidal tendencies, and breast-feeding. Must make certain patient is opioid free before administering naltrexone. Always give naloxone challenge test before using, except in patients showing clinical signs of opioid withdrawal.

SPECIFIC PATIENT/FAMILY EDUCATION

- Know that this drug will help facilitate abstinence from alcohol and block the effects of narcotics.
- Wear a medical identification tag to alert emergency personnel that you are taking this drug.
- Avoid use of heroin or other opiate drugs; small doses may have no effect, but large doses can cause death, serious injury, or coma.
- Report any signs and symptoms of adverse effects.
- Notify other health care providers that you are taking this drug.
- Keep appointments for follow-up blood tests and treatment program.

Adequate Nutrition and Supplemental Vitamins

Poor nutrition and vitamin deficiencies are often symptoms of alcohol dependence. Multivitamins and adequate nutrition are essential for patients who are severely malnourished, but other vitamin replacement may be necessary for certain individuals. Thiamine (vitamin B_1) may be needed when a patient is in withdrawal, to decrease ataxia and other symptoms of deficiency. It is usually given orally, 100 mg four times daily, but can be given intramuscularly or by intravenous infusion with glucose. Folic acid deficiency is corrected with administration of 1.0 mg orally, four times daily. Magnesium deficiency also is found in those with long-term alcohol dependence. Magnesium sulfate, which enhances the body's response to thiamine and reduces seizures, is given prophylactically for patients with histories of withdrawal seizures. The usual dose is 1.0 g intramuscularly, four times daily for 2 days.

STIMULANTS

Cocaine

Cocaine is an alkaloid found in the leaves of the *Erythroxylon coca* plant that is native to western South America, where for hundreds of years natives have known the powerful intoxicating effects of chewing the coca leaves. Cocaine is made from the leaves into a coca paste that is refined into cocaine hydrochloride, a crystalline form (white powder appearance), which is commonly inhaled or "snorted" in the nose, injected intravenously (with water), or smoked. The smokeable form of cocaine, often called *free-base cocaine*, can be made by mixing the crystalline cocaine with ether or sodium hydroxide.

After cocaine is inhaled or injected, the user experiences a sudden burst of mental alertness and energy ("cocaine rush") and feelings of self-confidence, being in control, and sociability, which last 10 to 20 minutes. This high is followed by an intense let-down effect ("cocaine crash"), in which the person feels irritable, depressed, and tired, and craves more of the drug. Although it has not been proven that cocaine is physically addictive, it is clear that users experience a serious psychological addiction and pattern of abuse. Although cocaine users typically report that the drug enhances their feelings of well-being and reduces anxiety, cocaine also is known to bring on panic attacks in some individuals. Long-term cocaine use leads to increased anxiety.

Severe anxiety, along with restlessness and agitation, is also among the major symptoms of cocaine withdrawal. Increased use of cocaine is associated with stress and drug craving (Fox, Talih, Malison, Anderson, Kreek, & Sinha, 2005). Users quickly seek more cocaine or other drugs, such as alcohol, marijuana, or sleeping pills, to rid themselves of the terrible effects of crashing. Withdrawal causes intense depression, craving, and drug-seeking behavior that may last for weeks. Individuals who discontinue cocaine use often relapse.

Crack cocaine, often called "crack," is a form of free-base cocaine produced by mixing the crystal with water and baking soda or sodium bicarbonate and boiling it until a rock precipitant remains. The hardened crystal is then broken into pieces ("cracked") and smoked in cigarettes or water pipes. This extremely potent form produces a rapid high and intense euphoria and an even more dramatic crash. It is extremely addictive because of the intense and rapid onset of euphoric effects, which leave users craving more.

Cocaine emerged as the popular drug of the 1990s and was characterized as the drug of the wealthy, the young, upwardly mobile professionals or celebrities, and those in high-profile social circles. Then crack cocaine emerged as a cheap street drug, and it became available to all socioeconomic circles. Crack quickly became one of the leading addictive drugs of the 1990s, causing serious national health concerns.

Biologic Responses to Cocaine

Cocaine is absorbed rapidly through the blood–brain barrier and is readily absorbed through the skin and mucous membranes. Cocaine acts as a potent local anesthetic when applied directly to tissue, preventing both the generation and conduction of nerve impulses by inhibiting the rapid influx of sodium ions through the nerve membrane. Peak intoxication occurs rapidly with intravenous injection or inhalation. Injecting releases the drug directly into the bloodstream and heightens the intensity of its effects. Smoking entails inhalation of cocaine vapor or smoke into the lungs, where absorption into the bloodstream is as rapid as by injection. The resulting increased levels of dopamine in the synaptic cleft cause euphoria and, in excess, psychotic symptoms. Dopamine and dopamine metabolite levels are depleted by prolonged cocaine use. This absence of dopamine (which normally inhibits prolactin secretion) increases prolactin levels in the blood. Cocaine use increases norepinephrine levels in the blood, causing tachycardia, hypertension, dilated pupils, and rising body temperatures. Dopamine and dopamine metabolite levels are depleted by prolonged cocaine use. Serotonin excess contributes to sleep disturbances and anorexia.

Cocaine Intoxication

Intoxication causes CNS stimulation, the length of which depends on the dose and route of administration. With steadily increasing doses, restlessness proceeds to tremors and agitation, followed by convulsions and CNS depression. In lethal overdose, death generally results from respiratory failure. A toxic psychosis is also possible and may be accompanied by physical signs of CNS stimulation (tachycardia, hypertension, cardiac arrhythmias, sweating, hyperpyrexia, and convulsions).

There is a potential dangerous interaction between cocaine and alcohol. Taken in combination, the two drugs are converted by the body to cocaethylene, which has a longer duration of action in the brain and is more toxic than either drug alone. Notably, this mixture of cocaine and alcohol is the most common two-drug combination that results in drug-related death (NIDA, 2006).

Cocaine Withdrawal

Long-term cocaine use depletes norepinephrine, resulting in the "crash" when use of the drug is discontinued and causing the user to sleep 12 to 18 hours. Upon awakening, withdrawal symptoms may occur, characterized by sleep disturbances with rebound REM sleep, anergia (lack of energy), decreased libido, depression with possible suicidality, **anhedonia**, poor concentration, and cocaine craving. Treating cocaine addiction is complex and involves assessing the psychobiological, social, and pharmacologic aspects of abuse. There is no current evidence supporting the clinical use of antidepressants, carbamazepine, disulfiram, or lithium in treating cocaine dependence (deLima, deOlivera Soceres, Reisser, & Farrell, 2002).

• NCLEXNOTE

NCLEXNOTE

In cocaine withdrawal, patients are excessively sleepy because of the norepinephrine depletion. Recovery is difficult because of the intense cravings. Nursing interventions should focus on helping patients solve problems related to managing these cravings.

Amphetamines

Amphetamines were first synthesized for medical use in the 1880s. Amphetamines (Biphetamine, Delcobase, Dexedrine, Obetrol) and other stimulants, such as phenmetrazine (Preludin) and methylphenidate (Ritalin), act on the CNS and peripheral nervous system. They are used to treat attention-deficit hyperactivity disorder in children, narcolepsy, depression, and obesity (on a short-term basis). Some people abuse these drugs to achieve the effects of alertness, increased concentration, a sense of increased energy, euphoria, and appetite suppression. Amphetamines are indirect catecholamine agonists and cause the release of newly synthesized norepinephrine. Like cocaine, they block the reuptake of norepinephrine and dopamine, but they do not affect the serotonergic system as strongly. They also affect the peripheral nervous system and are powerful sympathomimetics, stimulating both α and β receptors. This stimulation results in tachycardia, arrhythmias, increased systolic and diastolic blood pressures, and peripheral hyperthermia. The effects of amphetamine use and the clinical course of an overdose are similar to those of cocaine. Amphetamine abuse may be treated with pharmacologic agents similar to those used for cocaine, such as antidepressants and dopaminergic agonists. Amphetamine withdrawal symptoms are not as pronounced as those of cocaine withdrawal.

Methamphetamine

Methamphetamine is a potent central nervous system stimulant that releases excess dopamine. Highly addictive, it comes in many forms and can be smoked, snorted, orally ingested, or injected. A brief, intense sensation, or rush, is reported by those who smoke or inject methamphetamine. Oral ingestion or snorting produces a long-lasting high instead of a rush, which can continue for as long as half a day. Also known as Meth, Speed, Ice, Chalk, Crank, Fire, Glass, and Crystal, this illegal substance is cheap, easy to make, and has devastating consequences. According to the 2003 National Survey on Drug Use and Health, 12.3 million Americans age 12 and older have tried methamphetamine at least once in their lifetimes (5.2% of the population), with the majority between 18 and 34 years of age.

Methamphetame was developed early in this century from its parent drug, amphetamine, as a decongestant and bronchial inhaler. When used to produce a rush or a high, high levels of dopamine are released, contributing to the drug's toxic effects—including damage to nerve terminals. High doses can elevate body temperature and stimulate seizures. Long-term effects include dependence and addiction psychosis (paranoia, hallucinations), mood disturbances, repetitive motor activity, stroke, weight loss, and extensive tooth decay (NIDA, 2005c) (see Figure 25.2). Methamphetamine is often used in a "binge and crash" pattern. Tolerance occurs within minutes, and the pleasurable effect disappears even before the drug con-

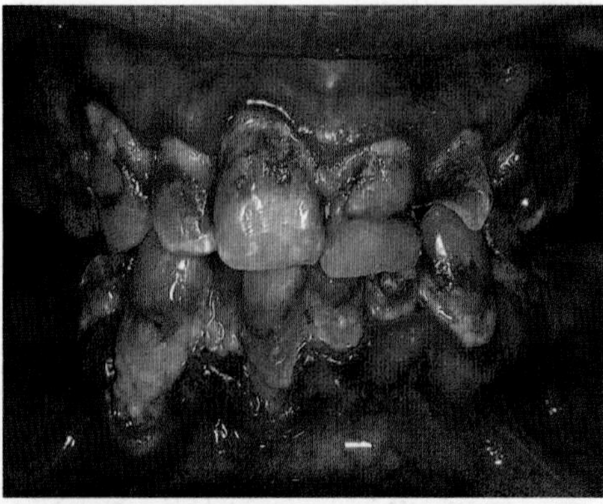

FIGURE 25.2. Severe tooth decay caused by abuse of methamphetamine.

centration in the blood falls significantly. Once assessed, referral to a drug treatment program is necessary.

MDMA

MDMA (3–4 methylenedioxymethamphetamine), or Ecstasy, is known as a "club drug" because it is used by teens and young adults as part of the nightclub, bar, and rave scenes. MDMA, similar in structure to methamphetamine, causes serotonin to be released from neurons in greater amounts than normal. Once released, this serotonin can excessively activate serotonin receptors. Scientists have also shown that MDMA causes excess dopamine to be released from dopamine-containing neurons. Alarmingly, research in animals has demonstrated that MDMA can damage and destroy serotonin-containing neurons. MDMA can cause hallucinations, confusion, depression, sleep problems, drug craving, severe anxiety, and paranoia. In high doses, MDMA can cause a sharp increase in body temperature (malignant hyperthermia), leading to muscle breakdown, kidney and cardiovascular failure, and death.

Nicotine

Nicotine, the addictive chemical mainly responsible for the high prevalence of tobacco use, is the primary reason tobacco is named a public health menace. Smoking is more prevalent among people with alcoholism, polysubstance users, and psychiatric patients than among the general population (Breslau, Novak, & Kessler, 2004). Nicotine stimulates the central, peripheral, and autonomic nervous systems, causing increased alertness, concentration, attention, and appetite suppression. It is readily absorbed and is carried in the bloodstream to the liver, where it is partially metabolized. It is also metabolized by the kidneys and is excreted in the urine.

Nicotine acts as an agonist of the nicotinic cholinergic receptor sites and stimulates autonomic ganglia in both the parasympathetic and sympathetic nervous systems, resulting in increased release of norepinephrine or acetylcholine. The release of epinephrine by nicotine from the adrenal medulla increases fatty acids, glycerol, and lactate levels in the blood, thereby increasing the risk for atherosclerosis and cardiac muscle pathology.

Other medical complications of nicotine use are numerous. Smoking either cigarettes or cigars can cause respiratory problems, lung cancer, emphysema, heart problems, and peripheral vascular disease. In fact, smoking is the largest preventable cause of premature death and disability. Cigarette smoking kills at least 400,000 people in the United States each year and makes countless others ill. The use of smokeless tobacco is also associated with serious health problems (NIDA, 2000).

Repeated use of nicotine produces both tolerance and dependence. Recent research has shown that nicotine addiction is extremely powerful and is at least as strong as addictions to other drugs, such as heroin and cocaine; 70% of those who quit relapse within a year (NIDA, 2000).

Nicotine Withdrawal and Replacement Therapy

Nicotine withdrawal is marked by mood changes (craving, anxiety, irritability, depression) and physiologic changes (difficulty in concentrating, sleep disturbances, headaches, gastric distress, and increased appetite). Nicotine replacements such as transdermal patches, nicotine gum, nasal spray, and inhalers have been used successfully to assist in withdrawal by reducing the craving for tobacco. Patches are rotated on skin sites and help maintain a steady blood level of nicotine. Products such as Habitrol, Nicoderm, and ProStep are used daily, with the decrease in strength of nicotine occurring during a period of 6 to 12 weeks.

The use of this medication should be accompanied by social support and education to enhance the commitment to abstain from tobacco. Symptoms of excessive nicotine released by the patches can resemble withdrawal symptoms. People with cardiovascular disease and peripheral vascular disease may not be candidates for this therapy because increased cardiac stimulation and peripheral vasoconstriction are common side effects. Smoking while using transdermal patches will enhance negative cardiovascular side effects. Patients who do smoke during therapy should not use patches (Ludvig & Eisenberg, 2002).

Caffeine

Caffeine is a stimulant found in many drinks (coffee, tea, cocoa, soft drinks), chocolate, and over-the-counter medications, including analgesics, stimulants, appetite suppressants, and cold relief preparations. Currently, regular daily consumption is widespread throughout the world, with use by more than 80% of the adults in the United States (Griffiths & Vernotica, 2000). Doses of less than 200 mg, found in one to two cups of percolated coffee, stimulate the cerebral cortex and increase mental acuity. At a dose of 300 mg, caffeine can cause tremors, poor motor performance, and insomnia (Bonnet, Balkin, Dinges, Roehrs, Rogers, & Wesensten, 2005). Doses exceeding 500 mg (more than five cups of coffee) increase the heart rate; stimulate respiratory, vasomotor, and vagal centers and cardiac muscles, resulting in increased force of cardiac contraction; dilate pulmonary and coronary blood vessels; and constrict blood flow to the cerebral vascular system.

Psychiatric symptoms such as panic, schizophrenia, or manic-depressive symptoms can be exacerbated by caffeine in higher doses (APA, 2000).

Symptoms of caffeine intoxication can include five or more of the following: restlessness, nervousness, excitement, insomnia, flushed face, diuresis, gastrointestinal disturbance, muscle twitching, rambling flow of thought and speech, tachycardia or cardiac arrhythmia, periods of inexhaustibility, and psychomotor agitation (APA, 2000).

Caffeine withdrawal syndrome has been described as headache, drowsiness, and fatigue, sometimes with impaired psychomotor performance, difficulty concentrating, craving, and psychophysiologic complaints, such as yawning or nausea. Patients with caffeine dependence can be supported in their efforts at withdrawal by learning about the caffeine content of beverages and medication, using decaffeinated beverages, and managing individual withdrawal symptoms.

CANNABIS (MARIJUANA)

Marijuana is the common name for the plant *Cannabis sativae*, also known as hemp. Marijuana's active ingredient is D-9-tetrahydrocannabinol (THC). Hashish, the resin found in flowers of the mature *C. sativae* plant, is its strongest form, containing 10% to 30% THC.

Marijuana is fat soluble and is absorbed rapidly after being smoked or taken orally. After ingestion, THC binds with an opioid receptor in the brain—the μ receptor. This action engages endogenous brain opioid receptors, which are associated with enhanced dopamine activity because THC blocks dopamine reuptake. THC can be stored for weeks in fat tissue and in the brain and is released extremely slowly. Long-term use leads to the accumulation of cannabinoids in the body, primarily the frontal cortex, the limbic areas, and the brain's auditory and visual perception centers. In other areas of the brain, it exerts cardiovascular effects, results in ataxia, and causes increased psychotropic effects. Marijuana use impairs the ability to form memories, recall events, and shift attention from one thing to another. It disrupts coordination of movement, balance, and reaction time. Studies show that 6% to 11% of fatal-accident victims have positive THC test results (NIDA, 2005a).

Marijuana is usually smoked and causes relaxation, euphoria, at times dyscoria (abnormal pupillary reaction or shape), spatial misperception, time distortion, and food cravings. It causes relaxation and drowsiness, unlike other hallucinogens, and is often associated with decreased motivation after long-term use. Effects begin immediately after the drug enters the brain and last from 1 to 3 hours.

Controversies Surrounding Marijuana Use

Controversy surrounds the use and effects of marijuana, matters of ongoing debate both in the medical world and in legal circles. Some evidence suggests that marijuana can be useful in the treatment of certain disorders such as epilepsy, postoperative pain, headache, and other types of pain, asthma, glaucoma, muscle spasms in people with cerebral palsy, and poor appetite in patients with cancer and weight loss or chemotherapy-related nausea and vomiting.

Some believe that long-term effects of marijuana use produces amotivational syndrome, described as changes in personality characterized by diminished drive, decreased ambition, lessened motivation, apathy, shortened attention span, distractibility, poor judgment, impaired communication skills, introversion, magical thinking, derealization, depersonalization, decreased capacity to carry out complex plans or to prepare realistically for the future, a peculiar fragmentation in the flow of thought, habit deterioration, and progressive loss of insight. They attribute this syndrome to the long-term effects of THC on the brain and to the slow release of stored THC in fat tissue. Others disagree and maintain that heavy marijuana use has no effect on motivation, learning, or perception and that these characteristics are not the result of marijuana use but rather are part of the causes (DeMarce, Stephens, & Roffman, 2005). Many believe that legitimizing the use of marijuana for medical reasons could possibly legitimize its use for recreational purposes as well. Until published medical research confirms or refutes its medical uses, the controversy will continue.

HALLUCINOGENS

The term **hallucinogen** refers to drugs that produce euphoria or dysphoria, altered body image, distorted or sharpened visual and auditory perception, confusion, incoordination, and impaired judgment and memory. Severe reactions may cause paranoia, fear of losing one's mind, depersonalization, illusions, delusions, and hallucinations. Hallucinogens typically affect the autonomic and regulatory nervous systems first, increasing heart rate and body temperature and slightly elevating blood pressure. The individual may experience dry mouth, dizziness, and subjective feelings of being hot or cold. Gradually, the physiologic changes fade, and perceptual distortions and hallucinations become prominent. Intense mood and sexual behavior changes may occur; the user may feel unusually close to others or distant and isolated. The true content of hallucinogenic drugs purchased on the street is always in doubt; they are often misidentified or adulterated with other drugs. There are more than 100 different hallucinogens with substantially different molecular structures. Psilocybin (mushroom), D-lysergic acid diethylamide (LSD), mescaline, and numerous amphetamine derivatives are just a few hallucinogens.

LSD

During the 1960s, LSD became a popular recreational drug associated with the antiestablishment movement of peace, free love, and sex that characterized the "hippies" and the "Woodstock generation." Acute LSD psychological toxicity, or so-called "bad trips" during which users felt extreme anxiety or fear and experienced frightening hallucinations, were often reported or experienced by users. These experiences are characteristically panic reactions that develop when individuals feel that the hallucinogenic experience will never end or when they have difficulty distinguishing drug effects from reality (NIDA, 2005a).

LSD binds very tightly to the serotonin receptor, causing a greater than normal activation of the receptor. Because serotonin has a role in many of the brain's functions, activation of its receptors by LSD produces widespread effects, including rapid emotional swings, altered perceptions, and, if taken in a large enough dose, delusions and visual hallucinations.

DEPRESSANTS AND SEDATIVES

Rohypnol and GHB (gamma-hydroxybutyrate) are predominately CNS depressants and are considered "club drugs." Often colorless, tasteless, and odorless, the drugs can be ingested unknowingly. Known also as "date rape" drugs when mixed with alcohol, they can be incapacitating, causing a euphoric, sedative-like effect and producing an "anterograde amnesia," which means individuals may not remember events they experience while under the influence of these drugs.

Benzodiazepines

Sedative-hypnotic drugs and anxiolytic (antianxiety) agents are medications that induce sleep and reduce anxiety (see Chapters 8 & 21). More prescriptions are written for these drugs than for any other class of drugs in the United States. If both prescriber and patient consider carefully the risks of these drugs, they can be a useful, safe, and appropriate treatment (Mueller et al., 2005). Patients who abuse prescription medications are often somnolent, have a clouded mental state, or may feel hyperactive or anxious after using the medication, yet continue to use it without reporting its distressing side effects. They often take the next dose ahead of time, may exceed the prescribed daily dosage, may lobby for a higher dose or a stronger medication, may supplement medication with alcohol or other drugs, or may obtain prescriptions for the same medication from several physicians.

Biologic Responses to Benzodiazepines

Barbiturates (amytal, nembutal, seconal, phenobarbital) were the first class of drugs used to treat sleep disturbances and anxiety, but benzodiazepines (Ativan, Halcion, Librium, Valium, Xanax) have largely replaced barbiturates because of their comparative safety with regard to potential toxicity and addictive qualities. Benzodiazepines modulate gamma-aminobutyric acid (GABA) transmission and interact with specific receptor sites in the brain. GABA is the most abundant inhibitory neurotransmitter in the brain. Benzodiazepines, by displacing an endogenous binding inhibitor, increase GABA's affinity for its receptor and thus enhance GABA function (see Chapter 7). Benzodiazepines act in a manner similar to alcohol and other sedative hypnotics, making neuronal membranes more permeable to K^+ and Cl^- and closing Na^+ and Ca^{++} channels, which causes CNS depression. Although benzodiazepines increase total sleep time, they decrease the duration of REM sleep (see Chapter 6).

Benzodiazepine Withdrawal

Withdrawal symptoms may begin to emerge as long as 8 days after cessation of a long-acting benzodiazepine. Often, patients combine these drugs with alcohol, which is extremely dangerous and can put patients at risk for overdose, causing coma or death. The combination of benzodiazepines and alcohol also complicates withdrawal treatment because the patient may seem to improve after the alcohol withdrawal syndrome subsides, only to have similar symptoms emerge as the benzodiazepine withdrawal syndrome appears.

The severity of symptoms during benzodiazepine withdrawal depends on the duration and dosage of regular use; symptoms include the following:

- Anxiety rebound—tension, agitation, tremulousness, insomnia, anorexia
- Autonomic rebound—hypertension, tachycardia, sweating, hyperpyrexia
- Sensory excitement—paresthesias, photophobia, hyperacusis (sensitivity to sound), illusions
- Motor excitation—hyperreflexia, tremors, myoclonus, fasciculation (visible muscle contraction), myalgia, muscle weakness, tonic–clonic convulsions
- Cognitive excitation—nightmares, delirium, depersonalization, hallucinations

Two methods of withdrawal are currently used. The first is to use the same medication in decreasing doses, and the second is to substitute an equivalent medication and reduce the dose slowly.

DISSOCIATIVE ANESTHETICS

A dissociative anesthetic reduces (or blocks) signals to the conscious mind from other parts of the brain. Users report a trancelike experience, as well as a feeling of being "out of body" and detached from their environment. Ketamine is associated with increased heart rate and blood pressure, impaired motor function, memory loss, numbness, and vomiting. At high doses, delirium, depression, respiratory depression and arrest can occur.

PCP (phencyclidine) causes altered perception of body image but rarely produces visual hallucinations. PCP (angel dust) can also cause effects that mimic the primary symptoms of schizophrenia, such as delusions and mental turmoil. People who use PCP for long periods of time have memory loss and speech difficulties. PCP is associated with panic, aggression, and violence (NIDA, 2005b).

Acute Intoxication of PCP

Often, patients can present at psychiatric emergency departments in acute states of intoxication or in dissociated states, and they may be combative. Intoxication can last 4 to 6 hours, with an extensive period of de-escalation. The primary goals of intervention are to reduce stimuli, maintain a safe environment for the patient and others, manage behavior, and observe the patient carefully for medical and psychiatric complications. Instructions to the patient should be clear, short, and simple, and delivered in a firm but nonthreatening tone.

OPIATES AND MORPHINE DERIVATIVES

The term *opiate* refers to any substance that binds to an opioid receptor in the brain to produce an agonist action. Derived from poppies, **opiates** are powerful drugs that have been used for centuries to relieve pain. They include opium, heroin, morphine, and codeine. Even centuries after their discovery, opiates are still the most effective pain relievers. They also cause CNS depression and sleep or stupor. Although heroin has no medicinal use, other opiates, such as morphine and codeine, are used to treat pain related to illnesses (e.g., cancer) and medical and dental procedures. When used as directed by a clinician, opiates are safe and generally do not produce addiction. However, opiates also possess very strong reinforcing properties and can quickly trigger addiction when used improperly. Commonly abused opiates are codeine, fentanyl, heroin, morphine, oxycodone, and hydrocodone (NIDA, 2000).

Two important effects produced by opiates are pleasure (or reward) and pain relief. The brain itself also produces substances known as endorphins that activate the opiate receptors. Research indicates that endorphins are involved in many functions, including respiration, nausea, vomiting, pain modulation, and hormonal regulation (NIDA, 2000). Opiates cause tolerance and physical dependence that appear to be specific for each receptor subtype. Tolerance develops particularly to the analgesic, respiratory depression, and sedative actions of opiates. Often, a 100% increase in dose is used to achieve the same physical effects when tolerance exists. Physical dependence can develop rapidly. When use of the drug is discontinued, after a period of continuous use, a rebound hyperexcitability withdrawal syndrome usually occurs. Table 25.5 describes the onset, duration, and symptoms of mild, moderate, and severe withdrawal symptoms.

Heroin is an illegal, highly addictive drug that is the most abused and the most rapidly acting of the opiates. Typically sold as a white or brownish powder or as the black sticky substance known as "black tar heroin" on the streets, it is frequently "cut" with other substances, such as sugar, starch, powdered milk, quinine, and strychnine or other poisons. It can be sniffed, snorted, and smoked but is most frequently injected, which poses risks for

Table 25.5 Severity of Opiate Withdrawal Syndrome

Initial Onset and Duration	Mild Withdrawal	Moderate Withdrawal	Severe Withdrawal
Onset: 8–12 h after last use of short-acting opiates. 1–3 d after last use for longer-acting opiates, such as methadone	Physical: yawning, rhinorrhea, perspiration, restlessness, lacrimation, sleep disturbance	Physical: dilated pupils, bone and muscle aches, sensation of "goose flesh," hot and cold flashes	Physical nausea, vomiting, stomach cramps, diarrhea, weight loss, insomnia, twitching of muscles and kicking movements of legs, increased blood pressure, pulse, and respirations
Duration: Severe symptoms peak between 48 and 72 h. Symptoms abate in 7–10 d for short-acting opiates. Methadone withdrawal symptoms can last several weeks.	Emotional: increased craving, anxiety, dysphoria	Emotional: irritability, increased anxiety, and craving	Emotional: depression, increased anxiety, dysphoria, subjective sense of feeling "wretched"

transmission of HIV and other diseases from the sharing of needles or other injection equipment. One of the most detrimental long-term effects of heroin is addiction itself, which causes neurochemical and molecular changes in the brain. Heroin also produces profound degrees of tolerance and physical dependence, which are powerful motivating factors for compulsive use and abuse. Once addicted, heroin users gradually spend more and more time and energy obtaining and using the drug, until these activities become their primary purpose in life (NIDA, 2005a).

Opiate Intoxication or Overdose

Emergency treatment of opiate intoxication is initiated with an assessment of central nervous functioning, specifically arousal and respiratory functioning. Naloxone (Narcan), an opioid antagonist, is given to reverse the respiratory depression, sedation, and hypertension. In the presence of physical dependence on opioids, Narcan will produce withdrawal symptoms that are related to the dose of Narcan and the degree and type of opioid dependence. When administered intravenously, the effect is generally apparent within 2 minutes. When administered intramuscularly, the effect is more prolonged.

Opiate Withdrawal

Ideally, opiate detoxification is achieved by gradually reducing an opiate dose over several days or weeks. Many treatment programs include administering low doses of a substitute drug that can help satisfy the drug craving without providing the same subjective high, such as methadone. If opiates are abruptly withdrawn ("cold turkey") from someone who is physically dependent on them, severe physical symptoms occur including body aches, diarrhea, tachycardia, fever, runny nose, sneezing, sweating, yawning, nausea or vomiting, nervousness, restlessness or irritability, shivering or trembling, abdominal cramps, weakness, and increased blood pressure.

Maintenance Treatment

Methadone maintenance is the treatment of opiate addiction with a daily, stabilized dose of methadone. Methadone is used because of its long half-life of 15 to 30 hours. Methadone is a potent opiate and is physiologically addicting, but it satisfies the opiate craving without producing the subjective high of heroin (see Box 25.4).

Detoxification is accomplished by setting the beginning methadone dose and then slowly reducing it during the next 21 days. Treatment programs determine the

BOX 25.4

Drug Profile: Methadone (Dolophine)

DRUG CLASS: Narcotic agonist, analgesic

RECEPTOR AFFINITY: Binds to opioid receptors in the CNS to produce analgesia, euphoria, sedation; the receptors mediating the effects of the endogenous opioids are thought to be enkaphalins, endorphins.

INDICATIONS: Detoxification and temporary maintenance treatment of narcotic addiction; relief of severe pain.

ROUTE AND DOSAGE: Available in 5-, 10-, and 40-mg tablets, oral concentrate.

Adults: Detoxification: Initially 15–30 mg. Increase to suppress withdrawal signs. 40 mg/d in single or divided dose is usually adequate stabilizing dose; continue stabilizing dose for 2–3 days, then gradually decrease dosage. Usual maintenance dose is 20–120 mg/d in single dosing. Individual dosage as tolerated.

HALF-LIFE (PEAK EFFECT):
PO 90–120 min
IM 1–2 h
SC 1–2 h

SELECTED ADVERSE REACTIONS: Light-headedness, dizziness; sedation, nausea, vomiting, facial flushing, peripheral circulatory collapse, arrhythmia, palpitations, urethral spasm, urinary retention, respiratory depression, circulatory depression, respiratory arrest, shock, cardiac arrest

WARNINGS: Never administer in the presence of hypersensitivity to narcotics, diarrhea caused by poisoning (before toxins are eliminated), bronchial asthma, chronic obstructive pulmonary disease. Use caution in the presence of acute abdominal conditions, cardiovascular disease. Increased effects and toxicity of methadone if taken concurrently with cimetidine, ranitidine. Methadone hydrochloride tablets are for oral administration only and *must not* used for injection. It is recommended that methadone hydrochloride tablets, if dispensed, be packaged in child-resistant containers and kept out of the reach of children to prevent accidental injection.

SPECIFIC PATIENT/FAMILY EDUCATION

- Take drug exactly as prescribed.
- Avoid use of alcohol.
- Take drug with food and lying quietly—should minimize the nausea.
- Eat small, frequent meals to treat nausea and loss of appetite.
- If experiencing dizziness and drowsiness, avoid driving a car or performing other tasks that require alertness.
- Administer mild laxative for constipation.
- Report severe nausea, vomiting, constipation, shortness of breath, or difficulty breathing. Methadone products, when used for treatment of narcotic addiction, shall be dispensed only by approved hospital and community pharmacies and maintenarce programs approved by the FDA and designated state authority.

dose of methadone that will block subjective feelings of craving and will not cause somnolence or intoxication in patients. The initial dose of methadone is determined by the severity of withdrawal symptoms and is usually 20 to 30 mg orally. If, after 1 to 2 hours, symptoms persist, the dosage can be raised and then should be re-evaluated daily during the first few days of treatment. Initial doses of greater than 40 mg can cause severe discomfort as the detoxification proceeds.

Patients receive this dose daily in conjunction with regular drug abuse counseling focused on the elimination of illicit drug use; on lifestyle changes, such as finding friends who do not use drugs or achieving stability in one's living situation; strengthening social supports; and structuring time into pursuits that do not involve drug use. After illicit drug use ceases for a period of time, major lifestyle changes have been made, and social supports are in place, patients may gradually detoxify from methadone with continuing support through community support groups, such as Narcotics Anonymous.

The length of methadone treatment varies for each patient. When to begin detoxification from methadone varies widely, depending on the patient's commitment to abstinence, lifestyle changes that have occurred, and strong peer group support, all of which are needed to sustain the patient during methadone detoxification, when increased cravings often occur. Methadone treatment, combined with behavioral therapy and counseling, has been used effectively and safely to treat opioid addiction for more than 40 years. Combined with behavioral therapy and counseling, methadone enables patients to stop using heroin (Marion, 2005).

Like methadone, L-acetyl-α-methadol (LAAM) is a synthetic opiate that can be used to treat heroin addiction. LAAM, taken orally, can block the effects of heroin for as long as 72 hours with minimal side effects. It has a longer duration of action than methadone, permitting dosing just three times per week, thereby eliminating the need to take doses home over weekends (Oliveto et al., 2005).

Naltrexone has also been used successfully to treat opiate addiction. It binds to opiate receptors in the CNS and competitively inhibits the action of opioid drugs, including those with mixed narcotic agonist–antagonist properties, thereby blocking the intoxicating effects. It is contraindicated in pregnant patients and in patients with allergy to narcotic antagonists. If a patient should require analgesia while taking naltrexone, a nonopioid agent is recommended. Should an opiate-dependent individual take naltrexone before he or she is fully detoxified from opiates, withdrawal symptoms may result (see Table 25.3).

In October 2002, the U.S. Food and Drug Administration (FDA) approved sublingual buprenorphine tablets for treating opioid dependence. In clinical trials, buprenorphine taken three times a week effectively treated opioid addiction. An inexpensive drug, buprenorphine could lower costs to the health care system while providing treatment for many more patients with addiction. Discontinuing buprenorphine use does not require tapering, as does methadone, which makes it easier to stop treatment (Jones, 2004.)

INHALANTS

Inhalants are organic solvents, also known as *volatile substances*, that are CNS depressants. When inhaled, they cause euphoria, sedation, emotional lability, and impaired judgment. Intoxication can result in respiratory depression, stupor, and coma. Inhalants typically are used by young individuals; low cost, universal availability, and ease of access are important factors in promoting their use as well as increasing the risk for other drug use (Storr et al., 2005).

Most inhalants are common household products that give off mind-altering chemical fumes when sniffed. They include the following:

- *Adhesives:* airplane glue, polyvinyl chloride cement, rubber cement
- *Aerosols*: paint, hair spray, analgesics, asthma sprays, deodorants, air fresheners
- *Anesthetics*: nitrous oxide, halothane, enflurane, isoflurane, ethyl chloride
- *Solvents*: paint and nail polish removers, paint thinners, correction fluids, lighter fluid, petroleum
- *Cleaning agents*: dry cleaning fluid, spot removers, degreasers, computer cleaners
- *Food products*: whipped cream and cooking oil sprays
- *Nitrites*: amyl, butyl, isopropyl nitrite

The chemical structure of the various types of inhalants is diverse, making it difficult to generalize about their effects. However, the vaporous fumes can change brain chemistry and may permanently damage the brain and CNS. Magnetic resonance imaging scans of users demonstrate severe changes in cerebral white matter (Bale et al., 2005).

Inhalant Intoxication

Inhalants are easily absorbed through the lungs and are widely distributed in the body, reaching the highest concentrations in fat tissue and the nervous system, where the most profound effects are exhibited. Mild intoxication occurs within minutes and can last as long as 30 minutes. Often, the drugs are inhaled repeatedly to maintain an intoxicated state for hours. Initially, the person experiences a sense of euphoria, but as the dose increases, confusion, perceptual distortions, and severe CNS depression appear. Inhalant users are also at risk for *sudden sniffing death*, which can occur when the inhaled fumes take the place of oxygen in the lungs and central nervous system, causing the user to suffocate. Inhalants can also cause death by disrupting the normal heart rhythm, which can lead to cardiac arrest (Bale et al., 2005).

Chronic neurologic syndromes can result from long-term use. Long-term inhalant use is linked to widespread brain damage and cognitive abnormalities that can range from mild impairment to severe dementia. In recent studies, considerably more inhalant users than cocaine users had brain abnormalities, and their damage was more extensive. Inhalant users also performed significantly worse on tests of working memory and of the ability to focus attention, plan, and solve problems. A withdrawal syndrome is reported, similar to alcohol withdrawal but milder, with primary symptoms of anxiety, tremors, hallucinations, and sleep disturbance (Wu, Schlenger, & Ringwalt, 2005).

STEROIDS

"Anabolic steroids" is the name for synthetic substances related to the male sex hormones (androgens). Developed in the late 1930s to treat hypogonadism, they are also used to treat delayed puberty, some types of impotence, and wasting of the body caused by HIV infection or other diseases. They promote growth of skeletal muscle and the development of male sexual characteristics. There are more than 100 different types; to be used legally, all require a prescription. Some dietary supplements such as dehydroepiandrosterone (DHEA) and androstenedione (Andro) can be purchased in commercial health stores. They are often used in the belief that large doses can convert into testosterone or a similar compound in the body that will promote muscle growth, but this belief has not been proven. In 2004, 1.9% of 8th graders, 2.4% of 10th graders, and 3.4% of 12th graders had taken anabolic steroids at least once in their lives. Few data exist about the extent of steroid use by adults. Although use among men is higher than among women, use among women is growing (NIDA, 2005).

Case reports and small studies indicate that anabolic steroids, in high doses, increase irritability and aggression. Some steroid users report that they have committed aggressive acts, such as physical fighting, armed robbery, or using force to obtain something, committing property damage, stealing from stores, or breaking into a house or building, and that they engage in these behaviors more often when they take steroids than when they are drug free. Other behavioral effects include euphoria, increased energy, sexual arousal, mood swings, distractibility, forgetfulness, and confusion.

With time, anabolic steroid use is associated with increased risk for heart attacks and strokes, blood clotting, cholesterol changes, hypertension, depressed mood, fatigue, restlessness, loss of appetite, insomnia, reduced libido, muscle and joint pain, and severe liver problems, including hepatic cancer. Males can have reduced sperm production, shrinking of the testes, and difficulty or pain in urinating. There can be undesirable body changes: breast enlargement in men and masculinization of women's bodies. Both sexes can experience hair loss and acne. Intravenous or intramuscular use of the drug and needle sharing puts users at risk for HIV, hepatitis B and C, and infective endocarditis, as well as bacterial infections at injection sites (NIDA, 2005).

NURSING MANAGEMENT: HUMAN RESPONSE TO SUBSTANCE RELATED DISORDERS

In psychiatric and substance-dependence treatment programs, the assessment process is, in part, a treatment intervention. Often, patients are in denial about the severity of the problem and about the emotional, social, legal, vocational, or other consequences of it.

Assessment Issues

The assessment is crucial to understanding level of use, abuse, or dependence and to determining the patient's denial or acceptance of treatment. Assessment is often detailed and may involve family members and loved ones. Box 25.5 gives examples of typical behaviors exhibited by individuals in each level of use, abuse, dependence, and addiction. Box 25.6 is an example of a nursing assessment guide that can be used to obtain information about an individual's substance use history. Usually, nurses encounter individuals during crisis when they seek professional help. These situations offer an opportunity to explore the denial that keeps their addiction thriving. The nurse's approach should be caring, matter-of-fact, gentle, and direct. Approaches that are punitive or attempt to elicit feelings of guilt or shame are destructive to the therapeutic relationship (see Nursing Care Plan 25.1).

Denial of a Problem

Denial can be expressed in a variety of behaviors and attitudes and may not be expressed as an overt denial of the problem. For example, patients may admit to a problem, even thank you for helping them to realize they have a problem, but insist they can overcome the problem on their own and do not need outside help.

KEY CONCEPT Denial is the patient's inability to accept his or her loss of control over substance use or the severity of the consequences associated with the substance dependence.

The following characteristics are typical of a person who has alcoholism and who is in denial:

BOX 25.5

Behaviors in Substance Use, Abuse, Dependence, and Addiction

Substance Use
- Does not have possible danger or potential legal problems
- Engages in use to enhance social situations and interaction
- Is not intended to result in intoxication
- Has control of the amount and frequency of use
- Exhibits socially acceptable behavior while using

Prescription Medication Use
- Use is for the dose, frequency, and indications prescribed
- Use is for the particular episode of the condition for which it was prescribed
- Use is coordinated among prescribing physicians

Substance Abuse
- Use for intoxication or feeling of being "high"
- Use that interferes with normal life functions (e.g., producing sleep when inappropriate, excitability or irritability interfering with social interaction)
- Potential harm to self or others (e.g., driving while intoxicated, use of injection drug equipment)
- Use that has legal consequences (i.e., all use of illicit drugs)
- Use resulting in socially unacceptable behavior (e.g., public drunkenness, verbal or physical abuse)
- Use to alter normal feeling states such as sadness or anxiety

Prescription Medication Abuse
- Use is at a higher dose and greater frequency than prescribed
- Use is for indications other than prescribed or for self-diagnosed condition
- Use results in feeling tired or having a clouded mental state or feeling "hyperactive" or nervous

Substance Dependence
- Supplementing medication with alcohol or drugs
- Soliciting more than one physician for the same medication
- Inability to control the amount and frequency of use
- Tolerance to larger amounts of the substance
- Withdrawal symptoms when stopping use
- Severe consequences from alcohol or drug use

Substance Addiction
- Drug craving
- Compulsive use
- Presence of aberrant drug-related behaviors
- Repeated relapse into drug use after withdrawal

- Confusion about severity of drinking history: "I went out drinking with friends last week and didn't have any problems; I don't get drunk all the time."
- Difficulty reconciling early positive experiences of alcohol use with current problems: "I used to drink with my buddies after work to unwind. We had a great time. Those were some good times…"
- Confusion regarding the definition of *alcoholic*: "Well, I don't have withdrawal symptoms, so I can't be an alcoholic."

BOX 25.6

Substance Abuse Evaluation

Drug/Last Use **Pattern of Use (Amount, route, first use, frequency, and length of use)**

Alcohol:
Stimulants:
Opiates:
Sedative-hypnotics and anxiolytic agents:
Hallucinogens:
Marijuana:
Inhalants:
Nicotine:
Caffeine:

Dependency Indicators

1. Tolerance (increasing use of drug or alcohol with the same level of intoxication): ____
2. Withdrawal symptoms: a. Shakes? Tremors? ____ b. Cramps, diarrhea, or rapid pulse? ____
   c. Feeling paranoid, fearful? ____ d. Difficulty sleeping? ____
3. Consequences of use (presenting problems, persistent or recurrent emotional, social, legal, or other problems):
   ____
4. Loss of control of amount, frequency, or duration of use: ____
5. Desire or efforts to decrease use or control use: ____
6. Preoccupation (increasing focus or time spent on use and obtaining substances): ____
7. Social, vocational, recreational activities affected by use: ____
8. Previous alcohol/drug abuse treatment: ____

Nursing Diagnoses:

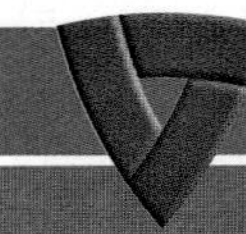

Nursing Care Plan 25.1

Patient With Alcoholism

JG is a 55-year-old veteran with a 25-year history of alcohol dependence. He is the youngest of three children born of "blue-collar" parents who valued hard work. His mother is still living with JG's older sister, but his father died of cirrhosis, a complication of years of alcohol abuse. JG has two children who are married with children, living in other states. He rarely sees them. He has been drinking as much as 1 quart of vodka per day for 3 years since sustaining a work-related back injury. He has a history of binge drinking on weekends. He denies other drug use.

Recently, his wife moved out of the house after 28 years of marriage. An argument about his drinking ended in a physical fight. She had to be treated in the emergency room for a broken arm. Their relationship had progressively deteriorated over the years. JG was sexually impotent due to excessive drinking, and she had moved into the spare bedroom. He was admitted to the hospital emergency department at a Veteran's Administration medical center with a gash above his right eye from a fall he sustained while intoxicated, 2 weeks after his wife left him. His wife returned to care for him.

JG began to have symptoms of alcohol withdrawal and became anxious shortly after admission. He requested hospital admission for alcohol detoxification and was transferred to a detoxification and brief treatment unit.

Setting: Inpatient Detoxification Unit, Veterans Administration Medical Center

Baseline Assessment: First admission, last drink 7 PM. Admission vital signs: T 99.2°F, HR 98, R 20, BP 140/88 on admission to the ER. He has a history of withdrawal seizures and hallucinosis. He had a blood alcohol level (BAL) of 0.15 mg%, becoming increasingly anxious and restless. He was given diazepam 10 mg PO at that time.

Four hours after admission, vital signs were T 99.8°F, HR 110, R 22, BP 152/100. He continued to be anxious and was tremulous, diaphoretic, and nauseous. Diazepam 20 mg PO stat was given.

Associated Psychiatric Diagnosis

Axis I: Alcohol withdrawal with hallucinations; alcohol abuse
Axis II: None
Axis III: Unspecified back injury
Axis IV: Social problems (social withdrawal); occupational problems (work-related injury)
Axis V: GAF = Current 60; Potential 75

Medications

Thiamine
Folic acid
Multivitamins
Diazepam 10 mg q2h for elevated BP, HR, and tremors
Haloperidol 5.0 mg IM PRN for hallucinations or agitation

Nursing Diagnosis 1: Risk For Injury

Defining Characteristics

Sensory deficits
Balance and equilibrium deficits
Lack of awareness of hazards

Related Factors

Altered cerebral function secondary to alcohol withdrawal
Potential withdrawal seizures resulting from magnesium deficiency or hypoglycemia
Anxiety

Outcomes

Initial

1. Prevent falls and other physical injuries.

Discharge

2. Relate an intent to practice selected prevention measures such as maintaining sobriety, removing loose throw rugs, using adequate lighting.

Interventions

Interventions	Rationale	Ongoing Assessment
Identify stage of alcohol withdrawal and severity of symptoms. Monitor gait and motor coordination, presence of tremors, mental status, electrolyte balance, and seizure activity.	The more severe the reactions, the more likely that disorientation, confusion, and restlessness increase. As the patient moves from stage I to III, he becomes at higher risk for a fall or injury.	Determine whether JG is becoming more disoriented, increasing his risk for injury.

Continued

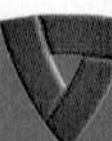

Nursing Care Plan 25.1 *(Continued)*

Interventions

Interventions	Rationale	Ongoing Assessment
Institute seizure precautions (bed in low position, padded side rails).	Withdrawal seizures usually occur within 48 hours after last drink.	Monitor for seizure activity.
Orient patient to surroundings and call light, maintain consistent physical environment.	Disorientation often occurs as blood alcohol level drops. These symptoms can last several days.	Determine JG's level of orientation to surroundings. Determine whether he can use call light.
Avoid sudden moves, loud noises, discussion of patient at bedside, and lighting that casts shadows downward.	Decreased environmental stimulation helps calm the patient, which in turn promotes optimal CNS responses.	Observe reactions to loud noises and monitor room environment.

Evaluation

Outcomes (at 3 days)	Revised Outcomes	Interventions
Gait steady, patient hydrated. No seizure activity. Patient oriented.	Maintain current level of orientation.	Continue to monitor for any signs of disorientation.

Nursing Diagnosis 2: Disturbed Thought Process

Defining Characteristics	Related Factors
Hallucinations (auditory, visual, and tactile) Inaccurate interpretation of stimuli Confusion and disorientation	Physiologic changes secondary to alcohol withdrawal

Outcomes

Initial	Discharge
1. Recognize changes in thinking/behavior. 2. Identify situations that occur before hallucinations/delusions.	3. Maintain reality orientation.

Interventions

Interventions	Rationale	Ongoing Assessment
Encourage communication that enhances the development of the nurse–patient relationship and promotes JG's sense of integrity.	The therapeutic relationship is important to individuals with alcohol withdrawal because of their fear of withdrawal symptoms and need for reassurance and support.	Monitor the development of the nurse–patient relationship.
Assess for the presence of any hallucinations through observation and interview.	Hallucinations can occur when patients are withdrawing from alcohol. If hallucinations are severe, patient may experience delirium tremens.	Assess patient frequently to determine the presence of hallucinations.
Administer haloperidol 5.0 mg IM PRN for hallucinations or agitation.	Administering an antipsychotic eliminates or reduces the occurrence of hallucinations.	Observe for hypotension. Instruct patient to avoid getting out of bed quickly to prevent falling.
JG had one episode of hallucinations. It occurred 8 h after admission with no identifiable precipitating event.	Continue to maintain reality orientation.	Continue to monitor for hallucinations.

Continued

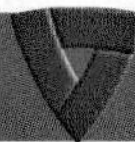

Nursing Care Plan 25.1 *(Continued)*

Nursing Diagnosis 3: Anxiety

Defining Characteristics	Related Factors
Physiologic: increased heart rate, elevated blood pressure, increased respiratory rate, diaphoresis, trembling, nausea Emotional: apprehension about alcohol withdrawal, nervousness, losing control after back injury Cognitive inability to concentrate, lack of awareness of surroundings	Physiologic changes secondary to alcohol withdrawal

Outcomes

Initial	Discharge
1. Identify an increase in physiologic and psychological comfort. 2. Maintain stable vital signs.	3. Describe anxiety as it relates to fear of detoxification process and use of alcohol.

Interventions

Interventions	Rationale	Ongoing Assessment
Demonstrate an accepting attitude by being calm and informing JG of any treatment.	A calm attitude of the nurse can help relax a patient.	Observe JG's reaction to the explanations and initiation of any treatments.
Include the patient in decision making regarding his care.	Empowering the patient in decision making helps him gain control over his situation.	Monitor decisions in terms of feasibility.
Administer diazepam 10 mg q2h for elevated BP, HR, and tremulousness PRN.	Diazepam can reduce physiologic impact of alcohol withdrawal.	Monitor vital signs, level of anxiety, and patient's sense of control.
Explain that anxiety is a symptom of withdrawal and is usually time limited.	Knowledge that the anxiety will decrease will help patient deal with the current anxiety.	Monitor whether or not JG understands that his discomfort will disappear.
Observe sleeping behavior.	Sleep is often disturbed. Sleep deprivation contributes to anxiety.	Monitor quality of sleep.

Evaluation

Outcomes	Revised Outcomes	Interventions
JG was able to refocus and redirect attention when exhibiting mild anxiety, sleeping about 6 hours.	None.	None.
Identified an increase in apprehension as his BP increased. Given diazepam as ordered.	Relate an increase in apprehension when it occurs.	Assess patient for apprehension and a change in vital signs.
JG discussed his fears of the detoxification process. Expressed mixed feelings about continuing treatment.	Comply with treatment regimen.	Encourage patient to follow up with treatment once he is detoxified.

- Relief when they compare themselves with others and find the others in worse condition: "They are the alcoholics, not me!"
- A delusion that drinking can be self-controlled: "If I search hard enough or long enough, I will find a way to control and enjoy drinking."
- Confusion or trouble accepting that behavior is different when intoxicated: "I couldn't have done that, that's just not like me."

This quandary about the nature of the problem has often been met with confrontation by nurses and other professionals in the past. Argumentation, presenting evidence of addiction, and lecturing often fail to elicit admission of a problem or induce behavior change.

Motivation for Change

Motivation is a key predictor of whether individuals will change their substance use behavior (Abreu-Villaca, Queiroz-Gomez, Dal Monte, Fiqueiras, & Manhaes, 2006; U.S. DHHS, 1999).

• NCLEXNOTE

Motivational approaches are priority interventions for patients with substance use disorders. They help patients recognize a problem and develop change strategies.

KEY CONCEPT Motivation involves recognizing a problem, searching for a way to change, and then beginning and sticking with the change strategy (Miller, 2004). Ambivalence about substance use is normal and can be resolved by working with patients' own concerns about their use of alcohol and other drugs. Motivation is fluid and can be modified. Experiences such as increased distress levels, critical life events, a period of evaluation or appraisal of one's life, recognizing negative consequences of use, and positive and negative external incentives for change can all influence a patient's commitment to change.

Techniques that enhance motivation are associated with increased success in treatment, higher rates of abstinence, and successful follow-up treatment (Vansteenkiste & Sheldon, 2006). Motivational interviewing is a method of therapeutic intervention that seeks to elicit self-motivational statements from patients, supports behavioral change, and creates a discrepancy between the patient's goals and their continued alcohol and other drug use (Miller, 2004). The acronym FRAMES summarizes elements of brief interventions with patients using motivational interviewing (see Box 25.7).

BOX 25.7

F.R.A.M.E.S.—Effective Elements of Brief Intervention

Feedback
Provide patients with personal feedback regarding their individual status, such as personal alcohol and other drug consumption relative to norms, information about elevated liver enzyme values, and so forth.

Responsibility
Emphasize the individual's freedom of choice and personal responsibility for change. General themes are as follows:

1. It's up to you; you're free to decide to change or not.
2. No one else can decide for you or force you to change.
3. You're the one who has to do it if it's going to happen.

Advice
Include a clear recommendation or advice on the need for change, typically in a supportive and concerned, rather than in a judgmental, manner.

Menu
Provide a menu of treatment options, from which patients may pick those that seem more suitable or appealing.

Empathic Counseling
Show warmth, support, respect, and understanding in communication with patients.

Self-efficacy
Reinforce self-efficacy, or an optimistic feeling that he or she can change.

Countertransference

Countertransference is the total emotional reaction of the treatment provider to the patient (see Chapter 6). Patients with substance-related disorders can generate strong feelings and reactions in nurses and other health care providers (Table 25.6). These feelings can be generated by overt unpleasant behaviors of the substance-dependent persons, such as lying, deceit, manipulation, or hostility, or these feelings may be more subconscious and stem from past experiences with people with alcoholism or addicts or even from dealing with situations in the care provider's own family.

Codependence

The concept of **codependence** emerged out of studies of women's relationships with husbands who abused alcohol. Today, the scope of codependency includes both men and women who grew up in any type of dysfunctional family system where substance abuse may or may not have been a problem. Codependency has also been described as "enabling," in which an individual in a relationship with an alcohol abuser inadvertently reinforces the drinking behavior of the other person (Stafford, 2001). The codependency label is controversial and is viewed by some as an oversimplification of complex emotions and behaviors of family members. Mental health professionals should be careful not to use it as a catch-all diagnosis and to take special care to assess and plan interventions that address each person's particular situation, problems, and needs.

Nursing Diagnoses

There are several nursing diagnoses that could be generated for persons using and abusing substances. The type of substance and the patient's addiction will be considered in the formation of the nursing diagnoses. For example, a person who is newly diagnosed with

Table 25.6 Patient Behaviors and Countertransference Reactions

Patient Behavior	Common Nursing Reaction
Behaves as a victim	Feels a sense of helplessness, increased need to give advice and "fix" the situation and the patient; shows anger toward the patient for not being able to take care of the situation himself or herself
Is intrusive, hostile, belittling	Can be frightened, withdraw from patient, express anger overtly, or be passive-aggressive (i.e., suggesting discharge to the team or ignoring legitimate requests)
Does everything right, is insightful, pleasant, and so forth	Congratulates self on therapeutic interventions; can become bored or complacent
Relapses into drug or alcohol use	Feels angry, personally betrayed; withdraws from other patients; doubts own abilities
Asks personal questions about staff qualifications or prior drug or alcohol abuse	Reveals personal information, resents the intrusion, and may regret divulging information
Is silent or divulges minimal information	Tries harder, doubts own therapeutic ability, is angered by patient's resistance
Tries to "bend" or ignore milieu and group rules	May permit program rule infractions; may feel pressured, angry, or passive-aggressive
Insists that no one can help him or her	Feels pressure to be the one who can help; may feel angry and inept or helpless

Adapted from Imhoff, J. E. (1991). Countertransference issues in alcoholism and drug addiction. *Psychiatric Annals, 21*(5), 292–306.

alcoholism will be assessed differently than one who has multiple attempts at treatment for cocaine addiction. One common nursing diagnosis is Ineffective Denial (see Figure 25.3).

Nursing Interventions and Treatment Modalities

Several treatment modalities are used in most addiction treatment (pharmacologic modalities were discussed earlier), including 12-step–program-focused, cognitive or psychoeducational, behavioral, group psychotherapy, and individual and family therapy. Discharge planning and relapse prevention are also essential components of successful treatment and are incorporated into most programs. See Table 25.7 and Box 25.8 for different approaches to chemical dependency treatment.

Because substance-dependent patients differ greatly, no one type of treatment program will work for every individual. Often, several approaches can work together,

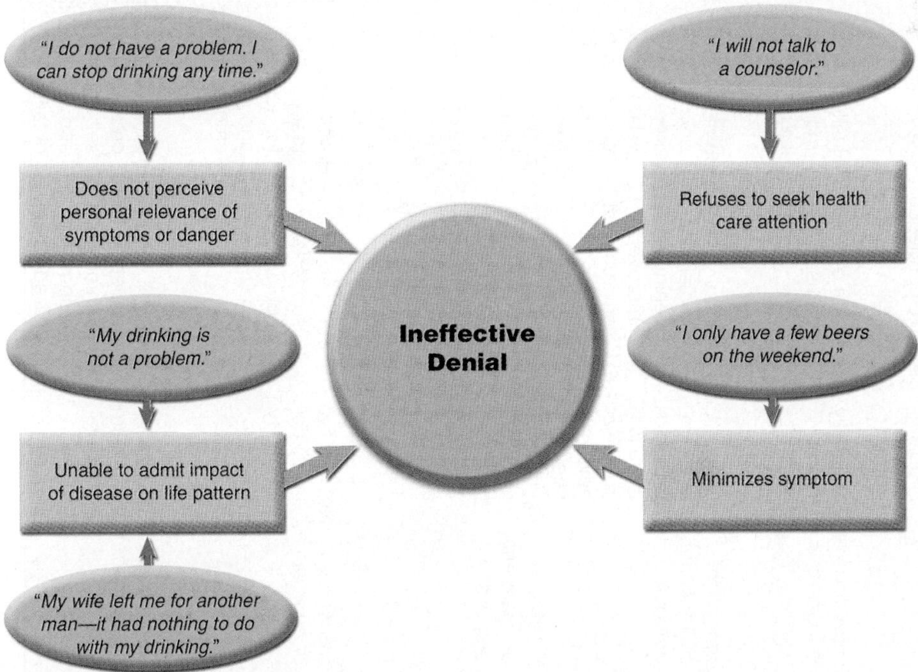

FIGURE 25.3. Nursing diagnosis concept map: Ineffective Denial.

Table 25.7 Treatment Approaches to Chemical Dependence

Approach	Psychiatric	Social	Moral	Learning	Disease	12-Step	Dual Diagnosis	Bio–Psychosocial	Multivariant
Conception of etiology	Symptom of underlying emotional problem	Society and environment cause dependence	Person is morally weak—can't say "no"	Abuse is a learned, reinforced behavior	Probably caused by genetic or biologic factors	Combination of disease concept and "spiritual bankruptcy"	Both a primary substance dependence and a mental health disorder	Biologic basis, with social and psychological influences	Many different causes; may be different for each individual
Conception of patient	Emotionally disturbed	Victim of circumstance	"Hustler," morally deficient	Has distorted thinking, poor coping skills	Has a chronic progressive disease	Has an allergy and is powerless over substances	Has both mental and substance abuse disorder	Has deficiencies in all three interacting areas	Has multiple issues to be assessed and addressed
Conception of treatment outcome	Emotional conflicts are resolved; there is increased emotional health	Improved social functioning or improved environment	Moral recovery, increased willpower, control, and responsible behavior	Patient learns new ways of thinking and new coping skills	Abstinence, arresting disease progression, and beginning of recovery process	Abstinence, ongoing spiritual recovery	Improvement in both mental health and substance abuse disorders	Improvement in mental and physical health, utilization of social supports	Particular issues for individual addressed, and improvement occurs
Conception of treatment process	Psychotherapy, medication to treat "cause" of substance abuse	Removal of environmental influences and increasing coping responses to it	"Street addict" behavior and manipulation confronted	Cognitive therapy techniques and coping skills taught	Is treated as a primary disease, reinforces patient is an addict and has illness	Use 12 steps, seeking spiritual support, making amends, serving others in need	Concurrent treatment of both disorders	Concurrent treatment of all issues	Treatment strategies are matched with individual patient needs
Advantages of approach	Not punitive, treats comorbidity	Stresses social supports and coping skills	Holds person responsible for actions and making amends	Not punitive, teaches new coping skills	Not punitive, stresses support and education	Widespread success, emphasis is on quality of life and spiritual growth	Treats both mental health disorder and dependency, minimizing relapse potential	Utilizes different modalities; is more inclusive	Treatment matched to individual's needs
Disadvantages of approach	Focus is only on treatment of mental disorder	Blames "ills of society"—the person not responsible for addiction	Punitive, increases low self-esteem and sense of failure	Places emphasis on control of use	Minimizes mental health disorders; discounts return to social use	Self-help group, not a treatment program	Not inclusive enough; does not include social or other issues	Does not match patient and specific interventions	Logistical problems can occur in its implementation

BOX 25.8

Principles of Addiction Treatment

The National Institute on Drug Abuse in 2005 published a review of the research literature that outlined the principles that characterize effective approaches to drug addiction treatment. The following are the summary of these principles:

1. *No single treatment is appropriate for all individuals.*
   - Matching treatment settings, interventions, and services to each individual's particular problems and needs is critical to his or her ultimate success in returning to productive functioning in the family, workplace, and society
2. *Treatment needs to be readily available.*
   - Because individuals who are addicted to drugs may be uncertain about entering treatment, taking advantage of opportunities when they are ready for treatment is crucial. Potential treatment applicants can be lost if treatment is not immediately available or is not readily accessible
3. *Effective treatment attends to multiple needs of the individual, not just his or her drug use.*
   - To be effective, treatment must address the individual's drug use and any associated medical, psychological, social, vocational, and legal problems.
4. *An individual's treatment and services plan must be assessed continually and modified as necessary to ensure that the plan meets the person's changing needs.*
   - A patient may require varying combinations of services and treatment components during the course of treatment and recovery. In addition to counseling or psychotherapy, a patient at times may require medication, other medical services, family therapy parenting instruction, vocational rehabilitation, and social and legal services. It is critical that the treatment approach be appropriate to the individual's age, gender, ethnicity, and culture.
5. *Remaining in treatment for an adequate period of time is critical for treatment effectiveness.*
   - The appropriate duration for an individual depends on his or her problems and needs. Research indicates that for most patients, the threshold of significant improvement is reached at about 3 months in treatment. After this threshold is reached, additional treatment can produce further progress toward recovery. Because people often leave treatment prematurely, programs should include strategies to engage and keep patientsin treatment.
6. *Counseling (individual and/or group) and other behavioral therapies are critical components of effective treatment for addiction.*
   - In therapy, patients address issues of motivation, building skills to resist drug use, replace drug-using activities with constructive and rewarding non–drug-using activities, and improve problem-solving abilities. Behavioral therapy also facilitates interpersonal relationships and the individual's ability to function in the family and community.
7. *Medications are an important element of treatment for many patients, especially when combined with counseling and other behavioral therapies.*
   - Methadone and levo-alpha-acetylmethadol (LAAM) are very effective in helping individuals addicted to heroin or other opiates to stabilize their lives and reduce their illicit drug use. Naltrexone is also an effective medication for some opiate addicts and some patients with co-occurring alcohol dependence. For persons addicted to nicotine, a nicotine replacement product (such as patches or gum) or an oral medication (such as bupropion) can be an effective component of treatment. For patients with mental disorders, both behavioral treatments and medications can be critically important.
8. *Addicted or substance-dependent individuals with coexisting mental disorders should have both disorders treated in an integrated way.*
   - Because addictive disorders and mental disorders often occur in the same individual, patients presenting for either condition should be assessed and treated for the co-occurrence of the other type of disorders.
9. *Medical detoxification is only the first stage of addiction treatment and by itself does little to change long-term drug use.*
   - Medical detoxification safely manages the acute physical symptoms of withdrawal associated with stopping drug use. Although detoxification alone is rarely sufficient to help addicts to achieve long-term abstinence, for some individuals, it is a strongly indicated precursor to effective drug addiction treatment.
10. *Treatment does not need to be voluntary to be effective.*
    - Strong motivation can facilitate the treatment process. Sanctions or enticements in the family employment setting or criminal justice system can increase significantly treatment entry, retention rates, and the success of drug treatment interventions.
11. *Possible drug use during treatment must be monitored continuously.*
    - Lapses to drug use can occur during treatment. The objective monitoring of a patient's drug and alcohol use during treatment, such as through urinalysis or other tests, can help the patient withstand urges to use drugs. Such monitoring can also provide early evidence of drug use so that the individual's treatment plan can be adjusted. Feedback to patients who test positive for illicit drug use is an important element of monitoring.
12. *Treatment programs should provide assessment for HIV/AIDS, Hepatitis B and C, tuberculosis and other infectious diseases, and counseling to help patients modify or change behaviors that place themselves or others at risk for infection.*
    - Counseling can help patients avoid high-risk behavior. Counseling can also help people who are already infected manage their illness.
13. *Recovery from drug addiction can be a long-term process and frequently requires multiple episodes of treatment.*
    - As with other chronic illnesses, relapse to drug use can occur during or after successful treatment episodes. Addicted individuals may require prolonged treatment and multiple episodes of treatment to achieve long-term abstinence and fully restored functioning. Participation in self-help support programs during and after treatment is often helpful in maintaining abstinence.

National Institute on Drug Abuse (2005). *Principles of drug addiction treatment: A research-based guide* (pp. 1–3). Rockville, MD: National Institute on Drug Abuse.

whereas others may be inappropriate. Treatment programs usually combine many different interventions to provide a comprehensive approach based on the individual's needs. Nursing interventions vary depending on the nature of the current problems and their severity. For a patient who is being detoxified, physical interventions (e.g., monitoring vital signs and neurologic functioning) are necessary. When the substance use disorder is secondary to other physical or psychiatric problems, education of patient and family may be a priority.

Assessment and interventions should include culturally relevant data such as unique physiological responses to substances, behavioral responses to dependence, and social expectations and sanctions. Staff who are knowledgeable about cultural differences and issues are integral to successful treatment.

Therapeutic Interactions

A variety of nursing interventions are used in the care of persons using substances. It is critical that the nurse establish a therapeutic relationship with these patients (Box 25.9). There are several general guidelines for establishing therapeutic interactions with patients in chemical dependence treatment programs:

- Encourage honest expression of feelings.
- Listen to what the individual is really saying.
- Express caring for the individual.
- Hold the individual responsible for behavior.
- Provide consequences for negative behavior that are fair and consistent.
- Talk about specific actions that are objectionable.
- Do not compromise your own values or nursing practice.
- Communicate the treatment plan to the patient and to others on the treatment team.
- Monitor your own reactions to the patient.

Confrontation, pointing out the inconsistencies in thoughts, feelings, and actions, can promote the person's experience of the natural consequences of one's behavior. Learning from previous behavior and its consequences is how change occurs. Confrontation can be very threatening to patients and should occur within the context of a trusting relationship. The levels of confrontation should support the patient in using the feedback received to grow in the recovery process (Box 25.10).

Brief Intervention

Within the alcohol and other drugs field, **brief intervention** is a highly developed, researched, and accepted approach. There is a growing body of evidence that

BOX 25.9

Therapeutic Dialogue: The Patient With Alcoholism

Ineffective Approach

Nurse: I would like to talk with you about your problem with alcoholism.

Patient: Alcoholism! It's not that bad. Everyone gets loaded!

Nurse: You tell why you were drinking. Your wife left you. You drink a quart of vodka a day. Your blood alcohol level was 0.15% when you were admitted.

Patient: So what! I do have some problems, or I wouldn't be here. But, I'm not an alcoholic. (denial)

Nurse: Do you know what an alcoholic is?

Patient: Sure I do. My father was one. He was a useless bum. I'm not anything like him.

Nurse: It sounds like you are a lot like him.

Patient: I think I need to rest now. My back is killing me. (avoidance)

Effective Approach

Nurse: I would like to talk with you about what happens when you drink.

Patient: It's not that bad. Everyone gets loaded!

Nurse: What concerns do you have about your drinking?

Patient: I'm not really concerned. My wife is. She thinks I drink too much. I even quit once for her.

Nurse: What does she tell you about that?

Patient: Well, she nags me a lot, and says it costs too much money, but I can stop whenever I want. Her nagging only made me drink again.

Nurse: It sounds as if she is concerned about this, but you have your doubts about how serious it is. Your wife is invited to our family education group so that she can learn about alcohol abuse. Family therapy is also available.

Patient: I have a lot of problems besides alcohol. I never use drugs. I only drink because it relaxes me and makes it easier to deal with stress.

Nurse: Many people drink to help them cope with stress. Sometimes the drinking itself can cause stress. While you are here, do you think it would be useful to look at the stress in your life and how it relates to your drinking?

Patient: Yes. But I only drink when things get too out of hand. My health is pretty good.

Nurse: We can provide information about your health and alcohol use. In order to evaluate what information may be helpful, I would like to get a little more information about your drinking.

Critical Thinking Challenge

- What effect did the nurse have on the patient in using the word *alcoholism* in the first interaction?
- Discuss what communication approaches the nurse used in the second scenario to engage the patient in disclosing problems with alcohol and his relationship with his wife. How does this nurse's approach vary from the one in the first interaction?

BOX 25.10

Levels of Confrontation

I. Inform
  A. To inform someone about the general consequences of an anticipated behavior (e.g., warning nonsmokers about the health risks of smoking)
  B. To inform someone about the general consequences of their behavior (e.g., educating drinker about the health consequences of drinking)
  C. To inform someone about the personal consequences of their behavior (e.g., to give feedback on their liver function tests; other health consequences)
  D. To inform someone emphatically about the consequences of either behavior (e.g., attack therapy). This form of confrontation is used much less today in treatment settings because it can have a negative effect on the therapeutic relationship and can be abusive
II. Experience
  A. To experience the consequences of their behavior in their natural environment (e.g, loss, job loss, separation, family disaffection, legal fees, and sentences)
  B. To experience the consequences of their behavior in a designed environment that generates those consequences immediately and dramatically (e.g, a therapeutic community or interactional group therapy)

indicates brief interventions are more effective than no treatment, and there are indications that they are as effective as more intensive interventions (O'Connor & Whaley, 2002).

Screening and brief intervention are two separate skills that can be used together to reduce risky substance use. "Screening" involves asking questions about alcohol or drug use. A "brief intervention" is a negotiated conversation between professional and patient designed to reduce alcohol and drug use.

Not everyone who is screened will need a brief intervention, and not everyone who needs a brief intervention will require treatment. In fact, the goals of screening and brief intervention are to reduce risky substance use before people become dependent or addicted.

Brief intervention is effective because:

- Research indicates that brief interventions are an appropriate response to clients presenting at a general health or community setting and who are unlikely to need, seek, or attend specialist treatment
- It may be all the client may want—to be given clear concise information by a professional
- It is an important part of the overall approach of Harm Reduction

Brief intervention is most successful when working with people who:

- are experiencing few problems with their drug use
- have low levels of dependence
- have a short history of drug use
- have stable backgrounds
- are unsure or ambivalent about changing their drug use

It is recommended that brief intervention at a minimum include:

- Advising how to reduce client's drug use
- Providing harm reduction information and/or self-help manuals that are relevant to the client
- Giving the client relevant information about
  - the consequences of a drug conviction on travel and employment
  - consequences of further or heavier drug charges
- Discussing harm reduction strategies especially those relating to
  - Overdose
  - Violence
  - Driving under the influence
  - Safe practices (e.g., safe injecting, safe sex)
- Offering and arranging a follow-up visit

Cognitive and Cognitive-Behavioral Interventions and Psychoeducation

Cognitive approaches to addiction hypothesize that if a patient can change the way he or she thinks about a situation, both the emotional reaction to it and the behavioral response will change. Psychoeducational materials, groups, and one-on-one interactions with nurses also impart information to reduce knowledge deficits related to alcohol and drug dependence (see Box 25.11). Cognitive-behavioral therapy is a brief treatment that is structured and focused on immediate problems. It

BOX 25.11

Psychoeducation Checklist: Substance Abuse

When caring for the patient and family with substance abuse, be sure to include the following topic areas in the family's teaching plan:

- Psychopharmacologic agents, if used, including drug action, dosage, frequency, and possible adverse effects
- Manifestations of intoxication, overdose, and withdrawal
- Emergency medical system activation
- Nutrition
- Coping strategies
- Structured planning
- Safety measures
- Available treatment programs
- Family therapy referral
- Self-help groups and other community resources
- Follow-up laboratory testing, if indicated

enables patients to examine the thinking process that leads to decisions to use substances, analyze distortions in thinking, and develop rational responses to these distortions (see Chapter 11).

Enhancing Coping Skills

Improving coping skills is thought to be one component of preventing relapse into alcohol and drug use. Coping skills include the ability to use thought, emotion, and action effectively to solve interpersonal and intrapersonal problems and to achieve personal goals. Groups in addiction treatment programs that also have a relapse prevention component look at coping skills that are needed when drug and alcohol cravings are triggered. The skills listed in Table 25.8 are often taught as coping strategies for dealing with alcohol and drug cravings. Patients role play new behaviors and learn from the feedback they receive from other group members. They also increase their sense of competency to use these skills in real-life situations. A lengthier discussion of relapse prevention groups appears in Chapter 34.

Group Therapy and Early Recovery

Isolation and alienation from friends and family are common themes in chemically dependent patients. In addition, thinking that has become distorted is left unchallenged without contact with others; thus, change is difficult. When a patient enters a group that is working with the goals of continuing recovery, numerous healing advantages can occur.

Groups in treatment settings focus on immediate goals of maintaining sobriety and not on childhood issues. The emphasis is on using problem solving and other skills to deal with stressful events that threaten abstinence (Yalom & Leszes, 2005). This type of support group is also extremely effective in outpatient treatment settings. After a period of successful abstinence, group therapy focuses more on traditional psychotherapy work.

Individual Therapy

Often, individual therapy is helpful, particularly in conjunction with group therapy or family therapy. In addiction treatment settings, counselors meet with individuals to maintain focus on the goals and objectives of their treatment, to review the fears and anxieties that often arise in early recovery, and to devise new and healthy responses and solutions to stressful and difficult situations.

Family Therapy 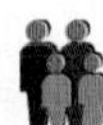

Family therapy, a vital part of addiction treatment, can be used in several beneficial ways to initiate change and help the family when the substance-dependent person is unwilling to seek treatment. Behavioral couples therapy for people with alcoholism can improve family functioning, reduce stressors, smooth marital adjustment, and lessen domestic violence and verbal conflict. When the substance-dependent person seeks help, family therapy can help stabilize abstinence and relationships. Often, inpatient substance abuse treatment programs have family education and group therapy components that help meet these goals. Family therapy can also help to maintain long-term recovery and prevent relapse. Goals of family therapy should be realistic and obtainable. Action plans must be specific and organized into manageable increments. Target dates should be realistic so that pressure is minimal, yet there is motivation to act in a timely manner. Planning for the future is very difficult as long as alcohol or drug abuse continues.

Harm-Reduction Strategies

Harm reduction, a community health intervention designed to reduce the harm of substance use to the individual, the family, and society, has replaced a moral or criminal approach to drug use and addiction. It recognizes that the ideal is abstinence but works with the individual regardless of his or her commitment to

Table 25.8 Skills Training Group Topics

Interpersonal	Intrapersonal
Starting conversations	Managing thoughts about alcohol
Giving and receiving compliments	Problem solving
Nonverbal communication	Increasing pleasant activities
Receiving criticism	Relaxation training
Receiving criticism about drinking	Awareness and management of anger
Drink and drug refusal skills	Awareness and management of negative thinking
Refusing requests	Planning for emergencies
Close and intimate relationships	Coping with persistent problems
Enhancing social support networks	

BOX 25.12

The Twelve Steps

1. We admitted we were powerless over alcohol, that our lives had become unmanageable.
2. We came to believe that a Power greater than ourselves could restore us to sanity.
3. We made a decision to turn our will and our lives over to the care of God *as we understood Him.*
4. We made a searching and fearless moral inventory of ourselves.
5. We admitted to God, to ourselves, and to another human being the exact nature of our wrongs.
6. We were entirely ready to have God remove all these defects of character.
7. We humbly asked Him to remove our shortcomings.
8. We made a list of all persons we had harmed, and became willing to make amends to them all.
9. We made direct amends to such people wherever possible, except when to do so would injure them or others.
10. We continued to take personal inventory and, when we were wrong, promptly admitted it.
11. We sought through prayer and meditation to improve our conscious contact with God as we understood Him, praying only for knowledge of His will for us and the power to carry that out.
12. Having had a spiritual awakening as a result of these steps, we tried to carry this message to alcoholics and to practice these principles in all our affairs.

Alcoholics Anonymous World Services, Inc. (1979). *Alcoholics Anonymous.* New York: Author.

reduce use. The goal is to reduce the potential harm of the associated behavior. Harm reduction initiatives range from widely accepted designated driver campaigns to controversial initiatives such as provision of condoms in schools, safe injection rooms, needle exchange programs, and heroin maintenance programs.

Twelve-Step Programs

Alcoholics Anonymous (AA) was the first 12-step, self-help program (see Box 25.12 for a list of these steps). AA is a worldwide fellowship of people with alcoholism who provide support, individually and at meetings, to others who seek help. The program steps include spiritual, cognitive, and behavioral components. Many treatment programs discuss concepts from AA, hold meetings at the treatment facilities, and encourage patients to attend community meetings when appropriate. They also encourage continuing use of AA and other self-help groups as part of an ongoing plan for continued abstinence.

Twelve-step programs do not solicit members, engage in political or religious activities, make medical or psychiatric diagnoses, engage in education about addiction to the general population, or provide mental health, vocational, or legal counseling (http://www.alcoholics-anonymous.org/). Alternative peer support groups differ from these programs in their approach. Four such groups in the United States are Women for Sobriety, Moderation Management, Men for Sobriety, and S.M.A.R.T. Recovery. For an additional discussion of 12-step programs and mental health patients, see Chapter 34.

CHEMICAL DEPENDENCY AND PROFESSIONAL NURSES

Although accurate epidemiologic data specific to nursing is scarce, extrapolations from national data reveal an estimated prevalence of chemical dependency for nursing professionals of approximately 10% to 15% (Raia, 2004a). Trinkoff and Storr (1998) found differences based on specific nursing specialties. Emergency and critical care nurses were more than three times as likely to use marijuana or cocaine as nurses in other specialty areas. The prevalence among certain advanced practice specialties, particularly nurse anesthesia, approaches 15% (Quinlan, 2002; Bell, McDonogh, Ellison, & Fitzhugh, 1998). Alcohol is the most abused drug, followed by controlled substances. Oncology and administration nurses were twice as likely to engage in binge drinking and psychiatric nurses were most likely to use nicotine. As a result of addictions, nursing licenses can be suspended. This often results from the late identification of the nurse with abuse and dependency problems. The lack of collegial response as well as insufficient education may be factors in the late identification of peers with problems. A nurse is as susceptible to addiction as is any other individual. In 2002, drug and alcohol-related issues were identified in a number of complaints against nurses (National Council of State Boards of Nursing, 2002).

The nursing profession, as other professions, is highly reluctant to identify the addicted nurse until the disease is well advanced. In addiction, in order to maintain standards of the profession, the practice of nurses who do not respond to treatment must be addressed promptly and appropriately. Some states have mandatory reporting laws to enforce, and hospitals are not always compliant with mandatory reporting. According to the nurse practice acts, any nurse who knows of any health care provider's incompetent, unethical, or illegal practice *must* report that information through proper channels (Box 25.13). In 1982, the ANA House of Delegates adopted a national resolution to provide assistance to impaired nurses. The **peer assistance programs** strive to intervene early, to reduce hazards to patients, and increase prospects for the nurse's recovery. The program offers consultation, referral,

BOX 25.13

Using Reflection: An Impaired Nurse

Incident: A nurse finds her roommate (also a nurse) using a controlled substance that was missing from the hospital. The roommate begs her friend not to turn her in—she is afraid that she will lose her license. The roommate promises to never use illegal substances again. The nurse reports her roommate to the hospital, but feels that she has betrayed her friend.

Reflection: Reflecting on the incident, the nurse realized that it was very unlikely that her roommate would stop using substances, especially when she has access to the substances. Ultimately the nurse protected patients from neglect or harm.

and monitoring for nurses whose practice is impaired, or potentially impaired, due to the use of drugs or alcohol, or psychological or physiological condition.

A referral can be made confidentially by the employer, Employee Assistance Program, coworker, family member, friend, or the nurse her or himself. If the nurse is willing to undergo a thorough evaluation to determine the extent of the problem and any treatment needed, all information is kept confidential from the Board of Nursing, and the nurse does not face disciplinary action against his or her nursing license. Some signs of chemical dependency in nurses are listed below:

- Mood swings; inappropriate behavior at work; frequent days off for implausible reasons; noncompliance with acceptable policies and procedures; deteriorating appearance; deteriorating job performance; sloppy, illegible charting; errors in charting; alcohol on breath; forgetfulness; poor judgment and concentration; lying; and volunteering to be the med nurse.
- Other characteristics of chemically dependent nurses include high achievement, both as a student and a nurse, volunteering for overtime and extra duties, no drug use until prescribed following surgery or a chronic illness, and family history of alcoholism or addiction.

Of course, any of these characteristics may be symptoms of a number of other problems besides chemical dependency.

MOVIE viewing GUIDES

SUMMARY OF KEY POINTS

- The *DSM-IV-TR* classifies substance use disorders related to the following categories: alcohol, cocaine, amphetamines and other stimulants, cannabis (marijuana), hallucinogens, phencyclidine, opiates, sedative-hypnotics and anxiolytics, inhalants, nicotine, and caffeine.
- Addiction is a condition of continued use of substances despite adverse consequences, Use is defined as using legal substances within the bounds of sociably acceptable circumstances and behavior that does not pose any harm or risk to the individual or others. Dependence is physiological dependence with tolerance, withdrawal, or impairment. Addiction also includes symptoms of tolerance and withdrawal syndromes.
- Accurate and comprehensive assessment is crucial in planning addiction treatment interventions. Evaluation should consider all substances for pattern of use, including factors of tolerance; withdrawal symptoms; consequences of use; loss of control over amount, frequency, or duration of use; desire or efforts to cease or control use; social, vocational, and recreational activities affected by use; and history of previous addiction treatment. Comprehensive evaluation also includes investigating family and social support systems.
- Denial of a substance use disorder is the individual's attempt to avoid accepting its diagnosis and can be exhibited by attempts to rationalize the substance use, minimize the harmful results, deflect attention from one's own problem to society's or someone else's, or blame childhood experiences.
- Nurses should use a nonconfrontational approach when dealing with patients in denial of their problem. Motivational interviewing approaches are most effective, using empathy and a nonjudgmental approach and helping the patient to realize the discrepancy between life goals and engaging in substance use, thus motivating patients to change their self-destructive behaviors and make personal choices regarding treatment goals.
- Several effective modalities are used in addiction treatment, and many programs combine several modalities, which can include 12-step programs, social skills groups, psychoeducational groups, group therapy, and individual and family therapies. There is no one best treatment method for all people.
- In addressing culturally diverse populations, addiction programs should provide staff who are knowledgeable about cultural differences and issues and programs that are responsive to those differences and specialized needs of cultural and ethnic groups.
- Substance use disorders have many social and political ramifications. Even the profession of nursing is not immune to substance use disorders among its members.

CRITICAL THINKING CHALLENGES

1 Jeff H., a 35-year-old cocaine-dependent patient, has entered a rehabilitation program. What goals do you

believe would be realistic to achieve by the end of his projected 30-day inpatient stay?

2 You are working in an orthopedic unit, and Mary L. has been admitted for treatment for a fractured femur. She has been drinking recently and has a blood-alcohol level of 0.08%. What further information in the following areas would you need to plan her care?
   a. Medical
   b. Alcohol and drug use related
   c. Other psychosocial issues

3 Medical use of marijuana has been approved in California. What is your opinion of this legislation? What are the advantages and disadvantages of this public policy?

4 Normal adolescent behavior is often similar to that associated with substance abuse. How would you differentiate this normal behavior from possible substance abuse or dependence?

5 John M. has sought treatment for depression and job stress. He came to your psychiatric assessment unit smelling of alcohol. He believes that he does not have a drinking problem, but a job problem. What interventions would you use for possible alcohol abuse or dependence?

6 Sylvia G. has been abusing heroin intravenously heavily for 2 years. She has come into the hospital with an abscess on her leg. What symptoms would you expect to observe as she experiences withdrawal from opiates? What medications would likely be used to ease these symptoms?

7 After Sylvia G. is free of withdrawal symptoms, she expresses interest in obtaining drug treatment. What are her options? How would you describe them to her?

8 Raymond L. has been treated for hypertension at your clinic. You notice that he complains of peripheral neuropathy and has an unsteady gait. What other medical signs would corroborate alcoholism?

9 What laboratory test results would help confirm a diagnosis of alcoholism?

Clean and Sober: 1989. Daryl Poynter, played by Michael Keaton, is a real estate broker with a substance-abuse problem that he denies. He embezzles company money and becomes involved with a woman's death. He decides to hide out in a 21-day detoxification program that promises total discretion and privacy. He is directly confronted with his addiction.

VIEWING POINTS: This film is realistic in its portrayal of the detoxification process and the denial that many experience regarding their addictions. Trace Daryl Poynter's thinking process as he struggles with accepting his addiction. What events led to his relapse?

REFERENCES

Abreu-Villaca, Y., Queiroz-Gomez, E., Dal Monte, A. P., Figueiras & Manhaes, C. C. (2006). Contrasting predictors of readiness for substance abuse treatment in adults and adolescents: a latent variable analysis of DATOS and DATO-A participants. *Drug and Alcohol Dependence, 80*(1), 63–81.

Alcoholics Anonymous. Retrieved March 31, 2006 from http://www.alcoholics-anonymous.org/en_information_aa.cfm.

Alcoholics Anonymous World Services, Inc. (1979). *Alcoholics Anonymous.* New York: Author.

American Psychiatric Association (APA). (2000). *The diagnostic and statistical manual of mental disorders* (4th ed., text revision). Washington, DC: Author.

Amodia, D. S., Cano, C., & Eliason, M. J. (2005). An integral approach to substance abuse. *Journal of Psychoactive Drugs, 37*(4), 363–371.

Anthony, J. C., & Helzer, J. E. (1995). Epidemiology and drug dependence. In M. Tsuang, M. Tohen, & G. Zahner (Eds.), *Textbook in psychiatric epidemiology* (pp. 361–407). New York: Wiley-Liss.

Bale, A. S., Tu, Y., Carpenter-Hyland, E. P., Changler, L. J. P., Changler, L. J., & Woodward, J. J. (2005). Alterations in glutamatergic and gabaergic ion channel activity in hippocampal neurons following exposure to the abused inhalant toluene. *Neuroscience, 130*(1), 197–206.

Ballesteros, J., Gonzalez-Pinto, A., Querajeta, I., & Cerino, J. C. (2004). Brief interventions for hazardous drinking delivered in primary care and equally effective in men and women. *Addiction, 99*(1), 3–4.

Bell, D. M., McDonough, J. P., Ellison, J. S., & Fitzhugh, E. C. (1999). Controlled drug misuse by certified registered nurse anesthetists. *AANA Journal, 67*(2), 133–140.

Bonnet, M. N., Balkin, T. J., Dinges, D. F., Roehrs, T., Rogers, N. L., & Wesensten, N. J. J. (2005). The use of stimulants to modify performance during sleep loss: a review of sleep deprivation and Stimulant Task Force of the American Academy of Sleep Medicine. *Sleep, 28*(9), 1163–1187.

Breslau, N., Novak, S. P., & Kessler, R. C. (2004). Psychiatric disorders and stages of smoking. *Biological Psychiatry, 55*(1), 69–76.

Collins, R. L., & McNair, L. D. (2002). Minority women and alcohol use. *Alcohol Research & Health, 26*(4), 251–256.

DeLima, M. S., deOlivera Soceres, B. G., Reisser, A. A., & Farrell, M. (2002). Pharmacological treatment of cocaine dependence: A systematic review. *Addiction, 97*(8), 931–949.

Delva, J., Wallace, J. M., O'Malley, P. M., Bachman, G., Johnston, L. D., & Schulenberg, J. E. (2005). The epidemiology of alcohol, marijuana, and cocaine use among Mexican American, Puerto Rican, Cuban American, and Other Latin American eighth-grade students in the United States: 1991–2002. *American Journal of Public Health, 95*(4), 696–702.

DeMarce, J. M., Stephens, R. S. & Roffman, R. A. (2005). Psychological distress and marijuana use before and after treatment: testing cognitive-behavioral matching hypotheses. *Addictive Behaviors, 30*(5), 1055–1059.

Ehlers, C. L., Giler, D. A., Wall, T. L., Phillips, E., Feiler, H., & Wilhelmsen, K. C. (2004). Genomic screen for loci associated with alcohol dependence in Mission Indians. *American Journal of Medical Genetics. Part B. Neuropsychiatric Genetics, 129*(1), 110–115.

Fox, H. C., Talih, M., Malison, R., Anderson, G. M., Kreek, M. J., & Sinha, R.(2005). Frequency of recent cocaine and alcohol use affects drug cravings and associated responses to drug-related cues. *Psychoneuroendocrinology, 30*(9), 880–891.

Fu, Q., Heath, A., Bucholz, K. K., Nelson, E., Goldberg, J., Lyons, M. J., et al. (2002). Shared genetic risk of major depression, alcohol dependence, and marijuana dependence: Contribution of antisocial personality disorder in men. *Archives of General Psychiatry, 59*(12), 1125–1132.

Green, C., Perrin, N., & Polen, R. (2004). Gender differences in the relationships between multiple measures of alcohol consumption and physical and mental health. *Alcohol Clinical Experimental Research, 28*(5), 754–764.

Griffiths, R. R. & Vernotica, E. M. (2000). Is caffeine a flavoring agent in cola softdrinks? *Archive of Family Medicine, 9*(8) 727–734.

Hanson, D. J. (2003). Center on alcohol marketing and youth: Its objectives and method. http://www.alcoholfacts.org/CAMY.html. Retrieved January 31, 2006.

Hendriks, H. F., & van Tol, A. (2005). Alcohol. *Handbook of Experimental Pharmacology, 170*, 339–361.

Hester, R. K. (2003). Treating alcohol problems: Toward an informed eclecticism. In R. K. Hester & W. R. Miller (Eds.), *Handbook of Alcoholism Treatment Approaches: Effective Alternatives* (3rd ed., pp 1–12I). Boston, MA: Allyn & Bacon.

Holdcraft, L. C., Iacono, W., Green, C. A., Perrin, N. A., & Polen, M. R. (2004), Gender differences in the relationships between multiple measures of alcohol consumption and physical and mental health. *Alcohol Clinical Experimental Research, 28*(5), 754–764.

Holmila, M., & Raitasalo, K. (2005). Gender differences in drinking: why do they still exist? *Addiction, 100*(12), 1763–1769.

Imhoff, J. E. (1991). Countertransference issues in alcoholism and drug addiction. *Psychiatric Annals, 21*(5), 292–306.

Jones, H. E. (2004). Practical considerations for the clinical use of buprenorphine. *Science & Practice Perspectives*, 4–23.

Kalbag, A. S., & Levin, F. R. (2005). Adult ADHD and substance abuse: diagnostic and treatment issues. *Substance Use and Misuse, 40*(13–14): 1955–1981, 2043–2048.

Leavitt, S. B. (2002). Evidence for the efficacy of naltrexone in the treatment of alcohol dependence (alcoholism). *Addiction Treatment Forum*: Mundilean, IL. www.atforum.com. Retrieved April 18, 2007.

Ludvig, J., & Eisenberg, M. (2002). Smoking cessation: Options for patients. *Perspectives in Cardiology*, October, p. 39–41.

Marion, I. J. (2005). Methadone treatment at forty. *Clinical Perspective-Methadone Treatment*, 25–31. Retrieved on April 10, 2006, from www.drugabuse.gov/PDF/Perspectives/vol3no1/Methadone.pdf.

Marmorstein, N. R., & Iacono, W. G. (2005). Longitudinal follow-up of adolescents with late-onset antisocial behavior: a pathological yet overlooked group. *Journal of American Academy Child Adolescent Psychiatry, 44*(12):1284–1291.

McCaul, M. E., Wand, G. S., Eissenberg, T., Rohde, C. A., & Cheskin L. J. (2000). Naltrexone alters subjective and psychomotor responses to alcohol in heavy drinking subjects. *Neuropsychopharmacology, 22*(5), 480–492.

Miller, W. R. (2004). Motivational interviewing in the service of health promotion. *Art of Health Promotion in American Journal of Health Promotion, 18*(3), 1–10.

Miller, W. R., & Hester, R. K. (2003). Treating alcohol problems: Toward an informed eclecticism. In R.K. Hester & W. R. Miller (Eds.), *Handbook of Alcoholism Treatment Approaches: Effective Alternatives* (3rd ed., pp 1–12). Boston, MA: Allyn & Bacon.

Mueller, T. I., Pagano, M. E., Rodrigueal, B. F., Bruce, S. E., Stout, R. L., & Keller, M. B. (2005). Long-term use of benzodiazepines in participants with comorbid anxiety and alcohol use disorders. *Alcohol Clinical Experimental Research, 29*(8), 1411–1418.

National Council of State Boards of Nursing (2002). *Commitment to public protection through excellence in nursing regulations.* Retrieved January 20, 2006, from http://www.ncsbn.org/fdf/ResearchFinal Aggregate Report/pdf.

National Institute on Drug Abuse. (2005a). InfoFacts:LSD. http://www.nida.nih.gov/Infofacts/index.html.

National Institute on Drug Abuse. (2005b). Hallucinogens and dissociative drug. Research report series. Retrieved March 28, 2006, from www.nida.nih.govb/Research Reports/Halucinogens/halluc2.html.

National Institute on Drug Abuse. (2005c). Methamphetamine abuse and addiction. Research report series Retrieved March 28, 2006 from www.nida.nih.govb/Research Reports/Halucinogens/halluc2.html.

National Institute on Drug Abuse (2005). Steroids (anabolic-androgenic reactions). Available at www.nidanih.gov. Retrieved March 31, 2006.

National Institute on Drug Abuse (NIDA). (2005). *Principles of drug addiction treatment: A research-based guide* (pp. 1–3). Rockville, MD: Author.

National Institute on Drug Abuse (NIDA), National Institutes of Health. (2000). Available at http://www.drugabuse.gov/Infofax. (Marijuana 13551).

National Institute on Drug Abuse (2006). Research report series cocaine abuse and addiction, http://www.drugabuse.gov/ResearchReports/Cocaine/cocaine3.html.

Nielsen, A. L. (2000). Examining drinking patterns and problems among Hispanic groups: Results from a national survey. *Journal of Studies on Alcohol, 61*(2), 301–310.

O'Connor, M. J. & Whaley, S.E (2007). Brief intervention for alcohol use by pregnant women. *American Journal of Public Health, 97*(2), 252–8.

Office of Applied Studies/Substance Abuse and Mental Health Services Administration (OAS/SAMHSA). (2003, January). Narcotic analgesics. *The D.A.W.N. Report.* Available at https://dawninfo.samhsa.gov/default.asp.

Oliveto, A., Poling, J., Sevarino, K. A., Gonsai, K. R., McCance-Katz, E. F., Stine, S. M., & Kosten, T. R. (2005). Efficacy of dose and contingency management procedures in LAAM-maintained cocaine-dependent patients. *Drug and Alcohol Dependence, 79*(2), 157–165.

Quinlan, D. (2002). *A Professional Study and Resource Guide for the CRNA.* Park Ridge, Illinois: AANA Press.

Raia, S. (2004). The problem of impaired practice. *New Jersey Nurse, 34*(7): 8.

Substance Abuse and Mental Health Services Association. (2005). *Results from the 2004 National Survey on Drug Use and Health: National findings* (Office of Applied Studies, NSDUH Series H-28, DHHS Publication No. SMA 05-4062). Rockville, MD.

Stafford, L. L. (2001). Is codependency a meaningful concept? *Issues in Mental Health Nursing 22*, 273–286.

Storr, C. L., Westergaard, R., Anthony, J., Storr, C. L., Westergaard, R., & Anthony, J.C. (2005). Early onset inhalant use and risk for opiate initiation by young adults. *Drug and Alcohol Dependence, 78(3)*, 253–261.

Trinkoff, A. M., & Storr, C. I. (1998). Substance use among nurses: differences in specialties. *American Journal of Public Health, 88*(4), 581–585.

U.S. Department of Health and Human Services. (2000). *Healthy people 2010: Understanding and improving health, (2nd ed.).*Washington, DC: U.S. Government Printing Office.

Vansteenkiste, M., & Sheldon, K. M. (2006). There's nothing more practical than a good theory: integrating motivational interview with self-determination theory. *British Journal of Clinical Psychology, 45*(Pt. 1), 63–68.

Wilhelmsen, K.C., & Ehlers, C. (2005). Heritability of substance dependence in a native American population. *Psychiatric Genetics, 15*(2), 101–107.

Winstanley, C. A., Eagle, D. M., & Robbins, T. W. (2006). Behavioral models of impulsivity in relation to ADHD: Translation between clinical and preclinical studies. *Clinical Psychology Review, 26*(4): 379–395.

Wu, P., Hoven, C. W., & Fuller, C J. (2003). Factors associated with adolescents receiving drug treatment findings from the national household survey on drug abuse J Behavioural Health Service Research *30*(2), 190–201.

Wu, L. T., Schlenger, W. E., Ringwalt, C L, (2005). Use of nitrate exhalants (poppers) among American youth. *Journal of Adolescent Health. 37*(1), 52–60.

Yalom, I., & Leszes, M. (2005). *The theory and practice of group psychotherapy* (5th ed.).New York: Basic Books.

Zilberman, M., Tavares, H., & el-Guebaly, N. (2003). Gender similarities and differences: the prevalence and course of alcohol- and other substance-related disorders. *Journal of Addictive Disorders, 22*(4), 61–74.

CHAPTER 26

Sleep Disorders

Nancy Anne Hilliker

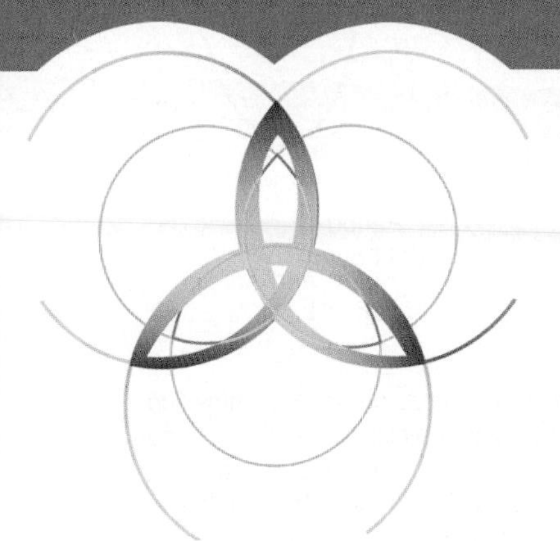

KEY CONCEPTS

- sleep-wake cycle
- insomnia
- rhythm

LEARNING OBJECTIVES

After studying this chapter, you will be able to:

- Describe the major features of sleep.
- Discuss the role of circadian rhythms in sleep.
- Distinguish among primary sleep disorders.
- Discuss biopsychosocial aspects of sleep disorders.
- Perform a sleep history during a patient's assessment.
- Formulate a model nursing care plan for patients with sleep disorders.

KEY TERMS

• cataplexy • circadian rhythm • chronotherapy • chronopharmacotherapy • desynchronized • dyssomnias • hypnagogic hallucinations • larks • luminotherapy • multiple sleep latency test (MSLT) • night terrors • non–rapid-eye-movement sleep (NREM) • owls • parasomnias • polysomnography • rapid-eye-movement sleep (REM) • relaxation training • sleep architecture • sleep debt • sleep diary • sleep disorders • sleep efficiency • OK sleep latency • sleep paralysis • sleep restriction • sleepiness • slow-wave sleep • somnambulism • stimulus control • synchronized

Sleep is a recurrent, altered state of consciousness that occupies nearly one third of our lives and occurs for sustained periods. The functions of sleep are unclear, but the consequences of disturbed sleep are well known and include impaired alertness and performance. Many Americans are severely sleep deprived. The percent of adults who reported sleeping 8 or more hours dropped from 38% in 2001 to 26% in 2005 (National Sleep Foundation, 2005). Sleepiness has been responsible for catastrophic disasters such as the Exxon Valdez oil spill, the nuclear meltdown at Chernobyl in the Ukraine, and the Three Mile Island disaster in the United States.

Sleep disorders are ongoing disruptions of normal waking and sleeping patterns and lead to excessive daytime sleepiness, inappropriate naps, chronic fatigue, and the inability to perform safely or properly at work, school, or home (American Psychiatric Association [APA], 2000). They are more common in women, and their prevalence increases with age in both genders. Because of these effects, insufficient sleep and sleep disorders are recognized as public health issues.

Understanding sleep, sleep disturbances, and sleep disorders is crucial for mental health practitioners today. This chapter presents a discussion of normal sleep rhythms and patterns, sleep disorders and their distinguishing characteristics, and nursing diagnoses and interventions appropriate for use in patients with sleep problems.

SLEEP

Sleep, necessary for human survival, can be viewed from both behavioral and physiologic perspectives. Behaviorally, sleep is a state of decreased awareness of environmental stimuli and a relative state of unconsciousness with no memory of the state. Sleep, different than a coma, can be disrupted and reversed quite easily. Theoretical concepts associated with sleep include conditioning, hyperarousal, stress response, predisposing personality traits, and attitudes and beliefs about sleep (National Institutes of Health [NIH], 2005). Sleep is usually preceded by a period of **sleepiness** or the urge to fall asleep.

From a physiologic perspective, dopamine, GABA, adenosine, histamine, hypocretin, melatonin, and cortisol seem to all play a role in changing sleep states (Mignot et al., 2002). Wakefulness is maintained by the reticular activating system in the brain. As the cycle of the reticular activating system dwindles, neurotransmitters that promote sleep take over (see Chapter 7).

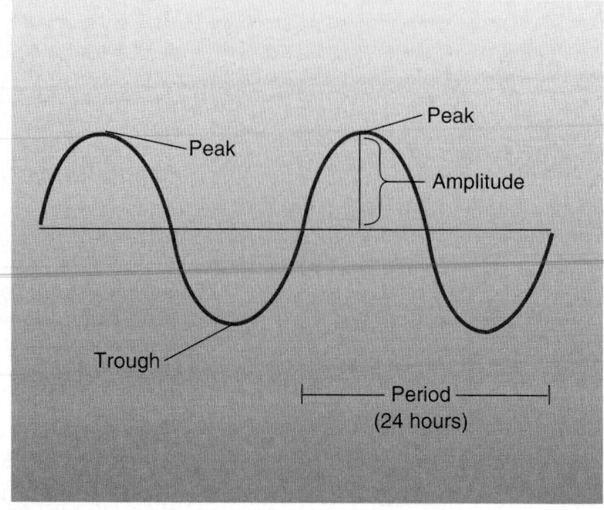

FIGURE 26.1. Circadian body rhythms. Circadian body rhythms fluctuate in patterns. The *peak* is the point at which the rhythm reaches its maximum, and the *trough* is the point at which the rhythm reaches its minimum. The *period* is the time it takes to complete a cycle. *Amplitude* is the extent of the peak and is half the distance from peak to trough.

Pattern of Sleep

Sleep is a patterned activity and is one component of the biphasic 24 hour sleep–wake cycle.

> **KEY CONCEPT Sleep–wake cycle** is an endogenously generated rhythm close to 24–25 hours synchronized with the day/night cycle. The release of the hormones melatonin and cortisol promotes wakefulness during the day and induces sleep at night.

Sleep latency is the time period measured from "lights out," or bedtime, to the beginning of sleep. **Sleep architecture** is the pattern of NREM and REM which are in about a 90- to 110-minute cycle. Sleep occurs in stages and the timing of sleep is regulated by circadian rhythms. **Sleep efficiency** is the ratio of total sleep time to nocturnal time in bed.

Circadian Rhythm

> **KEY CONCEPT Rhythm** is movement with a cadence, a measured flow that occurs at regular intervals, with a cycle of coming and going, ebbing and rising, to return at the start point and begin again.

Nearly all physiologic and psychological functions fluctuate in a pattern that repeats itself in a 24-hour cycle, called **circadian rhythm** (see Figure 26.1). The biologic clock that regulates our circadian rhythms is located in the *suprachiasmatic nucleus*, an area of the hypothalamus which lies on top of the optic chiasm. About the size of the letter "V" on this page, the suprachiasmatic nucleus is a boomerang-shaped cluster of nerve cells. Peripheral cells also contribute to the regulation of circadian rhythms. When two or more rhythms reach their peak at the same time, they are **synchronized** in phase with each other; if they reach their peak at different times, they are **desynchronized.**

Most physiologic functions reach their lowest levels during the middle of the sleep period. For example, body temperature follows a predictable pattern from lowest, in the early morning, to highest, in the mid-evening. Manual dexterity, reaction time, and simple recognition appear to coincide with the circadian rhythm of body temperature. Most circadian rhythms continue even when humans are unaware of the time of day. Natural age-related changes in circadian sleep rhythms generally regulate people as they get older toward morning alertness and productivity, and sleepiness at night.

Larks and Owls

Surveys show that most people (55%) are "early birds" or **larks** and are more alert and perform best in the early morning. Evening people or **owls** make up 41% of the population and are more alert and perform better during the late evening hours (National Sleep Foundation, 2005). The owls have a natural tendency to stay up late, which can be further reinforced by personal preference or necessity, such as having a job that requires either early morning or late night alertness. They are also at higher risk for insomnia or sleep apnea. Morning orientation is usually reinforced or imposed when people get a regular daytime job (see Box 26.1).

BOX 26.1

Using Reflection: Lark or Owl?

Incident: A nurse manager was very upset by a new staff nurse who was consistently late for work and seemed "drugged" in the morning. Yet, the staff nurse was reportedly the life of the party at night. The manager was ready to perform disciplinary actions.

Reflection: The nurse manager reflected on the staff nurse's behavior, which was consistent with an Owl's circadian rhythm. After discussion with the nurse, the manager assigned the staff nurse to the evening shift; performance improved dramatically.

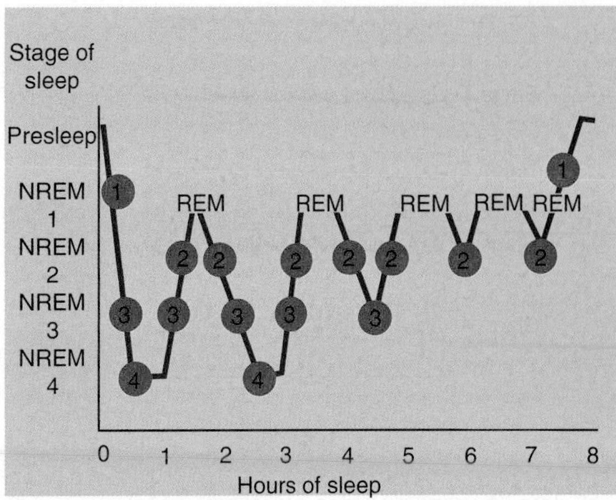

FIGURE 26.3. Hours of sleep. In typical sleep architecture in normal young adults, non–rapid-eye-movement (NREM) and rapid-eye-movement (REM) sleep stages cycle every 90 to 110 minutes through the night. Wakefulness accounts for less than 5% of the night's sleep pattern (presleep to NREM 1). Slow-wave sleep dominates the first third of the night during NREM stages 3 and 4. REM sleep occurs in four to six separate episodes throughout the night (20%–25% of sleep) and dominates the last third of the night's sleep. (Modified from Biddle, C., & Oaster, T. R. F. (1990). *Journal of the American Association of Anesthetists, 58*(1), 36.)

Stages of Sleep

Sleep is a two-phase cycle: **non–rapid-eye-movement (NREM)** and **rapid-eye-movement (REM)** (see Figure 26.2). During an 8-hour sleep period, the cycle of NREM and REM sleep repeats itself five or six times. This cycle changes as the night progresses. In the first cycle, the amount of REM sleep is brief. With each succeeding cycle, the amount of time spent in REM sleep lengthens until it seems to dominate at the end of the sleep period. Conversely, NREM is most prominent during the initial cycle but declines throughout the night (see Figure 26.3).

Non–Rapid-Eye-Movement Sleep

Non–rapid-eye-movement sleep occurs about 90 minutes after falling asleep and consists of four substages. Light sleep is characteristic of stages 1 and 2, in which the person is easily aroused. A person aroused from stage 1 sleep may even deny having been asleep, such as dozing while watching television and awakening minutes later during a loud commercial. Stage 1 accounts for only 2% to 5% of a night's sleep and is a transition between relaxed wakefulness and sleep. Stage 2 comprises about 45% to 55% of sleep. During Phase 1 and 2, an electroencephalogram shows an alpha rhythm gradually being replaced by a theta rhythm. Sleep spindles or "k complexes" occur in stage 2 (see Figure 26.4).

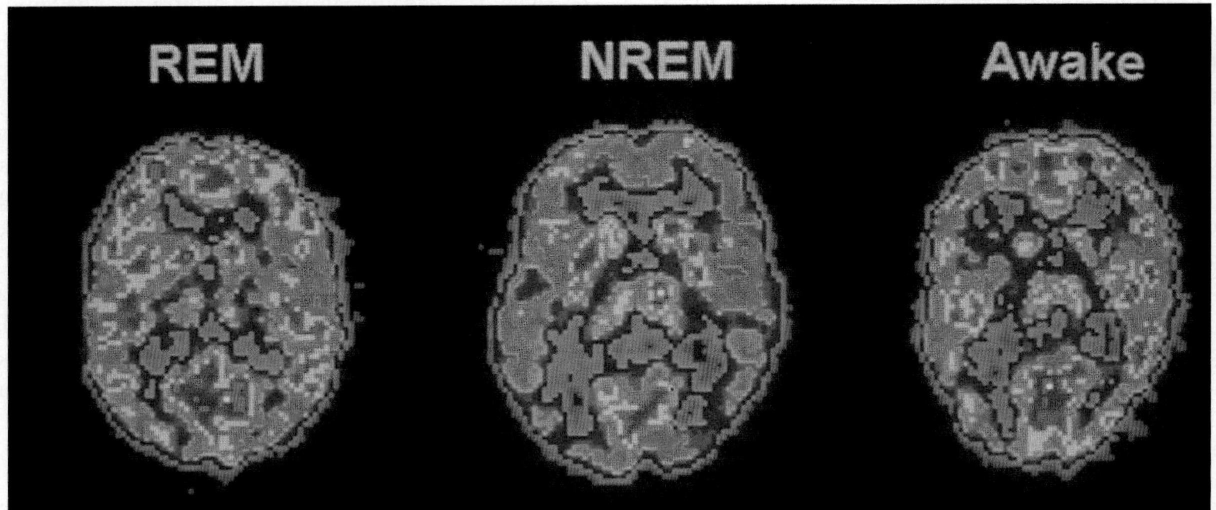

FIGURE 26.2. Brain activity during sleep-wake cycle. The brain is as active in rapid-eye-movement (REM) or dreaming sleep as when awake but is metabolically less active in slow-wave or non–rapid-eye-movement (NREM) sleep. (Courtesy of Monte S. Buchsbaum, MD, the Mount Sinai Medical Center and School of Medicine, New York, NY.)

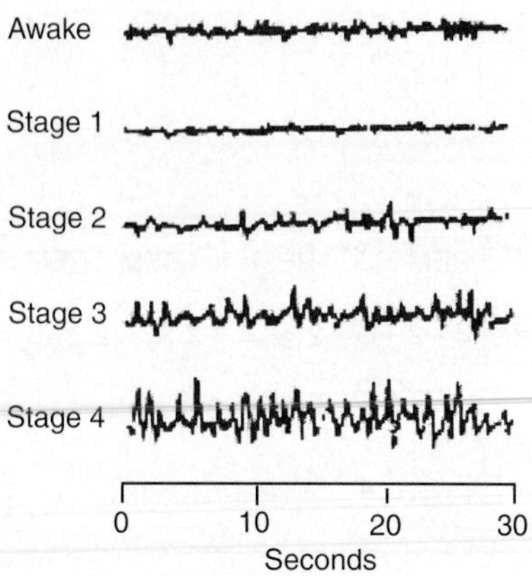

FIGURE 26.4. Brain waves during stages of non–rapid-eye-movement (NREM) sleep. Brain waves during wakefulness and stages 1, 2, 3, and 4 and duration of wakefulness. (Porth, C. M. (2005). *Pathophysiology: Concepts of altered health states.* Philadelphia: Lippincott Williams & Wilkins.)

Slow-wave sleep, or the deepest state of sleep, characterizes stages 3 and 4. Slow-wave sleep is believed to have a restorative function, although the exact mechanism for this is unclear. It may serve to conserve energy because metabolism and body temperature decrease during this part of sleep. These stages make up 10% to 23% of sleep. EEG findings show high-amplitude waves, slow waves, or delta waves. The difference between stages 3 and 4 is the amount of delta waves seen, with stage 3 demonstrating 20% to 50% of delta waves and stage 4 showing more than 50% of delta waves.

Rapid-Eye-Movement Sleep

Rapid-eye-movement sleep is a state characterized by bursts of rapid eye movements. REM sleep occurs in four to six separate episodes and makes up about 20% to 25% of a night's sleep. Although REM sleep is a deep sleep and muscles seem to be at rest, EEG findings demonstrate an active brain. More blood flows to the brain, and brain temperature increases. Brain waves resemble a mixture of wakeful and drowsy patterns. Although vivid dreaming is the outstanding feature reported by adults when awakened out of REM sleep, people also report dreams when they awaken from NREM sleep.

During REM sleep, nerve impulses are blocked within the spinal cord. Muscle tone diminishes to the point of paralysis of the head and neck as well as the longer muscle groups. Only stronger impulses are relayed, producing muscular twitches, eye movements, and impulses controlling heart rate and respiration. Breathing and heart rate become irregular.

This type of sleep also has a circadian rhythm that closely coincides with the body temperature rhythm. The greatest amount of REM sleep is seen when the body temperature cycle is at its lowest. Temperature regulation is impaired; that is, people do not sweat or shiver during REM sleep. Patterns of hormone release, kidney function, and reflexes change. Females have clitoral engorgement and an increase in blood flow to the vagina. Males have penile erections.

The function of REM sleep continues to be debated. Several theories have been put forth, such as REM sleep may stimulate brain growth or consolidate memory, but only limited evidence supports any of these hypotheses. Furthermore, REM sleep deprivation does not affect personality variables, as popularly believed. The function of REM sleep and dreaming remains a fundamental mystery.

Gender

Women are at greater risk for insomnia and other sleep problems than men. Sleep in women is influenced by the sex hormones, which vary throughout the life cycle (Soares & Murray, 2006). In The National Sleep Foundation's Women and Sleep Poll ($N = 1{,}012$), 53% of women experienced one or more symptoms of insomnia during the previous month (National Sleep Foundation, 2005).

Age

Sleep patterns change dramatically over the course of the life span. Newborns need 17 to 18 hours of sleep each day, which occurs in 3- to 4-hour episodes throughout the day. By 6 months, 12 hours at night and two 1- to 2-hour naps each day are needed. After age 5, children gradually need less sleep. The preadolescent needs about 10 hours of sleep each night, and napping is rare. A teenager's sleep need is only slightly less, at about 9 hours and 15 minutes. During young adulthood, about 8 hours of sleep is needed; napping is arbitrary. The amount of sleep needed and sleep architecture typically remain unchanged during the middle-aged years. Poor sleep is associated with menopause.

For older adults, the need for sleep does not decrease, but the ability to sleep does. Older people spend more time in bed, sleep less, wake more often during the night, and take longer to fall asleep than younger adults. Sleep becomes more fragmented in older adults, with an increase in the number of sleep stage shifts, arousals, and awakenings. Some sleep requirements are met by daytime napping. Further, temperature rhythm in older people peaks earlier; early morning arousals may reflect early rise of body temperature. Elderly people are at risk for sleep disorders (Cooke & Ancoli-Israel, 2006).

Environment

A person can be sleepy but may stay awake if in a stimulating environment with bright lights or a lot of activity.

In contrast, a sleepy person in a quiet place or engaged in sedentary activity cannot resist the urge to fall asleep. Sleepiness is a physiologic state, and although a stimulating environment can temporarily forestall it, once these stimuli are removed, the urge to sleep will persist. Even when someone who is chronically sleep deprived does not feel sleepy, the tendency to fall asleep is much greater and may manifest by causing the person to doze off while sitting in lectures or during the monotonous operation of machinery or driving.

Lifestyles

Many factors can cause disrupted sleep patterns, such as traveling across time zones, emotional stress or anxiety, or changing the sleep–wake pattern because of shift work. When traveling across time zones or working night shifts (and sleeping during the day), one's regular sleepiness–alertness rhythm may persist for several days. Even when daytime sleep is improved with a nighttime sedative, which produces longer and less fragmented sleep, sleepiness in the early morning hours usually continues to be profound for the first two to three nights. This extreme sleepiness significantly decreases after a 4- to 6-day reversal of the sleep–wake cycle.

Changes in Normal Sleep

Normal sleep is sensitive to changes, and the body responds when deprived of certain phases of sleep, particularly REM sleep and slow-wave sleep. Certain activities, such as early rising or alcohol intake before bedtime, or some medications, such as central nervous system (CNS)-acting drugs, can suppress REM sleep. Fragmented sleep interrupts the restorative function of a good night's sleep. Not only does insufficient sleep cause daytime sleepiness, but disturbed sleep affects daytime alertness and performance as well. The restorative biologic processes associated with sleep require an adequate amount of sleep for the completion of these processes. A **sleep debt** occurs when there is recurrent long-term sleep deprivation. Basic restoration is interrupted or does not happen.

When individuals are deprived of REM sleep, there is a subsequent "rebound effect," wherein the lost REM sleep is made up during the next sleep period. The body makes up for this lost REM sleep by earlier occurrence of REM sleep during the next night. The occurrence of REM at sleep onset implies REM deprivation. If sleep onset is delayed until the time of peak phase of REM sleep's circadian rhythm, REM sleep will predominate during those early sleep hours.

Slow-wave sleep does not appear to have a circadian determinant, but it is more sensitive to the amount of previous sleep obtained. When one is deprived of both REM and slow-wave sleep, the body prefers to make up the slow-wave before the REM sleep.

PRIMARY SLEEP DISORDERS

Primary sleep disorders are subdivided into **dyssomnias**, which are disorders of initiating or maintaining sleep or excessive sleepiness, and **parasomnias**, which are disorders of particular physiologic or behavioral reactions during sleep.

Dyssomnias

Dyssomnias are characterized by disturbances in the amount, quality, or timing of sleep, and include primary insomnia, primary hypersomnia, narcolepsy, breathing-related sleep disorders, and circadian rhythm sleep disorder. Primary insomnia will be highlighted in this chapter.

Primary Insomnia

KEY CONCEPT Insomnia refers to difficulty falling asleep, trouble maintaining sleep, or waking up too early. Complaints of disturbed sleep occur when there is adequate opportunity and circumstances for sleep (NIH, 2005).

Primary insomnia is diagnosed when daytime fatigue, difficulty with concentration, and poor mood are present and there is no indication of another disorder. Patients usually deny fighting sleep or falling asleep unintentionally during the day (see Box 26.2). The hallmark symptom of primary insomnia is the patient's intense focus and anxiety regarding the inability to fall asleep or maintain sleep. Ideally, a sleep disorder is diagnosed through measuring the physiologic changes that occur during sleep. **Polysomnography,** usually performed at night during sleep, monitors many body functions including brain wave activity, eye movements, muscle activity, heart rhythm, breathing function, and respiratory effort (see Figure 26.5). Polysomnography may show poor sleep continuity, increased stage 1 and decreased slow-wave sleep, and an increased amount of EEG alpha wave activity while asleep. Clinical evaluation includes oral and nasal airflow, respiratory effort, oxyhemoglobin saturation, and electromyogram of limb muscle activity.

Clinical Course

There are few studies describing the course of primary insomnia. This disorder can last for short periods in some patients and for decades in others. Limited data show that symptoms are usually of long duration (NIH, 2005).

BOX 26.2

Key Diagnostic Characteristics for Primary Insomnia 307.42

Diagnostic Criteria

- Difficulty initiating or maintaining sleep or nonrestorative sleep for at least 1 month
- Clinically significant distress or impairment in social, occupational, or other areas of functioning because of sleep disturbance
- Not occurring exclusively during course of another mental disorder, narcolepsy, breathing-related sleep disorder, circadian rhythm sleep disorder, or a parasomnia
- Not a direct physiologic effect of a substance or a medical condition

Target Symptoms and Associated Findings

- History of light or easily disturbed sleep before development of more persistent sleep problems
- Anxious concern with general health and increased sensitivity to daytime effect of mild sleep loss
- Interpersonal, social, and occupational problems developing because of anxiety about sleep
- Problems with inattention and concentration
- Inappropriate use of medications, such as hypnotics, alcohol, or caffeine

Associated Physical Examination Findings

- Fatigued and haggard appearance

Associated Laboratory Findings

- Poor sleep continuity, increased stage 1 sleep, decreased stages 3 and 4 sleep, increased muscle tension, or increased amounts of electroencephalogram alpha activity during sleep
- Elevated scores on psychological or personality inventories

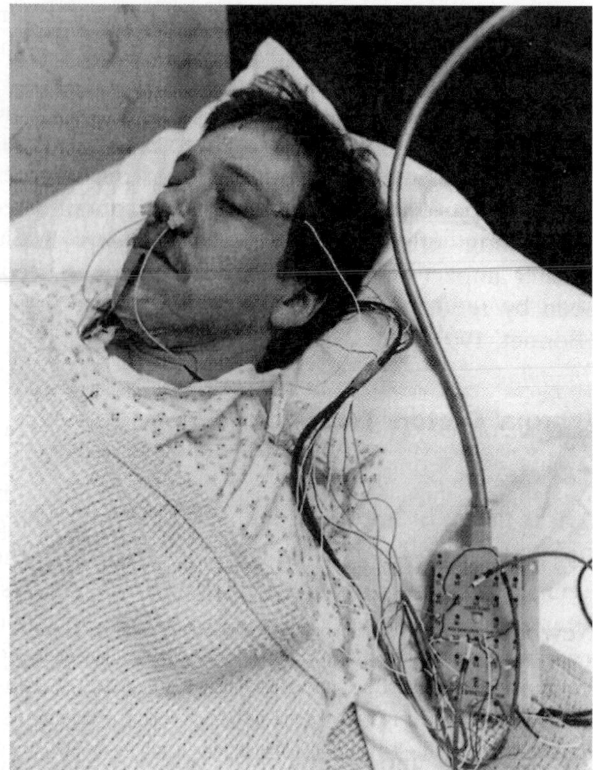

FIGURE 26.5. Polysomnography study. A patient undergoing polysomnography has electrodes affixed or taped to the scalp, face, chest, and legs.

Epidemiology

Of all sleep-related problems, insomnia is the most prevalent, with estimates ranging from 30% to 35%; the prevalence of chronic or severe insomnia is estimated to range from 10% to 15% (Sateia, 2002). It is estimated that 15% to 25% of the individuals with chronic insomnia are diagnosed with primary insomnia. There is a greater prevalence of insomnia among older people. There is also a higher prevalence among divorced, separated, and widowed adults. Observational studies have found a greater prevalence among women, especially among those who are postmenopausal (NIH, 2005).

Individuals at risk for developing primary insomnia often describe themselves as "light sleepers" before persistent sleep problems developed. They have a tendency to be more easily psychologically or physiologically aroused at night. They tend to develop sleep-preventing associations and behaviors in an attempt to control their insomnia (Harvey, 2002). Although initially insomnia may be precipitated by stressful situations and tension, this inability to fall asleep and stay asleep persists after the crisis or stressful situation has passed.

Comorbidities

Medical conditions, including arthritis, heart failure, pulmonary and gastrointestinal disorders, Parkinson's disease, stroke, and incontinence, affect sleep and increase the prevalence of insomnia. Several psychiatric disorders such as depression and bipolar disorder have strong relationships with insomnia. The extent to which treatment for these conditions ameliorates insomnia remains unclear (NIH, 2005).

Etiology

Many factors affect sleep, but there are no definitive studies that support a specific etiology for sleep disorders. Work is needed to examine those factors that correlate with insomnia along with the importance of family history for a systematic search for specific genes (NIH, 2005) (see Figure 26.6).

Interdisciplinary Treatment

Sleep disorders are best treated by clinicians specializing in this area, but primary and mental health care professionals should be able to identify sleep disturbances and

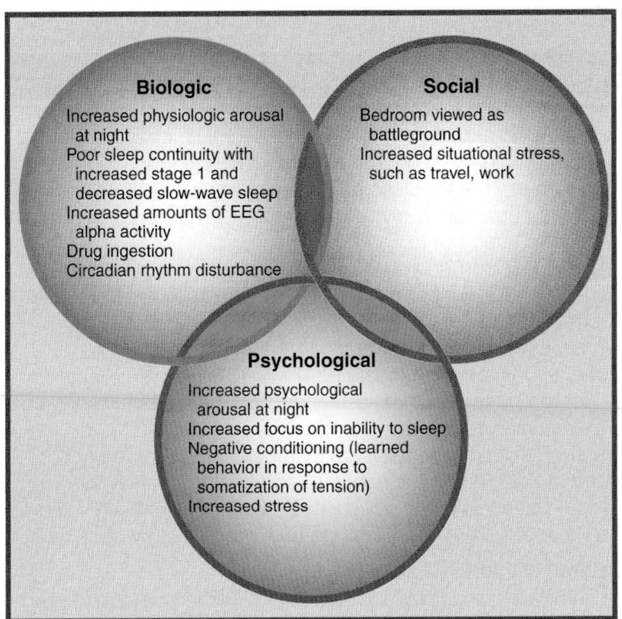

FIGURE 26.6. Biopsychosocial etiologies of primary insomnia.

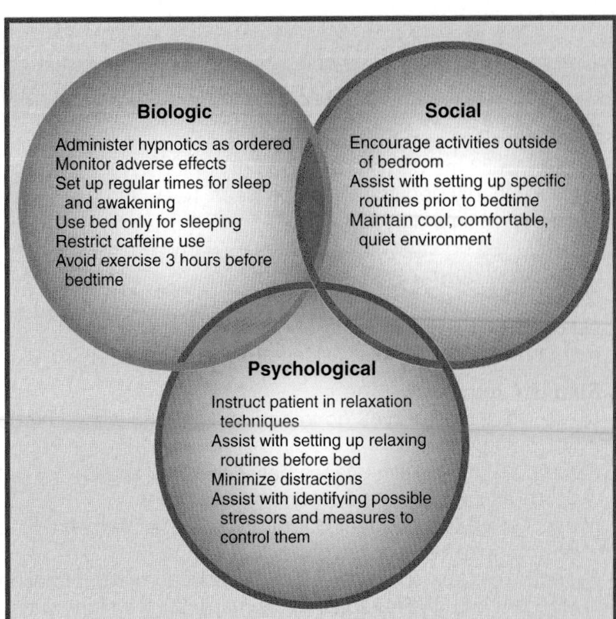

FIGURE 26.7. Biopsychosocial interventions for patients with primary insomnia.

provide education and interventions for normalizing sleep. The most common treatments for chronic insomnia are over-the-counter (OTC) antihistamines, alcohol, and prescription medications.

Priority Care Issues

Safety is a priority for people with primary insomnia. Sleep deprivation can lead to accidents, falls, and injuries, especially in the older patient. Sedating medication could potentially increase falls (Curry, Eisenstein, & Walsh, 2006).

Family Response 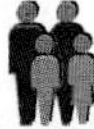

Living with a family member with insomnia is challenging. Irritability, complaints of sleeplessness, and chronic fatigue interfere with quality interpersonal relationships. Family members become weary of living with someone who never sleeps.

NURSING MANAGEMENT: HUMAN RESPONSE TO PRIMARY INSOMNIA

Primary insomnia usually involves a combination of approaches, as illustrated in Figure 26.7.

Biologic Domain

Biologic Assessment

The assessment of a patient's sleep pattern is a part of every psychiatric nursing assessment (see Chapter 10). If a patient has a sleep disorder, a detailed sleep history should be included in the assessment process. During the patient interview, the description, duration (when problem began), stability (every night?), and intensity (how bad is it?) should be determined (see Box 26.3). A sleep history includes sleeping pattern during health, current sleeping patterns, medical problems, current medications (including OTC and supplements), current life events, use of alcohol and caffeine, and emotional and mental status that might be affecting sleep (see Box 26.4 and Box 26.5). A **sleep diary** or a person's written account of the sleep experience is useful in determining the extent of the sleep problem (Nadolski, 2005). The diary may cover a few days to several weeks. A simple diary is typically a daily record of the patient's bedtimes, rising times, estimated time to fall asleep, number and length of awakenings, and naps. More complicated sleep diaries involve recording the amount and time of alcohol ingestion, ratings of fatigue, medication, and stressful events.

Nursing Diagnoses for the Biological Domain

The nursing diagnosis usually applied to the patient with a sleep disorder is Sleep Pattern Disturbance, Insomnia or Sleep Deprivation (Fig. 26.8). The diagnosis is made when a disruption of sleep time causes discomfort or interferes with lifestyle (see Nursing Care Plan 26.1).

Interventions for the Biologic Domain

Nonpharmacologic health-promoting interventions are the first choice before administering pharmacologic agents (Yang, Spielman, & Glovinsky, 2006). Sleep hygiene strategies are effective and should be encour-

BOX 26.3

Therapeutic Dialogue: Sleep Assessment

Ineffective Approach

Nurse: What time do you go to bed at night?

Patient: Oh, my bedtime varies between 10 PM and 2 AM.

Nurse: What time do you get up?

Patient: I get up anywhere between 6 AM and noon.

Nurse: How do you sleep during the night?

Patient: OK.

Nurse: OK?

Patient: Yeah, no problems sleeping.

Effective Approach

Nurse: What time do you go to bed at night and what time do you get up?

Patient: Oh, my bedtime varies between 10 PM and 2 AM. I get up anywhere between 6 AM and noon.

Nurse: Let's be more specific. During a week's time, what time do you go to bed each night?

Patient: Well, this semester I have a morning clinical rotation Monday through Thursday. I'm usually up til midnight writing my care plan. On Friday, I'm usually so exhausted that I go to bed around 10 PM. Saturday nights I go out with my friends and get to bed around 2 AM. On Sunday night, I usually get to bed around 11 PM.

Nurse: What time do you get up each day of the week?

Patient: On the mornings that I have clinicals, I have to get up around 5:30 AM to be at the hospital by 6:45 AM. On Friday I get up at 7 AM for class. Saturday morning, I get up around 8 AM so I can go to my part-time job. On Sunday, I get up at 9 AM so I can get to church.

Nurse: How long do you take to fall asleep?

Patient: That's gotten much better. I fall asleep in 15 minutes or so.

Nurse: Do you take any naps?

Patient: Outside of my lectures, I don't have time to nap. I'm just too busy with my classes and clinicals, homework, job, and social life.

Nurse: Before this semester, how much sleep did you get?

Patient: That was last summer, I had an afternoon job then so I could sleep as much as I wanted. I bet I got 8 or even 9 hours of sleep every night. It was great. I wasn't sleepy back then.

Critical Thinking Challenge

- Compare the quality and quantity of elicited data in the two scenarios.
- What conclusions could be drawn from the first scenario?
- Are the conclusions different for the second scenario? Explain.

aged (see Box 26.6). The goal is to normalize sleep patterns to improve well-being.

Activity, Exercise, and Nutritional Interventions

Exercise promotes sleep, but regular exercise should be planned for earlier in the day and never within 2 to 3 hours of going to bed. Bedtime routines are important. The patient should engage in a quiet, relaxing activity in preparation for sleep, such as listening to soft music, taking a warm bath, reading for pleasure, or watching television in another room (providing the show is not alarming).

BOX 26.4

Sleep History

Perception of sleep problem
Sleep schedule (time of retiring and arising)
Problems with falling asleep and maintaining sleep
Quality of sleep
Daytime sleepiness and impact of the sleep disorder on daytime functioning
General emotional and physical problems
Sleep hygiene (e.g., eating and drinking before retiring)
Sleep environment (bed comfort, room temperature, noise, light)

Adapted from Porth, C. M. (Ed.). 2005. Sleep and sleep disorders. *Pathophysiology: Concepts of altered health states* (pp. 259–277). Lippincott Williams & Wilkins: Philadelphia.

Patients suffering from insomnia should be counseled not to eat anything heavy for several hours before retiring. Spicy foods, alcohol, and caffeine should be avoided. If they insist on a bedtime snack, warm milk is appropriate for most patients. Milk contains L-tryptophan, an essential amino acid that is a precursor to serotonin, one of the neurotransmitters involved in sleep. L-Tryptophan allows more rapid onset of sleep and lowers the sensitivity to external stimuli during sleep. L-Tryptophan competes with other amino acids for transport into the brain. Therefore, eating an additional snack with milk may diminish the sleep effects of L-tryptophan.

Thermoregulation

Patients should be encouraged to evaluate the temperature of the room. Generally a cooler environment enhances sleep.

Pharmacologic Interventions

Benzodiazepine Receptor Agonists (BzRA)

The BzRA hypnotics have U.S. Food and Drug Administration (FDA) approval for insomnia. They include the benzodiazepines (triazolam, temazepam, estazolam, quazepam, and flurazepam) and the nonbenzodiazepines (zolpidem, zolpidem-extended release, zaleplon, and eszopiclone) (see Table 26.1). All of these medications bind to benzodiazepine receptors and exert

BOX 26.5

Medications and Other Substances and Their Effects on Sleep

Alcohol
- Increases TST during the first half of the night
- Decreases TST during the second half
- Decreases REM sleep during the first half of the night
- Withdrawal from chronic use of alcohol causes a decrease in TST, increased wakefulness after sleep onset, and REM rebound.

Amphetamines
- Disrupt sleep–wake cycle during acute use
- Decrease TST
- Decrease REM sleep
- Withdrawal may cause REM rebound.

Antidepressants (Tricyclics and MAOIs)
- Sleep effects vary with sedative potential
- Increase slow-wave sleep
- Decrease REM sleep

Barbiturates
- Increase TST
- Decrease WASO
- Decrease REM sleep
- Withdrawal may cause decrease in TST and REM rebound.

Benzodiazepines
- Drugs vary in onset and duration of action.
- Decrease SL
- Increase TST
- Decrease WASO
- Decrease REM sleep
- Daytime sedation may occur with long-acting drugs.

β-Adrenergic blockers
- Decrease REM sleep
- Increase WASO, nightmares
- Daytime sedation may occur

Caffeine
- Increases SL
- Decreases TST
- Decreases REM sleep

L-Dopa
- Vivid dreams and nightmares

Lithium
- Increases slow-wave sleep
- Decreases REM sleep

Opioids
- Effects vary with specific agents
- Increase WASO
- Decrease REM sleep
- Decrease slow-wave sleep

Phenothiazines
- Increase TST
- Increase slow-wave sleep

Steroids
- Increase WASO

MAOI, monoamine oxidase inhibitors; REM, rapid-eye-movement; SL, sleep latency; TST, total sleep time; WASO, wake after sleep onset.

their effects by facilitating GABA effects. GABA, the most common inhibitory neurotransmitter, must be present at the benzodiazepine receptor for the BzRA to exert its effect. All of these medications are absorbed rapidly and reduce sleep latency at recommended doses (Curry et al., 2006). Benzodiazepines slightly decrease REM sleep but greatly suppress slow-wave sleep. Nonbenzodiazepine hypnotics, which provide immediate relief, are often used for short-term treatment of insomnia. The margin of safety is wide. The most common side effects are headache, dizziness, and residual sleepiness (see Box 26.7). There is agreement among sleep experts that the BzRAs are safe and efficacious. The safety of their long-term use has not been established (NIH, 2005). The BzRAs are Schedule IV controlled substances by federal regulation. These drugs have abuse and dependence potential and have produced withdrawal signs and symptoms following abrupt discontinuation. The risk for residual sedation on the day after using hypnotic medication is determined by the dose and rate of elimination (Curry et al., 2006).

Melatonin Receptor Agonist

Melatonin has been shown to shift circadian rhythm, decrease body temperature, alter reproductive rhythm, enhance immune function, and decrease alertness. Normally, levels of melatonin increase with decreasing exposure to light. Ramelteon (Rozerem), indicated for insomnia, is a melatonin receptor agonist with high affinity for melatonin receptors (MT_1 and MT_2). This activity is believed to be related to its sleep-promoting properties (see Box 26.8). Ramelteon has a low abuse potential and is not a controlled substance.

Off-label Use of Sedating Antidepressants

Antidepressants have a potent effect on sleep and are used off-label to treat many sleep problems. For example, trazodone (Desyrel) is often taken at bedtime to improve sleep as well as mood. Most antidepressants decrease REM sleep and are thought to treat depression by depriving REM sleep (Lam, 2006). The efficacy and safety of antidepressants for insomnia have not been established and their use is not recommended (Mendelson, 2005).

Over-the-Counter Medications and Supplements

Sleeping pills bought OTC are usually antihistamines (Holcomb, 2006). The most common agents are doxylamine (Unisom) and diphenhydramine (Benadryl). These histamine-1 antagonists have a CNS effect that

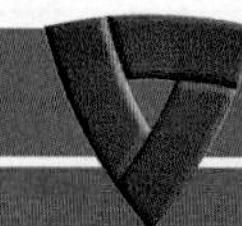

Nursing Care Plan 26.1

Insomnia

MT is a 20-year-old student who is majoring in nursing. He presents himself at Student Health Services with a complaint of insomnia. In assessing his problem, the nurse ascertains that MT takes 2 to 3 hours to fall asleep. During this interim of wakefulness, he lies in bed, calm but somewhat restless. He has had no prior difficulty with insomnia. His problem falling asleep occurs 3 nights a week—Monday, Wednesday, and Friday. He exercises vigorously during his physical education class (7–9 PM) on these three evenings. He denies any sleep problems during spring break, when he took a trip. The patient drinks 1 cup of coffee in the morning and denies the use of other stimulants. He reports that as a consequence he has had some irritability and difficulty concentrating on the days following a "bad night." He has tried an over-the-counter sleep medication, but does not remember the name of it. When he took these sleeping pills, he was able to fall asleep better, but found them to be costly. He would like a prescription for sleeping medication that would be covered by student health insurance.

Setting: Outpatient Student Health Service

Baseline Assessment: A 20-year-old man who presents with difficulty initiating sleep. After vigorous evening exercise, he takes 2–3 hours to fall asleep. Strengths: intelligence, motivated for treatment, adequate insurance coverage, good physical health.

Associated Psychiatric Diagnoses	Medications
Axis I: Primary insomnia Axis II: None Axis III: None Axis IV: None Axis V: GAF = Current 85 Potential 90	None

Nursing Diagnosis 1: Insomnia

Defining Characteristics	Related Factors
Difficulty falling asleep, estimated sleep latency of 2–3 hours, three nights a week Mood alterations Poor concentration	Changes in usual sleep environment Poor sleep hygiene

Outcomes

Initial	Discharge
1. Describe factors that prevent or inhibit sleep. 2. Identify strategies to improve sleep hygiene.	3. Report an optimal balance of rest and activity.

Interventions

Interventions	Rationale	Ongoing Assessment
Teach patient good sleep hygiene habits	Discussion of good sleep hygiene is the first treatment strategy.	Monitor MT's reports of estimated sleep latency.
Instruct patient to keep a sleep diary for 1 week—including bedtime, sleep latency, rising time, naps, caffeine intake, time of exercise.	Keeping a sleep diary can give insight into insomnia problems by identifying alerting influences in relation to disturbed sleep.	Exercise before sleep appears to be the primary factor that could be causing insomnia on Monday, Wednesday, and Friday. Monitor other sleep hygiene issues.
Reassure patient that short-term insomnia will resolve when the factors that caused the problem are eliminated.	Anxiety about insomnia is a predisposing factor to the development of primary insomnia.	Determine MT's level of anxiety about the insomnia.

Continued

Nursing Care Plan 26.1 (Continued)

Interventions

Interventions	Rationale	Ongoing Assessment
Determine whether it is possible to adjust schedule so that vigorous exercise occurs several hours before sleep.	Physical exercise raises basal metabolism, which may interfere with sleep.	Determine whether it is possible to adjust course schedule.
Problem solve with MT how to adjust sleep schedule to avoid insomnia.	Problem solving allows the patient to learn how to consider alternative strategies.	Evaluate whether strategies are reasonable.

Evaluation

Outcomes	Revised Outcomes	Interventions
After readjustment of exercise schedule, Matthew was able to resume normal sleep.	None	None

includes sedation, diminished alertness, and slowing of reaction time. These drugs also produce anticholinergic side effects, such as dry mouth, accelerated heart rate, urinary retention, and dilated pupils. Drowsiness lasts from 3 to 6 hours after a single dose. Next-morning hangover can be a problem. Diphenhydramine decreases sleep latency and improves quality of sleep for those with occasional sleep problems, but is not as effective as benzodiazepines for chronic sleep disturbances (Kirkwood & Melton, 2006).

Exogenous melatonin has long been available OTC and has been shown to have mild sleep-promoting properties when given outside the period of usual secretion. Studies of melatonin administration during the night do not show significant effects and do not support its use in insomnia (Buscemi et al., 2004).

Valerian, a nutritional supplement, is used as a medicinal herb in many cultures. The mechanism of action is not fully understood and is believed to inhibit GABA reuptake. Valerian extract is reported to be an inhibitor of cytochrome P450 3A4. Valerian may be useful for sleeplessness, but there is not enough evidence to confirm this (National Center for Complementary and Alternative Medicine, 2006).

Administering and Monitoring Medication

Sleeping medications are commonly used in all settings. These medications are usually given nightly for a short period to establish a wake–sleep pattern. Rebound insomnia can occur if a drug is abruptly discontinued. When it does occur, the insomnia usually lasts only one night. This effect can be minimized or prevented by giving the lowest effective dose and tapering before discontinuing (Curry et al., 2006). Nurses should observe for confusion, memory problems, excessive sedation, and falls, especially in the elderly.

Drug-to-Drug Interactions

Sleep medications generally have increased depressive effects when given with other CNS depressants. Because most sleep medications are metabolized by the CYP 3A family, drugs that inhibit or induce these enzymes have the potential to interact. Medications that inhibit 3A include oral contraceptives, isoniazid, fluvoxamine, and verapamil (see Chapter 8). Cimetadine may increase plasma concentration of BzRAs, requiring a lower initial dose. CYP 3A4 inducers such as carbamazepine may reduce the effectiveness of the BzRAs (Stahl, 2006). Grapefruit juice should be avoided with these drugs. Ramelteon should not be given with fluvoxamine.

Teaching Points 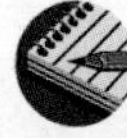

Pharmacological agents should complement sleep hygiene practices. These medications can be useful on a short-term basis, but rarely should be needed long term. Alcohol use should be very limited when taking sleeping medications. The nurse should emphasize that hypnotic medications are to be used only for a short time. Patients should use these medications when there is adequate time for sleeping, at least 8 hours, with the exception of Zaleplon, which is short-acting and can be used as long 5 or more hours to bedtime. The BzRAs should be taken at bedtime and ramelteon within 30 minutes of bedtime. Patients should be instructed about the safe use of these medications and possible side effects.

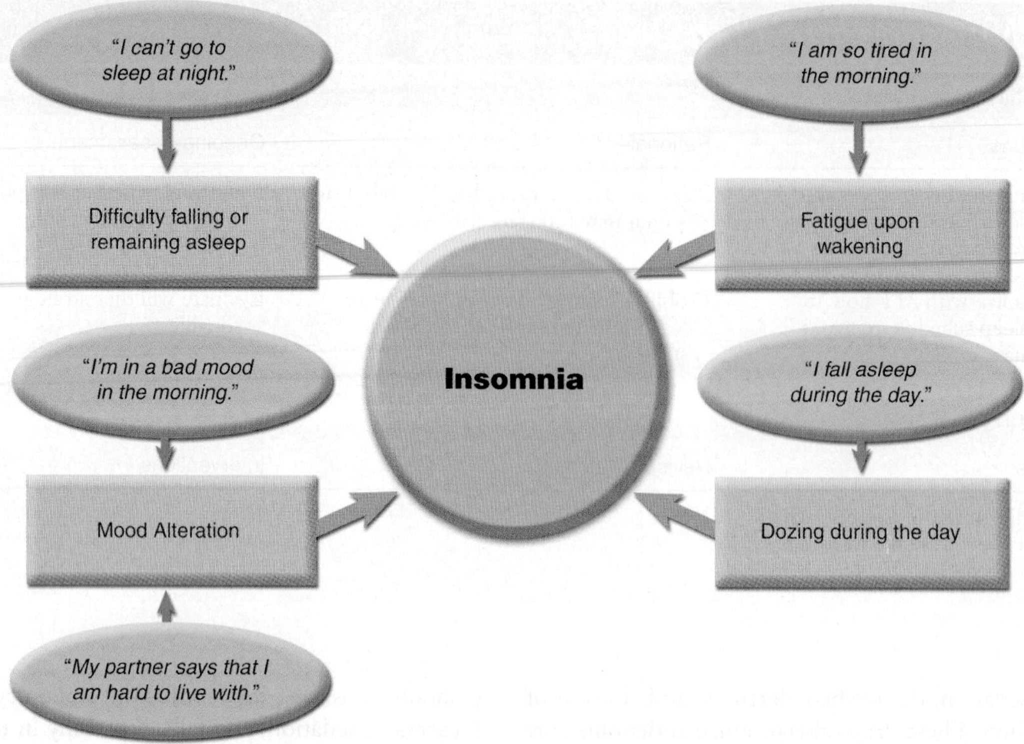

FIGURE 26.8. Nursing diagnosis concept map: Insomnia

Psychosocial Domain

Psychosocial Assessment

The assessment includes evaluating the behavioral and social factors related to sleep problems. Recent changes in relationships, particularly a divorce or death of a loved one, can significantly interfere with sleep. A recent move, travel, and addition of a new family member can also negatively impact sleep. Fatigue and stress increase when individuals assume caregiving roles in addition to working as professional caregivers. See Box 26. 9. Shift work compromises the circadian rhythms and contributes to insomnia.

Nursing Diagnoses for the Psychosocial Domain

The obvious nursing diagnoses are sleep deprivation and Insomnia (as discussed earlier). However, there

BOX 26.6

Sleep Hygiene Tips

Nurses are often involved in helping patients to develop and maintain good sleep habits that reinforce the patient's ability to fall asleep. Teaching Tips include the following:

1. The most important healthy sleep habit is *keeping regular bedtimes and rising times.* Even if sleep is very poor, get up and out of bed at a regular, consistent time. "Sleeping in" can disturb sleep the following night. For most, time in bed should not exceed 8 hours.
2. Avoid naps.
3. Abstain from alcohol. Although alcohol may shorten sleep latency, there tends to be an alerting effect when it wears off.
4. Refrain from caffeine after midafternoon. Avoid nicotine before bedtime and during the night. Although many claim that neither affects their sleep, caffeine and nicotine are strong stimulants and fragment sleep.
5. Exercise regularly, but not within 3 hours of bedtime. Exercising 6 hours before bedtime tends to strengthen the circadian rhythms of body temperature and sleepiness.
6. Use the bedroom for sleeping; avoid doing nonsleep activities there. Promote the bedroom as a stimulus for sleep, not for studying, watching television, or socializing on the telephone.
7. Set a relaxing routine to prepare for sleep. Avoid frustrating or provoking activities before bedtime.
8. Provide for a comfortable environment. Slightly cool ambient temperature is better than a warm one. Reduce the amount of light and noise.

Table 26.1 Hypnotics: Benzodiazepine Receptor Agonists (BzRA)

	Dosage	Half-life	CYP Metabolism/Excretion
Estazolam (ProSom)	1–2 mg	10–24 h	3A/renal
Flurazepam (Dalmane)	15–30 mg	48–120 h	hepatic/renal
Temazepam (Restoril)	15–30 mg	8–20 h	UGT2B7*,2C19, 3A4 /renal
Triazolam (Halcion)	0.125–0.25 mg	2.4 h	3A4/renal
Quazepam (Doral)	7.5–15 mg	48–120 h	Hepatic/renal
Zolpidem (Ambien)	5–10 mg	1.4–3.8 h	3A4, 2C9/renal
Zolpidem ER (Ambien)	6.25–12.5	2.8 h	3A4, 2C9/renal
Zaleplon (Sonata)	5–20 mg	1 h	3A4/renal
Eszopiclone (Lunesta)	1–3 mg	6 h	3A4, 2E1

*UGT = uridine 5"-diphosphate glucuronosyltransferase

may be other important problem areas such as Social Isolation, Spiritual Distress, Relocation Stress Syndrome, Impaired Parenting, Caregiver Role Strain and Grieving.

Interventions for the Psychosocial Domain

The nurse can help the patient develop bedtime rituals and good sleep hygiene. Bedtime should be at a regular hour, and the bedroom should be conducive to sleep. Preferably, the bedroom should not be where the individual watches television or does work-related activities. The bedroom should be viewed as a room for resting and sleep (see Box 26.6).

Behavioral interventions include stimulus control, sleep restriction, and relaxation therapy. **Stimulus control** is a technique used when the bedroom environment no longer provides cues for sleep but has become

BOX 26.7

Drug Profile: Zaleplon (Sonata)

DRUG CLASS: Sedative/hypnotic (pyrazolopyrimidine nonbenzodiazepine hypnotic). It is readily absorbed and metabolized with only about 1% of zaleplon eliminated in the urine.

RECEPTOR AFFINITY: Zaleplon acts at the GABA-benzodiazepine receptor complex.

INDICATION: Treatment of onset and/or maintenance insomnia

ROUTES AND DOSING: Zaleplon is available in 5 mg and 10 mg capsules. It should be taken at bedtime or after a nocturnal awakening with difficulty falling back to sleep (but at least 4 hours prior to the desired rise time).

Adults: The recommended starting dose is 10 mg with a maximum of 20 mg. An initial dose of 5 mg should be considered in adults with low body weight. Doses of over 20 mg have not been sufficiently studied.

Geriatric: Initially, 5 mg is recommended as a starting dose. Elderly individuals should not exceed a 10 mg dose.

HALF-LIFE (PEAK PLASMA CONCENTRATION): 1 hour (1 hour)

SELECTED ADVERSE REACTIONS: abdominal pain, headache, dizziness, depression, nervousness, difficulty concentrating, back pain, chest pain, migraine, conjunctivitis, bronchitis, pruritus, rash, arthritis, constipation, dry mouth

WARNINGS: Zaleplon should not be administered to patients with severe hepatic impairment. Zaleplon potentiates the psychomotor impairments of ethanol.

BOX 26.8

Drug Profile: Ramelteon (Rozerem)

DRUG CLASS: Sedative/hypnotic. It is readily absorbed and metabolized with median peak concentrations occurring 0.5–1.5 hours after fasted oral administration.

RECEPTOR AFFINITY: Ramelteon is a melatonin receptor agonist with high affinity for MT_1 and MT_2. No appreciable affinity for the GABA receptor complex.

INDICATION: Treatment of insomnia characterized by difficulty with sleep onset.

ROUTES AND DOSING: The recommended dose is 8 mg. It should be taken at 30 minutes before bedtime. It should not be taken with or immediately after a high-fat meal. Patients should be advised to use caution if they consume alcohol in combination with ramelteon.

Adults: The recommended starting dose is 10 mg, with a maximum of 20 mg. An initial dose of 5 mg should be considered in adults with low body weight. Doses of over 20 mg have not been sufficiently studied.

Geriatric: No differences in safety or efficacy were observed between elderly and younger adults.

HALF-LIFE (PEAK PLASMA CONCENTRATION): 1–2.6 hours.

SELECTED ADVERSE REACTIONS: Somnolence, dizziness, nausea, fatigue, headache, and insomnia.

WARNINGS: Ramelteon should not be used by patients with severe hepatic impairment. It should not be used in combination with fluvoxamine.

BOX 26.9

***Research for Best Practice:* Multiple Care-Giving Roles**

Scott, L. D., Hwang, W., & Rogers, A. D. (2006). The impact of multiple care giving roles on fatigue, stress, and work performance among hospital staff nurses. The Journal of Nursing Administration, 36(2), 86–95.

The Question: Does fatigue and stress of full-time hospital staff nurses caring for aging family members differ from fatigue and stress experienced by those caring for children younger than 18 years living at home?

Methods: Full time hospital staff nurses (n = 393) recorded daily information concerning their work hours, errors, sleep/wake patterns, perceptions of fatigue, alertness, stress, and periods of drowsiness and sleep episodes while on duty for 28 days.

Findings: Fatigue and stress levels were significantly higher among nurses caring for both children and elders. However, nurses providing elder care at home were more fatigued, sleep deprived, and likely to make errors at work.

Implications: Restorative sleep is important for nurses involved in dual care roles. Overtime should be limited.

BOX 26.10

***Psychoeducation Checklist:* Sleep Disorders**

When teaching patients with sleep disorders, be sure to include the following topics:

- Maintenance of a sleep log
- Foods that are okay to eat before going to bed
- Foods to avoid before going to bed
- Importance of developing a bedtime ritual and good sleep habits
- Use of sleep medications for short-term only
- Avoidance of caffeine 6 hours before bedtime
- Avoidance of cigarette smoking 1 hour before bedtime and during nighttime awakenings
- Sleeping 7 to 8 hours per night
- Maintenance of a regular sleep schedule, especially a consistent rising time
- An occasional "bad night" happens to nearly everyone.
- Avoidance of alcohol as it disrupts sleep and is a poor hypnotic.
- Daytime sleepiness as a symptom of sleep disorders.
- How to do relaxation exercises
- Bedroom rituals
- Appropriate family support

the cue for wakefulness. Patients are instructed to avoid behaviors in the bedroom incompatible with sleep, including watching television, doing homework, and eating. This allows the bedroom to be re-established as a stimulus for sleep.

Another behavioral intervention is **sleep restriction.** Patients often increase their time in bed to provide more opportunity for sleep, resulting in fragmented sleep and irregular sleep schedules. Patients are instructed to spend less time in bed and avoid napping.

Relaxation training is used when patients complain of difficulty relaxing, especially if they are physically tense or emotionally distressed. A variety of procedures to reduce somatic arousal can be used—progressive muscle relaxation, autogenic training, and biofeedback. Imagery training, meditation, and thought stopping are attention-focusing techniques that center on cognitive arousal (see Chapters 10 and 11).

Teaching Patients 

Psychoeducation interventions are crucial for patients with sleep disorders. An explanation of the sleep cycle and the factors that influence sleep are important for these patients. For those with insomnia, teaching about avoiding foods and beverages that interfere with sleep should be highlighted (see Box 26.10).

Teaching Families 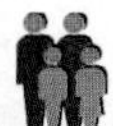

Family and friends should be encouraged to support the new habits the patient is trying to establish. Patients, spouses, and friends must understand that activities engaged in just before sleep can greatly affect sleep patterns and sleep difficulties, such as socializing, drinking alcohol, or engaging in stimulating activities. Relaxing activities before bedtime are crucial, and family and friends can help create a conducive sleep environment.

Evaluation

The primary treatment outcome is the establishment of a normal sleep cycle. Changes in diet and behavior should be evaluated for their impact on the individual's sleep. Environmental modifications, such as change in lighting, decreased stimulation, or modification in room temperature, can be monitored for any changes affecting the sleep cycle.

Primary Hypersomnia

The essential characteristic of primary hypersomnia is excessive sleepiness for at least 1 month, demonstrated by either daytime sleep episodes or sleeping extended periods at night. Sleepiness occurs on an almost daily basis. This diagnosis is reserved for individuals who have had other causes of daytime sleepiness (e.g., narcolepsy, obstructive sleep apnea [OSA] syndrome) ruled out (see Table 26.2).

Clinical Course

People with primary hypersomnia typically sleep 8 to 12 hours per night. They fall asleep easily and sleep through the night but often have difficulty awakening in the morning. Sometimes they are confused or even combative on awakening. They often have problems meeting morning obligations. They also exhibit poor concentration and memory and excessive daytime sleepiness, taking naps that may last an hour or more without feeling refreshed after awakening. They may even describe dangerous situations, such as being sleepy while driving or operating heavy machinery.

The **multiple sleep latency test** (MSLT) is a standardized procedure using polysomnography during daytime testing. This test measures sleep variables during a 20-minute period, which is repeated every 2 hours, 5 times during the day (Bonnet, 2006). The faster a person falls asleep during testing, the greater the physiologic sleep tendency. Polysomnography shows short sleep

Table 26.2 Key Diagnostic Characteristics for Sleep Disorders

Disorder	Diagnostic Characteristics and Target Symptoms
Primary hypersomnia	Excessive sleepiness for at least 1 month occurring almost daily Prolonged sleep episodes Daytime sleep episodes: nodding off unintentionally or napping Significant distress or impairment in social, occupational, or other areas of functioning Not accounted for by insufficient sleep Not a direct physiologic effect of a substance or general medical condition
Narcolepsy	Irresistible attacks of refreshing sleep occurring daily over at least a 3-month period Brief episodes of sudden bilateral loss of muscle tone precipitated by intense emotion (cataplexy) Dream-like hallucinations while falling asleep (hypnagogic hallucinations) Voluntary muscle paralysis at beginning or end of sleep episodes Not a direct physiologic effect of a substance or general medical condition
Breathing-related sleep disorder	Disruption in sleep leading to excessive sleepiness or insomnia Report of loud snoring Report of apparent apneic episodes during sleep
Circadian rhythm sleep disorder	Persistent or recurrent pattern of disrupted sleep leading to excessive sleepiness or insomnia Mismatch between sleep–wake cycle and environment Mismatch between circadian sleep–wake cycle Significant distress or impairment in functioning Not a direct physiologic effect of a substance or general medical condition
Nightmare disorder	Repeated awakenings from major sleep periods Detailed recall of extended and extremely frightening dreams Generally occur during second half of sleep period Rapid orientation and alertness on awakening from the frightening dreams Significant distress or impairment in functioning
Sleep terror disorder	Recurrent episodes of abrupt awakenings Usually occur during the first third of major sleep episode Intense fear and autonomic arousal during episode Onset with a panicked scream Tachycardia, rapid breathing, and sweating Unresponsive to attempts to comfort person during episode Significant distress or impairment in functioning Not a direct physiologic effect of a substance or general medical condition
Sleepwalking disorder	Repeated episodes of rising from the bed during sleep and moving about Usually occur during the first third of sleep episode Blank staring facial expression during episode Relatively unresponsive to attempts to communicate with person Great difficulty to awaken Amnesia for the episode on awakening No impairment of mental activity or behavior within several minutes after awakening Short period of confusion or disorientation Significant distress or impairment in functioning Not a direct physiologic effect of a substance or general medical condition

latency, a normal to long sleep duration, and normal sleep architecture. Subjective symptoms of sleepiness are recognized as heavy eyelids, loss of initiative, reluctance to move, and yawning or slowed speech. Sleepiness can vary from mild to severe.

Nursing Management of Hypersomnia

The nursing assessment for the patient with hypersomnia is similar to the one for insomnia, but the focus is on excessive sleepiness. The following are examples of assessment questions.

- Have you ever nodded off unintentionally?
- When did your sleepiness begin?
- Do you suddenly find yourself awakening feeling refreshed? Or paralyzed for a second? Does anyone in your family have unusual sleepiness?

Interventions stress the importance of sleep hygiene and helping the patient establish normal sleep patterns. If medications are given, the most commonly prescribed stimulants for treating excessive daytime sleepiness are dextroamphetamine (Dexedrine), methylphenidate (Ritalin, Concerta), and pemoline (Cylert). These agents increase the patient's ability to stay awake and perform. Amphetamines have a euphoric effect and are an abused drug. Stimulant medications often do not provide relief. In some cases, however, serotonin antagonists such methysergide are used off-label.

Sleepy people often self-medicate with caffeine. A cup of brewed coffee contains about 100 to 150 mg of caffeine. An ounce of chocolate contains 25 mg of caffeine. Peak plasma concentration is reached 30 to 60 minutes after consumption, and duration of effect is 3 to 5 hours in adults. Caffeine improves psychomotor performance, particularly tasks involving endurance, vigilance, and attention. Alertness significantly increases for 7.5 hours when 300 mg of caffeine is ingested at 11 PM. High doses, especially in people who are not habitual users, may reduce performance because side effects (irritability, anxiety, jitteriness) interfere.

Narcolepsy

The overwhelming urge to sleep is the primary symptom of narcolepsy. This irresistible urge to sleep occurs at any time of the day, regardless of the amount of previous sleep. Falling asleep often occurs in inappropriate situations, such as while driving a car or reading a newspaper. These sleep episodes are usually short, lasting 5 to 20 minutes, but may last up to an hour if sleep is not interrupted. Typically, people with narcolepsy have two to six sleep attacks a day and frequently report dreaming. They usually feel alert after a sleep attack, only to fall asleep unintentionally again several hours later (see Box 26.11).

BOX 26.11

Clinical Vignette:* *Is it Sleepiness or Narcolepsy

Jill is a 27-year-old college student and single mother of two young children, ages 10 and 3 years old. Jill had difficulty staying awake during high school classes. She attributed this problem to "boring teachers" and dropped out of school when she was a junior. She has earned her GED and now attends a local community college majoring in computer science. Although she enjoys her studies, she continues to fall asleep during classes. Because of her busy schedule, she gets about 6 hours of sleep each night. Her tendency to nod off is more frequent. She has had a couple of frightening episodes at bedtime, seeing things dance around her bed and not being able to move. She recalls an incident of laughing at a great joke, then feeling her face droop for several seconds.

What Do You Think?

- Which symptoms of narcolepsy does Jill have?
- If Jill increases her nighttime sleep, will her symptoms improve?
- What approaches will help Jill with controlling her daytime sleepiness?

Clinical Course

Narcolepsy is a chronic disorder that usually begins in young adulthood, between the ages of 15 and 35 years. Excessive sleepiness is the first symptom to appear. Disrupted nocturnal sleep sometimes develops in individuals in their forties or fifties. The severity of sleepiness remains stable over the lifetime. Narcolepsy has no cure. Treatment is designed to control symptoms and depends on the clinical presentation and severity. A secondary sleep disorder, such as sleep apnea, should be considered if sleepiness increases.

Narcolepsy is distinguished by a group of symptoms known as the narcolepsy tetrad: daytime sleepiness, cataplexy, hypnagogic hallucinations, and sleep paralysis. The symptom of daytime sleepiness is found in all individuals with narcolepsy, but existence of the other three symptoms varies (see Box 26.11). Only about 15% of individuals with narcolepsy have all four symptoms.

- **Cataplexy** is the bilateral loss of muscle tone triggered by a strong emotion, such as laughter. This muscle atonia can range from subtle (drooping eyelids) to dramatic (buckling knees). Eye and respiratory muscles are not affected. Cataplexy usually lasts only seconds. Individuals are fully conscious, oriented, and alert during the episode. Prolonged episodes of cataplexy may lead to sleep episodes. The frequency and severity generally increase with sleep deprivation.
- **Hypnagogic hallucinations** are intense dreamlike images that occur when an individual is falling asleep and usually involve the immediate environment. Most

hallucinations are visual, but some can be auditory, such as hearing one's name called or a door slammed.

- **Sleep paralysis**, the inability to move or speak when falling asleep or waking up, is often described as terrifying and is accompanied by a sensation of struggling to move or speak. Although the diaphragm is not involved, patients may also complain of not being able to breathe. These episodes are usually brief, lasting only a few seconds to minutes, and usually terminate spontaneously or when someone touches the individual.

Epidemiology

Narcolepsy is found in about 50 of 100,000 individuals. It is more common than other well-known neurologic disorders (e.g., multiple sclerosis, myasthenia gravis, or Huntington's chorea).

Etiology

The cause of narcolepsy involves a deficiency of hypocretin, a hypothalamic peptide that may be linked to chromosome 6 in the class II human leukocyte antigen (Mignot, Taheri, & Nishino, 2002). Hypocretin neurons are part of the neurologic system that wakes and maintains wakefulness. Injury to the CNS or immunologic factors may also play a part in the development of narcolepsy.

Nursing Management of Narcolepsy

The nursing assessment is similar to the disorder previously discussed. In general, sleepiness is treated with CNS stimulants. Methylphenidate, dextroamphetamine, modafinil, and pemoline are the most frequently prescribed stimulants. Cataplexy is treated with tricyclic antidepressants because these drugs suppress REM sleep. Gamma-hydroxybutyrate is also effective in decreasing cataplexy attacks (U.S. Xyprem Multicenter Study Group, 2003).

Patient education focuses on factors that can make symptoms worse, such as sleep deprivation and alcohol consumption. Patients need to develop strategies to manage symptoms. Naps can be integrated into their daily routines, for example, taking naps at lunch or work breaks, scheduling a short nap before the evening meal, or engaging in activities to sustain alertness while driving.

Breathing-Related Sleep Disorders

Breathing-related sleep disorders are a broad class of sleep disorders that includes obstructive sleep apnea syndrome (OSA), central sleep apnea syndrome, and central alveolar hypoventilation syndrome. Nocturnal polysomnography is used to diagnose these breathing disorders. OSA syndrome is the most commonly diagnosed breathing-related sleep disorder.

Obstructive Sleep Apnea Syndrome

OSA syndrome is characterized by excessive snoring during sleep and episodes of sleep apnea (cessation of breathing) that disrupt sleep and cause daytime sleepiness. The hallmark symptoms are snoring and daytime sleepiness. Often, snoring is so loud and disturbing that partners choose separate bedrooms for sleeping.

Clinical Course

Apneic episodes, which last from 10 seconds up to several minutes, cause restless sleep and abrupt awakenings with feelings of choking or falling out of bed; some people even leap out of bed to restore breathing. Typically, patients with OSA demonstrate 100 to 600 respiratory events per night during polysomnographic measurement. The person does not later recall the awakening. These brief awakenings deprive essential sleep, resulting in excessive daytime sleepiness that may reach the same degree of pathologic sleepiness found in narcolepsy. Unlike narcolepsy, naps tend to be unrefreshing.

There is an increased amount of stage 1 sleep and decreased amounts of slow-wave and REM sleep. Esophageal reflux, or heartburn, is a common complaint. Genitourinary symptoms include nocturia (three to seven trips to the bathroom), nocturnal enuresis, and impotence. Bradycardia in association with tachycardia is often seen in association with apneic events. Other cardiac arrhythmias are also seen, specifically sinus arrhythmias, premature ventricular contractions, atrioventricular block, or sinus arrest. Onset of sleepiness may coincide with weight gain. About two thirds of apnea patients are obese (20% over ideal body weight).

Epidemiology

Conservative estimates give the overall prevalence of OSA as 3.5% of the general population. The incidence of OSA increases for older populations, however, especially for those older than 50 years of age (Lavie, 2002). This disorder can occur in male or female patients of all age groups (Ray & Bower, 2005). OSA is most common in middle-aged overweight men. In general, the female-to-male ratio is about 1:8, although women are more likely to develop this syndrome after menopause. Men are twice as likely to snore as women. Snoring occurs in about 60% of men between the ages of 41 and 64 years (APA, 2000).

Etiology

An obstruction or collapse of the airway causes apnea, or cessation of breathing. In most cases, the site of obstruction is in the pharyngeal area, specifically the supraglottic airway. Vibrations of the soft, pliable tissues found in the pharyngeal airway cause the snoring sounds that occur during breathing.

Interdisciplinary Treatment

There are surgical and nonsurgical treatments for OSA syndrome. The most commonly performed surgical procedure to treat OSA is the uvulopalatopharyngoplasty. This procedure involves the removal of redundant soft palate tissue, the uvula, and tonsillar pillars. The surgery usually eliminates snoring and is judged to be about 50% effective in reducing the amount of sleep apnea. Currently, the most effective nonsurgical treatment is continuous positive airway pressure. This treatment takes place during sleep and involves wearing a nose mask that is connected by a long tube to an air compressor. Airway patency is maintained with air pressure. Although this method of treatment is highly effective, compliance can be a problem (Weaver et al., 2003).

Other nonsurgical treatments are recommended depending on the severity of OSA. For obese patients with less severe OSA, weight loss may help. For others whose apnea is mild, changing sleeping position from supine to lateral can help control the severity of OSA. There has also been some effort in devising an oral appliance to reduce snoring and the occurrence of apnea.

Circadian Rhythm Sleep Disorder

The chief feature of a circadian rhythm sleep disorder is the mismatch between the individual's internal sleep–wake circadian rhythm and the timing and duration of sleep (Buysse, 2005). People with these disorders complain of insomnia at particular times during the day and excessive sleepiness at others. This diagnosis is reserved for those individuals who present with marked sleep disturbance or significant social or occupational impairment (see Box 26.12). The *DSM-IV-TR* identifies a broad group of subtypes:

- *Delayed sleep phase type*: Individuals with delayed sleep phase type or "owls" tend to be unable to fall asleep before 2 to 6 AM; hence, their whole sleep patterns shift and they have difficulty rising in the morning.
- *Jet lag type*: Jet lag occurs after travel across time zones, particularly in coast-to-coast and international travel. The normal endogenous circadian sleep–wake cycle does not match the desired hours of sleep and wakefulness in a new time zone. Individuals traveling eastward are more prone to jet lag because it involves resetting one's circadian clock to an earlier time—it is easier to delay the endogenous clock to a later time period than adjust it to an earlier one.
- *Shift work type*: The endogenous sleep–wake cycle is normal but is mismatched to the imposed hours of shift work. Rotating shift schedules are disruptive because any consistent adjustment is prevented.

BOX 26.12

Clinical Vignette: Psychiatric Misdiagnosis in Teenager

A 14-year-old male was referred for evaluation for a complaint of daytime sleepiness. Prior to the referral, this patient suffered from major difficulties in functioning for 4 years. Conflicts with parents, teachers, and peers were noted. He was described by a licensed child psychologist as "extremely introverted with severe narcissistic traits, poverty of thought with persecutory content, and self-destruction that led to a paralyzing anxiety, anhedonia, social isolation and withdrawal." An assessment of his learning abilities showed difficulties with written language and poor memory. He also had above-average abilities in verbal comprehension and abstract reasoning. After dropping out of school at age 12, he was sent to an inpatient child psychiatry center. After 3 months of evaluation he was diagnosed as having atypical depressive disorder with possible schizotypal personality.

The patient underwent polysomnography. No primary sleep disorders were found. Three weeks monitoring with a wrist actigraph (a device which differentiates sleep and waking) suggested a circadian rhythm disorder. Oral temperature and melatonin secretion levels were measured during a 24-hour period and revealed the desynchronization of the temperature and melatonin rhythms. Treatment was begun with oral melatonin (5 mg at 8 PM). Follow-up actigraphy after 6 months showed the patient to be fully entrained to the normal 24 hour cycle. The patient returned to school. After one semester, the patient showed excellent grades. His parents reported improvement in his relationship with family and peers. Evaluation by licensed psychiatrists found no evidence of psychopathology; none of the previously described diagnoses were present (Dagan & Ayalon, 2005).

What Do You Think?

What symptoms of circadian rhythm sleep disorder did the patient experience?
How did melatonin improve the patient's sleep cycle?

Compared with day- and evening-shift workers, night- and rotating-shift workers have a shorter sleep duration and poorer quality of sleep. They may also be sleepier while performing their jobs. This disorder is further exacerbated by insufficient daytime sleep resulting from social and family demands and environmental disturbances (traffic noise, telephone). Because of the job requirements of the profession, nurses often suffer from this disorder. Further, 20% of the U.S. work force is engaged in shift work and thereby at risk for circadian rhythm disorders.

Etiology

Circadian rhythm disorders are caused by the dissociation of the internal circadian pacemaker and conventional time. The cause might be intrinsic, such as genetic factors called "clock genes" (Archer et al., 2003), or extrinsic, as in jet lag and shift work. Each results in overwhelming daytime sleepiness and overflowing wakefulness at night.

Epidemiology

There are no data regarding the prevalence of circadian rhythm disorders in the general population. Prevalence of circadian rhythm disorders among patients diagnosed at sleep disorder centers accounts for 2% or less of the total patients diagnosed. However, this is a gross underestimate given that jet lag, a circadian rhythm disorder, affects nearly everyone traveling over three time zones.

Interdisciplinary Treatment

Chronotherapy, frequently used for delayed sleep phase, manipulates the sleep schedule by progressively delaying bedtime until an acceptable bedtime is attained. A 27-hour day is imposed on successive days by delaying bedtime and rising time by 3 hours. Thereafter, strict adherence (within 1 hour) to the final schedule must be maintained.

Luminotherapy (light therapy) is used to manipulate the circadian system (Phipps-Nelson, Redman, Dijk, & Rajaratnam, 2003). Light is measured in lux units of illumination; indoor light is about 150 lux. Therapeutic light has a potency of 2,500 to 10,000 lux and is produced by commercially prepared light boxes.

Chronopharmacotherapy resets the biologic clock by using short-acting hypnotics to induce sleep. Small amounts of hypnotics can produce high-quality sleep in people who wish to reset their circadian schedule after long transmeridian flights. Conversely, for night-shift workers, caffeine taken while working at night improves alertness and performance. However, caffeine should be used judiciously by night-shift workers because they become quickly tolerant to the effects after a few nights.

Parasomnias

Parasomnias are characterized by abnormal physiologic or behavior events that occur in relationship to sleep or to specific sleep stages, or during transition from sleep to wakefulness. These disorders include nightmare disorder, sleep terror disorder, and sleepwalking disorder and involve activation of the autonomic nervous system, motor system, or cognitive processes during sleep or sleep–wake transitions. Individuals present with a complaint of unusual behavior during sleep. These disorders will be presented individually followed with a discussion of the nursing management.

Nightmare Disorder

The repeated occurrence of frightening dreams that fully awaken an individual is the essential characteristic of nightmare disorder. Typically, the individual can recall detailed dream content that involves physical danger (e.g., attack or pursuit) or perceived danger (e.g., embarrassment or failure). On awakening, the individual is fully alert and experiences a persisting sense of anxiety or fear. Many people have difficulty returning to sleep. Multiple same-night nightmares may be reported. Some people avoid sleep because of their fear of nightmares. Consequently, people may report that excessive sleepiness, poor concentration, and irritability disrupt their daytime activities. The occurrence of nightmares may be more serious than previously suspected.

Epidemiology

The actual prevalence of nightmare disorder is unknown. In adults, at least 50% of the population reports occasional nightmares. Women are more likely to report nightmares than men. In children, there is no difference between boys and girls. Nightmares often begin in children between the ages of 3 and 6 years, and most children outgrow them. Nightmares induced by medication are not considered part of nightmare disorder.

Etiology

The cause of nightmares is unknown. Intriguing evidence provokes a debate as to whether nightmares are a symptom or an adaptive reaction to pathophysiologic factors. Negative emotions, primarily fear, are the most common dream emotions. Brain imaging demonstrates increased metabolic activity during REM sleep in the most primitive regions of the brain, the paralimbic and limbic regions. Many classes of drugs trigger nightmares, including catecholaminergic agents, beta-blockers, some antidepressants, barbiturates, and alcohol. Additionally, withdrawal from barbiturates and alcohol causes REM rebound and more vivid dreaming.

Clinical Course

Nightmares occur in REM sleep almost exclusively. They most often occur during the second half of the night, when REM sleep dominates. Polysomnography demonstrates abrupt awakenings from REM sleep. In most cases, the REM sleep episode lasts for at least 10 minutes. Tachycardia and tachypnea may be evident.

Interdisciplinary Treatment

Traditionally, psychotherapy aimed at conflict resolution has been the treatment of choice. More recent therapies involving cognitive and behavioral interventions as well as desensitization and relaxation techniques have gained support. For example, one technique is teaching patients (while awake) to visualize and change their remembered nightmares and rehearse similar scenarios. This technique reduces nightmare distress and frequency.

Sleep Terror Disorder

The essential characteristic of sleep terror disorder is the repetition of episodes of sleep terrors with screaming, fear, and panic, causing clinical distress or impairing social, occupational, or other areas of functioning. Diagnostic considerations may also include the potential for injury to self or others.

Sleep terrors are frightening to the person and to anyone witnessing them. These sleep terrors, also called **night terrors,** or *pavor nocturnus*, usually occur in the first third of the night and may last 1 to 10 minutes. Often, individuals abruptly sit up in bed screaming; others have been known to jump out of bed and run across the room. Other symptoms include rapid heart rate and breathing, dilated pupils, and flushed skin. Usually, the person having a sleep terror is inconsolable and difficult to awaken completely. Efforts to awaken the individual may prolong the episode. Once awake, most are unable to recall the dream or event that precipitated such a response. A few report a fragmentary image. Often, the individual does not fully awaken and cannot recall the episode the next morning (Giglio, Undevia, & Spire, 2005).

Epidemiology

The actual prevalence of this disorder is not known. Episodes of sleep terrors are common in children (up to 6% prevalence) and peak between the ages of 5 and 7 years (Broughton, 2000). This condition usually resolves or diminishes in adolescence. However, sleep terrors can also occur in adults. At any age, the frequency of episodes varies, and they may occur several times a night over several nights.

Etiology

There is little evidence that sleep terrors indicate any significant underlying psychiatric disease or psychological problems. The most important factor is genetic predisposition. Individuals often report a family history of either sleep terrors or sleepwalking. The exact mode of inheritance is not known. Fever and sleep deprivation can increase the frequency of episodes. There is also some evidence (Espa et al., 2002) that breathing-related sleep disorders are associated with night terrors.

Clinical Course

Polysomnography shows that sleep terrors usually begin during slow-wave NREM sleep. Although sleep terrors most often occur during the first third of the night, when slow-wave sleep dominates, episodes also occur later during slow-wave sleep.

Sleepwalking Disorder

Waking up is a neurologic event. Arousal happens through a complex series of processes using several neurotransmitters. An arousal disorder is one that interrupts these processes or does not allow their completion and occurs when an individual is partially awake yet partially asleep. Sleepwalking, also called **somnambulism**, is a classic arousal disorder. It is considered to be a milder form of sleep terrors. Repeated episodes of complex motor behavior during sleep are the essential characteristic of sleepwalking disorder.

Sleepwalking involves episodes of mild to complex behaviors during sleep. Mild forms (sometimes called *confusional arousals*) consist of sitting up in bed and mumbling incoherently. More complex behavior may involve getting out of bed, walking around outside the house, and even driving an automobile. While sleepwalking, people typically have a blank stare, are relatively unresponsive to conversation, and are difficult to awaken. If individuals do not awaken, they are unable to recall the episode the following morning. Often, they awaken to find themselves in a different place from where they went to sleep. If awakened during the episode, there is a brief period of confusion, followed by a full recovery. Episodes usually happen during the first third of the night. Contrary to popular opinion, sleepwalking (and sleeptalking) are not enactments of the individual's dream.

Sleep-related violence has been documented in people with NREM sleep somnambulism, REM sleep behavior disorder, and epileptic discharges during sleep. Violence during sleep is an area of controversy for the legal system; the jury's willingness to accept sleep disorders as a defense has not always been consistent.

Epidemiology and Etiology

Sleepwalking is common in children. It occurs in 40% of children and peaks at about age 11 to 12 years. There appears to be some genetic predisposition: those patients with relatives who sleepwalk are more likely to sleepwalk themselves. Genetic typing shows an association with the *DQBI* gene, which is also implicated in narcolepsy (Lecendreux et al., 2000). Sleep deprivation appears to dramatically increase the frequency of sleepwalking episodes. Internal stimuli (a full bladder) or external stimuli (noise) can precipitate an episode. Sleep deprivation, fever, and stress may increase the likelihood of an episode.

Clinical Course

Polysomnography shows EEG elements of both wakefulness and NREM sleep. Because it usually occurs during slow-wave sleep, sleepwalking most often happens during the first third of the night. Sleepwalking rarely occurs during daytime naps.

BOX 26.13

General Safety Precautions for Sleepwalkers and Their Families

Ensure adequate sleep. The occurrence of sleepwalking dramatically increases after sleep loss. Although a regular sleep schedule is important, making up for lost sleep is more important (Birkenmeier, 2000).

- Anticipate sleepwalking when there is a significant sleep loss. Alert family members to be aware of the likelihood of sleepwalking for the first 2 hours after the sleepwalker goes to bed.
- Keep a sleep log to identify how much sleep is needed to prevent a sleepwalking event.
- Install noise devices on the sleepwalker's door to alert others that the sleepwalker is up.
- Deadbolt locks should be installed on doors leading outside. Windows should be secured so that they cannot be opened more than 8 inches.
- When the sleepwalker is spending the night away from home, alert appropriate individuals to the possibility that sleepwalking may occur. Ensure adequate sleep the preceding night.

Interdisciplinary Treatment

Patients are instructed to take precautions regarding possible sleepwalking episodes (see Box 26.13). Treatment might also include medications, such as benzodiazepines. Hypnosis supplemented by psychotherapy has also been useful, at least on a short-term basis. Because sleepwalking tends to occur out of slow-wave sleep, benzodiazepines are used to treat patients who show a potential for injury or harm.

Nursing Management of Parasomnias

Although polysomnography is used to diagnose or confirm a sleep disorder, the evaluation of a response to a parasomnia also involves a careful sleep history. Episodes of parasomnias are often unrealized by the patient but can be described in detail by the partner. Family members may clarify the degree of sleepiness that the patient may want to deny. Sleep histories and diaries should be used.

Nursing interventions will range from referring to sleep specialists to patient education about the disorders and strategies in dealing with these disorders. In some instances, nurses will care for patients in the inpatient environment who have one of these parasomnias. In this instance, nurses will develop care plans that address the individual patient's needs. In the instances of sleepwalking, staff should be alert to the safety issues and the patient protected from injury during sleepwalking episodes.

SUMMARY OF KEY POINTS

- The normal sleep–wake cycle runs in about a 24-hour pattern called circadian rhythm. Most body systems follow a circadian rhythm and are often associated with the sleep–wake cycle, such as the release of the hormones melatonin and cortisol, which help promote wakefulness during the day and sleepiness at night.
- Polysomnography is clinical testing used to diagnose or confirm sleep disorders. Results of polysomnography describe a person's sleep architecture (timing and distribution of sleep stages) and any abnormalities occurring during sleep.
- Assessment includes a thorough sleep history, including current sleep patterns, previous sleep patterns before sleep difficulties, medical problems, current medications, current life events, and emotional and mental status as well as an assessment of the details of the sleep complaint, including description, duration, stability, and intensity of the problem.
- Biologic nursing interventions for sleep disorders focus on nonpharmacologic approaches such as exercise, nutrition, activity, thermoregulation, and pharmacologic interventions. Pharmacologic agents include those prescribed, OTC, and nutritional/herbal supplements.
- Psychosocial nursing interventions for sleep disorders include educating patients about good sleep hygiene, instructing patients in relaxation exercises and sleep-inducing activities, providing patients with nutritional counseling regarding foods and substances to avoid, and educating family members and friends regarding the importance of encouraging new sleep habits for patients.
- Primary sleep disorders are ongoing disruptions of normal waking and sleeping patterns and are subdivided into dyssomnias and parasomnias.
- Primary insomnia is a sleep disorder characterized by difficulty falling asleep or staying asleep. It involves behaviors that perpetuate this abnormal sleep and rest pattern. Although insomnia is often precipitated by feelings of stress or tension, these patients develop sleep-preventing associations and behaviors that persist long after the crisis or stressful situation has passed.
- OSA syndrome is a commonly diagnosed breathing-related sleep disorder. It is characterized by excessive snoring during sleep and episodes of apnea (cessation of breathing), which disrupt sleep and cause daytime sleepiness.
- Parasomnias are characterized by abnormal physiologic or behavioral events that occur during sleep or transition from sleep to wakefulness and include nightmare disorder, sleep terror disorder, and sleepwalking disorder. The etiology of these disorders is unknown,

but there appears to be some genetic predisposition. These disorders cause unrestful sleep and can jeopardize daytime activities because of excessive sleepiness, poor concentration, and irritability.

CRITICAL THINKING CHALLENGES

1 Discuss the relationship of circadian rhythm and sleep.
2 Identify the stages of sleep and briefly describe each one.
3 How does sleep architecture change throughout the life cycle? Highlight the usual sleep pattern of each age group.
4 Compare the sleep problems individuals with primary insomnia experience with those individuals with primary hypersomnia experience.
5 How does hypersomnia differ from narcolepsy?
6 Develop nursing interventions for a 24-year-old professional truck driver who experiences insomnia at home.
7 A 55-year-old airline pilot has developed difficulty with sleep and attributes his insomnia to jet lag. Develop a list of assessment questions that could be used in exploring the pilot's sleep patterns.

The Cabinet of Dr. Caligari: (1919). This is the first of many movies suggesting that mental health professionals are odd. In this film, the director of an asylum becomes a part of a patient's delusion. The content of the delusion involves Dr. Caligari hypnotizing a sleepwalker who then murders another man.

VIEWING POINTS: When did you realize that Dr. Caligari was not directing the murders? Is there doubt at the end of the movie as to the innocence of Dr. Caligari? Is it realistic that crimes can be committed during periods of sleepwalking?

Insomnia: (1997). This movie is a compelling thriller that occurs in a state of perpetual light. The setting is north of the Arctic Circle in the middle of summer, where it is daylight 24 hours a day. Jonas Engstrom (Stellan Skarsgard) and Erik Vik (Sverre Anker Ousdal) are cops from Oslo brought into a small town to help with a murder investigation. Things go wrong, and Engstrom finds himself trapped in a web of deceit. His guilty conscience and the never-ending light keep him awake at night, and the lack of sleep makes him increasingly desperate and prone to error.

VIEWING POINTS: How did the lack of sleep impact Engstrom's ability to make sound decisions? If the setting of this movie were in an area that had normal nighttime darkness, would the outcome have been different? Does Engstrom's symptom presentation meet the *DSM-IV-TR* criteria of primary insomnia? If you were conducting a sleep assessment, what nursing diagnosis would be generated from the data?

REFERENCES

American Psychiatric Association. (2000). *Diagnostic and statistical manual of mental disorders* (4th ed., text revision). Washington, DC: Author.

Archer, S. N., Robilliard, D. L., Skene, D. J., Smits, M., Williams, A., Arendt, J., & von Schantz, M. (2003). A length polymorphism in the circadian clock gene Per3 is linked to delayed sleep phase syndrome and extreme diurnal preference. *Sleep, 26* (4), 413–415.

Biddle, C., & Oaster, T. R. F. (1990). The nature of sleep. *Journal of the American Association of Nurse Anesthetists, 58* (1), 36.

Birkenmeier, N. (2000). *General safety precautions for sleepwalkers and their families.* Chesterfield, MO: Unity Sleep Medicine and Research Center.

Bonnet, M. H. (2006). ACNS Clinical Controversy: MSLT and MWT have limited clinical utility. *Journal of Clinical Neurophysiology, 23* (1), 50–58.

Broughton, R. (2000). The Berger Lecture: Chronobiology of sleep/wake and of sleepiness/alertness states in normal and sleep disordered human subjects. *Supplements to Clinical Neurophysiology, 53,* 9–18.

Buscemi, N., Vandermeer, B., Pandya, R., Hootonk M., Tjosvold, F., Hartling, L., et al. (2004). Melatonin for treatment of sleep disorders. Summary. Evidence Report/Technology Assessment. No. 108. AHRQ Publication No. 05-E002-1. Rockville, MD: Agency for Healthcare Research and Quality.

Buysse, D. J. (2005). Diagnosis and assessment of sleep and circadian rhythm disorders. *Journal of Psychiatric Practice, 11* (2), 102–115.

Cooke, J. R., & Ancoli-Israel, S. (2006). Sleep and its disorders in older adults. *Psychiatric Clinics of North America, 28,* 1077–1093.

Curry, D. T., Eisenstein, R. D., & Walsh, J. K. (2006). Pharmacologic management of insomnia: past, present, and future. *Psychiatric Clinics of North America, 29,* 871–893.

Dagan, Y. & Ayalon, L. (2005). Case study: Psychiatric misdiagnosis of non-24-hours-sleep-wake schedule disorder resolved by melatonin. *Journal of American Academy of Child and Adolescent Psychiatry, 44* (12), 1271–1275.

Espa, F., Dauvilliers, Y., Ondze, B., Billiard, M., & Besset, A. (2002). Arousal reactions in sleep walking and night terrors in adults: The role of respiratory events. *Sleep, 25* (8), 871–875.

Giglio, P., Undevia, N., & Spire, J. P. (2005). The primary parasomnias: A review for neurologists. *The Neurologist, 11* (2), 90–97.

Harvey, A. (2002). Identifying safety behaviors in insomnia. *Journal of Nervous and Medical Disease, 190* (1), 16–21.

Holcomb, S. S. (2006). Recommendations for assessing insomnia. *Nurse Practitioner, 31* (2), 55–60.

Kirkwood, C. K., & Melton, S. T. (2006). Insomnia. In R. R. Berardi, L. A. Kroon, J. H. McDermott, G. D. Newton, M. A. Oszko, N. G. Popovich, et al. (Eds.). *Handbook of nonprescription drugs: An interactive approach to self-care* (pp. 995–1009). American Pharmacists Association: Washington, DC.

Lam, R. W. (2006). Sleep disturbances and depression: a challenge for antidepressants. *International Clinical Pharmacology, 21* (suppl. 1), S25–S29.

Lavie, P. (2002). Sleep apnea in the presumably healthy working population revisited. *Sleep, 25* (4), 380–385.

Lecendreux, M., Mayer, G., Bassetti, C., et al. (2000). HLA* class II association in sleepwalking. *Sleep, 23* (Suppl 2), A13.

Mendelson, W. B. (2005). A review of the evidence for the efficacy and safety of trazodone in insomnia. *Journal of Clinical Psychiatry, 66* (4), 469–476.

Mignot, E., Lammers, G. J., Ripley, B., et al. (2002). The role of cerebrospinal fluid measurement in the diagnosis of narcolepsy and other hypersomnias. *Archives of Neurology, 59,* 1553–1562.

Mignot, E., Taheri, S., & Nishino, S. (2002). Sleeping with the hypothalamus: Emerging therapeutic targets for sleep disorders. *Nature* (Neuroscience Suppl, 5), 1071–1075.

Nadolski, N. (2005). Getting a good night's sleep: diagnosing and treating insomnia. *Plastic Surgical Nursing, 25* (4), 167–173.

National Center for Complementary and Alternative Medicine. (2006). Valerian: Herbs at a Glance. National Insitutes of Health. U.S. Department of Health and Human Services: Washington, DC. Retrieved on January 8, 2007, from http://nccam.nih.gov.

National Sleep Foundation. (2005). *Sleep in America Poll 2005*. National Sleep Foundation: Washington, DC.

National Institutes of Health. (2005). NIH State-of-the-Science Conference Statement on Manifestations and Management of Chronic Insomnia in Adults. June 13-15, 2005. *NIH Consens Sci Statements 2005, 22* (2), 1–30.

Phipps-Nelson, J., Redman, J. R., Dijk, D. J., & Rajaratnam, S. M. (2003). Daytime exposure to bright light, as compared to dim light, decreases sleepiness and improves psychomotor vigilance performance. *Sleep, 26* (6), 695–700.

Sateia, M. J. (2002). Epidemiology, consequences and evaluation of insomnia. In T. L. Lee-Chiong, M. J. Sateia, & M. A. Carskdadon (Eds.) *Sleep medicine* (pp. 151–160). Philadelphia: Hanley & Belfus.

Soares, C. M., & Murray, B. J. (2005). Sleep disorders in women: Clinical evidence and treatment strategies. *Psychiatric Clinics of North America, 29*, 1095–1113.

Ray, R. M., & Bower, C. M. (2005). Pediatric obstructive sleep apnea: the year in review. *Current Opinion in Otolaryngology & Head & Neck Surgery, 13* (6), 360–365.

Stahl,. S. J. (2006). *Essential psychopharmacology: The prescriber's guide*. Cambridge University Press: New York.

U.S. Xyprem Multicenter Study Group. (2003). A 12-month, open-label, multicenter extension trial of orally administered sodium oxybate for the treatment of narcolepsy. *Sleep, 1*, 3–5.

Weaver, T., Maislin, G., Dinges, D. F., Younger, J., Cantor, C., McCloskey, S., & Pack, A. I. (2003). Self-efficacy in sleep apnea: Instrument development and patient perceptions of obstructive sleep apnea risk, treatment benefit, and volition to use continuous positive airway pressure. *Sleep, 26* (6), 727–732.

Yang, C., Spielman, A. J., & Glovinsky, P. (2006). Nonpharmacologic strategies in the management of insomnia. *Psychiatric Clinics of North America, 29*, 895–919.

UNIT VI
Children and Adolescents

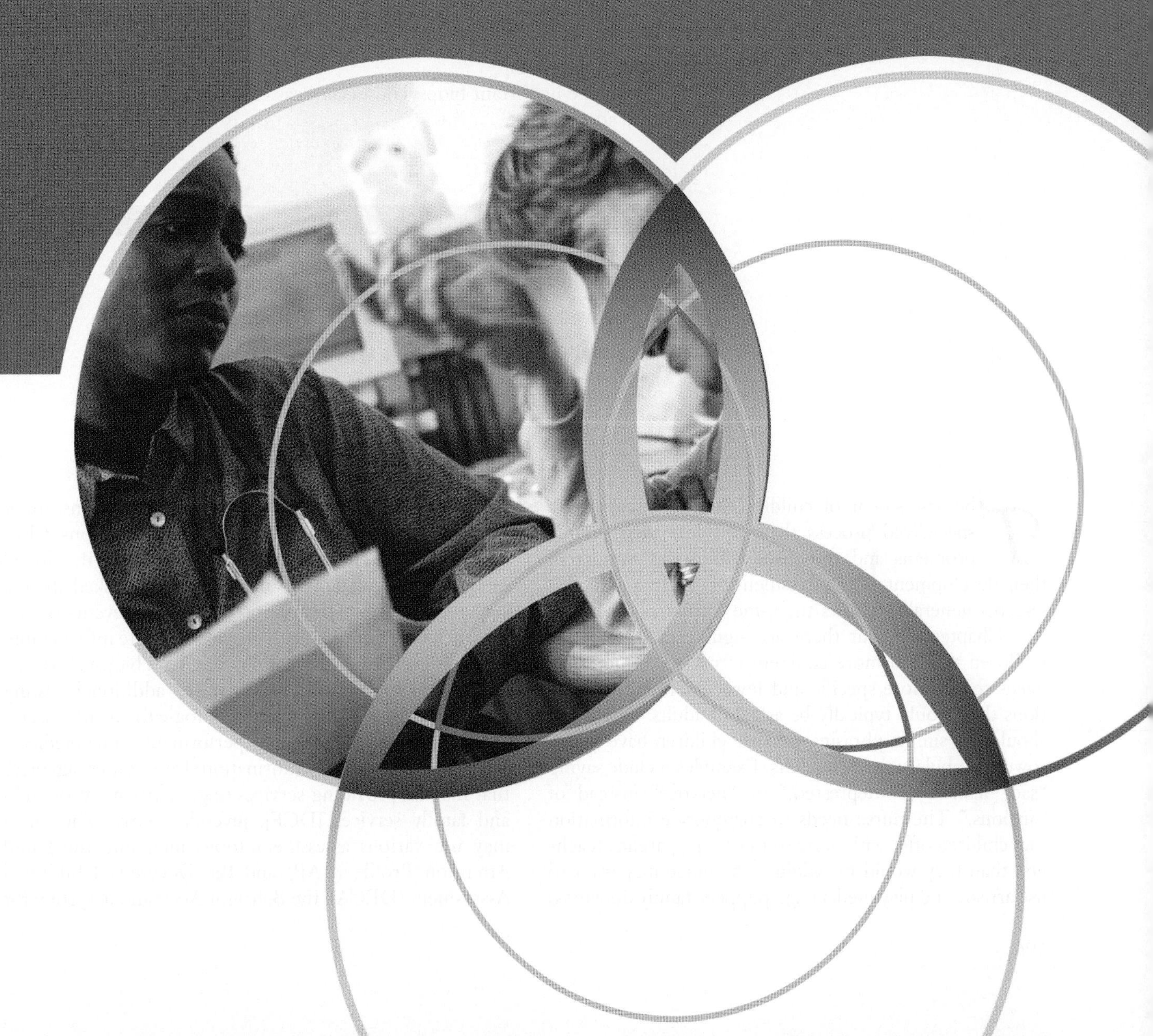

CHAPTER 27

Mental Health Assessment of Children and Adolescents

Vanya Hamrin, Catherine Gray Deering, and Lawrence Scahill

LEARNING OBJECTIVES

After studying this chapter, you will be able to:

- Define the assessment process for children and adolescents.
- Discuss techniques of data collection used with children and adolescents.
- Discuss the synthesis of biopsychosocial assessment data for children and adolescents.
- Delineate important biopsychosocial areas of assessment for children and adolescents.

KEY TERMS

• assortative mating • attachment • attachment disorganization • developmental delays • egocentrism • maturation • temperament • mental status examination

The assessment of children and adolescents is a specialized process that considers their unique problems and responses within the context of their development. The assessment of children and adolescents generally follows the same format as for adults (see Chapter 10), but there are significant differences. Children think in more concrete terms; thus, the nurse needs to ask more specific and fewer open-ended questions than would typically be asked of adults. The nurse should use simple phrasing because children have a narrower vocabulary than do adults. Examples include saying "sad" instead of "depressed," or "nervous" instead of "anxious." The nurse needs to corroborate information that children offer with more sources (e.g., parents, teachers) than they would for adults. The nurse may want to use artistic and play media (e.g., puppets, family drawings) to engage children and evaluate their perceptions, inner worlds, fine motor skills, and intellectual functions. Children have a less specific sense of time and a less developed memory than do adults. When children are asked about a sequence of events or specific times when events occurred, they may not be able to provide accurate information.

A comprehensive evaluation includes a biopsychosocial history; mental status examination; additional testing (e.g., cognitive or neuropsychological) if necessary; records of the child's school performance and medical–physical history; and information from other agencies that may be providing services (e.g., department of child and family services [DCF], juvenile court). The nurse may use various assessment tools, including the Child Attention Profile (CAP) and the Devereux Childhood Assessment (DECA), the Behavior Assessment System for

Children (BASC), the Child Behavior Checklist (CBCL), or the Children's Depression Inventory (CDI).

• NCLEXNOTE

NCLEXNOTE Whenever assessing children or adolescents, developmental level will frame the assessment and implementation of the management plan.

DATA COLLECTION IN THE CLINICAL INTERVIEW

The clinical interview is the primary assessment tool used in child and adolescent psychiatry. A unique set of skills is necessary for interviewing children and adolescents. How the nurse obtains mental health information depends on the developmental level of each child, specifically considering the child's language, cognitive, social, and emotional skills. For example, the nurse should simplify questions for young children or children with developmental delays (e.g., mental retardation, Asperger's syndrome, pervasive developmental disorder) so that these children can understand and respond appropriately.

The assessment interview may be the initial contact between the child and parent or guardian and the nurse. The first step is to establish a treatment alliance, and the second is to assess the interactions between the child and parent.

Treatment Alliance

The nurse can establish rapport by greeting the child or adolescent in a friendly, polite, open manner and putting him or her at ease. Speaking clearly and at a normal volume and using friendly, reassuring tones are essential measures. The nurse can establish a treatment alliance by recognizing the child's individuality and showing respect and concern for that child. The nurse should demonstrate sensitivity, objectivity, and confidentiality. The child will be more forthcoming if he or she feels that the nurse is listening carefully and is interested in what he or she has to say.

Child and Parent Observation

Because the child's primary environment is with the parent, child–parent interactions provide important data about the child–parent attachment and parenting practices. The nurse's observations focus on both the child alone and the child within the family. The nurse can actually make some of these observations while the family is in the waiting area, including:

- How the child and parent talk to each other, including how frequently each initiates conversation
- How the parent disciplines the child
- How attached the parent and child appear
- How the child and parent separate
- If the parent and child play together
- How the child gets the parent's attention, and how responsive the parent is to the child's attention-seeking initiatives
- How the parent and child show affection to each other

Interviewing Techniques

To get an accurate picture of the child, the nurse should interview the child and parent individually because each can provide unique meaningful information. Research has shown that when parent and child are interviewed separately in a structured interview about the child's psychopathology, they rarely agree on the presence of diagnostic criteria, regardless of the diagnostic type (Jensen et al., 1999). Generally, children provide better information about internalizing symptoms (e.g., mood, sleep, suicide ideation), and parents provide better information about externalizing symptoms (e.g., behavior disturbances, oppositionality, relationship with parents).

Discussion with the Child

After talking with the parent and child together, the nurse should ask to speak with the child alone for awhile. Young children may fear separating from their parents. The nurse can reassure children by showing them where the waiting area is and telling them that, if they get scared, the nurse will accompany them to check on their parents. Introducing a toy or game or allowing the child to hold a transitional object may help. Remember that observing how the child separates from the parent is part of the data needed to complete the assessment.

Adolescents may act indifferent or even hostile when the nurse asks to speak with them alone. Teens tend to be skeptical that adults can really understand their experience, suspicious that they will be blamed for their problems, and fearful that their thoughts and feelings are abnormal. The nurse should be patient with adolescents and say something like, "I can see you're pretty angry about being here. What are you particularly angry about? Perhaps there is some way I can help you" (Lewis, 2002). Another useful and reassuring question is, "During the last few minutes, you've been quiet. I'm wondering what you are feeling." Or the nurse may ask, "It can be uncomfortable to tell personal information to someone you don't know. Do you feel this way?" (Sattler, 1998).

To begin the initial assessment of a child, the nurse introduces himself or herself and explains briefly what they will be doing. For children younger than 11 years of age, the nurse should explain that he or she helps worried or upset children by talking, playing, and giving advice to them and their parents. The nurse should then ask about the child's understanding of why he or she is there. This question often helps to identify children's misperceptions (e.g., believing the nurse is going to give them an injection, thinking they have done something bad) that could create barriers to working with them. When conducting the child interview the nurse will need to get several releases of information from the child's guardian to obtain the corroborating reports, such as the child's physical assessment from the pediatrician or pediatric nurse practitioner; the school's report about the child's academic and behavioral performance including their report card, behavior at school, peer interactions, and adult interactions; and records of diagnosis and treatment from any previous psychiatric provider.

The nurse must adapt communication to the child's age level (Box 27.1). The challenge is to avoid using overly complex vocabulary or talking down to children. Young children often express themselves more easily in the context of play than through adult-like conversation. For example, a child may re-enact a conversation that he had with a sibling or parent using puppets. Children respond well to third-person conversation prompts, such as "Some kids don't like being compared to their brothers and sisters," or "I know a kid who was so sad when he lost his dog that he thought he would never be happy again."

Early in the interview, the goal is to explain the nurse's purpose, elicit any concerns the child may have about what is happening, and establish rapport with the child by engaging in unthreatening discussion. Many adults rarely ask children about things that truly interest them but expect children to respond readily to adult conversation. The nurse can establish a high degree of credibility simply by taking note of and asking about things that are obviously important to children (e.g., a sport they participate in, a rock group displayed on a shirt, a toy they have brought with them). However, children have an uncanny natural "radar" for phony adult behavior. Attempts to establish rapport work only when the nurse is genuinely interested in the child's life.

BOX 27.1

Strategies for Interviewing Children

- Use a simple vocabulary and short sentences tailored to the child's developmental and cognitive levels.
- Be sure that the child understands the questions and that you do not lead the child to give a particular response. Phrase your questions so that the child does not receive any hint that one response is more acceptable than another.
- Select the questions for your interview on an individual basis, using judgment and discretion and considering the child's age and developmental level.
- Be sure that the manner and tone of your voice do not reveal any personal biases.
- Speak slowly and quietly, and try to allow the interview to unfold, using the child's verbalizations and behavior as guides.
- Use simple terms (e.g., "sad" for "depressed") in exploring affective reactions, and ask the child to give examples of how he or she behaves or how other people behave when emotionally aroused.
- Assume an accepting and neutral attitude toward the child's communications.
- Learn about children's current interests by looking at Saturday morning television programs, talking with parents, visiting toy stores, looking at children's books, and visiting day care centers and schools to observe children in their natural habitat (Sattler, 1998).

Discussion with the Parents

After meeting alone with the child, the nurse should spend some time alone with the parents and ask for a detailed description of their view of the problem. When alone, parents may feel comfortable discussing their children in depth and sharing frustrations with their behavior. Parents need this opportunity to speak freely without being constrained by concern for the child's feelings. In some cases, it would be detrimental for the child to hear the full force of the parents' complaints and feelings, such as helplessness, anger, or disappointment. Parents need the nurse to allow them to express their feelings without passing judgment. This is the nurse's opportunity to enlist the help of parents as partners in the child's evaluation and treatment. This time is also good for filling in any gaps in the history and clarifying the data obtained from the interview with the child.

Parents need the chance to describe the presenting problem in their own words. The nurse can encourage them by asking general questions, such as, "What brings you here today?" or "How have things been in your family?" The nurse should then reflect his or her understanding of the problem, showing empathy and respect for both parent and child. Asking any other family members about their view of the problem is always a good idea to clarify discrepant points of view, obtain additional data, and communicate awareness that different family members experience the same problem in different ways.

Building Rapport

To reduce anxiety about the evaluation, the nurse must develop rapport with the family members. Establishing rapport can be facilitated by maintaining appropriate eye contact; speaking slowly, clearly, and calmly with friendliness and acceptance; using a warm and expressive tone; reacting to communications from interviewees objectively; showing interest in what the interviewees are saying; and making the interview a joint undertaking (Sattler, 1998). Suggestions for building rapport with children and adolescents are also addressed in each of the developmental sections that follow. The information in Box 27.2 can serve as a guide to asking specific questions during a comprehensive assessment.

Preschool-Aged Children

When interviewing preschool-aged children, the nurse should understand that these children may have difficulty putting feelings into words and that their thinking is very concrete. For example, a preschool-aged child might assume that a tall container holds more water than a wide container, even if both containers hold the same amount of fluid.

The nurse can achieve rapport with preschool-aged children by joining their world of play. Play is an activity by which the child transforms an experience from real life into a symbolic, nonliteral representation. Play encourages verbalizations, promotes manual strength, teaches rules and problem-solving, and helps children master control over their environment (Moore-Taylor, Menarchek-Fetkovich, & Day, 2000). With children younger than 5 years of age, the nurse may conduct the assessment in a playroom. Useful materials are paper, pencils, crayons, paints, paint brushes, easels, clay, blocks, balls, dolls, doll houses, puppets, animals, dress-up clothes, and a water supply. The nurse must inform preschool-aged children about any rules for the play. For example, the nurse must tell the child that the nurse must ensure safety, so that there will be no hitting in the playroom.

BOX 27.2

Semi-Structured Interview With School-Aged Children

Precede the questions below with a preliminary greeting, such as the following: "Hi, I am (your name and title). You must be Tom Brown. Come in."

For All School-Aged Children

1. Has anyone told you about why you are here today?
2. (If yes) Who?
3. (If yes) What did he (she) tell you?
4. Tell me why *you* think you are here. (If child mentions a problem, explore it in detail.)
5. How old are you?
6. When is your birthday?
7. Your address is. . .?
8. And your telephone number is. . .?

School

9. Let's talk about school. What grade are you in?
10. What is your teacher's name?
11. What grades are you getting?
12. What subjects do you like the best?
13. And what subjects do you like least?
14. What subjects give you the most trouble?
15. And what subjects give you the least trouble?
16. What activities are you in at school?
17. How do you get along with your classmates?
18. How do you get along with your teachers?
19. Tell me how you spend a usual day at school.

Home

20. Now, let's talk about your home. Who lives with you at home?
21. Tell me a little about each of them.
22. What does your father do for work?
23. What does your mother do for work?
24. Tell me what your home is like.
25. Tell me about your room at home.
26. What chores do you do at home?
27. How do you get along with your father?
28. What does he do that you like?
29. What does he do that you don't like?
30. How do you get along with your mother?
31. What does she do that you like?
32. What does she do that you don't like?
33. (Where relevant) How do you get along with your brothers and sisters?
34. What do (does) they (he/she) do that you like?
35. What do (does) they (he/she) do that you don't like?
36. Who handles the discipline at home?
37. Tell me about how they (he/she) handle (handles) it.

Interests

38. Now, let's talk about you. What hobbies and interests do you have?
39. What do you do in the afternoons after school?
40. Tell me what you usually do on Saturdays and Sundays.

Friends

41. Tell me about your friends.
42. What do you like to do with your friends?

Moods and Feelings

43. Everybody feels happy at times. What things make you feel happiest?
44. What are you most likely to get sad about?
45. What do you do when you are sad?
46. Everybody gets angry at times. What things make you angriest?
47. What do you do when you are angry?

Fears and Worries

48. All children get scared sometimes about some things. What things make you feel scared?
49. What do you do when you are scared?

(Continued on following page)

BOX 27.2

Semi-Structured Interview With School-Aged Children (continued)

50. Tell me what you worry about.
51. Any other things?

Self-Concerns

52. What do you like best about yourself?
53. Anything else?
54. What do you like least about yourself?
55. Anything else?
56. Tell me about the best thing that ever happened to you.
57. Tell me about the worst thing that ever happened to you.

Somatic Concerns

58. Do you ever get headaches?
59. (If yes) Tell me about them. (How often? What do you usually do?)
60. Do you get stomach aches?
61. (If yes) Tell me about them. (How often? What do you usually do?)
62. Do you get any other kinds of body pains?
63. (If yes) Tell me about them.

Thought Disorder

64. Do you ever hear things that seem funny or usual?
65. (If yes) Tell me about them. (How often? How do you feel about them? What do you usually do?)
66. Do you ever see things that seem funny or unreal?
67. (If yes) Tell me about them. (How often? How do you feel about them? What do you usually do?)

Memories and Fantasy

68. What is the first thing you can remember from the time you were a very little baby?
69. Tell me about your dreams.
70. Which dreams come back again?
71. Who are your favorite television characters?
72. Tell me about them.
73. What animals do you like best?
74. Tell me about these animals.
75. What animals do you like least?
76. Tell me about these animals.
77. What is your happiest memory?
78. What is your saddest memory?
79. If you could change places with anyone in the whole world, who would it be?
80. Tell me about that.
81. If you could go anywhere you wanted to right now, where would you go?
82. Tell me about that.
83. If you could have three wishes, what would they be?
84. What things do you think you might need to take with you if you were to go to the moon and stay there for 6 months?

Aspirations

85. What do you plan on doing when you become an adult?
86. Do you think you will have any problem doing that?
87. If you could do anything you wanted when you become an adult, what would it be?

Concluding Questions

88. Do you have anything else that you would like to tell me about yourself?
89. Do you have any questions that you would like to ask me?

For Adolescents

These questions can be inserted after number 67.

Sexual Relations

1. Do you have any special girlfriend (boyfriend)?
2. (If yes) Tell me about her (him).
3. What kind of sexual concerns do you have?
4. (If present) Tell me about them.

Drug and Alcohol Use

5. Do your parents drink alcohol?
6. (If yes) Tell me about their drinking. (How much, how frequently, and where?)
7. Do your friends drink alcohol?
8. (If yes) Tell me about their drinking.
9. Do you drink alcohol?
10. (If yes) Tell me about your drinking.
11. Do your parents use drugs?
12. (If yes) Tell me about the drugs they use. (How much, how frequently, and for what reasons?)
13. Do your friends use drugs?
14. (If yes) Tell me about the drugs they use.
15. Do you use drugs?
16. (If yes) Tell me about the drugs you use. (Sattler, 1998)

When observing the child in a free play setting, the nurse should pay attention to initiation of play, energy level, manipulative actions, tempo, body movements, tone, integration, creativity, products, age appropriateness, and attitudes toward adults. In addition, themes of play, expression of emotions, and temperament are important to observe. The nurse must allow children to direct and initiate these themes. When evaluating the young child's peer relationships through play therapy in a play group or school setting, observe play settings and themes, initiation of play, response to peer initiations of play, integration of affect and action during play, resolution of conflicts, responses to suggestions of others during play, and the ability to engage in role taking and role reversals. In Bratton and colleagues' (2005) meta-analysis, they found including parents in the play therapy and using a humanistic approach produced the greatest positive effect over other forms of play therapy (Bratton, Ray, Rhine, & Jones, 2005).

The nurse's roles are to be a good listener; to use appropriate vocabulary; to tolerate a child's anxious, angry, or sad behavior; and to use reflective comments about the child's play. Through play, the nurse can assess the child's sensorimotor skills, cognitive style, adaptability, language functioning, emotional and behavioral responsiveness, social level, moral development, coping styles, problem-solving techniques, and approaches to perceiving and interpreting the surrounding world. Lidz (2003) devel-

BOX 27.3

LIDZ Assessment Tool

Child's Name: __________ Birth Date: ______ Age: ____
Assessor: ______________ Date of Assessment: ______
Describe typical play style/sequence.
Describe range of levels of play from lowest to highest level with age estimates and within contexts of independent/facilitated, familiar/unfamiliar, single/multiple toys.
Describe language and evidence of self-talk and internalized speech.
Describe interpersonal interactions with assessor and facilitator (if not assessor).
Describe content of any play themes.
What held the child's attention the longest? (For how long?)
And what were the child's toy/play preferences?
Describe the child's affective state during play.
Implications of above for intervention:

Lidz, C. S. (2003). *Early childhood assessment.* Hoboken, NJ: Wiley & Sons, Inc.

oped a tool that the clinician can use to assess preschoolers' play (see Box 27.3). Analyzing children's perceptions of fairy tales can provide the clinician with clues to culture, problems, solutions, and elements of mental functioning (Lebuffe & Naglieri, 1999; Trad, 1989).

Drawings are also used in child assessment to illuminate the child's intellect, creative talents, neuropsychological deficits, body image difficulties, and perceptions of family life (Fig. 27.1). Types of drawings used in child assessments are free drawings, self-portraits, the kinetic family drawing, tree, person, house drawing, and a picture of someone of the opposite sex (Cepeda, 2000). The Devereux Early Childhood Assessment (DECA) instrument measures protective factors of attachment, self-control, and initiative in children 2 to 5 years of age. The DECA tool is used in the preschool classroom setting with the goal of promoting positive resilience in children.

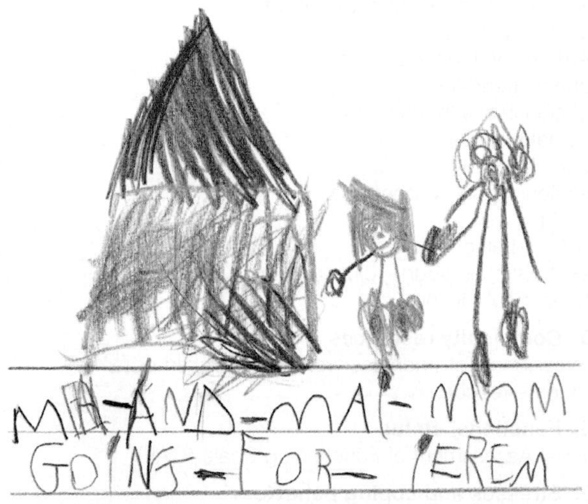

FIGURE 27.1. Me and my mom going for ice cream. Drawing and writing by a 5-year-old girl.

School-Aged Children

Unlike preschool-aged children, school-aged (5 to 11 years) children can use more constructs, provide longer descriptions and make better inferences of others, and acquire more complete conceptions of various social roles. Children in middle school are more capable of verbal exchange and can tolerate limited periods of direct questioning (see Box 27.4). The nurse can establish rapport with school-aged children by using competitive board games, such as checkers and playing cards. A therapeutic game helpful in assessing the child's perceptions, cognition, and emotions and in establishing rapport between clinician and child is the thinking–feeling–doing game. In this game, the clinician and child take turns drawing cards that pose hypothetical situations and ask what a person might think, feel, or do in such scenarios. For example, one card might say, "A boy has something on his mind that he is afraid to tell his father. What is he scared to talk about?" Another might read, "A girl heard her parents fighting. What were they fighting about? What was the girl thinking while she listened to her parents?"

Adolescents

Adolescents have an increased command of language concepts and have developed the capacity for abstract and formal operations thinking. Their social world is also more complex. Some early adolescents tend to assume that their subjective experiences are real and congruent with objective reality, which can lead to egocentrism. Egocentrism includes the concepts of the imaginary audience (others are watching them) and the personal fable (they are special and unique and omnipotent) (Rycek, Stuhr, McDermott, Benker, & Swartz, 1999). Egocentrism is a preoccupation with one's own appearance, behavior, thoughts, and feelings. For example, a preteen may think that he caused his parents to divorce because he fought with his father the day before the parents announced their decision to separate. Because teenagers have a heightened sense of self-consciousness, they may be preoccupied during the interview with applying makeup or other self-grooming tasks.

During early adolescence, cognitive changes include increased self-consciousness, fear of being shamed, and demands for privacy and secrecy. An adolescent's willingness to talk to a nurse will depend partly on his or her perception of the degree of rapport between them. The nurse's ability to communicate respect, cooperation, honesty, and genuineness is important. Rejection by the adolescent, even outright hostility, during the first few

BOX 27.4

Biopsychosocial Psychiatric Nursing Assessment of Children and Adolescents

1. Identifying information
Name
Sex
Date of birth
Age
Birth order
Grade
Ethnic background
Religious preference
List of others living in household

2. Major reason for seeking help
Description of presenting problems or symptoms
When did the problems (symptoms) start?
Describe both the child's and the parent's perspective.

3. Psychiatric history
Previous mental health contacts (inpatient and outpatient)
Other mental health problems or psychiatric diagnosis (besides those described currently)
Previous medications and compliance
Family history of depression, substance abuse, psychosis, etc., and treatment

4. Current and past health status
Medical problems
Current medications
Surgery and hospitalizations
Allergies
Diet and eating habits
Sleeping habits
Height and weight
Hearing and vision
Menstrual history
Immunizations
If sexually active, birth control method used
Date of last physical examination
Pediatrician or nurse practitioner's name and telephone number

5. Medications
Prescription (dosage, side effects)
Over-the-counter drugs

6. Neurologic history
Right handed, left handed, or ambidextrous
Headaches, dizziness, fainting
Seizures
Unusual movement (tics, tremors)
Hyperactivity
Episodes of weakness or paralysis
Slurred speech, pronunciation problems
Fine motor skills (eating with utensils, using crayon or pencil, fastening buttons and zippers, tying shoes)
Gross motor skills and coordination (walking, running, hopping)

7. Responses to mental health problems
What makes problems (symptoms) worse or better?
Feelings about those experiences (what helped and did not help)
What interventions have been tried so far?
Major loss or changes in past year
Fears, including punishment

8. Mental status examination
See Box 27.5

9. Developmental assessment
Mother's pregnancy, delivery
Child's Apgar score
Physical maturation
Psychosocial
Language
Developmental milestones: walking, talking, toileting

10. Attachment, temperament/significant behavior patterns
Attachment
Concentration, distractibility
Eating and sleeping patterns
Ability to adjust to new situations and changes in routine
Usual mood and fluctuations
Excitability
Ability to wait, tendency to interrupt
Responses to discipline
Lying, stealing, fighting, cruelty to animals, fire-setting

11. Self-concept
Beliefs about self
Body image
Self-esteem
Personal identity

12. Risk assessment
History of suicidal thoughts, previous attempts
Suicide ideation, plan, lethality of plan, accessibility of plan
History of violent, aggressive behavior
Homicidal ideation

13. Family relationships
Relationship with parents
Deaths/losses
Family conflicts (nature and content)
Disciplinary methods
Quality of sibling relationship
Sleeping arrangements
Who does the child relate to or trust in the family?
Relationships with extended family

14. School and peer adjustment
Learning difficulties
Behavior problems at school
School attendance
Relationship with teachers
Special classes
Best friend
Relationships with peers
Dating
Drug and alcohol use
Participation in sports, clubs, other activities
After-school routine

15. Community resources
Professionals or agencies working with child or family
Day care resources

16. Functional status
Global Assessment of Functioning Scale (GAF)

17. Stresses and coping behaviors
Psychosocial stresses
Coping behaviors (strengths)

18. Summary of significant data

interactions is not uncommon, especially if the teen is having behavior problems at home, at school, or in the community. The nurse should be patient and avoid jumping to conclusions. Hostility or defiance may be a test of how much the teen can trust the nurse, a defense against anxiety, or a transference phenomenon (see Chapter 6).

Adolescents are likely to be defensive in front of their parents and concerned with confidentiality. At the start of the interview, the nurse should clearly convey to the adolescent what information will and will not be shared with parents. Adolescents generally prefer a straightforward, candid approach to the interview because they often distrust those in authority. Mentioning to adolescents that they do not have to discuss anything that they are not ready to reveal is also a good idea, so that they will feel in control while they gradually build trust.

BIOPSYCHOSOCIAL PSYCHIATRIC NURSING ASSESSMENT OF CHILDREN AND ADOLESCENTS

As discussed, the comprehensive assessment of the child or adolescent includes interviews with the child and parents, child alone, and parents alone. After completing these components, the nurse should bring the child and parents back together to summarize his or her view of their concerns and to ask for feedback regarding whether these perceptions agree with theirs. The nurse must give the family a chance to share additional information and ask questions. Then, the nurse should thank them for their willingness to talk and give them some idea of the next steps. Use of an assessment tool is helpful in organizing data for mental health planning and intervention.

When interviewing both child and parents, directly asking the child as many questions as possible is generally the best way to get accurate, first-hand information and to reinforce interest in the child's viewpoint. Asking the child questions about the history of the current problem, previous psychiatric experiences (both good and bad), family psychiatric history, medical problems, developmental history (to get an idea of what the child has been told), school adjustment, peer relationships, and family functioning is particularly important. If necessary, the nurse can ask some or all of these same questions of the parents to verify the accuracy of the data, attain supplemental information, or both. Keep in mind that developmental research shows moderate to low correlation between parent and child reports of family behavior.

Biologic Domain

Nurses should include a thorough history of psychiatric and medical problems in any comprehensive assessment. A physical assessment is necessary to rule out any medical problems that could be mistaken for psychiatric symptoms (e.g., weight loss resulting from diabetes, not depression; drug-induced psychosis). Pharmacologic assessment should include prescription and over-the-counter (OTC) medications. Nurses should ask about any allergies to food, medications, or environmental triggers.

Genetic Vulnerability

The line between nature and nurture is not always clear. Characteristics that appear to be inborn may influence parents and teachers to respond differently toward different children, thus creating problems in the family environment. A phenomenon called assortative mating, the tendency for individuals to select mates who are similar in genetically linked traits such as intelligence and personality style, may contribute to the genetic transmission of psychiatric disorders. Research increasingly shows that major psychiatric disorders (e.g., depression, anxiety disorder, schizophrenia, bipolar disorder, substance abuse) run in families. Thus, having a parent or sibling with a psychiatric disorder usually indicates increased risk for the same or another closely related disorder in a child or adolescent. In addition, many childhood psychiatric disorders, such as autism, mental retardation, developmental learning disorders, some language disorders (e.g., dyslexia), attention-deficit hyperactivity disorder (ADHD), Tourette's syndrome, and enuresis (bed wetting), appear to be genetically transmitted (Faraone et al. 2005; Spence 2004; von Gontard et al., 2001; Finucane, Haas-Givler, & Simon, 2003; Abelson et al., 2005). Certain disorders (e.g., attention-deficit hyperactivity disorder [ADHD], enuresis, stuttering) are more common in boys than in girls.

Neurologic Examination

A full neurologic evaluation is beyond the scope of practice for a baccalaureate-level or master's-level nurse without specific neuropsychiatric training. However, a screening of neurologic soft signs can help establish a database that will clarify the need for further neurologic consultation. The nurse should ask the brief neurologic screening questions suggested in Box 27.4 directly of the child and also should note any soft signs of neurologic dysfunction, such as slurred speech, unusual movements (e.g., tics, tremors), hyperactivity, and coordination problems. The nurse can ask young children to hop on one foot, skip, or walk from toe to heel to assess their gross motor coordination and to draw with a crayon or pencil or play pick-up-sticks or jacks to assess their fine motor coordination.

Psychological Domain

Children can usually identify and discuss what improves or worsens their problems. The assessment may be the first time that someone has asked the child to explain his or her view of the problem. It is also a perfect opportunity to discuss any life changes or losses (e.g., death of grandparents or pets, parental divorce) and fears, especially of punishment.

Mental Status Examination

The mental status examination is essential in formulating a diagnosis. It can provide initial data that alerts the clinician to obtain further cognitive, neurological, or psychological testing. The mental status examination of children combines observation and direct questioning (Box 27.5). The nurse should note any areas where the child or adolescent is symptomatic or has difficulty with the task. A mental status examination should be obtained on subsequent visits so that improvements or changes in the patient's functioning can be noted.

The nurse should note the child's general appearance, including level of attractiveness. Although it perhaps should not be so, social-psychological research shows

BOX 27.5

Mental Status Examination

Appearance
Provide a head to toe assessment: describe head shape and size (Down's syndrome, fragile X syndrome, Turner's syndrome, fetal alcohol syndrome), eyes (clarity, gaze, glasses, eye contact), height, weight, cleanliness, facial expressions, mannerisms, ears, hearing, skin (bruising could indicate physical abuse), gait, posture, nutritional status (possible eating disorder).

Evaluate dress: Is it appropriate for the weather? Does the child wear shirts with logos or groups? Does the child appear older or younger looking? Inquire about symptoms of physical illness.

Motor activity
Use the following descriptors to assess motor activity: calm, psychomotor retardation, akathisia, agitated, hyperalertness, tics, muscle spasms, nail biting, hyperactivity, anxiety, restlessness, and/or compulsions.

Self-Concept
Ask about play, favorite stories, and three wishes. Ask the child to draw a self-portrait, describe best- and least-liked qualities. Ask what he or she imagines doing for an occupation when grown up. Also evaluate planning ability and sense of a future.

Behavior
Observe for temper tantrums, attention span, separation from family member, self-care activities, dressing, toileting, feeding, oppositionality, compliance, etc.

Social Interaction
How does the child relate to the examiner? Is the child wary, submissive, attentive, friendly, manipulative, approval seeking, conforming, hostile, or guarded?

Assess the child's relationships with parent or guardian, siblings, and friends.

General Intelligence
Assess general vocabulary, fund of knowledge, alertness, orientation, concentration, memory, calculations, organization, abstract reasoning creativity, spontaneity, and frustration tolerance. Ask about school, including regular or special education, grades and grade retention.

Fund of Knowledge
Ask child: How many legs does a dog have? How many pennies in a nickel? Have child identify body parts, draw a person, name colors, count as high as possible, and inquire about letter identification (younger children).

Inquire about the time. How many states are in the United States? Who was George Washington? How many days are in a week? What are the seasons of the year? (middle-schoolers) What does the stomach do? Who is Charles Darwin? (teenagers).

Orientation
Ask questions such as: How old are you?

Who is the current president of the United States?

Do you know who was the president before our current president?

What are two major news events in the last month? (Older children)

What is the year, seasons, date, day, and month?

Where are we? (country, state, city, clinic)

Recent memory
Ask the child to repeat a memory phrase; remember three to five objects that you say or show and then recall them in a few minutes.

What school do you currently attend? What did you have for breakfast or lunch today?

Remote memory
Ask questions such as: What did you do last weekend? What was your last birthday like? What is your address and telephone number? Who was your first best friend? How old were you when you learned to ride a bike? What was the name of your kindergarten teacher?

Abstract reasoning and Analogies
Ask what is meant by a stitch in time saves nine; a rolling stone gathers no moss; a bird in the hand is worth two birds in a tree; too many cooks spoil the broth.

Which object does not belong in this group: fish, tree, rock? Why?

Assess the similarity about objects such as peaches and lemons, oceans and lakes, a pencil and typewriter, a bicycle and a bus.

To evaluate comparative ability ask: Complete this sentence: An engine is to an airplane as an oar is to a ______.

Arithmetic calculations
Provide simple addition and subtraction questions based on the child's age. Ask older children multiplication and division problems.

Count backwards 20 to 1 for younger children.

(Continued on following page)

BOX 27.5
Mental Status Examination (continued)

Ask how many quarters are in $3.50 or if you buy something that cost $2.50 and you have $5 dollars, how much change will you receive.

Writing and spelling ability
Ask a 1st or 2nd grader to spell cat, hat, bad, old, dog. Ask a 3rd or 4th grader to spell words like clock, face, house, or flower. Ask older children to write a sentence such as "The grass is greener on the mountains," etc.

Reading
Have the child read a paragraph from an age-appropriate book.

Reading begins in 1st grade. Children should demonstrate basic reading skills by the end of 2nd grade.

Gross motor skills
Assess level of activity, type of activity, and any unusual gestures or mannerisms and compulsions

Have the patient walk, jump, hop on one foot, and walk heel to toe, throw a ball, balance and climb stairs.

By age 3, a child should walk up stairs with alternating feet, pedal a tricycle, jump in one place, and broad jump.

By age 4, a child can balance on one foot for 5 seconds, catch a bounced ball two of three times.

By age 5, a child can do heel-to-toe walking.

By age 6, a child should jump, tumble, skip, hop, walk a straight line, skip rope with practice, ride a bicycle.

By age 7, a child should skip and play hopscotch, run and climb with coordination.

By age 9, a child should have highly developed eye–hand coordination.

Fine motor skills
Have the child draw a picture or self-portrait as well as pick up sticks.

Have the child copy a design that you have drawn. Ask the child to draw a circle (age 3), an ×(age 3 to 4), a square (age 5), a triangle (age 6), a diamond (age 7), and connecting diamonds (age 8).

At age 3, a child should unbutton front buttons, copy a vertical line, copy a circle, build an eight-block tower.

By age 4, he should copy a cross, button large buttons.

By age 5, he should dress himself with minimal assistance, color within lines, draw a three-part human.

By age 6, a child should be able to draw a six-part human.

By age 7, a child should print well and begin to write script.

By age 8, a child should demonstrate mature handwriting skills.

Attention span
Ask the patient to follow a series of short commands. Observe motor activity, attention, concentration, impulsivity, hyperactivity, outbursts, and organization.

Observe the child's ability to stay on task and focus during the course of the interview.

Tasks include: counting backwards by 7, spelling the word *world* backwards, and saying the letters of the alphabet backward.

Insight and judgment
Ask the child to provide a solution to a hypothetical situation such as what would you do if you found a stamped envelope lying on the ground? What would you do if a policeman stopped you for driving your bike through a red light? What would you do if you saw two children fighting on the school ground? Assess the child's ideas about the current problem and the solutions tried so far. Assess if child can make use of assistance. Evaluate how impaired child is in activities of daily living: attending school, attending recreational activities, making friends, self-care activities, etc.

Comprehension
Read a few pages or paragraphs from a short book or newspaper article and ask the child to relate what happened in the story.

Mood and feelings
Affect is the child's emotional tone. Evaluate the child's range of emotions, intensity and appropriateness.

Assess for any mood swings, crying, anxiety, depression, anger, hostility, hyperalertness, lability, pressured speech. Assess mood by asking how many times a week do you feel sad, how often do you cry? What makes you sad, angry, anxious, etc. Risk assessment questions include: Have you ever felt like hurting yourself or someone else? Do you have a plan to hurt yourself? Have you ever done anything to hurt yourself in the past?

Thought process and content
Were there any recurrent themes?

Observe the child's patterns of thinking for appropriateness of sequence, logic, coherence, and relevance to the topics discussed. Does the child talk about age-appropriate topics; is there any thought blocking, or disturbance in the stream of thinking, repetition of words, circumstantial or tangential thinking, perseverations, preoccupations, obsessive thoughts, actions, or compulsive behaviors, any grandiose reasoning, ideas of reference, any paranoia (feelings of being watched or followed, controlled, manipulated, and ritual or checking routines)?

Evaluate the child's perceptions for hallucinations (false perceptions or false impressions or experiences), and delusions (false beliefs that contradict social reality, such as hears voices, sees images or shadowy figures, smells offensive odors, tastes offensive flavors, feels worms crawling on skin). Assess hallucinations in all five senses: auditory, visual, tactile, gustatory, and olfactory. Assess for command hallucinations, which tell the patient to do something.

Speech and language
Note any speech impediments and incongruence between verbal and nonverbal communication.

Show a pencil and a watch and ask the patient to name them.

Have the patient repeat "no ifs ands or buts"

Assess communication skills: expressive language, vocabulary, and the ability to understand what you are saying (receptive language); check voice quality, articulation, pronunciation, fluency, rhythm, rate, and ease of expression and volume.

Assess comprehension by giving the child a task. Assess coherence for flight of ideas, loose associations, word salad (meaningless, disconnected word choices), neologisms, clang associations (words that rhyme in a nonsensical way), echolalia (repetition of another person's words), thought blocking, perseveration, irrelevance, and vagueness. Check for aphasia by listening for an omission or addition of letters, syllables, and made-up words or misuse or transposition of words.

that the appearance and attractiveness of both children and adults strongly influence their social relationships (Sugiyama, 2005). The nurse also should note the following:

- Does he or she seem to have difficulty focusing on the interview, sitting still, refraining from impulsive behavior, and listening without interrupting? (possible signs of ADHD)
- Does the child seem underactive, lethargic, distant, or hopeless? (possible signs of depression)
- Are there problems with speech patterns, such as rate (overly fast or slow), clarity, and volume, and any speech dysfluencies (e.g., stuttering, halting) [possible mood disorders (e.g., depression, mania), language disorders, psychotic processes, and anxiety disorders (see Chapter 26)].

When assessing thought processes, keep in mind that young children are in the concrete operations stage; middle-schoolers can begin to use logic and understand conversations. Adolescents should be able to demonstrate abstract thinking and think hypothetically, although they may appear to be self-conscious and introspective. Assessment of preteens and adolescents should address substance use and sexual activity because responses may provide useful information about high-risk behavior or substance abuse. In addition, the nurse should inquire about any obsessions or compulsions (e.g., worries about germs, severe hand washing).

Developmental Assessment

Children respond to life's stresses in different ways and in accord with their developmental level. Knowing the difference between normal child development and psychopathology is crucial in helping parents view their children's behavior realistically and respond appropriately. The key areas for assessment include maturation, psychosocial development, and language.

Maturation

Healthy development of the brain and nervous system during childhood and adolescence provides the foundation for successful functioning throughout life. Such development, called **maturation**, unfolds through sequential and orderly growth processes. These processes are biologically and genetically based but depend on constant interactions with a stimulating and nurturing environment. If trauma or neglect impairs the process of normal biologic maturation, **developmental delays** and disorders that may not be fully reversible can result. For example, babies born with fetal alcohol syndrome experience permanent brain damage, often resulting in mental retardation, learning disabilities, behavior disorders, and delays in language (Cone-Wesson, 2005). A pregnant woman's use of crack cocaine deprives the fetus of nutrients and oxygen, leading to developmental delays, speech and language problems, deformities, and behavior disorders (e.g., impulsivity, withdrawal, hyperactivity). The nurse can assess for developmental delays by asking questions from specific sections of the mental status examination:

- *Intellectual functioning*: Evaluate the child's creativity, spontaneity, ability to count money and tell time, academic performance, memory, attention, frustration tolerance, and organization.
- *Gross motor functioning*: Ask the child to hop on one foot, throw a ball, walk up and down the hall, and run.
- *Fine motor functioning*: Ask the child to draw a picture or pick up sticks.
- *Cognition*: The nurse can evaluate the child's general level of cognition by assessing the child's vocabulary, level of comprehension, drawing ability, and responsiveness to questions. Testing, such as the Wechsler Intelligence Scale for Children (WISC-III), provides measures of intelligence quotient (IQ). A psychologist usually performs such tests. The nurse can request cognitive testing if he or she has concerns about developmental delays or learning disabilities.
- *Thinking and perception*: Evaluate level of consciousness; orientation to date, time, and person; thought content; thought process; and judgment.
- *Social interactions and play*: Assess the child's organization, creativity, drawing capacity, and ability to follow rules. Children experiencing developmental delays may remain engaged solely in parallel play, instead of moving to reciprocal play. They may consistently play with toys designed for younger children, draw crude body pictures, or display receptive or expressive language problems.

Psychosocial Development

Assessment of psychosocial development is very important for children with mental health problems. Various theoretical models are available from which to choose; the most commonly used model is Erikson's stages of development. When considering this model, the nurse should examine the child's gender and cultural background for appropriateness. The nurse also may use the Baker Miller's model for girls (see Chapter 6).

Language

At birth, infants can emit sounds of all languages. Maturation of language skills begins with babbling, or the utterance of simple, spontaneous sounds. By the end of the first year, children can make one-word statements, usually naming objects or people in the environment. By age 2 years, they should speak in short, telegraphic sentences consisting of a verb and noun (e.g., "want cookie"). Between ages 2 and 4 years, vocabulary and sentence structure develop rapidly. In fact, the preschooler's ability to produce language often surpasses motor development, sometimes causing temporary stuttering when the child's mind literally works faster than the mouth.

Language development depends on the complex interaction of physical maturation of the nerves, development of head and neck musculature, hearing abilities, cognitive abilities, exposure to language, educational stimulation, and emotional well-being. Social needs create a natural inclination toward communication, but the child needs reinforcement to develop correct pronunciation, vocabulary, and grammar.

Before a diagnosis of a communication disorder (i.e., impairment in language expression, comprehension, or both) can be made, the child must be tested to rule out hearing, visual, or other neurologic problems. Brain damage, especially to the left hemisphere (dominant for language in most individuals), can seriously impair the development of communication abilities in children. Any child who has experienced brain damage from anoxia at birth, congenital trauma, head injury, infection, tumor, or drug exposure should be closely monitored for signs of a communication disorder. Before the age of 5 years, the brain has amazing plasticity, and sometimes other intact areas of the brain can take over functions of damaged areas, especially with immediate speech therapy. Genetically based disorders such as autism cause language delays that are sometimes permanent and severe. Children with language delays need particular encouragement to communicate properly because they tend to compensate by using nonverbal signals (Tanguay, 2000).

The nurse must recognize normal variations in child development and assess lags in the development of vocabulary and sentence structure during the critical preschool years. Delays in this area can seriously affect other areas, such as cognitive, educational, and social development. Many children who receive psychiatric treatment have speech and language disorders that are sometimes undetected, either leading to or compounding their emotional problems. Cantwell and Baker (1991) studied 600 consecutive child referrals to an urban community clinic for speech and language disorders and found the psychiatric prevalence was 50% for any diagnosis, 26% for behavior disorders, and 20% for emotional disorders. The most common individual psychiatric diagnoses were ADHD (19%), oppositional defiant disorder (7%), and anxiety disorders (10%). Beitchman, Cohen, Konstantareas, & Tannock (1996) found that children with receptive language disorders also had a high prevalence of ADHD (59%).

Children's Rating Scales

A number of children's rating scales can assist in the assessment of various psychiatric disorders. The Behavior Assessment System for Children (BASC), developed by Reynolds and Kamphouse (1998), is a tool to measure behaviors and emotions in children ages 2 to 18 years. The scales include a teacher rating scale, parent rating scale, and a 180-item self-report of personality. The scale evaluates several dimensions, including attitude to school, attitude toward teachers, sensation seeking, atypicality, locus of control, somatization, social stress, anxiety, depression, sense of inadequacy, relations with parents, interpersonal relations, self-esteem, and self-reliance. The Child Behavior Checklist (CBCL), developed by Achenbach and Edelbrock (1983), is a 113-item self-report tool to identify forms of psychopathology and competencies that occur in children ages 4 to 16 years. This instrument provides scores on internalizing and externalizing behaviors.

Several scales are useful for diagnosing specific problems in children and adolescents. The Children's Depression Inventory (CDI), developed by John March (1997), is a 27-item self-rated symptom orientation scale for children ages 7 to 17 years that is useful for diagnosing physical symptoms, harm avoidance, social anxiety, and separation/panic disorder. The pediatric anxiety rating scale (PARS) developed by the Rupp Anxiety Study Group is a clinician-administered, 50-item semistructured interview to assess severity of anxiety in children ages 6 to 17 years (Riddle et al., 2001). The SNAP-IV, developed by James Swanson (1983), is a 90-item teacher and parent rating scale containing items from the Conners questionnaire for measuring inattention and overactivity; it is useful for diagnosing ADHD (inattentive and impulsive types) and oppositional defiant disorder. The Children's Yale-Brown Obsessive Compulsive Scale, developed by Goodman et al. (1989), is a 19-item scale that can help diagnose childhood obsessive-compulsive disorder in children 6 to 17 years of age.

Attachment

Studies of **attachment** show that the quality of the emotional bond between the infant and parental figures provides the groundwork for future relationships. The need to touch and be close to a parental figure appears biologically driven and has been demonstrated in classic studies of monkeys who bonded with a terry-cloth surrogate mother (Harlow, Harlow, & Suomi, 1971). A secure attachment is based on the caretaker's consistent, appropriate response to the infant's attachment behaviors (e.g., crying, clinging, calling, following, protesting). Children who have developed a secure attachment protest when their parents leave them (beginning at about age 6 to 8 months), seek comfort from their parents in unfamiliar situations, and playfully explore the environment in the parent's presence. When parents are unresponsive to a child's attachment behaviors, the child may develop an insecure attachment, evidenced by clinging and lack of exploratory play when the parent is present, intense protest when the parent leaves, and indifference or even hostility (Thompson, 2002) when the parent returns (Ainsworth, 1989).

Secure attachments in early childhood produce cooperative, harmonious parent–child relationships, in which the child is responsive to the parents' socialization efforts and likely to adopt the parents' viewpoints, values, and goals. Securely attached young children also socialize competently and are popular with well-acquainted peers during the preschool years, and have warm relationships with important adults in their lives. Securely attached children see themselves and others constructively and have relatively sophisticated emotional and moral understanding (Thompson, 2002).

Although the importance of the parent's responsiveness is unquestionable in determining the development of a secure attachment, the process works both ways. Some babies seem to encourage attachment naturally with their parents by responding positively to holding, cuddling, and comforting behaviors. Others, such as those with developmental delays or autistic disorders, may respond less readily and even reject parental attempts at bonding.

Attachment Theories

Bowlby's early studies (1969) of maternal deprivation formed the initial framework for attachment theory, based on the notion that the infant tends to bond to one primary parental figure, usually the mother. Although this pattern is common, recent studies show that children make multiple attachments to parents and other caregivers, but high-quality, intense bonds remain essential for healthy development. Contemporary nursing theories, such as Barnard's parent–child interaction model, have stressed the importance of the interaction between the child's spontaneous behavior and biologic rhythms and the mother's ability to respond to cues that signal distress (Baker et al., 1994). Doyle, Markiewicz, Brendgen, Lieberman, and Voss (2000) studied 216 parents' attachment style and marital adjustment and found that mothers' anxious attachment style uniquely predicted that children's attachment to both mother and father would be insecure. Child–mother attachment was associated uniquely with perceived global self-worth and physical appearance for both younger and older children, whereas child–father attachment was associated uniquely with child-perceived school competence and only for older children with global self-worth. Although most attachment research has been done with mothers, the father's role in child development has become better understood through research done during the past two decades. Fathers' emotional support tends to enhance the quality of mother–child relationships and facilitates positive adjustment by children, whereas when fathers are unsupportive and marital conflict is high, children suffer (Cummings & O'Reilly, 1997).

Fathers play an important role in children's play, which affects the quality of the child's attachment. Playful interactions involving emotional arousal provide an especially good opportunity to learn how to get along with peers by reinforcing turn taking, affect regulation, and acceptable ways of competing. Fathers are important as role models who assist in their sons' identity formation and serve as models of gender-appropriate behavior, particularly around aggressive behavior (DeKlyen, Speltz, & Greenberg, 1998). Biller and Lopez-Kimpton's (1997) review of the literature found that children who have active, committed, and involved fathers generally perform better cognitively, academically, athletically, and socially than do children who do not benefit from such involvement. All these data support the importance of including the father in the mental health assessment of his child.

Disrupted Attachments

Disrupted attachments may result from deficits in infant attachment behaviors, lack of responsiveness by caregivers to the child's cues, or both and may lead to reactive attachment disorder, feeding disorder, failure to thrive, or anxiety disorder. A **reactive attachment disorder** is a state in which a child younger than 5 years of age fails to initiate or respond appropriately to social interaction and the caregiver subsequently disregards the child's physical and emotional needs. Attachment disorder behaviors are related to attention and conduct problems (O'Connor and Rutter 2000). **Attachment disorganization** is a consequence of extreme insecurity that results from feared or actual separation from the attached figure. Disorganized infants appear to be unable to maintain the strategic adjustments in attachment behavior represented by organized avoidant or ambivalent attachment strategies, with the result that both behavioral and physiological dysregulation occurs. Preschoolers with disorganized attachment manifest behaviors of fear, contradictory behavior, and/or disorientation/disassociation in the caregivers' presence.

Temperament and Behavior

Temperament is a person's characteristic intensity, activity level, threshold of responsiveness, rhythmicity, adaptability, energy expenditure, and mood. According to research findings, temperamental differences can be observed early in life, suggesting that they are at least partly biologically determined, and patterns of temperament can be correlated with emotional and behavioral problems (Signoretta, Maremmani, Liquori, Perugi, & Akiskal, 2005). One basic aspect of temperament, the tendency to approach or avoid unfamiliar events, appears moderately stable over time and has been associated with distinct, apparently genetically based, physiologic profiles in 2-year-old children (Caspi & Silva, 1995; Schwartz, Snidman, & Kagan, 1999; Snidman, Kagan, Riordan, & Shannon, 1995). When looking at the cerebral asymmetry of the brain in children with inhibited compared to uninhibited temperaments, Davidson (1994) found that inhibited children in the third year of life showed greater EEG activation on the right frontal area under resting conditions.

The classic New York Longitudinal Study (Thomas, Chess, & Birch, 1968) identified three main patterns of temperament seen in infancy that often extend into childhood and later life:

- **Easy temperament**, characterized by a positive mood, regular patterns of eating and sleeping, positive approach to new situations, and low emotional intensity
- **Difficult temperament**, characterized by irregular sleep and eating patterns, negative response to new stimuli, slow adaptation, negative mood, and high emotional intensity
- **Slow-to-warm-up temperament**, characterized by a negative, mildly emotional response to new situations that is expressed with intensity and initially slow adaptation but evolves into a positive response

On the positive side, an easy temperament can serve as a protective factor against the development of psychopathology. Children with easy temperaments can adapt to change without intense emotional reactions. Difficult temperament places children at high risk for adjustment problems, such as with adjustment to school or bonding with parents.

Temperament has a major influence on the chances that a child may experience psychological problems; however, temperament is not unchangeable, and environmental influences can change or modify a child's emotional style (Tomlinson, Harbaugh, & Anderson, 1996). Children who respond positively to the environment continue in this pattern. Children who have other temperaments may develop positive temperaments at a later time.

The concept of temperament provides an excellent example of the interaction between biologic–genetic and environmental factors in producing child psychopathology. Although a child may be born with a particular temperament, longitudinal studies show that the temperament itself is less influential than the "goodness of fit" (Chess & Thomas, 2002) between the child's temperament and the reactions of parents and significant others. Difficult children in particular may evoke negative reactions in parents and teachers, thereby creating environments that exacerbate their biologically based behavior problems, initiating a vicious cycle. Vanden Boom and Hoeksma (1994) found that infants with difficult temperaments received less sensitive caring than did other children, and parents of 2-year-old children with difficult temperaments often resorted to angry, punitive discipline.

Difficult temperament that persists beyond 3 years of age is correlated with the development of child psychopathology. Rettew and colleagues (2004) found temperament problems such as low persistence were found in 156 children with ADHD, and high novelty seeking was found in children with oppositional defiant disorder. Many parents of children with difficult temperaments blame themselves for their children's behavior. Parents may compare the child with a difficult temperament to children with easier temperaments and wonder what they have done wrong or attribute negative motives to the child. The nurse can help parents accept biologically based differences in their children and learn to adapt their behavior to each child's needs to improve "fit." Linder (1993) developed a worksheet to assist the clinician in evaluating the child's temperament during play that is divided into measures of activity level, adaptability, and reactivity (see Box 27.6).

Self-Concept

For young children, eliciting their view of themselves and the world is helpful. One technique is asking them what they would wish for if they had three wishes. Answers can be revealing. An inability to wish for anything beyond a nice meal or place to live may reflect hopelessness, whereas wishes to conquer the world or put one's teacher in jail may indicate feelings of grandiosity. Another technique is to tell a story and ask the child to make up an ending for it. For example, a baby bird fell out of a nest—what happened to it? The nurse may design stories to elicit particular fears or concerns that may be relevant for the individual child.

Drawings also provide an excellent window into the child's internal world (Fig. 27.2). Asking the child to draw a picture of a person can provide data about the child's self-concept, sexual identity, body image, and developmental level. By age 3 years, children should be able to draw some facial features and limbs, but their drawings may have an "x-ray" quality, in which clothing is transparent and the body can be seen underneath. Older children should produce more sophisticated drawings, unless they are resistant to the task. After the child has finished the drawing, the nurse can ask what the person in the drawing is thinking and feeling, using this device to assess the child's mental processes. For example, one adolescent with school phobia drew a person fully dressed, in great

BOX 27.6

Social-Emotional Observation Worksheet

Name of child: ______ Date of birth: ______ Age: ______
Name of observer: ______ Discipline or job title: ______ Date of assessment: ______

On the following pages, note specific behaviors that document the child's abilities in the social-emotional categories. Qualitative comments should also be made. The format provided here follows that of the Observation Guidelines for Social-Emotional Development in Transdisciplinary Play-Based Assessment. It may be helpful to refer to the guidelines while completing this form.

1. Temperament
   A. Activity level
      1. Motor activity:
      2. Specific times that are particularly active
         a. Beginning, middle, or end:
         b. During specific activities:
   B. Adaptability
      1. Initial response to stimuli
         a. Persons:
         b. Situations:
         c. Toys:
      2. Demonstration of interest or withdrawal (*circle one*):
         a. Smiling, verbalizing, touching
         b. Crying, ignoring or moving away, seeking security
      3. Adjustment time:
      4. Adjustment time after initially shy or fearful response (*circle one*):
         a. Self-initiation b. Adult as base of security c. Resists; stays uninvolved
   C. Reactivity
      1. Intensity of stimuli for discernible response:
      2. Type of stimulation needed to interest child (*circle those that apply*):
         a. Visual, vocal, tactile, combination
         b. Object, social
      3. Level of affect and energy:
      4. Common response mode:
      5. Response to frustration:

From Linder, T. W. (1993). *Transdisciplinary play-based assessment: A functional approach to working with young children* (revised ed.). Baltimore: Paul H. Brookes Publishing Co., Inc.

detail, but with no feet. When asked about the drawing, he said that the boy could not go anywhere because his mother was afraid to let him leave home.

Other ways to assess children's self-concepts include asking them what they want to do when they grow up, what their best subjects are in school, what things they are really good at, and how well-liked they are at school. Before concluding the individual interview with a child, the nurse should always ask if the child has any other information to share and whether he or she has any questions.

Risk Assessment

The nurse must ask the child about any suicidal or violent thoughts. The best way to assess these areas is to ask straightforward questions, such as, "Have you ever thought about hurting yourself? Have you ever thought about hurting someone else? Have you ever acted on these thoughts? Have you thought about how you would do it? What did you think would happen if you hurt yourself? Have you ever done anything to hurt yourself before?" Contrary to popular belief, even young children attempt suicide, and they are capable of violent acts toward other children, adults, and animals. When a child shares the intent to commit a suicidal or violent act, the nurse must remind him or her that they will have to discuss this concern with the parent to keep the child and others safe. Substance abuse disorders across the life span account for more deaths, illness, and disabilities than any other preventable health condition. Screening for potential use and abuse of substances is becoming a priority in mental health assessment of adolescents. House (2002) developed an interview protocol that can be useful in identifying substance abuse problems in youth (see Box 27.7).

Social Domain

Family Relationship

Children depend on adults to create a safe, nurturing, and appropriate environment to support their development.

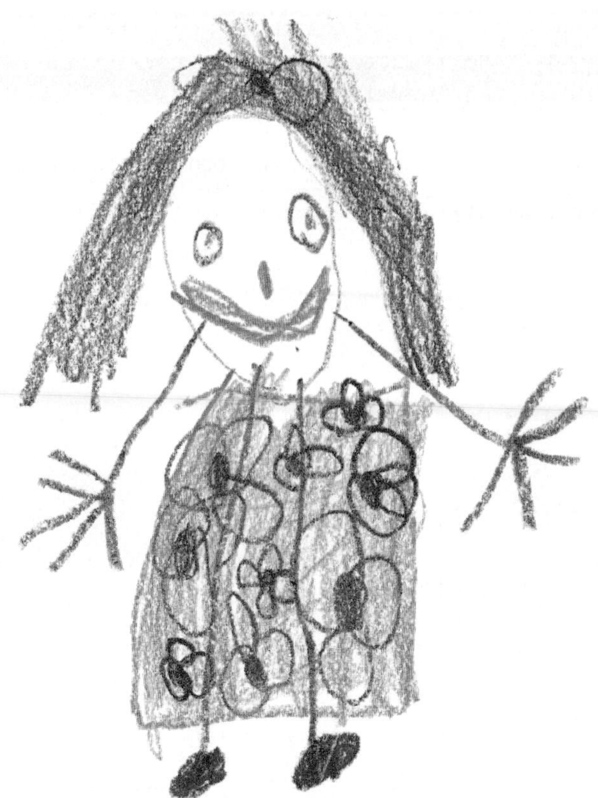

FIGURE 27.2. Self portrait of a girl, age 5.

The nurse should assess the quality of the home, including living space, sleeping arrangements, safety, cleanliness, and child care arrangements, either through a home visit or by discussing these issues with the family. When gathering a family history, a genogram and timeline are useful tools to map family members' birth order and medical and psychiatric histories; family roles, norms, boundaries, strengths, and family subgroups; birth dates, deaths, and relationships; stage in the family cycle; and critical events. To understand fully the family's values, goals, and beliefs, the nurse must consider the family's ethnic, cultural, and economic background throughout the assessment. A comprehensive family assessment should be considered (see Chapter 13).

School and Peer Adjustment

The child's adjustment to school is also significant. Often, children are referred for a mental health assessment as a result of changes in behavior at school. Falling grades, loss of interest in normal activities, decreased concentration, or withdrawal from or aggression toward peers may indicate that the child is experiencing emotional problems. It is very important that the nurse obtain signed permission from the parents to talk to the child's teacher for his or her observations of the child. The nurse may want to observe the child in school, if feasible, to see how the child functions there. The parent can request a treatment planning conference in which the teacher, parent, and nurse discuss the child's school performance and plan ways to promote the child's emotional, cognitive, and social functioning in school. Suggestions may range from having the child tested for learning disabilities to designing behavior plans that include rewards for improved functioning, such as computer time at the end of the day.

Community

Blyth and Leffert (1995) undertook a cross-sectional, longitudinal study of 112 different communities comprising a total of 300 youths in grades 9 through 12. The study showed that youth in healthy communities were more likely to attend religious services, to feel their schools were places of caring and encouragement, to be involved in structured activities, and to remain committed to their own learning. Assessing the child's economic status, access to medical care, adequate home environment, exposure to environmental toxins (e.g., lead), neighborhood safety, and exposure to violence is important because these community factors place the child at risk.

Children and adolescents function better if they are linked to community supports, such as churches, recreational programs, park district programming, and after-school programming. The Big Brother/Big Sister program fosters mentoring relationships for children. A parent or child may call the local Big Brother/Big Sister organization to request a mentor for the child. The mentor may perform a wide range of services, from taking a child to community events, helping with homework, or talking about how the child can achieve his or her dreams and goals. Some towns offer community-based juvenile justice programs to rehabilitate children who have had an altercation with the legal system. Juvenile justice programs provide support, such as individual and family counseling and prosocial recreational activities; teach children how to make positive choices about spending free time; and closely monitor their behaviors.

Religious and Spiritual Assessment of Children

There is a growing body of research suggesting that religious and spiritual practices may promote both physical and mental health (Sloan, Bagieila, & Powell, 1999; Seeman, Dubin, & Seeman, 2003). Barnes, Plotnikoff, Fox, & Pendleton (2000) linked religious identification to a number of health-enhancing behaviors such as decreased drinking, drug use, adolescent pregnancy, and violence. Spiritual assessment of our clients is an integral part of a mental health assessment. The Joint Commission Accreditation of Health Care Organizations (JCAHO) requires that each psychiatric evaluation include spiritual assessment questions.

BOX 27.7

Practice Note 0.1 An Interview Protocol for Reviewing Chemical Use in Youths

As with other topics, questions about substance use are interactive—the answers given determine to some extent the subsequent questions. However, certain topics and areas should be addressed irrespective of the previous responses. In the sample questions below, those marked with an asterisk should always be asked.

"Now I'd like to ask you about your experience with cigarettes, alcohol, and other drugs."
*"When was the last time you smoked tobacco?"
"Have you ever smoked? Tell me about that."
"How old were you when you first smoked a cigarette?"
"How many cigarettes do you smoke a day now?"
  "How long have you smoked this much?"
"Where do you usually do your smoking?"
"Where do you usually get your cigarettes from?"
"What kind of problems has smoking caused for you?"
  "How do your parents feel about your smoking?"
  "Have you gotten into trouble at school for smoking?"
  "Have you lost any friends or had problems with friends over smoking?"
*"What other tobacco products have you used?"
*"When was the last time you drank any alcohol?"
  "How much alcohol did you drink? What kinds of alcohol were you drinking? What happened afterward?"
  "Who was with you the last time you were drinking? What happened?"
  "How about the time before that? Tell me about that."
"What is the most alcohol you have ever drunk? What happened?"
"How do you get alcohol?"
"What kinds of problems have drinking caused for you?"
  "How do your parents feel about your drinking?"
  "Have you ever gotten into problems at school due to drinking?"
  "Have you ever gotten into legal problems due to drinking?"
  "Have you had problems with your friends because of drinking?"
  "What is the worst thing that has happened while you were drinking?"
"How old were you the first time you drank alcohol? When did most of your friends start drinking? How does your drinking compare with other kids in your classes at school or other kids your age?"
"How has your drinking changed over the past year?"
*"When was the last time you used any marijuana?"
  "How old were you when you first tried marijuana?"
  "How often have you used marijuana in the past month?"
  "What's usually going on when you use marijuana?"
*"What other drugs have you used?
  "When was the first time you used ______?"
  "When was the last time you used ______?"
  "How many times have you used ______?"
  "Where did you get the ______? How did you know that's what it was?"
  "How did the ______ affect you?"
  "What other drugs have you used?"
"What has been the biggest effect you have gotten using ______?"
  "What has been the worst thing about using ______?"
*"Have you ever 'huffed' or inhaled something to get high? Tell me about that."
*"Have you ever used another person's prescription medications? Tell me about that."
*"How many people do you regularly do things with—hang out, party with, talk to?"
  "How many of your friends smoke tobacco occasionally?"
  "How many of your friends smoke tobacco regularly?"
  "How many of your friends drink alcohol occasionally?"
  "How many of your friends drink alcohol regularly?"
  "How many of your friends smoke marijuana occasionally?"
  "How many of your friends smoke marijuana regularly?"
  "What other drugs do your friends use?"
  "How has drug use affected your friends?"

From House, A. (2002). *The first session with children and adolescents: conducting a comprehensive mental health evaluation.* New York: Guilford Press. Used with permission.

Questioning a patient's spiritual life should include interviewing strategies that are unbiased and facilitate understanding of the client's spiritual values. Questions can include, but are not limited to the following items: the child's and family's specific faith background, level of activity with that group, support received from spiritual practices, religious rituals of importance, and religious influences on life style and health choices. Sexson (2004) suggests that in the child interview, appropriate questions would include "Where is God?" and what does the child think about God and God's involvement in his or her life? Hart and Schneider (1997) recommend asking what the child might ask or say to God if they could talk to God.

Functional Status

Functional status is evaluated in children and adolescents using the Global Assessment of Functioning (GAF) scale, which tallies behaviors related to school, peers, activity level, mood, speech, family relationships, behavioral problems, self-care skills, and self-concept. The GAF scale ranges from 0 to 100; the lower the score, the higher the level of impairment, indicated by psychiatric symptoms and level of general functioning. For example, a score of 30 may indicate that the child is severely homicidal or suicidal and has made previous attempts; that hallucinations or delusions influence the child's behavior; or that the child has serious impairment in communication or judgment. Moderate impairment scores usually fall in the range of 51 to 69. Indications of moderate impairment include difficulty in one area, such as school phobia, that hinders school attendance or performance, while the child is functioning well within other areas, such as with family and peers. Children in this category are not homicidal or suicidal and usually respond well to outpatient interventions. A score of 70 to 100 usually indicates that the child is functioning well in relation to school, peers, family, and community. The GAF is always measured at the initial assessment so that treatment can be evaluated in terms of symptom improvement.

Stresses and Coping Behaviors

Biologic, behavioral, and personality predispositions; family; and community environment may affect a child's ability to cope with stressful life events. Stressful experiences for children include the death of a loved person or pet, parental divorce, violence, physical illness (especially chronic illness), mental illness, social isolation, racial discrimination, neglect, and physical and sexual abuse.

Evaluation of Childhood Sexual Abuse

There are several special considerations in interviewing an abused child. First, the nurse must establish a safe and supportive environment in which to conduct the evaluation. Second, the nurse needs to understand the forensic implications of assessment, so that the interview format will be acceptable for disclosure in a court hearing. The American Academy of Child and Adolescent Psychiatry (1997) offers practice guidelines for evaluating children who may have been abused. If the child reports abuse, the nurse has a legal responsibility to report the abuse to the child protection agencies. The nurse must use the same language and vocabulary that the child uses to describe the abuse or anatomical terms and ask nonleading questions. Nursing professionals who regularly interview children who have been abused may have special training in the use of anatomically correct dolls to obtain information about the abuse. The use of anatomically correct dolls is beneficial because it does not overstimulate or distress the child, assists in identifying and naming specific body parts, increases verbal productivity during the examination, helps to prompt memory, and is useful with immature, language-impaired, or cognitively delayed children (Cepeda, 2000). White (2000) provides a detailed chapter on the use of these dolls in interviewing preschoolers. Some questions that may be asked in forensic evaluation of a child for sexual abuse are presented in Box 27.8.

The number of stressful events that a child experiences, the supports that the child has in place, and the child's

BOX 27.8

Assessing Possible Sexual Abuse of a Child

1. Have you ever been touched on any part of your body?
2. Have you ever touched a part on anybody else's body?
3. Have you ever been hurt on any part of your body?
4. Have you ever hurt a part on anybody else's body?
5. Has anyone done something you didn't like to your body?
6. Have you ever been asked to do something you didn't like to someone else's body?
7. Has anyone put anything on or in any part of your body?
8. Have you ever been without your clothes?
9. Has anyone else asked you to take off your clothes?
10. Have you seen anyone else without clothes?
11. Has anyone asked you not to tell something about your body?
12. Has anyone said that something bad might happen to you or to someone else if you told some secret about your body?
13. Has anyone ever kissed you?
14. Has anyone ever kissed you when you didn't want them to?
15. Has anyone ever taken your picture?
16. Has anyone ever taken your picture without your clothes on?

From White, S. (2000). Using anatomically detailed dolls in interviewing preschoolers. In K. Gitlin-Weiner, A. Sandgrund, & C. Schaefer (Eds.), *Play diagnosis and assessment* (2nd ed., pp. 210–227). New York: Wiley & Sons, Inc. Used with permission.

developmental stage may also influence his or her ability to cope with stressors. Werner (1989) performed a longitudinal study of 500 Hawaiian youths considered to be at high risk for mental health problems because they were born into poverty, homelessness, or families whose parents had little education or were alcoholic, mentally ill, or headed by a single parent. Other risk factors included low birth weight, difficult temperament, mental retardation, childhood trauma, exposure to racism, poor schools, and community and domestic violence. One third of the children born at risk did not experience mental health problems by age 18 years. Protective factors that were identified in these children were:

- Individual attributes, such as resilience, problem-solving skills, sense of self-efficacy, accurate processing of interpersonal cues, positive social orientation, and activity level
- A supportive family environment, including bonding with adults in the family, low family conflict, and supportive relationships
- Environmental supports, including those that reinforce and support coping efforts and recognize and reward competence

Doll and Lyon's (1998) review of the literature about resilience found that children who show resilience in the face of adversity typically have good intellectual functioning, positive-easygoing temperament, positive social orientation, strong self-efficacy, achievement orientation with high expectations, positive self-concept, faith, high rate of involvement in productive activities, close affective relationship with at least one caregiver, effective parenting, access to positive extrafamilial models, and strong connections with prosocial institutions. Bernard (2004) advocates that emotional resilience can be taught to children using rational emotive educational strategies such as distraction techniques, diversion, seeking social support, exercise, and using rational thought processes.

SUMMARY OF KEY POINTS

- Mental health assessment of children and adolescents includes evaluating the child's biologic, psychologic, and social factors.
- Assessment of children and adolescents differs from assessment of adults in that the nurse must consider the child's developmental level, specifically addressing the child's language, cognitive, social, and emotional skills. Establishing a treatment alliance and building rapport are essential to obtaining a good mental health history.
- The mental status examination includes observations and questions about the child's appearance, motor activity, self-concept, behavior, social interaction, general intelligence, fund of knowledge, attention span, insight and judgment, comprehension, mood and feelings, thought process and content, speech and language, orientation, memory, reasoning, writing and spelling, reading, and motor skills. Assessment of the child and caregiver together provides important information regarding child–parent attachment and parenting practices.
- The three main types of temperament include the easy temperament, difficult temperament, and slow-to-warm-up temperament. Temperament can be evaluated by assessing the child's sleep and eating habits, mood, emotional intensity, and responses to new stimuli.
- A child's self-concept can be evaluated using tools such as play, stories, asking three wishes, and asking the child to draw a picture of himself or herself.
- If a child reveals suicidal ideation in the interview, the nurse must determine whether the child has a plan, let the parent know the child is suicidal, and make a plan to keep the child safe, such as an inpatient hospitalization.
- If a child reports to the nurse neglect or physical or sexual abuse, the nurse must by law report the child's disclosure to the state DCF.
- Protective factors that promote resiliency in children are the ability to problem solve, a sense of self-efficacy, accurate processing of social cues, supportive family environment, and environmental supports that promote coping efforts and recognize and reward competence.

CRITICAL THINKING CHALLENGES

1 An adolescent is hostile and refuses to talk in an interview. How would you respond?
2 What are some strategies for building rapport with children?
3 A child reports that he is suicidal. What would be your next question? What measures would you take next?
4 What are some techniques and media for obtaining information about a child's inner world, such as self-concept, sexual identity, body image, and developmental level?
5 Explain why it may be detrimental to interview a child in front of his or her parent. Why may it be detrimental to interview a parent in front of his or her child?
6 Why is obtaining the mental health histories of parents relevant to the child's mental health assessment?
7 What are useful tools in obtaining a family history from the child and parent?

8 Anatomically correct dolls are used in what specific type of child assessment?

9 Describe five characteristics of the resilient child.

10 What types of questions would you ask to inquire about a child's spiritual life?

REFERENCES

Abelson, J. R., Kwan, K. Y., O'Roak, B. J., Baek, D. Y., Stillman, A. A., Morgan, T. M., et al. (2005). Sequence variants in SLITRK1 are associated with Tourette's syndrome. *Science, 310*(5746), 317–320.

Achenbach, T. M., & Edelbrock, C. (1983). *The child behavior checklist: Manual for the child behavior checklist and revised child behavior profile.* Burlington, VT: Queen City Printers.

Ainsworth, M. D. S. (1989). Attachments beyond infancy. *American Psychologist, 44,* 709–716.

American Academy of Child and Adolescent Psychiatry. (1997). Practice parameters for the forensic evaluation of children and adolescents who may have been physically or sexually abused. *Journal of the American Academy of Child and Adolescent Psychiatry, 36*(10 Suppl.), 37S–56S.

Baker J. K., Borchers, D. A., Cochran, D. T., et al. (1994). Parent–child interaction model (of Kathryn Barnard). In A. Marriner-Tomey (Ed.), *Nursing theorists and their work.* St. Louis: Mosby.

Barnes, L. P., Plotnikoff, G. A., Fox, K., Pendleton, S. (2000) Spirituality, religion, and pediatrics: intersecting worlds of healing. *Pediatrics 104*(6), 899–908.

Beitchman, J. H., Cohen, N. J., Konstantareas, M. M., & Tannock, R. (Eds.). (1996). *Language, learning, and behavior disorders: Developmental, biological, and clinical perspectives.* New York: Cambridge University Press.

Bernard (2004). Emotional resilience in children: Implications for rational emotive education. *Journal of Cognitive and Behavioral Therapies, 4*(1) 39–52.

Biller, H., & Lopez-Kimpton, J. (1997). The father and the school-aged child. In M. Lamb (Ed.), *The role of the father in child development* (3rd ed., pp. 143–161). New York: John Wiley & Sons, Ltd.Wiley & Sons Inc..

Blyth, D. A., & Leffert, N. (1995). Communities as contexts for adolescent development: An empirical analysis. *Journal of Adolescent Research, 10*(1), 64–87.

Bowlby, J. (1969). Attachment (Vol. 1 of *Attachment and loss*). New York: Basic Books.

Bratton, S., Ray, D., Rhine, T., & Jones, L. (2005) The efficacy of play therapy with children: a meta-analytic review of treatment outcomes. *Professional Psychology: Research and Practice 36*(4), 376–390.

Cantwell, D. P., & Baker, L. (1991). *Psychiatric and developmental disorders in children with communication disorders.* Washington, DC: American Psychiatric Press.

Caspi, A., & Silva, P. A. (1995). Temperamental qualities at age 3 predict personality traits in young adulthood: Longitudinal evidence from a birth cohort. *Child Development, 66,* 486–498.

Cepeda, C. (2000). *The concise guide to the psychiatric interview of children and adolescents.* Washington, DC: American Psychiatric Press, Inc.

Chess, S., & Thomas, A. (2002). Temperament and its clinical applications. In M. Lewis (Ed.), *Child and adolescent psychiatry: A comprehensive textbook* (3rd ed.). Philadelphia. PA: Lippincott Williams & Wilkins.

Cone-Wesson, B. (2005). Prenatal alcohol and cocaine exposure. Influences on cognition, speech, language and hearing. *Journal of Communication disorders, 38*(4), 279–302.

Cummings, E. M., & O'Reilly, A. (1997). Fathers in family context: Effects of marital quality on child adjustment. In M. Lamb (Ed.), *The role of the father in child development* (3rd ed.). New York: Wiley. John Wiley & Sons, Ltd.

Davidson, R. J. (1994). Asymmetric brain function, affective style, and psychopathology. *Developmental Psychopathology, 6,* 741–758.

DeKlyen, M., Speltz., M., & Greenberg, M. (1998). Fathering and early onset conduct problems: Positive and negative parenting, father–son attachment, and the marital context. *Child and Family Psychology Review, 1,* 3–21.

Doll, B., & Lyon, M. A. (1998). Risk and resilience: Implications for delivery of educational and mental health services in the schools. *School Psychology Review, 27*(3), 348–363.

Doyle, A., Markiewicz, D., Brendgen, M., Lieberman, M., & Voss, K. (2000). Child attachment security and self-concept: Associations with mother and father attachment style and marital quality. *Merrill-Palmer Quarterly, 46*(3), 514–539.

Faraone, S. V., Perlis, R. H., Doyle, A. E., Smoller, J. W., Goralnick, J. J., et al. (2005). Molecular genetics of attention-deficit/hyperactivity disorder. *Biological Psychiatry, 57*(11):1313–1323.

Finucane, B., Haas-Givler, B., & Simon, E. (2003). Genetics, mental retardation and the forging of new alliances. *American Journal of Medical Genetics, 117*(1), 66–72.

Goodman, W. K., Price, L. H., Rasmussen, S. A., Mazure, J. C., Fleischmann, R. L., Hill, C. L., et al. (1989). The Children's Yale-Brown Obsessive Compulsive Scale (CYBOCS) I. Development, use, and reliability. *Archives of General Psychiatry, 46,* 1006–1011.

Harlow, H. F., Harlow, M. K., & Suomi, S. J. (1971). From thought to therapy: Lessons from a private laboratory. *American Scientist, 59*(5), 538–549.

Hart, D. S., & Schneider, D. (1997). Spiritual care for children with cancer. *Seminars in Oncology Nursing, 13*(4), 263–270.

House, A. (2002). *The first session with children and adolescents: Conducting a comprehensive mental health evaluation.* New York: Guilford Press.

Jensen, P. S., Rubio-Stipec, M., Canino, G., Bird, H. R., Dulcan, M. K., et al. (1999). Parents and child contributions to diagnosis of mental disorder: Are both informants always necessary? *Journal of the American Academy of Child and Adolescent Psychiatry, 38*(12), 1569–1579.

Lebuffe, P. A., & Naglieri, J. (1999). *Devereux early childhood assessment. The Devereux Foundation.* Lewisville, NC: Kaplan Press.

Lewis, M. (2002). Psychiatric assessment of infants, children and adolescents. In M. Lewis (Ed.), *Child and adolescent psychiatry: A comprehensive textbook* (2nd ed.). Baltimore: Williams & Wilkins.

Lidz, C. S. (2003). *Early childhood assessment.* Hoboken, NJ: John Wiley & Sons, Ltd.

Linder, T. W. (1993). *Transdisciplinary play-based assessment: A functional approach to working with young children* (Revised ed.). Baltimore: Paul H. Brookes Publishing Co.

March, J. (1997). *Multidimensional anxiety scale for children.* North Tonawanda, NY: Multi-Health Systems, Inc.

Moore-Taylor, K. M., Menarchek-Fetkovich, M., & Day, C. (2000). In K. Gitlin-Weiner, A. Sandgrund, & C. Scafer (Eds.), *The play history, interview play diagnosis and assessment* (2nd ed.) New York: John Wiley & Sons, Ltd.

O'Connor, T., & Rutter, M. (2000). Attachment disorder behavior following early severe deprivation: Extension and longitudinal follow-up. *Journal of the American Academy of Child and Adolescent Psychiatry, 39*(6), 709–712.

Rettew, D., Copeland, W., Stanger, C., & Hudziak, J. (2004). Associations between temperament and DSM-IV externalizing disorders in children and adolescents. *Journal of Developmental and Behavioral Pediatrics, 25*(6), 383–391.

Reynolds, C. R., & Kamphouse, R. W. (1998). *Behavior assessment system for children (BASC).* Circle Pines, MN: American Guidance Service.

Riddle, M. A., Reeve, E. A., Yaryura-Tobias, J. A., Yang, H. M., Claghorn, J. L., et al. (2001). Fluvoxamine for children and adolescents with obsessive-compulsive disorder: a randomized, controlled, multicenter trial. *Journal of the American Academy of Child and Adolescent Psychiatry, 40*(2):222–229.

Rycek, R., Stuhr, S., McDermott, J., Benker, J., Swartz, M. (1999). Adolescent egocentrism and cognitive functioning during late adolescence. *Adolescence, 33*(132), 745–749.

Sattler, J. (1998). *Clinical and forensic interviewing of children and families.* San Diego: Jerome Sattler Publisher.

Schwartz, C., Snidman, N., & Kagan, J. (1999). Adolescent social anxiety as an outcome of inhibited temperament in childhood. *Journal of the American Academy of Child and Adolescent Psychiatry, 38*(8), 1008–1015.

Seeman, T. D., Dubin, L. F., & Seeman, M. (2003). Religious/spirituality and health: a critical review of the evidence for biological pathways. *American Psychology, 58*(1), 58–63.

Sexson, S. (2004). Religious and spiritual assessment of the child and adolescent. *Child and Adolescent Psychiatric Clinics, 13,* 35–47.

Signoretta, S., Maremmani, I., Liquori, A., Perugi, G., Akiskal, H. (2005). Affective temperament traits measured by the TEMPS-I and emotional-behavioral problems in clinically-well children, adolescents, and young adults. *Journal of Affective Disorders, 85*(1–2), 169–180.

Sloan, R. B., Bagieila, E., Powell, T. (1999). Religion, spirituality, and medicine: viewpoint. *Lancet, 353,* 664–667.

Snidman, N., Kagan, J., Riordan, L., & Shannon, D. C. (1995). Cardiac function and behavioral reactivity. *Psychopathology, 32,* 199–207.

Spence, SJ. (2005). The genetics of autism. *Seminars in Pediatric Neurology. 11*(3):196–204.

Sugiyama, L. (2005) Physical attractiveness in adaptionist perspective. In Buss, D. (Ed.), *The handbook of evolutionary psychology* (pp. 292–343). Hoboken, NJ: John Wiley & Sons, Ltd.

Swanson, J. M. (1983). *The SNAP-IV.* Irvine, CA: University of California, Irvine.

Tanguay, P. (2000). Pervasive developmental disorders: A 10-year review. *Journal of the American Academy of Child and Adolescent Psychiatry, 39,* 1079–1095.

Thomas, A., Chess, S., & Birch, H. G. (1968). *Temperament and behavior disorders in childhood.* New York: New York University Press.

Thompson, R. (2002). Attachment theory and research. In M. Lewis (Ed.), *Child and adolescent psychiatry: A comprehensive textbook* (3rd ed.). Philadelphia: Lippincott Williams & Wilkins.

Tomlinson, P., Harbaugh, B., & Anderson, K. (1996) Children's temperament at 3 months and 6 years old: stability, reliability and measurement issues. *Issues in Comprehensive Pediatric Nursing 19*(1), 33–47.

Trad, P. (1989). *The preschool child assessment, diagnosis and treatment.* New York: John Wiley & Sons, Ltd.

Vanden Boom, D. C., & Hoeksma, J. B. (1994). The effect of infant irritability on mother–infant interaction: A growth curve analysis. *Developmental Psychology, 30,* 581–590.

von Gontard, A., Schaumburg, H., Hollmann, E., Eiberg, H., & Rittig S. (2001). The genetics of enuresis: A review. Journal of Urology, 166, 238-243.

Werner, E. E. (1989). High-risk children in young adulthood: A longitudinal study from birth to 32 years. *American Journal of Orthopsychiatry, 59,* 72–81.

White, S. (2000). Using anatomically detailed dolls in interviewing preschoolers. In K. Gitlin-Weiner, A. Sandgrund, & C. Schaefer (Eds.), *Play diagnosis and assessment* (2nd ed., pp. 210–227). New York: John Wiley & Sons, Ltd.Wiley & Sons, Inc.

CHAPTER 28

Mental Health Promotion with Children and Adolescents

Catherine Gray Deering and Lawrence Scahill

LEARNING OBJECTIVES

After studying this chapter, you will be able to:

- Describe protective factors in the mental health promotion of children and adolescents.
- Identify risk factors for the development of psychopathology in childhood and adolescence.
- Analyze the role of the nurse in mental health promotion with children and families.

KEY CONCEPTS

- grief in childhood
- invincibility fable

KEY TERMS

• attachment • bibliotherapy • child abuse and neglect • developmental delay • early intervention programs • family preservation • fetal alcohol syndrome • formal operations • normalization • protective factor • psychoeducational programs • resilience • risk factor • social skills training

Children and adolescents respond to the stresses of life in different ways according to their developmental levels. This chapter examines the importance of childhood and adolescent mental health, discusses the effects of common childhood stressors, identifies stressors that create risk for psychopathology, and provides guidelines for mental health promotion and risk reduction. Nurses are in a key position to identify and intervene with children and adolescents at risk for psychopathology by virtue of their close contact with families in health care settings and their roles as educators. Knowing the difference between normal child development and psychopathology is crucial in helping parents to view their children's behavior realistically and to respond appropriately.

Childhood and Adolescent Mental Health

Supportive social networks and positive childhood and adolescent experiences maximize the mental health of children and adolescents. Children are more likely to be mentally healthy if they have normal physical and psychosocial development, an easy temperament (adaptable, low intensity, positive mood), and secure **attachment** at an early age. These three areas are considered in the mental health assessment of children (see Chapter 27). **Developmental delays** not only slow the child's progress but also can interfere with the development of positive self-esteem. Children with an easy temperament can adapt to change without intense emotional reactions. A secure attachment helps the child test the world without fear of rejection.

• NCLEXNOTE

Attachment and temperament are key concepts in the behavior of children and adolescents in any health care setting. Apply these concepts to any pediatric patient.

Common Childhood Problems

Loss is an inevitable part of life. All children experience significant losses, the most common being death of a grandparent, parental divorce, death of a pet, and loss of friends through moving or changing schools. Learning to mourn losses can lead to a renewed appreciation of the precious value of life and close relationships.

DEATH AND GRIEF

Vast research shows that both children and adults who experience major losses are at risk for mental health problems, particularly if the natural grieving process is impeded. The grieving process differs somewhat between children and adults (Table 28.1).

KEY CONCEPT Grief in childhood differs from grief in adulthood. Children tend to grieve in stages. They begin without understanding the full effects of the loss and experience some numbness or dulling of emotional pain. This stage progresses to a greater acceptance of the reality of the loss, which leads to more intense psychological pain. Finally, they undergo a reorganization of identity to incorporate the loved person, which may involve engaging in new activities and interests (Van Epps, Opie, & Goodwin, 1997).

Children's responses to loss reflect their developmental level. As early as age 3 years, children have some concept of death. For example, the death of a goldfish provides an opportunity for the child to grasp the idea that the fish will never swim again. However, not until about age 7 years can most children understand the permanence of death. Before this age, they may verbalize that someone has "died" but in the next sentence ask when the dead person will be "coming back." Even adolescents sometimes flirt with death by driving dangerously or engaging in other risky behaviors, as if they believe they are immune to death. This phenomenon is known as the invincibility fable because adolescents view themselves in an egocentric way, as unique and invulnerable to the consequences experienced by others.

KEY CONCEPT Invincibility fable is an aspect of egocentric thinking in adolescence that causes teens to view themselves as immune to dangerous situations, such as unprotected sex, fast driving, and drug abuse.

If the concept of death is difficult for adults to grasp, they should be particularly sensitive to the child's struggle to understand and cope with it. Most children closely watch their parents' response to grief and loss and use

Table 28.1 Grieving in Childhood, Adolescence, and Adulthood

Children	Adolescents	Adults
• View death as reversible: do not understand that death is permanent until about age 7 years	• Understand that death is permanent but may flirt with death (e.g., reckless driving, unprotected sex) due to omnipotent feelings	• Understand that death is permanent: may struggle with spiritual beliefs about death
• Experiment with ideas about death by killing bugs, staging funerals, acting out death in play	• May be fascinated by death, enjoy morbid books and movies, listen to rock music about death and suicide	• May try not to think about death, depending on cultural background
• Mourn through activities (e.g., mock funerals, playing with things owned by the loved one); may not cry	• Mourn by talking about the loss, crying, and reflecting on it, sometimes becoming dramatic (e.g., overidentifying with the lost person, developing poetic or romantic ideas about death)	• Mourn through talking about the loss, crying, reviewing memories, and thinking privately about it
• May not discuss the loss openly, but express grief through regression, somatic complaints, behavior problems, or withdrawal	• Often withdraw when mourning or seek comfort through peer groups; may feel parents do not understand their feelings	• Usually discuss loss openly, depending on level of support available; may feel there is a "time limit" on how long it is socially acceptable to grieve
• Need repeated explanations to fully understand the loss; it may be helpful to read children's books that explain death	• Need permission to grieve openly because they may believe they should act strong or take care of the adults involved; need acceptance of their sometimes extreme reactions	• Need friends, family, and other supportive people to listen and allow them to mourn for however long it takes; need opportunities to review their feelings and memories

fantasy to fill the gaps in their understanding. In many cases, family members take turns grieving, with children sensing that their parents are so overwhelmed by their own emotional pain that they cannot bear the children's grief, and adults taking turns being strong for each other.

Loss and Preschool-Aged Children

The preschool-aged child may react more to the parents' distress about a death than to the death itself. Young children who depend totally on their parents may be frightened when they see their parents upset. Anything the parent can do to alleviate the child's anxiety, such as reassuring him or her that the parent will be okay and continuing the child's routine (e.g., normal bedtimes, snacks, play times) will help the child to feel secure. Because preschool-aged children have limited ability to verbalize their feelings, they may need to express them through fantasy play and activities, such as mock funerals. Books that explain death, such as *Charlotte's Web by* E. B. White, may also be helpful. Parents should take care not to use euphemisms that could fuel misconceptions of death, such as "He went to sleep" or "Jesus took him." Young children may interpret these messages literally and fear going to sleep (because they might die) or focus their natural, grief-related anger on the irrational idea that the person deliberately has not returned. The best approach is to explain honestly that the person has died and is not coming back, elicit the child's understanding and questions about what has happened, and then repeat this process continually as the child gradually begins to grasp the reality of the situation. The decision of whether to take a small child to a funeral may be particularly complex. Figure 28.1 enumerates some factors to consider.

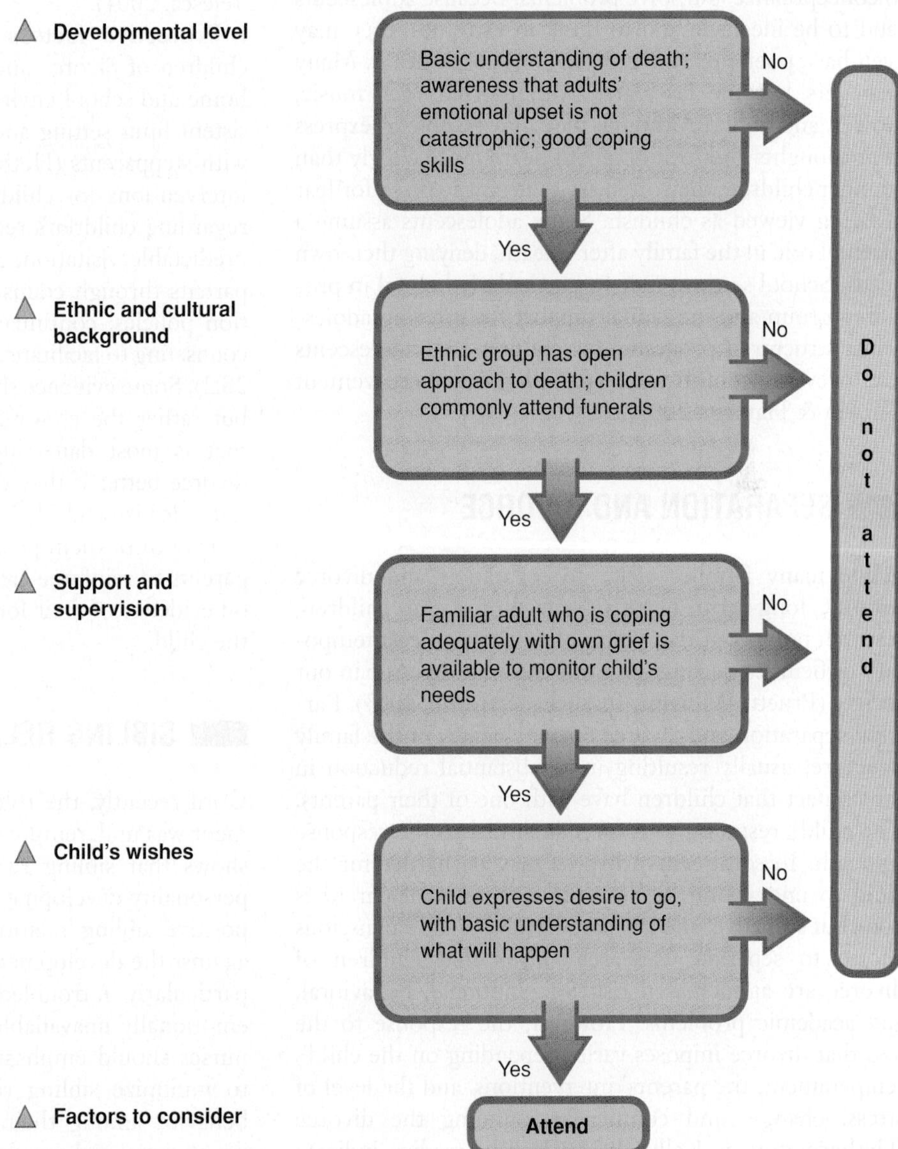

FIGURE 28.1. Decision tree: should a child attend a funeral?

Loss and School-Aged Children

School-aged children understand the permanence of death more clearly than do preschoolers, but they may be unable to express their feelings in a grown-up way. Children in this age group may express their grief through somatic complaints, regression, behavior problems, withdrawal, and even hostility toward parents. They may think that others expect them to cry and react with immediate emotional intensity to the death; when they do not react this way, they feel guilty.

Loss and Adolescents

Adolescents who are in Piaget's stage of formal operations can better understand death as an abstract concept. **Formal operations** is the period of cognitive development characterized by the ability to use abstract reasoning to conceptualize and solve problems. Because adolescents tend to be idealistic and to think in extremes, they may even have poetic or romantic notions about death. Many teenagers become fascinated with morbid rock music, movies, and books. Although they may be able to express their thoughts and feelings about death more clearly than younger children, they often are reluctant to do so for fear of being viewed as childish. Some adolescents assume a parental role in the family after a death, denying their own needs. School settings may be particularly helpful in providing group and individual support for grieving adolescents; structured programs for children and adolescents can prevent complicated (pathological) bereavement (Kirwin & Hamrin, 2005).

SEPARATION AND DIVORCE

While many families adapt to separation and divorce without long-term negative effects for the children, research points out that youth often show at least temporary difficulties dealing with this common stressor in our society (Pruett, Williams, Insabella, & Little, 2003). Parental separation and divorce create changes in the family structure, usually resulting in a substantial reduction in the contact that children have with one of their parents. The child's response to divorce is similar to the response to death. In some ways, divorce may be harder for the child to understand because the noncustodial parent is gone but still alive, and the parents have made a conscious choice to separate. Research shows that children of divorce are at increased risk for emotional, behavioral, and academic problems. However, the response to the loss that divorce imposes varies depending on the child's temperament, the parents' interventions, and the level of stress, change, and conflict surrounding the divorce (Hetherington & Kelly, 2002). Recent studies indicate that a major change in socioeconomic status, that is, moving from dual-earner status to single-parent family status, may account for much of the variation in levels of distress among divorcing families (Jeynes, 2002; Sun & Li, 2002).

The first 2 or 3 years after the couple's breakup tend to be the most difficult. Typical childhood reactions include confusion, guilt, depression, regression, somatic symptoms, acting-out behaviors (e.g., stealing, disobedience), fantasies that the parents will reunite, fear of losing the custodial parent, and alignment with one parent against the other. After an initial adjustment period, children usually accept the reality of the situation and begin coping adaptively. Most divorced parents eventually remarry to new partners, which often imposes another period of coping difficulties for the children. Children with stepparents and stepsiblings are at renewed risk for emotional and behavioral problems as they struggle to cope with the new relationships (Reifman, Villa, Amans, Rethinam, & Telesca, 2001).

Protective factors against emotional problems in children of divorce and remarriage include a structured home and school environment with reasonable and consistent limit setting and a warm, supportive relationship with stepparents (Hetherington & Kelly, 2002). Helpful interventions for children of divorce include education regarding children's reactions; promotion of regular and predictable visitation; reduction of conflict between the parents through counseling, mediation, and clear visitation policies; continuance of usual routines; and family counseling to facilitate adjustment after remarriage (Table 28.2). Some evidence shows that it is not the divorce itself but rather the continuing conflict between the parents that is most damaging to the child. Parents manage divorce better if they can remember that children naturally idealize and identify with both parents and need to view both of them positively. Therefore, it is helpful for parents to reinforce each other's good qualities and focus on evidence of their former partner's love and respect for the child.

SIBLING RELATIONSHIPS

Until recently, the role of siblings in a child's development was underemphasized. A growing body of research shows that sibling relationships significantly influence personality development. Moreover, research shows that positive sibling relationships can be protective factors against the development of psychopathology (Fig. 28.2), particularly in troubled families in which the parents are emotionally unavailable (Kramer & Bank, 2005). Thus, nurses should emphasize that whatever parents can do to minimize sibling rivalry and maximize cooperative behavior among their children will benefit their children's social and emotional development throughout life.

Table 28.2 Play Therapy with a 4-Year-Old whose Parents are Divorcing

Patient Statement	Nurse Response	Analysis and Rationale
(Child smashes two cars together and makes loud, crashing sound.)	That's a loud crash. They really hit hard.	Child may be expressing anger and frustration nonverbally through play. Nurse attempts to establish rapport with child by relating at child's level, using age-appropriate vocabulary.
Crrrash!	I know a boy who gets so mad sometimes that he feels like smashing something.	Child is engrossed in fantasy play, typical of preschoolers. Children often use toys as symbols of human figures (animism). Nurse uses indirect method of eliciting child's feelings because preschoolers often do not express feelings directly. Reference to another child's anger helps to normalize this child's feelings.
Yeah!	Sounds like you feel that way sometimes, too.	Child is beginning to relate to nurse and sense her empathy. Nurse reflects the child's feelings to facilitate further communication.
Yeah, when my mom and dad fight.	It's hard to listen to parents fighting. Sometimes it's scary. You wonder what's going to happen.	Child is experiencing frustration and helplessness related to family conflict. Nurse expresses empathy and attempts to articulate child's feelings because preschool children have a limited ability to identify and label feelings.
My mom and dad are getting a divorce.	That's too bad. What's going to happen when they get the divorce?	Child has basic awareness of the reality of parents' divorce, but may not understand this concept. Nurse expresses empathy and attempts to assess the child's level of understanding of the divorce.
Dad's not going to live in our house.	Oh, I guess you'll miss having him there all the time. It would be nice if you all could live together, but I guess that's not going to happen.	Preschool child focuses on the effects the divorce will have on him (egocentrism). Child seems to have a clear understanding of the consequences of the divorce. Nurse articulates the child's perspective and reinforces the reality of the divorce to avoid fueling child's possible denial and reconciliation fantasies.
(Silently moves cars across the floor.)	What do you think is the reason your parents decided to get a divorce?	Child expresses sadness nonverbally. Nurse further attempts to assess the child's understanding of the circumstances surrounding the divorce.
Because I did it.	What do you mean—you did it?	Child provides clue that he may be feeling responsible. Nurse uses clarification to fully assess child's understanding.
I made them mad cause I left my bike in the driveway and Dad ran over it.	How? Do you think that's why they're getting the divorce?	Child uses egocentric thinking to draw conclusion that his actions caused the divorce. Nurse continues to clarify the child's thinking. The goal is to elicit the child's perceptions so that misperceptions can be corrected.
Yeah, they had a big fight.	They may have been upset about the bike, but I don't think that's why they're getting a divorce.	The nurse goes on to explain why parents get divorced and to provide opportunities for the child to ask questions.
Why?	Because parents get divorced when they're upset with *each other*—when they can't get along—not when they're upset with their children.	

Sibling rivalry begins with the birth of the second child. Often, this event is traumatic for the first child who, up until then, was the sole focus of the parents' attention (Kramer & Ramsburg, 2002). The older sibling usually reacts with anger and may reveal not-so-subtle fantasies of getting rid of the new sibling (e.g., "I dreamed that the new baby died"). Parents should recognize that these reactions are natural and allow the child to express feelings, both positive and negative, about the baby while reassuring the child that he or she has a very special place in the family. Allowing the older child opportunities to care for the baby and reinforcing any nurturing or affectionate behavior will promote positive bonding.

Some sibling rivalry is natural and inevitable, even into adulthood. However, intense rivalry and conflict between siblings correlates with behavior problems in children (Moser & Jacob, 2002). One factor that can exacerbate this problem is differential treatment of children. Although it is natural and appropriate for parents to use different methods to manage children with different per-

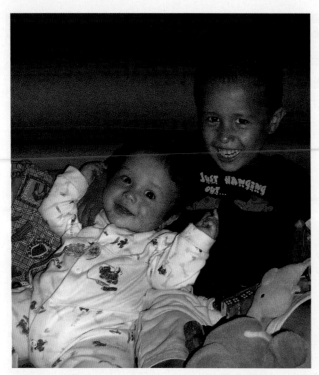

FIGURE 28.2. Sibling relationships significantly influence personality development.

sonalities, parents must be sensitive to their children's perceptions of their behavior and emphasize each child's strengths. Helping each child to develop a separate identity based on unique talents and interests can minimize rivalry and perceptions of favoritism.

Children with emotionally disturbed siblings are at increased risk for mental health problems. Nurses should be alert to behavior problems and include siblings in family interventions (Sharpe & Rossiter, 2002).

PHYSICAL ILLNESS

Many children experience a major physical illness or injury at some point during development. The experience of hospitalization and intrusive medical procedures is at least acutely traumatic for most children. The likelihood of lasting psychological problems resulting from physical illness depends on the child's developmental level and previous coping mechanisms, the family's level of functioning before and after the illness, and the nature and severity of the illness. As with any major stressor, the perception of the event (i.e., meaning of the illness) will influence the family's ability to cope.

Common childhood reactions to physical illness include regression (e.g., loss of previous developmental gains in toilet training, social maturity, autonomous behavior), sleep and feeding difficulties, behavior problems (negativism, withdrawal), somatic complaints that mask attempts at emotional expression (e.g., headaches, stomach aches), and depression. Infants and children younger than school age are particularly vulnerable to separation anxiety during illness and may regress to earlier levels of anxiety about strangers, becoming fearful of health care providers. Young children often have magical thinking about the illness, and their tendency to process information in concrete terms may lead to misperceptions about the illness and treatment procedures (e.g., dye = die; stretcher = stretch her) (Deering & Cody, 2002). Adolescents may be concerned about body image and maintaining their sense of independence and control.

Nurses must remember that parents are the primary resource to the child and the experts who know the child's needs and reactions. Thus, nurses must maintain a collaborative approach in working with parents of physically ill children. If the child is a sick infant, nurses should take care to allow the normal attachment process between parents and the infant to unfold, despite health care professionals' efforts to assume some parenting functions. Parents who view their children as physically and emotionally fragile will feel disempowered in decision making and limit setting and may develop helpless or overprotective styles of dealing with their children.

Many parents react with guilt to their child's illness or injury, especially if the illness is genetically based or partially the result of their own behavior (e.g., drug or alcohol abuse during pregnancy). Parents may project their guilt onto each other or health care professionals, lashing out in anger and blame. Nurses should view this behavior as part of the grieving process and help parents to move forward in caring for their children and regaining competence. Teaching parents how to care for their children's medical problems and reinforcing their successes in doing so will help.

Chronic physical illness in childhood presents a unique set of challenges. Although studies show that most children with chronic illnesses and their families are remarkably resilient and adjust to the stressors and regimens involved in their care (LeBlanc, Goldsmith, & Patel, 2003), research shows that children with chronic health conditions are three to four times more likely to experience psychiatric symptoms than are their healthy peers (Lewis & Vitulano, 2003). Conditions that affect the central nervous system (CNS) (e.g., infections, metabolic diseases, CNS malformations, brain and spinal cord trauma) are particularly likely to result in psychiatric difficulties. Nurses who understand pathophysiologic processes are in a unique position to assess the interaction between biologic and psychological factors that contribute to mental health problems in chronically ill children (e.g., lethargy from high blood sugar levels or respiratory problems; mood swings from steroid use). Inactivity and lack of sensory stimulation from hospitalization or bed rest may contribute to neurologic deficits and developmental delays. The major challenge for a chronically ill child is to remain active despite the limitations of the illness and to become fully integrated into school and social activities. Children who view themselves as different or defective will experience low self-esteem and be more at risk for depression, anxiety, and behavior problems. Studies show that parental perceptions of the child's vulnerability predict greater adjustment problems, even after controlling for age and disease severity (Anthony, Gil, & Schanberg, 2003). Educating parents and helping them to foster maximum independence within the limitations of the child's health problem is the key.

ADOLESCENT RISK-TAKING BEHAVIORS

Adolescence is a time of growing independence and, consequently, experimentation. Emotional extremes prevail. To adolescents, the world seems great one day and terrible the next; people are either for them or against them. Adolescents are struggling to consolidate their abilities to control their impulses and react to the many "crises" that may seem trivial to adults but are very important to teens. Biologic changes (e.g., onset of puberty, height and weight changes, hormonal changes), psychological changes (increased ability for abstract thinking), and social changes (dating, driving, increased autonomy) are all significant. The primary developmental task of identity formation leads teenagers to test different roles and struggle to find a peer group that fits their unfolding self-image.

During this process, many adolescents experiment with risk-taking behaviors, such as smoking, using alcohol and drugs, having unprotected sex, engaging in truancy or delinquent behaviors, and running away from home. Although most youths eventually become more responsible, some develop harmful behavior patterns and addictions that endanger their mental and physical health. Adolescents whose psychiatric problems have already developed are particularly vulnerable to engaging in risky behaviors because they have limited coping skills, may attempt to self-medicate their symptoms, and may feel increased pressure to fit in with other teens. Moreover, research shows that risky behaviors tend to be interrelated (Eggert, Thompson, Randell, & Pike, 2002).

Several approaches to mental health promotion with adolescents are recommended. First, intervening at the peer group level through education programs, alternative recreation activities, and peer counseling is most successful (Box 28.1). Adolescents are skeptical of authority figures and tend to take cues from one another. Nurses working with teenagers find it helpful to use a discussion approach that encourages questioning and argument, as opposed to talking down to or "talking at" teenagers (Deering & Cody, 2002).

Second, research has shown that training in values clarification, problem solving, social skills, and assertiveness

BOX 28.1

Research for Best Practice: Long-term Effectiveness of a Psychoeducational Program

Puskar, K. R., Sereika, S., & Tusaie-Mumford, K. (2003). Effect of the Teaching Kids to Cope (TKC) Program on outcomes of depression and coping among rural adolescents. Journal of Child and Adolescent Psychiatric Nursing, 16(2), 71–80.

THE QUESTION: This study investigated the long-term effectiveness of a psychoeducational program developed by a group of psychiatric nurses, using a 10-session format focusing on self-esteem, stress, and coping skills in high school students. The goal of the program was to prevent depression, suicide, and other mental health problems by teaching cognitive behavioral strategies for coping with common adolescent stressors.

METHODS: The nurses intervened with students (n = 89) from three rural high schools in southwestern Pennsylvania. They randomly assigned the students to the cognitive behavioral intervention (n = 46) versus a control group (n = 43) and measured the outcomes immediately after the intervention, at 6 months, and at 12 months' follow-up.

FINDINGS: The results showed that the psychoeducational program produced significant improvement in the range of coping skills and the incidence of depressive symptomatology, which was maintained at the 1-year follow-up. Four major themes emerged from the group sessions among the high school students: (1) confidentiality struggles (ambivalence about sharing personal information), (2) issues of daily living (questioning their ability to meet the demands of the adolescent experience), (3) identity issues (struggles to define themselves in terms of family and peer relationships, risk-taking behaviors, and career choices), and (4) affect regulation (emotional reactivity and depression).

IMPLICATIONS FOR NURSING PRACTICE: This study is an excellent example of outcome-focused research in preventive mental health. The nurses used both quantitative data (objective measures of depressive symptoms and coping skills) and qualitative data (transcribed tapes of the group sessions to identify themes and to examine the personal meaning of the intervention). Because this was a randomized, controlled, experimental study, it offers strong support for the effectiveness of a carefully designed psychoeducational approach.

The research project was funded by the National Institutes of Health and the National Institute for Nursing Research. It is part of a continuing series of interventions and studies designed by this team of nurse researchers who argue that helping teens to develop better coping skills is a cost-effective way to prevent later mental health problems.

helps give adolescents the skills to cope with situations in which they are pressured by their peers (Botvin, 2000). Social psychological research shows that if just one person can find the strength to express an unpopular viewpoint in a group and decline to participate in a destructive activity, others will quickly follow. It takes enormous courage, as well as concrete knowledge and practice with assertiveness, to speak up in these situations.

A third type of intervention is a program that uses team efforts by teachers, parents, community leaders, and teen role models. These programs help at-risk youth by building self-esteem, setting positive examples, and working to involve the youth in community activities. Approaches that have not proved effective include mere education about dangerous activities without behavior training and programs that provide inadequate training for the professionals implementing them.

Risk Factors for Childhood Psychopathology

POVERTY AND HOMELESSNESS

An estimated 16.7 % of children in the United States live in poverty (U.S. Department of Commerce, 2003), and a disproportionate number of children from minority groups live in poverty. The effects of poverty on child development and family functioning are numerous and pervasive. Lack of proper nutrition and access to prenatal and mother-infant care place children from poor families at risk for physical and mental health problems. Children from poor rural areas often lack access to educational and other resources. Urban children living in ghetto areas are vulnerable to violent crime, crowded living conditions, and drug-infested neighborhoods (Leventhal & Brooks-Gunn, 2000). Although crime, drug abuse, gang activity, and teenage pregnancy are seen in adolescents from all socioeconomic backgrounds, children living in poverty may be more vulnerable to these problems because they may view their options as limited. Thus, they may have an increased need to maintain a tough image and struggle more for a sense of control over their environment. The obstacles inherent in overcoming the effects of poverty can seem insurmountable to young people.

A major focus of preventive nursing interventions for disadvantaged families involves simply forming an alliance that conveys respect and willingness to work as an advocate to help patients gain access to resources. In terms of Maslow's need hierarchy, families living in poverty may be more focused on survival needs (e.g., food, shelter) than self-actualization needs (e.g., insight-oriented psychotherapy for themselves or their children). Unless the nurse can work as a partner with the family and address the issues most pressing for the family with an active, problem-solving approach, other types of intervention may be fruitless. At the same time, it is inappropriate to assume that poor families will be resistant to or unable to benefit from psychotherapy or other mental health interventions.

Homelessness in children and teens may result from loss of shelter for the entire family, running away, or being thrown out of their homes. Chapter 30 reviews in detail mental health issues related to homelessness, but some mention of the specific effects of homelessness on youth deserves mention here. Research reveals an increased risk for physical health problems (e.g., nutrition deficiencies, infections, chronic illnesses), mental health problems (particularly developmental delays in language, fine or gross motor coordination, and social development; depression; anxiety; disruptive behavior disorders), and educational underachievement in homeless youth. Many homeless youth have been physically and/or sexually abused, leading to elevated rates of externalizing disorders for boys and internalizing disorders for girls (Cance et al., 2000). For adolescents, running away from abusive conditions at home often thrusts them onto the street and into environments where staying alive and developing self-reliance are a daily struggle (Rew, 2003). The living conditions of many shelters place children at risk for lead poisoning and communicable diseases and make the regular sleep, feeding, play, and bathing patterns important for normal development nearly impossible. Nurses working with homeless families need to be aware of the effects of this lifestyle on children because they have a limited ability to speak for themselves and because their needs are often overlooked. Studies show that the demands of parenting often overwhelm parents in homeless shelters. The unstable nature of their living conditions limits the ability of these parents to nurture their children (Gorzka, 1999).

Typically, runaway youth have experienced extreme stress in the course of their lives even before they run away, with most fleeing temporary living arrangements (e.g., foster homes, friends, relatives) (Warren, Gary, & Moorhead, 1997). Thus, their runaway experience serves only to compound an already chronic history of trauma and disruption. The key is to prevent the conditions that preceded the runaway behavior.

CHILD ABUSE AND NEGLECT

Early recognition and reduction of risk factors are the keys to preventing **child abuse and neglect** (Box 28.2).

Risk factors for child abuse and neglect include high levels of family stress, drug or alcohol abuse, a stepparent or parental boyfriend or girlfriend who is unstable or unloving toward the child, and lack of social support for the parents. In addition, young children (particularly those younger than 3 years) and children with a history of

BOX 28.2

Research For Best Practice: Screening for Abuse

Murray, S. K., Baker, A. W., & Lewin, L. (2000). Screening families with young children for child maltreatment potential. Pediatric Nursing, 26, 47–54.

THE QUESTION: What tools are effective in assessing risk for child abuse and neglect in families with children aged 3 years and younger?

METHODS: The nurses who developed a screening assessment tool undertook a comprehensive review of the literature on risk factors for child maltreatment and combined these data with ideas from other screening and research tools.

FINDINGS: The result was a 19-question interview protocol that can be administered in 5 minutes or less. The researchers' goal was to provide a tool that could be used efficiently in primary care settings because other available tools are more cumbersome and impractical. The nurse researchers piloted the instrument in a primary care clinic, and the nurses who administered it reported that it was concise and easy to use. The tool includes an interview screening protocol with carefully worded questions designed to avoid accusatory attitudes and with a scoring guide that indicates the need for referral to community resources.

IMPLICATIONS FOR NURSING PRACTICE: The nurses who developed this tool assert that assessment of risk for abuse and neglect should be a standard of practice in child health care programs. Screening for possible risk for maltreatment allows nurses to identify families who are most in need of tracking and preventive intervention. This maximizes the efficient use of resources by both families and health care providers; however, assessment tools must be brief and designed with specific, helpful questions that both experienced and novice professionals can adapt. Because primary care providers may be a family's only formal source of support in the early years of child rearing, this is a key setting for assessment. The development of this tool is a useful contribution to nursing practice, and it provides the potential to intervene with families early enough to make a difference.

prematurity, medical problems, and severe emotional problems are at high risk because they place great demands on the parents. Abuse has a well-known intergenerational pattern, such that children who are abused and neglected are more likely to repeat this behavior when they become parents (Helfer, Kemper, & Kongman, 1997).

Table 28.3 lists signs of physical and sexual abuse in children. Research clearly documents that child abuse is a risk factor for later psychopathology, especially depression and substance abuse (Putnam, 2003). Nurses should be aware that they are legally mandated to report any reasonable suspicion of abuse and neglect to the appropriate authorities in their given state. Mandated reporting laws are designed to allow the state to investigate the possibility of abuse, provide protection to children, and link families with the support and services that they need to

Table 28.3 Signs of Possible Child Abuse

Sexual Abuse	Physical Abuse
• Bruises or bleeding in genitals or rectum	• Bruises or lacerations, especially in clusters on back, buttocks, thighs, or large areas of torso*
• Sexually transmitted disease (e.g., HIV, gonorrhea, syphilis, herpes genitalis)	• Fractures inconsistent with the child's history
• Vaginal or penile discharge	• Old and new injuries at the same time
• Sore throats	• Unwilling to change clothes in front of others: wears heavy clothes in warm weather
• Enuresis or encopresis	• Identifiable marks from belt buckles, electrical cords, or handprints
• Foreign bodies in the vagina or rectum	• Cigarette burns
• Pregnancy, especially in a young adolescent	• Rope burns on arms, legs, face, neck, or torso from being bound and gagged
• Difficulty in walking or sitting	• Adult-size bite marks
• Sexual acting out with siblings or peers	• Bald spots interspersed with normal hair
• Sophisticated knowledge of sexual activities	• Shrinking at the touch of an adult
• Preoccupation with sexual ideas	• Fear of adults, especially parents
• Somatic complaints, especially abdominal pain and constipation	• Apprehensive when other children cry
• Sleep difficulties	
• Hyperalertness to environment	• Scanning the environment, staying very still, failing to cry when hurt
• Withdrawal	• Aggression or withdrawal
• Excessive daydreaming or seeming preoccupied	• Indiscriminant seeking of affection
• Regressed behavior	• Defensive reactions when questioned about injuries
	• History of being taken to many different clinics and emergency rooms for different injuries

*Note: Because many injuries do not represent child abuse, a careful history must be taken.

reduce the risk for further abuse. Nurses are immune from liability for reporting suspected abuse, but they may be held legally accountable for not reporting it. The decision to report abuse sometimes poses an ethical dilemma for nurses as they try to balance the need to maintain the family's trust against the need to protect the child. This decision is further complicated by the knowledge that, if temporary out-of-home placement is necessary, the quality of the placement may not be optimum, and the child and family may suffer in the process of the separation.

Experts recommend that nurses report abuse in the presence of the parents, preferably with the parent initiating the telephone call, and that the professional should explain the reporting as necessary to provide safety for the child and to obtain services for the family. If the parents cannot be present when the report is made, the nurse should, at minimum, notify the family that the report was made and explain why to minimize damaging the professional relationship. A major protective factor against psychopathology stemming from abuse and neglect is the establishment of a supportive relationship with at least one adult, who can provide empathy, consistency, and possibly, a corrective experience (e.g., a foster parent or other family member) for the child (Taussig, 2002).

Preventing child abuse and neglect occurs with any intervention that supports the parents with physical, financial, mental health, and medical resources that will reduce stress within the family system. Early intervention and family support programs are considered the cornerstone of preventive efforts. Nurses working with abused children should resist the temptation to view the child as the only victim. Remembering that most abusive parents were abused themselves as children and, therefore, may have limited coping mechanisms or little access to positive parental role models will help the nurse maintain empathy toward the parents. Once state agencies intervene to establish the child's safety, a family systems approach that is supportive of the whole family unit is most effective.

OUT-OF-HOME PLACEMENT

The tendency to blame parents and view out-of-home placement as a refuge for children has sharply declined in recent years. This change in attitudes results from public awareness of the deficiencies in the foster care system, greater support for parents' rights, and increased knowledge of the biologic basis for many of the disorders of parents and children that lead to out-of-home placement. **Family preservation** involves efforts made by professionals to preserve the family unit by preventing the removal of children from their homes by providing support and education to secure the attachment between children and parents. Today children are removed from their homes only as a last resort. Family support services are designed to assist families with access to resources and education regarding child rearing, to monitor and facilitate the development of the bond between child and caregiver, and to increase the caregiver's confidence in his or her abilities (MacLeod & Nelson, 2000).

However, despite recent trends toward family preservation, an increasing number of children are placed in foster homes, group homes, or residential treatment centers—in many cases for months to years. Factors leading to the increased number of children in out-of-home placement include increased willingness of the public and professionals to report child abuse and neglect, the epidemic proportions of substance abuse and cases of AIDS, and the increasing number of families living in poverty, which may lead to abuse, neglect, and homelessness. About 50% of children in out-of-home placement are adolescents, but the numbers of infants and young children are growing, particularly those with serious physical and emotional problems, who pose particular challenges for placement (Zenah et al., 2001). Infants who are abandoned by drug-abusing parents and children with HIV whose parents are sick or deceased need permanent out-of-home placements, which are often difficult to find.

The adjustment to an out-of-home placement can be viewed through the conceptual framework of Bowlby's stages of coping with parental separation. According to Bowlby (1960), the child initially responds to separation from parents with protest (crying, kicking, screaming, pleading, and attempting to elicit the parent's return). The child then moves to a state of despair (listlessness, apathy, and withdrawal, which lead to some acceptance of caregiving by others, but a reluctance to reattach fully). Finally, the child experiences detachment if the child and new parent cannot manage to form an emotional bond. Because children often experience multiple placements, the potential for a disrupted attachment may be great by the time the child faces the prospect of a permanent family. After repeatedly undergoing separation and mourning, the child learns that rejection is inevitable and may automatically maintain distance from a new caregiver.

Typical coping styles seen in children exposed to multiple placements include detachment, diffuse rage, chronic depression, antisocial behavior, low self-esteem, and chronic dependency or exaggerated demands for nurturing and support. Sometimes these symptoms develop into attachment disorders that can be difficult to treat (O'Connor, Bredenkamp, & Rutter, 1999). It takes a very committed and resilient parent to continue caring for a child who does not reinforce attempts at caregiving and who exhibits these kinds of significant emotional and behavior problems.

SUBSTANCE-ABUSING FAMILIES

Children whose parents are alcoholic live in an unpredictable family environment, coping with stress that may disrupt their ability to perform in school and lead to other emotional problems (Casa-Gil & Navarro-Guzman, 2002). Many individuals with alcoholism become polysubstance abusers, addicted to other drugs as well. The codependency movement, which emphasizes the effects of addiction on family members, and groups such as Adult Children of Alcoholics (ACOA) and Al-Anon have brought increasing attention to the effects of parental substance abuse on child development. Any review of this topic must examine the role of biologic-genetic mechanisms and environmental mechanisms in creating increased risk for psychological problems among children of those who abuse substances.

Biologic factors affecting children of those who abuse substances include **fetal alcohol syndrome,** nutritional deficits stemming from neglect, and neuropsychiatric dysfunction related to overstimulation or understimulation (Kaemingk & Paquette, 1999). Genetic factors are at least partly responsible for the well-documented increased risk for substance abuse among children whose parents abuse substances. Recent studies are beginning to link a family history of anxiety disorders and alcoholism with genetically transmitted anxiety disorders, which may be a precursor to alcohol abuse. The precise mechanism of family transmission of alcoholism remains unknown. Recent studies suggest that children of those who abuse substances may inherit a predisposition to a nonspecific form of biologic dysregulation that may be expressed phenotypically, either as alcoholism or some other psychiatric disorder (e.g., hyperactivity, conduct disorder, depression), depending on the individual's developmental history.

Children of those who abuse substances are at high risk for both substance abuse and behavior disorders (Mylant, Ide, Cuevas, & Meehan, 2002). Moreover, some evidence shows that other factors related to addiction, such as family stress, violence, divorce, dysfunction, and other concurrent parental psychiatric disorders (e.g., depression, anxiety), are as important as the alcoholism itself in increasing this risk (Ritter, Stewart, Bernet, Coe, & Brown, 2002). The experience of growing up in a substance-abusing family is marked by unpredictability, fear, and helplessness because of the cyclic nature of addictive patterns.

The literature on children of parents who are alcoholic has described several typical roles that children assume, including the "hero" (overly responsible children who may ignore their own needs to take care of parents and other children), "scapegoat" (problem children who divert attention away from the parent with alcoholism), "mascot" (family clowns who relieve tension and mask feelings through joking), and "lost child" (children who suffer in silence but may exhibit difficulties at school or in later life) (Veronie & Freuhstorfer, 2001). These roles, combined with the enabling behaviors of other family members who attempt to cover up and minimize the effects of the addiction, may become so rigid and effective in masking the problem that children of substance abusers may not come to the attention of mental health professionals until after the parent stops drinking and family roles are disrupted.

Even for children who do not experience significant psychopathology, the experience of growing up in a substance-abusing family can lead to a poor self-concept when children feel responsible for their parents' behavior, become isolated, and learn to mistrust their own perceptions because the family denies the reality of the addiction. Despite the well-documented risk for children in substance-abusing families, there is no uniform pattern of outcomes, and many children demonstrate resilience (Harter, 2000). **Resilience** is the phenomenon by which some children at risk for psychopathology—because of genetic and/or experiential circumstances—attain good mental health, maintain hope, and achieve healthy outcomes (Masten, 2001). Again, individual protective factors and preventive interventions are paramount.

Intervention Approaches

Mental health promotion with children, adolescents, and their families encompasses the full range of preventive

> **FAME AND FORTUNE**
>
> *The Resilience of Dave Pelzer*
>
> **Public Persona**
>
> Dave Pelzer entered the U.S. Air Force at age 18 years and managed to develop into a dedicated, sensitive human being who worked to help other children as a juvenile hall counselor, youth service worker, and adviser to foster care and youth service boards. He is now a noted author with a fifth book recently published and a busy speaking schedule. Dave has appeared on numerous television shows, including "Oprah." He is especially admired for his sense of humor, intriguing outlook on life, and sense of personal responsibility. Undoubtedly these personal qualities served as protective factors contributing to his mental health throughout childhood and into his current life.
>
> **Personal Realities**
>
> Dave Pelzer is a survivor of extreme physical and emotional abuse by his alcoholic mother. He is the author of five internationally best-selling books (best known for *A Child Called It*) that chronicle his experience of abuse, foster placement, and rescue by teachers who reported his abuse and got him the help he needed at the age of 12 years. Although Dave endured years of torture, he is a wonderful example of resilient coping.

efforts discussed in Chapter 3. The new millennium began with the Surgeon General's first-ever Report on Mental Health, which concluded with a national action plan emphasizing preventive interventions with children, calling on families as essential partners in this effort (Raphael, 2001). The overall philosophy of nursing is to advocate for the least restrictive type of intervention possible. This means focusing on interventions that allow maximal autonomy for the child and family, that keep the family unit intact, if possible, and that provide the appropriate level of care to meet the needs of the child and family. A continuum of modalities of care is available to children and families (Fig. 28.3).

Professional nursing emphasizes an interdisciplinary approach in which the nurse acts as coordinator, case manager, and advocate to establish linkages with physicians and nurse practitioners, teachers, speech and language specialists, social workers, and other professionals to develop and implement a comprehensive biopsychosocial plan of intervention (Box 28.3). A view of parents as partners should be foremost. In the past, parents were viewed as the culprits in creating children's mental health problems and were treated as patients themselves. Recent insights into the biologic and genetic origins of psychiatric disorders have contributed to a shift from blaming parents to seeking their collaboration in treatment.

Psychoeducational programs are a particularly effective form of mental health intervention. These programs are designed to teach parents and children basic coping skills for dealing with various stressors. Among other techniques, they use the process of **normalization** (i.e., teaching families what are normal behaviors and expected responses) and provide families with information about normal child development and expected reactions to various stressors so that they will feel less isolated, know what to expect, and put their reactions into perspective. For example, if families learn that anger is a natural part of grieving, they will be less likely to view it as abnormal and more likely to accept and cope with it constructively. Parallel curricula can be established, with concurrent psychoeducational groups for adults and children. Most foster care agencies now provide a program of education and training for prospective foster parents to help them know what to expect and how to help the child adjust to placement.

Social skills training is one psychoeducational approach that has been useful with youth who have low self-esteem, aggressive behavior, or a high risk for sub-

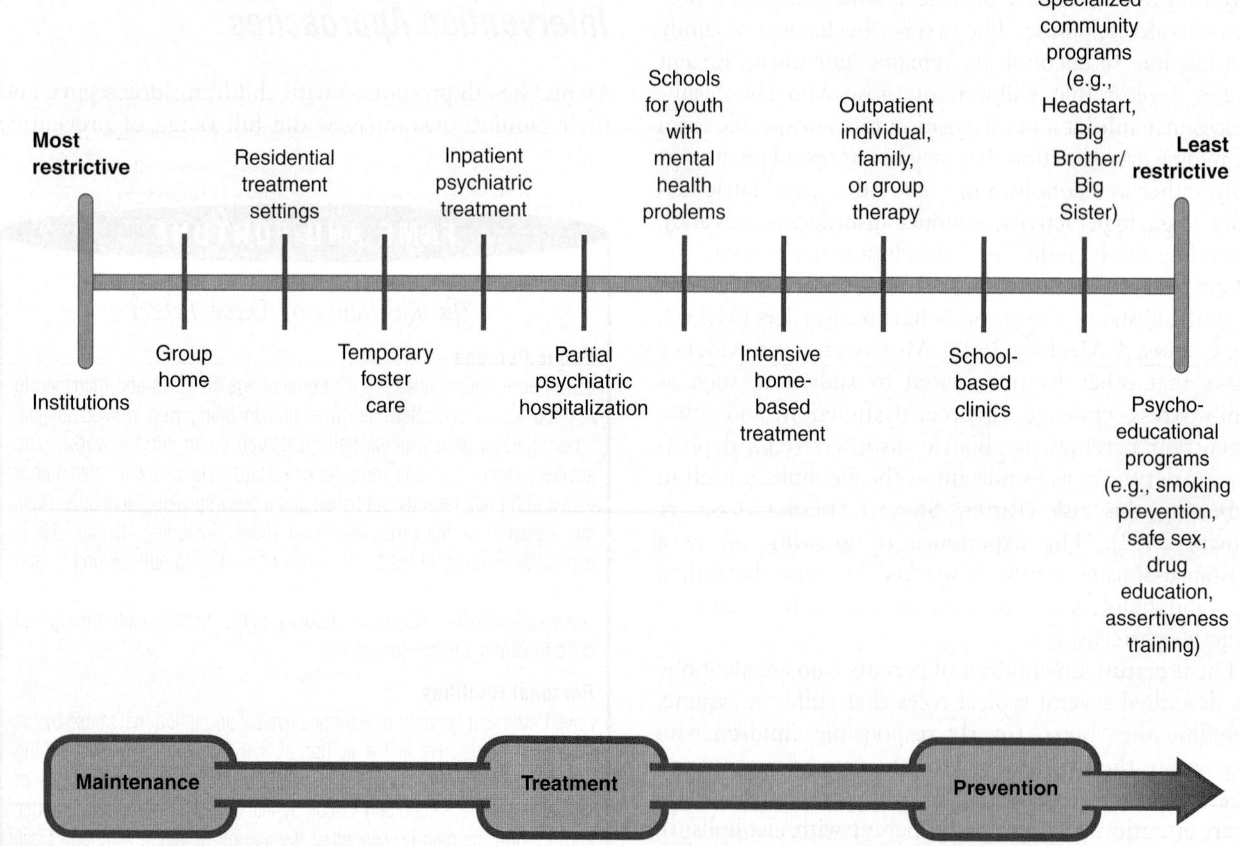

FIGURE 28.3. The continuum of mental health care for children and adolescents.

BOX 28.3

Clinical Vignette: Preventive Interventions with an Adolescent in Crisis

Ben and Rita were just transferred to a second foster home after being removed from their mother's care when she relapsed on cocaine and left them unattended. The plan is for the two children to return to their mother's home after she completes a 30-day drug treatment program. Ben, a high school freshman, is in the school nurse's office asking for aspirin for another headache.

The nurse notices that Ben's nose looks inflamed, he is sniffling, and he seems more "hyper" than usual. In a concerned tone of voice, she asks him if he's been using cocaine and he snaps back, "Just because my mother's a coke head doesn't give you the right to suspect me!" When the nurse gently says, "Tell me about what's been happening with your mother; I had no idea," Ben responds less defensively and explains the situation about the foster home and his mother's drug problem. He says that if it weren't for Rita, his younger sister, he would have run away by now. His foster parents are "making him" go to school, but he's going to drop out as soon as he returns to live with his mother. The only thing that he likes about school is playing basketball, and the basketball coach, who is his gym teacher, wants him on the team.

After a lengthy talk with Ben, the nurse finishes the assessment interview and concludes that he is at risk for drug abuse, running away, and dropping out of school. He is also showing symptoms of depression, which he may be attempting to medicate with cocaine. Protective factors for Ben include his strong attachment to his sister, his ability and willingness to express his thoughts and feelings, his interest in basketball, and a positive relationship with the basketball coach.

The nurse develops a plan with Ben to attend the weekly drug and alcohol discussion group at the school, so that he can talk with other teens from substance-abusing families and learn coping skills to prevent addiction. The nurse contacts the basketball coach, who agrees to find a student mentor who can shoot hoops with Ben and help him come up with a plan to stay in school, maybe find a part-time job, and join the basketball team. Ben agrees to check in regularly with the nurse to report how the plan is working and revise it if needed. The nurse feels optimistic that with support from his peers, coach, mentor, and herself, Ben can overcome what is probably a genetically based risk for depression and addiction. Ben shows signs of resilience. He is motivated to "keep his act together for Rita," capable of forming positive attachments, and willing to seek help when he knows where to find it.

stance abuse (Cavell, Ennett, & Meehan, 2001). Social skills training involves instruction, feedback, support, and practice with learning behaviors that help children to interact more effectively with peers and adults. When combined with assertiveness training, social skills training can be particularly helpful in providing children with coping skills to resist engaging in addictive or antisocial behaviors and to prevent social withdrawal under stress. Social skills training may be particularly helpful for children who are bullies or who are rejected by their peers (Fopma-Loy, 2000).

Bibliotherapy involves the use of books and other reading materials to help individuals cope with various life stressors. It is a particularly potent form of intervention because it empowers families to learn and develop coping mechanisms on their own. A wide variety of books are available to help children understand issues such as death, divorce, chronic illness, stepfamilies, adoption, and birth of a sibling. In addition, many mental health organizations and public health agencies have pamphlets designed to educate parents about various physical and psychological problems. In addition to providing concrete information and advice, these reading materials help to reduce anxiety by pointing out common reactions to the various stressors so that families do not feel alone.

Support groups are available for just about every kind of stressor that a family can experience, including substance abuse, death, divorce, and coping with a chronic illness. Both parents and children in groups can experience Yalom's (2005) healing effects of group therapy, including group cohesiveness, universality (awareness of the normalcy and commonality of one's reactions), catharsis, hope, and altruism (being able to help others).

Finally, **early intervention programs,** possibly the most important form of primary prevention available to children and families, offer regular home visits, support, education, and concrete services to those in need. Research supports the effectiveness of these programs, which may be the key to preventing the placement of children outside the home (Gimpel & Holland, 2003; Tomlin & Viehweg, 2003). The assumption underlying these programs is that parents are the most consistent and important figures in children's lives, and they should be afforded the opportunity to define their own needs and priorities. With support and education, parents will be empowered to respond more effectively to their children.

Historically, nurses have been underused in school-based mental health efforts, although schools are good locations for other early intervention programs because they are physically near the families they serve and are less intimidating than mental health centers. Programs can be targeted for very young children before symptoms have time to develop. Studies show that by fourth grade, a large number of young children already use some kind of substance (e.g., inhalants, which are toxic). So prevention efforts may be crucial in the early grades (Finke et al., 2002).

In conclusion, undertaking interventions to promote the mental health of children and adolescents is time and effort well spent. Many adult mental health problems can be prevented, coped with more effectively, or at least reduced in their scope and severity through focused intervention with children and families. Children lack the power and voice to fight for their own needs, making them one of the most vulnerable groups in society. By virtue of their close interaction with families, nurses are in a key position to identify the mental health needs of children and intervene, particularly in times of crisis. The feeling that comes from making a difference can be fulfilling and long-lasting.

SUMMARY OF KEY POINTS

- Nurses working with children and adolescents are in a key position to identify risk and protective factors for psychopathology and to intervene to reduce risk.
- Nurses who are aware of normal developmental processes can educate parents about their children's behaviors, help them better understand their children's reactions to stress, and decide when intervention may be warranted.
- If the process of normal biologic maturation in childhood is disrupted through trauma or neglect, developmental delays and disorders can occur, some of which may have irreversible effects.
- From early infancy, children exhibit different kinds of temperaments that are at least partially biologically determined.
- Studies of attachment show that the quality of the emotional bond between the child and parental figure is an important determinant of the success of later relationships.
- Research shows that children who experience major losses, such as death or divorce, are at risk for developing mental health problems.
- Sibling relationships have significant effects on personality development. Positive sibling relationships can be protective factors against the development of mental health problems.
- Medical problems in childhood and adolescence may cause psychological problems when illness leads to regression or lack of full participation in family, school, and social activities.
- Striving for identity and independence may lead adolescents to participate in high-risk activities (e.g., drug use, unprotected sex, smoking, delinquent behaviors) that may lead to mental health problems.
- Poverty, homelessness, abuse, neglect, and parental alcoholism all create conditions that undermine a child's ability to make normal developmental gains and contribute to vulnerability for various emotional and behavioral problems.
- Children who experience disrupted attachments because of out-of-home placements may have difficulty forming close relationships with their new parents and trusting others.
- Family support services and early intervention programs are designed to prevent removal of the child from the family as a result of abuse or neglect and to maintain a strong, nurturing family system.
- Psychoeducational approaches, such as training opportunities, group experiences, and bibliotherapy provide children and families with the information and skills to promote their own mental health.

CRITICAL THINKING CHALLENGES

1. Analyze a case of a family that is grieving a loss and compare the parents' and children's reactions. Include an evaluation of how each child's reactions differ, depending on his or her developmental level.
2. Watch a movie or read a book that provides a child's view of death, divorce, or some other loss and consider how adults may be insensitive to the child's reactions.
3. Examine your own developmental history and pinpoint periods when stressful life events might have increased risk for emotional problems for you or other family members. What protective factors in your own personality and coping skills and in the environment around you helped you to maintain your good mental health?
4. What aspects of life are more stressful for children than for adults (i.e., how is it different to experience life as a child)?
5. Examine how your own social and cultural background may either facilitate or create barriers to your ability to interact with families from other ethnic groups or those who are poor or homeless.
6. Allow yourself to reflect on how your own judgmental attitudes might interfere with your ability to communicate effectively with families who have abused or neglected their children.
7. Why is the process of normalization of feelings such a powerful intervention with children and families? What kinds of mental health issues, developmental processes, or both would benefit from teaching related to normal reactions? How can nurses incorporate this kind of intervention into their practice roles?
8. How can nurses expand their roles to have maximal effects on primary, secondary, and tertiary mental health intervention with children and families?

Antwone Fisher. 2002. This is the true story of a young naval officer who grew up in the foster care system and endured horrible abuse. The autobiography, called *Finding Fish*, gives an even more detailed, riveting account of this young man's ability to overcome his abusive childhood, find his biological family, and grow into a loving husband and father.

VIEWING POINTS: Explain how Antwone's violent outbursts in the Navy may have developed as an outcome of his childhood experiences of loss, abuse, and poverty. What do you think allowed Antwone to ultimately express his anger more constructively and use psychotherapy as a healing relationship? How could the social workers and other professionals have intervened differently to advocate for Antwone?

Because of Winn Dixie (2005). This is a heart-rending account of a 10-year-old girl who overcomes her loneliness after moving to a small town by adopting a dog and reaching out to people in her new community. The movie explores such issues as parental separation, single parenting, substance abuse, and childhood grieving.

VIEWING POINTS: Describe how Opal's grieving process is typical of school-aged children and how it differs from that of her father. What aspects of her coping demonstrate resilience? Explain the importance of Opal's dog, Winn Dixie, in the healing process for this family. Discuss how pets may play a key role in the mental health of children. How is the relationship with a pet similar and different from the role of a sibling?

My Girl. 1991. This story lovingly portrays a young girl coping with her mother's death. It provides a thoughtful general analysis of death because the family runs a funeral parlor.

VIEWING POINTS: How is the depiction of the child's grieving process in this film typical of childhood mourning? What aspects of it appear to be uniquely influenced by her family and the circumstances? How could the adults in the film have been more sensitive to the child's fears and anxieties about death?

To Kill a Mockingbird. 1962. The narrator of this beautiful film is a young girl growing up in the South before the Civil Rights Movement. The story illustrates several important factors that can influence a child's development, including single-parent families, cultural factors, the effects of abuse and alcoholism, and the child's attempt to reconcile good and evil forces in the world.

VIEWING POINTS: How effective is this single-parent family in coping with life stresses and developmental changes? What aspects of the family's functioning appear particularly strong? Compare Scout and Jem's upbringing to that of the young woman from the family with alcoholism. In what ways does this young girl appear to be at risk for developing mental health problems?

The Breakfast Club. 1985. This funny, poignant portrayal of adolescence is told through the eyes of several teens from different backgrounds brought together when they are assigned to all-day Saturday detention. It illustrates the heightened sense of drama that typifies adolescence, identity concerns, and peer relationship struggles.

VIEWING POINTS. Which of these adolescents do you consider to be most at risk for having mental health problems? State the reasons for your choice. What are some factors that appear to be contributing to the risk-taking and acting-out behaviors among these adolescents?

REFERENCES

Anthony, K. K., Gil, K. M., & Schanberg, L. E. (2003). Parental perceptions of child vulnerability in children with chronic illness. *Journal of Pediatric Psychology, 28*(3), 185–190.

Botvin, G. J. (2000). Preventing drug abuse in schools: Social and competence enhancement approaches targeting individual-level etiologic factors. *Addictive Behaviors, 25*(6), 887–897.

Bowlby, J. (1960). Grief and mourning in infancy and early childhood. *Psychoanalytic Study of the Child, 15*, 9–52.

Brody, G. H. (1998). Sibling relationship quality: Its causes and consequences. *Annual Review of Psychology, 49*, 1–24.

Cance, A. M., Paradise, M., Ginzler, J. A., Embry, L., Morgan, C. J., Lohr, Y., & Theofelis, J. (2000). The characteristics and mental health of homeless adolescents: Age and gender differences. *Journal of Emotional & Behavior Disorders, 8*(4), 230–239.

Casa-Gil, M. J., & Navarro-Guzman, J. I. (2002). School characteristics among children of alcoholic parents. *Psychological Reports, 90*(1), 341–348.

Cavell, T., Ennett, S. T., & Meehan, B. T. (2001). Preventing alcohol and substance abuse. In J. N. Hughes, A. M. LaGreca, & J. C. Conoley (Eds.), *Handbook of psychological services for children and adolescents* (pp. 133–160). Oxford: Oxford University Press.

Deering, C. G., & Cody, D. J. (2002). Communicating effectively with children and adolescents. *American Journal of Nursing, 102*(3), 34–42.

Deering, C. G., & Cody, D. J. (2002). Communicating with children and adolescents. *American Journal of Nursing, 104*(13), 34.

Eggert, L. L., Thompson, E. A., Randell, B. P., & Pike, K. (2002). Preliminary effects of brief school-based prevention approaches for reducing youth suicide: Risk behaviors, depression, and drug involvement. *Journal of Child and Adolescent Psychiatric Nursing, 15*(2), 48–64.

Finke, L., Williams, J., Ritter, M., Kemper, D., Kersey, S., Nightenhauser, J., Autry, K., Going, C., Wulfman, G., & Hail, A. (2002). Survival against drugs: Education for school-age children. *Journal of Child and Adolescent Psychiatric Nursing, 15*(4), 163–169.

Fopma-Loy, J. (2000). Peer rejection and neglect of latency age children: Pathways and group psychotherapy model. *Journal of Child and Adolescent Psychiatric Nursing, 13*, 29–38.

Gimpel, G. A. & Holland, M. L. (2003). Emotional and Behavioral problems of Young Children: Effective Interventions in the Preschool and Kindergarden Years. New York: Guilford Press.

Gorzka, P. (1999). Homeless parents' perceptions of parenting stress. *Journal of Child and Adolescent Psychiatric Nursing, 12*, 7–16.

Harter, S. (2000). Psychosocial adjustment of adult children of alcoholics: A review of recent empirical literature. *Clinical Psychology Review, 20*(3), 311–337.

Helfer, M. E., Kemper, S., & Kongman, R. D. (1997). *The battered child.* Chicago: University of Chicago Press.

Hetherington, E. M., & Kelly, J. (2002). *For better or for worse: Divorce reconsidered.* New York: WW Norton.

Jeynes, W. (2002). *Divorce, family structure, and the academic success of children.* New York: Haworth Press.

Kaemingk, K., & Paquette, A. (1999). Effects of prenatal alcohol exposure on neuropsychological functioning. *Developmental Neuropsychology, 15,* 111–140.

Kirwin, K. M., & Hamrin, V. (2005). Decreasing risk of complicated bereavement and future psychiatric disorders in children. *Journal of Child and Adolescent Psychiatric Nursing, 18*(2), 62–78.

Kramer, L. & Bank, L. (2005). Sibling relationship contributes to individual and family well-being. *Journal of Family Psychology, 19*(4), 483–485.

Kramer, L., & Rambsburg, D. (2002). Advice given to parents on welcoming a second child: A critical review. *Family Relations: Interdisciplinary Journal of Applied Family Studies, 51*(1), 2–14.

LeBlanc L. A., Goldsmith, T., & Patel, D. R. (2003). Behavioral aspects of chronic illness in children and adolescents. *Pediatric Clinics of North America, 50*(4), 859–878.

Leventhal, T., & Brooks-Gunn, J. (2000). The neighborhoods they live in: The effects of neighborhood residence on child and adolescent outcomes. *Psychological Bulletin, 126,* 309–337.

Lewis, M., & Vitulano, L. A. (2003). Biopsychosocial issues and risk factors in the family when the child has a chronic illness. *Child & Adolescent Psychiatric Clinics of North America, 12*(3), 389–399.

MacLeod, J., & Nelson, G. (2000). Programs for the promotion of family wellness and the prevention of child maltreatment: A meta-analytic review. *Child Abuse & Neglect, 24*(9), 1127–1149.

Masten, A. S. (2001). Ordinary magic: Resilience processes in development. *American Psychologist, 56*(3), 227–238.

Menke, E. M. (1998). The mental health of homeless school-age children. *Journal of Child and Adolescent Psychiatric Nursing, 11,* 87–98.

Moser, R. P., & Jacob, T. (2002). Parental and sibling effects in adolescent outcomes. *Psychological Reports, 91*(2), 463–479.

Murray, S. K., Baker, A. W., & Lewin, L. (2002). Screening families with young children for child maltreatment potential. *Pediatric Nursing, 26,* 47–54.

Mylant, M. L., Ide, B., Cuevas, E., & Meehan, M. (2002). Adolescent children of alcoholics: Vulnerable or resilient? *Journal of the American Psychiatric Nurses Association, 8*(2), 57–64.

O'Connor, T. G., Bredenkamp, D., & Rutter, M. (1999). Attachment disturbances and disorders in children exposed to early severe deprivation. *Infant Mental Health Journal, 20*(1), 10–29.

Pruett, M. K., Williams, T. Y., Insabella, G., & Little, T. D. (2003). Family and legal indicators of child adjustment to divorce among families with young children. *Journal of Family Psychology, 17*(2), 169–180.

Putnam, F. W. (2003). Ten-year research update review: Child sexual abuse. *Journal of the American Academy of Child & Adolescent Psychiatry, 42*(3), 269–278.

Raphael, S. (2001). A national action agenda for children's mental health. *Journal of Child and Adolescent Psychiatric Nursing, 14*(4), 193–198.

Rew, L. (2003). A theory of taking care of oneself grounded in experiences of homeless youth. *Nursing Research, 52*(4), 234–241.

Ritter, J., Stewart, M., Bernet, C., Coe, M., & Brown, S. A. (2002). Effects of childhood exposure to familial alcoholism and family violence on adolescent substance use, conduct problems, and self-esteem. *Journal of Traumatic Stress, 15*(2), 113–122.

Reifman, A., Villa, L. C., Amans, J. A., Rethinam, V., & Telesca, T. Y. (2001). Children of divorce in the 1990's: A meta-analysis. *Journal of Divorce and Remarriage, 35*(1–2), 27–36.

Sharpe, D., & Rossiter, L. (2002). Siblings of children with a chronic illness: A meta-analysis. *Journal of Pediatric Psychology, 27*(8), 699–710.

Slomkowski, C., Rende, R., Conger, K. J., Simons, R. L., & Conger, R. D. (2001). Sisters, brothers, and delinquency: Evaluating social influence during early and middle adolescence. *Child Development, 72*(1), 271–283.

Sun, U., & Li, Y. (2002). Children's well-being during parents' marital disruption process: A pooled time-series analysis. *Journal of Marriage and the Family, 64*(2), 472–488.

Taussig, H. N. (2002). Risk behaviors in maltreated youth placed in foster care: A longitudinal study of protective and vulnerability factors. *Child Abuse & Neglect, 26*(11), 1179–1199.

Tomlin, A. M., & Viehweg, S. A. (2003). Infant mental health: Making a difference. *Professional Psychology: Research and Practice, 34*(6), 617–625.

U.S. Department of Commerce News. (September 26, 2003). www.census.gov/Press-Release/www/2003/cb03-153.html

Van Epps, J., Opie, N. D., & Goodwin, T. (1997). Themes in the bereavement experience of inner city adolescents. *Journal of Child and Adolescent Psychiatric Nursing, 10,* 25–36.

Veronie, L., & Freuhstorfer, D. B. (2001). Gender, birth order and family role identification among children of alcoholics. *Current Psychology: Developmental, Learning, Personality, Social, 20*(1), 53–67.

Warren, J. K., Gary, F. A., & Moorhead, M. S. (1997). Runaway youths in a Southern community: Four critical areas of inquiry. *Journal of Child and Adolescent Psychiatric Nursing, 10*(2), 26–35.

Yalom, I. D., with Leszcz, M. (2005). *The theory and practice of group psychotherapy* (5th ed.) New York: Basic Books.

Zenah, C. H., Larrieu, J. A., Heller, S. S., Valliere, J., Hinshaw-Fuselier, S., Aoki, Y., & Drilling, M. (2001). Evaluation of a preventive intervention for maltreated infants and toddlers in foster care. *Journal of the American Academy of Child & Adolescent Psychiatry, 40*(2), 214–221.

CHAPTER 29

Psychiatric Disorders Diagnosed in Childhood and Adolescence

Lawrence Scahill, Vanya Hamrin, Catherine Gray Deering, and Maryellen Pachlar

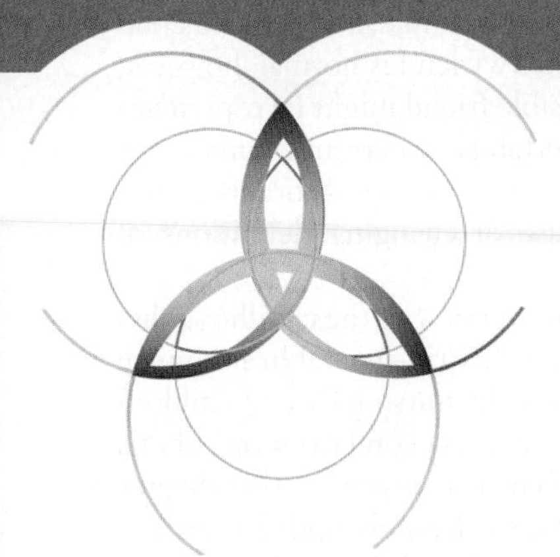

KEY CONCEPTS

- attention
- autistic disorder
- developmental delay
- hyperactivity
- impulsiveness
- pervasive developmental disorders
- tics

LEARNING OBJECTIVES

After studying this chapter, you will be able to:

- Identify the disorders usually first diagnosed in infancy, childhood, or adolescence, according to the *Diagnostic and Statistical Manual of Mental Disorders*, 4th edition, Text revision *(DSM-IV-TR)*.
- Differentiate between mental retardation and pervasive developmental disorders.
- Identify the biopsychosocial dimensions of the developmental disorders of childhood.
- Discuss the nursing care of children with pervasive developmental disorders.
- Compare the disruptive behavior disorders: attention-deficit hyperactivity disorder, oppositional defiant disorder, and conduct disorder.
- Relate the assessment data of children with attention-deficit hyperactivity disorder to the development of nursing diagnoses, interventions, and evaluation of outcomes.
- Identify the steps involved in fundamental behavior modification interventions, such as "time out," for children.
- Discuss the epidemiology, etiology, psychopharmacologic interventions, and nursing care of children with disorders of mood and anxiety.
- Discuss the epidemiology, etiology, psychopharmacologic interventions, and nursing care of children with tic disorders.
- Discuss behavioral intervention strategies for the treatment of encopresis.

KEY TERMS

• ascertainment bias • autism • communication disorders • concordant • dyslexia • encopresis • enuresis • externalizing disorders • internalizing disorders • learning disorder • mental retardation • phonologic processing • school phobia • stereotypic behavior

The understanding of child psychiatric disorders has benefited from advances in several related fields, including developmental biology, neuroanatomy, psychopharmacology, genetics, and epidemiology. Before the introduction of the third edition of the American Psychiatric Association's (APA's) *Diagnostic and Statistical Manual of Mental Disorders* (*DSM-III*) in 1980, clinicians based their diagnostic decisions on subjective impressions, rather than on clearly defined diagnostic criteria. Because the clinician's theoretic orientation directly influenced these subjective impressions, psychiatric diagnoses were notoriously unreliable.

The aims of any diagnostic system are to (1) foster communication between clinicians, (2) provide insight concerning etiology, and (3) predict long-term outcomes. Thus, a reliable method for making psychiatric diagnoses is necessary for ongoing research efforts concerning the etiology and outcome of childhood disorders. Because they are categorical in nature without clear categorical boundaries, current psychiatric diagnoses for children and adolescents provide only limited explanations of a condition's etiology or outcomes. However, the clear diagnostic criteria and the multiaxial system introduced by *DSM-III* facilitate communication among clinicians. This chapter uses criteria from the current *Diagnostic and Statistical Manual of Mental Disorders* (4th edition, Text revision) (*DSM-IV-TR;* APA, 2000) in defining childhood disorders. *The DSM-IV-TR* contains 10 categories of disorders, as listed in Table 29.1. Despite their limitations, the *DSM-III* and *DSM-IV-TR* represent major steps forward in defining psychiatric disorders of childhood.

Child psychopathology can be classified according to several broad categories: developmental disorders, disruptive behavior disorders, mood and anxiety disorders, tic disorders, and psychotic disorders. The prevalence of child psychiatric disorders varies across these categories. For example, child schizophrenia is rare, whereas attention-deficit hyperactivity disorder (ADHD) is relatively common. In cited estimates of prevalence for psychiatric disorders of childhood, the numbers usually include adolescents; however, it should be noted that some of these disorders vary with age; for example, depression is more common in adolescents than in younger children. Gender ratio may also vary with some disorders according to age. For example, depression is probably more common in boys in children younger than 12 years of age but is more common in girls during adolescence.

A report by the Surgeon General estimates that 10% of all 9- to 17-year-olds have serious emotional disturbances with extreme functional impairment (Satcher, 2001). These percentages translate into an estimated 8 million American children younger than 18 years with a psychiatric disorder. Of these, only 20% are receiving appropriate treatment. This discrepancy appears to be the result of limited access to treatment facilities, either because of financial constraints or because appropriate mental health services for children are simply unavailable (Satcher). Psychiatric problems are less easily diagnosed in children than they are in adults. One factor contributing to this difference is that sometimes the symptoms of disorders are difficult to distinguish from the turbulence of normal growth and development. For example, a 4-year-old child who has an invisible imaginary friend is normal; however, an adolescent with an invisible friend might be experiencing a hallucination. The certainty of current estimates for the frequency of the various psychiatric disorders is also inconsistent, partly because of changing definitions of these disorders.

This chapter presents an overview of the childhood disorders that the generalist psychiatric–mental health nurse may encounter and discusses the nursing care of children with these problems. Because it is beyond the scope of this text to present all child psychiatric disorders, this chapter focuses on developmental disorders, disruptive behavior, mood and anxiety, and tic disorders. It highlights in detail ADHD. It also briefly describes childhood schizophrenia and elimination disorders.

• NCLEXNOTE

NCLEXNOTE All of the psychiatric disorders of childhood and adolescence should be viewed within the context of growth and development models. Safety and self-esteem are priority considerations.

Developmental Disorders of Childhood

Under the primary influences of genes and environment, development may be said to proceed along several pathways, such as attention, cognition, language, affect, and social and moral behavior. The developmental disorders of childhood include several conditions that are etiologically unrelated; however, their common feature is a significant delay in one or more lines of development. Some of these developmental pathways and developmental delays are closely interwoven. For example, a language delay can interfere with a child's social development and contribute to behavior problems (Paul, 2002). The *DSM-IV-TR* classifies developmental disorders in several categories, including mental retardation, pervasive developmental disorders, and specific developmental disorders. It places mental retardation on Axis II and records pervasive developmental disorders and specific developmental disorders on Axis I. This is a change from the *DSM-III*, which could be a source of confusion when reading child psychiatric literature or past medical records.

Table 29.1 Disorders Usually First Diagnosed in Infancy, Childhood, or Adolescence

Disorder	Characteristics
Mental Retardation	
Mild Moderate Severe Profound Severity unspecified	Significantly below-average intellectual functioning (IQ about 70 or below) with onset before age 18 years and concurrent impairments in adaptive functioning
Learning Disorders	
Reading disorder Mathematics disorder Disorder of written expression Learning disorders not otherwise specified	Academic functioning substantially below that expected given the person's chronologic age, measured intelligence, and age-appropriate education
Motor Skills Disorders	
Developmental coordination disorder	Motor coordination substantially below that expected given the person's chronologic age and measured intelligence
Communication Disorders	
Expressive language disorder Mixed receptive–expressive language disorder Phonologic disorder Stuttering Communication disorder not otherwise specified	Significant delay or deviance in speech or language
Pervasive Developmental Disorders	
Autistic disorder Asperger's disorder Pervasive developmental disorder not otherwise specified Rett's disorder Childhood disintegrative disorder	Severe deficits in multiple areas of development; these include impairment in reciprocal social interaction, impairment in communication, and the presence of stereotyped behavior, restricted interests, and activities
Attention-Deficit and Disruptive Behavior Disorders	
Predominantly inattentive type Predominantly hyperactive–impulsive type Combined type	Prominent symptoms of inattention and/or hyperactivity–impulsivity
Conduct disorder	A pattern of behavior that violates the basic rights of others or major age-appropriate societal norms or rules
Oppositional defiant disorder	A pattern of negativistic, hostile, and defiant behavior
Feeding and Eating Disorders of Infancy or Early Childhood	
Pica Rumination disorder Feeding disorder of infancy or early childhood	Persistent disturbances in feeding and eating
Tic Disorders	
Tourette's disorder Chronic motor or vocal tic disorder Transient tic disorder Tic disorder not otherwise specified	Vocal or motor tics
Elimination Disorders	
Encopresis	Repeated passage of feces into inappropriate places
Enuresis	Repeated voiding of urine into inappropriate places
Other Disorders of Infancy, Childhood, or Adolescence	
Separation anxiety disorder	Developmentally inappropriate and excessive anxiety concerning separation from home or those to whom the child is attached
Selective mutism	A consistent failure to speak in specific social situations despite speaking in other situations
Reactive attachment disorder of infancy or early childhood	Markedly disturbed and developmentally inappropriate social relatedness that occurs in most contexts and is associated with physical and/or emotional neglect
Stereotypic movement disorder	Repetitive, seemingly driven, and nonfunctional motor behavior that markedly interferes with normal activities and at times may result in bodily injury

Data from American Psychiatric Association (2000). *Diagnostic and statistical manual of mental disorders* (4th ed., text revision)(pp.39–41). Washington, DC: Author.

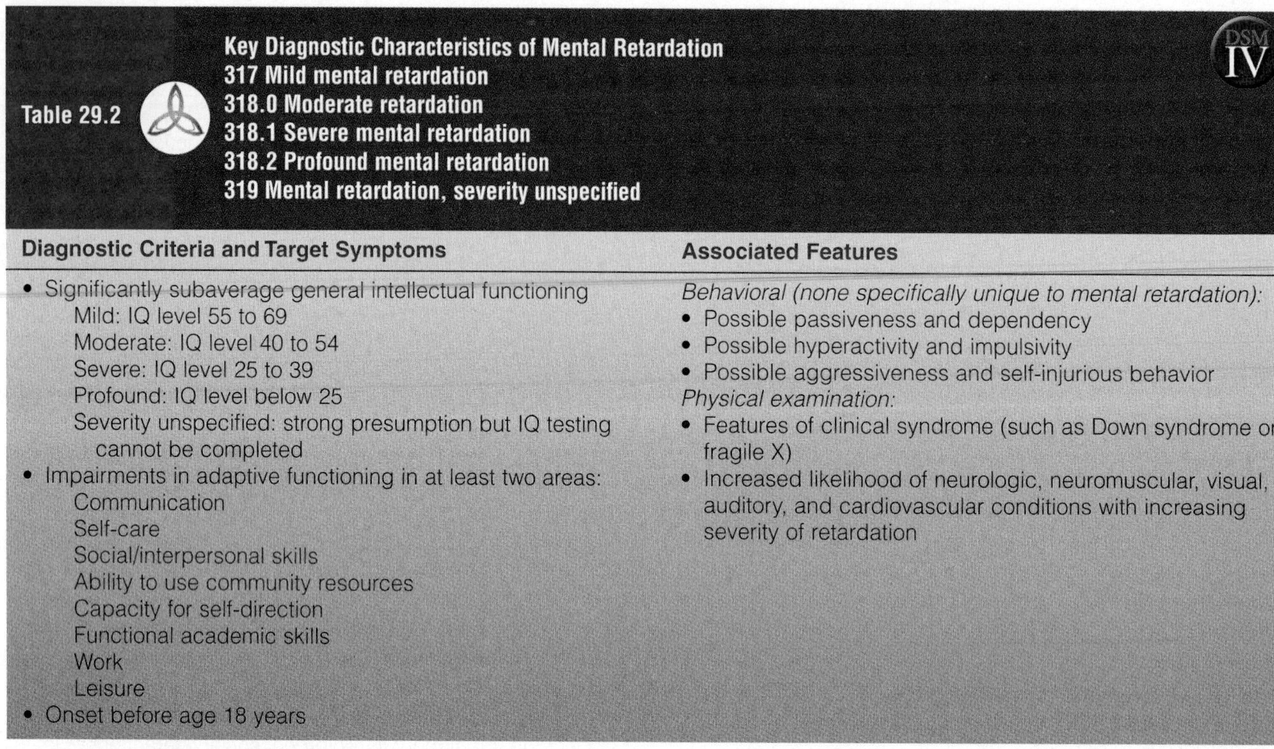

Table 29.2 — DSM IV

Key Diagnostic Characteristics of Mental Retardation
317 Mild mental retardation
318.0 Moderate retardation
318.1 Severe mental retardation
318.2 Profound mental retardation
319 Mental retardation, severity unspecified

Diagnostic Criteria and Target Symptoms	Associated Features
• Significantly subaverage general intellectual functioning Mild: IQ level 55 to 69 Moderate: IQ level 40 to 54 Severe: IQ level 25 to 39 Profound: IQ level below 25 Severity unspecified: strong presumption but IQ testing cannot be completed • Impairments in adaptive functioning in at least two areas: Communication Self-care Social/interpersonal skills Ability to use community resources Capacity for self-direction Functional academic skills Work Leisure • Onset before age 18 years	*Behavioral (none specifically unique to mental retardation):* • Possible passiveness and dependency • Possible hyperactivity and impulsivity • Possible aggressiveness and self-injurious behavior *Physical examination:* • Features of clinical syndrome (such as Down syndrome or fragile X) • Increased likelihood of neurologic, neuromuscular, visual, auditory, and cardiovascular conditions with increasing severity of retardation

MENTAL RETARDATION

Mental retardation is defined by significantly below-average intelligence accompanied by impaired adaptive functioning (Table 29.2). The diagnosis is made through clinical assessment of behavioral features, historical accounts from parents and teachers, and performance on standardized tests (Moss & Racusin, 2002), such as the Stanford-Binet or the Wechsler Intelligence Scales for Children. Because intelligence tests have been standardized to a mean of 100 with a standard deviation of 15 points, the usual threshold for mental retardation is an intelligence quotient (IQ) of 70 or less (i.e., two standard deviations below the population mean). The emphasis is not only on intelligence, but also on adaptive behavior and developmental delays. Impaired adaptive functioning is primarily a clinical judgment based on the child's capacity to manage age-appropriate tasks of daily living. However, standardized assessments, such as the Vineland Adaptive Behavior Scales (Sparrow, Balla, & Cicchetti, 1984), are available to assist with determination of the child's capabilities.

Mental retardation is below average intelligence accompanied by impaired adaptive functioning.

Because the diagnosis of mental retardation includes deficits in adaptive functioning, the classification of an individual as mentally retarded is not necessarily lifelong. Some children may be diagnosed at school age as mentally retarded, but the diagnosis is no longer appropriate in some adults because their social skills and occupational functioning may have improved.

Epidemiology and Etiology

No large prevalence study for mental retardation comparable with the Epidemiological Catchment Area (ECA) program for mental disorders has been conducted within the general population. Using the intelligence threshold of an IQ below 70, the prevalence of mental retardation has been estimated at 2%, with a range from 1% to 2.5%. Nearly 90% of those who are mentally retarded are in the mildly retarded range (Volkmar, Klin & Paul, 2004). The rate of co-occurring psychiatric disorders is estimated at 25%, but the rate of nonspecific behavioral problems is much higher (Volkmar & Kiln, 2004). Estimates are that psychosis occurs in 5% to 12% of individuals who are mentally retarded. Some children display symptoms of pervasive developmental disorders (discussed later), such as poor eye contact, extreme difficulty in managing transitions, and repetitive behavior.

Mental retardation has no single cause. Recent evidence indicates that a substantial number of cases of mental retardation result from specific genetic abnormalities, such as fragile X syndrome, trisomy 21 (Down syndrome), and phenylketonuria (PKU). Many other cases appear to result from multifactorial causes, in which several genes combine with environmental factors (e.g., perinatal exposures) to produce the handicap.

BOX 29.1

History and Hallmarks of Childhood and Adolescent Disorders

- Maternal age and health status during pregnancy
- Exposure to medication, alcohol, or other substances during pregnancy
- Course of pregnancy, labor, and delivery
- Infant's health at birth
- Eating, sleeping, and growth in first year
- Health status in first year
- Interest in others in first 2 years
- Motor development
- Mastery of bowel and bladder control
- Speech and language development
- Activity level
- Response to separation (e.g., school entry)
- Regulation of mood and anxiety
- Medical history in early childhood
- Social development
- Interests

Nursing Management

The assessment of a child who is mentally retarded focuses on current adaptive skills, intellectual status, and social functioning. A developmental history is a useful way to gather information about past and current capacities (Box 29.1). The nurse compares these data with normal growth and development. Developmentally delayed children who have not had a psychological evaluation should be considered for referral. These children also require evaluation for other comorbid psychiatric disorders, which may be a challenge because of the child's cognitive limitations. Discussions about feelings and behavior may be too complex for these children.

The nurse also assesses the child's support systems (family, school, rehabilitative, and psychiatric) to ensure that the child's special needs have been identified and are being addressed. For example, a previous evaluation may have recommended occupational therapy to improve the child's motor coordination. However, the family may lack transportation to the recommended center for these services, requiring identification of an acceptable alternative that is closer to home. Individuals with mental retardation may also have a psychiatric disorder or serious behavioral problems. These patients may require carefully constructed behavioral care plans and administration of psychotropic medications (Volkmar, Klin, & Paul, 2004).

The complexity of the child and family's response to mental retardation and other comorbid conditions will determine the nursing diagnoses, planning, and implementation of nursing interventions. Some nursing diagnoses that may be appropriate include Ineffective Coping, Delayed Growth and Development, and Interrupted Family Processes. The overall goals are an optimal level of functioning for the family and eventual independent functioning within a normal social environment for the child. For many children with mental retardation, achieving independence in adulthood will be delayed but not impossible. Nursing interventions include promoting coping skills (interventions directed at building strengths, adapting to change, and maintaining or achieving a higher level of functioning), patient education, and parent education.

Continuum of Care

Children and families may require varying levels of interventions at different times throughout the life cycle. When a child is young, the family requires special academic support and, for some, residential services. The need for psychiatric intervention varies according to the severity of retardation, family functioning, and the existence of other disorders. Feelings of grief and loss in family members (especially parents) related to having a child with a disability may be relieved through family therapy. More specific parent training may be needed to deal with maladaptive behaviors in children with developmental disorders.

PERVASIVE DEVELOPMENTAL DISORDERS

Children with pervasive developmental disorders (PDDs) may or may not be mentally retarded, but they commonly show an uneven pattern of intellectual strengths and weaknesses. Children with PDDs may show a lifelong pattern of being rigid in style, intolerant of change, and prone to behavioral outbursts in response to environmental demands or changes in routine.

KEY CONCEPT Developmental delay means that the child's development is outside the norm, including delayed socialization, communication, peculiar mannerisms, and idiosyncratic interests.

KEY CONCEPT Pervasive developmental disorders are a group of syndromes marked by severe developmental delays in several areas that cannot be attributed to mental retardation.

Types

The *DSM-IV-TR* includes several categories of PDDs, but it is beyond the scope of this chapter to review all of them (Koenig & Scahill, 2001). This section focuses on autistic disorder and Asperger's disorder.

Autistic Disorder

Autistic disorder, or autism, has been a subject of considerable interest and research effort since its original description more than 50 years ago, when Leo Kanner (1943) described the profound isolation of these children and their extreme desire for sameness. Two features distinguish autism from other PDDs: early age of onset (before age 30 months) and severe disturbance in social relatedness. These children appear aloof and indifferent to others and often seem to prefer inanimate objects.

The impairment in communication is severe and affects both verbal and nonverbal communication (APA, 2000). Children with autism manifest delayed and deviant language development, as evidenced by *echolalia* (repetition of words or phrases spoken by others) and a tendency to be extremely concrete in interpretation of language. Pronoun reversals and abnormal intonation are also common. Other common features of autism categorized as **stereotypic behavior** include repetitive rocking, hand flapping, and an extraordinary insistence on sameness. The child may also engage in self-injurious behavior, such as hitting, head banging, or biting. In some children, their unusual interests may evolve into fascination with specific objects, such as fans or air conditioners, or a particular topic, such as Civil War generals.

KEY CONCEPT Autistic disorder is marked impairment of development in social interaction and communication with a restrictive repertoire of activity and interest.

Epidemiology and Etiology

As currently defined, autism affects between 10 and 20 people per 10,000 in the general population (Fombonne, 2003). It occurs in boys more often than girls, with the ratio ranging from 2:1 to 5:1. However, when girls are affected, they tend to be more severely impaired and have poorer outcomes (Volkmar, Klin, & Paul, 2004). About half of children with autism are mentally retarded, and about 25% have seizure disorders. Recent claims that the prevalence of autism is increasing are confounded by improved diagnosis in lower functioning (e.g., low IQ) and higher functioning children.

Numerous theories suggest various causes for autism, including genetics, perinatal insult, and impaired parent–child interactions (Volkmar et al., 2004). It was fashionable in the 1950s and 1960s to believe that the "indifference" of professional parents was a contributing cause of autism. This explanation is no longer seriously considered and almost certainly reflected an **ascertainment bias** (a bias that occurs when the method of identifying cases creates a sample that differs from the population it purports to represent) because professional families were more likely to use the services of major medical centers. It also represents a failure to recognize that the child's disability may have contributed to disturbed parent–child interactions, rather than being an effect of these interactions.

Low IQ and autism recur at a higher-than-expected rate in the siblings of children with autism, and monozygotic twins are more likely to be **concordant** (mutually affected) than are dizygotic twins, suggesting that genetic factors play a role in the disorder. Other proposed causes include perinatal complications, such as exposure to infectious agents or medications during gestation; prematurity; and gestational bleeding. The findings of minor physical anomalies in these children have led to a hypothesis of a first-trimester insult, but controlled studies fail to support a prominent role for perinatal complications in autism (Bolton et al., 1997). Biochemical studies have shown increased platelet serotonin levels, excessive dopaminergic activity, and alteration of endogenous opioids (Novotny, Evers, Barboza, Rawitt, & Hollander, 2003). Despite the substantial body of evidence pointing to a neurobiologic basis, the specific cause remains unknown and may result from multiple factors. Structural and functional imaging studies provide intriguing leads for future inquiry (Courchesne et al., 2003; Schultz et al., 1998; see Fig. 29.1).

Psychopharmacologic Interventions

No medication has proved effective at changing the core social and language deficits of autism. However, numerous psychiatric medications have been used to treat the associated behavioral difficulties in PDDs (see McDougle & Posey, 2003, for a detailed review). Medications can reduce the frequency and intensity of behav-

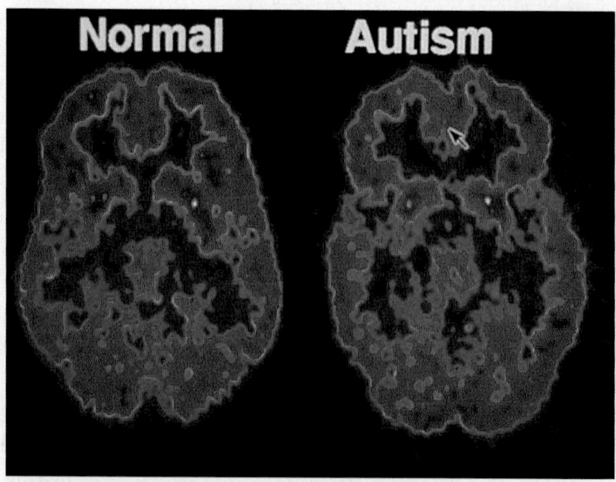

FIGURE 29.1. The patient with autism (*right*) may have decreased metabolic rates in the cingulate gyrus and other associated areas; however, wide heterogeneity in brain metabolic patterns is seen in patients with autism. (Courtesy of Monte S. Buchsbaum, MD, The Mount Sinai Medical Center and School of Medicine, New York, NY.)

ioral disturbances, including hyperactivity, agitation, mood instability, aggression, self-injury, and stereotypic behavior. Haloperidol has demonstrated efficacy in reducing hyperactivity, stereotypic behavior, and emotional lability (Scahill & Martin, 2005). Despite these reported benefits, haloperidol is associated with a range of side effects. Findings from a review of 224 children with autism treated with haloperidol showed that 12.5% had either tardive dyskinesia (n=5) or withdrawal dyskinesias (n=23) (Campbell et al., 1997). Given these findings, drug holidays every 6 to 12 months are often recommended to observe the child's continued need for medication. The less potent antipsychotics, such as chlorpromazine, tend to cause excessive sedation without clinical improvement.

Preliminary reports on the efficacy of the newer atypical antipsychotics in treating autism showed promise (see Koenig & Scahill, 2001; McDougle & Posey, 2003). A multisite placebo-controlled study showed that risperidone (Risperdal) was safe and effective for reducing aggression, tantrums, and self-injury in children with autism (Research Units on Pediatric Psychopharmacology [RUPP] Autism Network, 2002). These gains were stable over a 6-month follow-up period without having to increase the dose of medication. In the last phase of the study, children were randomly assigned to gradual withdrawal to placebo or continued treatment with risperidone under double-blind conditions. The group of children who switched over to placebo showed a significantly higher rate of relapse (i.e., return of tantrums, aggression, or self-injury) than the group who continued treatment with risperidone (RUPP Autism Network, 2005). Nonetheless, it is worth noting that not all children assigned to placebo substitution relapsed. This suggests that periodic attempts to withdraw a medication such as risperidone deserves consideration.

Methylphenidate (Ritalin) may reduce target symptoms of inattention, impulsivity, and overactivity in children and adolescents with PDD (Handen, Johnson, & Lubetsky, 2000). A multisite placebo-controlled study of methylphenidate was conducted in a group of 58 children with a diagnosis of PDD and symptoms of hyperactivity (RUPP, 2005). The study included three dose levels of methylphenidate and placebo. Once the most effective treatment dose was established, subjects completed an 8-week open-label trial of methylphenidate. Forty-four of the participants were rated as responders to treatment. Adverse effects included insomnia, decreased appetite, irritability, and increased self-injury. Although MPH appears useful in children with PDD and hyperactivity, this population appears more susceptible to adverse effects—even at the medium dose levels used in the study. Clinicians should start with low doses and increase at slower rates than used in typically developing children with ADHD and clinicians should not expect the same magnitude of benefit that is often observed in children with ADHD.

Several controlled studies of the opioid antagonist naltrexone found modest improvements in hyperactivity, but this was not supported in a recent study. Based on the demonstrated effectiveness of the SSRIs in children and adolescents with OCD, these medications are commonly used to reduce repetitive behavior in PDDs. The SSRIs have not been well studied in children with PDD; preliminary results suggest that a common adverse effect of the SSRIs in children with PDD is behavioral activation. This term refers to a set of behaviors such as insomnia, hyperactivity, increased impulsiveness, talkativeness and, occasionally, increased aggression. Furthermore, the best available evidence suggests that the SSRIs may only be moderately effective for repetitive behavior in PDD. Hollander and colleagues (2005) compared fluoxetine with placebo in a trial of 39 subjects aged 5 to 17. The medication was started at a low dose (e.g., 2.5 mg) and moved up gradually to an average dose of 10 mg per day at 4 weeks. The drug was well tolerated with a low frequency of activation, which is almost certainly due to the conservative dosing schedule. Although the study showed that fluoxetine was superior to placebo, there was only 10% improvement on average. Clearly, more study is needed (Scahill & Martin, 2005). There is also an open study showing that buspirone may reduce agitation and explosive outbursts in some individuals (Buitelaar, van der Gaag, & van der Hoeven, 1998), but these findings have not been replicated.

Continuum of Care

Autism is a chronic disorder usually requiring long-term care at various levels of intensity. Treatment consists of designing academic, interpersonal, and social experiences that support the child's development. Children with autism, even those who are severely affected, may be able to live at home and attend a special school for children with autism that uses behavioral modification. Other outpatient services may include family counseling, home care, and medication. As the child moves toward adulthood, living at home may become more difficult, given the appropriate need for greater independence. The level of structure required depends primarily on IQ and adaptive functioning.

Asperger's Disorder

Although Asperger's disorder was also described about 50 years ago, it was not included in *DSM-III* or *DSM-III-R*. It has been incorporated into *DSM-IV-TR* and is defined as severe and sustained impairment in social interaction and restricted, repetitive patterns of behavior, interests, and activities (APA, 2000). Children with Asperger's disorder have profound social deficits marked by inappropriate initiation of social interactions, inability to respond to usual social cues, and a tendency to be concrete in their interpretation of language. They also display stereotypic behaviors, such as rocking and hand flapping, and highly restricted areas of interest, such as train schedules, fans, air conditioners, dogs, or British royalty. Signs of developmental delay may not be apparent until preschool or school age, when social deficits become evident (Box 29.2). The differences in intelligence, language development, and age of clear onset suggest that Asperger's is distinguishable from autism. However, it may not be differentiated from autism in the literature (Volkmar et al., 2004).

Asperger's disorder is defined by severe and sustained impairment in social interaction and restricted, repetitive patterns of behavior, interests, and activities not associated with mental retardation. Communication deficits are less severe than in autism.

BOX 29.2

Clinical Vignette: Frank (Asperger's Disorder)

A pediatrician refers Frank, age 5 years 6 months, for an evaluation because of Frank's unusual preoccupation with ceiling fans and lawn sprinklers. According to his mother, Frank became interested in ceiling fans at age 3 years when he began drawing them, tearing pictures of them out of magazines, and engaging others in discussions about them. In the months before the evaluation, Frank also became fascinated by lawn sprinklers. These preoccupations so dominated Frank's interactions with others that he was practically incapable of discussing any other topics. He remained on the periphery of his kindergarten class and had few friends. Although he tried to make friends, his approaches were inept, and he had trouble reading others.

Frank was the product of a full-term uncomplicated pregnancy, labor, and delivery to his then 25-year-old mother. It was her first pregnancy, and both parents eagerly anticipated Frank's birth. As an infant, Frank was healthy but seemed to cry a lot and was difficult to comfort, causing his mother to feel inadequate and depleted. His motor development was also delayed, and at age 3 years, nonfamily members had difficulty understanding his speech. His articulation, however, was within normal limits at the time of consultation. Frank received regular pediatric care and had no history of serious illness or injury. There was no family history of mental retardation or psychiatric illness; results of genetic testing for chromosomal abnormality were negative.

In addition to his unusual preoccupations and social deficits, Frank resisted any change in his routine, was easily frustrated, and was prone to temper tantrums. His parents sharply disagreed about the nature of and appropriate response to his problems.

What Do You Think?

1. What effect do you think Frank's preoccupation may have on his family and their relationships?
2. What kind of teaching program would you develop if you were the nurse assigned to this family?

Epidemiology and Etiology

The prevalence of this disorder is difficult to determine because of shifts in its definition and lack of population data on the newly established diagnostic criteria. The current estimate is in the range of 1 to 3 per 10,000 (Fombonne, 2003). Asperger's disorder appears to be more common in boys. Although no genetic marker has been identified, the disorder often runs in families, with high recurrence in fathers (Volkmar et al., 2004; Volkmar, Klin, Schultz, Rubin, & Bronen, 2000).

Psychopharmacologic Interventions

Psychopharmacologic management is targeted to specific manifestations, such as compulsive behavior, or comorbid conditions, such as depression. Although no medication studies have been conducted on children with carefully diagnosed Asperger's, approaches to the treatment of depression and anxiety disorders would be the same as those used in typically developing young children.

Continuing Care

Asperger's disorder has been recognized only recently. As with autism, the family needs help in supporting the child's development and in managing symptoms.

NURSING MANAGEMENT: HUMAN RESPONSE TO PERVASIVE DEVELOPMENTAL DISORDER

Biologic Domain

Assessment

The assessment of children with PDDs is a complex endeavor (Koenig & Scahill, 2001). Biologic assessment should include a review of physical health and neurologic status, giving particular attention to coordination, childhood illnesses, injuries, and hospitalizations. The nurse should assess sleep, appetite, and activity patterns because they may be disturbed in these children. Lack of adequate sleep can increase irritability. Comorbid seizure disorders are common in autism, and depression is often seen concurrently with Asperger's. Thus, the nurse should consider these conditions in the assessment.

Youngsters with additional psychiatric disorders or seizures may be receiving multiple medications and require the care of several clinicians. Therefore, the assessment should include a careful review of current medications and treating clinicians.

Nursing Diagnoses for the Biologic Domain

Assessment data generate a variety of potential nursing diagnoses, including Self-Care Deficits, Impaired Verbal Communication, Disturbed Sensory Perceptions, Delayed Growth and Development, and Disturbed Sleep Pattern. Treatment outcomes need to be individualized to the child, family, and social environment.

Interventions for the Biologic Domain

In teaching self-care skills, the nurse needs to consider the child's current adaptive skills and language limitations. Developing a list of activities for the child to post in his or her bedroom may be effective for some children. Drawings or symbols may be useful for nonverbal children. Physical safety is an important concern for children who are cognitively delayed and may have impaired judgment.

As noted earlier, children with PDD may be treated with multiple medications in novel combinations (Martin, Van Hoof, Stubbe, Sherwin, & Scahill, 2003). In some cases, these unusual combinations are the result of careful management; in other cases, the combinations are the result of clinical mismanagement, perhaps because of poor coordination among treating prescribers. Consequently, the nurse should carefully review the target symptoms for each drug treatment with the parents. This review includes possible drug interactions that are especially important for this clinical population.

Psychological Domain

Assessment

Critical elements to evaluate include intellectual ability, communication skills, and adaptive functioning. Direct behavioral observation is critical to evaluate the child's ability to relate to others, to verify the selection of age-appropriate activities, and to watch for stereotypic behaviors. Children with PDD often need specific behavioral interventions to reduce the frequency of inappropriate or aggressive behavior. These interventions follow from a careful evaluation of the circumstances that precede or accompany the behavior and the usual consequences of the behavior (Volkmar et al., 2004). For example, a child may exhibit angry outbursts in response to routine transitions. If the tantrum is dramatic, the consequence may be that the transition does not take place. By structuring the environment and using visual cues to signal the end of one activity and the start of another, it may be possible to reduce the number and intensity of responses to transitions.

Nursing Diagnoses for the Psychological Domain

Assessment data generate a variety of potential nursing diagnoses, including Anxiety and Disturbed Thought Processes. Because of the long-term nature of these disorders, outcomes may change with time.

Interventions for the Psychological Domain

Managing the repetitive behaviors of these children will depend on the specific behavior and its effects on others or the environment. If the behavior, such as rocking, has no negative effects, ignoring it may be the best approach. If the behavior, such as head banging, is unacceptable, redirecting the child and using positive reinforcement are recommended. In some cases, especially in severely delayed children, these strategies may not work, and environmental alterations and perhaps protective headgear are needed.

Social Domain

Assessment

The nursing assessment is an ongoing process in which attention is given to establishing a positive relationship with the child and the family. The assessment should include a review of the child's capacity for self-care and maladaptive behaviors (Koenig & Scahill, 2001). Self-injury and aggression are sometimes present, and children may need to be protected from hurting themselves and others. Inquiry should also include the presence of perseverative behaviors and preoccupation with restricted interests. These odd behaviors may not necessarily cause a problem, but they often interfere with the child's relationships.

Another important domain to consider in the nursing assessment is the effects of the child's developmental delays on the family. Having a child with PDD is bound to influence family interaction, and responding to the child's needs may adversely affect family functioning. For example, sleep disruption in family members who care for these children may increase family stress.

Nursing Diagnoses for the Social Domain

Assessment data generate a variety of potential nursing diagnoses, including Social Isolation. The family may be grieving the loss of the normal child they had expected and are trying to cope with the multitude of problems inherent in raising a child with a disability. Because of the long-term nature of these disorders, the aims of treatment may change with time. However, throughout childhood the focus should be on the development of age-appropriate adaptive and social skills.

Interventions for the Social Domain

Planning interventions for youngsters with severe developmental problems considers the child, family, and community supports, such as schools, rehabilitation centers, or group homes. First and foremost, the various clinicians involved in the child's treatment should collaborate with the family toward the same general goals. As the number of clinicians and educators involved increases, the chance of fragmentation in treatment planning also increases. The nurse can serve as a case coordinator.

Promoting Interaction

Structuring interventions for social isolation should fit the child's cognitive, linguistic, and developmental levels. Interventions fostering nonverbal social interactions may be more useful than those based on speech. For higher functioning children, activities such as getting the mail, passing out snacks, or taking turns in the context of simple games can engage the child in social activities without requiring the use of their limited language skills. Structuring social interactions so that the child has to share a task with another, such as carrying a load of books, may help to boost confidence in relating to others.

Ensuring Predictability and Safety

When children with PDD are hospitalized, milieu management—a consistent, structured environment with predictable routines for activities, mealtimes, and bedtimes—is necessary for successful treatment. Changes in routine may provoke disorganization in the child with PDD, leading to emotional disequilibrium and explosive behavior. The safety of the inpatient unit offers an opportunity to try behavioral strategies, such as rewards for managing transitions. Health care professionals can pass on successful strategies to parents or primary caretakers.

Managing Behavior

Because children with PDD have difficulty relating to others, they should spend most of their time within the therapeutic environment of the unit. These children can learn social and communication skills, such as taking turns in conversation and warning the listener before changing the subject in the context of milieu. If a child requires isolation for control of aggressive or assaultive behavior, a brief "time out" followed by prompt reentry into unit activities is optimum.

Autism and related disorders are chronic conditions that call for extraordinary patience and determination. Unfortunately, lack of integration of medical, psychiatric, social, and educational services can add to the family's burden. Parents may manifest denial, grief, guilt, and anger at various points as they adjust to their child's disability. The nurse can offer parents the opportunity to express their frustrations and disappointments and can be alert for indications that parents are in need of additional assistance, such as parent support groups or respite care.

Residential care may be necessary in some cases. After making the decision to place a child into a residential facility, family members may experience guilt, loss, and a sense of failure concerning their inability to care for the child at home.

Supporting Family 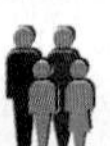

Family interventions include support, education, counseling, and referral to self-help groups. Whenever possible, the nurse provides education to help parents determine appropriate expectations for their child with PDD and to meet the child's special needs. The following are examples of potentially useful nursing interventions focusing on the family:

- Interpreting the treatment plan for parents and child
- Modeling appropriate behavior modification techniques
- Including the parents as cotherapists for the implementation of the care plan
- Assisting the family in identifying and resolving their sense of loss related to the diagnosis
- Coordinating support systems for parents, siblings, and family members
- Maintaining interdisciplinary collaboration

EVALUATION AND TREATMENT OUTCOMES

Evaluation of patient and family outcomes is an ongoing process. Short-term outcomes might consist of discrete behavioral improvements, such as reducing self-injurious behavior by 50%. The long-term goal is for the patient to achieve the highest level of functioning. The prognosis depends on the severity of the impairments, the interventions available, and the cognitive ability of the child. The use of standardized rating scales before and after treatment can improve the precision of outcome measurement (Arnold et al., 2000; RUPP Autism Network, 2002).

SPECIFIC DEVELOPMENTAL DISORDERS

In contrast to mental retardation and PDD, specific developmental disorders are characterized by a narrower range of deficits. These more discrete delays can occur in various developmental domains. However, some children have more than one specific developmental disorder, and some of these disorders may have a common etiology (Paul, 2002; Shaywitz, 2003).

Types

Specific developmental disorders are generally classified as learning, communication, and motor skills disorders. This section focuses primarily on learning and communication disorders.

Learning Disorders

Learning disorders (also called *learning disabilities*) are typically classified as verbal (reading and spelling) or nonverbal (mathematics). This distinction between verbal and nonverbal learning disorders comes from documented differences in their nature and etiology (Shaywitz, 2003).

Generally, learning disorders are defined as a discrepancy between actual achievement and expected achievement based on the person's age and intellectual ability. The definition varies depending on the source and state statute.

Reading disability, also called *dyslexia*, has been recognized for more than 100 years. It is defined as a significantly lower score for mental age on standardized tests in reading that is not the result of low intelligence or inadequate schooling. This relatively common problem affects about 5% of school-aged children, with some studies reporting higher prevalence. In clinical samples, dyslexia affects boys more often than girls; however, a large community-based sample of children with reading disorders found no gender difference. This discrepancy suggests that the observed difference in clinic samples may be related to biases in seeking treatment, rather than a true gender difference (Shaywitz, 2003).

Although it is clear that no single cause will provide a sufficient explanation for reading disability, the underlying problem appears to be a deficit in **phonologic processing,** which involves the discrimination and interpretation of speech sounds. A disturbance in the development of the left hemisphere is believed to cause this deficit. Both genetic and environmental factors have been implicated in the etiology of reading disability. Data from family studies show that reading disability is familial and that shared environmental factors alone cannot explain the high rate of recurrence in affected families. Additional evidence from twin studies indicates that specific weaknesses in phonologic processing are more likely to be observed in monozygotic twins than in dizygotic twins (Willcutt, Pennington, & DeFries, 2000).

Less is known about the prevalence of nonverbal learning disorder (mathematics disorder), with estimates of occurrence ranging from 0.1% to 1.0% of school-aged children, and no apparent difference between boys and girls. Mathematics disorder (which is manifested by significant delay in learning mathematics) appears to be a right-hemisphere disorder. Right-hemisphere dysfunction and math problems have been shown in fragile X syndrome and Turner's syndrome, both of which are genetic syndromes. Other reports from clinical populations have shown that acquired problems, such as early onset seizure disorders, can produce right hemisphere dysfunction and mathematic disability.

Communication Disorders

Communication disorders involve speech or language impairments. *Speech* refers to the motor aspects of speaking; *language* consists of higher-order aspects of formulating and comprehending verbal communication. A large community survey of 5-year-old children in Canada found a combined prevalence of 19% for speech and language disorders (Beitchman, Nair, Clegg, & Patel, 1986), suggesting they are fairly common in young school-aged children. However, available evidence also suggests that many communication deficits appearing at this age do resolve (Toppelberg & Shapiro, 2000). Nonetheless, speech and language disorders are also associated with psychiatric disability (Tomblin, Zhang, Buckwalter, & Catts, 2000). As with reading disability, there are undoubtedly multiple causes of speech or language handicap.

A delay in speech or language development can adversely affect the child's socialization and education. For example, peers may rebuff or tease a child with an articulation defect or stutter, contributing to withdrawal and a negative self-image. The resulting isolation could limit opportunities to negotiate rules, take turns, and learn cooperation. These same tasks could also be difficult for children with language delay. Moreover, language appears to play a role in the regulation of behavior and impulses. Not surprisingly, impaired language appears to be a risk factor for ADHD (Shaywitz, 2003; Toppelberg & Shapiro, 2000). Children with language delays may also be at greater risk for reading disability, which may share the same underlying phonologic defect (Tomblin et al., 2000; Willcutt et al., 2000).

NURSING MANAGEMENT: HUMAN RESPONSE TO SPECIFIC DEVELOPMENTAL DISORDER

Nursing assessment of children with a known specific developmental disorder includes (1) evidence of interference in daily life, (2) determination of the youngster's ability (and limitations) to communicate during the interview, (3) assessment of the child's perception about his or her disability, (4) observation for impaired learning and communication, and (5) past and current interventions for the learning or communication deficit, with data gathered through direct interview of the child and significant others such as parents. Several nursing diagnoses can be generated from these data, such as Impaired Verbal Communication and Social Isolation. For the child with learning disabilities, nurses can focus on building self-confidence and helping the family connect with guidance and educational resources that support the child's development into adulthood. For the child with communication disorders, the interventions focus on fostering social and communication skills and making referrals for specific speech or language therapy. Modeling appropriate communication in spontaneous situations with the child can be a useful intervention for some children. The following is an overview of nursing interventions for the child with specific developmental difficulties:

- Introduce strategies for increasing communication skills (e.g., initiating conversation, taking turns in conversation, facing the listener).
- Identify and develop specific intervention strategies for problems secondary to learning communication disorders, such as low self-esteem (Tomblin et al., 2000).
- Provide parental support for coping with the disorder.
- Maintain interdisciplinary medical, dental, speech therapy, and educational collaboration.
- Refer to learning or speech specialist for evaluation and assistance (Toppelberg & Shapiro, 2000).

CONTINUUM OF CARE

Children with learning disabilities obviously require careful psychoeducational and cognitive testing to identify their strengths and deficits. School or clinical psychologists usually perform this type of specialized testing. When a learning disability has been identified, the Education for the Handicapped Act (PL 94-142) mandates that public school systems provide remedial services in the least restrictive educational setting. Families occasionally need help in advocating for these services.

The same is true for children with communication disorders, although the services requested may be different. Speech pathologists conduct the diagnostic assessment of speech and language disorder. Nurses may be involved with formal screening for communication disorders (Tomblin et al., 2000). Services such as speech therapy (directed at the motor aspects of speaking) or social skills groups (directed at the social and interpersonal aspects of language) are often available in school districts and can be obtained if a speech or language disorder has been identified. For some children with communication disorders, the services offered by the school may be insufficient. In such cases, the nurse can help the family locate a facility that can provide these needed services.

Disruptive Behavior Disorders

The disruptive behavior disorders, which include ADHD, oppositional defiant disorder, and conduct disorder, are a group of syndromes marked by significant problems of conduct. Because these disorders are characterized by "acting out" behaviors, they are sometimes referred to as **externalizing disorders**. In contrast, disorders of mood (e.g., anxiety, depression) are classified as **internalizing disorders** because the symptoms tend to be within the child.

The disruptive behavior disorders are more common in boys and are associated with lower socioeconomic status, urban living (Scahill et al., 1999), learning disabilities (Shaywitz, 2003; Tomblin et al., 2000), and language delay (Toppelberg & Shapiro, 2000). These disorders are relatively common in school-aged children and are frequently presenting complaints in child psychiatric treatment settings.

ATTENTION-DEFICIT HYPERACTIVITY DISORDER

ADHD is a common disorder in school-aged children. It is almost certainly a heterogeneous disorder with multiple etiologies. The relatively high frequency of ADHD and associated behavior problems virtually guarantees that nurses will meet these children in all pediatric treatment settings.

Clinical Course and Diagnostic Criteria

ADHD is a persistent pattern of inattention, hyperactivity, and impulsiveness that is pervasive and inappropriate for developmental level (APA, 2000).

Parents and teachers describe children with ADHD as restless, always on the go, highly distractible, unable to wait their turn, heedless, and frequently disruptive. Indeed, it is often disruptive behavior that brings these children into treatment. The historical debate concerning the nature of ADHD is reflected in the labels used to describe it: organic brain syndrome, hyperkinetic impulse disorder, minimal brain dysfunction, hyperkinetic reaction of childhood, hyperkinesis, attention deficit disorder, and most recently, in *DSM-IV-TR*, attention-deficit hyperactivity disorder. This long list of terms also implies the various theories regarding the cause and the presumed site of the primary defect. The *DSM-IV-TR* represents yet another formulation of ADHD by defining ADHD as predominantly hyperactive type, predominantly inattentive type, or combined type (Table 29.3). Despite the historical shifts in terminology and the various proposals regarding the etiology of ADHD, the accumulated consensus during the past several decades is that three core symptoms define the disorder: inattention, impulsiveness, and hyperactivity.

Attention is a complex mental process that involves the ability to concentrate on one activity to the exclusion of others, as well as the ability to sustain focus. Children with ADHD are easily distracted and lack persistence in the performance of age-appropriate tasks, reflecting an inability to filter stimuli, sustain attention, or both. The inability to screen stimuli leaves the child unable to identify salient stimuli. The child may then treat all incoming stimuli with equal regard and respond to multiple incoming stimuli. Alternatively, it has been argued that the distractibility seen in ADHD is the result of stimulus-seeking behavior. Given the heterogeneity of ADHD, either of these models may be true for subgroups of affected children.

Both clinical observation and laboratory studies support the conclusion that children with ADHD are prone to impulsive, risk-taking behavior (Barkley, 1998).

KEY CONCEPT Attention is a complex process that involves the ability to concentrate on one activity to the exclusion of others and the ability to sustain that focus.

Table 29.3 Key Diagnostic Characteristics of Attention-Deficit Hyperactivity Disorder
314.10: Attention-deficit hyperactivity disorder, combined type
314.00: Attention-deficit hyperactivity disorder, predominantly inattentive type
314.01: Attention-deficit hyperactivity disorder, predominantly hyperactive–impulsive type
314.9: Attention-deficit hyperactivity disorder, not otherwise specified

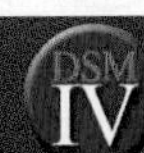

Diagnostic Criteria and Target Symptoms	Associated Features
• Symptoms of inattention (at least six) Lacks close attention to details; makes careless mistakes in activities Has difficulty sustaining attention Appears to not listen when spoken to directly Has difficulty following through on instructions; fails to finish work or activities Has difficulty organizing tasks and activities Has difficulty with tasks requiring sustained mental effort; commonly avoids, dislikes, or is reluctant to engage in them Loses items necessary for tasks Is easily distracted by outside stimuli Is often forgetful in daily activities • Symptoms of hyperactivity-impulsivity (at least six): Hyperactivity Fidgets or squirms Gets up when expectation is to remain seated Excessively runs about or climbs inappropriately Has difficulty with quiet leisure activities Often appears "on the go" or "driven by a motor" Talks excessively Impulsivity Blurts out answers before question completion Has difficulty awaiting turn Is interruptive or intrusive of others • Symptoms are maladaptive and inconsistent with developmental level, persisting for at least 6 months • Some symptoms present before age 7 years • Evidence of significant impairment in social, academic, or occupational functioning • Not exclusive during other psychiatric disorder; not better accounted for by another mental disorder	• Low frustration tolerance • Temper outbursts • Bossiness, stubbornness • Excessive and frequent insistence for requests to be met • Mood lability • Demoralization • Dysphoria • Rejection by peers • Low self-regard • Resentment and antagonism within family • Reduced vocational achievement

A fundamental question that some have raised is that impulsiveness may not be truly separate from distractibility or hyperactivity. Alternatively, some have argued that children with ADHD have an impaired capacity to learn through reinforcement, which predisposes them to impulsive behavior. Indirect support for this view comes from studies showing that animals with lesions of the frontal lobe are less able to make use of reinforcement without additional external structure and greater rewards (Barkley, 1998). In behavioral terms, children with ADHD often fail to consider the consequences of their actions, exercise poor judgment, and tend to have more than the usual lumps, bumps, and bruises because of their risk-taking behavior. They often require a high degree of structure and supervision.

KEY CONCEPT Impulsiveness is the tendency to act on urges, notions, or desires without adequately considering the consequences.

Although hyperactivity is a characteristic often associated with ADHD, controversy is long-standing about whether attention deficit can occur without overactivity. The decision by *DSM-IV-TR* to define ADHD as predominately hyperactive, predominately inattentive, or combined offers a compromise in the debate regarding attention-deficit disorder with or without hyperactivity. Even those who argue in favor of attention-deficit disorder without hyperactivity acknowledge that it is probably much less common than attention-deficit disorder with hyperactivity.

In many cases, it is the hyperactivity that prompts the search for treatment. Parents typically report that the child's hyperactivity was manifest early in life and evident in most situations. However, the child's overactivity may be more noticeable in the classroom because it is poorly tolerated there (Barkley, 1998).

KEY CONCEPT Hyperactivity is excessive motor activity, as evidenced by restlessness, inability to remain seated, and high levels of physical motion and verbal output.

Epidemiology and Risk Factors

Although prevalence estimates vary depending on the diagnostic criteria used, the sources of data, and the sampling procedure, ADHD is a common psychiatric disorder of childhood. The current estimate in school-aged children is about 6%, with a range of 2% to 14%. Boys are affected three to eight times more often than are girls (for a review, see Scahill & Schwab-Stone, 2000). Longitudinal studies that followed groups of children with ADHD into adulthood have shown that 30% to 40% continued to have problems with impulsiveness and inattention, although hyperactivity was less evident (Weiss & Weiss, 2002). Older adolescents and young adults with a history of ADHD were more likely to have multiple arrests, arrests for more serious offenses, and more car accidents than are individuals in the control group (Weiss & Weiss). Clearly, a substantial percentage of children do not "grow out of" ADHD. These findings bolster the connection between ADHD and antisocial behavior (see Chapter 20).

FAME AND FORTUNE

Kurt Cobain (1967–1994):
Songwriter, Guitarist, and Vocalist

Public Persona

Kurt Cobain was the multitalented leader of Nirvana, the "multiplatinum" grunge band that redefined the popular music sound of the 1990s. Thousands of fans idolized him and his music. He committed suicide at the age of 27.

Personal Realities

Kurt Cobain had emotional problems that began long before adulthood. During his childhood, he was a sickly bronchitic child. His parents divorced when he was 7 and he reported never feeling loved or secure again. He became increasingly difficult, antisocial, and withdrawn after his parent's divorce and was shuttled between relatives. After dropping out of school, he worked at various jobs and then embarked on a music career. He later developed stomach ulcers and colon problems. He began using heroin in the early 1990s and ultimately no longer wanted to live.

Etiologic Factors

Despite more than a half century of investigation, the etiology of ADHD remains unclear (Weiss & Weiss, 2002). Numerous environmental exposures, including perinatal insult, head injury, psychosocial disadvantage, lead poisoning, and diet (e.g., food allergies or sensitivity to food additives) have been proposed as potential causes. Although these hypotheses may explain some cases, none of these exposures alone is likely to account for a significant portion of children with ADHD (Weiss & Weiss). The claim that food additives or allergies cause ADHD has very limited data to support it (Weiss & Weiss).

Biologic Factors

Although the etiology of ADHD is uncertain, persuasive evidence from several lines of research has shown that the frontal lobe and functional connections with specific subcortical structures are dysregulated in patients with ADHD. For example, a structural magnetic resonance imaging (MRI) study of 57 boys with ADHD compared with those of 55 control subjects showed reduced volumes of the right dorsolateral frontal region and in selected regions of the basal ganglia (Castellanos et al., 1996). Using single-photon emission computed tomography (SPECT) to measure brain activity, Lou, Henriksen, and Bruhn (1990) found reduced blood flow in these same subcortical regions (caudate and putamen) of individuals with ADHD compared with those of control subjects. Additional evidence linking ADHD to dysfunction of the frontal lobe comes from a positron emission tomography (PET) scan study of adults who had a personal history of ADHD and were parents of children with ADHD. This study found hypoperfusion (decreased metabolic activity) in the frontal lobe of the adults with a history of ADHD compared with the control group (Zametkin et al., 1990). These investigators used similar techniques to evaluate frontal lobe functioning in a group of adolescents with ADHD. Although the findings were in the same direction, the difference between control subjects and the adolescents with ADHD was not statistically significant (Zametkin et al., 1993). More recently, Vaidya and colleagues (1998) showed differences in frontal-subcortical function during an attentional task. The difference between control subjects and subjects with ADHD was reduced when the subjects with ADHD received methylphenidate.

Genetic factors have also been implicated in the etiology of ADHD, and they clearly play a fundamental role for at least a subgroup of children. Several twin studies have shown that, although identical twins are not fully concordant for ADHD, they are far more likely to be mutually affected than are dizygotic twins (Levy et al., 1997). In this large twin study, investigators examined the concordance of ADHD symptoms in a large community sample of monozygotic and dizygotic twins across a wide range of symptoms, from none to severe (Levy et al.). In that study, roughly 82% of the monozygotic (MZ) twin pairs were mutually affected (concordant), compared with 38% in the dizygotic (DZ) twins. Moreover, the MZ twin pairs showed greater similarity on a parent rating of ADHD symptoms across the entire range (from no symptoms) when compared with the DZ twin pairs. These findings suggest that ADHD can be viewed as one or more heritable traits (e.g., attention and impulsiveness) on a continuum from mild to severe. Family genetic studies also support a prominent role for genetics in the etiology of ADHD. In the largest family study to date, Biederman and colleagues (1992) showed that ADHD is roughly six times more likely to affect biologic relatives of children with ADHD than biologic relatives of pediatric control subjects.

Psychological and Social Factors

Although genetic endowment clearly plays a fundamental role in the etiology of ADHD, environmental factors are also important. Psychosocial influences (family stress and marital discord) are associated with ADHD, but the direction of causality is difficult to determine (Scahill et al., 1999; Szatmari, Boyle, & Offord, 1989). Other psychosocial correlates that have been observed in large community samples (Scahill et al.; Szatmari et al.) and clinical samples (Biederman et al., 1995) are poverty, overcrowded living conditions, and family dysfunction.

NURSING MANAGEMENT: HUMAN RESPONSE TO ATTENTION-DEFICIT HYPERACTIVITY DISORDER

Biologic Domain

The nursing assessment for the biologic domain may be initiated either before or after the diagnosis of ADHD is made. In the school setting, the nurse may suspect ADHD and collect assessment data similar to that collected by the nurse in a psychiatric facility.

Assessment

In the school setting, the primary focus of the assessment is the impact of ADHD on classroom behavior and school performance. In the hospital, the nurse tries to determine the contribution of ADHD to the acute psychiatric problem. In both cases, the nurse collects assessment data through direct interview, observation of the child and parent, and teacher ratings. Because children with ADHD may have difficulty sitting through long sessions, interviews are typically brief. Parents and teachers are extremely important sources for assessment data. To this end, the nurse can make use of several standardized instruments (Box 29.3).

As with other psychiatric disorders with onset in childhood, the nursing assessment of children with ADHD begins with identification and exploration of the presenting problem. This typically entails a review of the child's developmental course, the onset and pattern of the current symptoms, factors that have worsened or improved the child's problems, and prior treatment or self-initiated efforts to remedy the situation. The association of ADHD and communication disorders suggests a need for careful consideration of language development and current language functioning. Medical history is also essential, consisting of perinatal course, childhood illnesses, hospital admissions, injuries, seizures, tics, physical growth, general health status, and timing of the child's last physical examination.

Behavior of these children is characteristically very active and can often be observed in the office. They cannot sit still. They fidget. Even in sleep, they may be more active than normal children. Thus, a careful assessment of eating, sleeping, and activity patterns is

BOX 29.3

Standardized Tools for ADHD Diagnosis

The Conners Parent Questionnaire is a 48-item scale that a parent completes about his or her child. Each item is a statement that the parent rates on a 4-point scale from 0 (not at all) to 3 (very much). The Conners Teacher Questionnaire is a 28-item questionnaire that the child's teacher completes according to the same 4-point scale as the Parent Questionnaire. Both questionnaires have been standardized by age and gender for a mean of 50 and a standard deviation of 10 (Conners, 1989; Goyette et al., 1978).

The ADHD Rating Scale is a recently developed measure that asks parents or teachers to respond directly to 18 items in the *DSM-IV-TR* criteria (see Barkley, 1998, for a description of this scale). A similar scale called the SNAP-IV is available on-line for free at www.adhd.net. The SNAP-IV was used as the primary outcome measure in the MTA Cooperative Group Study (1999).

The Child Behavior Checklist (CBCL) is a 118-item questionnaire that a parent completes. In addition to the 118 questions about specific behaviors and psychiatric symptoms, the CBCL also includes questions concerning the child's competence in social and academic spheres as well as age-appropriate activities. Normative data are available allowing the conversion of raw scores to standard scores for age and gender. There is also a teacher version of this scale.

*Note that the diagnosis of ADHD is not made on the basis of questionnaires alone. Data from these rating scales augment the information gathered through interview and observation. These questionnaires can be especially useful before and after initiating a treatment plan to measure change.

essential. Assessing daily food intake, typical diet, and frequency of eating will help identify any nutrition problems. Caffeinated products can contribute to hyperactivity. Sleep is often disturbed for children with ADHD and consequently the family. A detailed sleep assessment can provide points for interventions and help the interpretation of drug effects.

Nursing Diagnoses for the Biologic Domain

Depending on the severity of the responses, family situation, and school environment, several nursing diagnoses could be generated from the assessment data, including Self-Care Deficit, Risk for Imbalanced Nutrition, Risk for Injury, and Disturbed Sleep Pattern. The outcomes should be individualized to the child.

Interventions for the Biologic Domain

The planning of nursing interventions must be done within the context of the family, treatment setting, and school environment. With the parents, clinical team members, and school personnel, the nurse participates in designing a plan of care that fits the child's and family's needs. Medication can help the hyperactivity, impulsiveness, and inattention; therefore, teaching the parent, child, and school personnel about the importance of the medication in ADHD and the potential side effects is a place to begin. Explaining to the child that the medication improves concentration and the ability to sit still can help strengthen patient motivation.

Several medications may be used in the treatment of ADHD, although the stimulants are by far the most common (Table 29.4). Commonly used stimulants include methylphenidate, D-amphetamine, and D-, L-amphetamine. Although each of these medications has demonstrated efficacy in controlled studies, methylphenidate has received considerably more research effort and is typically the first medication tried in the treatment of ADHD (MTA Cooperative Group, 1999). In a study of 579 children with ADHD, the MTA project showed that carefully managed treatment with methylphenidate (MPH) produces a 50% improvement on average in ADHD symptoms. In the 2-year follow-up study, the MTA research group showed that these children were still doing better than baseline (MTA Cooperative Group, 2004). The investigators examined growth parameters in 540 of the original subjects at 24 months posttreatment. The data showed that medication was associated with reduced height (1 cm over 2 years) and weight (1 kg over 2 years) compared with those participants who were not treated with any medication. It should be noted that the stimulants are not effective in all cases; thus, alternatives to the stimulants may be prescribed for children who do not experience response to the stimulants or develop tics when taking them (Biederman & The ADHD Study Group, 2002; Scahill, Chappell, et al., 2001). Atomoxetine is one such

Table 29.4 Stimulant Medications Used in Treating ADHD

Medication	Total Daily Dosage*	Common Side Effects
Methylphenidate	10–60 mg in two or three divided doses	Loss of appetite, insomnia, rebound activation, increase in tics or compulsive behavior, psychotic reaction
D-Amphetamine	5–40 mg in two divided doses	Similar to methylphenidate
D, L-Amphetamine	5–40 mg in two divided doses	Similar to methylphenidate

*Dosage ranges similar for long-acting products Concerta, Metadate, and Adderall.

example. In a randomized, placebo-controlled study of atomoxetine (Michelson, et al., 2002) response rate for the medication group was 60% versus 30% for the placebo group. These results were observed with once-daily dosing. Common adverse events included gastrointestinal disturbances and fatigue.

Methylphenidate is a short-acting medication that peaks in about 90 minutes to 2 hours and has a total duration of action of about 4 hours. Thus, parents or teachers often describe a return of overactivity and distractibility as the first dose of medication wears off. This "rebound effect" can often be managed by moving the second dose of the day slightly closer to the first dose. Similar phenomena may be observed with the amphetamines, although the rebound typically occurs later because the duration of action is slightly longer than that for methylphenidate (see Box 29.4). To obviate the need for redosing during the day, several new long-acting formulations of methylphenidate and amphetamine compounds have been developed. The long-acting preparations of methylphenidate such as Concerta, Ritalin LA, and Metadate or the D,L-amphetamine compound, Adderall XR, trade once-daily convenience with reduced dosing flexibility due to the fixed dose (Rains & Scahill, 2004). Data from national surveys indicate significant regional differences in prescription of stimulant medication. These surveys also show a steady increase in stimulant prescribing during the decade of the 1990s. Nonetheless, claims that methylphenidate is overprescribed probably are not justified (Jensen, Edelman, & Nemeroff, 2003).

Psychological Domain

Assessment

Hyperactivity, impulsivity, and inattention are typically pervasive problems that are evident both at school and at home. Discipline is frequently an issue because parents may have difficulty controlling their child's behavior, which is disruptive and occasionally destructive.

Nursing Diagnoses for the Psychological Domain

Assessment of the psychological domain may generate several diagnoses, including Anxiety and Defensive Coping. The outcomes should be individualized to the child.

BOX 29.4

Drug Profile: Methylphenidate (Ritalin)

DRUG CLASS: CNS stimulant

RECEPTOR AFFINITY: The mechanisms of effect are not completely clear. At low doses, it provides mild cortical stimulation similar to that of amphetamines. This stimulation results from methylphenidate's ability to promote release and interfere with the reuptake of dopamine in the synaptic cleft. Main sites appear to be the cerebral cortex, striatum, and pons.

INDICATIONS: Treatment of narcolepsy, attention-deficit disorders, and hyperkinetic syndrome; unlabeled uses for treatment of depression in elderly patients and patients with cancer or stroke.

ROUTES AND DOSAGE: Available in 5- to 10-mg immediate release tablets and 20-mg sustained-release tablets (Ritalin-SR). Newer long-acting preparations such as Concerta and Metadate, in various dose strengths, are also available.

Adult dosage: Must be individualized; range from 10 to 60 mg/d orally in divided doses bid to tid, preferably 15 to 30 min before meals. If insomnia is a problem, drug should be administered before 6 PM.

Child dosage: The immediate-release formulation can be started at 5 mg twice or three times daily on a 4-hour schedule with weekly increases depending on response. Starting doses of the long acting preparations are equivalent to the total tid dose (e.g., 5 tid of short-acting would translate into 18 mg of Concerta). Usually given on a tid schedule, with the last dose being roughly half that of the first and second dose. Daily dosage of > 60 mg not recommended. Discontinue after 1 month if no improvement.

PEAK EFFECT: 1 h; *half-life:* 3–4 h for the immediate-release preparations.

SELECT ADVERSE REACTIONS: Nervousness, insomnia, dizziness, headache, dyskinesias (including tics), toxic psychosis, anorexia, nausea, abdominal pain, increased pulse and blood pressure, palpitations, tolerance, psychological dependence.

WARNING: The drug is discontinued periodically to assess the patient's condition. Contraindications include marked anxiety, tension and agitation, glaucoma, severe depression, and obsessive-compulsive symptoms. Use cautiously in patients with a personal or family history of tic disorders, seizure disorders, hypertension, drug dependence, alcoholism, or emotional instability.

SPECIFIC PATIENT/FAMILY EDUCATION

- Do not chew or crush sustained-release tablets—they must be swallowed whole.
- Take the drug exactly as prescribed; if insomnia is a problem, time and dose may need adjustment. The drug is rarely taken after 5 PM.
- Avoid alcohol and OTC products, including decongestants, cold remedies, and cough syrups—these could accentuate side effects of the stimulant.
- Keep appointments for follow-up, including evaluations for monitoring the child's growth and use of parent and teacher ratings to monitor benefit.
- Note that the prescriber may discontinue the drug periodically to confirm effectiveness of therapy.

Interventions for the Psychological Domain

As a complement to medication, behavioral programs based on rewards for positive behavior, such as waiting turns and following directions, can foster new social skills. Interventions may also include specific cognitive behavioral techniques in which the child learns to "stop, look, and listen" before doing. These approaches have been refined, and several useful treatment manuals are available (Barkley, 1997). In general, these manuals emphasize problem solving and development of prosocial behavior. Interactions with children can be guided by the following:

- Set clear limits with clear consequences. Use few words and simplify instructions.
- Establish and maintain a predictable environment with clear rules and regular routines for eating, sleeping, and playing.
- Promote attention by maintaining a calm environment with few stimuli. These children cannot filter extraneous stimuli and react to all stimuli equally.
- Establish eye contact before giving directions; ask the child to repeat what was heard.
- Encourage the child to do homework in a quiet place, outside of a traffic pattern.
- Assist the child to work on one assignment at a time (reward with a break after each completion).

Social Domain

Assessment

Dysfunctional interactions can develop within the family. Reviewing the problem behaviors and the situations in which they occur is a way to identify negative interaction patterns. These children are often behind in their work at school because of poor organization, off-task behavior, and impulsive responses. They can exhaust their parents, aggravate teachers, and annoy siblings with their intrusive and disruptive behavior. Because ADHD often occurs in the context of psychosocial adversity, it is important to review the family situation, including parenting style, stability of household membership, consistency of rules and routines, and life events, such as divorce, moves, deaths, and job loss. Identification of these factors can be useful in shaping a care plan that builds on potential strengths and mitigates the effects of environmental factors that may perpetuate the child's disruptive behavior. Data regarding school performance, behavior at home, and comorbid psychiatric disorders are essential for developing school interventions and behavior plans and establishing the baseline severity for medication.

Nursing Diagnoses for the Social Domain

Depending on the severity of the child's responses, family situation, and school environment, several nursing diagnoses could be generated from the assessment data, including Impaired Social Interaction, Ineffective Role Performance, and Compromised Family Coping. Short-term outcomes, such as decreasing the number of classroom ejections within a 2-week period, may be useful for one child, whereas reducing the frequency and amplitude of angry outbursts at home may be relevant to another child.

Interventions for the Social Domain

Family treatment is nearly always a component of cognitive behavioral treatment approaches with the child. This may involve parent training that focuses on principles of behavior management, such as appropriate limit setting and use of reward systems, as well as revising expectations about the child's behavior. School programming often involves increasing structure in the child's school day to offset the child's tendency to act without forethought and to be easily distracted by extraneous stimuli. Specific remediation is required for the child with comorbid deficits in learning or language. Some children may require small, self-contained classrooms.

EVALUATION AND TREATMENT OUTCOMES

Children may not notice any effects after taking medication, but people in their environment do. Often, within 1 to 2 weeks of initiating therapy, children with ADHD become more attentive, less impulsive, and less active. Parents and teachers are often the first to notice improvement. Useful tools for tracking changes in behavior are the Parent and Teacher Conners Questionnaires (Conners, 1989), the ADHD Rating Scale (Barkley, 1998), and the SNAP-IV (MTA Cooperative Group, 1999). With time, academic achievement also may improve (Fig. 29.2).

CONTINUUM OF CARE

Treatment of ADHD typically is conducted in outpatient settings. Optimal treatment is multimodal (includes several types of interventions), encompassing four main areas: individual treatment for the child, family treatment, school accommodations, and medication. The Multimodal Treatment of ADHD Study (MTA Cooperative Group, 1999) showed that well-managed medication is

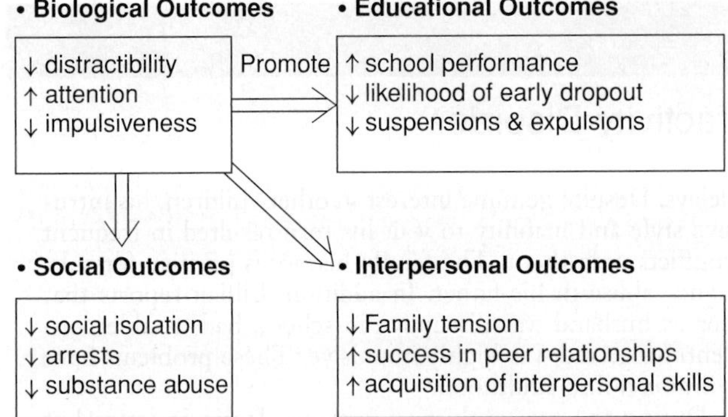

FIGURE 29.2. Long-term outcomes of optimal treatment for patients with attention-deficit hyperactivity disorder.

the most important intervention for the core symptoms of ADHD. Parent training and social skills training also help diminish disruptive and defiant behavior. See Nursing Care Plan 29.1.

OPPOSITIONAL DEFIANT DISORDER AND CONDUCT DISORDER

Oppositional defiant disorder is characterized by a persistent pattern of disobedience, argumentativeness, angry outbursts, low tolerance for frustration, and tendency to blame others for misfortunes, large and small. Conduct disorder is characterized by serious violations of social norms, including aggressive behavior, destruction of property, and cruelty to animals. Children with oppositional defiant disorder have trouble making friends and often find themselves in conflict with adults. This disorder is distinguishable from conduct disorder, which is characterized by more serious violations of social norms. Youngsters with conduct disorder often lie to achieve short-term ends, may be truant from school, may run away from home, and may engage in petty larceny or even mugging (Box 29.5).

The prevalence of conduct disorder is greater in boys and ranges from 6% to 16%, compared with a range of 2% to 9% in girls. Conduct disorder is one of the most frequently diagnosed disorders in children in mental health facilities. Individuals with conduct disorder are at greater risk for experiencing mood or anxiety disorders and substance-related disorders (APA, 2000). Other common comorbid conditions that may precede conduct disorder include specific developmental delays, such as learning disabilities and language delay, ADHD, and oppositional defiant disorder. Several reports from large community surveys, family studies, and studies of clinical samples confirm the high comorbidity among these disorders (Weiss & Weiss, 2002)

Children with ADHD, a learning disability, or a language deficit may frequently encounter failure and acquire a bitter and hostile attitude. Appropriate treatment focused on the ADHD or the specific developmental delay may foster more positive interactions and promote success at school. Success in these areas may lead to more positive behavior in some cases.

The etiology of oppositional defiant disorder and conduct disorder is complex. More attention has been paid to conduct disorder, probably because it is the more serious of the two. Models used to understand antisocial personality disorder (see Chapter 22) and aggressiveness (see Chapter 36) are useful in examining these childhood disorders, which appear to have both genetic and environmental components. For example, the risk for conduct disorder is increased in the offspring of individuals with conduct disorder. However, physical abuse by fathers, whether biologic or adoptive, also increases the risk for conduct disorder (Blackson et al., 1999).

NURSING MANAGEMENT: HUMAN RESPONSE TO OPPOSITIONAL DEFIANT DISORDER

Biologic Domain

Assessment

The nurse gathers data from multiple sources and domains, including biologic, psychological (mood, behavioral, cognitions), and social. These adolescents are at high risk for physical injury as a result of fighting and impulsive behavior. Sexual promiscuity is common, resulting in an increased frequency of pregnancy and sexually transmitted diseases.

Another important aspect of assessment of adolescents presenting with defiance or aggressive behavior is to rule out comorbid conditions that may partially explain or complicate their lack of behavioral control. These conditions include ADHD, learning disabilities, chemical dependency, depression, bipolar illness, or generalized anxiety. Young people who are chronically depressed may be irritable and easily frustrated. Given the tendency of adolescents to act out their frustration, chronic depression may exacerbate their behavior. Conduct problems can also elevate the risk for depression because young people who regularly elicit negative attention from parents and teachers and are constantly at odds with their environment may become despondent.

Nursing Diagnoses for the Biologic Domain

Typical nursing diagnoses in the biologic domain are Risk for Other-Directed Violence, Risk for Self-

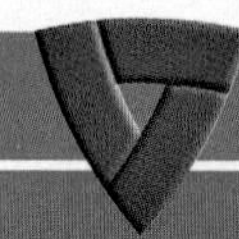

Nursing Care Plan 29.1

Attention-Deficit Hyperactivity Disorder

Jamie, age 6 years, comes to the primary health care clinic with his mother Lillian because of motor restlessness, distractibility, and disruptive behavior in the classroom. According to Lillian, Jamie had a reasonably good year in kindergarten, but early in the first grade, the teacher began to report disruptive behavior. On reflection, Lillian recalls that kindergarten was a half-day program with more activity. By contrast, Jamie is expected to sit in his seat and pay attention for longer periods in first grade.

Jamie's medical history is unremarkable. Lillian's pregnancy with Jamie was her first and unplanned. Although there were no complications during the pregnancy, the period was marked by significant marital discord, culminating in divorce before Jamie's first birthday. Jamie was born by cesarean section after a long, unproductive labor. He was healthy at birth and grew normally, with no developmental delays. Despite genuine interest in other children, his intrusive style and inability to wait his turn resulted in frequent conflicts with them. The family history is positive for substance abuse in his father. In addition, Lillian reports that her ex-husband was disruptive in school, had trouble concentrating, and was highly impulsive. These problems have continued into adulthood.

During the two evaluation sessions, Jamie is active but cooperative. His speech is fluent and normal in tone and tempo, but somewhat loud. His discourse is coherent, but at times he makes rather abrupt changes in conversation without warning his listeners. Psychological testing done at the school revealed average to above-average intelligence. Parent and teacher questionnaires concurred that Jamie was overactive, impulsive, inattentive, and quarrelsome, but not defiant.

Setting: Psychiatric Home Care Agency

Baseline Assessment: Jamie is a 6-year-old boy with prominent hyperactivity and disruptive behavior. He lives with Lillian, his single mother. These problems interfere with his interpersonal relationships and academic progress. Lillian is discouraged and feels unable to manage Jamie's behavior.

Associated Psychiatric Diagnosis

Axis I: Attention-deficit hyperactivity disorder
Axis II: None
Axis III: None
Axis IV: Problems with primary support (mother is exhausted)
Educational problems (failing in school)
Economic problems (mother in entry-level job with no health insurance)
Axis V: GAF = 52

Medications

Methylphenidate 5 mg at breakfast and lunch (i.e., at 8 AM and 12 noon), and then adding 5 mg at 4 PM. The likely dose would be 7.5 mg 8 AM & 12 noon & 5 mg at 7 PM.

Nursing Diagnosis 1: Impaired Social Interaction

Defining Characteristics

Cannot establish and maintain developmentally appropriate social relationships
Has interpersonal difficulties at school
Is not well accepted by peers
Is easily distracted
Interrupts others
Cannot wait his turn in games
Speaks out of turn in the classroom

Related Factors

Impulsive behavior
Overactive
Inattentive
Risk-taking behavior (tried to climb out the window to get away from Lillian)
Failure to recognize effects of his behavior on others.

Outcomes

Initial

1. Decrease hyperactivity and disruptive behavior.
2. Improve attention and decrease distractibility.
3. Decrease frequency of acting without forethought.

Discharge

4. Improve capacity to identify alternative responses in conflicts with peers.
5. Improve capacity to interpret behavior of age-mates.

Continued

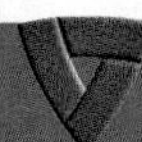

Nursing Care Plan 29.1 *(Continued)*

Interventions

Interventions	Rationale	Ongoing Assessment
Educate mother and teach about ADHD and use of stimulant medication.	Better understanding helps to ensure adherence; also parents and teachers often miscast children with ADHD as "troublemakers."	Determine extent to which parent or teacher "blames" Jamie for his problems.
Monitor adherence to medication schedule.	Uneven compliance may contribute to failed trial of medication.	Administer parent and teacher questionnaires; inquire about behavior across entire day.
Ensure that medication is both effective and well tolerated.	Stimulants can affect appetite and sleep and can cause "behavioral rebound" (Barkley, 1998).	Administer parent and teacher questionnaires; check height and weight; ask about sleep and appetite.

Evaluation

Outcomes	Revised Outcomes	Interventions
Jamie shows decreased hyperactivity and less disruption in the classroom.	Improve ability to identify disruptive classroom behavior.	Initiate point system to reward appropriate behavior.
Jamie shows improved attention and decreased distractibility.	Improve school performance.	Move to front of classroom as an aid to attention.
Mother and teacher attest to Jamie's decreased impulsive behavior.	Increase Jamie's capacity to recognize effects of his behavior on others.	Encourage participation in structured activities.
Jamie identifies alternative responses such as walking away until it is his turn.	Increase frequency of acting on these alternative approaches.	Inquire about social skills group at school, if available.
Jamie improves interpretation of motives and behaviors of others.	Improve acceptance by peers.	Encourage participation in community activities.

Nursing Diagnosis 2: Ineffective Coping (LILLIAN)

Defining Characteristics	Related Factors
Verbalizes discouragement and inability to handle situation with Jamie	Chronicity of ADHD More than average childrearing problems

Outcomes

Initial	Discharge
1. Verbalize frustration at trying to raise a child with ADHD alone. 2. Identify positive methods of interacting and disciplining Jamie that will support the parent–child relationship as well as meet Jamie's development needs.	3. Identify coping patterns that decrease the sense of frustration and increase parental competence. 4. Initiate a collaborative relationship with schoolteacher. 5. Identify sources of support in the community and begin to access these resources.

Interventions

Interventions	Rationale	Ongoing Assessment
Assess mother's discouragement and feelings about parenting, identifying specific problem areas.	Helping the mother verbalize her feelings and identify problem areas helps in formulating problem-solving strategies.	Assess the severity of the problems with which she is living.
Refer mother to Community Mental Health Center for free parenting class.	Parent training based on clear directives and rewards can be effective for decreasing impulsive and disruptive behavior.	Monitor mother's level of confidence and perceived change in Jamie's behavior.

Continued

Nursing Care Plan 29.1 (Continued)

Interventions

Interventions	Rationale	Ongoing Assessment
Refer mother to self-help organization.	Parent groups such as Children and Adults with Attention Deficit Disorder (CHAAD) can be sources of support and information.	Determine whether contact was made and whether it was helpful.
Make contact with school to enhance collaboration with mother.	Assess effectiveness of medication and other interventions, need feedback from teachers.	Determine whether mother has been able to contact teacher.

Evaluation

Outcomes	Revised Outcomes	Interventions
After four sessions, Lillian expresses her frustrations, but she has begun to identify different ways of relating to Jamie and his developmental needs.	None	None
Through attending the parenting class and joining a support group, Lillian begins to change her coping patterns, decrease her frustrations, and increase parental competence.	Complete parenting class; attend at least two support group meetings each month.	If necessary, refer for additional parent counseling.
Lillian initiates a collaborative relationship with Jamie's teacher.	Lillian and teacher mutually develop and implement behavior plans for home and school.	Have mother observe in the classroom; have mother visit highly structured classroom.

Directed Violence, and Impaired Verbal Communication. Although the outcomes are individualized for each patient, some outcomes for these patients are as follows:

- Maintenance of physical safety in the milieu (or other treatment setting)
- Decreased frequency of verbal and physical aggressive episodes

BOX 29.5

Clinical Vignette: Leon (Conduct Disorder)

Leon, a 14-year-old Hispanic boy, was admitted to the child psychiatric inpatient service from the emergency department after a fight with his mother. His mother reported that she and Leon had argued earlier in the evening and that he stormed out of the house screaming and vowing he would never return. Several hours later, Leon came back, yelling and demanding entry into the apartment. Leon's father was working. While his mother was getting up to open the door, Leon continued to yell and scream, waking the neighbors. This led to further arguing between Leon and his mother. Before long, the police were called, and Leon was taken to the emergency department.

The admission interview revealed that Leon had run away on several occasions and had even stayed away overnight. Although he strongly denied drug use, he had gotten drunk on several occasions. He had also been in several fights, the latest of which resulted in an expulsion from school. Three months before admission he was caught trying to steal a CD from a music store. More recently, he boasted that he and his friends had snatched a purse at an outdoor concert and had broken into a car to steal its contents. Leon's school performance has been declining; he was truant on several occasions and will probably have to repeat ninth grade.

Leon was born in Puerto Rico and is the oldest of three children. His family moved to the mainland shortly after his birth, and the primary language at home is Spanish. His father is employed as a janitor and speaks very little English. His mother works as a secretary and has achieved fairly good command of English. He has received no treatment except for consulation with the school social worker.

What Do You Think?

1. When conducting a nursing assessment, what would you want to learn about Leon's school performance?
2. What information could you provide Leon's parents about pharmacotherapy? About behavior management?

Interventions for the Biologic Domain

Children with oppositional defiant disorder or conduct disorder who also have specific developmental disorders should be placed in appropriate programs for remediation. If a diagnosis of ADHD or depression emerges from the evaluation, appropriate pharmacotherapy should be considered (see previous discussion of ADHD and after the discussion regarding depression).

Several medications have been used to treat extremely aggressive behavior, including antipsychotics, such as haloperidol and thioridazine; the anticonvulsant carbamazepine; the α-blocking agent propranolol; and the antimanic medication lithium carbonate. With the exception of haloperidol, most of these medications have limited support for their use in children and adolescents (Werry & Aman, 1998). More recently, several placebo-controlled studies have shown that low-dose risperidone therapy is effective for the treatment of aggression in children across a wide range of diagnostic groups (Aman et al., 2002; RUPP Autism Network, 2002).

Psychological Domain

Assessment

Adolescents with conduct problems are usually brought or coerced into the mental health system by family, school, or the court system because of fighting, truancy, speeding tickets, car accidents, petty crimes, substance abuse, or suicide attempts. These young people may be hostile, sarcastic, defensive, and provocative. At the same time, they may appear calm, outgoing, and engaging. Inconsistencies, distortions, and misrepresentations of the truth are common when interviewing these children, so obtaining a clear history may be difficult. Therefore, instead of asking if an event or behavior occurred, it may be better to ask when it occurred. A structured interview, such as the Diagnostic Schedule for Children (DISC), or self-reports, such as the Youth Self-Report (Achenbach, 1991), can aid the assessment. These adolescents are adept at changing the subject and diverting discussions from sensitive issues. They often use denial, projection, and externalization of anger as defense mechanisms when asked for self-disclosure. The assessment, which may take several sessions, should be conducted in a nonjudgmental fashion.

Nursing Diagnoses for the Psychological Domain

In the psychological domain, a typical nursing diagnosis is Ineffective Coping. Outcomes are individualized for each patient but can include the following:

- Increased personal responsibility for behavior
- Increased use of problem-solving skills as evidenced by decreased interpersonal conflicts
- Decreased rule violations and conflicts with authority figures

Interventions for the Psychological Domain

In planning interventions for patients with oppositional defiant disorder or conduct disorder, the focus is on problem behaviors. Therapeutic progress may be slow, at least partly because these patients often lack trust in authority figures.

Social Skills Training

The nurse should communicate behavioral expectations clearly and enforce them consistently. Consequences of appropriate and inappropriate actions also should be clear. Specific approaches for improving social and problem-solving skills are fundamental features for school-aged children and adolescents. Insofar as children and adolescents with conduct problems fail to recognize the adverse effects of their verbal and nonverbal behavior, their deficit can be formulated as an interpersonal problem. Social skills training teaches adolescents with these behavior disorders to recognize the ways in which their actions affect others. Training involves techniques such as role playing, modeling by the therapist, and giving positive reinforcement to improve interpersonal relationships and enhance social outcomes.

Problem-Solving Therapy

In contrast to social skills training, which proposes that problems of conduct are the result of poor interpersonal skills, problem-solving therapy conceptualizes conduct problems as the result of deficiencies in cognitive processes. These processes include assessment of situations, interpretation of events, and expectations of others that are congruent with behavior. As reviewed in Kazdin & Weisz (2003), these children often misinterpret the intentions of others and may perceive hostility with little or no cause. Problem-solving skills training teaches these children to generate alternative solutions to social situations, to sharpen thinking concerning the consequences of those choices, and to evaluate responses after interpersonal conflicts.

Social Domain

Assessment

High levels of marital conflict, parental substance abuse, and parental antisocial behavior often mark family history.

Nursing Diagnoses for the Social Domain

In the social domain, nursing diagnoses include Compromised Family Coping and Impaired Social Interaction. Some outcomes for these patients are as follows:

- Increased use of problem-solving skills as evidenced by decreased interpersonal conflicts
- Decreased rule violations and conflicts with authority figures

Interventions for the Social Domain

Parent education for preschool- and school-aged children with disruptive behavior problems appears to be the most effective psychosocial intervention.

Management Training

Parent training begins with educating parents about disruptive behavior disorders, focusing particularly on impulsiveness, impaired judgment, and self-control. Children with long-standing problems in these areas often elicit punitive responses and negative attributions about their behavior from their parents. Ironically, because these parental responses focus on the child's failure, they may contribute to the child's behavior problems. An important second step is to clarify parental expectations and interpretation of the child's behavior. Parent management training may be offered to a group of parents or to individuals (Kazdin & Weisz, 2003).

Educating Parents

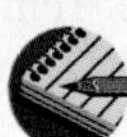

The aims of education are to provide parents with new ways of understanding their child's behavior and to promote improved interactions between parent and child. The most commonly presented techniques include the importance of positive reinforcement (praise and tangible rewards) for adaptive behavior, clear limits for unacceptable behavior, and use of mild punishment, such as time out (Box 29.6).

Family therapy is directed at assisting the family with altering maladaptive patterns of interaction or improving adjustment to stressors, such as changes in membership or losses. Multisystemic family therapy, which considers the child in the context of multiple family and community systems, has shown promise in the treatment of adolescents with conduct disorder (Henggeler et al., 1999).

> **BOX 29.6**
>
> ***Time Out***
>
> **Time Out Procedure**
> - *Labeling behavior:* Identify the behavior that the child is expected to perform or cease. The aim of this statement is to make clear what is required of the child. It typically takes the form of a simple declarative sentence: "Threatening is not acceptable."
> - *Warning:* In this step, the child is informed that if he or she does not perform the expected behavior or stop the unacceptable behavior, he or she will be given a "time out." "This is a warning: if you continue threatening to hit people, you'll have a time out."
> - *Time out:* If the child does not heed the warning, he or she is told to take a time out in simple straightforward terms: "take a time out."
> - *Duration:* The usual duration for a time out is 5 minutes for children 5 years of age or older.
> - *Location:* The child sits in a designated time-out chair without toys and without talking. The chair should be located away from general activity but within view. A kitchen timer can be used to mark the time, but the clock does not start until the child is sitting quietly in the designated spot.
> - *Follow-up:* The child is asked to recount why he or she was given the time out. The explanation need not be detailed, and no further discussion of the matter is required. Indeed, long discourse about the child's behavior is not helpful and should be avoided.

EVALUATION AND TREATMENT OUTCOMES

The nurse can review treatment goals and objectives to assess the child's progress with respect to verbal and physical aggression, socially appropriate resolution of conflicts, compliance with rules and expectations, and better management of frustration. As is true for the initial assessment, evaluation of treatment outcomes relies on input from parents, teachers, and other team members.

CONTINUUM OF CARE

Children and adolescents with disorders of conduct may be involved in many different agencies in the community, such as child welfare services, school authorities, and the legal system. Mental health services are requested when a child or adolescent's behavior is out of control or a comorbid disorder is suspected. Helping the youngster and the family negotiate their way through this maze of services may be an essential part of the treatment plan.

Disorders of Mood and Anxiety

ANXIETY DISORDERS

Anxiety is a universal human condition. Indeed, it may well be that common anxiety-provoking stimuli have biologically protective value. For example, a fear of snakes and the dark may have contributed to the survival of early humans through vigilance and avoidance behavior. Some degree of worry and specific fears is considered normal during the course of childhood (e.g., anxiety about strangers in the 1-year-old child). However, when the level of anxiety is excessive and hinders daily functioning, the diagnosis of an anxiety disorder may be appropriate. This section focuses on separation anxiety, a disorder diagnosed in childhood, and obsessive-compulsive disorder (OCD), a disorder that occurs in both adults and children (see Chapter 21).

SEPARATION ANXIETY DISORDER

Some have suggested that separation anxiety disorder is the childhood equivalent of panic disorder in adults. Although many children experience some discomfort on separation from their mothers or major attachment figures, children with separation anxiety disorder suffer great distress when faced with ordinary separations, such as going to school. In most cases, the mother is the focus of the child's concern, but this may not be so, especially if the mother is not the primary caregiver. The child may exhibit extraordinary reluctance or even refusal to separate from the primary caregiver. When asked, most children with separation anxiety disorder will express worry about harm or permanent loss of their major attachment figure. Other children may express worry about their own safety (Table 29.5).

A common manifestation of anxiety is **school phobia**, in which the child refuses to attend school, preferring to stay at home with the primary attachment figure. However, it should be noted that school phobia is a common presenting complaint in child psychiatric clinics and may be part of separation anxiety disorder, general anxiety disorder, social phobia, OCD, depression, or conduct disorder. In rare cases, school phobia can be a side effect of antipsychotic medication (see Scahill, Leckman, Schultz, Katsovich, & Peterson, 2003). The term *school phobia* was coined to distinguish it from truancy—whether it is a phobia in the usual sense is a matter of some debate. When another disorder such as depression is identified, it becomes the focus of treatment. In some cases, the school phobia may resolve when the primary disorder is successfully treated.

Separation anxiety disorder is excessive anxiety on separation from home or major attachment figure before age 18 years. It is manifested by acute distress, frequent nightmares about separation, and reluctance or refusal to separate. It lasts for at least 1 month, and causes clinically significant impairment in social or academic functioning.

Epidemiology and Etiology

The prevalence of separation anxiety disorder is estimated at 4% of school-aged children; thus, it is relatively common. Anxiety disorders run in families, and it appears that both environmental and genetic factors affect the risk for separation anxiety disorder. For example, it may emerge after a move, change to a new school, or death of a family member or pet. By contrast, recent

Table 29.5  Key Diagnostic Characteristics of Separation Anxiety Disorder 309.21 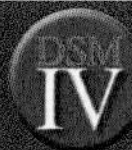

Diagnostic Criteria and Target Symptoms	Associated Findings
• Inappropriate and excessive anxiety about being away from home or primary attachment figure Excessive distress when separation occurs or is anticipated Persistent, excessive worry about losing or having harm come to attachment figures Persistent and excessive worry about an event that might cause separation from attachment figure Persistent reluctance or refusal to go to school or somewhere else because of separation anxiety Reluctance to be alone without attachment figures at home or without significant adults in other settings Persistent reluctance or refusal to go to sleep without being near attachment figure or sleep away from home Repeated nightmares about being separated Repeated complaints of physical symptoms when separated or when separation from attachment figures is anticipated • Duration of at least 4 weeks • Onset before age 18 years (for early-onset type: onset before age 6 years) • Not exclusively occurring during course of other psychotic disorder; not better accounted for by panic disorder with agoraphobia	• Social withdrawal, apathy • Difficulty concentrating • Fears of other situations, such as animals, monsters, accidents, and plane travel • Concerns about death and dying • School refusal and subsequent academic difficulties • Anger or lashing out with prospect of separation • Unusual perceptual experiences when alone • Demanding and needing constant attention and reassurance • Somatic complaints • Depressed mood • Other recurring worries that do not involve attachment figure

evidence suggests that traits such as shyness and behavioral inhibition (reluctance in new situations) are inherited (Koda, Charney, & Pine, 2003; Schwartz, Snidman, & Kagan, 1999). Furthermore, not only are children with an enduring "inhibited" temperament at greater risk for anxiety disorders themselves, but their immediate family members are also at greater risk for anxiety disorders compared with a psychiatric control group. Others have argued in favor of environmental determinants of separation anxiety, contending that anxious parents communicate to the child that the world is inhospitable and menacing to keep the child near. Available data suggest that the long-term outcome of childhood disorders is favorable in many cases but may evolve and take other forms in adulthood. For example, separation anxiety in childhood may re-emerge as panic disorder in adults (Koda et al., 2003).

Psychopharmacologic Interventions

The tricyclic antidepressant medication imipramine has been used as an adjunct to behavioral treatment or as a primary therapy for several years (Velosa & Riddle, 2000). However, in the largest controlled study to date, imipramine was no better than a placebo in managing separation anxiety (reviewed in Velosa & Riddle). In addition, some children display drowsiness and irritability when taking imipramine. Other side effects may include tachycardia, dry mouth, constipation, urinary retention, and dizziness. As a class of medications, the tricyclics can alter cardiac conduction; thus, baseline and follow-up electrocardiograms are recommended (King, Scahill, Lombroso, & Leckman, 2003). A recent multicenter study showed that the SSRI fluvoxamine is effective for reducing separation anxiety (RUPP Anxiety Study Group, 2001). The inconsistent results with the tricyclics and the positive results with fluvoxamine suggest that an SSRI would be a first-line treatment.

NURSING MANAGEMENT: HUMAN RESPONSE TO SEPARATION ANXIETY DISORDER

School phobia is often what prompts the family to seek consultation for the child. The onset of school refusal may be gradual or acute. Because school phobia can be a behavioral manifestation of several different child psychiatric disorders, it requires careful assessment. Issues to consider are whether the parents have been aware that the child is avoiding school (separation versus truancy); what efforts the family has used to return the child to school; the presence of significant subjective distress in the child with anticipation of going to school; and whether the school refusal occurs in the context of other behavioral, social, or emotional problems. The nurse should also review the purpose and dose of current medications.

The child's developmental history and response to new situations and prior separations provide essential background information for understanding the child's current separation anxiety. The assessment should also include a review of recent life events and the methods the family has used to promote the child's return to school. Finally, the family history with respect to anxiety, panic attacks, or phobias is also informative.

Most clinicians agree that the child should return to school as soon as possible because resistance to attending school invariably mounts the longer the child remains absent. Several therapeutic approaches are used in treating separation anxiety disorder, including individual psychotherapy, behavioral treatment, and pharmacotherapy. Although individual psychotherapy is a common treatment, data to support this approach are sparse. By contrast, evidence suggests that behavioral techniques can be effective in reducing separation anxiety. These techniques include flooding (rapid and forcible return to school) and desensitization in which the child is gradually returned to school (Labellarte & Ginsberg, 2003). To be successful, these techniques require close collaboration with the family and the school and may also include medication (Labellarte & Ginsberg).

OBSESSIVE-COMPULSIVE DISORDER

Obsessive-compulsive disorder (OCD) is characterized by intrusive thoughts that are difficult to dislodge (obsessions) and/or ritualized behaviors that the child feels driven to perform (compulsions). Historically, OCD was regarded as a neurosis, and the primary symptoms were viewed as the expression of unresolved sexual and aggressive impulses. Recent evidence from family genetic studies, pharmacologic trials, and neuroimaging studies has dramatically shifted the conceptualization of OCD (see Chapter 19). The notion that OCD is the manifestation of internal conflict concerning sexual and aggressive impulses has given way to a more biologic model (Murphy, Voeller, & Blier, 2003).

Epidemiology and Etiology

Until recently, OCD was considered uncommon in adults and even more rare in children; the multicenter ECA study estimated a 2% to 3% prevalence in the general population for adults. In addition, many of these adults reported that their symptoms began in childhood (Karno, Golding, Sorenson, & Burnam, 1988). A large community sample of high school students found a prevalence of about 2% (Flament et al., 1988). Thus, OCD is far more prevalent than previously supposed and can be expressed in childhood (Scahill et al., 2003).

Family genetic studies indicate that OCD recurs with a greater-than-expected frequency in the families of patients with OCD or Tourette disorder, suggesting an inherited vulnerability in some cases (Murphy et al., 2003). OCD has also been associated with other movement disorders, such as Sydenham's chorea (Murphy et al.). This observation led to speculation that autoimmune mechanisms may underlie some cases of OCD (Morshed et al., 2001; Taylor et al., 2002).

Regardless of etiology, most researchers now conceptualize OCD as a disorder of the basal ganglia (Murphy et al., 2003). Results from neuroimaging studies, which have shown functional abnormalities in the brain circuits connecting the frontal cortex and basal ganglia structures such as the caudate nucleus, strongly support this view (see Murphy et al. for a review). OCD is accompanied by anxiety disorders in some cases and tic disorders in others (Scahill et al., 2003).

Psychopharmacologic Interventions

Double-blind trials with clomipramine, fluoxetine, fluvoxamine, and sertraline have demonstrated the effectiveness of these agents in reducing symptoms of OCD in children and adolescents (DeVeaugh-Geiss et al., 1992; Geller et al., 2001; March et al., 1998; Riddle et al., 2001; POTS, 2004).

Sertraline was studied in a multisite trial of 112 subjects aged 7 to 17 by the Pediatric Obsessive-Compulsive Disorder Team (POTS, 2004). Participants were randomly assigned to receive cognitive-behavioral therapy (CBT) alone, CBT combined with sertraline, sertraline alone, or placebo for 12 weeks. All three treatments were superior to placebo. For those receiving sertraline, the drug was well tolerated and there were no reports of self-harm, suicidal ideation, or intent. Although combined treatment (medication plus CBT) was superior to CBT alone or sertraline alone, there were differences across sites. The results suggest that CBT was more effective at one of the study sites. This suggests that more work is needed to disseminate CBT in children and adolescents. Although the precise mechanism for their positive effects on OCD is not completely clear, these agents block the reuptake of serotonin in the brain. This property appears to be essential to the therapeutic effects of these agents because other antidepressants that do not block the reuptake of serotonin are not effective in treating OCD.

NURSING MANAGEMENT: HUMAN RESPONSE TO OBSESSIVE-COMPULSIVE DISORDER

Recurrent worries and ritualistic behavior can occur normally in children at particular stages of development. The first step in the assessment of OCD in children is to distinguish between normal childhood rituals and worries and pathologic rituals and obsessional thoughts (King & Scahill, 2001). Obsessional thoughts are recurrent, nagging, and bothersome. Although children may describe obsessions as occurring "out of the blue," external events may trigger obsessions. For example, a child may fear contamination whenever he or she is in contact with a certain person or object. Likewise, compulsions waste time, cause distress, and interfere with daily living (Box 29.7).

Several measures are now available to assist in the assessment of OCD in children. The Leyton Survey is a 20-item self-report used in both epidemiologic studies and clinical trials; high scores appear to be predictive of a clinical diagnosis of OCD (Flament et al., 1988). The Children's Yale-Brown Obsessive Compulsive Scale (CY-BOCS) is a semistructured interview designed to measure the severity of OCD once the diagnosis has been made. The CY-BOCS is a revision of the original adult instrument, and available evidence suggests that it is a reliable and valid measure of OCD severity in children (Scahill et al., 1997).

The severity of the child's and family's response to OCD will determine the appropriate nursing diagnoses. When the obsessions and compulsions emerge, these children or adolescents are in distress because of the disturbing and relentless nature of the symptoms. Parents may be pulled into the child's rituals (King & Scahill, 2001). Ineffective Coping, Compromised Family Coping, and Ineffective Role Performance are likely nursing diagnoses.

Treatment goals focus on reducing the obsessions and compulsions and their effects on the child's development. Behavior modification techniques have demonstrated benefit in reducing the primary symptoms of OCD in adults. However, behavior therapy has not been well studied in children and adolescents (Piacentini, 1999). Consistently effective OCD treatment techniques include exposure and response prevention (Piacentini). Exposure consists of gradual confrontation with events or situations that trigger obsessions and cause the urge to ritualize. According to the theory behind behavior therapy, repeated exposure works because the patient learns that the immediate anxiety will subside even if he or she does not complete the ritual. Response prevention complements exposure and consists of

BOX 29.7

Clinical Vignette: Kimberly and OCD

Kimberly, an 11-year-old fifth grader, comes for evaluation because her mother and teacher have become increasingly concerned about her repetitive behaviors. In retrospect, Kim's mother recalls first noticing repetitive rituals about 2 years before, but she did not become alarmed about these behaviors until recently when they began to interfere with daily living. At the time of referral, Kim exhibits complicated jumping rituals that involve a specific number of jumps and a particular manner of jumping. She also turns light switches off and on and performs complex movements, such as blinking in patterns and thrusting her arms back and forth a certain number of times. Her mother also reports Kim's near-constant request for reassurance about her own safety. In recent months, her incessant demands for reassurance have been more frequent and elaborate. For example, Kim's mother has to answer three times that everything is all right and then say. "I swear to it."

At the evaluation, Kim expresses fears that some ill fate, such as catastrophic illness or injury, will befall her. This fear is triggered by contact with any individual who seems sick, chance exposures to foul smells or dirt, or minor scrapes or bumps. Once the fear is triggered, she becomes increasingly anxious and consumed with the fear that she will develop an illness and die. Sometimes, her fears are specific, such as cancer or AIDS. Other times, her fears are more ambiguous, as evidenced by statements such as, "something bad will happen" if she doesn't complete the ritual. Kim acknowledges that the ritual is probably not related to the feared event, but she is reluctant to take a chance. If the ritual does not reduce her anxiety, she seeks reassurance from her mother.

Kim's medical history was negative for serious illness or injury, she was born after an uncomplicated pregnancy, labor, and delivery and achieved developmental milestones at appropriate times. Indeed, her mother could recall no unusual problems in the first few years of life except that Kim was typically anxious in new situations. Kim's mother reports a prior history of panic attacks, but the family history is otherwise negative for anxiety disorders, including obsessive-compulsive disorder.

instructing the patient to delay execution of the ritual. When exposure and response prevention are combined, the patient is confronted with a triggering stimulus such as dirt (exposure) but agrees not to do the hand washing for a brief period (response prevention) and tracks the anxiety level during the exercise. Successful cognitive behavioral treatment of children with OCD includes parents, both to include them in the treatment plan and to reduce parental involvement in the ritualized behavior. For example, the child may demand that the parent participate in a washing and checking ritual (Piacentini).

MOOD DISORDERS: MAJOR DEPRESSIVE DISORDER

The *DSM-IV-TR* includes several mood disorders, among them major depressive disorder, dysthymic disorder, bipolar I and bipolar II disorders, and cyclothymic disorder. Although these disorders occur in children and adolescents, they are less common in prepubertal children. These disorders are reviewed in detail in Chapter 18. Thus, this section is confined to a brief discussion of major depressive disorder in children and adolescents.

Depression is characterized by profound sadness, loss of interest in usual activities, loss of appetite with weight loss, sleep disturbance, loss of energy, feeling worthless or guilty, and recurrent thoughts of death or suicide. To meet *DSM-IV* criteria, these symptoms must be present on a daily basis and persist for at least 2 weeks (see Chapter 18).

Epidemiology

The prevalence of depression in children and adolescents is estimated at 1% to 5%, with adolescents being at the high end of this range and young children at the low end. Boys appear to be at higher risk for depression until adolescence, when depression becomes more common in girls.

NURSING MANAGEMENT: HUMAN RESPONSE TO MAJOR DEPRESSIVE DISORDER

The clinical picture of a child with depression may be similar to that of an adult, but children may not spontaneously express feelings of sadness and worthlessness. Thus, clinical experience is helpful when trying to elicit the symptoms of depression from young children. Reports from parents are important sources of information about changes in sleep patterns, appetite, activity level and interests, and emotional stability. In addition, quantitative measures, such as the Children's Depression Rating Scale and the Children's Depression Inventory, can assist in the assessment of childhood depression (Birmaher & Brent, 2003).

Nursing diagnoses for children or adolescents who are depressed are similar to those for adults, including Ineffective Coping, Chronic Low Self-Esteem, Disturbed Thought Processes, Self-Care Deficit, Imbalanced Nutrition, and Disturbed Sleep Pattern.

Treatment goals include improving the depressed mood and restoring sleep, appetite, and self-care. Interventions for responses to major depressive disorder in children and adolescents are also similar to those for adults. The psychiatric nurse develops a therapeutic relationship with the child and provides parent education and support. These children may act out their feelings, rather than discuss them. Thus, behavior problems may accompany depression. Developing sensitivity to the influence of environmental events on the child is important for the nurse, parents, and teachers (Box 29.8). These children are likely to be treated with an antidepressant medication and may also be in psychotherapy with a mental health specialist. Fluoxetine was studied in a National Institute of Mental Health-funded, multisite trial of 439 patients ages 12 to 17 years of age with major depression (Treatment for Adolescents with Depression Study [TADS], 2004). Subjects were randomly assigned to fluoxetine alone, CBT alone, fluoxetine plus CBT, or placebo. Fluoxetine alone or in combination with CBT was superior to placebo in reducing depression. Although fluoxetine plus CBT was better than fluoxetine alone, the difference was not statistically significant. Seven percent of all the patients receiving an SSRI (n = 216) expressed suicidal ideation compared with 4% of the 223 children in the non–drug-treated groups (i.e., CBT only and placebo groups). Six of the 216 (3%) fluoxetine-treated subjects exhibited mania, hypomania, or elevated mood symptoms compared with 1% (two of 223) subjects in the non–drug treatment groups.

The recent controversy surrounding the use of SSRIs in children reminds us that all treatments involve a risk–benefit equation. Given the modest benefit of the SSRIs and the potential for adverse behavioral effects, these medications merit careful monitoring in children and adolescents. Pediatric patients treated with an SSRI should be seen weekly for the first 4 weeks, biweekly during months 2 and 3, and then monthly for the next few months. Patient monitoring should focus on evidence of benefit and adverse effects including sleep problems, hyperactivity, sudden changes in mood or behavior, suicidal ideation, or self-injurious behavior (Scahill, Hamrin, & Pachler, 2005).

Tic Disorders and Tourette's Disorder

Motor tics are usually quick, jerky movements of the eyes, face, neck, and shoulders, although they may involve other muscle groups as well. Occasionally, tics involve slower, more purposeful, or dystonic movements. Phonic tics typically include repetitive throat clearing, grunting, or other noises, but may also include more complex sounds, such as words, parts of words, and, in a minority of patients, obscenities. Transient tics by definition do not endure over time and appear to be fairly common in school-aged children.

BOX 29.8

Questions, Choices, and Outcomes

Mrs. S has just returned with her son Jared to the child psychiatric inpatient services following an overnight pass. She reports that the visit did not go well due to Jared's anger and defiance. She remarked that this behavior was distressingly similar to his behavior before the hospitalization. She expressed additional concern because of the upcoming discharge from the hospital. After saying goodbye to Jared, she pulled the nurse aside and stated that she had decided to file for divorce.

Mrs. S indicated that she had not told her husband or the family therapist. When asked whether Jared knew about her decision, Mrs. S suddenly realized that he may have overheard her discussing the matter with her sister on the telephone during this home visit.

How should the nurse approach this situation?

Choice		*Possible Outcomes*
Discuss her hypothesis about Jared's behavior and his uncertainty	→	Mother can see relationship between Jared's behavior and her plan for divorce
	→	Mother ignores the nurse
	→	Mother is interested, but does not see the connection
Ignore the statement	→	Child and family did not learn about the connection between Jared's behavior and the events at home
Encourage mother to sort out her problems	→	The focus is then on mother's problems

Analysis

The best response is focusing on the possible relationship between Jared's recent behavioral deterioration and his uncertainty of his family's future. If the nurse ignores the statement or focuses on the mother's interpretation of Jared's behavior, the mother is less likely to appreciate the connection between pending divorce and Jared's behavior. The nurse should also emphasize the importance of discussing the matter in family therapy.

KEY CONCEPT Tics are sudden, rapid, repetitive, stereotyped motor movements or vocalizations.

Tic disorder is a general term encompassing several syndromes that are chiefly characterized by motor tics, phonic tics, or both. The *DSM-IV-TR* includes four tic disorders: Tourette's syndrome or disorder, chronic motor or vocal tic disorder, transient tic disorder, and tic disorder not otherwise specified. This section focuses on the most severe tic disorder, Tourette's disorder (Table 29.6). Because no diagnostic tests are used for this disorder, the diagnosis is based on the type and duration of tics present (Leckman, Peterson, King, Scahill, & Cohen, 2001). The typical age of onset for tics is about 7 years, and motor tics generally precede phonic tics. Parents often describe the seeming replacement of one tic with another. In addition to this changing repertoire of motor and phonic tics, Tourette's disorder exhibits a waxing and waning course. The child can suppress the tics for brief periods. Thus, it is not uncommon to hear from parents that their child has more frequent tics at home than at school. Older children and adults may describe an urge or a physical sensation before having a tic. The general trend is for tic symptoms to decline by early adulthood (Leckman et al., 1998).

Tourette's disorder is defined by multiple motor and phonic tics for at least 1 year.

Epidemiology and Etiology

The prevalence of Tourette's disorder is estimated to be between 1 and 10 per 1,000 in school-aged children, with boys being affected three to six times more often than girls (Scahill et al., 2005). The observation in the 1970s that the potent dopamine blocker haloperidol could reduce tics sparked interest in the biologic mechanisms, with particular focus on central dopaminergic systems.

The precise nature of the underlying pathophysiology is unclear, but the basal ganglia and functionally related cortical areas are presumed to play a central role (Mink, 2001). The basal ganglia, which consist of the caudate, putamen, and globus pallidus, are located at the base of the cortex and play an important role in planning and executing movement. This functional role is accomplished by means of parallel circuits that connect the basal ganglia to the cortex and the thalamus. To date, no specific lesions in the basal ganglia have been found in Tourette's disorder. Nonetheless, findings from neuroimaging studies are consistent with the presumption that a dysregulation of frontal cortical and basal ganglia circuits underlies Tourette's disorder (Peterson et al., 2001).

In the 1980s, data from family genetic studies suggested that Tourette's disorder is inherited as a single autosomal dominant gene. However, more recent studies suggest that the inheritance may involve more than a single gene (Tourette Syndrome Association, 1999; Walkup et al., 1996). The range of expression is presumed to be variable and includes Tourette's disorder, chronic motor or chronic vocal tics, and OCD. Twin studies have shown that monozygotic twins are far more likely to be concordant for Tourette's disorder than are dizygotic twins, further supporting the genetic hypotheses. However, even when monozygotic twins are concordant, the twins may not be equally affected. Thus, although substantial evidence supports a genetic etiology, environmental factors affect the expression of the gene (for a more complete review, see Walkup et al.).

Several neurochemical systems have been implicated in the etiology of Tourette's disorder, including dopamine systems, noradrenaline, endogenous opioids, and

Table 29.6  **Key Diagnostic Characteristics of Tourette's Syndrome 307.23** 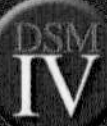

Diagnostic Criteria and Target Symptoms	Associated Findings
• Multiple motor tics and one or more vocal tics Sudden rapid recurrent, nonrhythmic, stereotyped motor movements or vocalizations Motor tics typically involving the head and other parts of body Vocal tics typically involving throat clearing, grunting, and occasionally words or parts of words • Tics occurring many times a day, present for at least 1 year Appear simultaneously or at different periods during the illness No tic-free period of more than 3 consecutive months • Onset before age 18 years • Not a direct physiologic effect of a substance or general medical condition	• Obsessions and compulsions • Hyperactivity, distractibility, and impulsivity • Social discomfort, shame, self-consciousness, and depressed mood • Impaired social, academic, and occupational functioning • Possible interference with daily activities if tics are severe

serotonin. The consistent observation that boys are more likely to be affected than girls has also led to speculation about the potential role of androgens in the pathophysiology of tic disorders. However, treatment strategies based on this theory appear to be ineffective (Peterson, Zhang, Anderson, & Leckman, 1998).

Psychopharmacologic Interventions

Two classes of drugs are commonly used in the treatment of tics: antipsychotics and α-adrenergic receptor agonists. Historically, the most commonly used antipsychotics included haloperidol and pimozide. These potent dopamine blockers are often effective at low doses. Attempts to eradicate all tics by increasing the dosages of these antipsychotics almost certainly results in diminishing therapeutic returns and additional side effects. The most frequently encountered side effects include drowsiness, dulled thinking, muscle stiffness, akathisia, increased appetite and weight gain, and acute dystonic reactions. Long-term use carries a small risk for tardive dyskinesia. Also, the atypical antipsychotics ziprasidone and risperidone have been evaluated for the treatment of tics in children and adolescents (Sallee et al., 2000; Scahill et al., 2003). Both were found to be superior to placebo.

The α_2-adrenergic receptor agonist clonidine (Catapres) has been used in treating Tourette's disorder for more than 20 years. Guanfacine (Tenex) is a newer α_2-adrenergic receptor agonist that has only recently been studied in children with Tourette's disorder. Both drugs were originally developed as antihypertensive agents, but their regulatory action on the brain's norepinephrine system led researchers to try these medications in patients with Tourette's disorder. Results from double-blind, placebo-controlled studies indicate that both are effective in reducing tics (King et al., 2003; Scahill, Chappell, et al., 2001). However, the level of improvement in tic symptoms is generally less than that observed with the antipsychotics. In the study by Scahill, Chappell, and colleagues, guanfacine was also effective in reducing symptoms of ADHD. (For additional discussion of pharmacotherapy in Tourette's disorder, see King et al.)

NURSING MANAGEMENT: HUMAN RESPONSE TO TIC DISORDER

Nursing assessment of a child with tics includes a review of the onset, course, and current level of the symptoms. The goals of the assessment are to identify the frequency, intensity, complexity, and interference of the tics and their effects on functioning; determine the child's level of adaptive functioning; identify the child's areas of strength and weakness in general and in school; and identify social supports for the child and family (Leckman et al., 2001). Another important aspect of the assessment is to determine the effects of the tic symptoms on the child and family. Some children and families adjust well; however, others are embarrassed or devastated and tend to withdraw socially. About half of school-aged children with Tourette's disorder have ADHD, and a substantial percentage have symptoms of OCD (Leckman et al.). Therefore, in addition to inquiring about tics, the nurse should assess the child's overall development, activity level, and capacity to concentrate and persist with a single task, as well as explore repetitive habits and recurring worries.

Nursing diagnoses could include Ineffective Coping, Impaired Social Interaction, Anxiety, and Compromised Family Coping. Children with Tourette's disorder typically have normal intelligence, although clinical samples may show a higher frequency of learning problems. These learning problems may include subtle problems of organization and planning or more severe problems with reading (Schultz et al., 1998). Handwriting, including both speed and legibility, is another common problem for these youngsters. The use of a computer can obviate difficulties with handwriting in some cases.

The approach to planning nursing interventions depends on the primary source of impairment: tics themselves, OCD symptoms, or the triad of hyperactivity, inattention, and poor impulse control. The nurse can provide counseling and education for the patient, education for the parents, and consultation for the school. Most children and their families need some education about Tourette's disorder. Individual psychotherapy with a mental health specialist (such as a psychologist or an advanced practice nurse) may be indicated for some children and adolescents with Tourette's disorder to deal with maladaptive responses to the chronic condition.

Before evaluation and diagnosis of Tourette's disorder, most families struggle with various explanations for the child's tics. Because tics fluctuate in severity with time and may be more prominent in some settings than in others, family members may have difficulty understanding their involuntary nature. Some parents may be convinced that the tics are deliberate and done to secure attention; others may judge that the tics are "nervous habits" indicative of underlying trouble. Such views require reconciliation with the currently accepted view that tics are involuntary. Some parents may conclude that the child is incapable of controlling any behavior because of Tourette's disorder. They may subsequently feel uncertain about setting limits. In these families, delineating the boundaries of Tourette's disorder can be helpful (Leckman et al., 2001).

On learning that this disorder is probably genetic, some parents may harbor guilt for having passed it on to their child. The nurse can assist such families by listening to these concerns and providing information about the natural history of Tourette's disorder—it is not a progressive condition, tics often diminish in adulthood, and it need not restrict what the child can achieve in life.

Teaching Points 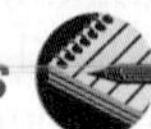

Teachers, guidance counselors, and school nurses may need current information about Tourette's disorder and related problems. Discussions with school personnel often include issues such as how to deal with tic behaviors that are disruptive in the classroom, how to manage teasing from other children, and how to handle medication side effects. A careful discussion of the boundaries of Tourette's disorder and tic symptomatology usually can resolve these matters. Teachers who understand the involuntary nature of tics can often generate creative solutions, such as excusing the child for errands. This maneuver allows the child to step out of the classroom briefly to release a bout of tics, thereby reducing stress. In some situations, a brief presentation about Tourette's disorder to the class will reduce teasing and help both teachers and classmates tolerate the tic symptoms (Leckman et al., 2001) (see Box 29.9).

Before initiating these interventions, it is essential to identify the child's needs and to pursue these strategies in collaboration with the family and other clinical team members. The Education for the Handicapped Act (Public Law 94–142) ensures that children with conditions such as Tourette's disorder are eligible for special education services, even if they do not meet full criteria for learning disability. Thus, if evidence shows that Tourette's disorder is hindering academic progress, parents can demand special education services for their child. Nurses can help families negotiate with the school to obtain appropriate services.

Childhood Schizophrenia

Childhood (early onset) schizophrenia is diagnosed by the same criteria as those used in adults (see Chapter 16). The difficulty in diagnosing a psychiatric disorder in children has led to years of debate and controversy regarding whether childhood schizophrenia differs from the adult type or is merely an early manifestation of the same disorder. For many years, it was believed that autism represented the childhood form of schizophrenia. However, in recent years autism and childhood schizophrenia have been differentiated (Volkmar et al., 2004). As currently defined, childhood schizophrenia (occurring before the age of 13 years) is rare, with an estimated 2 cases per 100,000 in the population. Other forms of psychosis, falling short of diagnostic criteria for schizophrenia, can occur in children. By way of comparison, the adult disorder, which usually has its onset in late adolescence, has a prevalence of 10 cases per 1,000 in the United States.

Childhood schizophrenia is usually characterized by poorer premorbid functioning than later onset schizophrenia. Common premorbid difficulties include social, cognitive, linguistic, attentional, motor, and perceptual delays (Volkmar et al., 2004). Taken together, these findings suggest that early-onset schizophrenia is a more severe form of the disorder.

BOX 29.9

Therapeutic Dialogue: *Tics and Disruptive Behaviors*

Ineffective Approach

Teacher: I see the tics. He jerks his head, makes faces, and flicks his hands.

Nurse: What do you do about them?

Teacher: What can I do? If he isn't disrupting the class, I leave him alone. Even when he is throwing spitballs.

Nurse: Spitballs! He shouldn't be allowed to throw spitballs.

Teacher: Oh, I thought that was a part of his problem.

Nurse: Well, throwing spitballs has nothing to do with tics.

Effective Approach

Teacher: I see the tics. He jerks his head, makes faces, and flicks his hands.

Nurse: He cannot help the tics that you are seeing. Tic disorders can exhibit a wide range of severity, from mild to severe and from simple to complex. Some complex tics may be difficult to distinguish from habits or rituals.

Teacher: What about things like throwing spitballs? When he does things like that, I try to ignore that behavior.

Nurse: Sounds like you give him the benefit of the doubt. (Validation) However, throwing a spitball is not a tic behavior.

Teacher: What should I do?

Nurse: How do you usually handle that type of behavior? (A modification of reflection)

Teacher: I'd ask him to stop and sometimes go into the hall.

Nurse: Disruptive behavior that is voluntary in a student with a tic disorder should be handled as you would handle any other child.

Critical Thinking Challenge

- Compare the responses of the nurse in these scenarios. What made the difference in the teacher's responsiveness to the nurse?

Nursing care for these children follows an approach similar to that used in treatment of PDDs. Antipsychotic medication is prescribed for symptoms (Kumra, 2000). Increasingly, clinicians are using the newer atypical antipsychotics, such as risperidone, olanzapine, and quetiapine (Kumra). To varying degrees, these medications have both dopamine-blocking and serotonin-blocking properties. This combined effect is presumed to decrease the risk for neurological side effects associated with the traditional antipsychotics (see Chapters 8 and 18 for more detailed description of the atypical antipsychotics).

Development of an individualized care plan for children with schizophrenia begins with a nursing assessment to identify functional problems specific to the child. Similarly, the recognition that childhood schizophrenia is a chronic and severe condition should guide the identification of outcomes. Goals should be realistic, and the nurse should pay special attention to the child's support systems. Parent education about the disorder, medications, and long-term management (including use of community resources) is an essential part of the treatment plan. Long-term management also requires monitoring of chronic antipsychotic therapy. Although the newer, atypical antipsychotic medications appear to have a lower risk for neurologic effects, other side effects such as weight gain also warrant careful monitoring (Martin et al., 2000).

Elimination Disorders

ENURESIS

Enuresis usually means involuntary bedwetting, although repeated urination on clothing during waking hours can occur (diurnal enuresis). For nocturnal enuresis, the *DSM-IV-TR* specifies that bedwetting occurs at least twice per week for a duration of 3 months and that the child is at least 5 years of age. Even without treatment, 50% of these children can achieve dryness by age 10 years.

Enuresis is the involuntary excretion of urine after the age at which the child should have attained bladder control.

Epidemiology and Etiology

The prevalence of nocturnal enuresis varies with age and gender, being most common in young boys—an estimated 15% of 5-year-old boys, 7% of boys aged 7 to 9 years, and 1% of 14-year-old boys have nocturnal enuresis (Mikkelsen, 2002; Reiner, 2003). The frequency in girls is about half that of boys in each age group. The etiology of enuresis is unknown, with probably no single cause. Most children with nocturnal enuresis are urologically normal. Some evidence has shown that at least some children with nocturnal enuresis secrete decreased amounts of antidiuretic hormone during sleep, which may play a role in enuresis (Reiner, 2003).

NURSING MANAGEMENT: HUMAN RESPONSE TO ENURESIS DISORDER

The nursing assessment should include the child's developmental history, the onset and course of enuresis, prior treatment, presence of emotional problems, and medical history. The nurse should also explore the family's home environment, family attitudes about the child's enuresis, and the family's medical history. Routine laboratory tests such as urinalysis and a urine culture are used to determine the presence of infection. The nurse should obtain baseline data regarding toileting habits, including daytime incontinence, urinary frequency, and constipation. He or she should refer children with persistent daytime enuresis for consultation with a urologist (Reiner, 2003).

In many cases, limiting fluid intake in the evening and treating constipation (if present) is sufficient to decrease the frequency of bedwetting.

Pharmacologic Interventions

If conservative methods fail, both drug and behavioral treatment have been beneficial for nocturnal enuresis. Imipramine (Tofranil), a tricyclic antidepressant, has shown efficacy in the treatment of enuresis (Reiner, 2003). The nasal spray preparation of desmopressin (DDAVP) has also shown promise, but beneficial effects may not endure (Hamano et al., 2000). DDAVP is a synthetic antidiuretic hormone that actually inhibits the production of urine. One review suggests that DDAVP helps about 25% of children who use it, with minimal risk for adverse effects (Harari & Moulden, 2000). Given its safety margin, DDAVP is preferred to imipramine.

Behavioral Interventions

The most effective nonpharmacologic treatment is the use of a pad and buzzer. In this form of behavioral treatment, the bed is equipped with a pad that sets off a buzzer if the child wets. The buzzer then wakes up the child, thereby reminding the child to void. Bedwetting can often be extinguished with this method in a relatively brief period.

ENCOPRESIS

Encopresis involves soiling clothing with feces or depositing feces in inappropriate places. Additional diagnostic criteria include that the child is older than 4 years, that the soiling occurs at least once per month, and that the soiling is not the result of a medical disorder, such as aganglionic megacolon (Hirschsprung's disease). The most common form of encopresis is fecal impaction accompanied by leakage around the hardened mass of stool. Because of the loss of muscle tone in the lower bowel, the child loses the usual urge to defecate and may not feel the leakage. Surprisingly, the child may not detect the smell of the stool because the olfactory apparatus becomes accustomed to the odor. If left untreated, this problem generally resolves independently by middle adolescence. Nonetheless, the social consequences may be substantial (Mikkelsen, 2002).

Epidemiology and Etiology

As with enuresis, encopresis is more common in boys, and the frequency of the condition declines with age. The current estimate of prevalence is 1.5% of school-aged children, with boys three to four times more likely to have encopresis than girls (Mikkelsen, 2002).

The reasons for withholding stool and starting the cycle of fecal impaction are unclear but are usually not the result of physical causes. However, as noted, once the fecal impaction occurs, there is a loss of tone in the bowel and leakage.

NURSING MANAGEMENT: HUMAN RESPONSE TO ENCOPRESIS DISORDER

The assessment includes a detailed interview with the child and parent regarding the pattern of the encopresis. A calm, matter-of-fact approach can help to reduce the child's embarrassment. A physical examination is also necessary; thus, collaboration with the child's primary care provider or consulting pediatric specialist is essential. The presence of encopresis does not necessarily signal severe emotional or behavioral disturbances, but the nurse should inquire about other psychiatric disorders. The diagnosis of encopresis is presumed given a history of intermittent constipation and soiling. Collaboration with primary care consultants often is helpful to rule out rare medical conditions, such as Hirschsprung's disease.

Teaching Points

Effective intervention begins with educating the parents and the child about normal bowel function and the self-perpetuating cycle of fecal impaction and leakage of stool around the hardened mass of feces. The short-term goal of this educational effort is to decrease the anger and recrimination that often complicate the picture in these families. Because encopresis often results in a loss of bowel tone, it may help to motivate children by emphasizing the need to strengthen their muscles. In many cases, cleaning out the bowel is necessary before initiating behavioral treatment. The bowel catharsis is usually followed by administration of mineral oil, which is often continued during the bowel retraining program. A high-fiber diet is often recommended.

The behavioral treatment program involves daily sitting on the toilet after each meal for a predetermined period (e.g., 10 minutes). The child and parents can measure the time with an ordinary kitchen timer, and the parents can encourage the child to read or look at picture books while sitting. They can give the child rewards in the form of stars, stickers, or points for complying with the retraining program and add bonuses for successful defecation. The family can tally stickers or points on a calendar, and the child can "cash in" collected points for small prizes (Mikkelsen, 2002; Reiner, 2003). All the disorders discussed in this chapter are summarized in Table 29.7.

Table 29.7 Summary of Diagnostic Characteristics

Disorder	Diagnostic Characteristics
Pervasive Developmental Disorder Not Otherwise Specified	• Impairment of reciprocal social interaction Marked impairment in use of nonverbal behaviors Failure to develop appropriate peer relationships Absence of spontaneously seeking to share enjoyment, interest, or achievements (e.g., pointing out things of interest) Lack of social or emotional reciprocity (oblivious to others, not noticing another's distress) • Repetitive and stereotypic behavior patterns and activities Preoccupation with pattern that is abnormal in intensity or focus Inflexible adherence to nonfunctional routines or rituals

(Continued)

Table 29.7 Summary of Diagnostic Characteristics (Continued)

Disorder	Diagnostic Characteristics
	Stereotypic, repetitive motor mannerisms Persistent preoccupation with idiosyncratic interests (e.g., train schedules, air conditioners)
Autism	• As listed above for pervasive developmental disorders • Severe impairment in communication Delay or total lack of spoken language Impaired ability to initiate or sustain a conversation Use of stereotypic, repetitive, or idiosyncratic language Lack of varied, spontaneous make-believe or social imitative play • Abnormal social interaction, use of language for social communication, or symbolic or imaginative play before age 3 years • Not better accounted for by another psychiatric disorder
Asperger's disorder	• As listed above for pervasive developmental disorders • Clinically significant impairment in social, occupational, or other areas of functioning • No general delay in language • Less likely to have delay in cognitive development or daily living skills • Over focus on an area of restricted interest is a prominent feature • Not better accounted for by another pervasive developmental disorder or schizophrenia
Learning Disorders	• Discrepancy between academic achievement and intellectual ability
Reading disorders	• Reading achievement substantially below that expected for age, intelligence, and education
Mathematics disorders	• Mathematic ability substantially below that expected for age, intelligence, and education
Disorders of written expression	• Writing skills substantially below that expected for age, intelligence, and education
Communication Disorders	• Interference with academic or occupational achievement or social communication
Expressive language disorder	• Deficits not explained by retardation or deprivation • Impairment of expressive language development Limited amount of speech Limited range of vocabulary Vocabulary errors Sentence structure problems Unusual word order Slow rate of language development Difficulty in communication, both verbally and with sign language • As listed above for communication disorders • Deficits cannot be explained by pervasive developmental disorder
Mixed receptive-expressive language disorder	• Impairment of receptive and expressive language development Markedly limited vocabulary Errors in tense Difficulty recalling words or appropriate-length sentences General difficulty expressing ideas Difficulty understanding words, sentences, or types of words or statements Multiple disabilities such as inability to understand basic vocabulary or simple sentences; deficits in sound discrimination, storage, recall, and sequencing • As listed above for communication disorders • Deficits not explained by pervasive developmental disorder
Phonologic disorder	• Failure to use appropriate developmentally expected speech sounds • Errors in sound production Substitution of one sound for another Omission of sounds • As listed above for communication disorders
Stuttering	• Disturbed fluency and timing patterns of speech Repetition of sounds and syllables Prolongation of sound Interjections Broken words Filled or unfilled pauses in speech Substitutions of words to avoid problematic sounds Production of words with an excess of physical tension Repetitions of monosyllabic whole word • As listed above for communication disorders

(Continued on following page)

Table 29.7 Summary of Diagnostic Characteristics (Continued)

Disorder	Diagnostic Characteristics
Disruptive Behavior Disorders Conduct disorder	• Significant impairment in social, academic, or occupational functioning • Not accounted for by antisocial personality disorder if older than 18 years • Repetitive and persistent behavior that violates the rights of others or major age-appropriate societal norms Aggression to people and animals Destruction of property Deceitfulness or theft Serious violations of rules • As listed above for disruptive behavior disorders
Oppositional defiant disorder	• Negativistic, hostile behavior pattern Loss of temper Frequently argumentative Active defiance or refusal to comply with adult requests or rules Deliberate annoyance of others Blaming of others for own mistakes or misbehavior Anger and resentment Spitefulness and vindictiveness • As listed above for disruptive behavior disorders • Not exclusive during course of psychotic or mood disorder
Anxiety Disorders Obsessive-compulsive disorders	See Chapter 22.
Mood Disorders Major depressive disorder	See Chapter 20.
Tic Disorders	• Single or multiple tics • Onset before age 18 years • Not due to substance (e.g., amphetamine) or general medical condition
Chronic motor or vocal tic disorder 307.22	• Motor or vocal tics • Occurring many times per day nearly every day or intermittently throughout more than 1 year; no tic-free period greater than 3 months As listed above for tic disorders
Transient tic disorder 307.21	• Motor or vocal tics • Occurring many times during the day for at least 4 weeks; not longer than 12 consecutive months
Tourette's disorder	• Motor and phonic tics lasting more than 12 months
Childhood Schizophrenia	See Chapter 19
Elimination Disorders Enuresis 307.6	• Repeated voiding into bed or clothes (involuntary or intentional) • Occurring twice a week for at least 3 consecutive months or significant impairment in social, academic, or other area of functioning • At least 5 years of age or developmental equivalent • Not a physiologic effect of a substance or general medical condition
Encopresis 307.7 without constipation and overflow incontinence 787.6 with constipation and overflow incontinence	• Repeated passage of feces into inappropriate places, such as clothing or floor • Occurring at least once a month for at least 3 months • At least 4 years of age or developmental equivalent • Not the physiologic effect of a substance or general medical condition except involving constipation

SUMMARY OF KEY POINTS

■ Improved methods of assessing and defining psychiatric disorders have enhanced appreciation for the frequency of psychiatric disorders in children and adolescents.

■ An estimated 8 to 10 million children and adolescents have a serious psychiatric disorder in the United States (10% of individuals younger than 18 years).

■ The developmental disorders include mental retardation, pervasive developmental disorders (PDDs), and specific developmental disorders. Mental retardation often complicates PDDs. Assessment findings should guide nursing management. Specific developmental disorders include communication disorders and learning disorders. These disorders are fairly common in the general population, but they are more common in children with other primary psychiatric disorders.

- Child psychiatric disorders can be divided into externalizing and internalizing disorders. Externalizing disorders include the disruptive behavior disorders: attention-deficit hyperactivity disorder (ADHD), oppositional defiant disorder, and conduct disorder. Internalizing disorders include depression and anxiety disorders.
- ADHD is defined by the presence of inattention, impulsiveness, and in most cases, hyperactivity. As currently defined, ADHD is the most common disorder of childhood. This heterogeneous disorder affects boys more often than girls.
- Effective treatment of ADHD often involves multiple approaches, including medication and parent training.
- Primary features of oppositional defiant disorder include persistent disobedience, argumentativeness, and tantrums.
- Conduct disorder is characterized by lying, truancy, stealing, and fighting.
- Assessment of children with disruptive behavior problems involves securing data from multiple sources, including the child, parents, and school personnel.
- Standardized rating instruments can assist data collection from multiple informants.
- Separation anxiety and obsessive-compulsive disorder (OCD) are relatively common anxiety disorders in school-aged children. (OCD becomes more common in adolescents.)
- Treatment of separation anxiety and OCD may include medication, behavioral therapy, or a combination of these treatments.
- Major depression in children is believed to be similar to major depression in adults.
- The efficacy of antidepressant medications is less well established in children and adolescents than in adults.
- Tourette's disorder is a tic disorder characterized by motor and phonic tics. Common comorbid conditions include ADHD and OCD.
- Childhood schizophrenia is a rare disorder.
- Elimination disorders include encopresis and enuresis. Behavioral therapy approaches are the most effective treatment for these disorders. Medication may also be used.

CRITICAL THINKING CHALLENGES

1 Discuss the distinguishing features of ADHD and conduct disorder.
2 What brain region is believed to play a fundamental role in the pathophysiology of Tourette's disorder?
3 Discuss the differences and similarities among mental retardation, pervasive developmental disorders, and learning disability.
4 Analyze how genetic and environmental factors may interact in the etiology of child psychiatric disorders.
5 Learning disabilities and communication disorders are more common in children with psychiatric disorders than in the general population. How might a learning disability or a communication disorder complicate a psychiatric illness in a school-aged child?
6 Compare and contrast nursing approaches for a child with ADHD with those used for a child with autistic disorder. How are they different? How are they similar?
7 Discuss the significance of the Education for the Handicapped Act. What are some of the implications for nurses working with children with a psychiatric disorder and their families?
8 How would you answer these questions from a parent: "What causes ADHD? Is it my fault?"

Rain Man: 1988. This classic film stars Dustin Hoffman as Raymond Babbitt, a man who has autism (savant). Tom Cruise plays his brother Charlie, a self-centered hustler who believes that he has been cheated out of his inheritance. Discovering Raymond in an institution, Charlie abducts Raymond in a last-ditch effort to get his fair share of the family estate. The story evolves around the relationship that develops as the brothers drive across the country.

Dustin Hoffman brilliantly portrays the behaviors and symptoms of high functioning autism, such as the monotone speech, insistence on sameness, and repetitive behavior.

VIEWING POINTS: Identify and describe Raymond's ritualistic behaviors. Identify the behaviors that depict extreme autistic isolation. Observe Raymond's language patterns and any distinct abnormalities. What happens when Raymond's rituals are interrupted?

REFERENCES

Achenbach, T. (1991). *Manual for the child behavior checklist and behavior profile*. Burlington, VT: University of Vermont.

American Psychiatric Association. (2000). *Diagnostic and statistical manual of mental disorders* (4th ed., text revision). Washington, DC: Author.

Arnold, L. E., Aman, M. G., Martin, A., Collier-Crespin, A., Vitiello, B., Tierney, E., et al. (2000). Assessment in multisite randomized clinical trials (RCTs) of patients with autistic disorder. *Journal of Autism Development, 30,* 99–111.

Barkley, R. A. (1997). *Defiant children: A clinician's manual for parent training.* New York: Guilford Press.

Barkley, R. A. (1998). *Attention deficit hyperactivity disorder: A handbook for diagnosis and treatment.* New York: Guilford Press.

Beitchman, J. H., Nair, R., Clegg, M., & Patel, P. G. (1986). Prevalence of speech and language disorders in 5-year-old kindergarten children in the Ottawa-Carleton Region. *Journal of Speech and Hearing Disorders, 51,* 98–110.

Biederman, J., Faraone, S. V., Keenan, K., et al. (1992). Further evidence for family-genetic risk factors in attention deficit disorder. *Archives of General Psychiatry, 49,* 728–738.

Biederman, J., Milberger, S., Faraone, S. V., et al. (1995). Family-environment risk factors for attention-deficit hyperactivity disorder. *Archives of General Psychiatry, 52,* 464–470.

Biederman, J., & the ADHD Study Group. (2002). Efficacy of atomoxetine versus placebo in school-age girls with attention-deficit/hyperactivity disorder. *Pediatrics, 110*(6), 75–79.

Birmaher, B., & Brent, D. (2003). Depressive disorders. In A. Martin, L. Scahill, D. S. Charney, & J. F. Leckman (Eds.), *Pediatric psychopharmacology: Principles and practice* (1st ed.; pp. 466–483). New York: Oxford.

Blackson, T. C., Butler, T., Belsky, J., et al. (1999). Individual traits and family contexts predict sons' externalizing behavior and preliminary relative risk ratios for conduct disorder and substance use disorder outcomes. *Drug and Alcohol Dependence, 56*(2), 115–131.

Bolton, P. F., Murphy, M., Macdonald, H., et al. (1997). Obstetric complications in autism: Consequences or causes of the condition? *Journal of the American Academy of Child and Adolescent Psychiatry, 36*(2), 272–281.

Buitelaar, J. K., van der Gaag, R. J., & van der Hoeven, J. (1998). Buspirone in the management of anxiety and irritability in children with pervasive disorders: Results of an open-label study. *Journal of Clinical Psychiatry, 59*(2), 56–59.

Campbell, M., Armenteros, J. L., Malone, R. P., et al. (1997). Neuroleptic-related dyskinesias in autistic children: A prospective, longitudinal study. *Journal of the American Academy of Child and Adolescent Psychiatric Nursing, 36,* 835–843.

Carroll, D. H., Scahill, L., & Phillips, K. (2002). Current concepts in body dysmorphic disorder. *Archives of Psychiatric Nursing, 16,* 72–79.

Carroll, D. H., Shyam, R., & Scahill, L. (2002). Cardiac conduction and antipsychotic medication: A primer on electrocardiograms. *Journal of Child and Adolescent Psychiatric Nursing, 15*(4), 170–177.

Castellanos, F. X., Giedd, J. N., Marsh, W. L., et al. (1996). Quantitative brain magnetic resonance imaging in attention-deficit hyperactivity disorder. *Archives of General Psychiatry, 53*(7), 607–616.

Conners, C. K. (1989). *Conners' rating scales manual.* North Tonawanda, NY: Multi-Health Systems.

Courchesne, E., Redcay, E., Morgan, J.T., Kennedy, D. P. (2005). Austism at the beginning; microstructural and growth abnormalities underlying the cognitive and behavioral phenotype of autism. *Development and Psychopathology* 17(3) 577–597.

DeVeaugh-Geiss, J., Moroz, G., Biederman, J., et al. (1992). Clomipramine hydrochloride in childhood and adolescent obsessive-compulsive disorder: A multicenter trial. *Journal of American Academy of Child and Adolescent Psychiatry, 31,* 45–49.

Flament, M. F., Whitaker, A., Rapoport, J. L., et al. (1988). Obsessive compulsive disorder in adolescence. *Journal of the American Academy of Child and Adolescent Psychiatry, 27,* 764–771.

Fombonne, E. (2003). Epidemiological surveys of autism and other pervasive developmental disorders. *Journal of Autism and Developmental Disorders, 33*(4), 365–382.

Ford, R. E., Greenhill, L. L., & Posner, K. (2003). Stimulants. In A Martin, L. Scahill, D. S. Charney, & J. F. Leckman (Eds.), *Pediatric psychopharmacology: Principles and practice* (1st ed.; pp. 255–263). New York: Oxford.

Geller, D. A., Hoog, S. L., Heiligenstein, J. H., Ricardi, R. K., Tamura, R., Kluszynski, S., Jacobsen, J. G., & Team TFPOS (2001). Fluoxetine treatment for obsessive-compulsive disorder in children and adolescents: A placebo-controlled clinical trial. *Journal of the American Academy of Child & Adolescent Psychiatry, 40,* 773–779.

Hamano, S., Yamanishi, T., Igarashi, T., et al. (2000). Functional bladder capacity as predictor of response to desmopressin and retention control training in monosymptomatic nocturnal enuresis. *European Urology, 37*(6), 718–722.

Handen, B. L., Johnson, C. R., & Lubetsky, M. (2000). Efficacy of methylphenidate among children with autism and symptoms of attention-deficit hyperactivity disorder. *Journal of Autism and Developmental Disorder, 30,* 245–255.

Harari, M. D., & Moulden, A. (2000). Nocturnal enuresis: What is happening? *Journal of Pediatrics and Child Health, 36*(1), 78–81.

Henggeler, S. W., Rowland, M. D., Randall, J., Ward, D. M., Pickrel, S. G., Cunningham, P. B., et al. (1999). Home-based multisystemic therapy as an alternative to the hospitalization of youths in psychiatric crisis: Clinical outcomes. *Journal of the American Academy of Child and Adolescent Psychiatry, 38*(11), 1331–1339.

Hollander, E., Phillips, A., Chaplin, W., Zagursky, K., Novotny, S., Wasserman, S., Iyengar, R. (2005). A placebo controlled crossover trial of liquid fluoxetine on repetitive behaviors in childhood and adolescent autism. *Neuropsychopharmacology, 30*(3), 582–589.

Jensen, P. S., Edelman, A., & Nemeroff, R. (2003). Pediatric psychopharmacoepidemiology: Who is prescribing? And for whom, how and why? In A. Martin, L. Scahill, D. S. Charney, J. F. Leckman (Eds.), *Pediatric psychopharmacology: Principles and practice* (1st ed.; pp. 701–711). New York: Oxford.

Kanner, L. (1943). Autistic disturbances of affective contact. *Nervous Child, 2,* 217–250.

Karno, M., Golding, J. M., Sorenson, S. B., & Burnam, M. A. (1988). The epidemiology of obsessive compulsive disorder in five US communities. *Archives of General Psychiatry, 45,* 1094–1099.

Kazdin, A. E., & Weisz, J. K. (2003). *Evidence-based psychotherapies for children and adolescents.* Guildford: New York.

King, R. A., & Scahill, L. (2001). Emotional and behavioral difficulties associated with Tourette syndrome. *Advances Neurology, 85,* 79–88.

King, R. A., Scahill, L., Lombroso, P. J., & Leckman, J. F. (2003). Tourette's syndrome and other tic disorders. In A. Martin, L. Scahill, D. S. Charney, J. F. Leckman (Eds.), *Pediatric psychopharmacology: Principles and practice* (1st ed.; pp. 526–542). New York: Oxford.

Koda, V. H., Charney, D. S., & Pine, D. S. (2003). In A. Martin, L. Scahill, D. S. Charney, J. F. Leckman (Eds.), *Pediatric psychopharmacology: Principles and practice* (1st ed.; pp. 138–149). New York: Oxford.

Koenig, K., & Scahill, L. (2001). Assessment of children with pervasive developmental disorders. *Journal of Child and Adolescent Psychiatric Nursing, 14,* 159–166.

Kumra, S. (2000). The diagnosis and treatment of children and adolescents with schizophrenia: 'My mind is playing tricks on me.' *Child and Adolescent Psychiatric Clinics of North America, 9*(1), 183–199.

Labellarte, M. J., & Ginsberg, G. S. (2003). Anxiety disorders. In A. Martin, L. Scahill, D. S. Charney, J. F. Leckman (Eds.), *Pediatric psychopharmacology: Principles and practice* (1st ed.; pp. 497-510). New York: Oxford.

Leckman, J. F., Peterson, B. S., King, R. A., Scahill, L., & Cohen, D. J. (2001). Phenomenology of tics and natural history of tic disorders. *Advances Neurology, 85,* 1–14.

Leckman, J. F., Zhang, H., Vitale, A., et al. (1998). Course of tic severity in Tourette syndrome: The first two decades. *Pediatrics, 102,* 14–19.

Levy, F., Hay, D. A., McStephen, M., et al. (1997). Attention-deficit hyperactivity disorder: A category or a continuum? Genetic analysis of a large-scale twin study. *Journal of the American Academy of Child and Adolescent Psychiatry, 36,* 737–744.

Lou, H. C., Henriksen, L., & Bruhn, P. (1990). Focal cerebral dysfunction in developmental learning disabilities. *Lancet, 335,* 8–11.

March, J. S., Biederman, J., Wolkow, R., et al. (1998). Sertraline in children and adolescents with obsessive-compulsive disorder: A multi-center randomized controlled trial. *Journal of the American Medical Association, 280,* 1752–1755.

Martin, A., Landau, J., Leebens, P., et al. (2000). Risperidone-associated weight gain in children and adolescents: A retrospective chart review. *Journal of Child and Adolescent Psychopharmacology, 10,* 259–268.

Martin, A., Van Hoof, T., Stubbe, D., Sherwin, T., & Scahill, L. (2003). Multiple psychotropic pharmacotherapy in children and adolescents: A study of Connecticut Medicaid managed care recipients. *Psychiatric Services, 54,* 72–77.

McDougle, C. J., & Posey, D. J. (2003). Autistic and other pervasive developmental disorders. In A. Martin, L. Scahill, D. S. Charney, & J. F. Leckman (Eds.), *Pediatric psychopharmacology: Principles and practice* (1st ed.; pp. 563–579). New York: Oxford.

Michelson, D., Allen, A., Busner, J., Casat, C., Dunn, D., Kratochvil, C., et al. (2002). Once daily atomoxetine treatment for children and adolescents with attention deficit hyperactivity disorder: a randomized, placebo-controlled study. *American Journal of Psychiatry*, 150(11), 1806–1901.

Mikkelsen, E. J. (2002). Modern approaches to enuresis and encopresis. In M. Lewis (Ed.), *Child and adolescent psychiatry: A comprehensive textbook* (3rd ed.; pp. 700–711). Philadelphia: Lippincott, Williams & Wilkins.

Mink, J. W. (2001). Neurobiology of basal ganglia circuits in Tourette syndrome: Faulty inhibition of unwanted motor patterns? *Advances in Neurology, 85*, 113–122.

Moss, N. E., & Racusin, G. R. (2002). Psychological assessment of children and adolescents. In M. Lewis (Ed.), *Child and adolescent psychiatry: A comprehensive textbook* (3rd ed.). Philadelphia: Lippincott Williams & Wilkins.

Morshed, S. A., Parveen, S., Leckman, J. F., Mercadante, M. T., Bittencourt Kiss, M. H., Miguel, E. C., et al. (2001). Antibodies against neural, nuclear, cytoskeletal, and streptococcal epitopes in children and adults with Tourette's syndrome, Sydenham's chorea, and autoimmune disorders [erratum appears in *Biol Psychiatry* 2001(Dec 15);50(12): following 1009]. *Biology Psychiatry, 50*(8), 566–577.

MTA Cooperative Group. (1999). A 14-month randomized clinical trial of treatment strategies for attention-deficit/hyperactivity disorder. *Archives of General Psychiatry, 56*, 1073–1086.

MTA Cooperative Group (2004). National Institute of Mental Health Multimodal Treatment Study of ADHD Follow-up: Changes in Effectiveness and Growth after the End of Treatment. *Pediatrics, 113*, 762–769.

Murphy, T. K., Voeller, K. K. S., & Blier, P. (2003). Neurobiology of obsessive-compulsive disorder. In A. Martin, L. Scahill, D. S. Charney, & J. F. Leckman (Eds.), *Pediatric psychopharmacology: Principles and practice* (1st ed.; pp. 150–163). New York: Oxford.

Novotny, S., Evers, M., Barboza, K., Rawitt, R., & Hollander, E. (2003). Neurobiology of affiliation: Implications for autism spectrum disorders. In A. Martin, L. Scahill, D. S. Charney, & J. F. Leckman (Eds.), *Pediatric psychopharmacology: Principles and practice* (1st ed.; pp. 195–209). New York: Oxford.

Paul, R. (2002). Disorders of communication. In M. Lewis (Ed.), *Child and adolescent psychiatry: A comprehensive textbook* (3rd ed.; pp. 612–621). Philadelphia: Lippincott, Williams & Wilkins.

Peterson, B. S., Staib, L., Scahill, L., Zhang, H., Anderson, C., Leckman, J. F., et al. (2001). Regional brain and ventricular volumes in Tourette syndrome. *Archives of General Psychiatry, 58*, 427–440.

Peterson, B. S., Zhang, H., Anderson, G. M., & Leckman, J. F. (1998). A double-blind, placebo-controlled, crossover trial of an antiandrogen in the treatment of Tourette's syndrome. *Journal of Clinical Psychopharmacology, 18*(4), 324–331.

Piacentini, J. (1999). Cognitive behavioral therapy of childhood OCD. *Child and Adolescent Psychiatric Clinics of North America, 8*(3), 599–616.

Pediatric Obsessive Compulsive Disorder Treatment Study (POTS) Team. (2004). Cognitive-behavior therapy, sertraline, and their combination for children with obsessive compulsive disorder: the Pediatric OCD Treatment Study (POTS) randomized controlled trial. *Journal of the American Medical Association, 292*(16), 1969–1976.

Rains, A., Scahill, L. (2004). New long-acting stimulants in children with ADHD. *Journal of Child and Adolescent Psychiatric Nursing, 17*(4), 177–179.

Reiner, W. G. (2003). Elimination disorders: Enuresis and encopresis. In A. Martin, L. Scahill, D. S. Charney, & J. F. Leckman (Eds.), *Pediatric psychopharmacology: Principles and practice* (1st ed.; pp. 686–698). New York: Oxford.

Research Units on Pediatric Psychopharmacology (RUPP) Anxiety Study Group. (2001). Fluvoxamine for the treatment of anxiety disorders in children and adolescents. *New England Journal of Medicine, 344*(17), 1279–1285.

Research Units on Pediatric Psychopharmacology (RUPP) Autism Network. (2002). Risperidone in children with autism and serious behavioral problems. *New England Journal of Medicine, 347*, 314–321.

Research Units on Pediatric Psychopharmacology (RUPP) Autism Network. (2005). Randomized, controlled, crossover trial of methylphenidate in pervasive developmental disorders with hyperactivity. *Archives of General Psychiatry, 62*, 1266–1274.

Riddle, M. A., Reeve, E. A., Yaryura-Tobias, J. A., et al. (2001). Fluvoxamine for children and adolescents with obsessive-compulsive disorder: A controlled multicenter trial. *Journal of American Academy of Child and Adolescent Psychiatry, 40*(2), 222–229.

RUPP Autism Network (2005). Risperidone treatment of autistic disorder: longer term benefits and blinded discontinuation after six months. *American Journal of Psychiatry, 162*:1361–1369.

Sallee, F. R., Kurlan, R., Goetz, C. G., et al. (2000). Ziprasidone treatment of children and adolescents with Tourette's syndrome: A pilot study. *Journal of the American Academy of Child and Adolescent Psychiatry, 39*(3), 292–299.

Satcher, D. (2001). *Report of the Surgeon General's Conference on Children's Mental Health*. National Institute of Mental Health. Bethesda, MD.

Scahill, L., Chappell, P. B., Kim, Y. S., et al. (2001). A placebo-controlled study of guanfacine in the treatment of attention deficit hyperactivity disorder and tic disorders. *American Journal of Psychiatry, 158*(7), 1064–1074.

Scahill, L., Hamrin, V., Pachler, M. (2005). The use of selective serotonin reuptake inhibitors in children and adolescents with major depression. *Journal of Child and Adolescent Psychiatry, 18*(2), 86–89.

Scahill, L., Kano, Y., King, R. A., Carlson, A., Peller, A., LeBrun, U., Rosario-Campos, M. C., & Leckman, J. F. (2003). Influence of age and tic disorders on obsessive-compulsive disorder in a pediatric sample. *Journal of Child and Adolescent Psychopharmacology, 13* (suppl 1): S7–S17.

Scahill, L., Leckman, J. F., Schultz, R. T., Katsovich, L., & Peterson, B. S. (2003). A placebo-controlled trial of risperidone in Tourette syndrome. *Neurology, 60*, 1130–1135.

Scahill, L., Martin, A. (2005). Psychopharmacology. In F. Volkmar, R. Paul, A. Kiln, D. Cohen (Eds.), *Handbook of autism and pervasive developmental disorders: volume two: assessment, interventions and policy*. (3rd ed.; pp 1102–1117). Hoboken: John Wiley & Sons, Inc.

Scahill, L., Riddle, M. A., McSwiggan-Hardin, M., et al. (1997). Children's Yale-Brown Obsessive Compulsive Scale: Reliability and validity. *Journal of the American Academy of Child and Adolescent Psychiatry, 36*, 844–852.

Scahill, L., & Schwab-Stone, M. (2000). Epidemiology of attention deficit hyperactivity disorder in school-age children. *Child and Adolescent Psychiatric Clinics of North America, 9*(3), 541–555.

Scahill, L., Schwab-Stone, M., Merikangas, K., Leckman, J., Zhang, H., & Kasl, S. (1999). Psychosocial and clinical correlates of ADHD in a community sample of young school-age children. *Journal of the American Academy of Child and Adolescent Psychiatry, 38*, 976–983.

Scahill, L., Sukhodolsky, D., Williams, S., Leckman, J. (2005). Public health significance of tic disorders in children and adolescents. *Advances in Neurology, 96*, 240–248.

Schultz, R. T., Carter, A. S., Gladstone, M., et al. (1998). Visual-motor integration functioning in children with Tourette syndrome. *Neuropsychology, 12*(1), 134–145.

Schwartz, C. E., Snidman, N., & Kagan, J. (1999). Adolescent social anxiety as an outcome of inhibited temperament in childhood. *Journal of the American Academy of Child and Adolescent Psychiatry, 38*(8), 1008–1015.

Shaywitz, S. E. (2003). *Overcoming dyslexia* (1st ed.). New York: Knopf.

Sparrow, S. S., Balla, D. A., & Cicchetti, D. V. (1984). *Vineland Adaptive Behavior Scales*. Circle Pines, MN: American Guidance Clinic.

Szatmari, P., Boyle, M., & Offord, D. R. (1989). ADHD and conduct disorder: Degree of diagnostic overlap and differences among correlates. *Journal of the American Academy of Child and Adolescent Psychiatry, 28*, 865–872.

Taylor, J. R., Morshed, S. A., Parveen, S., Mercadante, M. T., Scahill, L., Peterson, B. S., et al. (2002). An animal model of Tourette's syndrome. *Am J Psychiatry, 159*(4), 657–660.

Tomblin, J. B., Zhang, X., Buckwalter, P., & Catts, H. (2000). The association of reading disability, behavioral disorders, and language impairment among second-grade children. *Journal of Child Psychology and Psychiatry and Allied Disciplines, 41*(4), 473–482.

Toppelberg, C. O., & Shapiro, T. (2000). 10-year update review: Language disorders. *Journal of the American Academy of Child and Adolescent Psychiatry, 39*(2), 143–152.

Tourette Syndrome Association International Consortium for Genetics. (1999). A complete genome screen in sib pairs affected by Gilles de la Tourette syndrome. *American Journal of Human Genetics, 65*(5), 1428–1436.

The Tourette Syndrome Study Group. (1999). Short versus longer term pimozide therapy in Tourette's syndrome: A preliminary study. *Neurology, 52*, 874–877.

Treatment for Adolescents with Depression Study (TADS) Team. (2004). Fluoxetine, cognitive-behavioral therapy, and their combination for adolescents with depression: treatment for adolescents with depression study (TADS) randomized controlled trial. *Journal of the American Medical Association, 292*(7), 807–820.

Vaidya, C. J., Austin, G., Kirkorian, G., et al. (1998). Selective effects of methylphenidate in attention deficit disorder: A functional magnetic resonance study. *Proceedings of the National Academy of Sciences, 95*, 14494–14499.

Velosa, J. F., & Riddle, M. A. (2000). Psychopharmacologic treatment of anxiety disorders in children and adolescents. *Child and Adolescent Psychiatric Clinics of North America, 9*(1), 119–133.

Volkmar, F. R., Klin, A., & Paul, R. (2004). *Handbook of autism and pervasive developmental disorders* (3rd ed.). New York: Wiley.

Volkmar, F. R., & Klin, A. (2004). Behavioral and learning problems in school children related to cognitive test data. *Acta Paediatrica, 93*(7), 872–873.

Volkmar, F. R., Klin, A., Schultz, R. T., Rubin, E., & Bronen, R. (2000). Asperger's disorder. *American Journal of Psychiatry, 157*(2), 262–267.

Walkup, J. T., LaBuda, M. C., Singer, H. S., et al. (1996). Family study and segregation analysis of Tourette syndrome: Evidence of a mixed model of inheritance. *American Journal of Human Genetics, 59*, 684–693.

Weiss, M., & Weiss, G. (2002). Attention deficit hyperactivity disorder. In M. Lewis (Ed.), *Child and adolescent psychiatry: A comprehensive textbook* (3rd ed.; pp. 645–670). Philadelphia: Lippincott, Williams & Wilkins.

Werry, J. S., & Aman, M. G. (1998). *Practitioner's guide to psychoactive drugs for children and adolescents*. New York: Plenum Press.

Willcutt, E. G., Pennington, B. F., & DeFries, J. C. (2000). Twin study of the etiology of comorbidity between reading disability and attention-deficit/hyperactivity disorder. *American Journal of Medical Genetics, 96*(3), 293–301.

Zametkin, A. J., Liebenauer, L. L., Fitzgerald, G. A., et al. (1993). Brain metabolism in teenagers with attention-deficit hyperactivity disorder. *Archives of General Psychiatry, 50*, 333–340.

Zametkin, A. J., Nordahl, T. E., Gross, M., et al. (1990). Cerebral glucose metabolism in adults with hyperactivity of childhood onset. *New England Journal of Medicine, 323*(20), 1361–1366.

Acknowledgments

This work was supported in part by the following United States Public Health Service grants: Children's Clinical Research Center Grant RR06022; Program Project Grant MH49351 from the National Institute of Mental Health; Program Project Grant HD-03008 from the National Institute of Child Health and Human Development; Research Units on Pediatric Psychopharmacology; contract MH-70009 from the National Institute of Mental Health.

UNIT VII
Older Adults

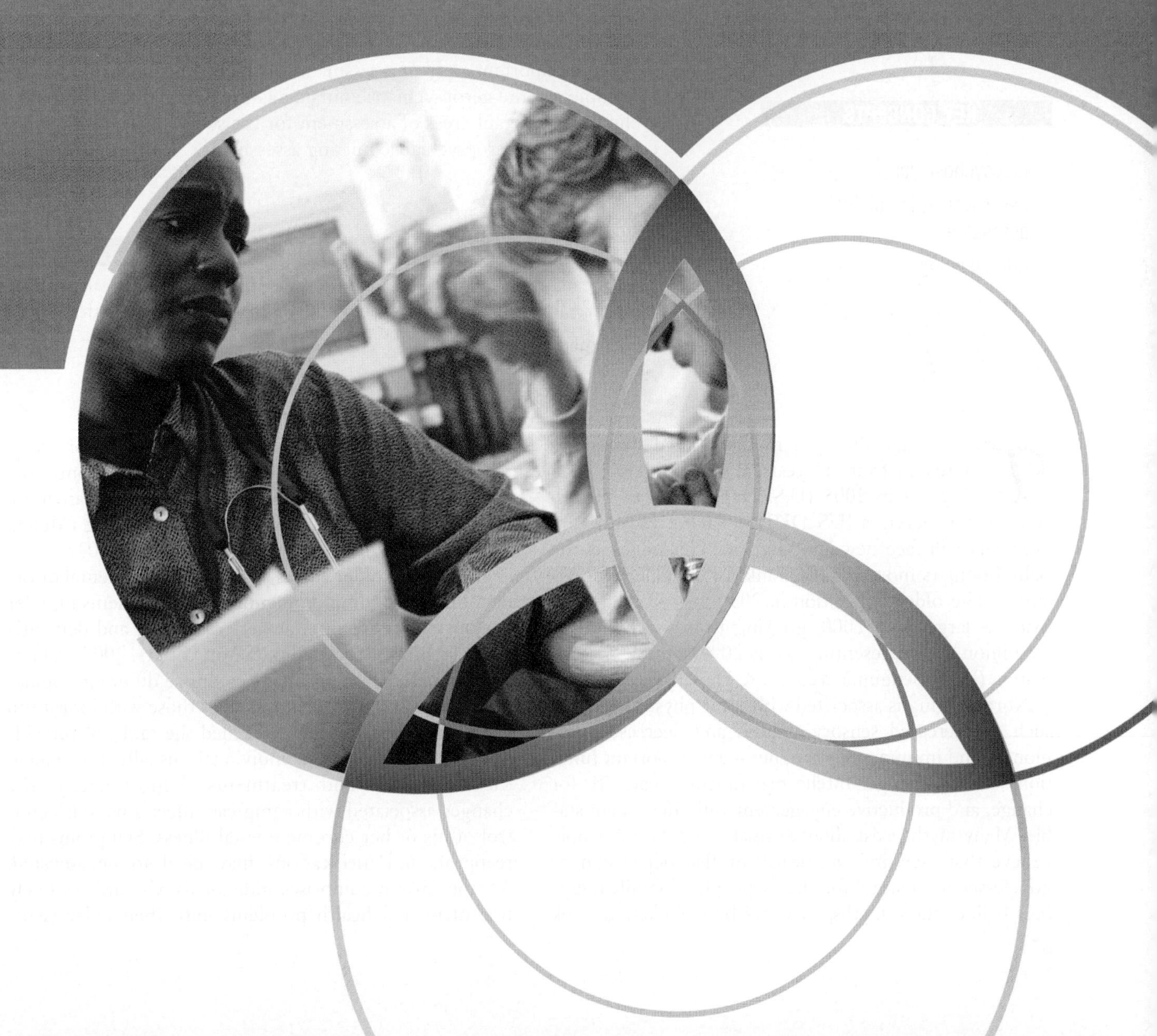

CHAPTER 30

Mental Health Assessment of the Elderly

Mary Ann Boyd and Mickey Stanley

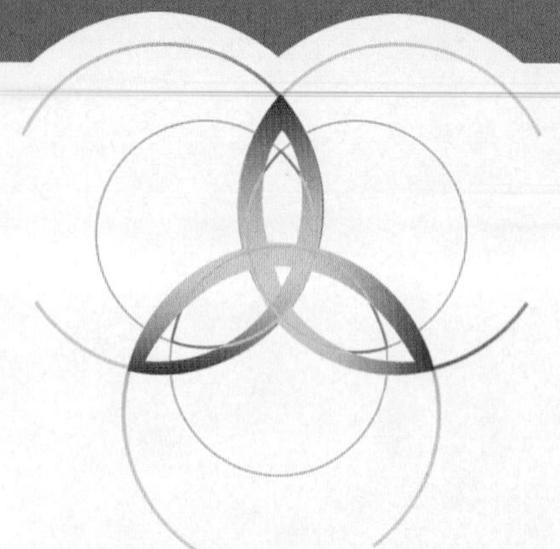

KEY CONCEPTS

- biopsychosocial
- geropsychiatric nursing assessment
- normal aging

LEARNING OBJECTIVES

After studying this chapter, you will be able to:

- Compare changes in normal aging with those associated with mental health problems in elderly people.
- Select various techniques in assessing elderly people who have mental health problems.
- Delineate important areas of assessment for the biologic domain in completing the geropsychiatric nursing assessment.
- Delineate important areas of assessment for the psychological domain in completing the geropsychiatric nursing assessment.
- Delineate important areas of assessment for the social domain in completing the geropsychiatric nursing assessment.

KEY TERMS

• dysphagia • functional activities • insomnia • instrumental activities • polypharmacy • xerostomia

The average life span in the United States has increased from 47 years in 1900 to more than 77 years in 2005 (U.S. Department of Health and Human Services [US DHHS], 2005). Health care providers will face new and increased challenges as the Baby Boomers move into the ranks of the elderly population. The older population in 2030 is projected to be twice as large as in 2000, growing from 35 million to 72 million and representing nearly 20% of the U.S. population (Wan, Sengupta, Velkoff, & DeBarros, 2005).

Normal aging is associated with some physical decline, such as decreased sensory abilities and decreased pulmonary and immune function, but many important functions do not change. Intellectual function, capacity for change, and productive engagement with life remain stable. Many myths exist about normal aging. Some people believe that "senility" is normal, or that depression or hopelessness is natural for elderly people. If family members believe these myths, they will be less likely to seek treatment for their elders with real problems. For example, although some normal cognitive changes contribute to a slower pace of learning, memory complaints are more likely related to depression than normal aging (Mehta, Yaffe, Langa, Sands, Whooley, & Covinsky, 2003).

One in four older adults has a significant mental disorder. The most common mental health problems in older persons are depression, anxiety disorders, and dementia (Bartels, Blow, Brockmann, & Van Citters, 2005). Elders with mental health problems comprise different population groups. One group consists of those with long-term mental illnesses who have reached the ranks of the elderly population. These individuals usually understand their disorders and treatments. Unfortunately, the changes associated with aging can affect a patient's control of his or her chronic mental illness. Symptoms may reappear, and medications may need to be adjusted. Another group comprises individuals who are relatively free of mental health problems until their elder years.

These individuals, who may already have other health problems, develop late-onset mental disorders, such as depression, schizophrenia, or dementia. For these individuals and their family members, the development of a mental disorder can be very traumatic.

Mental health problems in the elderly can be especially complex because of coexisting medical problems and treatments. Many symptoms of somatic disorders mimic or mask psychiatric disorders. For example, fatigue may be related to anemia, but it also may be symptomatic of depression. In addition, older individuals are more likely to report somatic symptoms, rather than psychological ones, making identification of a mental disorder even more difficult.

The purpose of this chapter is to present a comprehensive geropsychiatric–mental health nursing assessment process that serves as the basis of care for elderly people (discussed in Chapters 31 and 32). A mental health assessment is necessary when psychiatric or mental health issues are identified or when patients with mental illnesses reach their later years (usually about age 65 years). The assessment generally follows the same format as described in Chapter 10. However, the overall health care issues for the elderly can be very complex, so it follows that certain components of the geropsychiatric nursing assessment are unique. Thus, the geriatric assessment emphasizes some areas that are less critical to the standard adult assessment.

KEY CONCEPT Normal aging is associated with some physical decline, such as decreased sensory abilities and decreased pulmonary and immune function, but many important functions do not change.

TECHNIQUES OF DATA COLLECTION

The nurse assesses the patient using an interview format that may take a few sessions to complete. He or she also may rely on self-report standardized tests, such as depression and cognitive functioning tools. A wide variety of physiologic disorders may cause changes in mental status for older adults; thus, results of laboratory tests often are significant. For example, urinalysis can detect a urinary tract infection that has affected a patient's cognitive status. Box 30.1 contains a representative listing of common physiologic causes of changes in mental status. In addition, medical records from other health care providers are useful in developing a complete picture of the patient's health status.

An important source of patient data is family members, who often notice changes that the patient overlooks or fails to recognize. A patient with memory impairment may be unable to give an accurate history. By interviewing family members, the nurse expands the scope of the patient assessment. Moreover, the nurse has an opportunity to evaluate the caregivers themselves to determine whether they can care for the patient adequately and how they are coping with the situation. For example, a husband may be unable to care for his wife but is unwilling to admit it. If the nurse can establish rapport with the husband, the nurse may use the assessment interview as an opportunity to help the husband to examine his wife's care requirements realistically.

BOX 30.1

Changes That Affect Mental Status

- Acid–base imbalance
- Dehydration
- Drugs (prescribed and over-the-counter)
- Electrolyte changes
- Hypothyroidism
- Hypothermia and hyperthermia
- Hypoxia
- Infection and sepsis

BIOPSYCHOSOCIAL GEROPSYCHIATRIC NURSING ASSESSMENT

KEY CONCEPT A **biopsychosocial geropsychiatric** nursing assessment is the comprehensive, deliberate, and systematic collection and interpretation of biopsychosocial data that is based on the special needs and problems of elderly people to determine current and past health, functional status, and human responses to mental health problems, both actual and potential (Box 30.2).

At the beginning of the assessment, the nurse should determine the patient's ability to participate. A key component in a successful interview with an older adult is the formation of an atmosphere of respect for the person. Use of child-like language with the older adult signifies an ageist attitude and often results in poor results. For example, if a patient is using a wheelchair, he or she may have physical limitations that prevent full participation in the assessment. However, physical limitations should not be assumed to indicate decreased mental capacity. The patient must be able to hear the nurse. For a patient with compromised hearing, the nurse must attend to voice projection and volume. Shouting at the older patient is unnecessary. The nurse should remember to lower the pitch of his or her voice because higher-pitched sounds are often lost with presbyacusis (loss of hearing sensitivity associated with aging). The nurse should eliminate distracting noises, such as from a television or radio, and ensure that the patient's hearing aid is in place and turned on. Facing the patient and using distinct enunciation will

BOX 30.2

Biopsychosocial Geropsychiatric Nursing Assessment

I. Major reason for seeking help ______

II. Initial information

Name ______

Age ______ Current marital status ______

Gender ______ Caregiver's name ______

Living arrangements ______

III. Level of independence:

High (needs no help) ______

Moderate (lives independently, but needs some help with instrumental activities) ______

Low (relies on others for help in meeting functional and instrumental activities) ______

Physical limitations ______

Level of education completed ______

	Normal	Treated	Untreated
Physical functions: system review	☐	☐	☐
Activity/exercise	☐	☐	☐
Sleep patterns	☐	☐	☐
Appetite and nutrition	☐	☐	☐
Hydration	☐	☐	☐
Sexuality	☐	☐	☐
Existing physical illnesses	☐	☐	☐

List any chronic illnesses ______

Presence of pain (Use standardized instrument if pain is present.) No ______ Yes ______

Score ______ Treatment of pain ______

Medication (prescription and over-the-counter)	**Dosage**	**Side Effects**	**Frequency**

Significant Laboratory Tests	**Values**	**Normal Range**

IV. Responses to mental health problems

Major concerns regarding mental health problem ______

Major loss/change in past year: No ______ Yes ______

Fear of violence: No ______ Yes ______

Strategies for managing problems/disorder ______

V. Mental status examination

General observation (appearance, psychomotor activity, attitude) ______

Orientation (time, place, person) ______

(Continued on following page)

BOX 30.2

Biopsychosocial Geropsychiatric Nursing Assessment (continued)

Mood, affect, emotions (Geriatric Depression Scale should be used if evidence of depression)

Speech (verbal ability, speed, use of words correctly) ______

Thought processes (hallucinations, delusions, tangential, logic, repetition, rhyming of words, loose connections, disorganized) *(Describe content of hallucinations, delusions.)*

Cognition and intellectual performance *(Use standardized test scores as well as observations.)*

Attention and concentration ______

Abstract reasoning and concentration ______

Memory (recall, short-term, long-term) ______

Judgement and insight ______

(MMSE, CASI scores) ______

VI. Significant behaviors (psychomotor, agitation, aggression, withdrawn) *(Use standardized test if behaviors are problematic.)* ______

When did problem behavior begin? Has it gotten worse? ______

VII. Self-concept beliefs about self—body image, self-esteem, personal identity) ______

VIII. Risk assessment

Suicide: High ______ Low ______ Assault/homicide: High ______ Low ______

Suicide thoughts or ideation: No ______ Yes ______

Current thoughts or harming self ______ Plan ______

Means ______

Means available

Assault/homicide thoughts: No ______ Yes ______

What do you do when angry with a stranger? ______

What do you do when angry with family or partner? ______

Have you ever hit or pushed anyone? No ______ Yes ______

Have you ever been arrested for assault? No ______ Yes ______

Current thoughts of harming others ______

IX. Functional status *(Use standardized test such as FAQ.)* ______

X. Cultural assessment

Cultural group ______

Cultural group's view of health and mental illness ______

By what cultural rules do you try to live? ______

Special, cultural foods that are important to you ______

XI. Stresses and coping behaviors ______

Social support ______

Family members ______

Which members are important to you? ______

On whom can you rely? ______

Community resources ______

XII. Spiritual assessment ______

XIII. Economic status ______

XIV. Legal status ______

XV. Quality of life ______

Summary of significant data that can be used in formulating a nursing diagnosis:

SIGNATURE/TITLE ______ Date ______

help lip-reading patients understand what is being said. Sometimes, deafness is mistaken for cognitive dysfunction. If a patient's hearing is questionable, the nurse should enlist the help of a speech and language specialist. Generally, the pace of the interview should mirror the patient's ability to move through the assessment. Usually, the pace will be slower than the nurse uses with younger populations.

Biologic Domain

Collecting and analyzing data for assessment of the biologic domain includes areas similar to those discussed in Chapter 10. The assessment components include present and past health status, physical examination results, physical functioning, and pharmacology review. When focusing on the biologic domain, the nurse pays special attention to the patient's general physical appearance as well as any observable manifestations of illness. The nurse should assess how all physical problems affect the patient's mental well-being. For example, pain and immobility are physical problems that can negatively affect mental health. Low energy level may be immediately apparent. Women with obvious osteoporosis are experiencing pain most of the time. Men undergoing radiation for prostate cancer worry about sexual functioning and urinary incontinence. Assessment tools specific to these areas can be found in the "Try This" section of the Hartford Institute for Geriatric Nursing located at www.GeroNurseOnline.org.

Present and Past Health Status

A review of the patient's current health status includes examining health records and collecting information from the patient and family members. The nurse must identify chronic health problems that could affect mental health care. For example, the patient's management of diabetes mellitus could provide clues to the likelihood of complications such as retinopathy or neuropathy, which in turn will affect the patient's ability to follow a mental health treatment regimen. The nurse must document a history of psychiatric treatment.

Physical Examination

The psychiatric nurse reviews the physical examination findings, paying special attention to recent laboratory values, such as urinalysis, white and red blood cell counts, thyroid studies, and fasting blood glucose data (see Chapter 7). Results of neurologic tests could indicate compromise of the neuromuscular systems. Many psychiatric medications lower the seizure threshold, making a history of seizures, which can cause behavior changes, an important assessment component. The nurse should note any evidence of movement disorders, such as tremors, abnormal movements, or shuffling. If a patient has been taking conventional antipsychotics, the nurse should consider assessment for symptoms of tardive dyskinesia, using one of the appropriate assessment tools (see Chapter 18 for additional discussion of tardive dyskinesia).

The nurse should take routine vital signs during the assessment. He or she should note any abnormalities in blood pressure (i.e., hypertension or hypotension) because many psychiatric medications affect blood pressure. Generally, these medications may cause orthostatic hypotension, which can lead to dizziness, unsteady gait, and falls. A baseline blood pressure is needed for future monitoring of medication side effects. Lying, sitting, and standing blood pressures are especially useful in assessing for orthostatic hypotension.

Physical Functions

The nurse must consider the patient's physical functioning within the context of the normal changes that accompany aging and the presence of any chronic disorders. The nurse should note the patient's use of any personal devices, such as canes, walkers, wheelchairs, or oxygen, or environmental devices, such as grab bars, shower benches, or hospital beds. Specific areas to consider are nutrition and eating, elimination, and sleep patterns.

Nutrition and Eating

Assessment of the type, amount, and frequency of food eaten is standard in any geriatric assessment. The nurse should note any weight loss of more than 10 pounds. He or she must consider such nutrition changes in light of mental health problems. For example, is a patient's weight loss related to an underlying physical problem or to the patient's belief that she is being poisoned, which makes her afraid to eat?

Eating is often difficult for elderly patients, who may experience a lack of appetite. The nurse must assess eating and appetite patterns because many psychiatric medications can affect digestion and may impair an already compromised gastrointestinal tract. A common problem of elderly people who live in nursing homes is **dysphagia**, or difficulty swallowing. Dysphagia can lead to dehydration, malnutrition, pneumonia, or asphyxiation. People who have been exposed to conventional antipsychotics (e.g., haloperidol, chlorpromazine) may have symptoms of tardive dyskinesia, which can make swallowing difficult. Thus, the nurse should evaluate any patient who has been exposed to the older psychiatric medications for symptoms of tardive dyskinesia.

Xerostomia, or dry mouth, which is common in elderly people, also may impair eating. The nurse should pay particular attention to those who are currently receiving treatment for mental illnesses, particularly with medications that have anticholinergic properties. Dry mouth is also a side effect of many other anticholinergic medications, such as cimetidine, digoxin, and furosemide. Frequent rinsing with a nonalcohol-based mouthwash will help to correct the dry condition. Observe for the frequent use of candy or sugar-based gum for these clients, as dental caries and gum disease provide a portal of entry for sepsis in the older adult. Decreased taste or smell is common among elderly people and may reduce the pleasure of eating so that the patient may eat less. Making meal times social and relaxing experiences can help the patient compensate for some of the loss of pleasure associated with decreased taste or smell. Preparing favorite foods will also enhance the quality of meals and meal times.

The nurse also must determine the patient's use of alcohol. Alcoholism is a growing problem in the elderly population. A screening tool for alcohol use is important as patients and family members often conceal the problem due to the stigma associated with alcohol abuse. Estimates are that the prevalence of problem drinking in older adults ranges from 1% to 15%. The number of older adults in need of substance abuse treatment is estimated to more than double from 1.7 million in 2000 and 2001 to 4.4 million in 2020 (Bartels et al., 2005). There is a substantially increased mortality risk for heavy drinkers and slightly reduced risk for lighter drinkers. Limited data suggest a more favorable mortality experience for drinkers of wine than for drinkers of liquor or beer (Klatsky, Friedman, Armstrong, & Kipp, 2003). The use of the CAGE questionnaire may be helpful in this area (see Appendix G).

Elimination

The nurse must assess the patient's urinary and bowel functions. Elderly patients are more likely to experience constipation due to a change in eating or activity patterns or intentional reduction in fluid intake. Medications with anticholinergic properties can cause constipation, leading to fecal impaction. Abuse of laxatives is common among the elderly and requires evaluation. Although the addition of fiber is recommended for constipation, such measures may cause bloating and excessive gas production. Elderly patients are also more likely to experience urinary frequency because the strength of the sphincter muscles decreases. Because many older adults drink fewer fluids to manage urinary incontinence, fluid intake also becomes an important factor in assessing urinary functioning and constipation. The nurse should remember that urinary incontinence is not a normal age-related finding but a symptom of a disorder that requires follow-up and treatment.

Sleep

During the normal aging process, sleep patterns change, and patients often sleep less than they did when younger. The nurse must assess any recent changes in sleep patterns and evaluate whether they are related to normal aging or are symptomatic of an underlying disorder. **Insomnia**, the inability to fall or remain asleep throughout the night, may be the result of depression or can lead to an increased risk for depression and regular use of sleep medications. Patients with insomnia report that they cannot sleep at night and do not feel rested in the morning. They often sleep during the day. In a large 3-year study of 10,430 women, 70 to 75 years of age, more than 60% of them reported difficulty sleeping and 15% reported using sleep medications (Byles, Mishra, Harris, & Nair, 2003). Sleep problems are also often linked to the use of alcohol. If a patient reports sleep problems, the nurse should ask about the patient's use of alcohol, over-the-counter medications, and prescription drugs (Box 30.3).

BOX 30.3

Research for Best Practice: Health & Changes in Late-life Drinking

Moos, R. H., Brennan, P. L. Schutte, K. K., & Moos, B. S. (2005). Older adults' health and changes in late-life drinking patterns. *Aging & Mental Health, 9(1). 49-59.*

THE QUESTION: Is there an association between older adults' health-related problems and alchol consumption?

METHODS: Late-middle-aged community residents 55-65 years old (N=1291) were surveyed regarding their health and alcohol consumption and were followed for one year, four years, and then 10 years later.

FINDINGS: Those who had medical conditions, physical symptoms, medication use, and acute health events were more likely to abstain from drinking. However, overall health problems were related to drinking problems.

IMPLICATIONS FOR NURSING: Older adults with several health problems who consume more alchol are at elevated risk for drinking problems and should be targeted for brief interventions to help them curtail their drinking.

Pain

Elders are more likely to experience pain than younger adults because they are at increased risk for chronic illness and may be suffering from the consequences of a lifetime of injuries. For many elders, pain is a constant companion. The experience of chronic pain often contributes to unexplained behavior and personality changes. To assess pain, the nurse can use many pain instruments. One of the most popular is the Wong-Baker FACES Pain Rating Scale, initially developed for children but now used for all age groups (Fig. 30.1). This scale is especially useful in communicating with people whose cultures and languages are different from the nurse's. See Chapter 36 for further discussion of pain.

Assessment of pain is especially critical for those elders who are cognitively impaired and living in long-term care (LTC) institutions. Studies indicate that older adults, especially those with dementia in LTC, have untreated pain (Nygaard & Jarland, 2005).

Pharmacologic Assessment

One of the most important areas of the biologic domain is the pharmacologic assessment. **Polypharmacy**, defined as the use of duplicate medications, interacting medications, or drugs used to treat adverse drug interactions, is common in elderly people. The nurse must ask the patient and family to list all medications and times that the patient takes them. Asking family members to bring in all the medications the patient is taking, including over-the-counter medications, vitamins, and herbal supplements, allows for a careful assessment of polypharmacy. Because elderly people are more sensitive than younger people to medications, the possibility of drug-to-drug interactions is greater. When considering potential drug interactions, the nurse should ask the patient about his or her consumption of grapefruit juice, which contains narginin, a compound that inhibits the CYP3A4 enzyme involved in the metabolism of many medications (e.g., antidepressants, antiarrhythmics, erythromycin, and several statins).

Psychological Domain

Assessment of the psychological domain provides the nurse with the opportunity to identify limitations, behavior symptoms, and reactions to illness. The nurse assesses many of the same areas as in other adult assessments, but again, the emphasis may be different. The following discussion focuses on the responses of elderly patients to mental health problems, mental status examination, behavior changes, stress and coping patterns, and risk assessments.

Responses to Mental Health Problems

Many elderly patients are reluctant to admit that they have psychiatric symptoms, particularly if their culture stigmatizes mental illness, and may deny having mental or emotional problems. They may also fear that if they admit to any symptoms, they may be placed outside their home. If patients do not recognize or admit to having psychiatric symptoms, their vulnerability to being taken advantage of or injured increases.

Throughout the assessment, the nurse evaluates the patient's verbal reports, obvious symptoms, and family reports. If a patient flatly denies any psychiatric symp-

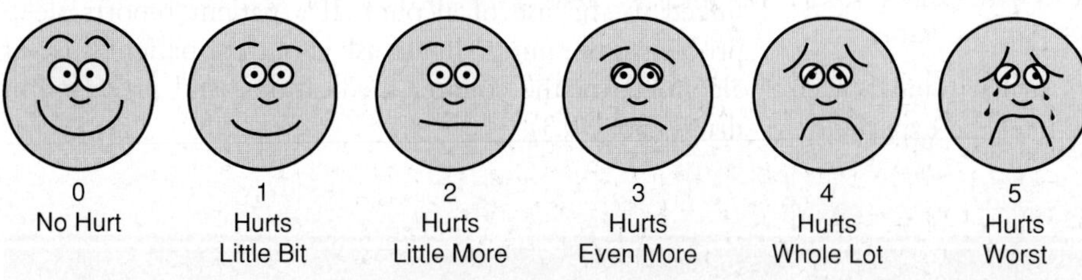

Wong-Baker FACES Pain Rating Scale

Each face represents a person who is happy or sad depending on how much or how little pain he/she has:

0 "a person who is very happy because he/she doesn't hurt at all"
1 "it hurts just a little bit"
2 "it hurts a little more"
3 "it hurts even more"
4 "it hurts a whole lot"
5 "it hurts as much as you can imagine, but you don't have to be crying to feel this bad"

Subject ID #:__________ Date:___/___/___ Visit #______

Pt. name:____________________

RA:____________________

FIGURE 30.1. Wong-Baker FACES Pain Rating Scale.

BOX 30.4

Therapeutic Dialogue: Assessment Interview

Tom, 79 years old, is being seen for the first time in a geropsychiatric clinic because of recent changes in his behavior and his accusations that family members are trying to steal his house and car. He locked his wife out of the house, accusing her of being unfaithful. When Susan, the psychiatric nurse assigned to his case, is conducting the assessment interview, Tom cooperates and is very pleasant until the nurse begins to assess the psychological domain.

Ineffective Approach

Nurse: Have there been times when you have had problems with any members of your family?

Patient: No. (Silence)

Nurse: Have you noticed that lately you have been getting more upset than usual?

Patient: No. Who has been talking to you?

Nurse: Your wife seems to think that you may be getting a little more upset than usual.

Patient: You are just like her. She keeps telling me something is wrong with me. (Getting very agitated)

Nurse: Please, Ím trying to help you. I understand that you locked your wife out of the house last week.

Patient: Leave me alone. (Gets up and leaves)

Effective Approach:

Nurse: How have things been going at home?

Patient: All right.

Nurse: (Silence)

Patient: Well, my wife and I sometimes argue.

Nurse: Oh. Most husband and wives argue. Any special arguments?

Patient: No. Just the usual. I donít pick up after myself enough. I don't dress right to suit her. But, lately, she's gone a lot.

Nurse: She is gone a lot?

Patient: Yeah! A lot.

Nurse: The way you say that, it sounds like you have some feelings about her being gone.

Patient: You're damned right I do—and you would, too.

Nurse: I'm missing something.

Patient: Well, if you must know, I think she's having an affair with the man next door.

Nurse: Really? That must upset you to think your wife is having an affair.

Patient: I am devastated. I feel so bad.

Nurse: Would you say that you are depressed?

Patient: Well, wouldn't you be? Yes, I'm feeling pretty low.

Critical Thinking Challenge

- How do the very first questions differ in the two interviews?
- What therapeutic techniques did the nurse use in the second interview to avoid the pitfalls the nurse encountered in the first scenario?
- How did the nurse in the second scenario elicit the patient's delusion about his wife's affair?
- From the data that the second nurse gathered, how many patient problems can be identified?

toms (e.g., depression, mood swings, outbursts of anger, memory problems), the nurse should respectfully accept the patient's answer and avoid arguments or confrontation (see Box 30.4). If the patient's family members contradict the patient's report or symptoms are obvious during the interview, the nurse can approach the issue while planning care. Nurses may need to use conflict resolution strategies in helping families and patients arrive at mutually agreed on reports.

Mental Status Examination

The areas of special interest in the mental status examination are mood and affect, thought processes, and cognitive functioning. The nurse should interpret the results in light of any accompanying physical problems, such as chronic pain, or life changes, such as loss of a spouse.

Mood and Affect

Depression in elderly people is common and associated with the following risk factors: loss of spouse, physical illness, low socioeconomic status, impaired functional status, and heavy alcohol consumption. In older people, other disorders may mask depression. When symptoms are present, they may be attributed to normal aging or atherosclerosis or other age-related problems. Older patients are less likely to report feeling sad or worthless than are younger patients. As a result, family members and primary care providers often overlook depression in elderly patients.

Depressive symptoms are much more common than a full-fledged depressive disorder, as characterized by the *Diagnostic and Statistical Manual of Mental Disorders, 4th edition, text revision* [*DSM-IV-R*] (APA, 2000). Rates vary by settings, with up to 24% in outpatient settings, 30% in acute care, and up to 43% to 85% in the LTC setting experiencing depressive symptoms (Butcher & McGonigal-Kenney, 2005). The term *late-onset depression* refers to the development of depression or depressive symptoms that impair functioning after 60 years of age. In late-onset depression, the risk for recurrence is relatively high (Bartels et al., 2005).

The Geriatric Depression Scale (GDS) is a useful screening tool with demonstrated validity and reliability (Hyer & Blount, 1984). The GDS was designed as a self-administered test, although it also has been used in observer-administered formats. One advantage of the test is its "yes/no" format, which may be easier for older adults than the Hamilton Rating Scale for Depression (HAM-D), which uses a scale from 0 to 4 (see Chapter 20). This tool is easy to administer and provides valuable informa-

BOX 30.5

Geriatric Depression Scale (Short Form)

1. Are you basically satisfied with your life?	Yes	No
2. Have you dropped many of your activities and interests?	Yes	No
3. Do you feel that your life is empty?	Yes	No
4. Do you often get bored?	Yes	No
5. Are you in good spirits most of the time?	Yes	No
6. Are you afraid that something bad is going to happen to you?	Yes	No
7. Do you feel happy most of the time?	Yes	No
8. Do you often feel helpless?	Yes	No
9. Do you prefer to stay at home rather than go out and do new things?	Yes	No
10. Do you feel you have more problems with memory than most?	Yes	No
11. Do you think it is wonderful to be alive now?	Yes	No
12. Do you feel pretty worthless the way you are now?	Yes	No
13. Do you feel full of energy?	Yes	No
14. Do you feel that your situation is hopeless?	Yes	No
15. Do you think that most people are better off than you are?	Yes	No
Score: —/15 One point for "No" to questions 1, 5, 7, 11, 13	Normal	3 ± 2
	Mildly depressed	7 ± 3
One point for "Yes" to other questions	Very depressed	12 ± 2

Adapted from Sheikh, J. I., & Yesavage, J. A. (1986). Geriatric Depression Scale (GDS): Recent evidence and development of a shorter version. In T. L. Brink (Ed.), *Clinical gerontology: a guide to assessment and intervention* (pp. 165–173). Binghamton, NY: Haworth Press.

tion about the possibility of depression (Box 30.5). If results are positive, the nurse should refer the patient to a psychiatrist or advanced practice nurse for further evaluation. Among nursing home residents, the usefulness of the GDS depends on the degree of cognitive impairment. Residents who are mildly impaired may be able to answer yes/no questions; however, moderately to severely impaired patients will be unable to do the same. The best validated scale for patients with dementia is the Cornell Scale for Depression in Dementia (CSDD) (Alexopoulos, Abrams, Young, & Shamoian, 1998). The CSDD is an interview-administered scale that uses information both from the patient and an outside informant.

Anxiety is another important mood for nurses to assess in elderly people because it can interfere with normal functioning. In dementia, anxiety is common (Lopez et al., 2003). The Rating Anxiety in Dementia (RAID) scale was developed as a global scale to assess anxiety in patients with dementia (Shankar, Walker, Frost, & Orrell, 1999). The domains that the RAID scale assesses include worry, apprehension and vigilance, motor tension, autonomic hyperactivity, and phobias and panic attacks.

Thought Processes

Thought processes and content are critical in the assessment of elderly patients. Can the patient express ideas and thoughts logically? Can the patient understand questions and follow the conversation of others? If the patient shows any indication of hallucinations or delusions, the nurse should explore the content of the hallucination or delusion. If the patient has a history of mental illness, such as schizophrenia, these symptoms may be familiar to family members, who can validate whether they are old or new problems. If this is the first time the patient has experienced these abnormal thought processes, the nurse should further evaluate the content. Suspicious and delusional thoughts that characterize dementia often include some of the following beliefs:

- People are stealing my things.
- The house is not my house.
- My relative is an impostor.

Cognition and Intellectual Performance

Cognitive functioning includes such parameters as orientation, attention, short- and long-term memory, consciousness, and executive functioning. Intellectual functioning, also considered a cognitive measure, is rarely formally assessed with a standardized intelligence test in elderly people. Considerable variability among individuals depends on lifestyle and psychosocial factors. Some changes in cognitive capacity may accompany aging, but important functions are spared. Normal cognitive changes during aging include a slowing of information processing and memory retrieval. Abnormalities of consciousness, orientation, judgment, speech, or language are not related to age but to underlying neuropathologic changes. Cognitive changes in elderly people are associated with delirium or dementia (see Chapter 32) or with schizophrenia (see Chapter 18).

BOX 30.6

Research for Best Practice:* *Cognitive Status: Documentation Versus Standardized Assessments

Souder, E., & O'Sullivan, P. S. (2000). Nursing documentation versus standardized assessment of cognitive status in hospitalized medical patients. Applying Nursing Research, 13(1), 29–36.

THE QUESTION: How does standard nursing documentation compare with standard assessment tests in identifying problems of cognitive function in older adults? Although the literature discusses the importance of assessing cognitive status, few studies have explored the concordance of nurses' documentation of cognitive status and standardized assessment.

METHODS: This study examined nurses' documentation of cognitive status in 42 medically hospitalized individuals (mean age, 51.9 years; SD,10.1 years) using various standardized measures.

FINDINGS: Although the chart review revealed no documentation of impaired cognitive status, it identified impaired performance in 24% to 67% of the cognitive measures.

IMPLICATIONS FOR NURSING: This study suggests nurses are missing cognitive impairment in hospitalized patients by limiting assessment of orientation. Use of a combination of several brief screening measures, such as the clock-drawing test and the standardized Mini-Mental State Examination (MMSE), would provide timely, effective, and inexpensive assessment of cognitive status (abstract). This article supports the use of standardized instruments in assessing cognitive status.

The assessment includes the number of years of education. An inverse relationship between Alzheimer's disease and the number of years of education exists. When assessing cognitive functioning, the nurse should use standardized instruments and not rely on observations or chart documentation (Box 30.6) (Souder & O'Sullivan, 2000).Two new easy to administer and easily accessible screening tools are the SLUMS (Saint Louis University Mental Status Examination) and AD8 (see Chapter 32). Evidence suggests that severe cognitive deterioration may occur in elderly people with schizophrenia. In assessing the cognitive status of this population, the Cognitive Abilities Screening Instrument (CASI) demonstrates specific assessment of nine domains: attention, concentration, orientation, long-term memory, short-term memory, language, visual construction (copying pentagons), fluency (naming four-legged animals), and abstraction and judgment (Sherrell, Buckwalter, Bode, & Strozdas, 1999). The CASI is a 25-item instrument test developed as a research instrument and piloted in Japan and the United States (Teng et al., 1994). The total score ranges from 0 (poor) to 100 (good), with a suggested cutoff of 74 for classifying dementia. Because it determines the level of cognitive impairment, the CASI could be used in establishing individualized care plans.

Behavior Changes

Behavior changes in elderly people can indicate neuropathologic processes and thus require nursing assessment. If such changes occur, it is most likely that family members will notice them before the patient does. Apraxia (inability to execute a voluntary movement despite normal muscle function) is not attributed to age but indicates an underlying disease process, such as Alzheimer disease, Parkinson's disease, or other disorders. Various other behavior problems are associated with psychiatric disorders in elderly people, including irritability, agitation, apathy, and euphoria. Other behaviors in elderly people who are experiencing psychiatric problems include wandering and aggressive behaviors.

The Neuropsychiatric Inventory (NPI) was developed in 1994 to assess behavior problems associated with dementia. The scale assesses 10 behavior problems: delusions, hallucinations, dysphoria, anxiety, agitation/aggression, euphoria, inhibition, irritability/lability, apathy, and aberrant motor behavior (Cummings et al., 1994). This very popular tool is used in many medication clinical trials. There are two versions. The standard version is used when the patient is still at home; the second is used when the patient is in a nursing home.

Stress and Coping Patterns

Identifying stresses and coping patterns is just as important for elderly patients as it is for younger adults. Unique stresses for elderly patients include living on a fixed income, handling declining health, losing partners and friends, and ultimately confronting death. Coping ability varies, depending on patients' unique circumstances. For example, some patients respond to stressful events with amazing adaptability, whereas others become depressed and suicidal.

Bereavement, a natural response to the death of a loved one, includes crying and sorrow, anxiety and agitation, insomnia, and loss of appetite. These symptoms, while overlapping with those of major depression, do not constitute a mental disorder. Only when these symptoms persist for 2 months or longer can a diagnosis of either adjustment disorder or major depressive disorder be made (American Psychiatric Association, 2000). Although bereavement is a normal response, the nurse must identify it and develop interventions to help the individual successfully resolve the loss. Bereavement is an important and well-established risk factor for depression. At least 10% to 20% of widows and widowers experience symptoms of depression during the first year of bereavement. Without interventions, depression can persist, become chronic, and lead to further disability. It also can lead to other serious health problems.

Risk Assessment

Suicide is a major mental health risk for the elderly. Suicide rates increase with age; the rate among older white men is six times that of the general population. The highest rates are for white men older than 85 years of age (68.2 per 100,000). Most elderly people who commit suicide have visited their primary care physician in the month before their death (Lantz, 2003).

When caring for the elderly patient with mental health problems, the nurse always should consider the patient's potential to commit suicide. Depression is the greatest risk factor for suicide. In assessing an elderly patient, the nurse should consider the following characteristics as indications of high risk for committing suicide:

- Depression
- Attempted suicide in the past
- Family history of suicide
- Firearms in the home
- Abuse of alcohol or other substances
- Unusual stress
- Chronic medical condition (e.g., cancer, neuromuscular disorders)
- Social isolation

• NCLEXNOTE

NCLEXNOTE Suicide assessment is a priority for the older adult experiencing mental health problems. It is important to carefully assess recent behavior changes and loss of support.

Social Domain

Assessment of the social domain includes determining the patient's interactions with others in his or her family and community. The nurse targets social support because it is so important to the well-being of the older adult's functional status, and because of the potential physical changes that can affect this area, and social systems, which encompasses all community resources.

Social Support

Remaining active throughout one's life is one of the best predictors of mental health and wellness in an elderly patient. People obtain their sense of self-worth through their interactions with others in their environment. A sense of "who one is" is closely tied to the roles that a person plays in life. When older adults relinquish such roles because of physical disabilities, become isolated from friends and family, or begin to sense that they are a burden to those around them, rather than contributing members of society, a sense of hopelessness and helplessness often follows.

The role of social support is critical to assess in this age group. Social support is a reciprocal concept, meaning that simply receiving assistance increases the person's sense of being a burden. Those elders who believe that they contribute to the welfare of others are most likely to remain mentally healthy. For this reason, pets are often "life savers" for older adults who live alone. Nothing can be more understanding and accepting of an older adult's behavior or disabilities than a beloved pet.

The nurse should assess the patient's number of formal and informal social contacts. The nurse should ask about the frequency of contacts with others (in person and through telephone calls, letters, and cards). Determining whether these contacts are actually satisfying and supporting to the patient is essential. If family members are important to the patient's well-being, the nurse should complete a more in-depth family assessment (see Chapter 13).

The nurse can use the following questions to focus on social support (Kane, 1995):

- In the past 2 weeks, how often would you say that others let you know that they care about you?
- In the past 2 weeks, how often has someone provided you with help, such as giving you a ride somewhere or helping around the house?
- Do you have any one special person you could call or contact if you needed help? Who?
- In general, other than your children, how many relatives do you feel close to and have contact with at least once a month?

For patients who are isolated with few social contacts, the nurse can develop interventions to improve social support.

Functional Status

As part of a complete assessment, the nurse will need to assess the older adult's functional status. **Functional activities** or activities of daily living (ADLs) are the activities necessary for self-care (i.e., bathing, toileting, dressing, and transferring). **Instrumental activities** of daily living (IADLs) include those that facilitate or enhance the performance of ADLs (i.e., shopping, using the telephone, using transportation). These aspects are critical to consider for any older adult living alone. The most common tools used to assess functional status are the Index of Independence in Activities of Daily Living and the Instrumental Activities of Daily Living Scale (Katz & Akpom, 1976). The Functional Activities Questionnaire (FAQ) measures an adult's functional abilities based on information from family members and caregivers. The older person is rated on 10 complex, higher order activities, such as writing checks, assembling tax records, and driving (Costa et al., 1996).

Social Systems

Community resources are essential to an older adult's ability to maintain mental health and wellness, as well as to his or her ability to remain at home throughout the later years. Senior centers are federally funded community resources that provide a wide array of services to the nation's elderly. They provide daily balanced meals at a nominal cost. In addition, they provide opportunities for socialization, which is key to combating loneliness and social isolation. Many senior centers provide annual influenza and pneumonia vaccination clinics and education on such topics as fall prevention, and recognition and prevention of elder abuse. Additional community resources that are specific to elderly people include geriatric assessment clinics and adult day care centers.

During the assessment, the nurse must determine which community resources are available and if the elderly patient uses them. Lack of transportation to and from these community resources may be a barrier to use. Most communities have buses available for elderly or handicapped individuals. The nurse may need to assist the elder in accessing this important resource.

Many elderly citizens rely on the Social Security Administration for their monthly income. For many elders, this financial support, although less than adequate in most instances, is their only source of income. In addition to Social Security, the federal government provides basic health care coverage in the form of the state-administered Medicare program. Together, these programs contribute to the patient's ability to live independently and receive health care. The nurse should assess a patient's sources of financial support. Sometimes, nurses are uncomfortable asking for financial information, fearing that they are invading the patient's privacy. However, such data are important for the nurse to determine whether a patient's resources adequately meet his or her needs. The source of financial support is also important. For example, a patient whose income is adequate and from personal resources is more likely to be independent than is the patient who depends on family members for income.

The nurse should ask the patient about accessible clinics, support groups, and pharmaceutical services. Information about available health care resources can provide useful data regarding the patient's ability to access services and can also provide potential referral sources. In urban areas that are likely to have adequate health care resources, cultural and language barriers may prohibit access. People who live in rural areas where health care resources are limited are less likely to enjoy the full range of health care resources than are those in urban areas. Even in rural areas with mental health services, the use of these services by elderly people with mental illnesses is low (Bartels, 2003). If elders are married and have insurance, they are more likely to seek mental health services.

Spiritual Assessment

Spiritual needs are basic for all age groups and are requirements for establishing meaning and purpose, love and relatedness, and forgiveness. The 1971 White House Conference on Aging affirmed that all people are spiritual, even if they do not rely on religious institutions or practice personal pieties (Fish & Shelley, 1978). Aging is a process that can bring one closer to understanding the finite nature of existence. With advanced age, many people begin to reflect on their successes and failures. During such reflection, many seek out God or a higher being to make sense of the past and establish hope for the future.

The process of spiritual assessment involves active listening, thoughtful observing, and sensitive questioning. The nurse may simply ask if the elder would find comfort from a visit from a spiritual leader. Many forms of religion use various rituals that are important to the elder's daily routine. The nurse should explore and honor these aspects to the extent possible.

Legal Status

A growing trend in the United States is to view the elderly as a special population whose rights deserve increased attention. Instances of elder abuse are far too common. Every nurse must consider himself or herself a patient advocate and be vigilant in recognizing the signs of neglect or abuse, such as unexplained injuries. At times, abuse can take the form of another individual usurping the rights of the older person. Unless the older person is determined to be incompetent, he or she has the same rights to personal decision making as any other adult, including the right to refuse treatment.

Quality of Life

Sense of quality of life is closely tied to values and beliefs. For many elders, quality of life is not reflected in material possessions or physical health. At this stage, quality of life is connected more with contentment over how the person has lived life and the extent to which his or her life has had meaning and purpose. Keeping close personal contacts with friends and family and having the opportunity to shares stories of lifetime experiences are essential to maintaining mental health and wellness for older adults. For elderly people, physical illnesses may affect the quality of life more than psychiatric disorders. The assessment of quality of life becomes especially important when assessing a patient living in a nursing home or isolated in his or her own home. The assessment of quality of life of the elderly is similar to that for younger adults (see Chapter 10).

SUMMARY OF KEY POINTS

- Normal aging is associated with some physical decline, but most functions do not change. Intellectual functioning, capacity for change, and productive engagement with life remain stable.
- Mental health assessments are necessary when elderly patients face psychiatric or mental health issues. The biopsychosocial geropsychiatric nursing assessment examines many sources of data, including self-reports, laboratory test results, and reports from family members.
- The biopsychosocial geropsychiatric nursing assessment is based on the special needs and problems of the elderly. This assessment examines current and past health, functional status, and human responses to mental health problems.
- Assessment of the biologic domain involves collecting data about past and present health status, physical examination findings, physical functions (i.e., nutrition and eating, elimination patterns, sleep), pain, and pharmacologic information.
- Assessment of the psychological domain includes the patient's responses to mental health problems, mental status examination, behavioral changes, stress and coping patterns, and risk assessment.
- When conducting an assessment, the nurse may find several tools useful. For patients with possible depression, the Geriatric Depression Scale (GDS) may be helpful. For patients with anxiety, nurses can use the Rating Anxiety in Dementia (RAID) scale.
- Coping with the stresses of aging varies among patients. Determining stresses and coping skills for dealing with stresses is important.
- Social support is critical to patients in this age group and requires assessment.
- Determination of the patient's ability to perform functional and instrumental activities of daily living is critical in the assessment of the elderly. The Functional Activities Questionnaire (FAQ) measures the functional abilities based on information from others.
- Social systems, spiritual assessment, legal information, and quality of life are components within the social domain that the nurse should consider.

CRITICAL THINKING CHALLENGES

1. The director of your church's senior center has asked you to be the guest speaker at the monthly meeting of the Retired Active Citizens group. The subject is to be "Maintaining Your Mental Health After Retirement." What key points will you touch on in your presentation? What activities or handouts will you use to highlight your talk?
2. When asking about current illnesses, a patient begins telling you her whole life story. What approach would you take to elicit the most important information needed to develop an individualized plan of care for your elderly patient?
3. A caregiver tells you that her mother has become suspicious of the neighbors and other family members. How would you assess this perceptual experience? What other data should you gather from this patient?
4. A caregiver brings a sack of medications to the patient's assessment interview. What information should you obtain from the caregiver regarding the patient's use of these medications?
5. A woman brings her father, who has a long history of frequent psychiatric hospitalizations for depression, to the clinic. The patient's wife recently died, and the daughter fears that her father is becoming depressed again. What approach would you use in assessing for changes in mood?
6. Obtain a listing of the social services available in your community. Examine the list for areas of duplication and omission of services needed by an older adult living alone in his or her own home.

On Golden Pond: 1981. In this classic film, Henry Fonda portrays a crotchety, retired professor named Norman Thayer. Norman is angry that he is 80 years old and scared that he may lose his cognitive abilities. His wife, played by Katherine Hepburn, provides support and encouragement in maintaining his independence. The story revolves around Norman's relationship with his estranged daughter (played by Jane Fonda) as they finally try to understand each other during Norman's later years.

VIEWING POINTS: Identify the physical impairments that are obvious throughout the movie. Identify specific memory problems that Norman experiences. Are these problems part of normal aging? If you were Norman Thayer's nurse, what key assessment areas would you explore?

REFERENCES

Alexopoulos, G. S., Abrams, R. C., Young, R. C., Shamoian, C. A. (1998). Cornell Scale for Depression in Dementia. *Biological Psychiatry, 23*, 271–284.

American Psychiatric Association (APA). (2000). *Diagnostic and statistical manual of mental disorders* (4th ed., text revision). Washington, DC: Author.

Bartels, S. J. (2003). Improving the United States' system of care for older adults with mental illness: Findings and recommendations for the Presidents' New Freedom Commission on Mental Health. *American Journal of Geriatric Psychiatry, 11*(5), 486–497.

Bartels, S.J., Blow, F.C., Brockmann, L.M., & Van Citters, A.D. (2005). *Substance abuse and mental health among older Americans: The state of the knowledge and future directions.* Older American Substance Abuse and Mental Health Technical Assistance Center. Substance Abuse and Mental Health Services Administration: Rockville, MD.

Butcher, H.K., McGonigal-Denney, M. (2005). Depression and dispiritedness in later life. *American Journal of Nursing 105(12)*, 52–61.

Byles, J. E., Mishra, G. D., Harris, M. A., & Nair, K. (2003). The problems of sleep for older women: Changes in health outcomes. *Age and Ageing, 32*(2), 123–124.

Costa, P. T., Williams, R. F., Somerfield, M., et al. (1996). *Recognition and initial assessment of Alzheimer's disease and related dementias.* No. 19, AHCPR Publication No. 97–0703. Rockville, MD: U.S. Department of Health and Human Services, Public Health Service, Agency for Health Care Policy and Research.

Cummings, J. L., Mega, M., Gray, K., Rosenberg-Thompson, S., Carusi, D. A., & Gornbein, J. (1994). The Neuropsychiatric Inventory: Comprehensive assessment of psychopathology in dementia. *Neurology, 44*(12), 2308–2314.

Fish, S., & Shelley, J. A. (1978). *Spiritual care: The nurse's role.* Downers Grove, IL: InterVarsity.

Hyer, L., & Blount, J. (1984). Concurrent and discriminant validities of the geriatric depression scale with older psychiatric inpatients. *Psychological Reports, 54*, 611–616.

Kane, R. A. (1995). Assessment of social functioning: Recommendations for comprehensive geriatric assessment. In Z. Rubenstein, D. Wieland, & R. Bernabei (Eds.), *Geriatric assessment technology: The state of the art* (pp. 91–110). New York: Springer.

Katz, S., & Akpom, A. (1976). A measure of primary sociobiological functions. *International Journal of Health Science, 6*, 493.

Klatsky, A. L., Friedman, G. D., Armstrong, M. A., & Kipp, H. (2003). Wine, liquor, beer, and mortality. *American Journal of Epidemiology, 158* (6), 585–595.

Lantz, M (2003). Suicide in late life. *Clinical Geriatrics, 11*(10), 26–28.

Lopez, O. L., Becker, J. T., Sweet, R. A., Klunk, W., Kaufer, D. I., Saxton, J., et al. (2003). Psychiatric symptoms vary with the severity of dementia in probable Alzheimer's disease. *Journal of Neuropsychiatry and Clinical Neuroscience, 15*(3), 346–353.

Mehta, K. M., Yaffe, K., Langa, K. M., Sands, L., Whooley, M. A., & Covinsky, K. E. (2003). Additive effects of cognitive function and depressive symptoms on mortality in elderly community-living adults. *The Journals of Gerontology Series A: Biological Sciences and Medical Sciences, 58*(5), M461–M467.

Nygaard, H. A., & Jarland, M. (2005). Are nursing home patients with dementia diagnosis at increased risk for inadequate pain treatment? *International Journal of Geriatric Psychiatry, 20*, 730–737.

Shankar, K. K., Walker, M., Frost, D., & Orrell, M. W. (1999). The development of a valid and reliable scale for rating anxiety in dementia (RAID). *Aging & Mental Health, 3*(1), 39–49.

Sheikh, J. I., & Yesavage, J. A. (1986). Geriatric Depression Scale (GDS): Recent evidence and development of a shorter version. In T. L. Brink (Ed.), *Clinical gerontology: A guide to assessment and interventions* (pp. 165–177). Binghamton, NY: Haworth Press.

Sherrell, K., Buckwalter, K., Bode, R., & Strozdas, L. (1999). Use of the Cognitive Abilities Screen Instrument to assess elderly persons with schizophrenia in long-term care settings. *Issues in Mental Health Nursing, 20*, 541–558.

Souder, E., & O'Sullivan, P. S. (2000). Nursing documentation versus standardized assessment of cognitive status in hospitalized medical patients. *Applying Nursing Research, 13*(1), 29–36.

Tabloski, P. A., & Church, O. M. (1999). Insomnia, alcohol and drug use in community-residing elderly persons. *Journal of Substance Use, 4*(3), 147–154.

Teng, E. L, Hasegawa, K., Homma, A., Imai, Y., Larson, E., Graves, A., et al. (1994). The Cognitive Abilities Screen Instrument (CASI): A practical test for cross-cultural epidemiological studies of dementia. *International Psychogeriatrics, 6*(1), 45–58.

U.S. Department of Health and Human Services (U.S. DHHS). (2005). *Health, United States, 2005.* Centers for Disease Control and Prevention, National Center for Health Statistics, DHHS Publication No. 2005–1232, Hyattsville, Maryland.

Wan, H., Sengupta, M., Velkoff, V. A., & DeBarros, K. A. (2005). *U.S. Census Bureau, Current Populations Reports, 65+ in the United States: 2005.* U.S. Government Printing Office: Washington, D.C.

CHAPTER 31

Mental Health Promotion with the Elderly

Mary Ann Boyd

LEARNING OBJECTIVES

After studying this chapter, you will be able to:

- Identify important biopsychosocial factors occurring in late adulthood.
- Identify risk and protective factors related to geriatric psychopathology.
- Analyze the nurse's role in mental health promotion with elders and their families.
- Discuss mental health prevention and promotion interventions that are especially effective with elderly patients.

KEY CONCEPT

- late adulthood

KEY TERMS

- gerotranscendence • middle-old • old-old • young-old

Elderly people are at somewhat greater risk than younger age groups for the development or recurrence of mental health problems. One in four older adults has a significant mental disorder. The most common mental health problems in older persons are depression, anxiety disorders, and dementia (Bartels, Blow, Brockmann, & Van Citters, 2005). Yet, despite the high prevalence of psychiatric disorders and mental health problems in later life, older people remain vastly underserved by the current mental health system.

ELDER MENTAL HEALTH

This chapter explains the effect of aging on mental health and identifies risk and protective factors related to geriatric psychopathology.

KEY CONCEPT Late adulthood can be divided into three chronological groups: young-old (ages 65–74 years), middle-old (ages 75–84 years), and old-old (age 85 years and older).

People 75 years and older are the most rapidly growing segment of the U.S. population (National Center for Health Statistics, 2006). The transition from young-old to old-old is more than a series of birthdays; it is a gradual biopsychosocial process that may be viewed as both positive and negative. From a positive perspective, the later years allow time for personal growth and development, providing an opportunity to do all the things that were impossible when work and family responsibilities took precedence. Traveling, visiting friends, and engaging in neglected hobbies enhance quality of life and improve well-being.

In late adulthood, changes in health status can lead to negative outcomes. A loss in physical functioning can lead to a loss in independence, which can result in an unplanned change in residence. Family relationships change, as once-dependent children grow into adulthood and become parents themselves. Friendships change and losses occur. Many elders retire from meaningful lifelong work and are faced with establishing new meaning in life.

In all health care settings, communication is an integral factor in nursing care. Communication with the elderly requires special attention to verbal interactions and environmental influences. Box 31.1 highlights many of the considerations necessary when interacting with the older adult.

BOX 31.1

Communicating with Elderly People

- Focus the person's attention on the exchange of communication; the older adult may need extra time to begin to process information.
- Face the elder when speaking to him or her.
- Minimize distractions in the room, including other people, objects in your hands, noise, and other activities.
- Reduce glare from room lighting by dimming too-bright lights. Conversely, avoid sitting in shadows.
- Speak slowly and clearly. Elders may depend on lip reading, so ensure that the individual can see you. Speak loudly, but do not shout.
- Use short, simple sentences and be prepared to repeat or revise what you have said.
- Limit the number of topics discussed at one time to prevent information overload.
- Ask one question at a time to minimize confusion. Allow plenty of time for the elder to answer and express ideas.
- Frequently summarize the important points of the conversation to improve understanding and comprehension.
- Avoid the urge to finish sentences.
- If the communication exchange is going poorly, postpone it for another time.

Biologic Domain

During the later years, changes in vital biologic structures and processes can occur in a particular organ or tissue or in the whole body. Changes may occur from disuse after the function of the organ has been fulfilled (e.g., the uterus or thymus gland) or from disuse associated with insufficient exercise or movement (e.g., in neuromusculoskeletal systems). Body fat increases (18%–36% in men, 33%–48% in women), total body water decreases (10%–15%), and muscle mass decreases. Distinguishing whether changes occur because of decreased physical activity, level of motivation, influence of societal expectations, or cumulative effects of disease is difficult.

When changes occur in the organ systems, functional capacity is often decreased. However, many older adults can integrate profound decrements in physical capacity without affecting the ability to function under normal conditions. It is only when functional reserves are needed, such as during an infection, that the absence of these reserves is observed. The following sections highlight significant biologic changes that occur in later adulthood.

Renal Changes

Even without disease, a predictable decline in glomerular filtration and tubular secretion occurs with aging. Renal blood flow decreases by as much as 10% every decade after age 40 years. Renal clearance is estimated to decrease by as much as 35% between the ages of 20 and 90 years. These changes result in decreased renal excretion, which is of particular concern because the kidneys excrete most drugs (Tiao, Semmens, Masarei, & Lawrence-Brown, 2002).

Gastrointestinal Changes

Blood flow in the liver tends to decrease with advancing age, decreasing as much as 40% to 50% by the age of 65 years. Reduced cardiac output is the major factor slowing blood flow through the liver. Reduced blood flow decreases the liver's opportunity to metabolize medications; consequently, medications may remain in the blood longer, increasing the risk for toxicity. As a result, fat-soluble drugs become sequestered in fatty tissue, rather than remaining in the circulating plasma. These factors increase the risk for accumulation and drug toxicity (Anantharaju, Feller, & Chedid, 2002).

Neurologic Changes

Nervous system changes that occur with aging include central and peripheral neuronal cell loss; slowed transmission of nervous impulses; slowed reaction time; diminished proprioception, balance, and postural control; poor thermoregulation; and altered sleep patterns. The effects of changes in the nervous system are confounded by changes in other systems, such as the cardiovascular system (e.g., decreased arterial elasticity) and respiratory system (e.g., diminished response to hypoxia and hypercapnia). Physiologic changes occurring with physical illness may precipitate altered mental status (e.g., delirium) or exacerbate symptoms of existing psychiatric illness (e.g., depression).

The brain, like most other body organs, undergoes changes with aging. Although brain weight begins to decline after the age of 30 years, visible atrophy is not apparent until about 60 years. Brain weight decreases by about 10% from early life to the ninth decade; this change is reflected in enlarged ventricles and widened sulci. Brain atrophy may result from a net loss of neurons (Scahill et al., 2003).

Sensory Changes

All five senses decline with age. This factor is important to remember when assessing psychiatrically ill elderly patients because diminished senses may affect attention and perception, potentially affecting interpretation of standard mental status examinations. Structural changes in the eye include rigidity of the iris, accumulation of yellow substance in the lens, and diminished lens elasticity. These changes result in decreased pupil size, alteration in color perception, presbyopia, impaired adaptation to darkness, and significant vision impairment in the presence of glare (Bakker, 2003). Auditory changes are noticeable as early as 40 years of age; however, age of onset varies, according to lifestyle (e.g., previous exposure to occupational noise). Cochlear neurons are lost, resulting in hearing loss that may affect performance on intelligence tests. Several other factors beyond loss of hearing can influence age-related differences in performance on intelligence tests. Research on taste, touch, and smell is sparse, but a uniform dulling of these senses occurs with aging. The rate of decline is highly variable among individuals.

Sexuality

Misinformation and attitudinal barriers continue to plague the study of sexuality in the aging individual. Several generalizations have emerged: older persons retain interest in sex; frequency of sexual activity is less than desired; and increasing problems with sexual performance are associated with increasing age in both men and women. Although several physical changes with aging affect sexual functioning, interest in and enjoyment of sexual activities can continue until one's death. Health, desire to remain sexually active, access to a partner, and a conducive environment contribute to positive sexual functioning.

Physiological changes in women include decreasing estrogen levels, alterations in the structural integrity of the vagina (e.g., decreased blood flow, decreased flexibility, diminished lubrication, and diminished response during orgasm), and decreased breast engorgement during arousal (Wright, 2001). The sexual response continues as in younger women, but with less intensity. Even with chronic illness, many older women remain interested in and satisfied with a variety of sexual activities. Although being older is often associated with decrease in sexual interest in women, sexual attitudes and knowledge are also important predictors of interest, participation, and satisfaction with sexual activity. In reality, sexual activity in aging women often depends on availability of a partner.

Physiological changes in men include a decline in testosterone production, increased time to achieve erection, less firm erections, decreased urgency for ejaculation, decreased sperm production, and a longer refractory period (i.e., the amount of time before the man can achieve another erection) (Wright, 2001). Problems with sexual performance in aging men are usually centered around erectile dysfunction.

In men, frequency and desired frequency for coitus declines as age increases. Men are more likely to be sexually active but less satisfied with their level of sexual activity than are women. As with women, partner availability and willingness influence the frequency of sexual activity.

Access to a conducive environment may be hindered if the parent resides with an adult child or in a nursing home. Although nursing home residents may remain interested in maintaining sexual relationships, the attitudes of the staff and physicians constitute an additional barrier for this population beyond those noted previously (Bauer, 1999; Gott & Hinchliff, 2003).

Psychological Domain

Cognitive Function

Changes in cognition are most likely accounted for by structural and functional changes in the brain (Rosenzweig & Barnes, 2003). These alterations are probably highly specific because aspects of cognitive decline are very specific (e.g., secondary memory), and many abilities are preserved. Moreover, external factors, including activity levels, socioeconomic status, education, and personality, may modify the development or expression of age-related changes in cognition (see Chapter 32).

Normal aging does not impair consciousness. Alertness is required for attention, but the alert patient may not necessarily be able to attend. Attention has two aspects: sustained attention (vigilance) and selective attention (ability to extract relevant from irrelevant information). Numerous studies indicate that elderly people perform well on tests of both sustained and selective attention. Earlier findings of poor performance on tests of selective attention have been attributed to lack of control for perceptual difficulties (e.g., vision and hearing deficits).

Slower reaction time may affect how quickly the elder responds to questions. Hurrying elders to answer questions may interfere with their ability to provide the correct answer. This has been labeled the *speed–accuracy* shift, by which the elderly person focuses more on accuracy than speed in responding. Caution tends to increase, whereas risk-taking behavior tends to decrease; older adults are more likely to make errors of omission (leave the answer out) than errors of commission (make a guess) (Zimprich, 2002).

Learning

Intelligence and personality are stable across the life span in the absence of disease; however, the learning abilities of older people may be more selective, requiring motivation ("How important is this information?"), meaningful content ("Why do I need to know this?"), and familiarity with the idea or content. Although age causes no differences in the ability to process knowledge to learn a skill, younger people are more likely to employ strategies to learn tasks. Level of education needs to be considered in evaluating responses on mental status examinations because it may represent socioeconomic status and occupation.

Memory

Other than overall intelligence, age-related memory alterations have been more widely studied than any other aspect of cognition. Memory loss is not a normal part of aging. To remember events, humans must first attend to information and process it. Older people may well dismiss information that is not important to them. Memory problems in later life are believed to result from encoding problems, or "getting" the information in the first place. This problem may be related to sensory problems, not paying attention, or a general failure to link the "to be remembered" information to existing knowledge through association or to strengthen the memory through repetition. However, it is important not to confuse decline with deficit. Although a decline in memory ability may be frustrating for the older individual, it does not necessarily hamper his or her ability to function daily. Threats to memory include medications, depression (impairs concentration and attention), poor nutrition, infection, heart and lung disease (lack of oxygen), thyroid problems (can cause symptoms of depression or confusion that mimic memory loss), alcohol use, and sensory loss (interferes with perception).

Development

Late-life adult developmental phenomena have not been well defined (see Chapter 6). Although Erik Erikson identified "integrity versus despair" as a developmental task specific to late adulthood, recently his wife published an extension of his theory that included old age as a ninth stage, **gerotranscendence** (Erikson & Erikson, 1997). Rather than emphasizing decrements in physical capacity for function, gerotranscendence theory provides for continued growth in dimensions such as spirituality and inner strength. The concept of gerotranscendence may be used in establishing health promotion interventions (Box 31.2).

Relationship Strains

As family relationships change, interpersonal relationship strains can develop. Disappointments with lifestyles of adult children and changes in caregiving responsibilities affect the quality of a long-time family relationship. In some instances, the young-old assume caregiving responsibilities for their old-old relatives. It is also common for grandparents to assume some caregiving responsibilities for their grandchildren. The well-being of grandmothers raising grandchildren in coparenting and custodial households depends on a variety of factors, including cultural ones. In a study of African American, Latino, and Caucasian grandmothers, a sample of 1,058 grandmothers raising or helping to raise school-aged grandchildren in Los Angeles were interviewed, and analyses were conducted within ethnic groups. African American grandmothers experienced equal well-being in coparenting and custodial families; however, if the stresses related to the parents' problems were removed by statistical control, they favored the custodial arrangement. Latino grandmothers had greater well-being in coparenting families, reflecting a tradition of intergenerational living. Caucasian custodial grandmothers experienced somewhat higher levels of affect (positive and negative), but showed no difference in other types of well-being. This implies that the cultural lens through which grandparenthood is viewed has a marked impact on the adaptation to custodial or coparenting family structures (Goodman & Silverstein, 2002).

BOX 31.2

Research for Best Practice: *Practical Application of Gerotranscendence Theory*

Wadensten, B., & Carlsson, M. (2003). Theory-driven guidelines for practical care of older people, based on the theory of gerotranscendence. Journal of Advanced Nursing, 41(5), 462–470.

THE QUESTION: The developmental process toward gerotranscendence can be obstructed or accelerated by life crises and grief, but elements in the culture can also facilitate or impede the process. Similarly, the caring climate can obstruct or accelerate the process toward gerotranscendence. This study was undertaken to find out what practical guidelines could be devised for use in the care of older people.

METHODS: The method of deriving guidelines from the theory was focus group interviews. The theory of gerotranscendence was used as a foundation for stimulating the discussions in the focus groups, as well as for organizing the proposals that emerged.

FINDINGS: Concrete guidelines at three levels, focusing on the individual, activity, and organization, were derived. The following guidelines were generated to support older people in their process toward gerotranscendence.

- Accept the possibility that behaviors resembling the signs of gerotranscendence are normal signs of aging.
- Reduce preoccupation with the body.
- Allow alternative definitions of time.
- Allow thoughts and conversations about death.
- Choose topics of conversation that facilitate and further older people's personal growth.
- Accept, create, and introduce new types of "activities."
- Encourage and facilitate quiet and peaceful places and times.

IMPLICATIONS FOR NURSING: These guidelines could support staff in their practical care of older people and could be used as a supplement to enrich current care. The guidelines should be used to promote development toward gerotranscendence.

Social Domain

Functional Status

Functional status, the extent to which a person can carry out independently personal care, home management, and social functions in everyday life in a way that has meaning and purpose, often changes during the later years (see Chapter 30). Estimates of the prevalence of functional dependency vary, but in general, studies show that difficulty in performing activities of daily living (ADLs) increases with advancing age, and that rates of dependency are significantly higher for women than for men, particularly for women who live alone (von Strauss, Aguero-Torres, Kareholt, Winblad, & Fratiglioni, 2003).

Retirement

The transition from a paid work role to a potentially less structured and purposeful pattern of living can lead to alterations in self-concept. Retirement is frequently characterized as a stressful life event that may bring psychological, social, and economic uncertainty. It is often associated with negative myths and stereotypes. Although retirement is potentially stressful, the average age of retirement decreased from age 66 years between 1955 and 1960 to age 63 years between 1985 and 1990. Today the average age for retirement is 58 (Korczyk, 2004; Taylor, Funk & Craighill, 2006). (Fig. 31.1).

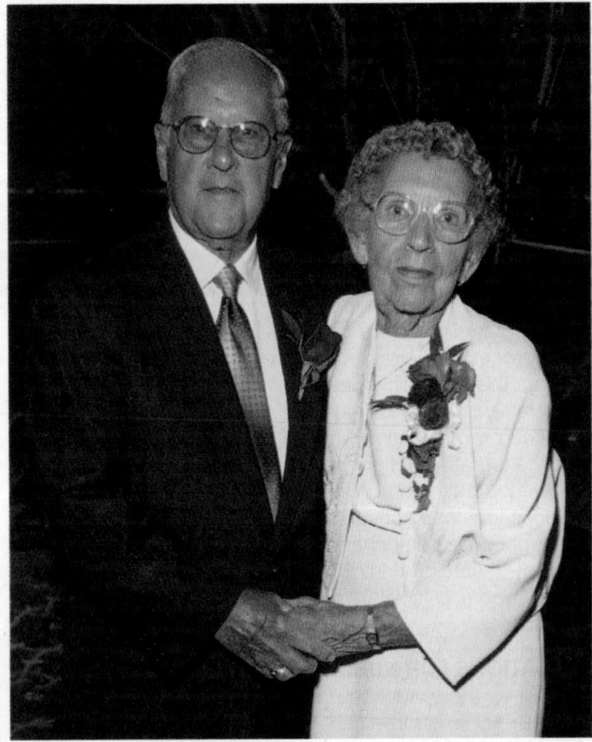

FIGURE 31.1. Most older adults do very well in retirement, finding time to enjoy social activity among friends, families, and community.

Retirement affects social roles, income, use of health services, and participation in leisure activities. Social security continues to provide the largest share of income for many older people (Wan, Sengupta, Velkoff, & DeBarros, 2005). The traditional "three-legged stool" on which retirement rests—Social Security, pensions, and savings/investments—excludes groups that have faced barriers to education, health, stable work history, or financial stability. Disproportionately, such groups include people of color, gays and lesbians, women, and immigrants (Stanford & Usita, 2002).

Cultural Impact

Wide cultural variations exist in family expectations of and responsibilities for the elderly. Some groups, such as Asian cultures, tend to highly value the experience and wisdom of their elderly, and family members feel a responsibility for their care. Based on the latest census, it is projected that between 2000 and 2030, the percentage of elders will increase by 328% for Hispanics, 285% for Asian and Pacific Islanders, 147% for American Indians and Aleuts, and 131% for African Americans, compared with 81% for Caucasians. Our communities are increasingly a reflection of multiple ethnic histories and value (Hayes-Bautista, Hsu, Perez, & Gamboa, 2002).

Social Activities

Health conditions may also prevent participation in home maintenance and leisure activities, especially walking, gardening, and active sports. Among serious health conditions in the years after retirement, lung disease and diabetes most seriously affect leisure activities. As age increases, participation decreases. Higher education levels are associated with increased participation in both formal and informal activities (Holmes & Dorfman, 2000).

Community Strains

Older adults can find themselves living in changing or deteriorating neighborhoods. With decreasing social support, they are often faced with either living in a familiar but increasingly socially isolated environment or moving to an unfamiliar place (Djernes, 2006). One major problem is housing and the proximity of home to social resources, such as church, community centers, shopping, health care, and related social services. Although most elders live in their own homes, relocating to smaller and more protective housing may be welcomed by some and fiercely resisted by others.

Residential Care

Various residential care models are in part a response to the medical model emphasized in most long-term care facilities and the need to develop alternatives to nursing home care. Residential care models include a spectrum of state-licensed residential living environments, such as foster care homes, family homes, personal care homes, residential care facilities, and assisted living arrangements.

For every person currently in institutional care, an estimated four others who require some form of long-term care are in the community. How and by whom will they be provided care? Approaches to this looming problem include the following:

- Reducing the need for home care by improving the health of older people
- Finding and paying for home care when disability and frailty preclude continued independence
- Ensuring better integration across the total continuum of care and coordination of different care providers who subscribe to a biopsychosocial view of health care that includes both medical and social components

Consumers should question residential providers about all aspects of services to determine whether the older adult's needs and abilities match the care provided in that facility, including staff training and staffing patterns, medication supervision, approaches to behavior management, activities provided, services available (e.g., care management, family support, counseling, day care), safety and security issues, provision of personal care with attention to dignity and privacy, health and nutrition concerns, and full disclosure of costs and funding and payment issues.

Assisted Living

The assisted living concept has emerged as an important long-term care alternative for the mentally and physically frail. Assisted living provides community-based, residential services for older persons and/or adults with physical disabilities who need help with ADLs. Assisted living services combine housing, personal services, and light medical or nursing care. Perhaps the most important feature of these assisted living facilities is the orientation toward the elderly resident that empowers the frail older adult by sharing responsibilities for care and ADLs, enhancing their choices and managing risks. The need for alternative long-term care strategies for this population is expected to continue, with the growing number of older adults in need of supportive services.

RISK FACTORS FOR GERIATRIC PSYCHOPATHOLOGY

Chronic Illnesses

Although the frequency of acute conditions declines with advancing age, about 80% of older adults have at least one chronic health condition; 50% have at least two. Poor physical health is a well-established risk factor for mental disorders. The major chronic conditions that cause activity limitation are arthritis, hypertension, heart disease, and respiratory disorders (Wan, Sengupta, Velkoff, & DeBarros, 2005). Chronic illnesses can reduce physiologic capacity and consequently increase functional dependency. In addition, during acute episodes of illness, many elders lose functional ability because they have limited reserves or cannot mobilize reserves to regain their premorbid performance levels.

Substance abuse is associated with poor health outcomes, higher health care utilization, and increased complexity of the course of the disorder. In addition, increased disability and impairment, compromised quality of life, increased caregiver stress, increased mortality, and higher risk of suicide are associated with substance abuse. The majority of older adults with substance abuse problems do not receive adequate treatment (Bartels, Blow, Brockmann, & Van Citters, 2005).

Polypharmacy

Polypharmacy, the use of several medications, is often associated with chronic illness and long-term drug therapy (see Chapter 30). Older persons consume an average of two to six prescription medications and two to three over-the-counter medications. Medication misuse can easily occur and in some combinations, lead to drug abuse (Blow, Bartels, Brockmann, & Van Citters, 2005). The aging process affects pharmacokinetics and the strength and number of protein-binding sites (see Chapter 8). These changes place the elderly person at increased risk for adverse drug reactions. In a review of literature, the reported prevalence of elderly patients using at least one inappropriately prescribed drug ranged from 40% of nursing home patients to 21.3% of community-dwelling patients (Liu & Christensen, 2002). Serious problems result when coordination of the care delivery and treatment regimen specific to prescribed medications is lacking. These problems are compounded when the patient uses over-the-counter drugs, herbal remedies, and home or folk remedies without considering their potential interaction with prescribed drugs. Nurses can follow the principles delineated in Box 31.3 to improve drug therapy in the elderly population.

Bereavement and Loss

The elder experiences many losses—friends and family members die, physical health is compromised, and social status is diminished. Loss of one's spouse, particularly when the relationship has been long and satisfying, constitutes a major life event. Women are more likely to lose their spouses and tend to be widowed at a younger age

BOX 31.3

Drug Therapy Interventions

- Minimize the number of drugs that the patient uses, keeping only those drugs that are essential. One third of the residents in one long-term care facility received 8 to 16 drugs daily.
- Always consider alternatives among different drug classifications or dosage forms that are more suitable for elderly patients.
- Implement preventive measures to reduce the need for certain medications. Such prevention includes health promotion through proper nutrition, exercise, and stress reduction.
- Most age-dependent pharmacokinetic changes lead to potential accumulation of the drug; therefore, medication dosage should start low and go slow.
- Exercise caution when administering medication with a long half-life or in an older adult with impaired renal or liver function. Under these conditions, the time may be extended between doses.
- Be knowledgeable of each drug's properties, including such factors as half-life, excretion, and adverse effects. For example, venlafaxine HCl (Effexor), a structurally novel antidepressant that inhibits the reuptake of serotonin and norepinephrine, requires regular monitoring of the patient's blood pressure.
- Assess the patient's clinical history for physical problems that may affect excretion of medications.
- Monitor laboratory values (e.g., creatinine clearance) and urinary output in patients receiving medications eliminated by the kidneys.
- Monitor plasma albumin levels in patients receiving drugs that have high binding affinity to protein.
- Regularly monitor the patient's reaction to all medications to ensure a therapeutic response.
- Look for potential drug interactions that may complicate therapy. Antacids lower gastric acidity and may decrease the rate at which other medications are dissolved and absorbed.
- Instruct patients to consult with their provider before taking any over-the-counter medications.

than are men. Consequently, women have more time to adjust and develop substitute social relationships to replace the spouse. Conversely, men tend to lose their wives at an older age, have fewer social networks to replace the spouse, and express feelings of loneliness and abandonment. Because of differences in longevity, men and women usually experience life events at different ages.

Regardless of gender differences, survivors are at higher risk for depression and face financial issues after the death of a loved one. Health care professionals should work closely with grieving survivors to help them understand that their lives will be displaced for some time. Support sessions on the grief process and financial and employment planning could become a standard part of care.

Poverty

Because retirement and widowhood are common events in late life, elders can be at higher risk for poverty than other age groups. Two groups of poor elderly include those who have lived in poverty all their lives and those who become impoverished in late life. Poverty may result from inadequate retirement income, illness and medical bills, discrimination against women in pension plans, and financial exploitation of older individuals. Health care costs probably are the largest contributor to economic insecurity in elderly people. Older women are more likely to live in poverty than older men (13% compared to 7%). Older people living alone have the highest poverty rates (Wan et al., 2005). Poverty has significant effects on the elderly population, including higher mortality rates, poorer health, lower health-related quality of life, lower likelihood of participating in health screening programs, and higher likelihood of using the emergency department for acute illness (Fleming, Evans, & Chutka, 2003).

Lack of Social Support and Suicide

A lack of social support has been linked to the rate of suicide in the elderly. After falls and motor vehicle collisions, suicide is the third leading cause of death from injury among people older than 65 years. Suicide rates are consistently higher among the elderly than any other age group. Of people 65 years of age or older, men account for 81% of suicides. Rates are the highest for divorced or widowed men (see Figure 31.2). Risk factors for suicide in elderly people include being Caucasian, male, widowed or divorced, retired or unemployed, living alone in an urban area, in poor health (including poor mental health), or lonely, and having a history of poor interpersonal relationships (Waern, Rubenowitz, & Wilhelmson, 2003). Older people make fewer attempts per successful suicide; firearms are the most common method of suicide by both men and women older than 65 years (Older Americans Substance Abuse & Mental Health Technical Assistance Center, 2006).

Shared Living Arrangements and Elder Mistreatment

Elder mistreatment can be defined as intentional actions that cause harm or create a serious risk of harm to a vulnerable elder by a caregiver or other person who stands in a trust relationship to the elder (Bonnie & Wallace, 2002). Estimates of occurrence of abuse and neglect vary from

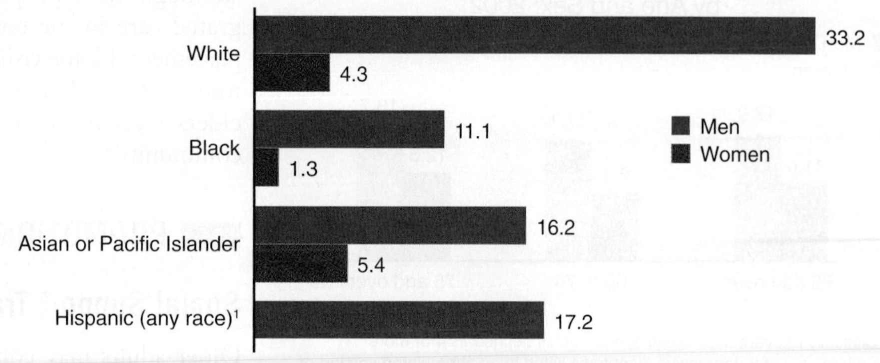

FIGURE 31.2. Suicide among people aged 65 and over by race and sex.

2% to 10%, but there are few available studies. Clinical and empirical evidence suggests that a shared living arrangement is a major risk factor for elder mistreatment, with the older person living alone at lowest risk. A shared living arrangement increases the opportunities for contact that can lead to conflict and mistreatment (Bonnie & Wallace, 2002).

PROTECTIVE FACTORS FOR MENTAL ILLNESS IN OLDER PERSONS

Protective factors in older persons are similar to those in younger adults. Evidence supports four protective factors including marriage, education, nutrition, and exercise.

The Marriage Effect

It has long been known that married people have lower mortality rates than unmarried at all ages. In the 65- to 74-year-old age group, the death rate per 100,000 for never-married people was 4,030 compared with 2,351 for married people. There are several possible explanations for the marriage advantage. Married people may be less likely to engage in high-risk and health-damaging behaviors. They may also be more likely to receive care and support when needed. They have shared economic resources and a large social network of relatives and friends who can provide vital support at older ages (Wan et al., 2005).

Physical Activity

There is emerging evidence that physical activity is related to positive mental health and may be a protective factor. There is a moderate amount of evidence that exercise can prevent the onset or worsening of depression (Blow et al., 2005). Structured exercise programs may enhance older persons' overall physical functioning and well-being (LIFE Study Investigators, 2006).

Education and Income

Education and income are directly related to physical activity and disability. Those with higher education and income are more likely to engage in physical activity and have the resources to provide care when needed. Conversely, those with less education and income are more likely to have ADL disabilities and difficulties in physical functioning (Wan et al., 2005).

Nutrition

Undernutrition is a greater problem in today's elderly than obesity. The prevalence of undernutrition appears to be high in the elderly (2% to 32%), especially those living in an institutionalized setting (1% to 83%) (Bhat, Chiu, & Jeste, 2005). Undernutrition can lead to low levels of micronutrients such as folic acid, vitamin B_{12}, and homocysteine, which in turn can lead to symptoms of depression. Essential fatty acids have to be obtained in the diet and may have biological effects through gene expression in various tissues. The prevalence of deficiencies in these nutritional factors appears to increase with age. Adequate nutrition is an important factor in maintaining mental health.

PREVENTION OF MENTAL ILLNESS

Preventing Depression and Suicide

Depression is one of the most common mental disorders of the elderly (see Chapter 20; see Figure 31.3). Because

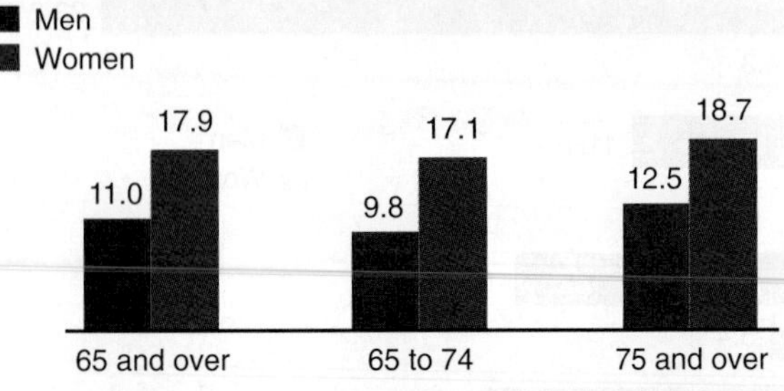

[1] "Clinically relevant depressive symptoms" is defined as 4 or more symptoms out of 8 depressive symptoms listed in an abbreviated version of the Center for Epidemiological Studies Depression (CES-D) scale adapted by the Health and Retirement Study. The CES-D scale is a measure of depressive symptoms and is not to be used as a diagnosis of clinical depression. A detailed explanation concerning the "4 or more symptoms" cut-off can be found in the following documentation:http://hrsonline.isr.umich.edu/userg/dr-005.pdf. Proportions are based on weighted data using the preliminary respondent weight from HRS-2002.

FIGURE 31.3. Depressive symptoms in people aged 65 and over by age and sex.

depression can lead to suicide, recognition and early intervention are the keys to avoiding ongoing depressive episodes. Early indications of symptomatology can be identified in primary care settings. Several preventive interventions are helpful, such as grief counseling for widows and widowers, self-help groups, and social activities.

Reducing the Stigma of Mental Health Treatment

The stigma of mental illness continues to interfere with the willingness of the elderly to seek treatment. Today's older Americans grew up during a time when institutionalization in asylums, electroconvulsive treatments, and other treatment approaches were regarded with fear. This fear can lead to denial of problems. Nurses can help reduce the stigma through education interventions and facilitation of access to services.

> **• NCLEXNOTE**
>
> Safety concerns are a priority. Carefully explore any suicidal ideation and develop a plan for prevention.

Monitoring Medication Side Effects

With the approval of new medications, the elderly will be able to treat health problems with pharmacologic agents that were not previously available. Side effects and drug interactions should be carefully monitored to detect untoward symptoms and delirium (see Chapter 32).

Avoiding Premature Institutionalization

Although many people require nursing home care, integrated care in the community can delay nursing home placement. Home visits that focus on assessment of symptoms and coordination of health care needs can result in elders receiving their mental health support within the community.

PROMOTION OF MENTAL HEALTH

Social Support Transitions

Older adults may compensate for loss of family by expanding friendship networks, and employment may become an important method of establishing a network in late life. The elder can be prepared for the transition by receiving information about internal developmental processes, sources of social support, and opportunities for personal growth and role supplementation.

Lifestyle Support

Lifestyle interventions, such as exercise promotion and nutrition counseling, are particularly important in late life because a tendency to slow down and become more sedentary usually accompanies aging. For many, retirement provides an opportunity to restructure the time that was previously spent working. Developing regular exercise habits can help maintain physical and psychological well-being. Self-help programs generally include components of exercise, nutrition, health screening, and health habits.

Self-Care Enhancement

Enhancing health self-care is a major area for mental health promotion. Education of elderly patients and their families is crucial to ensuring compliance and minimizing untoward effects of medications. Basic principles regarding neurobiologic changes in normal aging (as previously discussed) should be applied when designing teaching strategies. The nurse must consider the elder's pace of learning, as well as visual and hearing deficits. Education should include the reason for administering the drug and important side effects of the drug. The nurse should provide instructional aids, large-print labeling, and devices such as medication calendars that encourage compliance. The nurse should inform patients of the option to waive the requirements for childproof containers if they have trouble opening them.

Spiritual Support

Humanists suggest that the main purpose of life is to find meaning and that this can be accomplished through cre-ations (or accomplishments), experiences in the world, and attitude toward suffering (Frankl, 1963). In nursing, spirituality is recognized as a basic quality, inherent in all humans. The spiritual perspective includes three critical attributes:

- Connectedness (with other humans, nature, universal forces, or God)
- Beliefs in powers or forces beyond the self, and a faith that affirms life
- A creative energy

The spiritual perspective also can provide a path for the quest for the meaning of life and can organize and guide human values and motivations.

Spirituality can be extremely important to the elderly and can positively affect attitude, particularly as health declines (Lowry & Conco, 2002). Supporting contact with spiritual leaders important to the patient is an ongoing mental health promotion intervention. The nurse can also support a patient's spiritual growth by exploring the meanings that a particular life change has for the elder. In late life, existential issues such as experiencing losses, redefining meanings in existence, and living in the present become the standard, replacing the performance and future orientation that characterize earlier adulthood.

Community Services

More emphasis should be placed on community care options, services that provide both sustenance and growth. Examples of supportive services that foster independent community living include information and referral services, transportation and nutrition services, legal and protective services, comprehensive senior centers, homemaker and handyman services, matching of older with younger individuals to share housing, and use of the supports available through churches, community groups, or mental health and other community agencies (e.g., area agencies on aging) to maintain elderly individuals in the community for as long as possible. The availability and accessibility of these services vary greatly, and eligibility requirements may exist.

FAME AND FORTUNE

Grandma Moses (1860–1961):
Mental Health Idealized

Anna Mary Robertson was born in upstate New York, married when she was 27, and had 10 children (five living to adulthood). She was feisty and strong-willed. She did not begin painting until she was 75. Her work was discovered by a collector during the Depression. Her work was known as American primitive in the art world. She painted her scenes on pieces of wood that she first painted white. From age 75 until her death at age 101, she painted approximately 1600 paintings—250 of which were painted after her 100th birthday.

SUMMARY OF KEY POINTS

- Major changes in social roles with aging include retirement, loss of partner, and changes in residence.
- The brain changes with aging; these changes include a decline in weight and reduction in synapses.
- The nervous system has a considerable degree of plasticity and can sustain some structural losses without losing function.
- All five special senses (sight, hearing, touch, taste, and smell) decline with age.
- Intelligence and personality are stable throughout the life span; however, reaction time slows with age.
- Threats to memory in the elderly include medications, depression, poor nutrition, infection, heart and lung disease, thyroid problems, alcohol use, and sensory loss.
- Polypharmacy is prevalent in the elderly, particularly in nursing homes. Ongoing assessment of medication is needed to prevent inappropriate medication administration.
- Elderly people are at higher risk for poverty and suicide.
- Although older adults experience many physical changes, they can and have the desire to remain sexually active.
- Aging affects pharmacokinetics; it also affects the strength and number of protein-binding sites.
- Mental health protective factors include marriage, education, nutrition, and exercise.
- Residential care environments ideally emphasize family-oriented care that optimizes existing functional capacities.
- Assisted living is a supportive housing environment that provides routine nursing services within a philosophy of patient empowerment.

CRITICAL THINKING CHALLENGES

1 Compare the three late adulthood chronological groups in terms of age. Using the recommendations of Box 31.1, interview people representing each of the three chronological groups about their views of mental health.
2 Highlight normal biological changes that occur during the aging process.
3 Hypothesize why IQ tests and personality do not change with time.

4 Explain the concept of *gerotranscendence* and use the concept to explain differences between the young-old and the old-old.
5 Identify positive and negative perspectives of retirement.
6 Explain why chronic illnesses, polypharmacy, and poverty are all risk factors for mental health problems in later life.
7 Describe mental health promotion interventions that relate to social support transitions, lifestyle support, and self-care.

Driving Miss Daisy: 1989. This delightful film stars Jessica Tandy as Daisy Werthan, a cantankerous old woman. Morgan Freeman plays Hoke Colburn, Daisy's chauffeur. This beautiful story examines a relationship between two people who have more in common than just getting old. Driving Miss Daisy challenges some of the myths about getting old.

VIEWING POINTS: Identify the normal behaviors in the growth and development of the elderly. Observe the verbal and nonverbal communication of Daisy and Hoke. How do they support each other?

REFERENCES

Anantharaju, A., Feller, A., & Chedid, A. (2002). Aging liver: A review. *Gerontology, 48*(6), 343–353.

Bakker, R. (2003). Sensory loss, dementia, and environments. *Generations, 27*(1), 46–51.

Bartels, S. J., Blow, F. C., Brockmann, L. M., & Van Citters, A. D. (2005). *Substance abuse and mental health among older Americans: The state of the knowledge and future directions.* Older American Substance Abuse and Mental Health Technical Assistance Center. Substance Abuse and Mental Health Services Administration: Rockville, MD.

Bauer, M. (1999). Their only privacy is between their sheets: Privacy and the sexuality of elderly nursing home residents. *Journal of Gerontological Nursing, 25*(8), 37–41.

Bhat, R. S., Chiu, D., & Jeste, D. V. (2005). Nutrition and geriatric psychiatry: a neglected field. (Editorial). *Current Opinion in Psychiatry, 18*(6), 609–614.

Blow, F. C., Bartels, S. J., Brockmann, L. M., & Van Citters, A. D. (2005). *Evidence-based practices for preventing substance abuse and mental health problems in older adults.* Older American Substance Abuse and Mental Health Technical Assistance Center. Substance Abuse and Mental Health Services Administration: Rockville, MD.

Bonnie, R. J., & Wallace, R. B. (Eds). (2002*). Elder mistreatment: Abuse, neglect, and exploitation in an aging America.* Committee on National Statistics and Committee on Law and Justice. National Research Council. The National Academies Press: Washington, DC.

Djernes, J. K. (2006). Prevalence and predictors of depression in populations of elderly: a review. *Acta Psychiatrica Scandinavica, 113* (5), 372–387.

Erikson, E. H., & Erikson, J. M. (1997). *The Lifecycle Completed, Extended Version.* New York: WW Norton.

Fleming, K. C., Evans, J. M., & Chutka, D. S. (2003). A cultural and economic history of old age in America. *Mayo Clinic Proceedings, 78*(7), 914–921.

Frankl, V. (1963). *Man's search for meaning: An introduction to logotherapy.* New York: Pocket Books.

Goodman, C., & Silverstein, M. (2002). Grandmothers raising grandchildren: Family structure and well-being in culturally diverse families. *Gerontologist, 42*(5), 676–689.

Gott, M., & Hinchliff, S. (2003). How important is sex in later life? The views of older people. *Social Science Medicine, 56*(8), 1617–1628.

Hayes-Bautista, D. E., Hsu, P., Perez, A., & Gamboa, C. (2002). The 'browning' of the graying of America: Diversity in the elderly population and policy implications. *Generations, 26*(3), 15–24.

Holmes, J. S., & Dorfman, L. T. (2000). The effects of specific health conditions on activities in retirement. *Activities, Adaptation & Aging, 25*(1), 47.

Korczyk, S.M. (2004). Is early retirement ending? AARP Pulic Policy Institute: Washington, DC. Retrieved on December 6, 2006, from www.aarp.org.

LIFE Study Investigators (2006). Effects of a physical activity intervention on measures of physical performance: Results of the Lifestyle Interventions and Independence for Elders Pilot (LIFE-P) study. *Journal of Gerontology & Medical Sciences: 61* A; 1157–1165.

Liu, G. C., & Christensen, D. B. (2002). The continuing challenge of inappropriate prescribing in the elderly: An update of evidence. *Journal of the American Pharmaceutical Association,* 7(12), 634–638.

Lowry, L. W., & Conco, D. (2002). Exploring the meaning of spirituality with aging adults in Appalachia. *Journal of Holistic Nursing, 20*(4), 388–402.

National Center for Health Statistics (2006). *Health United States, 2006.* Superintendent of Documents. U.S. Government Printing Office: Washington, DC.

Older Americans Substance Abuse & Mental Health Technical Assistance Center (2006). *Suicide prevention for older adults, Fact Sheet.* U.S. Department of Health and Human Services, Substance Abuse and Mental Health Services Administration. Center for Substance Abuse Prevention. Retrieved November 22, 2006, from www.samhsa.gov.

Rosenzweig, E. S., & Barnes, C. A. (2003). Impact of aging on hippocampal function: Plasticity, network dynamics and cognition. *Progress in Neurobiology, 69*(3), 143–179.

Scahill, R. I., Frost, C., Jenkins, R., Whitwell, J. L., Rossor, M. N., & Fox, N. C. (2003). A longitudinal study of brain volume changes in normal aging using serial registered magnetic resonance imaging. *Archives of Neurology, 60*(7), 989–994.

Stanford, E., & Usita, P. M. (2002). Retirement: Who is at risk? *Generations, 26*(2), 45–48.

Taylor, P., Funk, C., & Craighill, P. (2006). *Working after retirement: The gap between expectations and reality.* Pew Research Center. A Social Trends Report. Retrieved on December 7, 2006, from http://pewresearch.org.

Tiao, J. Y., Semmens, J. B., Masarei, J. R., & Lawrence-Brown, M. M. (2002). The effect of age on serum creatinine levels in an aging population: Relevance to vascular surgery. *Cardiovascular Surgery, 10*(5), 445–451.

von Strauss, E., Aguero-Torres, H., Kareholt, I., Winblad, B., & Fratiglioni, L. (2003). Women are more disabled in basic activities of daily living than men only in very advanced ages: A study on disability, morbidity, and mortality from the Kungsholmen Project. *Journal of Clinical Epidemiology, 56*(7), 669–677.

Wadensten, B., & Carlsson, M. (2003). Theory-driven guidelines for practical care of older people, based on the theory of gerotranscendence. *Journal of Advanced Nursing, 41*(5), 462–470.

Waern, M., Rubenowitz, E., & Wilhelmson, K. (2003). Predictors of suicide in the old elderly. *Gerontology, 49*(5), 328–334.

Wan, H., Sengupta, M., Velkoff, V. A., & DeBarros, K. A. (2005). 65+ in the United States. *Current Population Reports,* pp. 23–209, U.S. Census Bureau. U.S. Government Printing Office: Washington, DC.

Wright, L. (2001). Sexuality-reproductive pattern: Normal changes with aging. In M. L. Maas, K. C. Buckwalter, M. D. Hardy, et al. (Eds.), *Nursing care of older adults: Diagnoses, outcomes, and interventions* (pp. 729–732). St. Louis: Mosby.

Zimprich, D. (2002). Cross-sectionally and longitudinally balanced effects of processing speed on intellectual abilities. *Experimental Aging Research,* 28, 231–251.

CHAPTER 32

Delirium, Dementias, and Related Disorders

Mary Ann Boyd, Linda Garand, Linda A. Gerdner, Bonnie J. Wakefield, and Kathleen C. Buckwalter

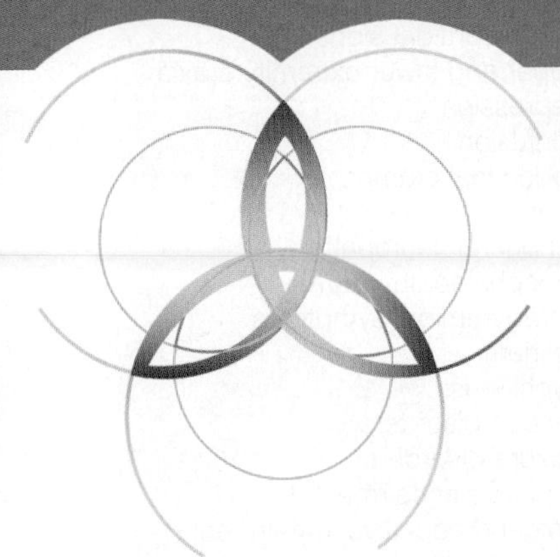

LEARNING OBJECTIVES

After studying this chapter, you will be able to:

- Distinguish the clinical characteristics, onset, and course of delirium and dementia.
- Integrate biologic, psychological, and social theories related to delirium and dementia.
- Analyze human responses to delirium and dementia, with emphasis on the concepts of impaired cognition and memory.
- Formulate nursing diagnoses based on a biopsychosocial assessment of patients with impaired cognitive function.
- Identify expected outcomes and interventions for patients with impaired cognition.
- Discuss nursing interventions used for patients with impaired cognition.
- Identify protective strategies for mental health promotion of cognitive functioning.

KEY CONCEPTS

- cognition
- delirium
- dementia
- memory
- cognitive reserve

KEY TERMS

• acetylcholine (ACh) • acetylcholinesterase (AChE) • acetylcholinesterase inhibitors (AChEI) • agnosia • aphasia • apraxia • beta-amyloid plaques • bradykinesia • catastrophic reactions • cortical dementia • disinhibition • disturbance of executive functioning • hyperkinetic delirium • hypokinetic delirium • hypersexuality • hypervocalization • illusions • impaired consciousness • mild cognitive Impairment • mixed variant delirium • neurofibrillary tangles • oligomers • oxidative stress • subcortical dementia • tau • validation therapy

The concept of cognition describes a relatively high level of intellectual processing in which perceptions and information are acquired, used, or manipulated. Cognition involves the perception of reality and an understanding of its representations. There are a number of cognitive functions such as the acquisition and use of language, the orientation of time and space, and the ability to learn and solve problems. Cognition also is the basis of judgment, reasoning, attention, comprehension, concept formation, planning, and the use of symbols, such as numbers and letters used in mathematics and writing.

KEY CONCEPT Cognition is based on a system of interrelated abilities, such as perception, reasoning, judgment, intuition, and memory that allow one to be aware of oneself and one's surroundings. Impairments in these abilities can result in a failure of the afflicted person to recognize that he or she is ill and in need of treatment.

Memory, a facet of cognition, refers to the ability to recall or reproduce what has been learned or experienced. It is more than simple storage and retrieval; it is a complex cognitive mental function that includes most areas of the brain, especially the hippocampus, which is believed to be essential to the transfer of some memories from short-term to long-term storage. Defects of memory are an essential feature of many cognitive disorders, particularly dementia.

KEY CONCEPT Memory is a facet of cognition concerned with retaining and recalling past experiences, whether they occurred in the physical environment or internally as cognitive events.

The disorders discussed in this chapter—delirium, dementia, and related cognitive disorders—are characterized by deficits in cognition or memory that represent a clear-cut deterioration from a previous level of functioning. Delirium is a disorder of acute cognitive impairment and can be caused by a medical condition (e.g., infection) or substance abuse, or it may have multiple etiologies. Dementia is characterized by chronic cognitive impairments and is differentiated by underlying cause, not by symptom patterns, which are often similar. Some dementias are irreversible and progressive, such as the Alzheimer type, but not all dementias are irreversible. For example, some organic compounds and chemicals, such as lead, aluminum, manganese, and toluene (one of the toxins in glue and paint) may produce symptoms of dementia (Table 32.1). Once evaluated and treated, the symptoms of dementia can resolve in many of these disorders (e.g., endocrine disorders).

KEY CONCEPT Delirium is a disorder of acute cognitive impairment and is caused by a medical condition (e.g., infection), substance abuse, or multiple etiologies.

KEY CONCEPT Dementia is characterized by chronic cognitive impairments and is differentiated by underlying cause, not by symptom patterns. Dementia can be further classified as cortical or subcortical to denote the location of the underlying pathology.

Cortical dementia results from a disease process that globally afflicts the cortex. **Subcortical dementia** is caused by dysfunction or deterioration of deep gray- or white-matter structures inside the brain and brain stem. Symptoms of subcortical dementia may be more localized and tend to disrupt arousal, attention, and motivation, but they can produce a variety of clinical behavioral manifestations. In this chapter, a type of cortical dementia, Alzheimer disease, is highlighted because it is the most prevalent form of dementia.

Table 32.1 Selected Compounds and Chemicals That May Produce Dementia

Substance	Related Symptoms
Arsenic	Headache Drowsiness Confusion
Mercury	Tremors Extrapyramidal signs Upper and lower extremity ataxia Depression Confusion
Lead	Abdominal cramps Anemia Peripheral neuropathy Encephalopathy (rare)
Manganese	Extrapyramidal symptoms Delirium
Aluminum	Myoclonus Speech disorders Seizure disorders Cognitive impairment
Toluene (methyl benzene)	Profound cognitive impairment Tremor Ataxia Loss of vision and hearing

DELIRIUM

Clinical Course of Delirium

Delirium is a disturbance in consciousness and a change in cognition that develops over a short time. It is usually reversible if the underlying cause is identified and treated quickly. It is a serious disorder and should always be treated as an emergency.

Emergency!

Individuals who are delirious arrive in the emergency room in a state of confusion and disorientation that developed during a period of a few hours or days. If delirium is not treated in a timely manner, irreversible neurologic damage can occur. About 25% of patients do not survive.

Diagnostic Criteria

Impaired consciousness is the key diagnostic criterion. The patient becomes less aware of his or her environ-

Table 32.2 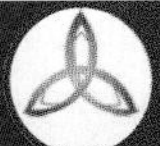 **Key Diagnostic Characteristics for Delirium Caused by a General Medical Condition 293.0** 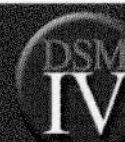

Diagnostic Criteria	Associated Findings
• Disturbance of consciousness Reduced clarity of awareness Decreased ability to focus, sustain, or shift attention • Developing over a short period of time—usually hours to days; fluctuating during the course of the day • Cognitive changes Memory deficit, disorientation, language disturbance Development of perceptual disturbance not better accounted for by a pre-existing, established, or evolving dementia • History, physical examination, or laboratory tests indicating change as a direct cause of physiologic effects of medical condition ***Etiologies*** • Substance intoxication delirium • Substance withdrawal delirium • Multiple etiologies (due to more than one medical condition, substance effect, or medication side effect) • Not otherwise specified	***Associated Behavioral Findings*** • Attention wandering • Perseveration • Easily distracted • Recent memory changes • Dysnomia, dysgraphia • Speech is rambling, irrelevant, incoherent • Misinterpretations, illusions, and hallucinations ***Associated Physical Findings*** • Daytime sleepiness • Nighttime agitation • Difficulty falling asleep • Restlessness, hyperactivity, or sluggishness and lethargy • Anxiety, fear, irritability, anger, euphoria, and apathy • Rapid unpredictable shifts from one emotional state to another ***Associated Laboratory Findings*** • Abnormal electroencephalogram

ment and loses the ability to focus, sustain, and shift attention. Associated cognitive changes include problems in memory, orientation, and language. The patient may not know where he or she is, may not recognize familiar objects, or may be unable to carry on a conversation. Another important diagnostic indicator is that the problem developed during a short period (compared with dementia, which develops gradually) (American Psychiatric Association [APA], 2000). Table 32.2 presents the diagnostic criteria of delirium caused by a general medical condition. Delirium is different from dementia, but the presenting symptoms are often similar. Impaired alertness, apathy, anxiety, disorientation, and hallucinations commonly occur (Turkel, Trzapacz, & Tavare, 2006). Table 32.3 highlights the differences between delirium and dementia.

• NCLEXNOTE

Delirium and dementia have similar presentations. Because delirium can be life-threatening, identifying the potential underlying cause for the symptoms is a priority.

Delirium in Special Populations

Children

Delirium can occur in children and may be related to medications (anticholinergic agents) or fever. Children seem to be especially susceptible to this disorder, probably because of their immature brain. Sleep–wake disturbance, fluctuating symptoms, impaired attention, irritability, agitation, mood lability, and confusion are typ-

Table 32.3 Differentiating Delirium From Dementia

Characteristics	Delirium	Dementia
Onset	Sudden	Insidious
24-h course	Fluctuating	Stable
Consciousness	Reduced	Clear
Attention	Globally disoriented	Usually normal
Cognition	Globally disoriented	Globally impaired
Hallucinations	Visual auditory	Possible
Orientation	Usually impaired	Often impaired
Psychomotor activity	Increased, reduced, or shifts	Often normal
Speech	Often incoherent, slow or rapid	Often normal
Involuntary movement	Often asterixis or coarse tremor	Rare
Physical illness or drug toxicity	One or both	Rare

Adapted from Bair, B. D. (2000). Presentations and recognition of common psychiatric disorders in the elderly. *Clinical Geriatrics, 8*(2), 26, 28–29, 33–34.

ical symptoms of delirium in children. However, delirium may be hard to diagnose and may be mistaken for uncooperative behavior (Turkel et al., 2006).

Older Adults

Although delirium may occur in any age group, it is most common among older adults. In this age group, delirium is often mistaken for dementia, which in turn leads to inappropriate treatment. In these adults, impaired memory, depressed mood, speech disturbances, delusions, and paranoia are typical (Turkel et al., 2006).

Epidemiology and Risk Factors

Statistics concerning prevalence are based primarily on elderly individuals in acute care settings. Estimated prevalence rates range from 10% to 50% of patients. Delirium is particularly common in elderly, postoperative patients. In some groups, such as those with dementia, the prevalence may be nearer to 90% (Curran & Wattis, 2006).

Pre-existing cognitive impairment is one of the greatest risk factors for delirium. Severe illness and age also put patients at higher risk for delirium. Male gender, alcohol abuse, lower levels of educational attainment, fracture, depression, and impaired vision have been identified as risk factors (Jones et al., 2006; Schuurmans, Duursma, & Shortridge-Baggett, 2001). Box 32.1 lists proposed risk factors for delirium, and Box 32.2 presents a vignette of a patient who experienced delirium after using an over-the-counter (OTC) sleeping medication.

Etiology

The etiology of delirium is complex and multifaceted. Because delirium is a fluctuating process, it is difficult to establish its onset or termination. Delirium in the older adult is associated with medications, infections, fluid and electrolyte imbalance, metabolic disturbances, or hypoxia/ischemia (Schuurmans et al., 2001). The probability of the syndrome developing increases if certain predisposing factors, such as advanced age, brain damage, or dementia, are also present. Sensory overload or underload, immobilization, sleep deprivation, and psychosocial stress also contribute to delirium.

Because delirium has multiple causes, a wide variety of brain alterations may also be responsible for its development. Delirium may result from a neuroanatomic abnormality such as stroke, but the majority of cases are caused by an imbalance of key neurochemicals such as dopamine, serotonin, cortisol, acetylcholine, glutamate, and GABA (Marcantonio et al., 2006).

Interdisciplinary Treatment and Priority Care Issues

Although delirium may be recognized and diagnosed in any health care setting, appropriate intervention requires

BOX 32.1

Risk Factors for Delirium

Advanced age
Pre-existing dementia
Functional dependence
Endocrine and metabolic disorders
Bone fracture
Infection (pneumonia, urinary tract)
Medications (anticholinergic side effects)
Changes in vital signs (including hypotension and hyper- or hypothermia)
Electrolyte or metabolic imbalance (dehydration, renal failure, hyponatremia)
Admission to a long-term care institution
Postcardiotomy
AIDS
Pain
Substance use and alcohol withdrawal

BOX 32.2

Clinical Vignette: Delirium

Mrs. Campbell, a widowed 72-year-old woman living in her own home, has been having trouble sleeping. Her daughter visits her and suggests that Mrs. Campbell try an over-the-counter sleeping medication. Mrs. Campbell has also been taking antihistamines for allergies and the antidepressant amitriptyline. Three nights later, a neighbor calls the daughter, concerned because she encountered Mrs. Campbell wandering the streets, unable to find her home. When the neighbor approached Mrs. Campbell to help her home, Mrs. Campbell began to scream and strike out at the neighbor.

The daughter visits immediately and discovers that her mother does not know who she is, does not know what time it is, appears disheveled, and is suspicious that people have been in her home stealing the things she cannot find. Mrs. Campbell does not recall taking any medication, but when her daughter investigates she finds that 10 pills of the new sleeping aid have already been used. Mrs. Campbell is irritable and refuses to go to the hospital, but over the course of a few hours, she appears to calm down, and her daughter is able to take her to see her doctor the following morning. After hearing the history, the doctor hospitalizes Mrs. Campbell, withholds all medication, and provides intravenous hydration. Within 3 days, Mrs. Campbell is again able to recognize her daughter, and her mental status appears to be greatly improved.

What Do You Think?

- Identify risk factors that may have contributed to Mrs. Campbell experiencing delirium.
- How could the addition of an OTC sleeping medication interact with the antihistamine and antidepressant to be responsible for Mrs. Campbell's delirium?

that the patient be admitted to an acute care setting for rigorous assessment and rapid treatment. Priority in care is identifying the underlying cause of the delirium. Interdisciplinary management of delirium includes two primary aspects: (1) elimination or correction of the underlying cause, and (2) symptomatic and supportive measures (e.g., adequate rest, comfort, maintenance of fluid and electrolyte balance, and protection from injury) (Potter, 2006).

When developing a treatment plan for a patient in whom delirium is suspected, close attention must be paid to correcting any organic or disease-related factors. If possible, the use of all suspected medications should be stopped and vital signs monitored at least every 2 hours. Close observation of the patient with particular regard to changes in vital signs, behavior, and mental status is required. Patients are monitored until the delirium subsides or until discharge. If the delirium still exists at discharge, it is critical that referrals for postdischarge follow-up assessment and care be implemented.

NURSING MANAGEMENT: HUMAN RESPONSE TO DELIRIUM

The best management is prevention or early recognition of delirium (see Box 32.3). If the patient is a child, the assessment process presented in Chapter 27 should be used. If the patient is an elderly person, the assessment in Chapter 30 should serve as a guide. Special efforts should be made to include family members in the nursing process.

BOX 32.3

Research for Best Practice: Educational Interventions Decrease Prevalence of Delirium

Tabet, N., Hudson, S., Sweeney, V., Sauer, J., Bryant, C., Macdonald, A., & Howard, R. (2005). An educational intervention can prevent delirium on acute medical wards. Age and Ageing, 34(2), 152–156.

THE QUESTION: Does education of the nursing and medical staff reduce the number of cases of delirium and increase its recognition?

METHODS: Single-blind case-control study of two acute medical units in a busy inner-city teaching hospital admitting 250 acute admissions over the age of 70. Nurses and physicians on one unit received a 1-hour formal presentation and group discussion, written management guidelines, and follow-up sessions. The other unit did not receive the educational interventions.

FINDINGS: The point prevalence of delirium was significantly reduced on the intervention unit compared to the control unit (9.8% vs 19. 5%, $P < 0.05$), and clinical staff recognized *significantly* more delirium cases than the control unit.

IMPLICATIONS FOR NURSING: Early recognition of symptoms can reduce the occurrence of delirium. Educational interventions can be helpful in increasing staff members' skill in detecting and preventing delirium.

Biologic Domain

Biologic Assessment

The onset of symptoms is typically signaled by a rapid or acute change in behavior. To assess the symptoms, the nurse needs to know what is normal for the individual. Caregivers, family members, or significant others should be interviewed because they can often provide valuable information. Family members may be the only resource for accurate information.

Current and Past Health Status

History should include a description of the onset, duration, range, and intensity of associated symptoms. Chronic physical illness, dementia, depression, or other psychiatric illnesses should be identified. Sorting out historic information may be particularly problematic when delirium accompanies acute illness, recent surgery, or infection.

Physical Examination and Review of Systems

If the patient is cooperative, a physical examination will be conducted in the emergency room. Vital signs are crucial. A review of systems must be conducted in each patient suspected of having delirium or other organic mental disorders. Laboratory data, including a complete blood count, glucose, blood urea nitrogen, creatinine, and electrolyte analyses; liver function and oxygen saturation, as well as fluid balance, signs of constipation, or a recent history of diarrhea, should be assessed in an attempt to discover an underlying cause.

Physical Functions

Functional assessment includes physical functional status (activities of daily living), use of sensory aids (eyeglasses and hearing aids), usual activity level and any recent changes, and pain assessment. Because sleep is often disturbed in patients with delirium, sleep patterns must be assessed, including what is typical for the individual and recent changes. Often, the sleep–wake cycle of the patient with delirium becomes reversed, with the individual attempting to sleep during the day and be awake at night. Sleep disturbances are a symptom of delirium, and sleep deprivation may add to the confusion. Restoration of a normal sleep cycle is extremely important.

Pharmacologic Assessment

A substance use history (including alcohol intake and smoking history) should be obtained (see Chapters 25 and 34). In addition, information regarding medication use must be obtained, with particular attention given to new medications or changes in dose of current medications. Table 32.4 lists some of the drugs that can cause delirium. Special attention should be given to combinations of these medications because drug interactions can cause delirium.

Information regarding OTC medications should be included in this assessment. OTC medications are often thought of as harmless, but several, such as cold medications, taken in sufficient quantities may produce confusion, especially in elderly patients.

Findings from the medication assessment are integrated with findings of the physical assessment, including such things as fluid and electrolyte balance, lack of adequate pain management, or serum drug levels, if available. For example, chronic pain may lead an individual to use more medication for pain relief than has been intended. Careful monitoring of the effectiveness of pain medications may lead to the use of a different medication that is more effective with less potential for misuse. Because many classes of medications have been associated with delirium, the focus is on changes in the type and number of medications and how medications relate to other findings in the history and physical assessment.

Nursing Diagnoses for the Biologic Domain

The nursing diagnoses typically generated from assessment data are Acute Confusion, Disturbed Thought Processes, or Disturbed Sensory Perception (visual or auditory) (NANDA-I, 2007). However, an astute nurse will also use nursing diagnoses based on other indicators, such as Hyperthermia, Acute Pain, Risk for Infection, and Insomnia.

Interventions for the Biologic Domain

Important interventions for a patient experiencing acute confusional state include providing a safe and therapeutic environment, maintaining fluid and electrolyte balance and adequate nutrition, and preventing

Table 32.4 Examples of Drugs That Can Cause Delirium

Class	Specific Drugs	Class	Specific Drugs
Anticholinergic	antihistamines	Cardiac	β-blockers
	chlorpheniramine (Ornade and Teldrin)		propranolol (Inderal)
	antiparkinsonian drugs (eg, benztropine [Cogentin], biperiden [Akineton], or trihexyphenidyl)		clonidine (Catapres)
			digitalis (Digoxin and Lanoxin)
			lidocaine (Xylocaine)
			methyldopa (Aldomet)
			quinidine
	atropine		procainamide (Pronestyl)
	belladona alkaloids	Sedative-hypnotic	barbiturates
	diphenhydramine (Benadryl)		benzodiazepines
	phenothiazines	Sympathomimetic	amphetamines
	promethazine (Phenergan)		phenylephrine
	scopolamine		phenylpropanolamine
	tricyclic antidepressants	Over-the-counter	Compoz
Anticonvulsant	phenobarbital		Excedrin P.M.
	phenytoin (Dilantin)		Sleep-Eze
	sodium valproate (Depakene)		Sominex
Antiinflammatory	corticosteroids	Miscellaneous	acyclovir (antiviral)
	ibuprofen (Motrin and Advil)		aminophylline
	indomethacin (Indocin)		amphotericin (antifungal)
	naproxen (Naprosyn)		bromides
Antiparkinsonian	amantadine (Symmetrel)		cephalexin (Keflex)
	carbidopa (Sinemet)		chlorpropamide (Diabinese)
Antituberculous	levodopa (Larodopa)		cimetidine (Tagamet)
	isoniazid		disulfiram (Antabuse)
	rifampin		lithium
Analgesic	opiates		metronidazole (Flagyl)
	salicylates		theophylline
	synthetic narcotics		timolol ophthalmic

Cozza, K.L, Armstrong, S.D, & Oesterheld, J.R. (2003). *Drug Interaction Principles for Medical Practice. Cytochrome P450s.* 2nd ed. American Psychiatric Association: Washington, DC

aspiration and decubitus ulcers, which are often complications. Other interventions relate to a particular nursing diagnosis focused on individual symptoms and underlying causes, for example, for patients with Insomnia, the Sleep Enhancement intervention is appropriate (Dochterman & Bulechek, 2004).

Safety Interventions

Behaviors exhibited by the delirious patient, such as hallucinations, delusions, illusions, aggression, or agitation (restlessness or excitability), may pose safety problems. The patient must be protected from physical harm by using low beds, guardrails, and careful supervision. The interventions Delirium Management and Fall Prevention may be implemented (Dochterman & Bulechek, 2004) for any patient at risk for falls.

Pharmacologic Interventions

The goal of psychopharmacologic management is treatment of the behaviors associated with delirium, such as symptoms of agitation, inattention, sleep disorder, and psychosis, so that the patient can be more comfortable. The decision to use medications should be based on the specific symptoms. Dosages are usually kept very low, especially with elderly patients. There is no consensus on the use of psychopharmacologic agents to control the symptoms of delirium, and limited studies have been conducted. Use of these medications usually relates to agitation, combativeness, or hallucinations. However, medication should be chosen in light of the potential side effects (particularly anticholinergic effects, hypotension, and respiratory suppression) and in light of making the delirium worse. For most patients with delirium, short-term (off-label) use of low doses of an antipsychotic agent, such as risperidone, appears effective and safe (Boettger & Breitbart, 2007). Benzodiazepines are also used, especially when the delirium is related to alcohol withdrawal. In some patients, these medications may further impair cognition because of the sedation. Also, in some cases, a paradoxical agitation may develop (Gleason, 2003).

Administering and Monitoring Medications

Patients experiencing delirium may resist taking medication because of their confusion. If medication is given, ideally it should be oral.

Monitoring and Managing Side Effects. Monitoring drug action and side effects is especially important because the cause of the delirium may not be known, and the patient may inadvertently be affected by the medication. Patients should be monitored for sedation, hypotension, or extrapyramidal symptoms. Although mental status often fluctuates during delirium, it may also be influenced by these medications, and any changes or worsening of mental status after administration of the medication should be reported immediately to the prescriber. Some side effects may also be confused with the symptoms of delirium. For example, akathisia (see Chapter 8), a side effect of antipsychotics may appear as agitation or restlessness. The patient's physical condition and concurrent medication regimen may also influence the bioavailability, metabolism, and elimination of these medications. Adequate hydration and nutrition must be maintained. When using antipsychotic medications, closely monitor the patient for symptoms of neuroleptic malignant syndrome (see Chapter 8). The appearance of these symptoms may be missed because many may be confused with those related to delirium.

Finally, the use of antipsychotic agents or other medications for treating symptoms related to delirium should be discontinued as soon as possible. These medications should not be stopped abruptly, but rather withdrawn gradually during a period of several days or weeks.

Identifying Drug Interactions. The etiology of delirium is often a drug–drug interaction. OTC sleeping, cold, or allergy medication may be the cause. If medication is the underlying cause, it is important to identify accurately which medications are involved before administering any other drugs. A consultation with a clinical pharmacist may also be helpful.

Teaching Points

To prevent future occurrences, the nurse needs to educate the patient and family about the underlying cause of the delirium. If the delirium is not resolved before discharge, family members need to know how to care for the patient at home.

Psychological Domain

Assessment

Psychological assessment of the individual with delirium focuses on cognitive changes revealed through the mental status examination as well as the resulting behavioral manifestations. Changes in mental status must be monitored frequently for early detection of delirium, especially in elderly patients. In addition, other factors, such as stressors and environmental change, may contribute to the symptoms.

Mental Status

Rapid onset of global cognitive impairment that affects multiple aspects of intellectual functioning is the hallmark of delirium. Mental status evaluation reveals several changes:

- Fluctuations in level of consciousness with reduced awareness of the environment
- Difficulty focusing and sustaining or shifting attention
- Severely impaired memory, especially immediate and recent memory

Patients may be disorientated to time and place but rarely to person. Environmental perceptions are often disturbed. The patient may believe shadows in the room are really people. Thought content is often illogical, and speech may be incoherent or inappropriate to the context. Mental status tends to fluctuate over the course of the day. During the same day, an individual with delirium may appear confused and uncooperative, whereas later, that person may be lucid and able to follow instructions. Nurses must continually assess the cognitive status of the individual throughout the day so that interventions may be modified accordingly. Calculations, orientation (especially to time), and recall are most affected in delirium, whereas naming and registration are relatively preserved.

Behavior

Delirious patients exhibit a wide range of behaviors, complicating the process of making a diagnosis and planning interventions. At times, the individual may be restless or agitated, and at other times lethargic and slow to respond. Delirium can be categorized into three types.

- **Hyperkinetic delirium** involves behaviors most commonly recognized as delirium (e.g., psychomotor hyperactivity, marked excitability, and a tendency toward hallucinations).
- **Hypokinetic delirium** is marked by lethargy, sleepiness, and apathy, and psychomotor activity decreases; this is the "quiet" patient for whom the diagnosis of delirium often is missed.
- **Mixed variant delirium** involves behavior that fluctuates between the hyperactive and hypoactive states.

Nursing Diagnoses for the Psychological Domain

The nursing diagnosis Acute Confusion is also associated with impaired cognitive functioning. Although the underlying cause of confusion is physiologic, nursing care should focus on the psychological domain, as well as the physical. Other typical nursing diagnoses related to the psychological domain include Disturbed Thought Process, Ineffective Coping, and Disturbed Personal Identity (NANDA-I, 2007).

Interventions for the Psychological Domain

Staff should have frequent interaction with patients and support them if they are confused or hallucinating. Patients should be encouraged to express their fears and discomforts that result from frightening or disconcerting psychotic experiences. Adequate lighting, easy-to-read calendars and clocks, a reasonable noise level, and frequent verbal orientation may reduce this frightening experience. If the patient wears eyeglasses or uses a hearing aid, these devices should be used. Including familiar personal possessions in the environment may also help. Interventions that may be useful for these individuals are discussed in detail later in the chapter (see the section on dementia).

Social Domain

Assessment

Discussion should be initiated with the family to determine whether the patient's behaviors are new. An assessment of living arrangements may provide information about sensory stimulation or social isolation. Cultural and educational background must be considered when the patient's mental capacity is evaluated. Individuals from certain ethnic backgrounds may not be familiar with the information used in tests of general knowledge (e.g., names of presidents, geographic knowledge), memory (e.g., date of birth in cultures that do not routinely celebrate birthdays), and orientation (e.g., sense of placement and location may be conceptualized differently in some cultures) (APA, 2000). Some cultural practices may involve using substances such as elixirs that contain chemicals that may exacerbate delirium. Assessment should address these practices.

Family Roles 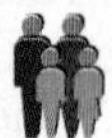

Family support for the individual and understanding of the disorder must be assessed. The behaviors exhibited by the person experiencing delirium may be frightening or at least confusing for family members. Some family members may actually contribute to the patient's increased agitation. Assessing family interactions and family members' ability to understand delirium is important. If feasible, family presence may help to calm and reassure the patient.

Nursing Diagnoses for the Social Domain

Several nursing diagnoses associated with the social domain can be generated. Interrupted Family Processes, Ineffective Protection, Ineffective Role Performance, and Risk for Injury are the most typical. Risk for Injury is a high-priority diagnosis because individuals with delirium are more likely to fall or injure themselves during a confused state (Nanda-I, 2007).

Interventions for the Social Domain

The environment needs to be safe to protect the patient from injury. A predictable, orienting environment will help to re-establish order to the patient's life. That is, a calendar, clocks, and other items may be provided to help orient the patient to time, place, and person. If the patient is agitated, de-escalation techniques should be used (see Chapters 10 and 38). Physical restraint should be avoided.

Support from Families 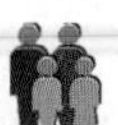

Families can be encouraged to work with staff to reorient the patient and provide a supportive environment. Families need to understand that important decisions requiring the patient's input should be delayed if at all possible until the patient has recovered. Although patients may be able to participate in decision making, they may not remember the decision later; therefore, it is important to have several witnesses present.

Evaluation and Treatment Outcomes

The primary treatment goal is prevention or resolution of the delirious episode with return to previous cognitive status. Outcome measures include

- correction of the underlying physiologic alteration
- resolution of confusion
- family member verbalization of understanding of confusion
- prevention of injury.

Resolution of confusion is the primary goal; however, the nurse makes important contributions to all four of these outcomes. The end result of delirium is either full recovery, incomplete recovery, incomplete recovery with some residual cognitive impairment, or a downward course leading to death.

Continuum of Care

The nurse may encounter patients with delirium in a number of treatment settings (e.g., home, nursing home, ambulatory care, day treatment, outpatient setting, hospital). Patients usually are admitted to an acute care setting for rapid evaluation and treatment of the underlying etiology. An abrupt change in cognitive status can also occur while the patient is hospitalized for another reason. Delirium often persists beyond discharge from the hospital. Discharge planning should routinely include family education and referrals to community health care providers. If the patient will return to a residential long-term care setting, communication with facility staff about the patient's hospital stay and treatment regimen is crucial. For more information on caring for patients with delirium, see Box 32.4.

BOX 32.4

Psychoeducation Checklist: Delirium

When caring for the patient with delirium, be sure to include the caregivers, as appropriate, and address the following topic areas in the teaching plan:

- Psychopharmacologic agents, if used, including drug action, dosage, frequency, and possible adverse effects
- Underlying cause of delirium
- Mental status changes
- Safety measures
- Hydration and nutrition
- Avoidance of restraints
- Decision-making guidelines

DEMENTIA OF THE ALZHEIMER TYPE

Clinical Course of Alzheimer Disease

Alzheimer disease (AD) is a degenerative, progressive neuropsychiatric disorder that results in cognitive impairment, emotional and behavioral changes, physical and functional decline, and ultimately death. Gradually, the patient's ability to carry out activities of daily living declines, although physical status often remains intact until late in the disease. Primarily a disorder of the older adult, AD has been diagnosed in patients as young as age 35 years.

Two subtypes have been identified: early onset AD (age 65 years and younger) and late-onset AD (age older than 65 years). Late-onset AD is much more common than early onset AD, but early-onset AD has a more rapid progression. AD is also routinely conceptualized in terms of three stages: mild, moderate, and severe. Signs and symptoms of AD change as the patient passes from one phase of the illness to another (Fig. 32.1). It is unclear whether all patients with AD pass through a specific sequence of deterioration and whether the staging of a patient at initial assessment has any prognostic implications in terms of speed of decline. Nevertheless, staging is a useful technique for determining the patient's current cognitive status and provides a sound basis for decisions in clinical management.

MOVIE viewing GUIDES

Diagnostic Criteria

The diagnosis of AD is made on clinical grounds, and verification is confirmed at autopsy by abnormal degen-

Dementia/Alzheimer

Stage	Mild	Moderate	Severe
Symptoms	Loss of memory Language difficulties Mood swings Personality changes Diminished judgment Apathy	Inability to retain new info Behavioral, personality changes Increasing long-term memory loss Wandering, agitation, aggression, confusion Requires assistance w/ADL	Gait and motor disturbances Bedridden Unable to perform ADL Incontinence Requires long-term care placement

FIGURE 32.1. Alzheimer disease progression.

erative structures, neuritic plaques, and neurofibrillary tangles. The essential features of AD are multiple cognitive deficits, especially memory impairment, and at least one of the following cognitive disturbances: **aphasia** (alterations in language ability), **apraxia** (impaired ability to execute motor activities despite intact motor functioning), **agnosia** (failure to recognize or identify objects despite intact sensory function), or a **disturbance of executive functioning** (ability to think abstractly, plan, initiate, sequence, monitor, and stop complex behavior).

The cognitive deficits must be sufficiently severe to impair occupational or social functioning and must represent a decline from a previously higher level of functioning (APA, 2000). These symptoms are common to all presentations of dementia, regardless of the underlying pathology. Table 32.5 lists essential symptoms of AD, along with other possible behavioral and psychological changes that may or may not be present. To make a diagnosis of AD, all other known causes of dementia must be excluded (e.g., vascular, AIDS, Parkinson's disease).

Mild Cognitive Impairment

When memory problems occur, but symptoms do not meet the diagnostic criteria for dementia, patients may be diagnosed with **mild cognitive impairment (MCI)**, which can be a transitional state between normal cognition and AD. MCI is thought to be related to multiple causes and some, but not all, progress to AD (Ganguli, Dodge, Shen, & DeKosky, 2004). MCI is classified into two subtypes: Amnesic (MCI-A) with memory impairments and Multiple Cognitive Domain (MCI-MCD) with other mild impairments, such as in judgment or language. Mild memory loss may or may not be present in MCI-MCD. Both subtypes progress to AD at the same rate, but are a consequence of different patterns of atrophy. Hippocampal atrophy characterizes the MCI-A subtype, whereas cortical atrophy is present in MCI-MCD (Becker et al., 2006).

Epidemiology and Risk Factors

In 2007, an estimated 5.1 million Americans had AD, and conservative projections estimate that by the year 2030, the number of cases of AD in the United States will be 7.7 million (Alzheimer Association, 2007). Dementia appears to affect all groups, but studies in the United States reveal a higher incidence in African Americans (10.5%) and Latinos (9.8%) than in Caucasians (5.4%) (Tang et al., 2001). Currently, AD follows heart disease, cancer, and stroke as the fourth leading cause of death among older adults in the United States (U.S. Centers for Disease Control and Prevention, 2007).

AD can run in families. Compared with the general population, first-degree biologic relatives of individuals with early onset AD are more likely to experience the disorder. So far, studies point toward genetically related risk factors only in familial AD, which accounts for only a small proportion of cases of AD (less than 5%) (Cummings, 2003). The hypothesis that low educational level may increase the risk for AD remains a matter of controversy. Studies show that the higher the education, the less the risk of cognitive decline (Bennett et al, 2003; Manly, Touradji, Tang, & Stern, 2003). Prior head injury leading to unconsciousness may represent a risk factor for the later development of AD especially in those who have a genetic susceptibility to dementia (Cooper, 2002).

Etiology

Researchers have yet to identify a definitive cause of AD. In general, the brain appears normal in the early phases of AD, but it undergoes widespread atrophy as the disease advances.

Beta-amyloid Plaques

One piece of the puzzle is partially explained by a leading theory that, in AD, beta-amyloid deposits destroy cholin-

Table 32.5  Key Diagnostic Characteristics for Dementia of the Alzheimer Type 290 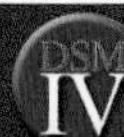

With early onset:
With delirium 290.11
With delusions 290.12
With depressed mood 290.13
Uncomplicated 290.10
With late onset:
With delirium 290.3
With delusions 290.20
With depressed mood 290.21
Uncomplicated 290.0

Diagnostic Criteria	Target Symptoms and Associated Findings
• Development of multiple cognitive deficits • Involvement of both memory impairment and one or more of the following cognitive disturbances: aphasia, apraxia, agnosia, or disturbance in executive functioning • Significant impairment in social or occupational functioning resulting from cognitive deficits; significant decline from previous level of functioning • Cognitive deficits not due to: other CNS conditions causing progressive deficits in memory or cognition; systemic conditions known to cause dementia; substance-induced conditions • Not occurring exclusively during course of a delirium • Not better accounted for by another Axis I disorder Early onset: age 65 y or less Late onset: over age 65 y	• Memory impairment • Cognitive disturbances ***Associated Behavioral Findings*** • Spatial disorientation and difficulty with spatial tasks • Poor judgment and poor insight • Little or no awareness of memory loss or other cognitive abnormalities • Unrealistic assessment of abilities; underestimation of risks involved in activities • Possible suicidal behaviors (usually in early stages when individual is more capable of carrying out a plan of action) • Possible gait disturbances and falls • Disinhibited behavior, such as inappropriate jokes, neglect of personal hygiene, undue familiarity with strangers, or disregard for conventional rules of social conduct • Delusions, especially ones involving persecution • Superimposed delirium ***Associated Physical Examination Findings*** • Few motor or sensory signs (in the first year of illness) • Myoclonus and gait disorder (later) • Seizure possible ***Associated Laboratory Findings*** • Brain atrophy (with computed tomography or magnetic resonance imaging) • Senile plaques, neurofibrillary tangles, granulovascular degeneration, neuronal loss, astrocytic gliosis, and amyloid angiopathy on microscopic examination

ergic neurons, in a manner similar to cholesterol causing atherosclerosis. It is hypothesized that **beta-amyloid plaques**—dense, mostly insoluble deposits of protein and cellular material outside and around neurons—gradually increase in number and are abnormally distributed throughout the cholinergic system. Plaques are partly made of a protein, beta-amyloid protein, which is a fragment snipped from a larger protein called amyloid precursor protein (APP) and apolipoprotein A (apoA) cores. When fragments of beta-amyloid peptides (ADDLs) clump together, they are called **oligomers**. As they become more insoluble, oligomers form plaques that cannot be easily moved away from the neurons. New evidence suggests that part of the reason that there is plaque build-up is that the receptors responsible for clearing beta-amyloid from the brain are inefficient (U.S. Department of Health and Human Services [USDHHS], 2005). Neuritic plaque densities are highest in the temporal and occipital lobes, intermediate in the parietal lobes, and lowest in the frontal and limbic cortex. Symptoms such as aphasia and visuospatial abnormalities are attributable to plaque formation (Cummings, 2003). Study continues as investigators examine the process by which APP releases beta-amyloid protein, how the fragments accumulate in the brain, and whether the plaques cause AD or are a by-product.

Neurofibrillary Tangles

Neurofibrillary tangles are made of abnormally twisted protein threads found inside the cell. The main component of the tangles is a protein called **tau.** A healthy neuron is supported by structures of microtubules that help transport nutrients and other substances from the body of the cell to ends of the axon and back. Tau helps stabilize the microtubules. In AD, tau separates from the microtubules because excess phosphate molecules have attached to it resulting in a phosphorylation process. Loose tau proteins tangle with each other, causing the characteristic neurofibrillary tangles. The microtubules disintegrate and the neuron's transport system collapses, which results in cell death (USDHHS, 2005). The neurofibrillary tangles are initially found in the limbic area and then progress to the cortex. Neurofibrillary tangles contribute to memory disturbance and psychiatric symptoms (Cummings, 2003) (Fig. 32.2).

Cell Death and Neurotransmitters

In patients with AD, neurotransmission is reduced, neurons are lost, and the hippocampal neurons degenerate. Several major neurotransmitters are affected. **Acetylcholine** (ACh) is associated with cognitive functioning, and disruption of cholinergic mechanisms damages memory in animals and humans (see Chapter 8). Cell loss in the nucleus basalis leads to deficits in the synthesis of cortical acetylcholine, but the number of ACh receptors is relatively unchanged. The reduced ACh is related to a decrease in *choline acetyltransferase* (a critical enzyme in the synthesis of ACh), especially in the forebrain. That is, there are fewer enzymes available to synthesize ACh, which leads to a reduction in cholinergic activity. Positron emission tomography (PET) scans, such as those in Figure 32.3, show changes in brain function.

Other neurotransmitters that are affected include norepinephrine and serotonin. Deficiencies in norepinephrine are associated with loss of cells in the locus ceruleus, and neuronal loss in the raphe nuclei leads to a loss of serotonergic activity (Cummings, 2003).

Genetic Factors

Approximately half of the cases of early onset AD appear to be transmitted as a pure genetic, autosomal dominant

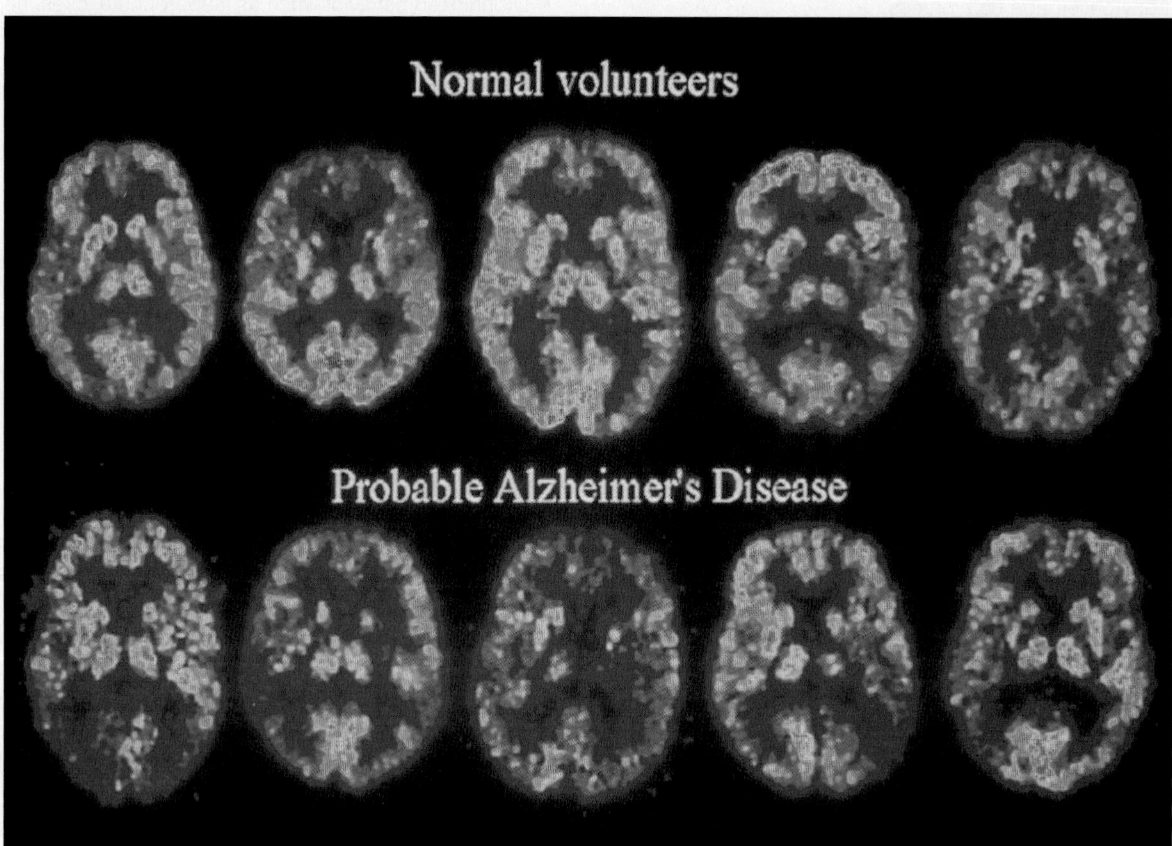

FIGURE 32.2. Series comparison of elderly control subjects (*top row*) and patients with AD (*bottom row*). Although there are some decreases in metabolism associated with age, in most patients with AD, there are marked decreases in the temporal lobe, an area important in memory functions. (Courtesy of Monte S. Buchsbaum, MD, The Mount Sinai Medical Center and School of Medicine, New York, NY.)

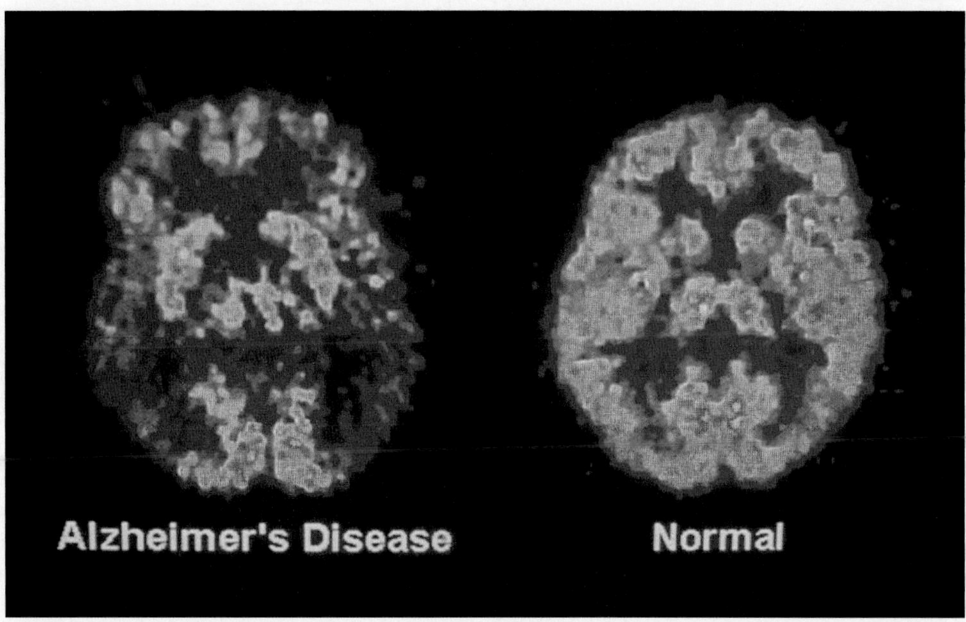

FIGURE 32.3. Metabolic activity in a subject with AD (*left*) and in a control subject (*right*). (Courtesy of Monte S. Buchsbaum, MD, The Mount Sinai Medical Center and School of Medicine, New York, NY.)

trait caused by mutations in genes on chromosomes 1 and 14 (Rogaeva, 2002; Suh & Checler, 2002). Mutations on chromosome 14 account for most cases of early onset familial AD (Taddei et al., 2002). Chromosome 21 is also associated with AD because amyloid plaques and neurofibrillary tangles accumulate consistently in older people with Down syndrome (trisomy 21) who have AD.

Oxidative Stress, Free Radicals, and Mitochondrial Dysfunction

Oxidative stress and mitochondrial dysfunction are being studied as factors in the development of AD. The mitochondria, the power plants for the cell, provide the energy a cell needs to carry out its functions. It is hypothesized that in AD brains, beta-amyloid prevents the normal functioning of the mitochondria. Damage to the mitochondria leads to a rapid increase in the formation of free radicals (highly reactive molecules). If unchecked, the build-up of these free radical molecules can lead to oxidative stress that damages other cellular molecules such as proteins, lipids, and nucleic acid (USDHHS, 2005).

Inflammation

Inflammation in the brain is one of the early hallmarks of AD. Epidemiological studies have linked the long-term use of nonsteroidal anti-inflammatory drugs (NSAIDs) with a decreased risk of AD. However, there are no clinical trials that show that NSAIDs prevent or delay progression of AD. Research is focusing on two kinds of glial cells, astrocytes and microglia, which respond to sites of injury. The astrocytes and microglia surround the beta-amyloid plaques, but fail to remove the plaques. Researchers are investigating why these glial cells do not remove the plaques (USDHHS, 2005).

Interdisciplinary Treatment

In designing services and interventions, the interdisciplinary team must keep in mind that AD has a progressively deteriorating clinical course and that the anatomic and neurochemical changes that occur in the brain are accompanied by impairments in cognition, sensorium, affect (facial expression representing mood), behavior, and psychosocial functioning. The nature and range of services needed by patients and families throughout the illness can vary dramatically at different stages.

Initial assessment of the patient suspected of having dementia has three main objectives: (1) confirmation of the diagnosis, (2) establishment of baseline levels in a number of functional spheres, and (3) establishment of a therapeutic relationship with the patient and family that will continue through subsequent phases of the disease. Treatment efforts currently focus on managing the cognitive symptoms, delaying the cognitive decline (e.g., memory loss, confusion, and problems with learning, speech, and reasoning), treating the noncognitive symptoms (e.g., psychosis, mood symptoms, agitation), and supporting the caregivers as a means of improving the quality of life for both patients and their caregivers.

Priority Care Issues

The priority of care will change throughout the course of AD. Initially, the priority is delaying cognitive decline and supporting family members. Later, the priority is protecting the patient from injury because of lack of judgment. Near the end, the physical needs of the patient are the focus of care.

• NCLEXNOTE

Needs and problematic behaviors of patients with dementia vary throughout the course of the disorder. Early in the disorder the nurse focuses on support, education, and cognitive interventions for depression. As the dementia progresses, priority care becomes safety interventions.

Family Response to Disorder 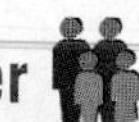

Families are the first to be aware of the cognitive problem, often before the patient, who can be unaware of the extent of memory impairment. When finally confirmed, the actual diagnosis can be devastating to the family. Unlike delirium, a diagnosis of AD means long-term care responsibilities, while the essence of a family member diminishes day by day. Most families keep their relative at home as long as possible to maintain contact and to avoid costly nursing home placement. The two symptoms that often result in nursing home placement are incontinence that cannot be managed and behavioral problems, such as wandering and aggression.

Especially in dementia, the needs of family members should also be considered. Caring for a family member with dementia takes its toll. Nearly one in four caregivers provide 40 hours a week or more of care. Seventy-one percent continue this intense caregiving for more than a year and 32% care for their loved one for more than 5 years (National Alliance for Caregiving and AARP, 2004). Caregivers' health often declines and directly affects their ability to provide care. An online survey of 528 caregivers in fair or poor health indicates that caregiving has made their own health worse. Seventy-five percent said that they did not feel they had a choice in their responsibility. Their most common health problems were (1) lack of energy and sleep (87%), (2) stress and/or panic attacks (70%), (3) pain, aching (60%), and (4) depression (52%) (Evercare & National Alliance for Caregiving, 2006).

NURSING MANAGEMENT: HUMAN RESPONSE TO ALZHEIMER DISEASE

The development and implementation of appropriate, effective, and safe nursing services for the care and support of patients with dementia and their families is a particular challenge because of the complex nature of the illness. Although AD is caused by biologic changes, the psychological and social domains are seriously affected by this disorder. The assessment of the patient with AD should follow the geropsychiatric nursing assessment in Chapter 30.

Biologic Domain

Assessment

The nursing assessment should include a medical history, current medication profile (prescription and OTC medications or home remedies), substance abuse history (including alcohol intake and smoking history), chronic physical or psychiatric illness, and a description of the onset, duration, range, and intensity of symptoms associated with dementia. The onset of symptoms in dementia is typically gradual, with insidious changes in behavior. To conduct a thorough assessment of the patient with dementia, the nurse needs to know what is typical for the individual; therefore, caregivers, family members, or significant others can be sources of valuable information.

Physical Examination and a Review of Body Systems

A review of body systems must be conducted on each patient suspected of having dementia. Specific biologic assessment parameters for a patient with dementia include vital signs, neurologic status, nutritional status, bladder and bowel function, hygiene (including oral hygiene), skin integrity, rest and activity level, sleep patterns, and fluid and electrolyte balance. The neurologic function of the patient with AD is usually preserved through the early and middle stages of the disease, although seizures, gait disturbances, and tremors may occur at any time. In the later stages of the disease, neurologic signs, such as flexion contractures and primitive reflexes, are prominent features.

Physical Functions

At first, limitations may primarily involve instrumental activities, such as shopping, preparing meals, and performing other household chores. Later in the disease process, basic physical dysfunctions occur, such as incontinence, ataxia, dysphagia, and contractures. Incontinence can be a major source of stress and a considerable burden to family caregivers. Evaluation of the patient's functional abilities includes bathing, dressing, toileting, feeding, nutritional status, physical mobility, sleep patterns, and pain.

Assessment of physical functions includes activities of daily living, recent changes in functional abilities, use of sensory aids (glasses and hearing aids), activity level, and assessment of pain. Eyeglasses and hearing aids may need to be in place before other assessments can be made.

Self-Care

Alterations in the central nervous system (CNS) associated with dementia impair the patient's ability to collect information from the environment, retrieve memories, retain new information, and give meaning to current situations. Therefore, patients with dementia often neglect self-care activities. Periodically, biologic assessment parameters need to be re-evaluated because patients with dementia may neglect activities such as bathing, eating, or skin care.

Sleep–Wake Disturbances

A variety of sleep disturbances occur in AD, such as waking up during the night, being drowsy during the day, and restless sleep (Tractenberg, Singer, & Kaye, 2006). There is a deterioration of the circadian sleep–wake patterns. Neurotransmitter dysregulation of melatonin in the pineal gland is thought to be one of the contributing factors to the sleep disturbance. Additionally, delays in the circadian phase of core body temperature also occur. Patients with dementia have frequent daytime napping and nighttime periods of wakefulness, with little rapid eye movement (REM) sleep. Lowered levels of REM sleep are associated with restlessness, irritability, and general sleep impairment (Meeks, Ropacki, & Jeste, 2006).

Activity and Exercise

One of the earliest symptoms of AD is withdrawal from normal activities. Motor activity is affected in the mild stages of AD and can lead to early problems in functional performance (Pettersson, Engardt, & Wahlund, 2002). As the disease progresses, the patient may just sit staring at a blank wall.

Nutrition

Eating can become a problem for a patient with dementia. Weight loss occurs in 40% of patients (Guérin et al., 2005). As the disease progresses, patients may lose the ability to feed themselves or recognize what is offered as food. Some patients with dementia are bulimic or hyperoral (eating or chewing almost everything possible and sometimes with an insatiable appetite). Other patients with dementia experience anorexia and have no appetite.

Pain

Assessment and documentation of any physical discomfort or pain the patient may be experiencing is a part of any geropsychiatric nursing assessment (see Chapter 30). Although AD is not usually thought of as a physically painful disorder, patients often have other comorbid physical diseases that may be painful. In the early stages of AD, the patient can usually respond to verbal questions regarding pain. Later, it may be difficult to assess objectively the comfort level, especially if the patient cannot communicate. Some patients in the end stage of dementia become hypersensitive to touch.

Pain can be assessed by obtaining vital signs, completing a physical assessment, and using one of the pain assessment scales. Sometimes, laboratory tests must be conducted to help identify the source of discomfort. Subtle behavioral changes, such as lethargy, anxiety, or restlessness, or more obvious physical signs, such as pyrexia, tachypnea, or tachycardia, may be the only indications of actual or impending illness. Observing for changes in patterns of nonverbal communication, such as facial expressions, may help the nurse identify indicators of pain. Hypervocalizations (disturbed vocalizations), restlessness, and agitation are other possible signs of pain.

Nursing Diagnoses for the Biologic Domain

The unique and changing needs of these patients present a challenge for nurses in all settings. A multitude of potential nursing diagnoses focusing on the biologic domain can be identified for this population. A sample of common nursing diagnoses include Imbalanced Nutrition: Less (or More) Than Body Requirements; Feeding Self-Care Deficit; Impaired Swallowing; Bathing/Hygiene Self-Care Deficit; Dressing/Grooming Self-Care Deficit; Toileting Self-Care Deficit; Constipation (or Perceived Constipation); Bowel Incontinence; Impaired Urinary Elimination; Functional Incontinence; Total Incontinence; Deficient Fluid Volume; Risk for Impaired Skin Integrity; Impaired Physical Mobility; Activity Intolerance; Fatigue; Insomnia; Pain; Chronic Pain; Ineffective Health Maintenance; and Impaired Home Maintenance.

Interventions for the Biologic Domain

The numerous interventions for the biologic domain vary throughout the course of the disorder. Initially, the patient requires simple directions for self-care activities and initiation of psychopharmacologic treatment. At the end of the disorder, total patient care is required.

Self-Care Interventions

Patients should be encouraged to maintain as much self-care as possible. Promotion of self-care supports cognitive functioning and a sense of independence. In the early stages, the nurse should maximize normal perceptual experiences by making sure that the patient and family have appropriate eyeglasses and working hearing aids. If eyeglasses and hearing aids are needed, but not used, patients are more likely to have false perceptual experiences (hallucinations). Ongoing monitoring of self-care is necessary throughout the course of AD. Oral hygiene can be a problem and requires excellent basic nursing care. Aging and many medications reduce salivary flow, which can lead to a painfully dry and cracking oral mucosa. Drugs that have xerostomia (dry mouth) as a side effect and are commonly prescribed for patients with progressive dementia include antidepressant, antispasmodic, antihypertensive, bronchodilator, and some antipsychotic agents. For patients with xerostomia, hard candy or chewing gum may stimulate salivary flow, or modification of the drug regimen may be necessary. Glycerol mouthwash can provide as much relief from xerostomia as artificial saliva.

During later stages of dementia, bathing can be problematic for the patient and nursing staff. Bath time is a high-risk time for agitation and aggression (Barrick, Rader, Hoeffer, & Sloane, 2002). A person-centered approach advocated by Hoeffer and colleagues increases the likelihood of positive outcomes for the patient and the caregiver (see Box 32.5). The person-centered approach focuses on personalizing care to meet residents' needs, accommodating to residents' preferences, attending to the relationship and interaction with the resident, using effective communication and interpersonal skills, and adapting the physical environment and bathing procedures to decrease stress and discomfort (Hoeffer et al., 2006).

Nutritional Interventions

Maintenance of nutrition and hydration are essential nursing interventions. The patient's weight, oral intake, and hydration status should be monitored carefully. Patients with dementia should eat well-balanced meals that are appropriate to their activity level and eating abilities, with special attention given to electrolyte balance and fluid intake. The hyperactive patient requires frequent feedings of a high-protein, high-carbohydrate diet in the form of finger foods (which they can carry while on the go). It may be wise to secure a fanny pack around the patient's waist with an assortment of nutritious finger foods appropriate for the patient who can no longer use eating utensils properly. Most patients with dementia prefer to feed themselves with their fingers rather than have someone feed them.

BOX 32.5

Research for Best Practice: Effects of Two Bathing Interventions

Hoeffer, B., Talerico, K. A., Rasin, J., Mitchell, C. M., Stewart, B. J., McKenzie, D., Barrick, A. L., Rader, J., & Sloane, P. D. (2006). Assisting cognitively impaired nursing home residents with bathing: effects of two bathing interventions on caregiving. Gerontologist, 46(4), 524–532.

THE QUESTION: Do certified nursing assistants (CNA) who receive training in a person-centered approach with showering and with the towel bath show improved caregiving behaviors (gentleness and verbal support) and experience greater preparedness (confidence and ease) and less distress (hassles) when assisting residents with bathing?

METHODS: Researchers used a crossover design and randomized 15 nursing homes into two treatment groups and a control group of five facilities each. In one treatment group, CNAs received person-centered training (showering, first 6 weeks; towel bath second 6 weeks); treatment group two reversed the order of the training. The control group used usual showering procedures without person-centered training.

FINDINGS: Data were analyzed from 37 CNAs assisting 69 residents. Compared with the control group, treatment groups significantly improved in the use of gentleness and verbal support and in the perception of ease.

IMPLICATIONS FOR NURSING: Person-centered approach with showering and with the towel bath can improve care given to residents who become agitated and aggressive during the bath and help the CNAs have a positive experience while bathing a resident.

When swallowing is a problem for the patient, thick liquids or semisoft foods are more effective than traditionally prepared foods. If a patient is likely to choke or aspirate food, less liquid (pureed) and more semisolid foods should be included in the diet because liquid flows into the pharyngeal cavity more quickly than does solid food.

The dining environment should be calm and food presentation appealing. If the patient eats only a small portion of food at one meal, reduce the presentation of food in terms of the amount and number of choices. One-dish meals (e.g., a casserole) are ideal. If the patient is stressed or upset, it is better to delay feeding because eating, chewing, and swallowing difficulties are accentuated.

As dementia progresses, intensive feeding efforts are needed to ensure adequate food and fluid intake. If food intake is low, vitamin and mineral supplements may be indicated. If weight loss cannot be stopped by skillful feeding or dietary adjustments, then enteral or parenteral feedings may be considered. The patient's quality of life is an important issue to consider when the family or other health care proxy must decide whether to use artificial feeding mechanisms. By inserting a feeding tube, the goal of sustaining weight can be met, but patient comfort may be jeopardized, especially if restraints are used to keep the tube in place. In fact, some patients with advanced dementia put inedible objects into their mouths, presumably because they fail to recognize the objects as nonfood items.

The patient with dementia should be presented food that is easy to chew (soft) and swallow and not too hot or cold. In the later stages of progressive dementia, some patients hoard food in their mouths without actually swallowing it; others swallow too rapidly or fail to chew their food sufficiently before attempting to swallow. The nurse needs to watch for swallowing difficulties that place the patient at risk for aspiration and asphyxiation. Swallowing difficulties may result from changes in esophageal motility and decreased secretion of saliva.

Supporting Bowel and Bladder Function

Urinary or bowel incontinence affects many patients with dementia. During middle phases of the disease, incontinence may be caused by the patient's inability to communicate the need to use the toilet or locate a toilet quickly; undress appropriately to use the toilet; recognize the sensation of fullness signaling the need to urinate or defecate; or apathy with lack of motivation to remain continent.

For the patient who is incontinent because of an inability to locate the toilet, orientation may be helpful. Signs and active training should help to modify disorientation in elderly patients. Displaying pictures or signs on bathroom doors provides visual cues; words should use appropriate terminology.

If the patient cannot recognize the need to void because of impaired sensory perception of fullness, increasing fluid intake can help to fill the bladder sufficiently to give a clear message of the need to urinate. In addition, getting to know the patient's habits and moods can help the nurse to identify signals that indicate a need to void. The patient can then be assisted to reach the bathroom in time. Positioning the patient near the toilet or placing a portable commode nearby may help if the patient cannot reach a toilet quickly. If the patient demonstrates dressing apraxia (cannot undress appropriately), clothing can be modified with easy-to-open fasteners in place of zippers or buttons. For nocturnal incontinence, other strategies may be effective. Limiting the amount of fluid consumed after the evening meal and taking the patient to the toilet just before going to bed or upon awakening during the night should reduce or eliminate nocturia.

Indwelling urinary catheters are contraindicated in patients with dementia because they are generally not well tolerated and because hand restraints are often used to prevent them from removing the catheter. In addition, indwelling urinary catheters foster the development of urinary tract infections and may compromise the patient's dignity and comfort. Urinary incontinence can be managed with the use of disposable, adult-size diapers that must be checked regularly and changed expeditiously when soiled.

Patients with dementia often experience constipation, although they may not be able to tell the nurse about this change. Therefore, subtle signs such as lethargy, reduced appetite, and abdominal distention need to be assessed frequently. Medications, decreased food and liquid intake, lack of motor activity, and decreased intestinal motility contribute to developing constipation. In such cases, the patient's diet should be rich in fiber, including bran or whole grains, vegetables, and fruit. Adequate oral intake (minimum of 1,500 to 2,000 mL/day) helps to prevent constipation. A gentle laxative such as milk of magnesia (1 to 2 tablespoons every other evening) is commonly used to promote bowel elimination. Enemas and harsher chemical cathartics should be avoided because they may increase pain or discomfort. Care must be taken to ensure that the patient does not become dehydrated in the process of treating constipation.

Sleep Interventions

Disturbed sleep cycles are particularly stressful to both family caregivers and nursing staff. Disturbed sleep is difficult to manage from a behavioral perspective, and the patient's overall level of health may suffer because sleep serves a restorative function. Sedative-hypnotic agents may be prescribed for a short time for restlessness or insomnia, but they may also cause a paradoxical reaction of agitation and insomnia (especially in elderly patients).

Sleep hygiene interventions are appropriate for patients with dementia, although morning and afternoon naps (or rest periods for patients who do not nap) may be the most effective intervention for a patient with altered diurnal rhythms. Morning naps are likely to produce REM sleep patterns and may help patients who are restless from a loss of REM sleep, whereas afternoon naps produce deep sleep and are suitable for restlessness associated with fatigue. Rest periods (in reclining chairs) in the morning and afternoon may help to eliminate late-day confusion (sundowning) and nighttime awakenings.

Activity and Exercise Interventions

Activity and exercise are important nursing interventions for patients with dementia. To promote a feeling of success, any activity or exercise plan must be culturally sensitive and adapted to the patient's functional ability and interests. The activity or exercise must be designed to prevent excess stress (both physical and psychological), which means that it must be individualized for each patient with dementia, based on their relative strengths and deficits. If the program of rest, activity, and exercise is truly individualized, the resultant feelings of value and competency will enhance the patient's morale and self-esteem.

Pain and Comfort Management

Nursing care of noncommunicative patients who have dementia and who also have pain can be challenging. Because of the difficulty in identifying and monitoring the pain, the patients are often undertreated. However, several measures may be used to assess the efficacy of pharmacologic interventions, such as decreased restlessness and agitation. Small doses of oral morphine solution appear to reduce discomfort during routine nursing procedures. The main side effect of morphine is constipation.

Relaxation

Approaching patients in a calm, confident, unhurried manner; maintaining a soothing, quiet environment; avoiding unnecessary noise or chatter around patients and lowering vocal tone and rate when addressing them, maintaining eye contact; and using touch judiciously are likely to promote a sense of security conducive to patient relaxation and comfort. Simple relaxation exercises can be used to reduce stress and should be performed by the patient.

Administering and Monitoring Medications

Because no medication can cure AD, psychopharmacologic interventions have two goals: restoration or maintenance of cognitive function and treatment of related psychiatric and behavioral disturbances that cause discomfort for the individual, interfere with treatment, or worsen the individual's cognitive status. Doses must be kept extremely low, and individuals should be monitored closely for any side effects or worsening of cognitive status. "Start low and go slow" is the principle guiding the administration of psychopharmacologic agents in elderly patients.

Often, convincing the patient to take the medication is one of the biggest nursing challenges. Patients may be unwilling, even though they previously agreed to take the drugs. The nurse will need to investigate and hypothesize the reason for the reluctance to take medication. It may be because of difficulty swallowing pills, paranoid ideas, or lack of understanding. The underlying reason for medication refusal will determine the strategy. If the patient has difficulty swallowing, most medications come in concentrate liquid form and can be easily swallowed. Some medications can also be mixed in food. If suspicion or paranoia is the reason, the nurse will need to try to identify the conditions under which the patient feels safe to take the medication, such as for a favorite nurse or relative.

Cholinesterase Inhibitors. **Acetylcholinesterase inhibitors** (AChEI) are the mainstay of pharmacologic treatment of dementia because they inhibit **acetylcholinesterase AChE**, an enzyme necessary for the breakdown of acetylcholine. Inhibition of AChE results in an increase in cholinergic activity. Because these medications have been shown to delay the decline in cognitive functioning, but generally do not improve cognitive function once it has declined, it is important that this medication be started as soon as the diagnosis is made. The primary side effect of these medications is gastrointestinal distress—nausea, vomiting, and diarrhea.

There are four cholinesterase inhibitors indicated for the treatment of mild to moderate AD. These drugs may help to delay or prevent symptoms from becoming worse. They include galantamine (Razadyne), donepezil (Aricept), rivastigmine (Exelon), and tacrine (Cognex). Aricept is also indicated for moderate to severe AD (see Table 32.6). Because the cholinesterase inhibitors can increase the risk of stomach ulcers, the prolonged use of NSAIDs with the AChEIs should be monitored closely. The cholinesterase inhibitors are oral medications usually taken once or twice a day. The earlier in the disease process these medications are initiated, the more likely they will delay cognitive decline. There are no special monitors for these medications. With cholinesterase inhibitors, patients should not be taking any anticholinergic medication (USDHHS, 2006).

NMDA Antagonists. Overstimulation of the *N*-methyl-D-aspartate (NMDA) receptor by glutamate (excitatory neurotransmitter) is considered to have a role in AD. In dementia, it is hypothesized that there is a chronic release of glutamate that causes a permanent increased intracellular calcium concentration that leads to neuronal degeneration. Memantine (Namenda) is an NMDA-receptor antagonist that has been shown to improve cognition and activities of daily living in patients with moderately severe to severe symptoms of dementia, as well as the mild to moderate symptoms (Reisberg et al., 2003) (see Box 32.6).

Antipsychotic Agents. Antipsychotic agents are often effective in reducing psychosis, agitation, or aggressive behaviors and are commonly used off-label in the moderate to severe stages of AD. Antipsychotics are not approved by the U.S Food and Drug Administration

Table 32.6 Cholinesterase Inhibitors

Drug	Dose	Common Side Effects	Drug–Drug Interactions
Galantamine (Razadyne): Prevents breakdown of acetylcholine and stimulates nicotinic receptors to release more acetylcholine in the brain.	4 mg, twice a day Titrate to 16-24 mg/day over 8 weeks.	Nausea, vomiting, diarrhea, weight loss	Some antidepressants such as paroxetine, amitriptyline, fluoxetine, fluvoxamine and other drugs with anticholinergic action may cause retention of excess Razadyne in the body. NSAIDs should be used with caution in combination with this medication.
Rivastigmine (Exelon) Prevents the breakdown of acetylcholine and buturylcholine in the brain	1.5 mg twice a day Titrate to 24 mg/day by increasing 3 mg/day every 2 weeks	Nausea, vomiting, weight loss, upset stomach, muscle weakness	None observed in laboratory studies; NSAIDs should be used with caution in combination with this medication
Donepezil (Aricept) Prevents the breakdown of acetylcholine in the brain	5 mg, once a day Increase after 4–6 weeks to 10 mg/day	Nausea, diarrhea, vomiting	None observed in laboratory studies. NSAIDs should be used with caution in combination with this medication
Tacrine (Cognex) Prevents the breakdown of acetylcholine in the brain. (Cognex is available, but no longer actively marketed by the manufacturer)	10 mg, four times a day (40 mg/day) Increase by 40 mg/day every 4 weeks to 160 mg/day (if liver enzyme functions remain normal)	Nausea, diarrhea, possible liver damage	NSAIDs should be used with caution in combination with this medication

Adapted from USDHHS (2006). Alzheimer's Disease Medications Fact Sheet. Alzheimer's Disease Education & Referral (ADEAR) Center, National Institute on Aging, National Institutes of Health, NIH Publication N. 03-3431. Retrieved on April 6, 2007, from http://www.nia.nih.gov/NR/rdonlyres/5178456B-4E16-4A71-A704-46637C6FE61B/5574/AD_Medications_FactSheet121906.pdf

for dementia-related psychosis and have a boxed warning for their use in this population. If atypical antipsychotics are used in elderly patients, the dosage should be much lower than in younger adults.

Antidepressant Agents and Mood Stabilizers. A depressed mood is common in patients with dementia, and they often experience response to psychotherapeutic intervention alone (individual or group therapy) or in combination with pharmacotherapy. Low doses of the selective serotonin reuptake inhibitors and other newer antidepressive agents are often used.

Antianxiety Medications (sedative–hypnotics). Antianxiety medications, also known as benzodiazepines, should be used with caution in elderly patients and, if used, should be administered on a short-term basis. An antianxiety medication may be considered in an emergency, but ideally, the patient should try a nonbenzodiazepine before being prescribed a benzodiazepine. In elderly people, the benzodiazepines can cause a paradoxical reaction.

Other Medications. Clinical observations indicate that elderly patients with defects in the cholinergic system are more vulnerable to the effects of anticholinergic drugs that can cause confusion and amnesia. Anticholinergic medications should be avoided in patients with AD if at all possible. See Box 32.7 for examples of medications that are commonly prescribed in elderly patients, all of which have anticholinergic receptor activity.

Psychological Domain

Psychological Assessment

Personality changes almost always accompany dementia and can take the form of either an accentuation or a marked alteration of a patient's previous lifelong character traits. The neural substrates underlying personality change in AD are not understood, but researchers have identified two contrasting patterns. One is marked by apathy, lack of spontaneity, and passivity. The other involves growing irritability, sarcasm, self-preoccupation, and intolerance of and lack of concern for others. Assessment of the psychological domain includes sexuality and spirituality.

Cognitive Status

The mental status assessment can be difficult for the patient with dementia because cognitive disturbance is the clinical hallmark of dementia. The use of any of the tools discussed in Chapter 8 can be used to determine

BOX 32.6

Drug Profile: Memantine (Namenda)

DRUG CLASS: NMDA receptor antagonist

RECEPTOR AFFINITY: Low to moderate affinity uncompetitive (open-channel) NMDA receptor antagonist, which binds preferentially to the NMDA receptor

INDICATIONS: For treatment of moderate to severe dementia of the Alzheimer type.

ROUTES AND DOSAGE: 5 mg, 10 mg tablets, and oral solution, 2 mL/mg
The dosage shown to be effective in controlled clinical trials is 20 mg/day. The recommended starting dose of Namenda is 5 mg once daily. The recommended target dose is 20 mg/day. The dose should be increased in 5 mg increments to 10 mg/day (5 mg twice a day), 15 mg/day (5 mg and 10 mg as separate doses), and 20 mg/day (10 mg twice a day). The minimum recommended interval between dose increases is 1 week.

HALF LIFE (PEAK EFFECT), terminal half-life 60–80 hours (peak effect 3–7 hours)

SELECT ADVERSE REACTIONS: Dizziness, headache, constipation; reduce dosage in patients with severe renal damage

PRECAUTIONS Avoid use during pregnancy, effect during lactation has not been determined.

May cause drowsiness or dizziness; use caution while driving or performing other activities requiring mental alertness

SPECIFIC PATIENT/FAMILY EDUCATION: Caregivers should be instructed in the recommended administration (twice per day for doses above 5 mg) and dose escalation (minimum interval of 1 week between dose increases).

- Advise patient or caregiver that this drug does not alter the Alzheimer process and that the efficacy of the medication may decrease over time.
- Instruct patient or caregiver to continue using other medications for dementia as prescribed by health care provider.
- Advise patient or caregiver to review the Patient Information.
- Advise patient or caregiver that doses greater than 5 mg are taken bid, without regard to meals, but to take with food if GI upset occurs.
- Teach preparation of oral solution (attach the green cap and plastic tube to new bottles of oral solution, withdraw prescribed dose using dosing syringe, and administer the dose).
- Advise patient or caregiver not to discontinue the drug or change the dose unless advised by health care provider.
- Caution patient or caregiver not to increase the dose of memantine if Alzheimer symptoms do not appear to be improving or appear to be getting worse, but to notify health care provider.
- Caution patient that memantine may cause drowsiness or dizziness and to use caution while driving or performing other activities requiring mental alertness or coordination until tolerance is determined.
- Instruct patient or caregiver not to use any prescription or OTC medications, dietary supplements, or herbal preparations unless advised by health care provider.
- Advise patient or caregiver that follow-up visits may be required to monitor therapy and to keep appointments.

mental status. However, family members should also be a part of any assessment, especially early in the disease process. The AD8 is a brief, sensitive measure that differentiates between those with and without dementia (Galvin et al., 2005; Galvin, Roe, Xiong, & Morris, 2006). The AD8 contains eight questions asking the family member to rate any change (yes or no) in memory, problem-solving abilities, orientation, and daily activities. The higher the number of changes, the more likely dementia is present (see Figure 32.4). If cognitive deterioration occurs rapidly, delirium should be suspected.

Memory. The most dramatic and consistent cognitive impairment is in memory. Patients with dementia appear mildly forgetful and repetitive in conversation. They misplace objects, miss appointments, and forget what they were just doing. They may lose track of a conversation or television story. Initially, they may complain of memory problems, but rapidly in the course of the illness, insight is lost and they become unaware of what is lost. Sometimes, they may confabulate, making what appears to be an appropriate explanation of why the information or object is missing. Eventually, all aspects of memory are impaired, and even long-term memories are affected. During the interview, short-term memory loss is usually readily evident by the patient's inability to recall three or four words given to him or her at the beginning of the assessment. Often, the earliest symptom of AD is the inability to retain new information.

Language. Language is also progressively impaired. Individuals with AD may initially have agnosia (difficulty finding a word in a sentence or in naming an object). They may be able to talk around it, but the loss is noticeable. Later, fluent aphasia develops, comprehension diminishes, and, finally, they become mute and unresponsive to directions or information.

Visuospatial Impairment. Deficits in visuospatial tasks that require sensory and motor coordination develop early, drawing is abnormal, and the ability to write may change. An inaccurate clock drawing is diagnostic of impairment in this area (see Figure 32.5).

BOX 32.7

Medications With Anticholinergic Effects

Amitriptyline (Elavil/Endep)
Captopril (Capoten)
Codeine
Cimetidine (Tagamet)
Citalopram (Celexa)
Digoxin (Lanoxin)
Diphenhydramine (Benadryl)
Dipyridamole (Trental)
Donepezil (Aricept)
Escitalopram (Lexapro)
Furosemide (Lasix)
Fluoxetine (Prozac)
Isosorbide (Ismotic)
Mirtazapine (Remeron)
Nifedipine (Procardia)
Oxybutynin ER (Ditropan XL)
Paroxetine (Paxil)
Phenytoin (Dilantin)
Prednisolone
Ranitidine (Zantac)
Theophylline (Bronkodyl)
Triamterene (Dyrenium) and hydrochlorothiazide (HCTZ)
Tolterodine (Detrol LA)
Warfarin (Coumadin)

Sequencing tasks, such as cooking or other self-care skills, become impaired. The individual becomes unable to complete complex tasks that require calculations, such as balancing a checkbook.

Executive Functioning. Judgment, reasoning, and the ability to problem solve or make decisions are also impaired later in the disorder, closer to the time of nursing home placement. It is hypothesized that as the disease progresses, the degeneration of neurons is spread diffusely throughout the neocortex.

Psychotic Symptoms

Delusional thought content and hallucinations are common in people with dementia. These psychotic symptoms differ from those of schizophrenia.

Suspiciousness, Delusions, and Illusions. During the early and middle stages of dementia, many patients are aware of their cognitive losses and compensate with hyperalertness. In a hyperalert state, one becomes aware of many environmental stimuli that are not readily understood. Suspiciousness is a variant of the hyperalert or hypervigilant state in which stimuli are interpreted as dangerous. **Illusions**, or mistaken perceptions, also occur commonly in patients with dementia. For example, a woman with dementia mistakes her husband for her father. He resembles her father in that he is roughly her father's age when he was last alive. If an illusion becomes a false fixed belief, it is a delusion.

As the disease progresses, delusions develop in 34% to 50% of the people with dementia. These characteristic delusions are different from those discussed in the psychotic disorders. Common delusional beliefs include the following:

- Belief that his or her partner is engaging in marital infidelity
- Belief that other patients or staff are trying to hurt him or her
- Belief that staff or family members are impersonators
- Belief that people are stealing his or her belongings
- Belief that strangers are living in his or her home
- Belief that people on television are real.

Hallucinations. Hallucinations occur frequently in dementia and are usually visual or tactile (they can also be auditory, gustatory, or olfactory). Visual, rather than auditory, hallucinations are the most common in dementia. A frequent complaint is that children, adults, or strange creatures are entering the house or the patient's room. These hallucinations may not seem unusual to the patient. If possible, the content and form of hallucination should be ascertained because this information may suggest a treatable disorder. For example, an auditory hallucination commanding the patient to commit suicide may be caused by a treatable depression, not dementia. In some cases, hallucinations may be pleasant, such as children being in the room; or they may frightening and uncomfortable.

Mood Changes

Recognition of coexisting (and often treatable) psychiatric disorders in patients with dementia is often ignored. A depressed mood is common and is reported in 40% to 50% of AD cases. A diagnosis of major depression is less common, occurring in 10% to 20% of patients with AD. A number of people with AD experience one or more depressive episodes with symptoms such as psychomotor retardation, anxiety, feelings of guilt and worthlessness, sadness, frequent crying, insomnia, loss of appetite, weight loss, and suicidal rumination. Depressive symptoms are most prevalent in the early stages of dementia, which may be attributed to the patient's awareness of cognitive changes, memory loss, and functional decline. However, dysphoric symptoms can occur at any stage, even in the most disoriented elderly patients. In more advanced stages of dementia, assessment of depression depends more on changes in behavior than on verbal complaints.

Anxiety. Moderate anxiety is a natural reaction to the fear engendered by gradual deterioration of intellectual function and the realization of impending loss of control over one's life. Failure to complete a task once regarded as simple creates a source of anxiety in the

Remember, "Yes, a change" indicates that there has been a change in the last several years caused by cognitive (thinking and memory) problems.	Yes, A change	No, No change	N/A, Don't know
1. Problems with judgment (e.g., problems making decisions, bad financial decisions, problems with thinking)			
2. Less interest in hobbies/activities			
3. Repeats the same things over and over (questions, stories, or statements)			
4. Trouble learning how to use a tool, appliance, or gadget (e.g., VCR, computer, microwave, remote control)			
5. Forgets correct month or year			
6. Trouble handling complicated financial affairs (e.g., balancing checkbook, income taxes, paying bills)			
7. Trouble remembering appointments			
8. Daily problems with thinking and/or memory			

The final score is a sum of the number of items marked "Yes, A change".

Based on clinical research findings from 995 individuals included in the development and validation samples, the following cut points are provided:
- 0-1: Normal cognition
- 2 or greater: Cognitive impairment is likely to be present

Interpretation of the AD8 (Adapted from Galvin, JE et al, The AD8, a brief informal interview to detect dementia, Neurology 2005; 58: 589-364)

Scores in the impaired range (see below) indicate a need for further assessment. Scores in the "normal" range suggest that a dementing disorder is unlikely, but a very early disease process cannot be ruled out. More advanced assessment may be warranted in cases where other objective evidence of impairment exists.

FIGURE 32.4. AD8 tool. (Used with permission from James E. Galvin, MD, MSc, Assistant Professor, Director of the Memory Diagnostic Center, Washington University School of Medicine, St. Louis, MO.)

patient with AD. As patients with AD become unsure of their surroundings and the expectations of others, they frequently react with fear and distress. It is thought that anxious behavior occurs when the patient is pressed to perform beyond his or her ability.

Catastrophic Reactions. **Catastrophic reactions** are overreactions or extreme anxiety reactions to everyday situations. Catastrophic responses occur when environmental stressors are allowed to continue or increase beyond the patient's threshold of stress tolerance. Behaviors indicative of catastrophic reactions typically include verbal or physical aggression, violence, agitated or anxious behavior, emotional outbursts, noisy behavior, compulsive or repetitive behavior, agitated night awakening, and other behaviors in which the patient is cognitively or socially inaccessible. Factors that contribute to catastrophic responses in patients with progressive cognitive decline include fatigue, change in routine (pace or caregiver), demands beyond the patient's abil-

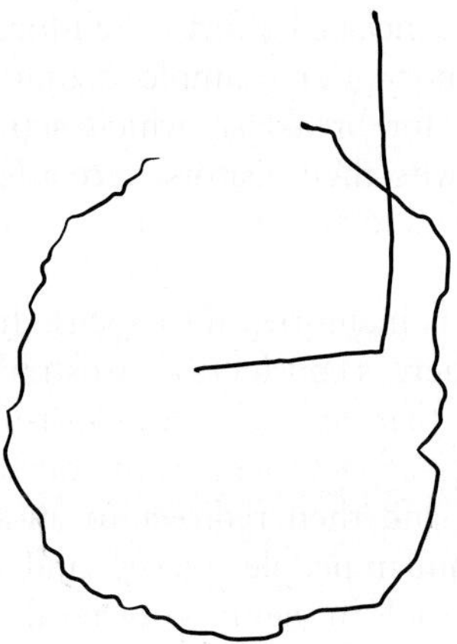

FIGURE 32.5. Clock drawing by a patient with moderate AD. The patient was asked to draw a clock at 3:00 PM.

ity, overwhelming sensory stimuli, and physical stressors, such as pain or hunger.

Behavioral Responses

Apathy and Withdrawal. Apathy, the inability or unwillingness to become involved with one's environment, is common in AD, especially in moderate to late stages. Apathy leads to withdrawal from the environment and a gradual loss of empathy for others. The lack of empathy is very difficult for families and friends to understand.

Restlessness, Agitation, and Aggression. Restlessness, agitation, and aggression are relatively common in moderate to later stages of dementia. Restlessness should be further evaluated to determine its underlying cause. If the restlessness occurs during medication change or adjustment, side effects should be suspected.

Agitation and aggressive physical contacts are among the most dangerous behavior management problems encountered in any setting. They often result in placement of a family member in a nursing home. Careful evaluation of the antecedents of the agitated behavior enable the nurse to plan nursing care that prevents future occurrences (see Box 32.8).

Aberrant Motor Behavior. Symptoms such as fidgeting, picking at clothing, wringing hands, loud vocalizations, and wandering may all be signs of such underlying conditions as dehydration, medication reaction, pain, or infection (suggesting delirium). One of the most difficult behaviors for which to determine an underlying cause is **hypervocalization,** the screams, curses, moans, groans, and verbal repetitiveness that are common in the later stages of disease in cognitively impaired elderly patients, often occurring during a hospitalization or nursing home placement. In the assessment of these hypervocalizations, it is important to identify when the behavior is occurring, antecedents of the behavior, and any related events, such as a family member leaving or a change in stimulation.

BOX 32.8

Research for Best Practice: ***Predicting when Agitation in a Nursing Home will Occur***

Kolanowski, A., & Litaker, M. (2006). Social interaction, premorbid personality, and agitation in nursing home residents with dementia. Archives of Psychiatric Nursing, 20(1), 12–20.

THE QUESTION: Is there a relationship between social interaction, premorbid personality trait of extraversion, and agitation?

METHODS: Researchers used a cross-sectional design with repeated measures to examine the temporal relationship between social interaction (high vs. low) and agitation as measured by their ranking on the trait of extraversion. The sample consisted of 30 persons, primarily female (77%), white (100%), and widowed (71%), with a mean age of 82.3 years. For 12 days, each subject was observed and videotaped under usual nursing home routines at the time when peak behavioral symptoms were exhibited. Staff rated the residents' social interaction and agitation.

FINDINGS: The most frequently observed agitated behaviors were pacing and aimless wandering, performing repetitious mannerisms, and restlessness. When social interaction occurred, it was associated with agitation. The higher levels of interacting with people and activity were significantly related to higher rates of agitation.

IMPLICATIONS FOR NURSING: Social interaction is important to monitor. Lack of interaction may lead to decline, but intense interaction may increase agitation and aggression.

Disinhibition. One of the most frustrating symptoms of AD is **disinhibition,** acting on thoughts and feelings without exercising appropriate social judgment. In AD, the patient may decide that he or she is more comfortable naked than with clothes. Or the patient may not be able to find his or her clothes and may walk into a room of people without any clothes on. This behavior is extremely disconcerting to family members and can also lead to nursing home placement.

Hypersexuality. A closely related symptom is **hypersexuality,** inappropriate and socially unacceptable sexual behavior. The patient begins talking and behaving in ways that are uncharacteristic of premorbid behavior. This behavior is very difficult for family members and nursing home staff.

Stress And Coping Skills. Patients with dementia seem extremely sensitive to stressful situations and often do not have the coping abilities to deal with the situation. A careful assessment of the triggers that precede stressful situations will help in understanding a provoking event.

Nursing Diagnoses for the Psychological Domain

A multitude of potential nursing diagnoses can be identified for the psychological domain of this population. A sample of common nursing diagnoses includes Impaired Memory; Disturbed Thought Processes; Chronic Confusion; Disturbed Sensory Perception; Impaired Environmental Interpretation Syndrome; Risk for Violence: Self-Directed or Directed at Others; Risk for Loneliness; Risk for Caregiver Role Strain; Ineffective Sexuality Patterns; Ineffective Individual Coping; Hopelessness; and Powerlessness (NANDA-I, 2007).

Interventions for the Psychological Domain

The therapeutic relationship is the basis for interventions for the patient and family with dementia. Care of the patient entails a long-term relationship needing much support and expert nursing care. Interventions should be delivered within the relationship context.

Cognitive Impairment

Validation Therapy. Validation therapy emerged in the 1970s as a method for communicating with patients with AD. It was developed as a contrast to reality therapy, which attempted to provide a here-and-now, factual focus to the interaction. **Validation therapy** focuses on the emotions and subjective reality of the patients. In validation therapy, individuals with cognitive impairment are viewed on one of four stages of a continuum: malorientation, time confusion, repetitive motion, and vegetation. The benefits of validation therapy for patients are reported as restoration of self-worth, less withdrawal from the outside world, communication and interaction with other people, reduction of stress and anxiety, help in resolving unfinished life tasks, and facilitation of independent living for as long as possible. These outcomes are highly desirable, but no substantive research supports its effectiveness (Neal & Briggs, 2003). Validation therapy is a useful model for nursing care of the patient with dementia. The nurse does not try to reorient the patient, but rather respects the individual's sense of reality.

Memory Enhancement. Interventions for progressive memory impairment should always be a part of the treatment plan. The sooner patients begin taking AChE inhibitors, the slower the cognitive decline. However, pharmacologic agents are only a small part of the intervention picture. The nursing goal is to maintain memory functioning as long as possible. The nurse should make a concerted effort to reinforce short- and long-term memory. For example, reminding patients what they had for breakfast, which activity was just completed, or who their visitors were a few hours ago will reinforce short-term memory. Encouraging patients to tell the stories of their earlier years will help bring long-term memories into focus. In the earlier stages of AD, there is considerable frustration when the patient realizes that he or she has short-term memory loss. In a matter-of-fact manner, the nurse should "fill in the blanks" and then redirect to another activity. Pictures of familiar people, places, and activities are also important tools in memory retrieval. Using scents (perfume, shaving lotions, spices, different foods) to stimulate memory retrieval and asking patients to relate memories are also useful. Formalized reminiscence groups also help patients relive their earlier experiences and support long-term memories.

Orientation Interventions. To enhance cognitive functioning, attempts should be made to remind patients of the day, time, and location. However, if the patient begins to argue that he or she is really at home or that it is really 1992, the patient need not be confronted by facts. Any confrontation could easily escalate into an argument. Instead, the nurse should either redirect the patient or focus on the topic at hand (see Box 32.9).

Maintaining Language. Losing the ability to name an object (agnosia) is frustrating. For example, the patient may describe a flower in terms of color, size, and fragrance but never be able to name it a flower. When this happens, the nurse should immediately say the name of the item. This reinforces cognitive functioning and prevents disruption in the interaction. Referral to speech therapists may also be useful if the language impairment impedes communication.

Supporting Visuospatial Functioning. The patient with visuospatial impairments loses the ability to sequence automatic behaviors, such as getting dressed or eating with silverware. For example, patients often put their clothes on backward, inside out, or with undergarments over outer garments. Once dressed, they become confused as to how they arrived at their current state. If this happens, the nurse should begin to place clothes for dressing in a sequence so that the patient can move from one article to the next in the correct sequence. This same technique can be used in other situations, such as eating, bathing, and toileting.

Interventions for Psychosis. Patients who are experiencing psychosis usually are prescribed an antipsychotic agent. Interventions associated with antipsychotic therapy were presented in earlier chapters.

BOX 32.9

Therapeutic Dialogue: The Patient With Dementia of the Alzheimer Type

Lois's daughter has told the home health agency nurse that on several occasions, Lois has been found cowering and fearful under the kitchen table, saying she was hiding from voices. The nurse also knows that Lois denies having any difficulty with her memory or her ability to care for herself.

Ineffective Approach

Nurse: I'm here to see you about your health problems.
Patient: I have no problems. Why are you here?
Nurse: I'm here to help you.
Patient: I do not need any help. I think there is a mistake.
Nurse: Oh, there is no mistake. Your name is Ms. W, isn't it?
Patient: Yes, but I don't know who you are or why you are here. I'm very tired, please excuse me.
Nurse: OK. I will return another day.

Effective Approach

Nurse: Hello, my name is Susan Miller. I'm the home health nurse and I will be spending some time with you.
Patient: Oh, alright. Come in. Sit here.
Nurse: Thank you.
Patient: There is nothing wrong with me, you know.
Nurse: Are you wondering why I am here? (open-ended statement)
Patient: I know why you are here. My children think that I cannot take care of myself.
Nurse: Is that true? Can you take care of yourself? (restatement)
Patient: Of course I can care for myself. When people get older they slow down. I'm just a little slower now and that upsets my children.
Nurse: You are a little slower? (reflection)
Patient: I sometimes forget things.
Nurse: Such as . . . (open-ended statement)
Patient: Sometimes, I cannot remember a telephone number or a name of a food.
Nurse: Does that cause problems?
Patient: According to my children, it does!
Nurse: What about you? What causes problems for you?
Patient: Sometimes the radio says terrible things to me.
Nurse: That must be frightening. (Acceptance)
Patient: It's terrifying. Then, my daughter looks at me as if I am crazy. Am I?
Nurse: It sounds like your mind is playing tricks on you. Let's see if we can figure out how to control the radio. (Validation)
Patient: Oh, OK. Will you tell my daughter that I am not crazy?
Nurse: Sure, I would be happy to meet with both you and your daughter if you would like. (Acceptance)

Critical Thinking Challenge

- How did the nurse's underlying assumption that the patient would welcome the nurse in the first scenario lead to the nurse's rejection by the patient?
- What communication techniques did the nurse use in the second scenario to open communication and set the stage for the development of a sense of trust?

Managing Suspicions, Illusions, and Delusions. Patients' suspiciousness and delusional thinking must be addressed to be certain that they do not endanger themselves or others. Often, delusions are verbalized when patients are placed in a situation they cannot master cognitively. The principle of nonconfrontation is most important in dealing with suspiciousness and delusion formation. No efforts should be made to ease the patient's suspicions directly or to correct delusions. Efforts should be directed at determining the circumstances that trigger suspicion or delusion formation and creating a means of avoiding these situations.

Frequent causes of suspicion are changes in daily routine and strangers. The common accusations that "Someone has entered my room," or "Someone has changed my room," can be managed by asking, "Do you want to see if anything is missing?" Such accusations usually arise when a patient cannot remember what the room looked like or when the room was rearranged or cleaned.

Patients with dementia often hide or misplace their belongings and later complain that the item is missing. It is helpful if the nurse and other caregivers pay attention to the patient's favorite hiding places and communicate this so that objects can be more easily retrieved. An outburst of delusional accusations after a social outing or other activity may indicate that the activity was too long, the setting too stimulating, there was too much activity, or the pace was too fast for the patient. All of these elements can be modified, or it may be necessary to exclude or significantly diminish the delusional patient's participation in overstimulating activities.

Patients with dementia have delusions that a spouse, child, or other significant person is an impostor. If this situation occurs, it is important to assert in a matter-of-fact manner, "This is your wife Barbara" or "I am your daughter Jenny." More vigorous assertions, such as offering various types of proof, tend to increase puzzlement as to why a person would go so far to impersonate the spouse or child.

When patients experience illusions, the nurse needs to find the source of the illusion and remove it from the environment if possible. For example, if a patient is watching a television program featuring animals and then verbalizes that the animal is in the room, switch the channel and redirect the conversation. Some patients with dementia may no longer recognize the reflection in the mirror as self and become agitated, thinking that a stranger is staring at them. Potentially misleading or disturbing stimuli, such as mirrors or art work, can be easily covered or removed from the environment.

Managing Hallucinations. Reassurance and distraction may be helpful for the hallucinating patient. For example, an 89-year-old patient with AD in a residential care facility would get up each night, walk to the nursing station, and whisper to the nurses, "There's a man in my bed who won't let me sleep. You should patrol this place better!" If the hallucination is not too disturbing for the patient, it can often be dismissed calmly with diversion or distraction. Because this patient did not seem too concerned by the man in her bed, the nurse may gently respond by saying, "I'm sorry you have to put up with so much. Just wait here (or come with me) and I'll make sure your room is ready for you." The nurse should then take the patient back to her room and help her into bed.

Frightening hallucinations and delusions usually require antipsychotic medications to dampen the patient's emotional reactions, but they can also be dealt with by optimizing perceptual cues (cover mirrors or turn off the television) and by encouraging patients to stay physically close to their caregivers. For example, one patient complained to her visiting nurse that she was being poisoned by deadly bugs that crawled up and down her arms and legs while she tried to sleep at night. Antipsychotic medication may help this patient sleep at night, and she would also likely benefit from reassurance and protection. Patients benefit more if nurses give them a specific intervention to help the hallucination, such as applying moisturizing lotion to her legs and arms to repel the bugs at night. The nurse does not have to agree with the patient's hallucination or delusion but should let the patient know that the feelings are justified based on the patient's perception of the threat.

Interventions for Mood Changes

Managing Depression. Psychotherapeutic nursing interventions for depression that accompanies dementia are similar to interventions for any depression. It is important to spend time alone with patients and to personalize their care as a way of communicating the patient's value. Encouraging expression of negative emotions is helpful because patients can talk honestly to a nonjudgmental person about their feelings. Although depressed patients with dementia are likely to be too disorganized to commit suicide, it is wise to remove potentially harmful objects from the environment (see Box 32.10).

Do not force depressed patients to interact with others or participate in activities, but encourage activity and exercise. One of the psychogenic aspects of depression is a sense of lowered worth related to the patient's actual decreased competence to work and to deal with the problems of daily living. Therefore, it may be helpful to involve the person in a simple repetitive task or project (such as folding linens or setting the table), especially one that involves helping someone else. Assist the patient to meet self-care needs while encouraging independence when possible.

Managing Anxiety. Cognitively impaired patients are particularly vulnerable to anxiety. Patients with dementia become unsure of their surroundings or of what is expected of them, and then tend to react with fear and distress. They may feel lost, insecure, and left out. Failure to complete a task once regarded as simple creates anxiety and agitation. Often, they cannot explain the source of their anxiety. The difficulty in developing interventions for the anxious patient with dementia is that the symptoms may also be a sign of underlying illnesses, such as depression, pain, infection, or other physical illnesses.

In many cases, lowering the demands, or perceived demands, on the patient will be conducive to promoting comfort. Although maintaining autonomy in any remaining function is a high priority in nursing care of the patient with dementia, it may decrease the patient's anxiety or stress level to have things done for him or her at certain points along the illness continuum. In addition, being sensitive to the pronounced startle reflexes and potential hypersensitivity to touch also helps reduce stress.

The threshold for stress is progressively lowered in AD and other progressive dementias. A healthy person

BOX 32.10

Clinical Vignette: *A Nurse's Dilemma*

It is 8 o'clock and you are working as a nurse on an inpatient general medical unit of a large urban hospital. A 72-year-old man is admitted to your unit with symptoms of disorientation to time and place, and he is intermittently exhibiting signs of agitation. He thinks you are his child, and he falls asleep while you ask him questions about his symptoms. When you ask him to sign a consent form and hand him a pen, he looks at you as if he didn't understand your request.

The patient's wife tells you that he has had trouble with his memory for the past 3 or 4 years but that her husband has been "acting strange for the past 4 days." The patient's wife denies any history of substance abuse or head injury, but states that her husband has been recently diagnosed as having dementia of the Alzheimer type.

What Do You Think?

- What assessment techniques would you use to determine whether this patient has dementia, delirium, or both?
- What nursing diagnosis would be included in the patient's plan of care?
- What nursing interventions would promote comfort and safety for this patient?

frequently uses cognitive coping strategies when under stress, whereas the person with dementia can no longer use many of these strategies. Effective nursing interventions include simplifying routines, making routines as consistent and predictable as possible, reducing the number of choices the patient must make, identifying areas in which control can be maintained, and creating an environment in which the patient feels safe. With any of the therapeutic interventions discussed, the nurse is reminded that each patient has relative strengths and weaknesses and that sound nursing judgment must be used in each situation.

Commonly used therapeutic approaches may exacerbate anxiety in a patient with dementia. For example, reality orientation is usually an effective intervention for acutely confused patients. Reality orientation is contraindicated in dementia because it is possible that the patient's disoriented behavior or language has inherent meaning. If the disoriented behavior or language is continuously neglected or corrected by the nurse, the patient's sense of isolation and anxiety may increase.

Another therapeutic intervention that may (or may not) be contraindicated in patients with dementia is providing the patient with information before a difficult or painful procedure. Anticipatory preparation for nonroutine events may produce anxiety because the patient is unable to retain information, use reasoning skills, or make sound judgments. Telling the patient that he or she is scheduled for an upcoming diagnostic test only communicates, on an emotional level, that something distressing is about to happen. A simple explanation immediately before the event may be more helpful.

Managing Catastrophic Reactions. If a patient reacts catastrophically, the nurse needs to remain calm, minimize environmental distractions (quiet the environment), get the patient's attention, and softly assure the patient that he or she is safe. Give information slowly, clearly, and simply, one step at a time. Let the patient know that you understand the fear or other emotional response, such as anger or anxiety.

As the nurse becomes skilled at identifying antecedents to the patient's catastrophic reactions, it becomes possible to avoid situations that provoke such reactions. Patients with AD respond well to structure but poorly to change. Attempts to argue or reason with them only escalate their dysfunctional responses.

Interventions for Behavior Problems

Managing Apathy and Withdrawal. As the patient withdraws and becomes more apathetic, the nurse is challenged to engage the patient in meaningful activities and interactions. To provide this level of care, the nurse must know the premorbid functioning of the patient. Close contact with family helps give the nurse ideas about meaningful activities.

Managing Restlessness and Wandering. Restlessness and wandering are major concerns for caregivers, especially in the community (home) or long-term care setting. The principal means of dealing with restless patients who wander into other patients' rooms or out the door is to have an adequate number of staff (or caregivers, in the home setting) to provide supervision, as well as electronically controlled exits. Wandering behavior may be interrupted in more cognitively intact patients by distracting them verbally or visually. Patients who are beyond verbal distraction can be distracted by physically joining them on their walk and then interrupting their course of action and gently redirecting them back to the house or facility. Many times, wandering is a result of a patient's inability to find his own room or may represent other agenda-seeking behaviors.

Managing Aberrant Behavior. When patients are picking in the air or wringing hands, simple distraction may work. Hypervocalizations are another story. Direct care staff tend to avoid these patients, which only makes the vocalizations worse. In reality, these vocalizations may have meaning to the patient. The nurse should develop strategies to try to reduce the frequency of vocalizations (Table 32.7).

Managing Agitated Behavior. Agitated behavior is likely to occur when patients are pressed to assist in their own care. A calm, unhurried, and undemanding approach is usually most effective. Attempts at reasoning may only aggravate the situation and increase the patient's resistance to care. If the nurse is unable to determine the source of the patient's anxiety, the patient's restless energy can often be channeled into activities such as walking. Relaxation techniques also can be effective for reducing behavioral problems and anxiety in patients with dementia.

Reducing Disinhibition. Anticipation of disinhibiting behavior is the key to nursing interventions for this problem. Disinhibition can take many forms, from undressing in a public setting, to touching someone inappropriately, to making cruel, but factual statements. This behavior can usually be viewed as normal by itself but abnormal within its social context. With keen behavioral assessment of the patient, the nurse should be able to anticipate the likely socially inappropriate behavior and redirect the patient or change the context of the situation. If the patient starts undressing in the dining room, offering a robe and gently escorting him or her to another part of the room might be all that is needed. If a patient is trying to fondle a staff member or another patient, having the staff member

Table 32.7 Messages; Meanings, and Management Strategies

Possible Underlying Meanings	Related Management Strategies
"*I hurt!*" (eg, from arthritis, fractures, pressure ulcers, degenerative joint disease, cancer)	• Observe for pain behaviors (eg, posture, facial expressions, and gait in conjunction with vocalizations) • Treat suspected pain judiciously with analgesics and nonpharmacologic measures (eg, repositioning, careful manipulation of patient during transfers and personal care, warm/cold packs, massage, relaxation)
"*I'm tired.*" (eg, sleep disturbances possibly related to altered sleep–wake cycle with day–night reversal, difficulty falling asleep, frequent night awakenings)	• Increase daytime activity and exercise to minimize daytime napping and promote nighttime sleep • Promote normal sleep patterns and biorhythms by strengthening natural environmental cues (eg, provide light exposure during the day, avoid bright, artificial lights at night), provide large calendars and clocks • Establish a bedtime routine • Reduce night awakenings: avoid excess fluids, diuretics, caffeine at bedtime, minimize loud noises, consolidate nighttime care activities (eg, changing, medications, treatments)
"*I'm lonely.*"	• Encourage social interactions between patients and their family, caregivers, and others • Increase time the patient spends in group settings to minimize time in isolation • Provide opportunity to interact with pets
"*I need . . .*" (eg, food, a drink, a blanket, to use the toilet, to be turned or repositioned)	• Anticipate needs (eg, assist patient to toilet soon after breakfast when the gastrocolic reflex is likely) • Keep patient comfort and safety in mind during care (eg, minimize body exposure to prevent hypothermia)
"*I'm stressed.*" (eg, Inability to tolerate sensory overload)	• Promote rest and quiet time • Minimize "white noise" (eg, vacuum cleaner) and background noise (eg, televisions and radios) • Avoid harsh lighting and busy, abstract designs • Limit patient's contacts with other agitated people • Reduce behavioral expectations of patient, minimize choices, promote a stable routine
"*I'm bored.*" (eg, lack of sensory stimulation)	• Maximize hearing and visual abilities (eg, keep external auditory canals free from cerumen plugs, ensure glasses and hearing aids are worn, provide reading material of large print, soften lighting to reduce glare) • Play soft, classical music for auditory stimulation • Offer structured diversions (eg, outdoor activities)
"*What are you doing to me?*" (eg, personal boundaries are invaded)	• Avoid startling patients by approaching them from the front • Always speak before touching the patient • Inform patients what you plan to do and why before you do it • Allow for flexibility in patient care
"*I don't feel well.*" (eg, a urinary or upper respiratory tract infection, metabolic abnormality, fecal impaction)	• Identify etiology through patient history, examination, possible tests (eg, urinalysis, blood work, chest radiograph, neurologic testing) • Treat underlying causes
"*I'm frustrated—I have no control.*" (eg, loss of autonomy)	• When possible, allow patient to make own decisions • Maximize patient involvement during personal care (eg, offer patient a washcloth to assist with bathing) • Treat patients with dignity and respect (eg, dress or change patient in private)
"*I'm lost.*" (eg, memory impairment)	• Maintain familiar routines • Label the patient's room, bathroom, drawers, and possessions with large name signs • Promote a sense of belonging through displays of familiar personal items, such as old family pictures
"*I feel strange.*" (eg, side effects from medications that may include psychotropics, corticosteroids, b-blockers, nonsteroidal antiinflammatories)	• Minimize overall number of medications; consider nondrug interventions when possible • Begin new medications one at a time; start with low doses, titrate slowly. Suspect drug reaction if patient's behavior (eg, vocal) changes • Educate caregivers about patient medications
"I need to be loved!"	• Provide human contact and purposeful touch • Acknowledge or verify patient's feelings • Encourage alternative, nonverbal ways to express feelings, such as through music, painting, or drawing • Stress a sense of purpose in life, acknowledge achievement, reaffirm that the patient is still needed

Clavel, D. S. (1999). Vocalizations among cognitively impaired elders. *Geriatric Nursing*, 20, 90–93.

leave the immediate area or redirecting the patient may alleviate the situation.

Social Domain

Social Assessment

Dementia interferes with a person's ability to interact socially as much as it disrupts intellectual functioning. The social domain assessment should include those areas explained in Chapter 30, including functional status, social systems, spiritual assessment, legal status, and quality of life (see Chapter 10). The Global Assessment of Functioning scale presented in Chapter 2 also can be used.

The patient's whole social network is affected by dementia, and the primary caregiver of a person with dementia (usually the partner or offspring in a community setting) is often considered a copatient. It is important to assess the family caregiver's ability to use supportive mechanisms to maintain his or her own integrity throughout the disease process.

The extent of the primary caregiver's personal, informal, and formal support systems must also be assessed, as well as personal resources, skills, and stressors. The assessment of the social domain provides objective data on the patient's social circumstances and impressions of the patient's family structure, sociocultural beliefs, attitudes toward health and disease, myths about dementia, patterns of communication, and degree of psychopathology (such as potential for abuse). If the patient still resides in the community, a home visit will prove useful because it gives the nurse information about the patient in the natural environment. From this assessment, the nurse can identify the situational and psychosocial stressors that affect the family and patient and can begin to develop interventions to strengthen coping strategies, including the ability to seek help from appropriate community resources.

Nursing Diagnoses for the Social Domain

Typical nursing diagnoses for the social domain are Deficient Diversional Activity; Impaired Social Interaction; Social Isolation; Risk for Loneliness; Caregiver Role Strain; Ineffective Coping; Hopelessness; and Powerlessness (NANDA-I, 2007). Outcomes are determined according to nursing diagnoses.

Interventions for the Social Domain

Safety Interventions

One of the primary concerns of the nurse should be patient safety. In the early stages of the illness, safety may not seem to be a prime issue because the individual is cognitively intact. However, early behaviors suggesting dementia are often related to safety, such as the patient getting lost while driving or going the wrong way on the highway. Patients may be prevented from driving even though they can continue to live at home. Safety continues to be an issue in the home when patients engage in unsupervised cooking, cleaning, or household tasks. Day care centers provide a structured, yet safe, environment for these individuals. Family members should be encouraged to assess continually the abilities of members to live at home safely.

During hospitalizations or nursing home care, the safety issues are different. There are more people with the patient, which presents more opportunity for wandering into unsafe areas. Most geropsychiatric units are locked, and in a dementia unit, there often is an electronic alarm system to alert staff of patients attempting to leave the secured floor. Staff and visitors need to be vigilant for perilous situations.

Environmental Interventions

The need for stimulation can also be an antecedent to catastrophic reactions. The need for stimulation varies from individual to individual and can change, depending on many factors, including cognitive intactness, alertness, emotional state, and physical state. The amount of stimulation received also influences each patient's behavior. Lack of stimulation or intense stimulation may cause emotional distress and aggression. Generally speaking, the more severe the dementia, the less stimulation can be integrated. The nurse should attempt to determine each patient's optimal level of stimulation at various times of the day. It may be that stimulating environments can be tolerated early in the morning but not in the afternoon when the patient is tired.

Socialization Activities

Overlearned social skills are rarely lost in patients with AD. It is not unusual for the patient with dementia to respond appropriately to a handshake or smile well into the disease process. Even patients who are no longer able to communicate coherently will carry on long discussions with people who are willing to listen and respond (to language that does not make sense). There is a strong risk for social isolation in patients with dementia because of communication difficulties. Reinforcing social remarks and gestures, such as eye contact, smiling, greetings, and farewells, can promote a sense of competency and self-esteem. Pet therapy and "stuffed animal" therapy can also enhance social interaction in cognitively impaired individuals. It is important to remember that patients with dementia do not lose their ability to laugh and play, and the psychosocial benefits of humor are well known.

The nurse who engages a patient with dementia in an activity is encouraged to (1) avoid confronting the patient with the disability; (2) allow the level of autonomy best tolerated by the patient; (3) simplify activities and directions to the point that they can be mastered (e.g., avoid directions such as "use right or left arm" because the patient may be unable to distinguish one from the other); (4) provide adequate structure or directions; and (5) recognize that instructions may not be carried out correctly. It is important to monitor the length of time, crowding, and noise level when the patient participates in a group activity because all of these factors may increase the patient's stress level.

Activities that elicit pleasant memories from an earlier time in the patient's life (reminiscence) may produce a soothing effect. Eliciting pleasant memories may be enhanced by gentle stimulation of the patient's senses, for example, viewing and discussing photo albums, looking at personal memorabilia, providing a favorite food item, playing a musical instrument, or listening to music the person preferred in younger years.

It may be useful to incorporate movement or dance along with a singing exercise. If the patient with dementia resists structured exercise, it may be because of a fear of falling or injury, or of demonstrating to others that his or her health is failing. Patients with dementia often forget how to move or how to coordinate their movements in relation to objects. Therefore, exercise should be light and enjoyable. Encourage the patient to take rest periods at intervals throughout the activity in an effort to minimize stress.

Home Visits

The goal of in-home and community-based long-term care services is to maintain patients in a self-determining environment that provides the most home-like atmosphere possible, allows maximum personal choice for care recipients and caregiver, and encourages optimal family caregiving involvement without overwhelming the resources of the family network. All services for patients with dementia and their families must be provided within a context of continuity of care, a concept that mandates access to a variety of health and supportive services over an unpredictable and changing clinical course.

The effectiveness of having nurses make home visits was recently demonstrated. In a randomized study, elderly residents with psychiatric disorders living in six public housing sites in Baltimore were identified by building staff. Residents in three of the buildings were assigned to receive nursing interventions by visiting nurses, whereas the residents in the other three did not. The interventions included patient counseling and education, liaisons with the patient's social worker, preparation of patient medication with monitoring of adherence and side effects, facilitation of care and support for patient physical health problems, discussion with home health care providers about medication, and monitoring of patient vital signs. Each patient was seen an average of five times. At the end of 26 months, patients receiving the interventions were significantly less depressed and had fewer psychiatric symptoms than did those who did not receive the intervention (Rabins et al., 2000).

Community Actions

Nurses working with patients with dementia are especially knowledgeable about all aspects of the illness and care. These nurses are often involved in local organizations, such as the Alzheimer Association. Issues of care and safety and reimbursement of services often require professional expertise and influence.

Family Interventions 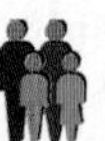

Caregivers are faced with extreme pressures. Caregivers are either spouses of the person with AD or children, usually a daughter, who also have other responsibilities, such as children and a job. The caregiver often feels isolated, frustrated, and trapped. The potential for patient abuse is significant, especially if agitated and aggressive behaviors are present in the relative. The use of home health nurses has been investigated relative to their impact on the burden and depression of elderly caregivers. The caregivers who used the home health services were significantly less burdened and less depressed than were those who did not use these services (Mignor, 2000).

It is important that the nurse recognize the need of the caregivers for support and relief from the 24-hour responsibility. Determining availability of family members or friends to assist with personal care of the patient should be included in the assessment (see Box 32.11). Caregivers should be encouraged to attend support groups and carve out personal time. Educational and training programs may help in understanding the complex nature of the disorder (Box 32.12). Community resources, such as day care centers, home health agencies, and other community services, can be an important aspect of nursing care for the patient with dementia.

Evaluation and Treatment Outcomes

The objectives of nursing interventions are to help the patient with dementia remain as independent as possible and to function at the highest cognitive, physical, emotional, spiritual, and social levels. The maximum level of functional ability can be promoted when nursing care is related to and based on the remaining abilities of the

BOX 32.11

***Psychoeducation Checklist:* Tips for Caregivers**

When caring for the patient with dementia, be sure to include the caregivers, as appropriate, and address the following topic areas in the teaching plan:

- Psychopharmacologic agents, if used, including drug action, dosage, frequency, and possible adverse effects
- Rest and activity
- Consistency in routines
- Nutrition and hydration
- Sleep and comfort measures
- Protective environment
- Communication and social interaction
- Diversional measures
- Community resources

BOX 32.12

***Research for Best Practice* Helping Families Provide Safe Care**

Gerdner, L. A., Buckwalter, K. C., & Reed, D. (2002). Impact of a psychoeducational intervention on caregiver response to behavioral problems. Nursing Research, 51(6), 363–374.

THE QUESTION: Because family members care for persons with Alzheimer disease (AD) who often lack adequate support and training for this all-consuming job, research was undertaken to determine the efficacy of a longitudinal, multisite, community-based intervention designed to teach home caregivers to manage behavioral problems in persons with AD.

METHODS: A psychoeducational nursing intervention was implemented for 132 caregiver/care recipient dyads. Family members were taught to modify the environment to compensate for the care recipients' cognitive and functional impairment, as well as their decreased tolerance to environmental stimuli. Interventions included lowering the temperature on the hot water heater to prevent inadvertent scalding, installing a toilet seat of contrasting color to facilitate visualization, and removing mirrors to eliminate misinterpretation of environmental stimuli. In addition, caregivers were encouraged to develop activities that would promote the care recipient's past interests and minimize television viewing. The comparison group (105) received routine information and referrals for case management, community-based services.

FINDINGS: These interventions had a positive impact on both the frequency of and response to problem behaviors among spouses who were caregivers.

IMPLICATIONS FOR NURSING: Family interventions are important for the person with dementia. Formally including these interventions in the treatment plan will help ensure the implementation of these strategies within families.

patient. Patients who receive diagnoses of AD or other types of dementia have a wide and varying range of functional abilities. As cognitive decline progresses, there is a tendency for caregivers to perform more and more tasks for the patient. It is essential to assess for strengths and to assist in the maintenance of existing skills. Adaptive and appropriate behaviors continue to some degree in people with dementia, even in the presence of increasing cognitive decline. It is important for nursing interventions to focus on more than the maintenance of optimal physical functional ability; interventions also must focus on meeting psychological, social, and spiritual needs of the patient with dementia.

Nurses can maintain quality of life if they protect a patient's overall well-being by balancing physical, mental, social, and spiritual health. Figure 32.6 illustrates the truly biopsychosocial aspects of the treatment of individuals with dementia by summarizing potential outcomes of nursing care.

Continuum of Care

Community Care

It is estimated that more than 7 of 10 people with AD live at home. Almost 75% of home care is provided by family and friends. Unpaid caregivers provide $83 billion economic worth (Alzheimer Association, 2007). Use of community-based services (e.g., home health aides, home-delivered meals, adult day care, respite care, caregiver support groups) often extends the amount of time an individual with AD or a related disorder can safely remain in the home. However, the progressive impair-

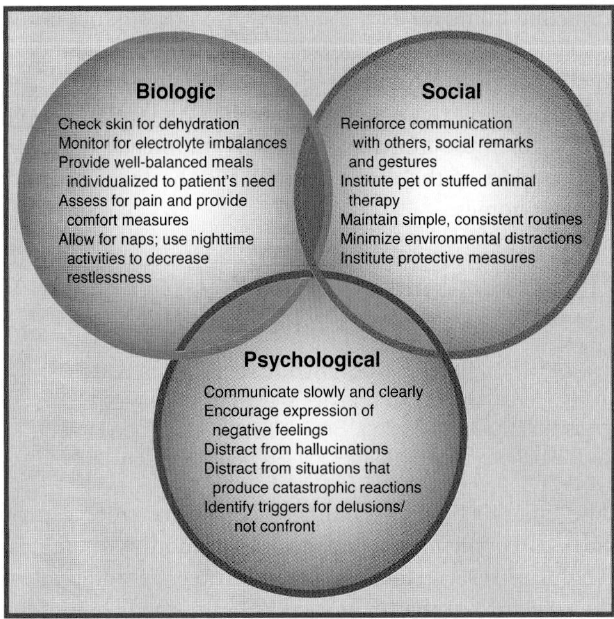

FIGURE 32.6. Biopsychosocial interventions for patients with dementia.

ment associated with dementia often culminates with placement in a long-term care facility. The nurse working in a physician's office or ambulatory setting may provide ongoing information about management and problem solving. The public health nurse may provide intermittent assessment and ongoing case management. Nurses working in programs designed specifically for patients with dementia, such as adult day care, also practice the role of educator. The nurse who is simply a neighbor or family member is often asked to advise about care of the person with dementia. The complex and interrelated problems often observed in patients with neuropsychiatric disorders will increasingly demand the attention of nurses in all health care settings. Cooperation among health care providers of different disciplines and in various settings is needed to meet the highly individualized needs of patients with neuropsychiatric deficits.

Inpatient-Focused Care

Comprehensive admission assessment, followed by the development of an individualized (and constantly updated) care plan that involves the patient, significant others, and a variety of health care professionals, is the foundation of an effective and efficient postdischarge plan. Attention to all aspects of this process is necessary to ensure that the goal of continuity of care is achieved. The hospital-based nurse may initiate family education and counseling as part of discharge planning. For more information on caring for the patient with dementia, see Nursing Care Plan 32.1.

Nursing Home Care

As the dementia progresses, many patients are placed in a nursing home for care. Nursing care in a nursing home is usually delivered by nurses' aides, who need support and direction. Interestingly, people with dementia require complex nursing care, but the skill level of people caring for these individuals often is minimal. Education and support of the direct caregiver is the focus of most nursing homes.

Mental Health Promotion

> **KEY CONCEPT: Cognitive reserve** refers to the brain's ability to operate effectively even when there is disruption in functioning. Brain structure and function buffer the effects of neuropathology (Richards & Deary, 2005).

The emerging understanding of cognitive reserve provides direction for mental health promotion strategies. Cognitive reserve focuses on the protective potential of the structure of the brain such as brain size, neural density, and synaptic connectivity and its function including the efficiency of the neural networks. It is hypothesized that there are factors that influence the development of cognitive reserve that range from early social and material environments, through inputs of education, occupation, socioeconomic environment to physical health, health behaviors, and degree of engaged lifestyle activity (Richards et al., 2005).

There are lifelong activities that help build and maintain cognitive reserve. Physical exercise, nutrition, stress management, and social engagement with family and friends are associated with positive cognitive outcomes. Levels of education and literacy are repeatedly shown to be related to higher cognitive functioning (USDHHS, 2005). Mental health promotion includes helping patients develop awareness of the importance of engaging in a lifestyle that supports the development of cognitive reserve.

OTHER DEMENTIAS

Dementia symptoms may occur as a result of a number of disorders and underlying etiologies. The subsequent sections provide a brief description of some of the dementias listed in the *Diagnostic and Statistical Manual of Mental Disorders*, 4th edition, text revision (*DSM-IV-TR*; APA, 2000). In each case, the classic symptoms of dementia (e.g., memory impairment with a number of other cognitive deficits) must be present. Nursing interventions for all dementias are similar to those described for individuals with AD.

Vascular Dementia

Vascular dementia (also known as *multi-infarct dementia*) is seen in about 20% of patients with dementia, most commonly people between the ages of 60 and 75 years. Slightly more men than women are affected. Vascular dementia results when a series of small strokes damage or destroy brain tissue. These are commonly referred to as "ministrokes" or transient ischemic attacks (TIAs), and several TIAs may occur before the affected individual becomes aware of the symptoms of vascular dementia. Most often, a blood clot or plaques (fatty deposits) block the vessels that supply blood to the brain, causing a stroke. However, a stroke can also occur when a blood vessel bursts in the brain.

The primary causes of stroke include high blood cholesterol levels, diabetes, heart disease, and high blood pressure. Of these, high blood pressure is the greatest risk factor for vascular dementia. It is essential that anyone who demonstrates symptoms of dementia or who has a history of stroke should have a complete physical examination that includes neurologic and neuropsychological evaluation, diet and medication history, review of recent

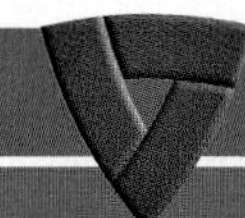

Nursing Care Plan 32.1

Patient With Dementia

LW is a 76-year-old widow who lives independently. Recently, her children have noticed that she is becoming more forgetful and seems to have periods of confusion. She has agreed to have someone help her during the day. Her oldest son lives with her and is with her during the evening and night. LW refuses to see a health care provider but did agree to go in for a routine checkup. Her daughter helped her get dressed and took her to the primary care office.

Setting: Primary care office

Baseline Assessment: A well-groomed woman is accompanied by her daughter. LW says there is nothing wrong, but daughter disagrees. A review of body systems reveals poor hearing and vision but is otherwise unremarkable. MMSE score is 19. Daughter reports that LW has become very suspicious of neighbors and has changed her locks several times.

Associated Psychiatric Diagnosis	Medications
Axis I: Probable dementia of the Alzheimer type Axis II: None Axis III: History of breast cancer, unilateral mastectomy Arthritis Axis IV: Social problems (suspiciousness) GAF = Current 70 Potential 70	Galantamine (Razadyne) 4 mg bid, titrate to 8 mg bid over 4 weeks.

Nursing Diagnosis 1: Impaired Memory

Defining Characteristics	Related Factors
Inability to recall information Inability to recall past events Observed instances of forgetfulness Forgets to perform daily activities—grooming	Neurocognitive changes associated with dementia

Outcomes

Initial	Long-term
Maintain or improve current memory	Delay cognitive decline associated with dementia

Interventions

Interventions	Rationale	Ongoing Assessment
Develop memory cues in home. Have clocks and calendars well displayed. Make lists for patients.	Maintaining current level of memory involves providing cues that will help patient recall information.	Contact family members for patient's ability to use memory cues.
Teach patient and family about taking an acetylcholinesterase inhibitor. Review expected effects, side effects, and adverse effects. Develop a titration schedule with family to decrease the appearance of side effects.	Confidence and self-esteem improve when a person looks well-groomed.	Monitor response to suggestions.
Observe patient for visuospatial impairment. If present, sequence habitual activities such as eating, dressing, bathing, etc.	Visuospatial impairment is one of the symptoms of dementia.	Observe for appropriate dress, bathing, eating, etc.

Evaluation

Outcomes	Revised Outcomes	Interventions
LW did have some improvement in memory. Suspiciousness and behavioral symptoms improved.	Continue maintaining memory.	Continue with memory cues and galantamine.

stressors, and an array of laboratory tests. Damage to the brain in vascular dementia is usually apparent using computed tomography scans or magnetic resonance imaging. At autopsy, multifocal lesions may be found, rather than the more generalized cortical atrophy characteristic of AD.

The behavior changes that result from vascular dementia are similar to those found in AD, such as memory loss, depression, emotional lability or emotional incontinence (including inappropriate laughing or crying), wandering or getting lost in familiar places, bladder or bowel incontinence, difficulty following instructions, gait changes such as small shuffling steps, and problems handling daily activities such as money management. However, these symptoms usually begin more suddenly, rather than developing slowly, as is the case in AD. Often, the neurologic symptoms associated with a TIA are minimal and may last only a few days, including slight weakness in an extremity, dizziness, or slurred speech. Thus, the clinical progression is often described as intermittent and fluctuating, or of step-like deterioration, with the patient's cognitive and functional status improving or plateauing for a period of time, followed by a rapid decline in function after another series of small strokes. The Hachinski Ischemia Score (Box 32.13) may be helpful in differentiating vascular dementia from AD and in summarizing the symptoms more closely related to vascular dementia.

Treatment aims to reduce the primary risk factors for vascular dementia, including hypertension, diabetes, and additional strokes. Interventions that reduce the tendency of the blood to clot and of platelets to aggregate include using medications and lifestyle changes, such as diet, exercise, and smoking cessation to control hypertension, high cholesterol, heart disease, and diabetes. Increasingly, physicians are recommending drugs such as aspirin to help prevent clots from forming in the small blood vessels. Occasionally, surgical procedures such as carotid endarterectomy may be needed to remove blockages in the carotid artery.

BOX 32.13

Hachinski Ischemia Score

Abrupt onset	2
Stepwise progression	1
Fluctuating course	2
Nocturnal confusion	1
Relative preservation of personality	1
Depression	1
Somatic complaints	1
Emotional incontinence	1
History of hypertension	1
History of stroke	2
Evidence of associated atherosclerosis	1
Focal neurologic symptoms	2
Focal neurologic signs	2
Alzheimer disease if scores total	4 or less
Vascular dementias if scores total	7 or more

Hachinski, V. C. (1983). Differential diagnosis of Alzheimer dementia: Multi-infarct dementia. In B. Reisberg (Ed.), *Alzheimer disease* (pp. 188–192). New York: Free Press/Macmillan.

Dementia Caused by Other General Medical Conditions

People of any age, race, or gender are at risk for dementia caused by a medical condition known to cause cerebral pathology. Elderly people are particularly vulnerable to the development of dementia caused by general medical conditions because so many older people are affected by one or more chronic medical illnesses. Strong relationships have been reported between chronic medical illness and the development of dementia. Of the conditions that cause dementia, about 10% are completely treatable, and about 25% to 30% cease to progress as long as treatment is initiated before irreversible brain damage has occurred. Finally, about 50% to 60% of patients with dementia continue to decline in spite of treatment.

Dementia Caused by AIDS

Dementia associated with AIDS has been called AIDS dementia complex (ADC). ADC has been observed in nearly two thirds of all patients with AIDS. AIDS is caused by human immunodeficiency virus-1 (HIV-1), which infects and destroys T lymphocytes as well as the central nervous system (CNS). HIV-1 directly invades the CNS and allows opportunistic infections of the CNS and other organ systems. Although there has been a proportional increase in ADC at AIDS diagnosis, survival after ADC has improved markedly in the era of highly active antiretroviral therapy (HAART) (Dore et al., 2003).

Dementia Caused by Head Trauma

When head trauma occurs in the context of a single injury, the resulting dementia is usually not progressive, but repeated head injury (e.g., from the sport of boxing) may lead to a progressive dementia. When the nurse observes progressive decline in intellectual functioning after a single incident of head trauma, the possibility of another superimposed process must be considered. Head injury associated with a prolonged loss of consciousness (days to months) may be followed by delirium or dementia or a profound alteration in personality.

The degree and type of cognitive impairment or behavioral disturbances demonstrated by a person with head trauma depend on the location and extent of the brain injury (as with other forms of dementia). Repeated head injuries, such as those sustained by young, healthy boxers, may lead to *dementia pugi listica*, or "punch-drunk syndrome." Although the exact mechanism of this disorder is unknown, it appears likely that early damage to neurons and their connections manifests later clinically, when the combination of normal neuronal cell loss and prior damage summate to reach a threshold of impaired cognitive function.

Dementia Caused by Parkinson's Disease

Parkinson's disease is a neurologic syndrome of unknown etiology, which manifests as a disorder of movement, with a slow and progressive course. Clinical manifestations of Parkinson's disease are **bradykinesia** (the slowing of body movements), rigidity, resting tremor, and postural changes. The person's gait is unstable, which results in frequent falls. Parkinson's disease may appear at any time after a person reaches 30 years of age, but the median age of onset is about 70 years of age. A subcortical dementia can be diagnosed in about 20% to 60% of patients with Parkinson's disease (APA, 2000). Although investigators do not know why, there is considerable pathologic overlap between Parkinson's disease and AD. Medical treatment of Parkinson's disease typically is with anticholinergics and dopamine agonists. It is important for nurses to know that in patients with dementia caused by Parkinson's disease, anticholinergic medications are likely to increase cognitive impairment (Katzenschlager, Sampaio, Costa, & Lees, 2003).

Dementia Caused by Huntington's Disease

Huntington's disease is a progressive, genetically transmitted autosomal dominant disorder characterized by choreiform movements and mental abnormalities. The onset is usually between the ages of 30 and 50 years, but onset occurs before 5 years of age in the juvenile form or as late as 85 years of age in the late-onset form. The disease affects men and women equally. A person with Huntington's disease usually lives for 15 to 20 years after diagnosis (APA, 2000). The dementia syndrome of Huntington's disease is characterized by insidious changes in behavior and personality. Typically, the dementia is frontal, which means that the person demonstrates prominent behavioral problems and disruption of attention.

Dementia Caused by Pick's Disease

Pick's disease is a rare form of dementia that is clinically similar to AD. The etiology of Pick's disease is unknown. Pick's disease particularly affects the frontal and temporal lobes of the brain (APA, 2000). The disorder usually manifests in individuals between the ages of 50 and 60 years, although it can occur among older individuals. Pick's disease is not readily distinguishable from AD until autopsy (APA, 2000), when the distinctive intraneuronal Pick's bodies can be identified microscopically.

Dementia Caused by Creutzfeldt-Jakob Disease

Creutzfeldt-Jakob disease is a rare, rapidly fatal brain disorder. Many of the symptoms seen in Creutzfeldt-Jakob disease are similar to those found in AD and other dementias. However, changes in the brain tissue are different in Creutzfeldt-Jakob disease and are best differentiated by surgical biopsy or on autopsy. Scientists speculate that Creutzfeldt-Jakob disease is caused by a "slow" and "unconventional" virus because it has a relatively long incubation period (3 years or more) before symptoms begin to appear. The precise mechanism by which the virus affects the brain is unknown (APA, 2000).

At present, there is no effective treatment for the disease, and nothing has been found to slow progression of the illness, although antiviral drug studies are ongoing. Because of its rapid clinical course, an important nursing role is assisting family members to understand and come to terms with the illness and to make decisions related to treatment setting and life-sustaining treatments. Creutzfeldt-Jakob disease progresses much more rapidly than most dementias, and death usually occurs within 1 year after onset, although some evidence suggests that extensive changes in the brain may be present before symptoms appear.

Only about 3,000 cases of Creutzfeldt-Jakob disease have been reported in the past 70 years, resulting in an annual incidence of about 1 per 1 million population. The disease strikes both men and women, most commonly between the ages of 50 and 75 years. Interestingly, there appears to be a genetic component to Creutzfeldt-Jakob disease (Cummings, 2003). Inhabitants of certain rural areas of the world, such as Slovakia and Chile, and Libyan-born Jews living in Israel have a much higher incidence of the disease. In the United States, about 15% of people with Creutzfeldt-Jakob disease have a positive family history of early-onset dementia (APA, 2000).

Person-to-person transmission of Creutzfeldt-Jakob disease is rare (but possible), and it can be transmitted from people to animals and between animals. Evidence indicates that the virus can be introduced into the nervous system of healthy patients during medical procedures, such as corneal transplantation, implantation of contaminated electrodes in the brain, and injection of contaminated growth hormones (a few health care workers exposed to the virus, probably through blood and spinal fluids, have experienced the disease). Because of the transmissible nature of Creutzfeldt-Jakob disease, and because the virus is not easily destroyed, strict criteria for the handling of infected tissues and other contaminated materials have been developed.

Substance-Induced Persisting Dementia

If dementia results from the persisting effects of a substance (e.g., drugs of abuse, a medication, or exposure to toxins), substance-induced persisting dementia is diagnosed. Other causes of dementia (e.g., dementia caused by a general medical condition) must always be considered, even in a person with a dependence on or exposure to a substance. For example, head injuries often result from substance use and may be the underlying cause of the dementia syndrome (APA, 2000).

Drugs of abuse are the most common toxins in young adults, and prescription drugs are the most common toxins in elderly people. In older patients, dementia results from use of long-acting benzodiazepines, barbiturates, meprobamate (Equanil), and a host of other drugs, depending on their dose and the length of time they have been used. Drugs such as flurazepam (Dalmane), with a half-life of more than 120 hours, accumulate rapidly in a person's body. Other drugs accumulate more slowly or require relatively high doses for toxicity to develop. A toxic etiology should be suspected in every patient with a probable diagnosis of dementia. The nurse should inquire about exposure to drugs and toxins (exposure to toxins at work sites, medication use, and recreational drug use) for each patient with dementia, and any substances known to be potentially injurious to the nervous system should be withdrawn if at all possible.

Most of the dementias in this category are related to chronic alcohol abuse. Understanding the cognitive deficits associated with chronic alcohol consumption is complicated. Alcoholic dementia is directly related to the toxic effects of alcohol, although the vitamin deficiencies associated with alcoholism (thiamine and niacin) are also known to be etiologically related to dementia. Individuals with alcoholism also have a high incidence of systemic illnesses that can affect cognition (e.g., cirrhosis, cardiomyopathy), and they are susceptible to repeated head injuries, which carry cognitive consequences of their own.

Much of our knowledge about cognitive deficits in individuals with alcoholism comes from the study of patients with Korsakoff's syndrome, which is a profound deficit in the ability to form new memories and is associated with a variable deficit in recall of old memories, despite a clear sensorium. Further careful examination reveals a flattening of drives, unconcern about incapacity, and profound apathy. Nonetheless, Korsakoff's syndrome does not qualify as a dementia; rather, it is considered an amnestic syndrome (or restricted deficit of memory). In alcohol-induced dementia, the cognitive deficits span a wider range of functioning than with Korsakoff's syndrome (see Chapter 25).

Chemicals and organic compounds that impair functioning of the CNS usually have their primary effects on other body systems: the gastrointestinal, renal, hepatic, blood-forming, and peripheral nervous systems. For example, metal poisonings generally produce gastrointestinal symptoms and peripheral neuropathy. Cognitive changes with poisoning tend to be more characteristic of delirium than dementia, with altered levels of consciousness a prominent feature. Table 32.1 lists some of the organic compounds or chemicals that can cause symptoms of dementia; related distinguishing symptoms are also included.

Many adolescents and indigent adults engage in the act of "huffing" because the cost of purchasing spray paint, hair spray, glue, and other aerosol products is relatively inexpensive (compared with illicit street drugs). The nurse is reminded to evaluate people who abuse drugs for signs of cognitive impairment because neural and cognitive symptoms tend to appear before permanent brain damage occurs. It is also important to realize that the patient's cognitive status may not immediately improve after discontinuation of use of the offending agent. The effects of drugs taken for a long period may be long lasting, and improvement may follow discontinuation of drug use only slowly. For example, in dementia associated with chronic alcoholism, cognition may improve only after many months of abstinence.

AMNESTIC DISORDER

Amnestic disorder is characterized by an impairment in memory that is caused either by the direct physiologic effects of a general medical condition or by the persisting effects of a substance (e.g., a drug of abuse, a medication, or exposure to a toxin) (APA, 2000). More specifically, amnestic disorder is diagnosed when there is severe memory impairment without other significant cognitive impairments (e.g., aphasia, apraxia, agnosia, or disturbances in executive functioning) or impaired consciousness, which would indicate a diagnosis of either delirium or dementia.

The amnestic disorders share a common symptom, memory impairment, but are differentiated by etiology. Amnestic disorders often occur as the result of pathologic processes. Traumatic brain injury, cerebrovascular events, or specific types of neurotoxic exposure (e.g., carbon monoxide poisoning) may lead to an acute onset of an amnestic disorder. Other conditions, such as prolonged substance abuse, chronic neurotoxic exposure, or sustained nutritional deficiency (e.g., thiamine deficiency) create a more insidious onset. The age of the patient and course of amnestic disorder may vary, depending on the pathologic process causing the disorder.

Amnestic disorder is characterized by an impaired ability to learn new information or an inability to recall previously learned information (short-term recall) or past events (long-term recall), with preservation of immediate recall (immediate-recall deficits are commonly associated with dementia) (APA, 2000). Although short-term and long-term memory are impaired in most patients who have a form of organic brain disease, the occurrence of memory impairment as a relatively circumscribed deficit is rare. Short-term or recent memory is usually more severely impaired than remote memory with an amnestic disorder, and no deficit may be observed when the patient is asked to recall events or dates that have been overlearned. Most patients with deficits in short-term recall are disoriented to place and time; therefore, disorientation is a common sign of amnestic disorder. However, in some forms of amnestic disorder, the patient may remember information from the very remote past better than more recent events (e.g., the patient may have a vivid memory of a hospital stay that occurred many years ago, but may have no idea that he or she is currently in the hospital) (APA, 2000).

Amnestic disorders are often preceded by an evolving and variable clinical picture, which includes confusion and disorientation, occasionally with attentional deficits that suggest a delirium (e.g., amnestic disorder caused by thiamine deficiency). Confabulation (filling gaps in memory with imaginary events) may be noted during the early stages of amnestic disorder but usually disappears with time. For this reason, it may be important for the nurse to obtain corroborating information from family members or other informants when gathering historical information on the patient. Most patients with a severe amnestic disorder lack insight into their memory deficits and may adamantly deny the presence of memory impairment despite evidence to the contrary. This lack of insight may lead to accusations against others or, in some instances, to agitation. Some individuals may acknowledge that they have memory problems but appear unconcerned. Apathy, lack of initiative, emotional blandness, or other changes in personality are not uncommon with amnestic disorder.

MOVIE viewing GUIDES

SUMMARY OF KEY POINTS

- Neuropsychiatric disorders, such as delirium and dementia, are characterized clinically by significant deficits in cognition or memory that represent a clear-cut change from a previous level of functioning. In some disorders, the loss of cognitive function is progressive, such as in AD. It is important to recognize the differences because the interventions and expected outcomes of the two syndromes are different.
- Delirium is characterized by a disturbance in consciousness and a change in cognition that develops over a short period of time. It requires rapid detection and treatment because in 25% of cases, it is a sign of impending death.
- Nursing assessment is critical in determining the onset of the confusion and disorientation. A thorough nursing assessment includes recent health status changes and practices such as OTC medications.
- Usually, delirium is caused by a combination of precipitating factors. The most commonly identified causes are medications, infections (particularly urinary tract and upper respiratory tract infections), fluid and electrolyte imbalance, and metabolic disturbances such as electrolyte imbalance or poor nutrition. Other important predisposing factors include advanced age, brain damage, pre-existing dementia, and biopsychosocial stressors.
- The primary goal of treatment of delirium is prevention or resolution of the acute confusional episode with return to previous cognitive status and interventions focusing on (1) elimination or correction of the underlying cause, and (2) symptomatic and safety and supportive measures.
- Dementia is characterized by the gradual onset of decline in cognitive function, especially memory, usually accompanied by changes in behavior and personality. There are numerous causes of the symptoms of dementia, some of which are reversible, such as hypoxia, carbon monoxide poisoning, and vitamin deficiencies.
- AD is an example of a progressive, degenerative dementia. Treatment efforts currently focus on reduction of cognitive symptoms (e.g., memory loss, confusion, and problems with learning, speech, and reasoning) in attempts to improve the quality of life for both patients and their caregivers.
- Research efforts continue to focus on understanding the relationship among the development of the beta-amyloid plaques, neurofibrillary tangles, and cell death.
- Nursing care of a person with dementia depends on the stage of the disease and the availability of family caregivers.
- Some of the psychosocial stressors known to precipitate delirium and contribute to worsening dementia include sensory overload or underload, immobilization, sleep deprivation, fatigue, pain or hunger, change in routine (pace or caregiver), or demands beyond the patient's ability.
- Educating and supporting families and caregivers through the progressive cognitive decline and behavior changes is essential to ensuring proper care.
- There are several mental health strategies (exercise, education, cognitive stimulation) that support and

protect a person's cognitive reserve. A healthy cognitive reserve is thought to be protective against neuropathologic insults.

■ Symptoms of dementia may occur as a result of a number of disorders, including vascular and amnestic disorders, head trauma, AIDS, and substance abuse and as a symptom of Parkinson's, Huntington's, Pick's, and Creutzfeldt-Jakob diseases.

CRITICAL THINKING CHALLENGES

1 What factors should the nurse consider in differentiating AD from vascular dementia?
2 Compare the defining characteristics and related risk factors of acute confusion with those for the NANDA diagnoses of Impaired Thought Processes and Sensory/Perceptual Disturbances. What are the differences and similarities between the recommended nursing interventions for delirium and dementia? What is the theoretic base for these similarities and differences?
3 Describe three ways in which medical disease can disrupt brain functioning, and relate these mechanisms to the neuropsychiatric disorders presented in this chapter.
4 Suggest reasons that older adults are particularly vulnerable to the development of neuropsychiatric disorders.
5 Compare the nursing care of a person with delirium versus one with dementia. What are the similarities and differences in the care?
6 The physical environment is particularly important to the patient with dementia. Every effort should be made to modify the physical environment to compensate for the cognitive and functional impairment associated with AD and related disorders, including safety measures and the avoidance of misleading stimuli. Visualize your last experience in a health care setting (hospital, nursing home, day care program, or home care setting). Identify environmental factors that could be misleading or stress producing to a person with impaired cognition (dementia), and identify ways to modify this environment to alleviate some of the stressors or misleading stimuli.

Iris. 2001. This film tells the story of British novelist Iris Murdoch (played by Judi Dench and Kate Winslet) and her relationship with her husband John Bayley (Jim Broadbent & Huh Bonneville) during the last 5 years of her life. Based on Bayley's memoir, *Elegy for Iris*, the film depicts Ms. Murdoch's decline into dementia and the stress associated with caregiving. This wonderful movie shows the suffering of AD, but also shows the strength of relationships. The film contrasts the start of their relationship when Iris was an outgoing, dominant individual and John was a timid, shy scholarly partner, with the two older adults who created a loving bond that provided the fabric of the last days of Iris' life.

VIEWING POINTS: Identify the symptoms of the progressive illness throughout the film. Were there any "breaking points" for the caregiver? Were there aspects of Iris' personality that were sustained throughout the course of her life that were evident at the end? What nursing interventions would have been helpful to support her cognitive functioning?

REFERENCES

Alzheimer Association (2007a). *Alzheimer Disease Facts and Figures.* Chicago: Author.

American Psychiatric Association. (2000). *Diagnostic and statistical manual of mental disorders* (4th ed., Text revision). Washington, DC: Author.

Bair, B. D. (2000). Presentations and recognition of common psychiatric disorders in the elderly. *Clinical Geriatrics, 8*(2), 26, 28–29, 33–34.

Barrick, A. L., Rader, J., Hoeffer, B., & Sloane, P. D. (Eds.). (2002). *Bathing without a battle: Personal care of individuals with dementia.* New York: Springer.

Becker, J. T., Davis, S. W., Hayashi, B. S., Meltzer, C. C., Toga, A.W., Lopez, O. L., & Thompson, P. M., et al. (2006). Three-dimensional patterns of hippocampal atrophy in mild cognitive impairment. *Archives of Neurology, 63*(1), 97–101.

Bennett, D. A., Wilson, R. S., Schneider, J. A., Evans, D. A., Mendes de Leion, C. F., Arnold, S. E., et al. (2003). Education modifies the relation of AD pathology to level of cognitive function in older persons. *Neurology, 60*(12), 1909–1915.

Boettger, S., & Breitbart, W. (2007). Atypical antipsychotics in the management of delirium: A review of the empirical literature. *Palliative & Supportive Care, 3*(3), 227–237.

Clavel, D. S. (1999). Vocalizations among cognitively impaired elders. *Geriatric Nursing, 20*, 90–93.

Cooper, B. (2002). Thinking preventively about dementia: a review. *International Journal of Geriatric Psychiatry, 17*(10), 895–906.

Cummings, J. L. (2003). *The neuropsychiatry of Alzheimer disease and related dementias.* London: Martin Dunitz, Ltd.

Curran, S., & Wattis, J. (2006). Hidden conditions. Detecting delirium. *Geriatric Medicine, 36*(10), 41, 47.

Dochterman, J. M., & Bulechek, G. M. (2004). *Nursing interventions classification* (NIC) (4th ed.). St. Louis: Mosby.

Dore, G. J., McDonald, A., Li, Y., Kaldor, J. M., Brew, B. J., & National HIV Surveillance Committee. (2003). Marked improvement in survival following AIDS dementia complex in the era of highly active antiretroviral therapy. *AIDS, 17*(10), 1539–1545.

Evercare, & National Alliance for Caregiving. (2006). Study of caregivers in decline: Findings from a national survey. Retrieved April 4, 2007, from http://www.caregiving.org/data/Caregivers%20in%20Decline%20Study-FINAL-lowres.pdf

Galvin, J. E., Roe, C. M, Powlishta, K. K., Coats, M. A., Muich, S. J., Grant, E., et al. (2005). The AD8: A brief informant interview to detect dementia. *Neurology, 65*(4), 559–564.

Galvin, J. E., Roe, C. M., Xiong, C., & Morris, J. C. (2006). Validity and reliability of the AD8 informant interview in dementia. *Neurology, 67*(11), 1942–1948.

Ganguli, M., Dodge, H. H., Shen, C., & DeKosky, S. T. (2004). Mild cognitive impairment, amnestic type: An epidemiologic study. *Neurology, 63*(1), 115–121.

Gerdner, L. A., Buckwalter, K. C., & Reed, D. (2002). Impact of a psychoeducational intervention on caregiver response to behavioral problems. *Nursing Research, 51*(6), 363–374.

Guérin, O., Andrieu, S., Schneider, M., Milano, M., Boulahssass, R., Brocker, P., & Vellas, B. (2005). Different modes of weight loss in Alzheimer disease: a prospective study of 395 patients. *American Journal of Clinical Nutrition, 82*(2), 435–441.

Gleason, O. C. (2003). Delirium. *American Family Physician, 67*(5), 1027–1034.

Hachinski, V. C. (1983). Differential diagnosis of Alzheimer dementia: Multi-infarct dementia. In B. Reisberg (Ed.), *Alzheimer disease* (pp. 188–192). New York: Free Press/Macmillan.

Hoeffer, B., Talerico, K. A., Rasin, J., Mitchell, C. M., Stewart, B. J., & McKenzie, D. (2006). Assisting cognitively impaired nursing home residents with bathing: effects of two bathing interventions on caregiving. *Gerontologist, 46*(4), 524–532.

Jones, R. N., Yang, F. M., Zhang, Y., Kiely, D. K., Marcantonio, E.R., & Inouye, S. K. (2006). Interrelationship of delirium and dementia: Does educational attainment contribute to risk for delirium? A potential role for cognitive reserve. *Journal of Gerontology A: Biological & Medical Sciences*, 61A(12), 1307–1311.

Katzenschlager, R., Sampaio, C., Costa, J., & Lees, A. (2003). Anticholinergics for symptomatic management of Parkinson's disease. *The Cochrane Database of Systematic Reviews* (2):CD003735.

Kolanowski, A., & Litaker, M. (2006). Social interaction, premorbid personality, and agitation in nursing home residents with dementia. *Archives of Psychiatric Nursing, 20*(1), 12–20.

Manly, J. J., Touradji, P. L., Tang, M. X., & Stern, Y. (2003). Literacy and memory decline among ethnically diverse elders. *Journal of Clinical and Experimental Neuropsychology, 25*(5), 6880–6890.

Marcantonio, E. R., Rudolph, J. L., Culley, D., Crosby, F., Alsop, D., & Inouye, S. K. (2006). Serum biomarkers for delirium. *Journal of Gerontology: Medical Sciences, 61A*(12), 1281–1286.

Meeks, T. W., Ropacki, S. A., & Jeste, D. V. (2006). The neurobiology of neuropsychiatric syndromes in dementia. *Current Opinion in Psychiatry, 19*(6), 581–586.

Mignor, D. (2000). Effectiveness of use of home health nurses to decrease burden and depression of elderly caregivers. *Journal of Psychosocial Nursing & Mental Health Services, 38*(7), 34–41.

National Alliance for Caregiving and AARP (2004). Caregiving in the U.S. Retrieved on April 4, 2007, from www.caregiving.org.

Neal, M., & Briggs, M. (2003). *Validation therapy for dementia. The Cochrane Database of Systematic Reviews* (2): (CD001394).

NANDA International. (2007). *Nursing diagnoses: Definitions & classification 2007-2008*. Philadelphia: Author.

Pettersson, A. F., Engardt, M., & Wahlund, L. (2002). Activity level and balance in subjects with mild Alzheimer disease. *Dementia & Geriatric Cognitive Disorders, 13*(4), 213–216.

Potter, J. (2006). The prevention, diagnosis and management of delirium in older people: concise guidelines. *Clinical Medicine: Journal of the Royal College of Physicians of London 6*(3), 303–308.

Rabins, P. V., Black, B. S., Roca, R., German, P., McGuire, M., Robbins, B., et al. (2000). Effectiveness of a nurse-based outreach program for identifying and treating psychiatric illness in the elderly. *Journal of the American Medical Association, 283*, 2802–2809.

Reisberg, B., Doody, R., Stöffler, A., Schmitt, F., Ferris, S., & Jörg Möbius, H. (2003). Memantine in moderate-to-severe Alzheimer disease. *New England Journal of Medicine, 343*(14), 1333–1334.

Richards, M., & Deary, I. J. (2005). A life course approach to cognitive reserve: A model for cognitive aging and development? *Annals of Neurology, 58*(4), 617–622.

Rogaeva, E. (2002). The solved and unsolved mysteries of the genetics of early-onset Alzheimer disease. *Neuromolecular Medicine, 2*(1), 1–10.

Schuurmans, M. J., Duursma, S. A., & Shortridge-Baggett, L. M. (2001). Early recognition of delirium: Review of the literature [Review]. *Journal of Clinical Nursing, 10*(6), 721–729.

Suh, Y. H., & Checler, F. (2002). Amyloid precursor protein, presenilins, and alpha-synuclein: Molecular pathogenesis and pharmacological applications in Alzheimer disease. *Pharmacological Reviews, 54*(3), 469–525.

Taddei, K., Fisher, C., Laws, S. M., Martins, G., Paton, A., Clarnette, R. M., et al. (2002). Association between presenilin-1 Glu318Gly mutation and familial Alzheimer disease in the Australian population. *Molecular Psychiatry*, 7(7), 776–781.

Tang, M. X., Cross, P., Andrews, H., Jacobs, D. M., Small, S., Bell, K., et al. (2001). Incidence of AD in African-Americans, Caribbean Hispanics, and Caucasians in northern Manhattan. *Neurology, 56*(1), 49–56.

Tractenberg, R. E., Singer, C. M., & Kaye, J. A. (2006). Characterizing sleep problems in persons with Alzheimer disease and normal elderly. *Journal of Sleep Research, 15*(1), 97–103.

Turkel S. B., Trzepacz P. T., & Tavare C. J. (2006). Comparing symptoms of delirium in adults and children. *Psychosomatics. 47*(4), 320–324.

U.S. Centers for Disease Control and Prevention, National Center for Health Statistics. Mortality Data From the National Vital Statistics System. Retrieved on March 26, 2007 from www.cdc.gov/nchs/deaths.htm

United States Department of Health and Human Services (U.S. DHHS). (2005). *National Institute on Aging, 2004-2005 Alzheimer Disease Progress Report.* National Institutes of Health Publication No. 05-5724.

USDHHS (2006). Alzheimer Disease Medications Fact Sheet. Alzheimer Disease Education & Referral (ADEAR) Center, National Institute on Aging, National Institutes of Health, NIH Publication No. 03-3431. Retrieved April 6, 2007, from http://www.nia.nih.gov/NR/rdonlyres/5178456B-4E16-4A71-A704-46637C6FE61B/5574/AD_Medications_FactSheet121906.pdf

UNIT VIII

Care of Special Populations

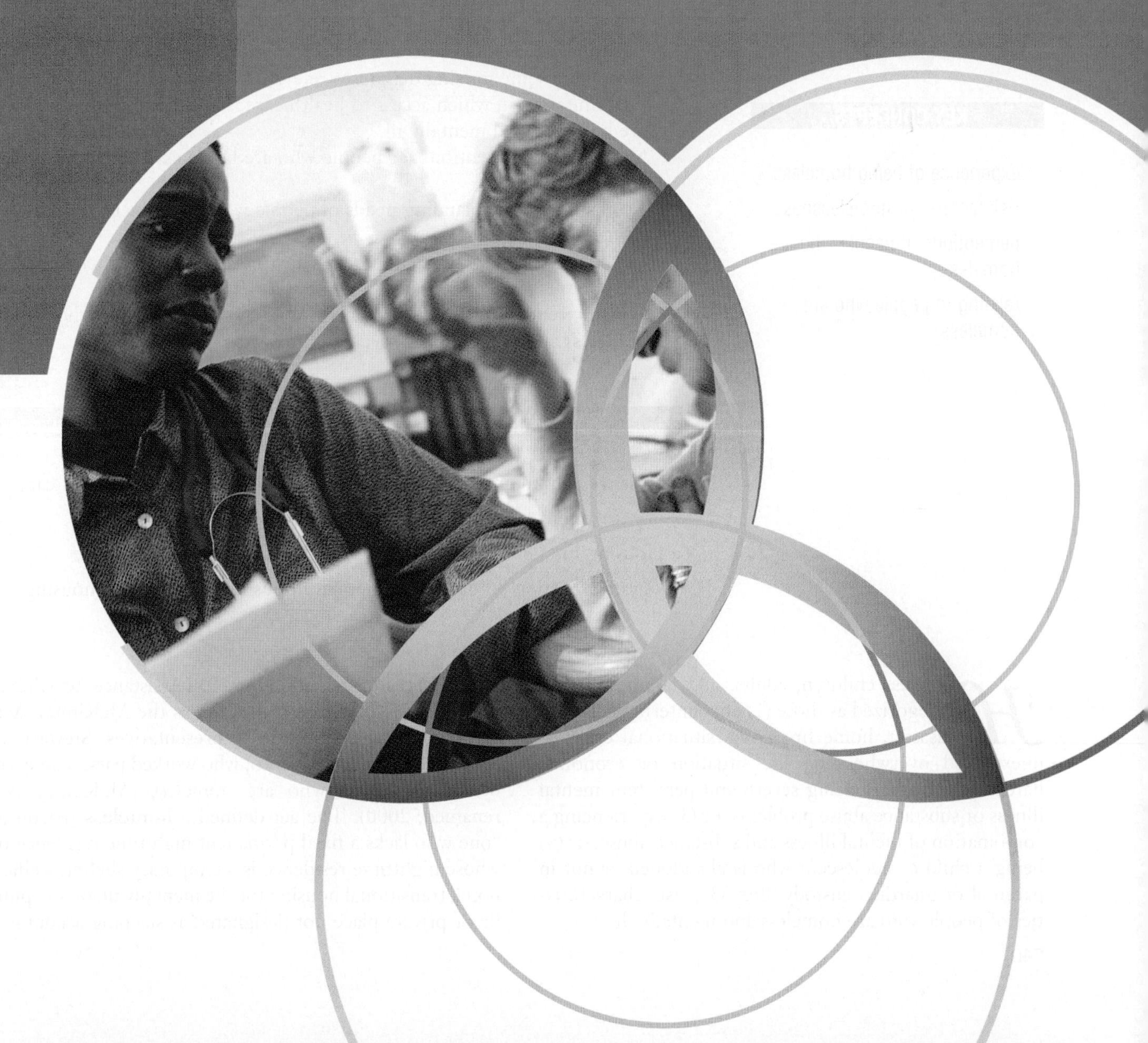

CHAPTER 33

Care of People Who are Homeless and Mentally Ill

Ruth Beckmann Murray, Richard Yakimo, and Marjorie Baier

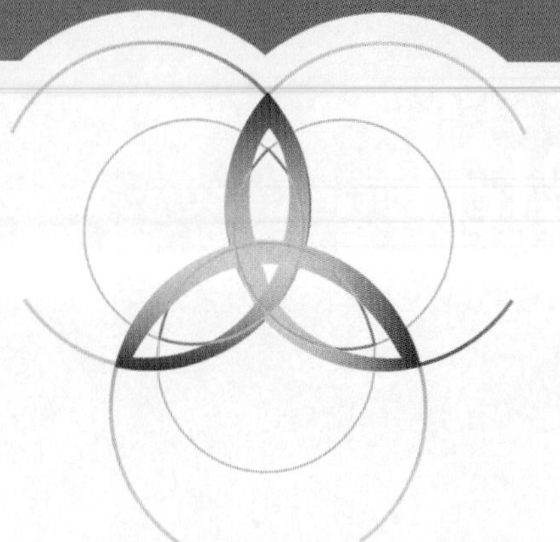

KEY CONCEPTS

- experience of being homeless
- risk factors for homelessness
- perceptions of people who are homeless
- relating to people who are homeless

LEARNING OBJECTIVES

After studying this chapter, you will be able to:

- Define the meaning of homelessness to the person and family.
- Describe risk factors for becoming homeless.
- Identify risk factors for developing mental illness or chemical dependence among people who are homeless.
- Differentiate characteristics of various populations who are homeless.
- Discuss personal and societal attitudes and beliefs about homelessness.
- Describe assessment of people who are homeless and mentally ill.
- Formulate some nursing diagnoses relevant to the homeless population.
- Examine ways in which access to health care is limited for people who are homeless and mentally ill.
- Summarize interventions for people who are homeless and have psychiatric disorders.
- Discuss discharge planning needs of people who are homeless and have psychiatric disorders.
- List major community resources to which nurses can refer members of the homeless population.
- Discuss trends that target improvement of services to people who are homeless and experiencing psychiatric disorders.

KEY TERMS

• assertive community treatment • case management • continuum of care • day treatment • deinstitutionalization • homeless • homelessness • Housing First • Oxford House • Safe Havens • Shelter Plus Care Program • Section 8 housing • supportive housing • transitional housing

Homeless children, adults, and families can be categorized as those (1) encountering a natural disaster, home fire, some situational crisis or unexpected overwhelming life situation or economic hardship; (2) experiencing severe and persistent mental illness or substance abuse problems; or (3) experiencing a combination of mental illness and substance abuse; or (4) being a child or adolescent who is abandoned or not in parental or guardian custody. Box 33.1 lists characteristics of people who are homeless and mentally ill.

The McKinney-Vento Homeless Assistance Act (Public Law 100–77, first passed in 1987 as the McKinney Act) was named in 2000 for Representatives Stewart B. McKinney and Bruce Vento, who worked passionately on behalf of people who are homeless (McKinney Act renamed, 2000). The act defined a **homeless** person as "one who lacks a fixed permanent nighttime residence or whose nighttime residence is a temporary shelter, welfare hotel, transitional housing for the mentally ill, or any public or private place not designated as sleeping accommo-

BOX 33.1

Characteristics of People Who are Mentally Ill and Homeless

- The seriously mentally ill are at greater risk for homelessness than the general population. Of the homeless population, about 30% are severely mentally ill, and 30% have concurrent substance abuse disorder or co-occurring illness.
- Fifteen percent (15%) of people treated for mental illness are homeless for at least 12 months; most average at least 6 months.
- Mental health problems increase with the duration of time the person is homeless.
- They are experiencing a new wave of "deinstitutionalization" because of denial of services or premature or unplanned discharge brought about by managed care and loss of Medicaid benefits.
- They have at least one psychiatric service encounter annually, usually in an emergency department rather than in-patient or out-patient units.
- They are homeless for longer periods, often years, than are those who are homeless and not mentally ill or substance abusing.
- They are more likely to be in poor physical health than other homeless people.
- They have more contacts with the legal system than other homeless or housed people.
- They are more likely to encounter employment barriers and less likely to benefit from societal economic growth.
- They are less likely to have contact with family or friends, especially if they come from higher-income households.
- Most are eligible for, but have difficulty obtaining, income maintenance such as Social Security Disability Insurance (SSDI), Veterans Affairs (VA) disability benefits, or other benefits.
- Most are willing to accept treatment after basic survival needs are met and a therapeutic relationship has been established.

From Caton et al., 2005; Folsom, et al., 2005; Latimer, 2005; Mahoney, 2005a, b; National Coalition for the Homeless, 2005c, d; Salkow & Fichter, 2003; Watts, 2003.

dations for human beings" (Interagency Council on the Homeless, 1994, p. 22).

The McKinney-Vento Homeless Assistance Act reflected concern in the United States about people who are homeless. This landmark legislation provided the first comprehensive federal funding program targeted specifically to address the health, education, and welfare needs of the homeless population. It allocated money for nontraditional crises and community services for chronically mentally ill people, alcohol and drug detoxification and treatment programs, psychosocial rehabilitation, families with children at risk for emotional disturbance because of homelessness, long-term case management, supportive housing, training of service providers, and research (Interagency Council on the Homeless, 1994). Subsequent revisions to the McKinney Act incorporated an approach called **continuum of care,** including emergency shelter, transitional or rehabilitative services, and permanent housing or supportive living arrangements. Because of the gap in services for people who are homeless and mentally ill, amendments were made to the McKinney Act in 1992 that included a provision for the creation of **safe havens,** which are a form of supportive housing that serves hard-to-reach people with severe mental illness (Center for Mental Health Services, 1997). The **Shelter Plus Care Program,** also a continuum of care program, allows for various housing choices and a range of supportive services funded by other sources (U.S. Department of Housing and Urban Development, 1998). The federal Health Care for the Homeless Program, a program to assist persons who are homeless and have acquired immunodeficiency syndrome (AIDS), expanded the focus of the original act by providing refuge in shelters for victims of domestic violence and for children in homeless families (Sullivan, Burnam, Koegel, & Hollenberg, 2000).

The McKinney-Vento Act Homeless Assistance Program of 2002 provided for the Emergency Shelter Grants Program; the Supportive Housing Program, which includes Transitional Housing, Supportive Housing, Supportive Services, and Safe Haven; the Shelter Plus Care Program, to provide long-term rental assistance for people who are homeless with mental illness, substance dependence, or human immunodeficiency virus (HIV)/AIDS; rental assistance through the Single Room Occupancy (SRO) and SRO/Section 8 Housing Program, and an emphasis on ensuring educational rights and protective measures to children and adolescents experiencing homelessness (Lowe, Slater, Welfley, & Hardie, 2002; McKinney-Vento Homeless Assistance Act, 2002).

Bipartisan legislation (S709/HR1471), known as the Services for Ending Long-Term Homelessness Act (SELHA), authorized federal funding through the U.S. Department of Housing and Urban Development (HUD) to finance permanent supportive housing targeted for chronically homeless people. This legislation complements housing funded under the McKinney-Vento Homeless Assistance Act (Shelter Plus Care and Subsidized Housing Program) and President Bush's "Samaritan Initiative," which centers on redirecting resources toward the development of permanent supportive housing. The focus is to provide coordinated, flexible, "wrap-around" services to housed individuals that lead to recovery from severe, persistent mental illness and co-occurring disorders and reintegration into community life.

The Bringing Home America Act (HR 4347), reintroduced by Julia Carson (D-IN) and nine cosponsors in November 2006, was based on research data, reported experiences of people who have been homeless, and information from service providers for the homeless. The bill includes housing production; support for living income; rental assistance (no more than 30% of income be spent on housing by low-income families or individuals); job training opportunities; civil rights (including right to vote) protection for persons without housing; emergency funds to prevent homelessness; and increased access to health care for this population (Bringing America Home, 2005, November).

This legislation would continue the work of the National Housing Trust Fund and Affordable Housing Trust Funds established in major U.S. cities to build and preserve 1.5 million units of rental housing for the lowest income and homeless families by 2010 to 2015. These efforts are in response to the data showing that, on average, U.S. families must earn almost $16.00 hourly, more than twice the minimum wage, to afford a two-bedroom apartment at fair market value (National Low Income Housing Coalition, 2006b).

This chapter explores issues relevant to individuals who are homeless who are also experiencing mental health problems. It presents nursing care measures for such individuals and suggests ways to improve services for the homeless population.

HOMELESSNESS

Homelessness is a word that evokes images and feelings in everyone. Without a consistent dwelling place, meeting basic needs is difficult. Homelessness means carrying all of one's possessions in a car, suitcase, bag, or shopping cart or storing necessities in a bus station locker or under the bed of a night shelter. It means no chest for treasured objects, no closet for next season's clothing, no pantry with food to eat, no place to entertain friends or have solitude, and no place for a child to play.

KEY CONCEPT The experience of being homeless for a long time results in a sense of depersonalization and fragmented identity, loss of self-worth and self-efficacy, and a stigma of being "nothing," "a bum," "lazy," and "stupid." However, most people who are homeless describe themselves as resourceful, independent, proud, and survivors (Murray, 1996).

Some people wrongly associate all homelessness with mental illness, violence, and alcohol or drug addiction (Murray, 1996). The person who is homeless for the first time or for a few months is more likely to describe positive personal feelings than the person who has been homeless for a long time, because the chances of recovering economic and social status are greater (Boydell, Goering, & Morrell-Bellai, 2000; Caton et al., 2005; Meadows-Oliver, 2005; Watts, 2003).

Biographies and research have presented descriptions of the tragedy and nightmare of being homeless (Banyard & Graham-Bermann, 1998; Boydell et al., 2000; Humphreys, 2000; Menke & Wagner, 1997; Meadows-Oliver, 2005; Murray, 1996; Sullivan, Burnam, Koegel, & Hollenberg, 2000; Watts, 2003). The person who is homeless is often engaged in hunting for shelter, food, and clothing and lacks consistent ways to meet basic needs. This lifestyle, plus grinding poverty and victimization, especially if the person is mentally ill, leave little energy for change or re-entrance into mainstream society. Panhandling, hustling, doing odd jobs, and selling plasma or aluminum cans are common sources of income, although some people who are homeless receive Social Security or veterans or pension benefits. The person becomes a victim of immediate circumstance—hunger, cold, or assault. The choices that people who are homeless make and the strategies that they pursue are affected by their need to subsist and to overcome fear, loss of freedom and privacy, resignation, loneliness, and depression (Murray, 1996; Sullivan et al., 2000). The longer a person is homeless, the more likely the person is to suffer mental illness or engage in substance use (Caton et al., 2005; Folsom, et al., 2005; North, Kyrich, Pollio, & Spitznagel, 2004).

The healthiest survivors have been those who seek support from other people, maintain hope for the future, and strive to have valued lives and selves. These people believe they are resourceful, can handle uncertainty, and can maintain health (Boydell et al., 2000; Caton et al., 2005; Folsom et al., 2005; Meadows-Oliver, 2005; Nyamathi, Leake, Keenan, & Gelberg, 2000). Homeless women who have children have described the need to keep going for the sake of and to avoid losing the children. They cite the importance of spiritual beliefs in developing inner resources, reducing distress, and enhancing the connection to self, others, and powers beyond the self (Humphreys, 2000; Meadows-Oliver, 2005; Menke & Wagner, 1997).

Historical Perspectives

Homelessness has not always been widespread in the United States. Housing was affordable for most people and was provided for the ill (Roman, 2002). The phenomenon of many mentally ill street people began in the mid-1900s. A public outcry followed a photographic essay in 1946 by *Life* magazine about deplorable conditions in state hospitals for the mentally ill. The introduction of chlorpromazine (Thorazine) in 1954 provided a simple means of reducing symptoms of psychosis. In 1958, President Dwight D. Eisenhower established the Joint Commission on Mental Illness and Health, which developed a nationwide plan for treating the mentally ill within their communities (Jones, 1983). President John F. Kennedy proposed this plan to Congress, and the "bold new approach to mental illness" resulted in federal legislation, the Mental Retardation Facilities and Community Mental Health Centers Construction Act of 1963. The goal of the act was to provide a complete array of neighborhood-located mental health services and to fund staffing. Furthermore, soon after the assassination of

President Kennedy, the civil rights movement gained momentum. Advocates for the chronically mentally ill claimed the right to the "least restrictive environment." Unfortunately, the vision of day and night care, halfway houses, group homes, home-visiting mental health teams, 24-hour crisis services, vocational and social programs, and sheltered workshops—all coordinated and implemented by a multidisciplinary treatment team—never fully materialized. Contributing factors included lack of federal or state funding, inadequate numbers of prepared professionals, and communities unprepared or unwilling to participate in the movement (Jones, 1983).

The **deinstitutionalization** of the population with mental illness during the late 1960s and 1970s was a major turning point in mental health care. In 1973, the National Institute of Mental Health defined *deinstitutionalization* of state mental hospitals as preventing inappropriate mental hospital admissions through the provision of community alternatives for treatment, releasing to the community all institutionalized patients who have been given adequate preparation for such a change and establishment and maintenance of community support systems for noninstitutional people receiving community mental health services (Jones, 1983). Because of deinstitutionalization, in the late 1960s and 1970s, the census of state hospitals declined from thousands to hundreds. However, cities were ill-prepared to handle the masses, and discharged patients and their families were given little or no preparation (Jones). The stigma against the mentally ill became greater as cities faced real social and financial consequences. Furthermore, people who were both homeless and severely, persistently mentally ill experienced fear, suspicion, caution, and disorganized thinking, which interfered with using available services and promoted a homeless lifestyle (Roman, 2002).

Most individuals who are currently homeless became homeless much more recently than the deinstitutionalization movement of the 1960s and 1970s. More accessible, integrated systems of care linking housing and mental health services are needed (Caton et al., 2005; Legislation to address, 2005; Mojtabai, 2005; National Coalition, 2005a; Roman, 2002; Watts, 2003). Trends in systems of care and services will be discussed later.

KEY CONCEPT Risk factors for homelessness are multiple. People prefer to have a home and to be part of a family or social group. People do not choose or purposefully maintain homelessness and living on the streets. Homelessness has no single cause. Many factors—unemployment, lack of skills, mental illness, substance abuse, domestic violence—typically combine, with time, to cause the person or family to lose permanent housing (Box 33.2). The series of events that results in having no home is the culmination of individual and environmental factors, including factors in the mental health system, society, and family or community (Box 33.3).

Homeless Populations

The homeless population includes people of all ages, economic levels, racial and cultural backgrounds, and geographic areas. People who are homeless are often chronically ill, jobless, or have recently lost all financial resources. Long-term homeless people may have lived in poverty for years with no home site. Among the homeless, educational level varies greatly, from less than an eighth-grade education to doctoral degrees.

Incidence

There is no easy way to determine how many people are homeless in the United States. Counting the homeless population is understandably difficult, given their mobility. In most cases, homelessness is a temporary circumstance, not a permanent condition. Studies of homelessness are complicated by problems of definition and methodology.

Researchers use different statistical methods to describe homelessness. Point-prevalence rate is a count of all the people who are homeless on a given day or during a given week. A second statistic, the period-prevalence rate, is the number of people who are homeless during a given period. Both methods are adjusted for the total population. Point-prevalence studies give just a "snapshot" of homelessness; consequently, they do not accurately identify people who are homeless intermittently. Point-prevalence counts are often criticized as misrepresenting the magnitude and nature of homelessness and the number of people who are chronically homeless. However, the period-prevalence rate may also misrepresent the magnitude and nature of homelessness because of the geographic mobility of some people who are homeless, who may be counted repeatedly or not at all (National Coalition for the Homeless, 2005b).

The best approximation of how many people are homeless has remained consistent: 2.3 to 3.5 million people (1% of the U.S. population), which includes 1.3 mil-

BOX 33.2

General Causes of Homelessness

- Poverty; history of childhood family instability
- Lack of affordable housing; doubling up with relatives or friends until situation is intolerable
- Mental illness or substance abuse and lack of needed services
- Low-paying jobs; unemployment
- Domestic violence; flight from a violent home or abandonment; youth age-out of services
- Eviction for not paying rent; multiple movers
- Prison release; having no money, job, or place to go
- Limited life coping skills; disturbing behavior
- Changes or reductions in public assistance programs

BOX 33.3

Risk Factors for Homelessness Among People With Serious Mental Illness

Individual Risk Factors

- The nature of mental illness, including unpredictable behavior, inability to manage everyday affairs, and inability to communicate needs, which results in conflicts with family, employers, landlords, and neighbors (Folsom et al., 2005; Lowe et al., 2002; Martens, 2001; National Coalition for the Homeless, 2005a; North et al., 2004; Salkow & Fichter, 2003; Sullivan et al., 2000).
- Concurrent mental illness and substance abuse disorders in youth and adults, with behaviors that place them at high risk for eviction, arrest, and incarceration in jails, or repeated admissions and short stays in mental hospitals (Caton et al., 2005; Folsom et al., 2005; Lowe et al., 2002; Min, Biegel, & Johnson, 2005; National Coalition for the Homeless, 2005a).
- Coexisting HIV or AIDS with severe persistent mental illness, chemical dependence, or both (Martens, 2001; Salkow & Fichter, 2003)
- Coexisting demographic and societal factors of poverty; single-parent family (usually female headed); dependent child; child in foster home; racial or ethnic minority; veteran status; single men and women; ex-offender released from jail or prison (Caton et al., 2005; Embry et al., 2000; Folsom et al., 2005; Lowe et al., 2002; McNeil, Binder, & Robinson, 2005; Meadows-Oliver, 2005; National Coalition for the Homeless, 2005a; North et al., 2004; Roman, 2002).
- Coexisting physical illness or developmental disability (Desai & Rosenheck, 2005; Martens, 2001)
- Exposure to traumatic events repeatedly, resulting in post-traumatic stress disorder and deficits in independent living skills (Mahoney, 2005a, b; Not getting over it, 2005; Reeves, Parker, & Konkle-Parker, 2005)
- Exposure to victimization (physical and sexual abuse), especially if a family member was the perpetrator (Bassuk et al., 1997; Embry, et al., 2000; Lowe et al., 2002; Sullivan, et al., 2000a)
- Inability to cope with or manage the requirements of community or group living home (Caton et al., 2005; Phelan & Link, 1999)
- Lack of high school education or equivalence (Bassuk et al., 1997; Caton et al., 2005; Lowe et al., 2002)

Environmental Risk Factors

- Mental Health System Factors (Folsom et al., 2005; Greenwood et al., 2005; Latimer, 2005; McCabe, Macnee, & Anderson, 2001; Mahoney, 2005a,b; National Coalition for the Homeless, 2005a,d; Roman, 2002; Rosenheck et al., 2003).
- Inadequate discharge planning with a lack of appropriate housing, treatment, and support services.
- Lack of funding for community-based services.
- Lack of integrated community-based treatment and support services for individual and group therapy, medication monitoring, and case management
- Lack of community-based crisis alternatives for housing, health care, and respite care for families, with risk for rehospitalization and loss of residence
- Lack of attention to consumer preferences for autonomy, privacy, and integrated regular housing

Societal Factors

- Lack of affordable housing; affluent economic times have caused housing prices to soar out of reach, to reduce construction of low-cost housing, and to create a tight rental market (Culhane, Metrauz, & Hadley, 2001; Greenwood et al, 2005; Legislation to address, 2005; Lowe et al., 2002; National Coalition for the Homeless, 2005a; Roman, 2002)
- Insufficient disability benefits; Social Security income recipients are below the federal poverty level (Caton et al., 2005; Culhane et al., 2001; Lowe et al., 2002; National Coalition for the Homeless, 2005a)
- Lack of coordination between mental health and substance abuse systems (McNiel et al., 2005; Min et al., 2005; Mojtabai, 2005; Rosenheck et al., 2003).
- Waiting lists to receive a subsidy that requires the person to pay only 30% of income for rent and utilities (Mojtabai, 2005; Rosenheck, 2000)
- Lack of job opportunities for disabled people (Lowe et al., 2002; National Coalition for the Homeless, 2005)
- *Family and community factors* (Caton et al., 2005; Culhane et al., 2001; Embry et al., 2000; Lowe et al., 2002; Meadows-Oliver, 2005; Nyamathi et al., 2000; Rosenheck, 2000; Watts, 2003)
- Stigma and discrimination; resistance to community housing for the mentally ill is widespread.
- Poor family relationships; willingness to help the ill person is exhausted as relatives cope with frightening or disturbing behavior and receive insufficient help from the community or medical profession.

lion children (39% of the total population), are likely to experience homelessness in a given year. Of these 1.3 million children who are under 18 years of age, 42% are children under age 5 years (Caton et al., 2005; National Coalition for the Homeless, 2005, a,b; Salkow & Fichter, 2003). The Weingert Center Institute for the Study of Homelessness reported in late 2005 that 406,033 people were homeless in 54 major U.S. cities and counties. Families accounted for 35% of the homeless population, and 22% of the population were chronically homeless individuals (National Low Income Housing Coalition, 2006a; Weingert Center, 2005). Among people who are mentally ill and homeless, those who became homeless prior to mental illness have the highest levels of disadvantage and disruption and the lowest General Assessment of Function (GAF) scores. Those who became homeless after becoming mentally ill have a higher prevalence of alcohol dependence. Mental illness may be a factor in initiating homelessness for some people, but other risk factors are also involved (Salkow & Fichter, 2003; Sullivan, Burnam, & Koegel, 2000). This same research methodology was implemented with homeless populations in 1980, 1990, and 2000 in St. Louis by North, Eyrich, Pollio, & Spitznagel (2004). They found a dramatic increase in prevalence in mood and substance use disorders from 1980 to 2000. The authors discuss possible risk factors for this changing incidence (see also Box 33.3).

An increasing number of people who are homeless are youth, women, and families headed by single parents. In rural areas, single mothers and children are the largest group of people who are homeless; people who are Caucasians, American Indians, and immigrants are also more likely to be among the rural homeless population. Fifty percent of all women and children who experience homelessness are fleeing from domestic violence. Studies show that men tend to report that their homelessness is caused by unemployment, alcohol and drug dependence, or imprisonment (National Coalition for the Homeless, 2005b). See Box 33.4 for more information about incidence.

Diverse Groups in the Homeless Population

Homelessness occurs in many groups of people. People with severe mental illness are at much higher risk for poverty and homelessness than are others. Symptoms of mental illness, such as impulsivity, hypersexuality, and poor judgment also may be related to risky sexual behaviors. Sexual risk-taking behaviors and drug use practices, such as sharing needles, contribute to a high rate of HIV infection among the homeless. Poverty also contributes to unsafe sexual behaviors because of unavailable condoms, shared sleeping sites, unplanned sexual contacts, and trading sex for other perceived needs (money, food, place to stay, illicit drugs). Furthermore, substance abuse or co-occurring substance use (cocaine, alcohol, other substances) with mental illness are stronger predictors than the sole presence of mental illness for HIV exposure risk (Salkow & Fichter, 2003).

Family homelessness, whatever its cause, has an especially adverse effect on children. Each year, about 20% of all children move from one residence to another, often because of decreasing family income (U.S. Bureau of the Census, 2000). The poorest children move two or three times within the year before becoming homeless and moving into a shelter (Buckner, Bassuk, Weinreb, & Brooks, 1999). According to Rosenheck, Bassuk, and Salomon (1999), homeless children are generally school-aged or younger. These children have high rates of both acute and chronic health problems and are more likely than children who are not homeless to be hospitalized, have delayed immunizations, and have elevated lead blood levels. In addition, they are at risk for developmental delays and emotional and behavioral difficulties. School attendance is disrupted frequently, and they are vulnerable to violence, either as victims or witnesses. The child who is homeless is more likely to experience homelessness in adulthood (Bassuk et al., 1997; Caton et al., 2005).

BOX 33.4

Incidence of Homelessness

The population who is homeless is estimated to consist of:

- Single men, 41%
- Families with children, 40%
- Families headed by single parent, 73%
- Single women, 14%
- Unaccompanied minors, 5%
- Adults, 25–34 years of age, 25%
- Adults, 55–64 years of age, 6%
- African Americans, 49%
- Caucasian, non-Hispanics, 35%
- Hispanics/Latinos, 13%
- American Indians, 2.9%
- Asians, 1%
- Veterans, 41% of homeless men; 10% of homeless population

From Folsom et al., 2005; National Coalition for the Homeless, 2005a,b; Salkow & Fichter, 2003.

Living in shelters is stressful for families for several reasons. Many shelters exclude men and adolescent boys older than 12 years; thus family members are separated. Overcrowding prevents privacy and promotes loss of personal control. Stressors of poverty and reduced social support compound the trauma of these experiences.

A history of abuse and assault is common among homeless mothers (Rosenheck et al., 1999). Homeless mothers have high lifetime rates of major depressive disorder, posttraumatic stress disorder, and substance use disorders. In addition, they have high rates of attempted suicide (Rosenheck et al.). Homeless women who have a social network, some cash assistance such as Social Security or welfare, or a housing subsidy are more likely to become and remain housed (Bassuk et al., 1997; Meadows-Oliver, 2005; Nyamathi et al., 2000).

Adolescents and runaway youth can become homeless because of strained family relationships, family dissolution, and instability of residential placements (Embry, Vander Stoep, Evens, Ryan, & Pollack, 2000; Greene, Enneth, & Ringwalt, 1997; Rosenheck et al., 1999). Homeless young people may resort to drug trafficking and prostitution to support themselves. They are at risk for physical and mental health problems, including substance abuse, HIV infection or AIDS, pregnancy, and suicidal behaviors. Because of their high rates of exposure to violence, they are more likely to experience posttraumatic stress disorder and depression. To compound their problems, they are less likely than other people who are homeless to use shelters because few available shelters will accept them and they often distrust and fear providers. Further, they have poor tenant skills and often little income so they cannot obtain rental housing.

More homeless people than sheltered people have been arrested or incarcerated. In one study, 16% of the inmates were homeless. When released, ex-offenders are cut off from their communities and are less likely to reestablish themselves after their release. They are at high risk for homelessness. Others with criminal records may have turned to crime after they became homeless to support themselves. Another group who have arrest records are mentally ill people who have been inappropriately jailed because of inadequacies in the mental health treatment system (McNiel, Binder, & Robinson, 2005; Rosenheck, et al., 2003).

Several other groups are at risk for homelessness or may experience homelessness at some point. About 10% of veterans who have been in combat are homeless and suffer posttraumatic stress disorder (acute or delayed), anxiety disorders, and major depression. They experience difficulty with re-entry into civilian life and employment (National Coalition for the Homeless, 2005c). New immigrants come to a specific location with the intention of setting up permanent residence. Economic problems or conflicts with the sponsoring family may jeopardize housing. Refugees are poor; they are involuntarily living outside their home countries because of persecution related to race, religion, nationality, social group membership, or political opinion. Mental health problems arise because of torture experiences, losses suffered in the country of origin, and culture shock and scapegoating experienced in the United States. Posttraumatic stress is common in this group; their physical health problems are often complex (Andrews & Boyle, 2003; DeSantis, 1997). Migrant workers and their families lack residential stability as they move from one geographic region to another for 6 to 9 months of the growing and harvest season. These laborers and their families may be U.S. citizens or foreign born. They are poor and typically lack adequate living quarters and health care. Physical health problems and depression are common in these families. After farm labor is completed, family members may be homeless until they can return to their place of origin or to a relative's home (DeSantis; Sandhaus, 1998).

Caton et al. (2005) studied 377 people who entered a homeless shelter and followed them at 6-, 12-, and 18-month intervals. Shorter duration of homelessness was associated with (a) younger age, (b) current or recent employment and earned income, (c) good coping skills, (d) adequate family support, (e) absence of substance abuse history, and (f) absence of arrest.

KEY CONCEPT Perceptions of people who are homeless depend largely on one's own feelings about people who are homeless and the mentally ill. Often people do not know how to respond to a person who is homeless and who asks for food, money, or interpersonal communication, because they hold common stereotypical beliefs about homelessness. Nurses and teachers, for example, who are accustomed to caring for others and giving attention to people who ask for it, can find themselves confronted by various myths when approached by a person who is homeless (Box 33.5). To respond appropriately, one must first examine these myths and one's own feelings about people who are homeless and mentally ill.

NURSING MANAGEMENT OF INDIVIDUALS AND FAMILIES WHO ARE HOMELESS

A holistic perspective is essential for assessing any person or family unit who is homeless because people and homelessness are complex and multifaceted. Avoid looking at people who are homeless as deficient. Rather, look at the unique individual, the person's or family's transactions with the environment, and the client's strengths.

KEY CONCEPT Relating to people who are homeless requires a gentle and compassionate approach.

The fast-paced, time-focused approach of the traditional health care system is unlikely to gather the needed information to intervene. In fact, the person may leave rather than be subjected to more depersonalization. Use the principles of a therapeutic relationship and therapeutic communication described in Chapter 10 to establish rapport and trust.

Biologic Domain

Assessment

The assessment must begin at the point of the person's need; often, it is a physical need or health problem (Box 33.6). Because of negative past experiences with the health care system or providers or because of mental illness or substance use, the person may not allow a thorough physical examination or may refuse to answer questions about history at the first visit. Realize that many people who are homeless consider themselves well as long as they can get where they need to go. The individual may believe that refusing to admit illness is adaptive behavior. Be aware of the many health problems that may be present (Box 33.7). The child or adolescent who is homeless may suffer any of those listed, plus diseases that are specific to their age group. If a homeless woman is pregnant, assess indications that she is at high risk for maternal or fetal complications.

Baseline and follow-up data for 7,213 homeless clients in a multisite program found 43.6% of the sample had need for medical care. Lack of medical care correlated with lower educational level, depressive and psychotic symptoms, and a high number of competing needs. The main factor in 36% of the clients receiving medical services during a 3-month period was a strong therapeutic alliance with the case manager (Desai & Rosenheck, 2005). People who are homeless are at higher risk of becoming ill, and age-adjusted mortality rates among the homeless population are 3.5 times higher than those of the general population because of lack of health screening and early or adequate treatment of disease (Salkow & Fichter, 2003).

BOX 33.5

Myths and Facts About Homeless People With Psychiatric Disorders

MYTH: People who are homeless are all alike.

FACT: People who are homeless come from all walks of life. Those with and without psychiatric illness share some characteristics. Being homeless is a leveling experience in that it is a sufficiently handicapping condition in itself to cause altered adaptation. Those with chronic substance abuse may have more difficulty in meeting basic needs than do those who are chronically mentally ill.

MYTH: Most people who are homeless are lazy, passive, and do not want to work.

FACT: People who are homeless and who loiter may be actively trying to survive by avoiding extreme weather, seeking monetary or other assistance, or trying to feel a part of mainstream society. Most desire work, even when physical or mental disabilities interfere.

MYTH: People who are homeless prefer being alone.

FACT: Peer relations with trusted people are preferred and essential to survival and meeting needs.

MYTH: People who are homeless are stupid and do not know how to manage life.

FACT: People who are homeless must be creative to secure resources and constantly change life ways to survive. However, the ability to think clearly is threatened under stress and in hostile environments.

MYTH: People who are homeless refuse to stay in a shelter because they are ill.

FACT: People who are homeless, including those with mental illness, do not use shelters for the following reasons: lack of shelter beds in an accessible area; difficulty in reaching the shelter; overcrowded or unpleasant conditions in specific shelters; restrictions on length of stay or criteria for admission; and availability of alternatives (Murray, 1996).

MYTH: Street dwellers are unwilling to accept services.

FACT: Most people who are homeless recognize the need for help; however, survival needs take priority over need for mental health treatment. Nontraditional approaches may be necessary to work with the person who is homeless and mentally ill.

MYTH: Most people who are homeless require acute, inpatient psychiatric care.

FACT: About 5% to 7% of adults who are mentally ill and homeless need inpatient care.

MYTH: Most people who are homeless, especially those who are mentally ill, are dangerous.

FACT: High visibility of this population lends itself to frequent reporting of minor crimes, such as loitering, panhandling, public misconduct, minor shoplifting, or efforts to protect self from dangerous others, which can result in a fight.

MYTH: Most people who are homeless are mentally ill or substance abusing.

FACT: Of the people who are homeless, about 23% are mentally ill and 32% are substance abusing.

MYTH: Homelessness is a monolithic problem that affects millions of people in the United States.

FACT: Between 200,000 and 250,000 people are estimated to be chronically homeless; most are homeless for a relatively short period of time.

From Lowe, et al., 2002; Folsom, et al., 2005; Latimer, 2005; McNiel, et al., 2005; National Coalition for the Homeless, 2005a,b,c,d; Roman, 2002; Watts, 2003.

Psychological Domain

Psychological Assessment

Behavior that looks like a mental illness may in reality be an expression of normal emotional or social needs. The person who is homeless may manifest the need to feel safe, secure, and respected and to be treated as a unique and valued person with overt distancing or aggressive behavior. Ask how long the person has been homeless and in what context (shelter, street, relatives); such variables can considerably affect behavior, feelings, and psychological function.

People who experience homelessness have their own way of being in the world. They feel

- heightened awareness of being labeled, on display, and judged or stigmatized by outer appearance
- that they are nothing, own nothing, and that health care providers and authorities expect certain behavior
- anxiety about having to be at a certain place at preset times to meet daily needs
- a sense of community with other homeless and ill people, as they go through rituals of waking, eating, lining up, and sharing facilities, space, and resources
- a sense of humor, amusement, aloofness, and optimism or faith about their ability to cope with a complicated lifestyle and to be hurt as little as possible (Boydell et al., 2000; Carter, Cuvar, McSweeney, Storey, & Stockmann, 2001; Herth, 1996; Jones, 1983; McCabe et al., 2001; Menke & Wagner, 1997; Sullivan, Burnam, Koegel, & Hollenberger, 2000).

Just as the physical examination may be incomplete, so may the mental status examination have to be done in part or over several visits. See Box 33.8 for information related to psychological assessment. Symptoms of schizophrenia may be difficult to differentiate from emotional responses to the stressors of a homeless lifestyle. Required hypervigilance may augment suspicion or paranoid beliefs. The need for constant awareness of possibilities for meeting basic needs can augment self-preoccupation. Blunted affect, lack of communication, loose associations, ambivalence, isola-

BOX 33.6

Assessment Tips for the Biologic Domain

- Use unobtrusive observation as a part of physical assessment. Some conditions will be immediately obvious. Other conditions may become apparent during the interview.
- Examine—look, touch, palpate, auscultate—the person to the extent that he or she allows. The person may resist anything more than a superficial conversation and observation. The nurse may need to perform initial palpation of the abdomen or auscultation of the lung through several layers of clothes. If the patient perceives the health care provider as too intrusive, the patient may leave the setting even though desperate for care.
- Listen carefully to what the patient does *not* say, and pay attention to nonverbal as well as verbal expressions. Avoid unnecessary directness and probing. Give the person time to answer questions. The blood test or urine screen may have to wait; a patient, nonintrusive manner may ensure that the person returns for needed tests or screening.
- Determine whether the person has been prescribed medications in the past. Often, the person who is homeless is not taking medications, even if they are prescribed and essential. The person may have difficulty keeping pills dry and easily retrievable, or paying for medications. A daily insulin injection, for example, may not seem practical.

tion, and uncertainty may be the result of life on the streets and in various places. Such symptoms or behaviors may be part of the homeless experience and reflect healthy coping mechanisms and creative survival techniques, rather than pathology.

BOX 33.7

Common Physical Health Problems Experienced by Homeless People

- Injuries, fractures, epistaxis, or edema from trauma, falls, burns, assault, gunshot wounds
- Influenza, colds, bronchitis, asthma, shortness of breath
- Hypothermia, hyperthermia
- Arthritis, musculoskeletal disorders, headaches, fatigue
- Diabetes mellitus
- Hypertension
- Cardiovascular and peripheral vascular diseases
- Malnutrition
- Pulmonary tuberculosis
- Infestations, such as lice or scabies
- Dermatitis, sunburn or frostbite, bruises
- Sexually transmitted diseases
- Hypothyroidism or hyperthyroidism
- Kidney or liver disease
- Cancer
- Epilepsy
- Impaired vision, glaucoma, cataracts
- Impaired hearing
- Dental caries, periodontal disease

Substance abuse must be ruled out because it is common among people who are homeless, including the mentally ill. Because people who are homeless, especially those with psychiatric disorders, are often victims of crime and violence, the incidence of posttraumatic stress disorder among them may be higher than in the general population. Homeless women are especially in danger of being assaulted, abused, and raped.

When the child or adolescent is homeless, ask about the educational history, if the youth is enrolled in school, and about perceived progress. Homeless children often have difficulty with school; the school district may change every time the parent changes shelters or moves from a temporary residence. Determine whether the child has behavioral or emotional problems and whether he or she needs special education services.

Homelessness places parents and children at risk for mental health problems; maternal depression may affect the mother–child relationship and create child behavior problems. Realize that homeless mothers and children also have great resilience. Homeless mothers are not necessarily depressed, nor do they have inadequate coping skills. Many homeless women, having made the decision to free themselves of a noxious relationship, are competent and resilient.

Social Domain

Social and Family Assessment 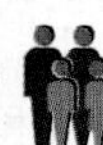

Cultural value differences exist between people who are homeless and people in the dominant American culture, to which most providers of health care subscribe. Thus, providers and the person who is homeless and needs health care may experience cultural conflict in their norms of health and illness, basic value systems and priorities, and perceptions about health care.

BOX 33.8

Assessment Tips for the Psychological Domain

- Observe for behavior that indicates hallucination and try to validate.
- Listen for delusions or denial over time; try to sense what purpose these serve.
- Observe and listen for what the person defines as a problem and potential solution and what he or she considers to be a strength or coping strategy; validate and reinforce when applicable.
- View the person and his or her situation from the individual's perspective; be a patient, nonthreatening listener. Such an approach encourages the person to return regularly; the nurse can then observe the patterns of behavior.
- Determine the extent of stability or integration of the person's sense of self, cognitive appraisals, and overt behavior. Lack of integration or stability indicates the need for continued monitoring and therapy.

Health care providers expect patients, including those who are homeless and mentally ill or chemically dependent, to problem solve, become more independent, and be future-oriented. These values affect assessment, treatment, and interactions with the person and can interfere with the nursing process and patient response to the health care system (Andrews & Boyle, 2003). Consider how the homeless ill patient perceives his or her everyday life and vary the assessment and therapy approach accordingly.

Homelessness is an expression of and response to certain family, societal, or environmental conditions, as well as to individual factors. See Box 33.9 for factors in the social and family assessment.

Spiritual Assessment

Listen for expressions that convey a spiritual faith, a connection to a transcendent being, or a belief system that helps the person endure. Questions about the spiritual dimension may convey an invitation to talk about an aspect of life that is often ignored but that may be very important to the person. Listening to values, beliefs, and preferred practices will help determine relevant therapy approaches.

Nursing Diagnoses for All Domains

Nursing diagnoses related to physical health status include impaired dentition, hypothermia or hyperthermia, imbalanced nutrition, acute or chronic pain, impaired skin integrity, and disturbed sleep patterns. Nursing diagnoses related to emotional health status include anxiety, risk for loneliness, powerlessness, chronic low self-esteem, and risk for self-mutilation or suicide. Nursing diagnoses related to social health status include compromised family coping, and social isolation. Nursing diagnoses related to cognitive status include decisional conflict, disturbed thought processes, and deficient knowledge (NANDA, 2007).

Interventions for All Domains

Interventions are to be directed at the social system, as well as at the individual or family level. Interventions should take advantage of community resources and the inner resources and support systems of the individual or family. Box 33.10 describes findings about factors that promote satisfaction with care.

Cost and lack of insurance are the biggest barriers to health and hospital care for the homeless. Another barrier is the inability of this population to carry out treatment recommendations; survival is their first priority. Compliance with medication and treatment regimens is difficult because successful treatment requires collaboration, monitoring, time for medication and other measures to be effective, and a secure place to keep medication. Mentally ill people who are homeless often cannot routinely get prescriptions filled. Medicine may be stolen. It is necessary for the person or family unit to have a place to keep medications that can be reached at the necessary times and to have access to primary care services for regular check-ups, assessment for adverse drug responses, and necessary blood monitoring.

BOX 33.9

Assessment Tips for the Social Domain

- Ask about support systems, people who could be helpful, and what services have been or could be used.
- Determine whether the person is isolated from the family, and if so, if it is by personal choice, rather than by family choice.
- Respect that the person who feels isolated may avoid talking about the biologic family.
- Explore if the patient views a homeless peer, local pastor, counselor, or another health care provider as "family" or as the support system.
- Convey genuine interest in the person and convey that others may also care. Questions may be the catalyst to re-establishing family ties.

• NCLEXNOTE

NCLEXNOTE

The priority for people who are homeless is meeting the basic needs—food, shelter, etc. Care for the response to the mental illness is secondary.

Interventions that improve quality of life include providing food, clothing, and assistance with housing, addressing physical health problems, and educating the person to decrease the risk of victimization (Sullivan, Burnam, Koegel, & Hollenberger, 2000). A trusting relationship with the care provider and ongoing follow-up care are also necessary (Carter et al., 2001). In a study of 1,302 women who were homeless and in shelters, modifying social support systems or networks was associated with improved mental health outcomes, less risky health behaviors, and greater continuing use of health services (Nyamathi et al., 2000).

People who have been homeless for several years have greater difficulty readjusting to stability and need more time for healing, depending on illness severity, comorbidity, and available support system (Murray, 1996). People who are homeless, including those with psychiatric disorders, become creative at surviving on the streets. Explore resources with the individual or family (see Box 33.11 for appropriate interventions).

Depending on the person's expression, the nurse may explore ways to meet spiritual needs. In one study, respondents listed the following as ways to meet spiritual needs (Murray, 1996): pray and put trust in God, hope that things will get better, obtain strength from religious beliefs and say these beliefs to self daily, seek

BOX 33.10

***Research for Best Practice:* Homeless Patients' Satisfaction With Health Care**

McCabe. S., Macnee, C., & Anderson, M. (2001). Homeless patients' experience of satisfaction with care. Archives of Psychiatric Nursing, 15, 78–85.

THE QUESTION: How satisfied are homeless people with health care?

METHODS: Three women and 14 men who were homeless from 4 weeks to 41 years were interviewed about their experiences of being homeless, what health is, satisfaction with health care, and dissatisfaction with health care.

FINDINGS: The researchers identified five themes from their in-depth interviews and analysis related to satisfaction with health care.

The first was that the people interviewed wanted health care providers not to give up on them, not to reject them if they were not compliant with treatment, and to be observant for potential health problems other than the problems for which they were seeking help.

The second theme was that they wanted to be treated with caring, empathy, acceptance, and respect. This included not feeling rushed and being addressed by name.

The third theme was trust. They wanted the health care providers to believe what they were told, to honor confidentiality, and to accept their need for privacy.

The fourth theme was that they did not want to be prejudged or considered as stereotypes.

Finally, the people interviewed wanted to be included in care decisions. They wanted to be respected for being able to prioritize their own health choices.

IMPLICATIONS FOR NURSING: Findings from this study illustrate the importance of treating people who are homeless with acceptance, respect, and trust. People who are homeless want to be seen as autonomous human beings with the ability to make important choices about their own health care. Psychiatric nurses need to be aware of their own feelings and behaviors and be vigilant for countertransference behaviors.

a religious worker and attend religious services, talk about the meaning of the life situation with someone who is understanding and caring, and read devotional material, such as the Bible or the Koran.

Discharge Planning

A crucial time for intervention occurs at discharge from inpatient or medical treatment. At this time, the nurse can assist in the patient's transition from institutional to community living by providing practical and emotional support. Nurses are in a key position to help patients re-establish family and other supportive relationships. Meadows-Oliver (2005) found that women who are homeless are likely to engage their children as a main social support; parents and other family members were perceived as unlikely to help. People with mental illness who have been homeless need assistance in using available resources, such as medical, psychiatric, substance abuse, emergency department treatment, and other outpatient psychiatric services. Adequate discharge planning includes linkages with intensive case management services.

In preparation for discharge, the nurse should make arrangements for transfer to transitional housing, if available. Provide the person with telephone numbers and directions for emergency shelters, lunch sites, day treatment programs, mental health hotlines, crisis lines (abuse, suicide), appropriate self-help or support groups, and relevant toll-free numbers. Some states fund cities to provide a Supportive Community Living Program (SCLP) that assists people who are mentally ill or substance abusing to receive funding for housing and utilities. Other services may also be available. Predischarge planning involves providing options to promote independent living. Whatever information is given should be legible; concise; able to fit in a pocket, purse, shoe, or boot; and as portable as possible. Bulky brochures or three-ring binders are impractical. The nurse must never assume the person's literacy level; the person may not admit inability to read. If the person is illiterate, the nurse must take the time to help him or her memorize essential information.

BOX 33.11

Interventions for People Who Are Homeless

- Provide a list with addresses and telephone numbers of shelters and luncheon sites that provide food; discourage rooting through dumpsters and panhandling.
- Provide a list of facilities that are safe, including shelters that provide clothing, a safe place to sleep, and opportunity for basic hygiene and laundry.
- Give information on city ordinances that forbid sleeping on park benches, in building doorways, on sidewalk grates, at bus or train stations, in vacant buildings, or in viaducts.
- Explore sources of income, such as gathering and selling aluminum cans or engaging in temporary day labor. Discourage selling blood or plasma.
- Assist the person directly or by referral to pursue entitlements, such as Social Security, veterans, or other benefits.
- Explore how to stay safe. Even in a night shelter, the person who is homeless may not be safe from assault. It is difficult for the person who is homeless to know who is trustworthy; carrying a bag or case is usually considered a marker for being robbed on the streets.
- Explore how to secure privacy, which is difficult to achieve, and how to cope with loneliness, which can be overwhelming.
- Give a list of names, addresses, and telephone numbers of agencies that offer services and socialization, such as the local mental health agency, the local chapter of National Alliance for the Mentally Ill, or the local Emotions Anonymous group.
- Give information about meetings of Alcoholics Anonymous, Narcotics Anonymous, or Cocaine Anonymous if the person is using substances.

TRENDS FOR IMPROVING SERVICES

Diverse services and integrated systems are essential to address all aspects of the life situations of people who are homeless and experiencing psychiatric disorders. Essential components include Safe Havens or stable shelters or residences; accessible outreach; integrated case management; accessible and affordable housing options; treatment and rehabilitation services; general health care services; vocational training and assistance with employment; income support; and legal protection. The agencies that provide these services must develop a physical and emotional atmosphere that conveys a sense of caring and community. Often, community agencies are located at one site, much like a shopping mall, so that the person or family does not have to travel to numerous separately located agencies to get needs met.

Emergency Services

Some agencies provide a street or mobile outreach program. As part of this program, a van travels the streets to areas where people who are homeless will be found outdoors. Food, warm coffee, hygiene kits, and a blanket are the first steps in building trust between staff and homeless persons. The person who is homeless may accept an offer to be driven to a local shelter for the night. Follow-up the next day by van or bicycle provides a way to recontact the individual and invite him or her to the agency programs or take him or her to other social service or health care services. Luncheon sites for the homeless are a basic step in emergency services. Some agencies have a health clinic on site for treatment of minor problems.

Emergency shelters typically provide refuge at night along with an evening meal and morning coffee. Shelters for homeless women and children usually allow them to remain during daytime hours as well. The child leaves the shelter for school; the mother may attend educational classes, counseling, day treatment, rehabilitation, or employment programs. Box 33.12 suggests additional ways to improve shelters.

Housing Services

The United States has a renewed commitment to assure that everyone has a roof over his or her head, can engage in an independent lifestyle, and has the opportunity to become employed. Policy makers at all governmental levels and leaders from the private sector are working together to end homelessness. This **Housing First** approach places people who are homeless, usually also experiencing severe mental illness, substance abuse, or release from prison, into affordable housing, including Section 8 and Oxford House units. Case management, living skills classes, and other services are provided as "wrap around" as needed. There is a direct relationship between the "Housing First" program and a decrease in psychiatric symptoms and chronic homelessness and an increase in a sense of independence, choice, and mastery of living skills (Culhane, Metraux, & Hadley, 2001, Greenwood, Schaefer-McDaniel, Winkel, & Tsemberis, 2005; Jason, Davis, Ferrari, & Bishop, 2001; Roman, 2002; Sperling, 2003).

Transitional housing may consist of a halfway house, short-stay residence or group home, or a room at a hotel designated for people who are homeless. Some agencies have a transitional home and stabilization center where the atmosphere and staff are a model for residents, who work on specific goals and a treatment plan. Sharing housekeeping tasks; obtaining psychiatric stabilization; and attending residence group meetings, social skills and budgeting classes, day treatment programs, and vocational training are steps to independent housing and employment. A holistic program reduces readmission to the hospital and re-entry to street dwelling.

The continuum of care approach to homelessness, sponsored by HUD, includes both the Safe Havens and Shelter Plus Care Programs mentioned at the beginning of this chapter. A Safe Haven, in addition to serving hard-to-reach people with severe mental illness who are on the streets and have been unwilling or unable to participate in traditional supportive services, meets the following criteria: it provides 24-hour residence for an unspecified duration, it provides private or semiprivate accommodations, and it limits overnight occupancy to 25 persons (U.S. Department of Housing and Urban Development, 2000). Shelter Plus Care provides long-term housing and supportive services for people who are homeless with disabilities, primarily those with serious mental illness, chronic problems with alcohol or drugs, or AIDS or related diseases (U.S. Department of Housing and Urban Development).

BOX 33.12

How Emergency Shelters Can Improve Services

- Extend hours to allow admission earlier in the afternoon and the opportunity to remain past 6 or 7 AM.
- Permit late entry to night shelters for those who have a temporary day job and who could not arrive before 6 or 7 PM because of work hours and bus transportation schedules.
- Maintain cleanliness and control vermin.
- Have adequate helpful staff and use effective security inside and outside the shelter.
- Provide a place to store belongings safely.
- Provide transportation from various points in the city to the night shelter or to needed health care services.
- Have policy that permits stay beyond 14 to 28 days, especially if the person is actively participating in recovery or employment programs.

From Murray, R. (1996). Needs and resources: The lived experience of homeless men. *Journal of Psychosocial Nursing, 34* (5), 18–24.

Other housing options are also available. **Oxford House** is a self-help, communal-living setting created to foster recovery in persons who are alcohol and substance abusing. The residents assume full responsibility for daily maintenance of the residence and for personal lifestyles and treatment management. Residents are expected to be employed, to be reducing need for government subsidies, and to engage in relapse prevention (Jason et al., 2001).

Section 8 housing has been helpful to this population for many years. Section 8 federally subsidized housing units are supervised or operated by the state or city, for which tenants are responsible for paying one third of the monthly income (e.g., Supplemental Security Income or Social Security Disability Insurance) toward rent. The difference between the tenant payment and the maximum fair market rental price is calculated as the federal Section 8 Housing contribution to the housing provider (Culhane et al., 2001; Sperling, 2003). Congress has been appropriating more of the McKinney-Vento Act funds for permanent supportive housing for people who are homeless and disabled. The emphasis in Congress and HUD is on establishing community housing programs (Culhane et al., 2001; Greenwood et al., 2005; Legislation to end, 2005; Roman, 2002). **Supportive housing,** permanently subsidized housing with attendant social services, was previously considered too expensive. However, New York City found that such programs for people who were mentally ill and homeless were a good investment. The person who is safely housed is less likely to use other acute care and publicly funded services, such as shelters, although case management services are needed. Use of acute psychiatric and medical services is reduced, and the person is less likely to be arrested or incarcerated. Housing retention rates remain at an average of 70% for the first year after placement. Altogether, such an approach provides a healthier and more humane alternative (Culhane et al.; Roman, 2002; Rosenheck, 2000; Sperling, 2003). The National Alliance for the Mentally Ill (NAMI) of Delaware has also collaborated actively with governmental and private agencies to establish quality housing for people who are homeless and mentally ill (Franz, 2003). Cost of cutting services is higher in the long term than the cost of providing them in the first place (North et al., 2004).

Case Management

Case management involves systematic assessment, planning, goal setting, counseling and other interventions, coordination of services, referral as necessary, and monitoring of the person's or family's needs and progress. It enhances self-care capability and quality of care along the continuum of care, decreases fragmentation, provides for cost containment, and reduces unnecessary duplication of services or hospitalization. The case manager is the gatekeeper and facilitator who may at first network with services on the person's or family's behalf and then encourage them to deal directly with other service providers to obtain bus passes and transportation, children's services and supplies, medical or obstetric care, or housing. The nurse is the ideal team member or case manager because of knowledge about both psychiatric and physical diseases and the ability to develop therapeutic relationships and stay connected with persons or families who are homeless and with the health care system.

Rehabilitation and Education

Day Treatment Programs

Day treatment provides a bridge between institutional and community care for severely mentally ill and substance-abusing people. Participation in structured day treatment programs can provide emotional and practical support and strengthen ties to community services and potentially to family and friends. A day treatment program can provide legal assistance, help with finding employment and independent housing, and a mailing address for people who are homeless. It can provide case management, assistance with goal setting and problem solving, and psychiatric or medical care. The day treatment program may incorporate adult basic education classes to increase literacy and survival skills, GED classes for those who want a high school diploma, and computer skills to improve employment options. A Living Skills Program typically includes content in nutrition, budgeting, parenting, household and family management, tenant responsibilities and rights, and employment readiness. Such classes are especially useful to women who will no longer be receiving welfare benefits. The person can receive assistance applying for government benefits, if qualified, and obtaining identification, such as a birth certificate, if needed. The informal environment of day treatment programs promotes a feeling of camaraderie, self-confidence, trust in staff, and aspirations to independent living. Such extensive services have been found to be effective (Caton et al., 2005; Greenwood et al., 2005; Latimer, 2005; Rosenheck, 2000).

Alcohol and Drug Treatment

The structure of some day treatment programs follows the 12-step model of Alcoholics Anonymous for people who abuse substances or have a dual diagnosis. Sobriety is the goal; the person attends daily meetings, receives necessary psychiatric and medical treatment, and participates in all the other activities and services available at the day treatment program. No one is terminated for relapse; the person is referred to more intensive services, including hospitalization, if necessary.

Employment Services

Job placement is most likely when an employment program teaches basic job-seeking skills (e.g., resume writing; interview skills; appropriate attire, hygiene, and behavior; and computer skills) and offers job training in settings that prepare the person for the real world and real jobs. Case management during employment training can increase self-confidence, teach the person budgeting skills and methods of coping with the stresses of regular employment, and link the person with community resources. It can also help to teach the person various skills for job retention and career development. The employment service should periodically follow up with both the employee and their employer to ensure a successful record and movement to independence.

Integrated Services

Assertive Community Treatment (ACT) programs focus on service delivery to this population by a transdisciplinary team of 10 to 12 specialists with a 1:10 staff–client ratio. A single, integrated, mobile staff team utilizes outreach, case management, practical assistance and support, and rehabilitation services to maximize the possibility that the most disabled consumers will live independently in the community and have quality of life. The team provides counseling and advocacy; monitors the person's management of housing, income, medication use, and leisure activities; and provides opportunities for employment if appropriate. Substance abuse management and physical health care are provided as needed. Research studies of more than 25 controlled trials link ACT programs to significant reduction in psychiatric symptoms, hospitalizations, and disability. Client and family satisfaction ratings have been high. Cost analysis reveals that the ACT model is no more expensive than standard care because of the above outcomes, consequent improved quality of life, and integration of the client into the community (Greenwood et al., 2005; Latimer, 2005; Mahoney, 2005a,b).

Ongoing social support groups, membership in day treatment programs, attendance at meetings of Alcoholics Anonymous, Narcotics Anonymous, or Cocaine Anonymous, or the local NAMI or Mental Health Association can help the person who was severely mentally ill or substance abusing to remain in the community and live independently or with family. Support groups foster peer socialization and problem solving, enhance self-esteem, and offer many activities, such as art and recreation therapy or legal assistance. An example of a support group is an Alumni Club for the "alumni" of a job-training center. The evening mental health, after-care program is attended by those who have become psychiatrically stabilized, are employed, and are living independently. A club-like setting provides a safe, friendly, substance-free environment for 7 evenings each week, year round. Case management, individualized treatment plans, and counseling continues for 6 months or longer. Alcoholics Anonymous meetings, self-improvement classes, and other educational opportunities are integrated with case management. Socialization, fun, and effective leisure activities result (Box 33.13). For a number of years, the Substance Abuse and Mental Health Services Administration (SAMHSA) and the Center for Substance Abuse Treatment (CSAT) have funded treatment programs for women and young children. Long-term stays have been found to predict positive treatment outcomes, including lower rates of drug use, criminal behavior, and unemployment. Improved parenting and mother–child relationships, less child abuse and neglect, improved developmental outcomes in children, and lowered costs for mother and infant health are other benefits. A minimum stay of 3 months is needed for the patient to benefit; a 12- to 24-month stay is optimal. Using a family-focused, interdisciplinary team approach can motivate mothers to stay in treatment (McComish, Greenberg, Ager, Chruscial, & Laken, 2000).

BOX 33.13

Community Resources to Aid People Who Are Homeless

The National Data Resource Center on Homelessness and Mental Illness
262 Delaware Avenue
Delmar, NY 12054
800–444–7415
www.nrchmi.com

VA Homeless Assistance Information
Department of Veterans Affairs (111C)
810 Vermont Avenue, NW
Washington, DC 20420
800–827–1000
www.va.gov/homeless

National Alliance for the Mentally Ill
200 North Glebe Road, Suite 1015
Arlington, VA 22203
800–950–6264
www.nami.org

National Coalition for the Homeless
1612 K Street, NW
Suite 1004
Washington, DC 20006
202–775–1322
www.nationalhomeless.org

Advocacy

Nurses can share experiences and research findings with the local chapter or national headquarters of NAMI and with state legislators and members of Congress who are involved in developing legislation and policies related to people who are homeless, mentally ill, and substance abusing. Continued advocacy is essential to convey the perceptions and needs of this population, to influence allocations for needed programs and services, and to end the social injustice of chronic homelessness.

Research

Philosophical and ethical issues are prominent in research with adults or youth who are homeless or homeless and mentally ill. Several authors discuss the concerns, risks, and challenges (Ensign, 2003; Fisher, Hoagwood, & Jensen, 1996; Ledbetter, 2002; Rew, Taylor-Seehafer, & Thomas, 2000; and Williamson & Prosser, 2002).

SUMMARY OF KEY POINTS

- People who are homeless are a heterogeneous, diverse group, some of whom are mentally ill or abusing substances.
- There are many risks for being homeless.
- People do not want to be homeless.
- The nursing assessment must be holistic; the nurse must listen to the person's perceptions and observe carefully.
- The person who is mentally ill or substance abusing and homeless may have various physical health problems.
- Intervention must be oriented to the person's or family's perceived needs, culturally sensitive, and compassionate.
- The person who is mentally ill and homeless may avoid traditional health care services.
- Nurses must incorporate new trends in providing and improving services for health care and social integration.

CRITICAL THINKING CHALLENGES

1. How do the effects of mental illness, substance abuse, and homelessness interact with one another?
2. What factors might interfere with the ability of the person who is mentally ill to participate in treatment?
3. What barriers to communication might the nurse experience when relating to the person who is homeless and mentally ill?

The Homeless Home Movie. 1997. This video profiles several different people who are homeless who struggle with homelessness during 1 year. They include a pregnant 15-year-old runaway; a couple who live in their car; a Vietnam veteran who lives outside all year; and a man bankrupted after his daughter's long fight with leukemia. This video is available for purchase at faculty and student rates from Media Visions, Inc., 8th Avenue South, South St. Paul, MN 55075.

VIEWING POINTS: Identify the similarities and differences in the lives of those who are homeless. Does your view of homelessness change after seeing this documentary?

West 47th Street: 2001, 2003. This documentary describes services offered by Fountain House, the original clubhouse for persons who are homeless and mentally ill, through the eyes of four clubhouse members. Fountain House has celebrated its 50th year of providing services and is the model for more than 300 clubhouses nationwide. This video is available for purchase from Lichtenstein Creative Media, 25 West 36th Street, 11th floor, New York, NY 10018.

VIEWING POINTS: Discuss the range of services needed for people who are homeless and mentally ill. Visit a clubhouse program in your community and compare the services with those of Fountain House.

REFERENCES

Andrews, M., & Boyle, J. (2003). *Transcultural concepts in nursing care* (4th ed.). Philadelphia: Lippincott Williams & Wilkins.

Banyard, V. L., & Graham-Bermann, S. (1998). Surviving poverty: Stress and coping in the lives of housed and homeless mothers. *American Journal of Orthopsychiatry, 68*(3), 479–489.

Bassuk, E., Buckner, J., Weinreb, L., Browne, A., Bassuk, S. S., Dawson, R., & Perloff, J. N. (1997). Homelessness in female-headed families: Childhood and adult risk and protective factors. *American Journal of Public Health, 87*, 241–248.

Boydell, K., Goering, P., & Morrell-Bellai, T. (2000). Narratives of identity: Re-presentation of self in people who are homeless. *Qualitative Health Research, 10*(1), 26–38.

Bringing America Home. (2005, November). Bill to end homelessness in America introduced in Congress. Retrieved on May 14, 2006, from www.bringingamericahome.org.

Buckner, J., Bassuk, E.L., Weinreb, L. F., & Brooks, M. G. (1999). Homelessness and its relation to the mental health and behavior of low income school age children. *Developmental Psychology, 35*, 246–257.

Carter, J., Cuvar, K., McSweeney, M., Storey, P., & Stockmann, C. (2001). Health-seeking behavior as an outcome of a homeless population. *Outcomes Management for Nursing Practice, 5*(3), 140–143.

Caton, C.L., Dominguez, B., Schanzar, B., Hasin, D.S., Shrout, P.E., Felix, A., et al. (2005). Risk factors for long-term homelessness: Findings from a longitudinal study of first-time homeless adults. *American Journal of Public Health, 95*, 1753–1759.

Center for Mental Health Services and Office of Special Needs Assistance Programs. (1997). *In from the cold: A tool kit for creating safe havens for homeless people on the street.* Washington, DC: U.S. Department of Housing and Urban Development.

Culhane, D., Metraux, S., & Hadley, T. (2001, May). The impact of supportive housing for homeless people with severe mental illness on the utilization of the public health, corrections, and emergency shelter systems. The New York–New York initiative. Housing Policy Debate: Fannie Mae Foundation; www.Fanniemaefoundation.org.

Desai, M. M., & Rosenheck, R. A. (2005). Unmet need for medical care among homeless adults with serious mental illness. *General Hospital Psychiatry, 27*, 418–425.

DeSantis, L. (1997). Building healthy communities with immigrants and refugees. *Journal of Transcultural Nursing, 9*(1), 20–31.

Embry, L.E., Vander Stoep, A.V., Evens, C., Ryan, K.D., & Pollack, A. (2000). Risk factors for homelessness in adolescents released from psychiatric residential treatment. *Journal of the American Academy of Child and Adolescent Psychiatry, 39*, 1293–1299.

Ensign, J. (2003). Ethical issues in qualitative health research with homeless youths. *Journal of Advanced Nursing, 43*(1), 43–50.

Fisher, C., Hoagwood, K., & Jensen, P. (1996). Casebook on ethical issues in research with children and adolescents with mental disorders. In Hoagwood, K., Jensen, P., & Fisher. C. (Eds.), *Ethical issues in mental health research with children and adolescents* (pp. 135–266). Mahwah, NJ: Lawrence Erlbaum Associates.

Folsom, D. P., Hawthorne, W., Lindamer, L., Gilmer, T., Bailey, D., Goldshan, G., et al. (2005). Prevalence and risk factors for homelessness and utilization of mental health services among 10,340 patients with serious mental illness in a large public mental health system. *American Journal of Psychiatry, 162*, 370–376.

Franz, R. (2003, Winter). A 'how-to' of housing: NAMI Delaware's success in establishing and maintaining community-based housing and supports. *NAMI Advocate*, pp. 14–16.

Greene, J., Enneth, S., & Ringwalt, C. (1997). Substance use among runaway and homeless youth in three national samples. *American Journal of Public Health, 87*, 229–235.

Greenwood, R., Schaefer-McDaniel, N., Wenkel, G., & Tsemberis, S. (2005). Decreasing psychiatric symptoms by increasing choice in services for adults with histories of homelessness. *American Journal of Community Psychiatry, 36*(3/4), 223–230.

Herth, K. (1996). Hope from the perspective of homeless families. *Journal of Advanced Nursing, 24*, 743–753.

Humphreys, J. (2000). Spirituality and distress in sheltered battered women. *Journal of Nursing Scholarship, 32*, 273–278.

Interagency Council on the Homeless. (1994). *Priority: Home! The federal plan to break the cycle of homelessness.* (HUD Publication No. 1454-CPD). Washington, DC: Author.

Jason, L. A., Davis, M. I., Ferrari, J. I., & Bishop, P. D. (2001). Oxford House: A review of research implications for substance abuse recovery and community research. *Journal of Drug Education, 31*(1), 1–27.

Jones, R. (1983). Street people and psychiatry: An introduction. *Hospital and Community Psychiatry, 34*, 807–811.

Latimer, E. (2005). Economic considerations associated with assertive community treatment and supported employment for people with severe mental illness. *Journal of Psychiatry Neuroscience, 30*(5), 355–360.

Ledbetter, B. (2002, April). Ethics in youth health research. *Youth and Society Newsletter, 4*, 3–4.

Lowe, E., Slater, A., Welfley, T., & Hardie, D. (2002, December). *A status report on hunger and homelessness in America's cities—2002: A 25-city survey.* Washington, DC: The United States Conference of Mayors.

Mahoney, D. (2005a). Assertive community treatment. *Clinical Psychiatry News, 33*(7), 46.

Mahoney, D. (2005b). Psychiatric first aid: A necessity. *Clinical Psychiatry News, 33*(10), 55–56.

Martens, W. H. (2001). A review of physical and mental health in homeless persons. *Public Health Review, 29*, 13–33.

McCabe, S., Macnee, C., & Anderson, M. (2001). Homeless patients' experience of satisfaction with care. *Archives of Psychiatric Nursing, 15*(2), 78–85.

McComish, J., Greenberg, R., Ager, J., Chruscial, H., & Laken, M. (2000). Survival analysis of three treatment modalities in a residential substance abuse program for women and children. *Outcomes Management for Nursing Practice, 4*(2), 71–77.

McKinney Act renamed. (2000, November 17). *Housing Assistance Council News, 29*(23). Retrieved on April 9, 2003, from *http://216.92.48.246/infoNews.php.*

McKinney-Vento Homeless Assistance Act. (2002, March 12). Homes & Communities. Washington, DC: U.S. Department of Housing and Urban Development, p. 1. Available online at www.hud.gov:80/offices/cpd/homeless/rulesandregs/laws/index.cfm.

McNiel, D, Binder, R., & Robinson, J. (2005). Incarceration associated with homelessness, mental disorder, and co-occurring substance abuse. *Psychiatric Services, 56*, 840–846.

Meadows-Oliver, M. (2005). Social support among homeless and housed mothers: An integrative review. *Journal of Psychosocial Nursing, 43*(2), 40–47.

Menke, E., & Wagner, J. (1997). The experience of homeless female-headed families. *Issues in Mental Health Nursing, 18*, 315–330.

Min, M. O., Biegel, D. E., & Johnson, S. A. (2005). Predictors of psychiatric hospitalization for adults with co-occurring substance and mental disorders as compared to adults with mental illness only. *Psychiatric Rehabilitation Journal, 29*, 114–121.

Mojtabai, R. (2005). Perceived reasons for loss of housing and continual homelessness among homeless persons with mental illness. *Psychiatric Services, 56*, 172–178.

Murray, R. (1996). Needs and resources: The lived experience of homeless men. *Journal of Psychosocial Nursing, 34*(5), 18–24.

NANDA International. (2005). *NANDA Nursing Diagnoses: Definition and classification: 2005–2006.* Philadelphia: Author.

National Coalition for the Homeless (2005a). *Why are people homeless? NCH fact sheet #1.* Available at www.nationalhomeless.org.

National Coalition for the Homeless (2005b). *How many people experience homelessness?* NCH fact *sheet #2.* Available at www.nationalhomeless.org.

National Coalition for the Homeless (NCH). (2005c). *Who is homeless? NCH fact sheet #3.* Available at www.nationalhomeless.org.

National Coalition for the Homeless (2005d). *Mental illness and homelessness. NCH fact sheet #5.* Available at www.nationalhomeless.org.

National Low Income Housing Coalition (2006a). Compilation of homeless counts in major U.S. cities. Retrieved on May 14, 2006, from www.nlihc.org/mtm/mtm10–46.html#22.

National Low Income Housing Coalition (2006b). National housing trust fund in your community. Retrieved on June 4, 2006, from www.nhtf.org.

North, C. S., Kyrich, K. M., Pollio, D. E., & Spitznagel, E. L. (2004). Are rates of psychiatric disorders in the homeless population changing? *American Journal of Public Health, 94*, 103–108.

Not getting over it: Post-traumatic stress disorder. *Harvard Women's Health Watch, 12*(7), 4–6.

Nyamathi, A., Leake, B., Keenan, C., & Gelberg, L. (2000). Type of social support among homeless women: Its impact on psychosocial resources, health and health behaviors, and use of health services. *Nursing Research, 49*(6), 318–326.

Phelan, J., & Link, B. (1999). Who are 'the homeless'? Reconsidering the stability and composition of the homeless population. *American Journal of Public Health, 89*(9), 1334–1388.

Reeves, R., Parker, J., Konkle-Parker, D. (2005). War-related mental health problems of today's veterans. *Journal of Psychosocial Nursing, 43*(7), 18–27.

Rew. L., Taylor-Seehafer, M., & Thomas, N. (2000). Without parental consent: Conducting research with homeless adolescents. *Journal of the Society of Pediatric Nurses, 5*, 131–138.

Roman, N. (2002). Why America can end homelessness in ten years. *Housing Facts and Findings: Fannie Mae Foundation, 24*(5), 3–8.

Rosenheck, R. (2000). Cost-effectiveness of services for mentally ill homeless people. The application of research to policy and practice. *American Journal of Psychiatry, 157*(10), 1563–1570.

Rosenheck, R., Bassuk, E., & Salomon, A. (1999). Special populations of homeless Americans. In L. B. Fosburg & D. L. Dennis (Eds.), *Practical lessons: The 1998 National Symposium on homelessness Research.* Retrieved on June 4, 2006, from www.aspe.hhs.gov/progsys/homeless/symposium/Toc.htm

Rosenheck, R. A., Resnick, S. G., & Morrissey, J. P. (2003). Closing service system gaps for homeless clients with a dual diagnosis: Integrated teams and interagency collaboration. *Journal of Mental Health Policy & Economics, 6*(2), 77–87.

Salkow, K., & Fichter, M. (2003). Homelessness and mental illness. *Current Opinion in Psychiatry, 16*, 467–471.

Sandhaus, S. (1998). Migrant health: A harvest of poverty. *American Journal of Nursing, 98*(9), 52–54.

Sperling, A. (2003, Winter). Locked out of housing: Lack of affordable housing, a barrier to recovery for many consumers. *NAMI Advocate*, pp. 12–13.

Sullivan, G., Burnam, A., & Koegel, P. (2000). Pathways to homelessness among the mentally ill. *Social Psychiatry & Psychiatric Epidemiology, 35*, 444–450.

Sullivan, G., Burnam, A., Koegel, P., & Hollenberg, J. (2000). Quality of life of homeless persons with mental illness: Results from the course-of-homelessness study. *Psychiatric Services, 51*(9), 1135–1141.

U.S. Bureau of the Census (2000). *Statistical abstract of the United States* (120th ed.). Washington, D.C.: U.S. Department of Commerce.

U.S. Department of Housing and Urban Development. (2000). *Continuum of care and HOPWA application* (Form HUD040076-CoC). Washington, DC: Author.

U.S. Department of Housing and Urban Development. (1998). *Understanding the shelter plus care program.* Washington, DC: Author.

Watts, J. (2003). The struggle to end homelessness. Publication of *Washington University in St. Louis, AQ4 75*(3), 14–19.

Weingart Center Institute for the Study of Homelessness and Poverty (2005, December). Homeless counts in major U.S. cities and counties. Retrieved on June 4, 2006, from www.weingart.org/center/pdf/200512-city-county-homeless-counts.pdf.

Williamson, G. R., & Prosser, S. (2002). Action research: Politics, ethics, and participation. *Journal of Advanced Nursing, 40*, 587–593.

CHAPTER 34

Issues in Co-Occurring Disorders

Mary Ann Boyd, Barbara G. Faltz, and Harvey Davis

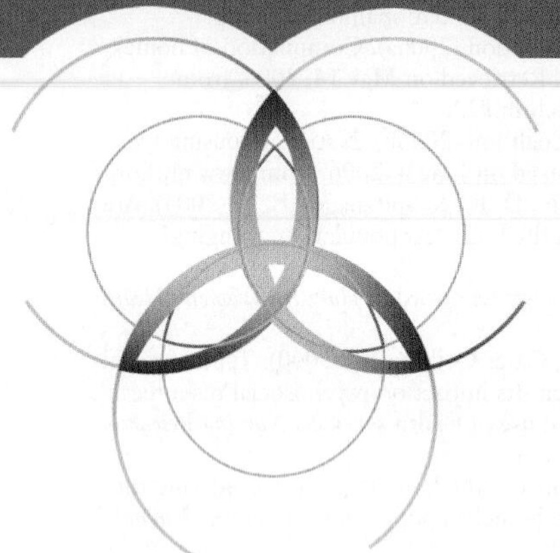

LEARNING OBJECTIVES

After studying this chapter, you will be able to:

- Define the term co-occurring disorders.
- Discuss the epidemiology of co-occurring disorders.
- Describe the cycle of relapse.
- Discuss patterns of substance abuse and other mental disorders.
- Analyze barriers to the treatment of patients with co-occurring disorders.
- Discuss stage-wise treatment for co-occurring disorders.
- Discuss the significance of an integrated treatment approach to co-occurring disorders.
- Describe nursing management of persons with co-occurring disorders.

KEY CONCEPTS

- co-occurring disorders
- relapse cycle

KEY TERMS

• assertive community treatment • case management • engagement • integrated treatment • motivational interventions • quadrants of care • relapse prevention • recovery • self-medicate • stage-wise treatment

KEY CONCEPT The term **co-occurring disorders** (COD) refers to the presence of co-morbid mental illness and a substance use disorder in the same person.

Mental illness and substance use disorder are each a primary mental disorder, even though they do not necessarily appear at the same time. A diagnosis of co-occurring disorders (COD) means that at least one disorder of each type can be established independently. People with COD respond to the interaction of two psychiatric illnesses, not just two discrete disorders. In many instances, the use of substances serves as a coping strategy for dealing with the psychiatric symptoms. Without alternative, effective coping behaviors, the patient will continue to **self-medicate** (using medication, usually over-the-counter or substances without professional prescription or supervision to alleviate an illness or condition). Persons with COD have poorer outcomes, such as higher rates of HIV infection, relapse, rehospitalization, depression, and suicide risk (Center for Substance Abuse Treatment, 2005).

The goal of treatment for patients with COD is a comprehensive recovery plan for the complex problems presented—one that offers the patient a way out of what can be a downward spiral of debilitation. Effective treatment of COD requires an integrated approach based on both an understanding of mental illness and addiction. **Integrated treatment**, coordinated substance abuse and mental health interventions, requires modifying traditional approaches to both the mental illness and addiction (Ziedonis, 2004).

This chapter presents the epidemiology and etiological patterns of COD and discusses specific mental illnesses and the adverse effects of concurrent substance use. It highlights methods of assessing COD and offers treatment strategies and nursing interventions to address this complex yet common presentation in psychiatric and substance use treatment settings. A complete discussion of related substance use disorders is provided in Chapter 25.

SUBSTANCE USE, MENTAL DISORDERS, AND RELAPSE

The problem of COD was inadvertently magnified during the community mental health reform movement when there was a rational movement toward deinstitutionalization of the mentally ill (see Chapter 1). Large numbers of mentally ill were left homeless, lost to local and state mental health systems. Their long-standing mental illnesses and protected life in a state hospital increased their vulnerability to exploitation by others, particularly the more astute and street-wise addicts. Along with homelessness came the increased use of drugs and alcohol (Hwang, 2001).

It is impossible to make any meaningful distinction between simple recreational use of a substance and actual substance use with this population because even small amounts of alcohol or other drugs can be damaging to people who have concurrent psychiatric problems. All substances of abuse exert profound effects on mental states, perception, psychomotor function, cognition, and behavior. The specific neurochemical and other biologic mechanisms that evoke these psychological features are discussed in Chapter 25. Table 34.1 lists the psychological effects of substances of abuse.

A frequent problem of this group is relapse, which leads to repeated hospitalizations or the "revolving door" phenomenon. When symptoms of the mental disorder are stabilized, the hospitalized patient is discharged. Once in the community, the patient fails to follow the therapeutic regimen and resumes the use of alcohol or drugs. Reappearance of symptoms leads to another episode of hospitalization. The relapse cycle is characterized by a pattern of decompensation, hospitalization, stabilization, discharge, and then decompensation (see Fig. 34.1).

KEY CONCEPT In the **relapse cycle,** re-emerging psychiatric symptoms lead to ineffective coping strategies, increased anxiety, substance use to avoid painful feelings, adverse consequences, and attempted abstinence, until psychiatric symptoms emerge once more and the cycle repeats itself.

EPIDEMIOLOGY

The pattern of alcohol and illicit drug use by the mentally ill varies, but it is now generally agreed that as many

Table 34.1 Psychological Effects of Substances of Abuse

Substance	Psychological Effects
Alcohol	Alcohol amnestic syndrome; dementia Agitation, anxiety disorders, sleep disorders Ataxia, slurred speech Withdrawal symptoms, which may include hallucinations, confusion, illusions, delusions; protracted withdrawal delirium can occur Depression, increased rate of suicide, disinhibition
Cocaine	Anxiety, agitation, hyperactivity, sleep disorders, delusions, paranoia, euphoria, internal sense of interest and excitement Rebound withdrawal symptoms, such as prolonged depression, somnolence, anhedonia
Amphetamines	Similar to cocaine but more prolonged Hyperactivity, agitation, anxiety, increased energy
Hallucinogens (MOMA Ecstasy) and phencyclidine	Hallucinations, delusions, paranoia, confusion Withdrawal can produce severe depression, somnolence Hallucinations, illusions, delusions, perceptual distortions, paranoia, rage, anxiety, agitation, confusion
Marijuana	Acute reactions: panic, anxiety, paranoia, sensory distortions, rare psychotic episodes; patients with schizophrenia use these reactions to distance themselves from painful symptoms and to gain control over symptoms Antimotivational syndrome: apathy, diminished interest in activities and goals, poor job or school performance, memory and cognitive deficits
Opiates	Confusion, somnolence Withdrawal can produce anxiety, irritability, and depression and can trigger suicidal ideation
Sedative-hypnotics	Confusion, slurred speech, ataxia, stupor, sleep disorders, withdrawal delirium, dementia, amnestic disorder, sleep disorders
Volatile solvents	Hallucinations, delusions, hyperactivity, sensory distortions, dementia

Adapted from Beauchamp, J. K., & Olson K. R. (2000). Drug overdoses and dependence. In R. M. Wachter, L. Goldman, H. Hollander (Eds.), *Hospital medicine.* Philadelphia: Lippincott Williams & Wilkins.

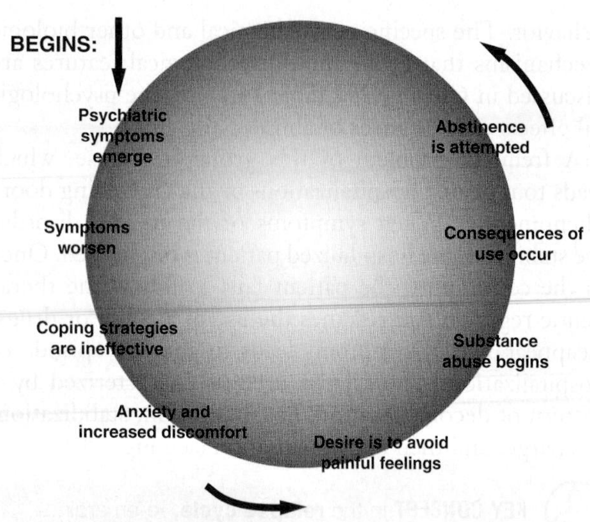

FIGURE 34.1. Relapse cycle.

as 50% of the mentally ill also have a substance abuse problem. Thirty-seven percent of alcohol abusers and 53% of drug users also have at least one serious mental illness. Of all people diagnosed with a mental disorder, 29% either abuse drugs or alcohol (National Alliance for the Mentally Ill [NAMI], 2007). The drug most commonly used is alcohol, followed by marijuana and cocaine. Prescription drugs such as tranquilizers and sleeping medicines may also be abused.

Risk for substance use varies among the mental disorders (see Table 34.2). Antisocial personality disorders, bipolar depression and disorders of childhood including conduct disorders, oppositional-defiant disorders, and attention-deficit disorders (see Chapter 29) are strongly associated with substance abuse disorders (Kessler, 2004).

ETIOLOGY

There is no one model that explains why mental disorders and substance abuse occur together so frequently. In one pattern of occurrence, the mental disorder precedes the substance abuse. As adolescents with emerging mental disorders are exposed to drug use, their disinhibition and impulsivity lead to drug experimentation. Substances of abuse are used to self-medicate the underlying mental disorders. In the second pattern, the substance abuse disorder appears first and leads to the mental disorder. For example, LSD or cocaine use may change the neurotransmission in the brain that results in panic attacks or psychosis. In the third pattern, there are common causes, either genetic or environmental, that lead to the onset or persistence of both disorders.

Current research is beginning to offer an explanation for the pattern where the symptoms of the mental disorder generally appear first followed by the substance use and abuse (Kessler, 2004). Psychiatric symptoms have long been associated with dysregulation of the monoamines and neuropeptides. Drugs of abuse (cocaine, alcohol, marijuana) temporarily potentiate neurotransmission in the brain's reward system, relieving the depression and anxiety for a short period of time. Self-administration of drugs of abuse temporarily masks or suppresses the aversive psychological effects of the dysregulated neuronal systems (Bruijnzeel, Repetto, & Gold, 2004).

Table 34.2 Major Psychiatric Disorders and Risks for Substance Abuse

Psychiatric Disorder	Increased Risk For Substance Abuse (%)
Antisocial personality disorder	15.5
Manic episode	14.5
Schizophrenia	10.1
Panic disorder	4.3
Major depressive episode	4.1
Obsessive-compulsive disorder	3.4
Phobias	2.4

From Mental Health America, Dual Diagnosis. Retrieved on February 21, 2007, from www.nmha.org/go/information.

BARRIERS TO TREATMENT

High morbidity rates point to the need for effective treatment of COD. Although it was recognized that integrated treatment should be the standard of care, data from the National Surveys on Drugs and Health on the use of treatment for adults with comorbid mental health and substance use problems found very low rates of substance abuse treatment (Harris & Edlund, 2005). These results raise concern about the barriers these patients often face in obtaining proper treatment. There are many well-documented social barriers such as homelessness, unemployment, and lack of social support for abstinence. The following discussion highlights some other barriers.

Nature of Co-Occurring Disorders

Patients often deny a problem with substances and do not seek treatment because they do not view themselves as needing it. They do not fully understand their mental illness or the effect of substance use on their mood or behavior. Even those who recognize their disorders are often reluctant to seek mental health treatment. It is confusing to be expected to abstain from alcohol and illicit drugs, yet be prescribed medication which also affects their thoughts and feelings. If they take the substance of choice, they experience fleeting moments of joy and escape, even though doing so will prompt a decline in overall function and worsen psychiatric symptoms. If they accept prescribed treatments, including medications, they will have higher levels of functioning and better treatment outcomes, but they lose their moments of joy and escape.

Staff Attitudes

Mental health professionals in psychiatric treatment programs are often frustrated in their efforts to assist substance-using patients. Behavior often associated with addiction, such as denial of substance use, manipulative behavior, and nonadherence with health-related protocols, is often regarded as a sign of treatment failure. This type of behavior can provoke hostility from the staff and can make planning for mental health recovery difficult.

Mental health professionals may have difficulty understanding the compelling nature of drug or alcohol cravings, may not understand differences in drug use patterns and behaviors associated with particular drugs of abuse, and may overdiagnose personality disorders in those who take drugs and commit crimes (Churchill, 2003). In addition, patients or their therapists may excuse substance use because of the patients' psychiatric symptoms.

Stigma

Drug-dependent patients may have the additional stigma of being regarded as criminals because they commit illegal acts every time they purchase, use, or distribute illicit drugs. Strong public feelings about alcohol-related motor vehicle accidents, negative experiences with family members or friends with drinking problems, and cultural biases against public intoxication can prejudice interactions with patients who are alcohol dependent (Kessler, 2004).

Health Issues

Numerous health hazards are associated with alcohol and drug abuse (see Chapter 25). Patients with COD are more likely than others to use emergency departments for primary health care, waiting until they can no longer ignore physical illness. They are more likely to be unclear about the medical plan they need to follow and to be noncompliant with health care directives. The use of alcohol and illicit substances in addition to medications prescribed for mental illness can lead to drug interactions and may exacerbate side effects of these medications. Homelessness can increase these patients' medical problems (Hwang, 2002), with inadequate nutrition, poor hygiene, and the adverse effects of exposure to the elements adding to their difficulties. Health care providers often become frustrated with patients' nonadherence and with what they see as behaviors that are difficult to manage. Their frustration may negatively affect the way they treat patients with COD. Because of the confusion about what is the primary and most immediate problem to treat, these patients are often underserved and only partially treated.

INTERDISCIPLINARY TREATMENT

Treatment programs designed for people whose problems are primarily substance abuse are generally not recommended for people who also have a mental illness. These programs tend to be confrontational and coercive and most people with severe mental illnesses are too fragile to benefit from them. Heavy confrontation, intense emotional jolting, and discouragement of the use of medications tend to be detrimental. These treatments may produce levels of stress that exacerbate symptoms or cause relapse.

The **quadrants of care** is a conceptual framework that classifies patients according to symptom severity, not diagnosis (see Figure 31.2). The quadrant can guide an individual's treatment and site of delivery of care. In an integrated treatment model, treatment for both disorders is combined in a single session or interaction or series of interactions.

Patients with COD enter treatment at various stages of recovery. Flexible treatment programs that can meet each patient's needs are the most effective. **Stage-wise treatment** moves the patient toward recovery through commonly recognized stages of treatment: engagement, persuasion or motivation, active treatment, and relapse prevention. This approach has proven useful because patients are at different stages (Drake et al., 2001). An integrated interdisciplinary team is needed in order to move patients to recovery.

Engagement

Engagement entails establishing a treatment relationship and enhancing motivation to make behavior changes and a commitment to treatment. Research has shown that engaged patients are more likely to stay in treatment and have positive outcomes (Drake, Mueser, Brunette, & McHugo, 2004). Patients who are abusing substances may experience repeated cycles of detoxification and relapse. Mentally ill patients may have prolonged cycles of "revolving-door" admissions and persistent medication nonadherence before acknowledging the need to engage in continuous treatment (Kertesz, Horton, Friedmann, & Samet, 2003). Each admission is a "window of opportunity." Relapse does not mean that a treatment intervention, the health care provider, or the patient has failed. Readmission and clear, realistic goals can further the patient's engagement in the treatment process. Effective programs emphasize a combination of empathic, long-term relationship building and the use of leverage and possible confrontation by family, other caregivers, or the legal system.

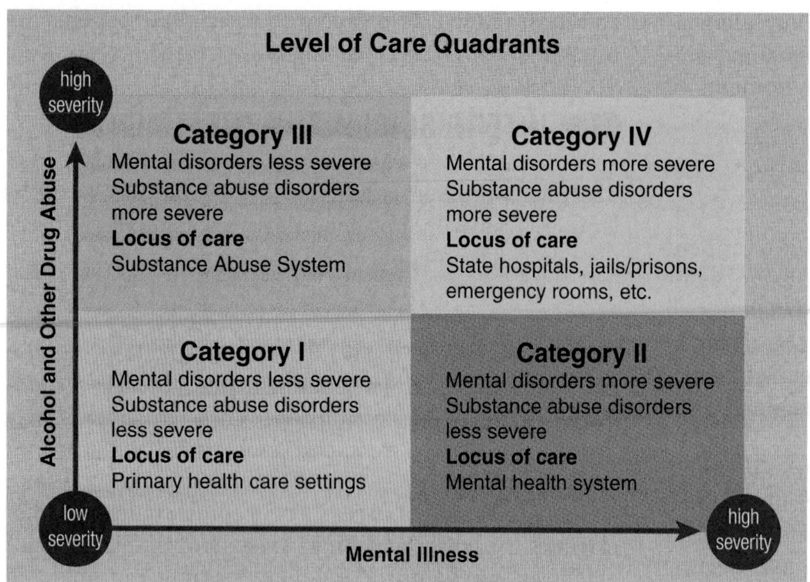

FIGURE 34.2. Level of care quadrants. From Center for Drug Abuse Treatment, 2005. Definition, terms and classification systems for co-occurring disorders.

Engaging patients with COD in treatment presents two main challenges. The first is developing relationships with people who tend to have difficulties in their relationships and with trusting authority figures. The second is patients' lack of motivation and the need to encourage them to enter drug and alcohol treatment programs.

Engagement in treatment is a process that may take many contacts with a patient and requires patience. Patients who struggle with authority and control issues must be convinced that the treatment team members have something to offer and are worth listening to before they will begin to trust them. The engagement process is enhanced if staff can deal with presenting crises concretely (e.g., provide help in avoiding legal penalties and obtaining food, housing, entitlements, relief from psychiatric symptoms, vocational opportunities, recreation, and socialization). Harm reduction may be a first step toward a goal of abstinence.

The process of engagement is often characterized by approach–avoidance behavior by the patient. Intake and assessment procedures may discourage the patient from engagement or be intolerable if they are protracted and begin with asking the patient numerous pointed personal questions. These procedures may have to be adjusted to tailor treatment and accommodate the needs or reactions of the patient with COD.

Motivational Interventions

Motivational interventions are useful in the COD patients (see Chapter 25). Typically, these interventions consist of one to several sessions delivered within a few weeks or less where the patient is motivated to become involved in treatment. One goal of this intervention is to increase engagement in treatment and help the patient identify his or her own goals (Drake et al., 2004).

Assertive Outreach

There are two models of assertive outreach that have been shown to be effective in reducing substance use (Essock et al., 2006). In the **case management** model, case managers are responsible for conducting outreach activities, linking patients with direct services, monitoring patients' progress through various milieus, educating patients about psychiatric and substance use disorders, reiterating treatment recommendations, and coordinating treatment planning across programs. In this model, case managers represent different disciplines and emphasize an interdisciplinary team approach. Team members carry their own individual caseloads, but discuss their patients and review cases together.

In **assertive community treatment,** the delivery of services are in the community (rather than a clinic), with shared caseloads, 24-hour responsibilities for patients, and direct provision of most services. This model was developed for patients with severe mental illness who do not use outpatient services, are prone to frequent relapses and rehospitalization, and have severe psychosocial impairment. This approach may be superior to case management in those settings characterized by high hospitalization use (Essock et al., 2006).

Relapse Prevention

Persons with COD are highly prone to relapse even after they have achieved full remission. Although many relapse factors are the same for those with mental disorders as with the general population such as interpersonal problems, negative emotions, social stresses, lack of involvement in more satisfying activities, and attempts to escape from painful experiences, there are additional factors that affect this population. Symptoms of the mental illness recur and there are inadequate treatment resources in many settings. Many people with mental illness live in extreme poverty, which forces them into high-crime, drug-infested neighborhoods, which makes them easy targets for crimes. Employment rates are low for this population, even though many want to work. Finally, the same neurobiologic dysfunctions may underlie both substance abuse and mental illness (Drake, Wallach, & McGovern, 2005).

Because persons with mental disorders face more challenges, emerging evidence suggests that **relapse prevention** for this population should be different than for the general population (Drake, Wallach, & McGovern, 2005). Relapse prevention needs to account for the pervasive cognitive and social dysfunctions that are inherent in many people with COD. There is usually a need for assistance in finding and maintaining housing and employment. Learning new skills may be difficult because of cognitive impairments that reduce the effectiveness of learning new skills. Social deficits can lead to isolation and victimization (Drake et al., 2005). Relapse prevention for COD involves the following:

- Living situations that provide meaningful opportunities and the acquisition of supports and skills
- Help in making fundamental changes, such as finding meaningful jobs and abstinent friends
- Long-term supports and relationships (new friendships with people who do not abuse substances)
- Specific and individualized treatments for specific problems
- Support for meeting spiritual needs and finding a sense of meaning in life
- Economic and political support in creating appropriate and decent housing (Drake et al., 2005).

NURSING MANAGEMENT

It is crucial for patients with COD to be thoroughly assessed for responses to both psychiatric and substance use disorders (Petrakis, Gonzalez, Rosenheck, & Krystal, 2002). In some cultural groups, recognition of psychiatric and substance abuse disorders is difficult because of the lack of access and stigma associated with COD. Nurses in nonpsychiatric, community settings may be the only health care professional contact that some groups have (see Box 34.1). Assessment should include determination of the patient's willingness to change or level of motivation for treatment.

It is important to delineate the relative contribution of each diagnosis to the severity of the current responses presented and to establish priorities accordingly. Because patients with COD often make unreliable historians or distort the reality of their mental health problems and the severity of their substance use, obtaining objective data is especially important. Ideally, one should obtain an objective history of the patient from family, significant others, board and care operators, other health care providers, or anyone familiar enough with the patient to provide an accurate history. Box 34.2 lists basic assessment tools and methods used for patients with COD. The following concepts are paramount when assessing persons with COD:

- Psychiatric and substance use disorders can coexist.
- Responses (psychosis, agitation) to both disorders can be similar.

BOX 34.1

Research for Best Practice: ***Comorbidity and Violence in Rural African American Women***

Boyd, M. B, Mackey, M. C., Phillips, K. D., & Tavakoli, A. (2006). Alcohol and other drug disorders, comorbidity and violence in rural African American women. Issues in Mental Health Nursing, 27(10), 1017–1036.

The Question: How do rural African American women (*N* = 142) with and without alcohol and other drug disorders (AOD) vary on drugs of abuse, Axis I psychiatric disorders, and adult and childhood victimization?

Methods: Women with AOD who live in rural counties were recruited at discharge from an inpatient facility. Women without AOD were voluntary participants from county health clinics serving the same counties. The presence of psychiatric disorders was based on the NIMH Diagnostic Interview Schedule. Four groups emerged: women with an AOD disorder only (*N* = 31), women with an AOD and a comorbid psychiatric disorder (*N* = 30); women with no psychiatric disorder (*N* = 58) and women with no AOD disorder but with other psychiatric disorders.

Findings: The most frequently abused drug for both groups of AOD women (with and without psychiatric disorders) was cocaine, followed closely by marijuana and alcohol. The group with co-occuring substance use and mental disorder drank more alcohol during the week and weekend than the AOD group with no other psychiatric disorder. The AOD women with a psychiatric disorder experienced greater violence and childhood and sexual abuse. The most common disorders for these women were PTSD and major depression.

Implications for Nursing: It is important that all nurses working in rural settings know the signs and symptoms of psychiatric disorders so they can identify women who need a more extensive evaluation and referral for treatment.

BOX 34.2

Assessment of Co-Occurring Disorders

Obtain history and physical examination, laboratory tests (e.g., liver function tests, complete blood count) to confirm medical indicators related to substance use and also to rule out medical disorders with psychiatric presentations

- Obtain substance use history and severity of consequences, and physical symptoms
  - Identify core cultural values; explore meaning of the symptoms
- Assess mental status examination and severity of symptoms (e.g., suicidal, homicidal, florid psychosis)
  - Explore social context—socioeconomic, environment, literacy, and support system

Interview with and assess family members, to verify or determine: (1) the accuracy of the patient's self-reported substance use or mental health history; (2) the patient's history of past mental health problems during periods of abstinence; and, if possible, (3) the sequence of the diagnoses (i.e., what symptoms appeared first)

- Conduct interviews with partner, friends, social worker, and other significant people in the patient's life
- Review court records, medical records, and previous psychiatric and substance use treatment
- Perform urine and blood toxicity screens; use of breath analyzer to test blood alcohol level

Revise initial assessment by observation of the patient in the clinical setting; full assessment of the underlying psychiatric problem may not be possible until there is a long (up to 6 months) period of total abstinence

- Observe patient for reappearance of psychiatric symptoms after a period of sobriety
- Assess patient's motivation to seek treatment, desire to change behavior, and understanding of diagnoses

- Substance use can mask other symptoms and syndromes.
- Psychiatric behaviors can mimic alcohol and other drug use problems.

• NCLEXNOTE

Patients with both mental illness and substance abuse disorders have responses to both disorders. Prioritizing nursing care will depend on the immediate issue, but responses to both disorders should be assessed.

Thought Disorders and Substance Use

Research shows a high percentage (47%-80%) of persons with schizophrenia will have a substance abuse disorder during their lifetime (Buckley, 2006; Westermeyer, 2006). There are a number of explanations for the increased rate of substance abuse in this disorder. One is that the use of substances (cocaine, amphetamines, marijuana, hallucinogens) triggers the onset of acute and chronic psychotic disorders (Caton et al., 2005). A neurobiologic model suggests that a dysregulated dopamine-mediated mesocorticolimbic network in patients with schizophrenia may also underlie substance use (Green, 2006) (see Chapter 18). Whereas all people are vulnerable to experiencing psychotic episodes from the use of various drugs, one psychotic episode increases susceptibility to subsequent episodes (Olson, 2004).

Assessing the needs of people with schizophrenia who are also chemically dependent is complicated by the changing interaction among psychotic symptoms, the antipsychotic effects of medications, and the side effects of medications. The patient with a psychotic disorder may have an altered thought process or delusional thinking and may experience auditory hallucinations. He or she may also be cognitively impaired and have poor memory. These patients can have negative symptoms, such as poor motivation and poor hygiene. They often have low self-esteem, poor social skills, and may have a general sense of not belonging to a community. Their sense of self in relation to the world may be altered.

As with all of the CODs, a multifaceted, integrated treatment approach is needed. Atypical antipsychotics continue to be the primary pharmacological agent for the treatment of comorbid schizophrenia with substance use. Not only do these agents treat the symptoms of schizophrenia, but they appear to reduce cue-trigger cravings of the substances and prevent relapse (Green, 2006). While monitoring side effects of antipsychotics, the nurse's attention needs to focus on liver functioning because drugs and alcohol are also metabolized by the liver. Relapse is frequently secondary to medication nonadherence, especially if patients experience side effects associated with the use of antipsychotics. Nursing interventions that focus on medication compliance may reduce the chances of relapse.

A confrontational interactive approach will not benefit this population and could even alienate patients. A more supportive approach is appropriate, in which relapses are treated as an expected part of the recovery process. Addressing relapse risk is part of treatment planning. Focus on examining behavior, feelings, and the thinking process that led to the relapse. The nurse must avoid blame and guilt-inducing statements.

Social skills training is needed to help the patient learn ways of avoiding peer pressure and social situations that could lead to substance use. The goal is to successfully interact in a sober living situation, develop problem-solving skills, and refine behaviors.

Mood Disorders and Substance Use

Substance use is more common in patients with bipolar depression than in those with any other Axis I diagnosis and may also contribute to treatment nonadherence and less positive outcomes (Kessler, 2004; Myrick, Cluver, Swavely, Peters, 2004). Mood disorders may be more prevalent among patients using opiates than among other drug users. Many who use substances self-medicate an underlying mood disorder. Because many of the symptoms of substance use are the same as those of mood disorders, it is difficult to differentiate between them. This is especially true in the case of stimulant use and bipolar disorder. It is often impossible to determine the presence of an underlying mood disorder until there has been a period of abstinence.

Screening for suicide ideation is a priority during the assessment of these individuals. Both mood disorders and substance abuse are related to suicide (see Chapters 17, 20, and 25). Depression during withdrawal from alcohol, cocaine, opiates, and amphetamines also puts patients at severe risk for suicide. A person's presenting behaviors may not have included depression, but depression may develop as the withdrawal syndrome unfolds. Hyperactivity often appears with stimulant use and at times with alcohol abuse. Patients may be treated for hypomania or bipolar disorder when they are in fact hyperactive. Symptoms usually improve as the person maintains abstinence.

Determining whether mood disorders are the cause or the effect of protracted substance use is difficult (Table 34.3). One important nursing assessment is to determine how drug use relates to mood states. Patients may be attempting to alleviate uncomfortable symptoms, such as depression or agitation, or to enhance a mood state, such as hypomania. Symptoms that persist during periods of abstinence are a clue to the degree that the mood disorder contributes to the presenting symptoms.

There is little research regarding pharmacological interventions for comorbid mood disorders and substance abuse. Consequently, treatment is similar to that of mood disorders without substance use or abuse. When a pharmacological agent is selected, attention is paid to its interaction with drugs and alcohol and its potential for abuse. The selective serotonin reuptake inhibitors (SSRIs) are frequently used for depression. Higher doses may be required because of the possibility that alcohol use may induce hepatic microsomal activity. In the bipolar disorders, mood stabilizers are used.

Patients with bipolar disorders can benefit from chemical dependency treatment if their medications are stabilized and they can tolerate group treatment approaches, focus on and complete simple goals, and follow simple ground rules in a treatment program. Evans and Sullivan (2001) suggest these guidelines for treatment:

- Limit responses in group sessions (e.g., to less than 5 minutes of total group time).
- Limit the length of responses to simple exercises.
- Work with patients to heal interpersonal relationships that may have become impaired as a result of manic episodes.
- Relate patients' substance use and manic episodes to out-of-control behavior for which ongoing treatment (recovery) plans are needed.

For patients who have depression and a substance use disorder, employing interventions centered on examining cognitive distortions (e.g., "I'll never get better, no one likes me, alcohol is my only friend") and cognitive therapy techniques can help improve mood. Use of positive self-talk can be helpful for both the depression and the substance use disorders. Working on unresolved grief can be appropriate. However, assignments that deal with patients' previous actions can evoke guilt, self-blame, and expressions of low self-esteem, thereby increasing depression (Evans & Sullivan, 2001).

Anxiety Disorders and Substance Use

Research is scant regarding the relationship of anxiety disorders to substance abuse. Because there are a variety of anxiety disorders with differing clinical symptoms and numerous substances of abuse, it is difficult to develop studies addressing all the anxiety disorders. Findings from one large 4-year study suggest that social phobia and panic disorder in adolescents and young adults pre-

Table 34.3 Drugs That Precipitate or Mimic Mood Disorders

Mood Disorders	During Use (Intoxication)	After Use (Withdrawal)
Depression and dysthymia	Alcohol, benzodiazepines, opioids, barbiturates, cannabis, steroids (chronic use), stimulants (chronic use)	Alcohol, benzodiazepines, opioids, barbiturates, cannabis, steroids (chronic use), stimulants (chronic use)
Mania and cyclothymia	Stimulants, alcohol, hallucinogens, inhalants, steroids (chronic and acute use)	Alcohol, benzodiazepines, barbiturates, opiates, steroids (chronic use)

dict alcohol disorders, while other anxiety disorders do not (Zimmerman et al., 2003). Posttraumatic stress disorder (PTSD) is of particular concern because it has been shown to increase the risk of substance use relapse and is associated with poor treatment outcomes (Rosenthal & Westreich, 1999).

The symptoms of anxiety may result from an anxiety disorder, such as panic attack, or may be secondary to drug or alcohol use, as part of a withdrawal syndrome. Symptoms are so subjectively disturbing that they can lead to drug or alcohol abuse as self-medication for the emotional pain; therefore, they require prompt evaluation and treatment. There are many unanswered questions regarding the relationship of the anxiety symptoms, stress, and changes in the HPA axis response to substance use. More research is sorely needed in this area.

Pharmacologic treatment of anxiety is difficult because the traditional medications used, the benzodiazepines, are themselves addicting. Long-term treatment of the anxiety disorders, particularly PTSD, with the SSRIs maintains and improves quality of life. For PTSD, other medications such as the atypical antipsychotics, non-SSRI antidepressants, and mood stabilizers also appear to result in improvements (Davis, Frazier, Williford, & Newell, 2006).

Comorbid anxiety disorders and substance abuse require psychosocial interventions along with pharmacological treatment. Cognitive behavior therapy has repeatedly been shown to be effective in treating COD patients with PTSD (Goldsmith & Garlapati, 2004). Patients with anxiety disorders should also pay particular attention to their physical health. Regular, balanced meals; exercise; and sleep are ways to decrease and manage stress levels. Patients should avoid excessive consumption of caffeine and sugars. If the patient has a fear of crowds, he or she may benefit from gradual desensitization techniques.

Personality Disorders and Substance Use

Personality disorders are frequently present in those who abuse alcohol and other substances. Antisocial personality disorder carries the highest risk of having a comorbid substance abuse problem (Hasin, Samet, Meydan, Matseonane, Waxman, 2006). In an earlier epidemiology study, lifetime prevalence rate of substance abuse in antisocial personality disorder was 83.6% for any substance use disorder, whereas borderline personality disorder had a 28% rate of substance dependence (Thomas, Melchert, & Banker, 1999).

The assessment of persons with comorbid personality disorders and substance abuse focuses on the problems related to the particular personality disorder as well as the substance use. Individuals with antisocial personality disorder are likely to have a family history of other psychiatric disorders and problems with hostility. Interventions should be individualized according to the disorder and are discussed in the next section.

INTERVENTIONS FOR PERSONS WITH CO-OCCURRING DISORDERS

The nurse who provides care to patients with COD faces numerous challenges. Nurses implement interventions according to their level of practice and knowledge. Comprehensive planning within a multidisciplinary team approach is highly successful in the care of such patients. The entire system is organized to care for persons with COD. (Center for Substance Abuse Treatment, 2005). Community organizations are valuable sources of support as well. Many of the interventions that are indicated for persons with COD are discussed in previous chapters (see Unit 5). The following discussion highlights interventions that are modified because of the special needs of this population.

Medication Management

One essential feature of COD treatment is medication management. Medication for a known mental disorder should never be discontinued on the grounds that the patient is using substances. Nonadherence with prescribed medications is associated with increased behavior problems after discharge and is a direct cause of relapse and rehospitalization. Impulsive behavior in response to transient exacerbations of psychotic symptoms, depressed mood, or anxiety symptoms may lead to relapse.

Treating a patient with COD can be as complex as the presenting symptoms. Errors in treatment can include treating temporary psychiatric symptoms resulting from withdrawal as if they were a permanent feature of the individual, withholding needed medication for a psychiatric disorder, or setting arbitrary limits on medication based on a belief that medication for all psychiatric symptoms should be suspended for a time. Benzodiazepines are not recommended in the ongoing treatment of patients with substance dependence (Minkoff, 2001).

Collaboration between the patient's prescriber and other treatment providers is important to minimize the possible misuse or abuse of prescription drugs such as forging prescriptions, acquiring drugs from nonmedical sources, frequent visits to emergency departments or seeking multiple prescribers. In addition, caution is essential in prescribing medications that can increase the patient's potential for relapse into abusing the drug of choice. The patient in recovery is often reluctant to use potentially mind-altering drugs, and the nurse should explore any concerns.

Substance Abuse Counseling

With the COD patient, substance abuse counseling is slower and less confrontational than in many traditional substance abuse programs. Content needs to be repeated frequently and motivation for treatment continually assessed (Drake et al., 2004).

Cognitive Behavioral Interventions

Cognitive behavioral interventions help patients to (1) analyze which situations are most likely to trigger relapses; (2) examine cognitive, emotional, and behavioral components of high-risk situations; and (3) develop cognitive, behavioral, and effective coping strategies and environmental supports. Role playing ways out of high-risk situations is a technique that these groups often use. Homework assignments help patients create relapse prevention plans that address new coping strategies for these high-risk situations.

Patient Education 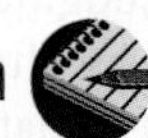

Patient education is an essential element in treating COD. Patients need to learn about their specific mental disorder, substance use and abuse, and their effects. Relapse prevention and recovery should be highlighted. Education can be conducted in individual sessions, but group sessions encourage interaction among patients. Sharing their experiences with their peers, patients can enhance these presentations.

Topics should be clear, relevant to the group members, and illustrated with charts, handouts, or appropriate films. Each session should be relatively short and not contain too many new or difficult concepts. Reinforcing and reviewing previous discussions can be helpful to remind patients of particularly relevant concepts. Box 34.3 lists some suitable topics for nurse-led discussion groups. Individual patient education can focus on areas of knowledge deficits and reinforce topics discussed in group settings. Group sessions can also assist patients in learning interpersonal skills (e.g., assertiveness) and problem-solving skills and in relapse prevention planning.

Mutual Self-Help Groups

Several mutual self-help groups are appropriate for many patients with COD. Peer-led self-help approaches specifically for persons with COD are being tried with some success (Dermatis et al., 2006). The most common groups are 12-step programs, such as Alcoholics Anonymous (AA) and Narcotics Anonymous (NA) (see Chapter 25). The advisability of a patient enrolling in a 12-step program needs to be evaluated on an individual basis. A health care provider familiar with 12-step concepts can often facilitate patients' attempts to use these programs. The numerous advantages of self-help groups make them a potentially powerful support for continued recovery. Alternative mutual self-help programs similar to 12-step programs are available in some geographic areas. Rational Recovery and Secular Organization for Sobriety are groups that downplay the concept of powerlessness and the spiritual aspects associated with 12-step programs.

Family Support and Education 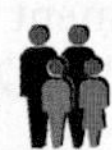

The families of patients with COD need education and support. Family psychoeducation interventions address mental illnesses, substance abuse, and their interactions. The focus of family support groups, such as those under the auspices of the National Alliance for the Mentally Ill, has been both to educate and to help the family cope with a mentally ill relative. AA and NA take a similar approach to providing peer support to families of substance users.

BOX 34.3

Topics for Education Groups for Patients with Co-Occurring Disorders

The effects of alcohol and drugs on the body
Alcohol, drugs, and medication—what can go wrong
- What is a healthy lifestyle?
- Triggers for relapse
- What is Alcoholics (or Narcotics) Anonymous?
- What is a sponsor in Alcoholics (or Narcotics) Anonymous?
- What is recovery from mental illness and substance abuse?
- What are tools of recovery?
- The disease of addiction
- The relapse cycle
- How to cope with feelings without using alcohol or other drugs
- Relapse prevention: what works?
- What are cognitive distortions?
- HIV prevention and education
- Leisure time management
- How to manage stress
- Relaxation training
- Assertiveness and recovery
- Common slogans to live by
- Pitfalls in treatment
- The process of recovery
- Creating a relapse prevention plan
- What are my goals? How does the use of alcohol and drugs affect them?

Coping with thoughts about alcohol and drugs
- Problem-solving basics
- Coping with anger
- Negative thinking and how to manage it
- Enhancing social support networks

These self-help groups aid family members in balancing confrontation of the problem, detachment from forcing a solution to it, and support of the treatment process.

CONTINUUM OF CARE

An integrated approach that combines mental health and substance abuse interventions at the clinical site has been shown to be the most effective (Drake et al., 2004). In an integrated system, the same team provides coordinated mental health and substance abuse interventions and guides the patient toward learning to manage these intertwined disorders. When the mental health/substance abuse systems are truly integrated, patient outcomes are positive.

Integration of mental health and substance abuse treatment systems has been difficult to achieve. Many treatment programs have some services integrated, but not all. For example, in a study of programs in the Department of Veterans Affairs, some key services were offered (assessment and diagnosis, crisis intervention, counseling targeted at psychiatric and at substance use problems, medications, patient education, HIV screening and counseling, family counseling and education) but there were many components missing (cognitive-behavioral treatment, assignment of a single case manager to each patient) (Timko, Dixon, & Moos, 2005).

When Hospitalization Is Necessary

Often, patients with COD can be treated effectively in community mental health settings if their symptoms are stable, they are following their treatment plan, they are compliant with the use of psychiatric medications, and they remain alcohol and drug free. Patients are hospitalized when they have a need for detoxification; exacerbation of comorbid psychiatric or medical disorders; suicide or homicidal ideation; or an illness that prevents abstinence or outpatient treatment.

Crisis Stabilization

Setting priorities is essential for hospitalized patients with COD. The first priorities are gathering data from a physical examination and nursing assessments, stabilizing psychiatric symptoms, and treating withdrawal symptoms (see Chapter 25). After these issues are addressed, the patient enters the rehabilitation phase of treatment for both diagnoses. Rehabilitative therapy is appropriate if the patient (1) can participate in a group process, (2) can focus attention on groups or reading material, (3) does not engage in behavior that is detrimental to the group process, (4) can listen to and receive feedback from others, and (5) can benefit from the group process.

Early Stages of Recovery From Substance Use

Many patients seeking alcohol or drug abuse treatment experience transitory cognitive impairment, which usually resolves within the first month of abstinence. Patients often experience difficulties with disorientation, clouding of consciousness, incoherent thoughts, memory loss, and delirium, which may hinder their ability to learn new concepts. These problems are a result of the neurobiological insult on the brain by these substances and psychosocial factors such as fear of legal or relationship difficulties, depression, grief, and feelings of guilt and shame (Petrakis et al., 2002). However, if Wernicke's syndrome, a reversible alcohol-induced amnestic disorder caused by a thiamine-deficient diet, or Korsakoff's psychosis, characterized by a loss of recent memory and confabulation (or filling in the blanks in memory by making up facts to cover this deficit) are present, cognitive problems may last longer. The patient with this condition is highly suggestible, has poor judgment, and cannot reason critically. Korsakoff's psychosis often follows Wernicke's encephalopathy and is also associated with prior peripheral neuropathy (see Chapter 25).

Psychological testing and other methods of assessment are necessary to determine whether the patient's cognitive functioning can improve and whether chemical dependency treatment can be used (Shivani, Goldsmith, & Anthenelli, 2002). It is also important to determine the extent of the mental disorder and the substance abuse. The nurse assesses the patient's abilities for self-care, independent living, impulse control, control of assaultiveness, direction taking, and development of new responses to new situations and ideas. The nurse must also evaluate changes in mental status during the past 6 months and examine previous treatment outcomes (Evans & Sullivan, 2001).

Intervention for patients with cognitive or memory impairment must consist of clear, direct, simple messages. The following points (Evans & Sullivan, 2001) illustrate this approach:

- Use reading material that is relevant to recovery and that can be referred to in short study sessions.
- For patients who have trouble grasping abstract concepts, read first-person accounts of addiction and recovery found in AA and NA literature.
- Concentrate on basic concepts of recovery, such as those in AA slogans, and on patients' need for continuing care after discharge.
- Show films with scenes illustrating relevant family problems or other problems related to substance use. Movies can be more effective than lectures.
- Avoid discussing extraneous issues and avoid theoretic or technical discussions.

BOX 34.4

Features of a Co-Occurring Disorders Outpatient Program

Community meeting and goal setting: Patients set small, realistic goals for themselves for the day, which aids them in their ultimate goal of better living in recovery.

Anger management and social communication: Patients learn appropriate ways to express anger and how to socialize with others.

Group therapy: Patients discuss interpersonal issues, get feedback from their peers, and learn problem-solving skills.

Dual recovery anonymous meetings: Patient-run meeting (a modified Alcoholics Anonymous meeting) addresses the specific needs of the patient with co-occurring disorders.

Leisure planning: Patients learn skills to enjoy leisure involving clean and sober fun.

Gardening, art therapy, music therapy, swimming: These methods provide alternatives to the use of alcohol and other drugs.

Health education: Patients learn about the effects of drugs and alcohol on the body and about other relevant medical topics.

Medication education: Patients learn about psychiatric medications, their uses, the side effects, and interactions with drugs or alcohol.

Relapse prevention planning: Patients talk about their last relapse; triggers, feelings, and stresses that contributed to the relapse; and the consequences and formulate relapse prevention plans.

Individual counseling: Patients receive individual counseling to develop goals and work on problem-solving techniques.

Psychiatric consultation: Patients are evaluated and followed up for medication and other psychiatric interventions.

Note: Patients are *not* discharged from the program if they are intoxicated. They are asked not to come to the program intoxicated but to return when they are sober to continue work on their recovery.

Social interaction skills and coping skills learned in treatment need to be reinforced in community settings to create or enhance a stable living situation and possible vocational opportunities. Active planning and intervention are needed for housing and employment, or deterioration may occur, despite gains made during hospitalization.

Recovery

Recovery from mental illness can be defined within the dimensions of hope, self-responsibility, and getting on with life beyond illness (Noordsy et al., 2002). To move toward recovery, establishing a positive social network is critical. Isolation and alienation from prior sources of support is a problem that most with comorbid mental disorders and substance use share. Some patients relate poorly to their families, others are overly dependent on them, and others have difficulty establishing and maintaining social relationships. Some patients' only "families" are peers within the drug subculture who reinforce substance-abusing behavior.

Compliance to an agreed-on treatment plan is integral to recovery. Box 34.4 presents features of a COD outpatient program. Opportunities to socialize, access to positive recreational activities, and a supportive peer group are stabilizing influences on patients who may otherwise drop out of treatment altogether. Part of a comprehensive relapse prevention plan is to establish or reinforce the patient's social support network so that he or she can obtain (1) opportunities for substance-free socializing, (2) crisis counseling to prevent readmission to a hospital, and (3) support for sobriety.

Supportive housing is also essential for patients with COD. Supportive housing is especially crucial for patients who are being discharged from the hospital because the risk for relapse is greatest during the first few months after discharge. Halfway houses for substance users may de-emphasize medication compliance, and housing designed for the chronically mentally ill may not emphasize abstinence enough. Thus, an important part of the multidisciplinary team approach to discharge planning for patients with COD is to help them find the best possible living situation.

Younger patients with severe mental illness may want and expect to find appropriate employment, but some of these patients may be unrealistic about potential professions. However, this desire can be a significant motivator and a useful tool in a treatment program. Referring patients to halfway houses or residential substance use treatment programs that stress vocational skill training can be beneficial. Use of community vocational rehabilitation services and of educational opportunities can be an important part of a discharge plan.

SUMMARY OF KEY POINTS

- In co-occurring mental illness and substance use disorder, each disorder is considered a primary disorder. They should be treated concurrently with an integrated approach.
- People with COD are high risk for relapse. The relapse cycle repeats itself without treatment.
- There is no one model that explains why mental disorders and substance abuse occur together so frequently. The most common pattern is the onset of the mental disorder followed by the problems with sub-

stance use leading to abuse. It appears that the substance use is an attempt to self-medicate the psychiatric symptoms.

- Barriers for treatment include homelessness, unemployment, and lack of social support. Other barriers include the complexity of the COD, staff attitudes, stigma, and health issues that interfere with treatment.
- Interdisciplinary treatment is through an integrated approach. Patients are moved towards recovery through engagement, motivation, assertive outreach and treatment, and relapse prevention.
- Nursing assessment of COD often depends on objective data obtained from interviews with family members, reviews of court records, laboratory test results, and physical examination findings. Assessment should include a determination of the willingness to change and motivation for treatment.
- Treatment and nursing care needs to be individualized within the context of the specific mental disorder and substances used.
- Interventions that are tailored to the special needs of the patient with a COD are medication management, substance abuse counseling, cognitive behavioral interventions, patient education, and family support and education. Participation in peer-led self-help groups has had some success.
- An ideal continuum of care is an integrated approach with one team coordinating the mental health and substance abuse interventions. Patients should not have to negotiate treatment with two separate systems. Hospitalization may be required during periods of crises. Most treatment occurs in the community where recovery is the goal.
- Recovery is a goal that can be defined in terms of hope, self-responsibility, and getting on with life.

CRITICAL THINKING CHALLENGES

1 An 18-year-old patient, newly diagnosed with schizophrenia, is relatively compliant with his medication and treatment. He was recently at a social event where he was experimenting with alcohol and marijuana. Develop a teaching plan for him that includes the risks of developing a substance abuse disorder.

2 A nurse in an emergency room recommends AA for every patient who is admitted for detoxification. Is that an appropriate referral for a person with comorbid mental disorder and substance abuse?

3 A community health nurse wants to refer a young woman who lives in a poor rural area to an integrated treatment program several miles away. Discuss the likelihood of the patient actually being able to access services. What barriers would she face and how could she have access to the care she needs?

4 How would you respond to a patient with COD who states, "Once my medication is stable, I will be able to drink again."

5 Compare traditional substance abuse approaches to an integrated treatment program.

6 A patient with a COD tells the nurse, "All chemicals are bad for you. I do not want to take my medication." Develop a response to this statement that reflects the use of engagement.

7 Explain the process of stage-wise treatment.

8 Discuss the differences in behavior of a person with schizophrenia who uses cocaine and a person with a mood disorder who uses marijuana.

9 Which COD concepts should be included in patient education?

Born on the Fourth of July: 1989. This wrenching, but true, account shows the experiences of Ron Kovic, played by Tom Cruise. Ron was a patriotic teen from a small town who volunteered to serve in Vietnam. During the war, he was shot in the spine, which left him paralyzed from the chest down. He returned home, bitterly alienated from his family, friends, and community. He faced a long and slow rehabilitation process. His depression and abuse of substances only compounded his physical problems. This movie depicts depression, PTSD, and substance dependence coexisting with major physical disabilities.

VIEWING POINTS: How does Ron express his depression? Is he using, abusing, or dependent on alcohol and drugs? How are you feeling throughout this movie? Do your feelings about the character change?

REFERENCES

Bruijnzeel, A. W., Repetto, M., & Gold, M. S. (2004). Neurobiological mechanisms in addictive and psychiatric disorders. *Psychiatric Clinics of North America, 27*(4), 661–674.

Buckley, P. F. (2006). Prevalence and consequences of the dual diagnosis of substance abuse and severe mental illness. *Journal of Clinical Psychiatry, 67*(suppl 7), 5–9.

Caton, C. L., Drake, R. E., Hasin, D. S., Dominguez, B., Shrout, P. E., Samet, S., & Schanzer, B. (2005). Differences between early-phase primary psychotic disorders with concurrent substance use and substance-induced psychoses. *Archives of General Psychiatry, 62*(5), 137–145.

Center for Substance Abuse Treatment (2005). *Substance abuse treatment for persons with co-occurring disorders.* Treatment Improvement Protocol (TIP) Series 42. DHHS Publication No. (SMA) 05-3922. Rockville, MD., Substance Abuse and Mental Health Services Administration.

Churchill, D. M. (2003). Toward an integrative approach to substance abuse: An inquiry into the recognition, diagnosis and treatment of substance abuse by social workers. *Dissertation Abstracts International, 63*(8-A), US: Univ Microfilms International.

Davis, L. L., Frazier, E. C., Williford, R. B., & Newell, J. M. (2006). Long-term pharmacotherapy for post-traumatic stress disorder. *CNS Drugs, 20*(6), 465–476.

Dermatis, H., Galanter, M., Trujillo, M., Rahman-Dujarric, D. Ramaglia, K., & LaGressa, D. (2006). Evaluation of a model for the treatment of combined mental illness and substance abuse: the Bellevue model for peer-led treatment in systems change. *Journal of Addictive Diseases, 25*(3), 69–78.

Drake, R. E., Essock, S. M., Shaner, A., Carey, K. B., Minkoff, K., Kola, L., et al. (2001). Implementing dual diagnosis services for clients with severe mental illness. *Psychiatric Services, 52*(4), 469–476.

Drake, R. E., Mueser, K. T., Brunette, M. F., & McHugo, G. J. (2004). A review of treatment for people with severe mental illnesses and co-occurring substance use disorders. *Psychiatric Rehabilitation Journal, 27*(4), 360–374.

Drake, R. E., Wallach, M. A., McGovern, M. P. (2005). Future directions in preventing relapse to substance abuse among clients with severe mental illnesses. *Psychiatric Services, 56*(10), 1297–1302.

Essock, S. M., Mueser, K. T., Drake, R. E., Covell, N. H., McHugo, G. J., Frisman, L. K., et al. (2006). Comparison of ACT and standard case management for delivering integrated treatment for co-occurring disorders. *Psychiatric Services, 57*(2), 185–196.

Evans, K., & Sullivan, J. (2001). *Dual diagnosis: Counseling the mentally ill substance abuser.* New York: Guilford Press.

Goldsmith, R. J., & Garlapati, V. (2004). Behavioral interventions for dual-diagnosis patients. *Psychiatric Clinics of North America, 27*(4), 709–725.

Green, A. I. (2006). Treatment of schizophrenia and comorbid substance abuse: Pharmacologic approaches. *Journal of Clinical Psychiatry, 67*(suppl 7), 31–35.

Harris, K. M., & Edlund, M. M. (2005). Use of mental health care and substance abuse treatment among adults with co-occurring disorders. *Psychiatric Services, 56*(8), 954–959.

Hasin, D., Samet, S., Meydan, J., Matseonane, K., & Waxman, B. A. (2006). Diagnosis of comorbid psychiatric disorders in substance users assessed with the psychiatric research interview for substance and mental disorders for DSM-IV. *The American Journal of Psychiatry, 163*(4), 689–696.

Hwang, S. (2001). Mental illness and mentality among homeless people. *Acta Psychiatrica Scandinavica, 103*(2), 81–82.

Hwang, S. (2002). Is homelessness hazardous to your health? Obstacles to the demonstration of a causal relationship. *Canadian Journal of Public Health, 93*(6), 407–410.

Kertesz, S. G., Horton, N. J., Friedmann, P. D., & Samet, J. H. (2003). Slowing the revolving door: Stabilization programs reduce homeless persons' substance use after detoxification. *Journal of Substance Abuse Treatment, 24*(3).

Kessler, R. C. (2004). The epidemiology of dual diagnosis. *Biological Psychiatry, 56*(10), 730–737.

Minkoff, K. (2001). Developing standard of care for individuals with co-occuring psychiatric and substance use disorders. *Psychiatric Services, 52*(5), 597–599.

Myrick, H., Cluver, J., Swavely, S., & Peters, H. (2004). Diagnosis and treatment of co-occurring affective disorders and substance use disorders. *Psychiatric Clinics of North America, 27*(4), 649–659.

National Alliance for the Mentally Ill. (2007). Dual diagnosis and integrated treatment of mental illness and substance abuse disorder. Retrieved on February 21, 2007, from www.NAMI.org.

Noordsy, D., Torrey, W., Mueser, K., Mead, S., O'Keefe, C., & Fox, L. (2002). Recovery from severe mental illness: an intrapersonal and functional outcome definition. *International Review of Psychiatry, 14*(4), 318–326.

Olson, W. (2004). Delirium tremens. In F. Ferri (Ed.), *Ferri's clinical advisor, 2004: Instant diagnosis and treatment.* St. Louis: Mosby.

Petrakis, I., Gonzalez, G., Rosenheck, R., & Krystal, J. (2002). Comorbidity of alcoholism and psychiatric disorders: An overview. *Alcohol Research and Health, 26*(2), 81–89.

Rosenthal, R. N., & Westreich, L. (1999). Treatment of persons with dual diagnosis of substance use disorders and other psychological problems. In *Addictions: A comprehensive guide* (pp. 439–476). New York: Oxford University Press.

Shivani, R., Goldsmith, R., & Anthenelli, R. (2002). Alcoholism and psychiatric disorders: Diagnostic challenges. *Alcohol Research and Health, 26*(2), 90–98.

Thomas, V., Melchert, T., & Banker, J. (1999). Substance dependence and personality disorders: Co-morbidity and treatment outcome in an inpatient treatment population. *Journal of Studies of Alcohol, 60,* 271–277.

Timko, C., Dixon, K., & Moos, R.H. (2005). Treatment for dual diagnosis patients in the psychiatric and substance abuse systems. *Mental Health Services Research,* 7(4), 229–242.

Westermeyer, J. (2006). Comorbid schizophrenia and substance abuse: A review of epidemiology and course. *American Journal on Addictions, 15*(5), 345–355.

Ziedonis, D. M. (2004). Integrated treatment of co-occurring mental illness and addiction: clinical intervention, program, and system perspectives. *Clinical Nurse Specialist Spectrum, 9*(12):892–904, 925.

Zimmermann, P., Wittchen, H.U., Höfler, M., Pfister, H., Kessler, R.C., & Lieb, R. (2003). Primary anxiety disorders and the development of subsequent alcohol use disorders: A four-year community study of adolescents and young adults. *Psychological Medicine, 22*(7), 1211–1222.

CHAPTER 35

Care of the Mentally Ill in Forensic Settings

Rhonda Kay Wilson

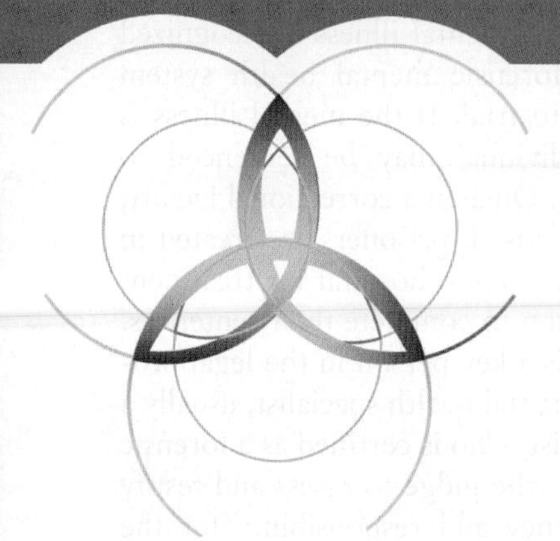

LEARNING OBJECTIVES

After studying this chapter, you will be able to:

- Define the mentally ill forensic populations.
- Discuss the stigma of mental illness and criminality.
- Describe legal outcomes for mentally ill patients in forensic settings.
- Assess personal attitudes in caring for persons with mental illness who have committed crimes.
- Identify the nursing challenges in forensic settings.
- Discuss rehabilitation and recovery once the mentally ill person no longer needs the forensic setting.

KEY CONCEPTS

- forensic
- fairness

KEY TERMS

• court process counseling • forensic examiner • fitness to stand trial • probation • unfit to stand trial (UST) • not guilty by reason of Insanity (NGRI) • guilty but mentally ill (GBMI) • conditional release

The term *forensic* has its roots in the Latin word "forensics," pertaining to forum. In ancient Rome, the forum was a marketplace where people gathered to purchase things and conduct business, including legal affairs. Today the term forensic refers to courts of law and legal proceedings.

KEY CONCEPT In mental health, the term **forensic** pertains to legal proceedings and mandated treatment of persons with a mental illness.

Forensic patients are treated in a variety of settings including county jails, correctional facilities, psychiatric hospitals, and the community. Treatment and psychiatric nursing care are regulated by the mental health and legal systems, two complex systems that are sometimes in conflict with each other. Nursing care is very challenging because the rules of the criminal justice system are often at odds with nursing practice standards.

FORENSIC POPULATION

People with a mental illness are more likely to be convicted of a crime than those without a mental illness. In one study, women with at least one psychiatric admission were 3.08 to 11.27 times more likely to be convicted of a crime and men were 2.29 to 7.5 times more likely to be convicted than their non–mentally ill counterpart (Schimmels, 2005). Prisoners have three times the prevalence of mental illness than the general population (Schimmels, 2005). In a survey of 22,790 prisoners in western countries, 3.7% of men (4% of women) had a psychosis, 10% of men (12% of women) had major depressive disorder, and 65% of men (42% of women) had personality disorders. In a Chicago study, it was found that 80% of the 1,272 women in jail studied had at least one psychiatric disorder and in North Carolina, 67% of the 805 women met criteria for a psychiatric diagnosis (Schimmels, 2005).

There are different views of mental illness and criminal behavior. Some people believe that people with mental illness commit criminal acts and it is their mental illness that causes their actions. Others believe that people engage in criminal behavior who happen to be mentally ill.

STIGMA AND CRIMINALITY

Forensic patients suffer the combined effects of the stigma of mental illness and criminality. Although stigma is an issue for all persons with a mental illness, it is magnified for those who have committed a crime. There is often reluctance on the part of mental health professionals to treat these patients, especially if murder and childhood sexual abuse are involved. Even if the worry is unfounded, clinicians express safety concerns for themselves and other patients and may refuse to care for these patients.

Delivery of coordinated mental health care services within a humane treatment network can be interrupted by conflict between the inpatient facility and the community. When non-forensic patients receive the maximum benefit from hospitalization, they are normally discharged into the community. For stigmatized forensic patients, the community often wants a more stringent discharge threshold and unrealistically expects the hospital to guarantee compliance with community rules and structure. These conflicting views can result in patients being discharged into community settings in a poorly coordinated fashion that sets them up for failure and another trip through the system (Box 35.1).

CRIMINAL JUDICIAL PROCESSES

There are two sides in any arrest and conviction: one side presented by the attorney of the accused and the other by the prosecution. It is important that the accused is able to work with an attorney. A basic concept underlying the criminal judicial process is one of fairness. The individual who is charged with a crime should know the legal rules and be able to explain the events surrounding the alleged crime or be "fit to stand trial."

KEY CONCEPT Fairness is a basic concept underlying the criminal judicial process.

Initiation of forensic psychiatric care ideally begins at the time of arrest. If the mental illness is recognized during the arrest, the forensic mental health system becomes involved prior to trial. If the mental illness is not recognized, the individual may be sentenced to prison without treatment. Once in a correctional facility, if a mental illness is diagnosed, prisoners are treated in prison or transferred to a mental hospital for treatment and then returned to prison to complete their sentences.

A **forensic examiner** is a key person in the legal process. The examiner is a mental health specialist, usually a psychiatrist or psychologist, who is certified as a forensic examiner and assigned by the judge to assess and testify to the patient's competency and responsibility for the crime including the mental state at the time of an offense. This testimony is based on interviews with the offender and a review of available records. The testimony directly influences the verdicts, judgments, sentencing, and damages of the defendant. For sex offenders, the examiner assesses the likelihood of recidivism and competence to stand trial.

Fitness to Stand Trial

Once a mental illness is diagnosed, the person's **fitness to stand trial** is determined. Fitness means that a person is able to consult with a lawyer with a reasonable degree of rational understanding of the facts of the alleged crime and of the legal proceedings as spelled out in the court case of Dusky vs. U.S. 1960 (Beran & Tommey, 1979, p. 12). In most states, when a mentally ill individual is found **unfit to stand trial (UST),** hospitalization in a forensic mental health facility follows. The goal of this hospitalization is to help the person become "fit" to stand trial, not to treat the mental illness. When fitness is attained, the court is notified and a hearing is held. If the court agrees that the individual is fit to stand trial, the case then goes to trial. If it is the court's opinion that the individual is still unfit, the individual is returned to the hospital.

An individual cannot be "unfit" forever. If fitness cannot be attained within 1 year, a hearing must be held at which facts of the alleged crime are presented to a judge who rules on the case. If the charges are dismissed, the judge could order a civil commitment (see Chapter 3). If there is sufficient evidence to convict, the individual could be sent back to the hospital for further treatment to attain fitness. The maximum length of this additional treatment is based on the severity of the charge. For mentally disordered sex offenders, states usually have

BOX 35.1

The Stigma of Mental Illness: Nowhere to Call Home

"But the insane criminal has nowhere to call home: no age or nation has provided a place for him. He is everywhere unwelcome and objectionable. The prisons thrust him out; the hospitals are unwilling to receive him; the law will not let him stay at his house; and the public will not permit him to go abroad. And yet humanity and justice, the sense of common danger, and a tender regard for a deeply degraded brother-man, all agree that something should be done for him . . . " Edward Jarvis, 1857.

special statutes for hospitalization and discharge (such as registration and community notification).

Not Guilty by Reason of Insanity

A possible outcome or disposition of a hearing or trial is **not guilty by reason of insanity (NGRI).** The accused is judged to not know right from wrong or to be unable to control his or her actions at the time of the crime. The rationale underlying this ruling is one of fairness. It is unfair to hold a person responsible if that individual does not know that the action is wrong or has control over his or her behavior.

After a finding of NGRI, the individual is ordered to a forensic facility for a psychiatric evaluation and the treatment recommendations are submitted to the court. Nearly all of those individuals found NGRI are also subject to involuntary commitment in a "secured" setting. Periodic reports of the individual's progress are sent back to the court. The patient cannot leave hospital grounds without court approval and only the committing court can discharge these individuals from the hospital.

Myths about the Insanity Plea

There are many misconceptions about the insanity plea. One is that the insanity defense provides a loophole through which criminals can escape punishment for illegal acts. In reality, the insanity defense is extremely difficult to employ, even in the cases of severely ill individuals. As a result, despite popular belief, the insanity defense is used in less that 1% of criminal cases (see Box 35.2).

Countless newspaper articles, talk shows, and news commentaries concerning the insanity defense have bombarded the public. Some of the cases have been highly publicized. One such case was that of John Hinckley, who attempted to assassinate President Ronald Reagan in 1981 and who was found NGRI. On psychiatric examination, Hinckley was found to be living in a "fantasy world with magical and grandiose expectations of impressing and winning over" his love, actress Jodie Foster (Goldstein, 1995, p. 309). Hinckley attempted to commit a historic deed that would make him famous and unite him with the love object of his delusions. His acquittal stimulated public cries for reform of the insanity defense. Within $2^1/_2$ years of John Hinckley's acquittal, 34 states changed their insanity defense statutes to limit its use or to prevent the premature release of dangerous people.

Despite its rarity, there continues to be a variety of strongly held opinions over whether the insanity defense is a way to "beat the rap" or results in unfair, lengthy hospitalizations for those stigmatized as "bad and mad." Many believe that hospitalizations are shorter than prison sentences. In reality, it is nearly certain that after an individual is judged NGRI, more time is spent in a mental hospital than if the person had been sentenced to a correctional facility.

BOX 35.2

The Case of Andrea Yates

In March 2002, Andrea Yates, age 37, was convicted of murder for drowning her children. She was sentenced to life in prison, despite past treatment for postpartum depression and psychosis, four hospitalizations, and two suicide attempts. Andrea Yates was found guilty because in her testimony to the police she stated that she knew the criminal justice system would punish her for her actions, implying that she knew the acts were wrong in the eyes of the law. Texas law does not recognize that for someone as ill as Andrea Yates, mental illnesses can create more powerful hierarchies of right and wrong than societal law.

Guilty but Mentally Ill

Different from NGRI, in which "not guilty" individuals are committed to the mental health system, **guilty but mentally ill (GBMI)** is a criminal conviction and the person is sent to the correctional system. Mental illness is considered a factor in the crime but not to the extent that the individual is incapable of knowing right from wrong or controlling their actions. The sentence for the GBMI is the same type of determinate sentence any inmate receives. Prior to release, every effort is made to ensure that patients will receive proper follow-up care in the community and close monitoring by parole staff.

Both NGRI or GBMI persons are treated for their mental disorders, but one is treated in jail and the other in a hospital. The conditions of release are different. Individuals with a GBMI are subject to the correctional system's parole decisions, whereas an NGRI individual is discharged from the hospital through the courts upon recommendations of the forensic mental health professionals.

Probation

Probation is a sentence of conditional or revocable release under the supervision of a probation officer for a specified time. For the mentally ill who have committed minor offenses, probation is sometimes used instead of jail as long as care in a treatment facility can be arranged. If treatment and rehabilitation are successful, criminal charges may be dropped and a prison record avoided. Probation is also used when a criminal has served time and continued monitoring is needed once released from the correctional facility.

Probation often includes requirements such as a mental health evaluation and an order to follow through with any recommended forms of treatment. It may include restrictions on certain activities such as the use of alcohol and other drugs, monetary fines, or mandatory community service. Successful completion of a probationary sentence for a person with a mental illness almost certainly depends on the ability and the willingness of a community mental health clinician to work cooperatively with the court and the assigned probation officer.

Forensic Conditional Release Program

In some states, patients who are judicially committed and found to be NGRI, incompetent to stand trial, or mentally disordered sex offenders are discharged through a forensic conditional release program. Patients whose psychiatric symptoms have been stabilized and are no longer considered a danger qualify for this program that is very similar to parole for inmates released from a correctional facility. In the forensic conditional release program, the patient is released but they must follow the conditions and criteria that are established by the program in order to maintain their discharged status. In states that do not have this program, the patient will remain an inpatient until the date expires or until the court grants them some form of conditional release. If the patient is granted a conditional release, the court will dictate the conditions of the release.

SELF-ASSESSMENT

Self-assessment is an ongoing process in which the nurse examines personal beliefs and attitudes about patients and crimes. It is the first step toward being an effective psychiatric nurse in a forensic setting. It is essential for the nurse to be aware of personal feelings about patients' crimes and to identify and recognize any bias toward these patients. A positive attitude toward people with mental illnesses including those who have committed a crime is basic to psychiatric nursing practice. At no time is it appropriate to convey a personal negative feeling toward the patient (Box 35-3).

If there is a negative attitude toward patients, the nurse should develop a plan to deal with the underlying feelings. In the mental health treatment environment, there are many skilled clinicians such as psychiatrists, social workers, and peers who can help the nurse talk through feelings and thoughts and assist the nurse to begin to work around or through the negativity. The nurse must want to change or explore this area in order to successfully resolve any issues he or she may have.

Some nurses have found that it is not necessary to know the details of the crime in order to work effectively with the forensic patient. The legal status and dangerousness of patients are important data, but it is not essential to know the actual crimes that patients committed.

Whereas some nurses develop biases against the patients, other nurses become too involved with patients in forensic facilities. It is essential to maintain professional boundaries and the nurse should seek assistance if he or she is unable to maintain these professional boundaries. The supervisor should be notified if the nurse finds him- or herself in a situation where professional boundaries have been broken. Together the employee and supervisor will decide the best course of action. In some cases the nurse will be relocated or change job assignments to avoid future contact with the patient; be referred to an Employee Assistance Program for counseling, or, if the breach of professionalism is too great, the employee may be encouraged to seek other employment for his or her safety and professional integrity.

BOX 35.3

The Importance of a Positive Attitude towards Patients

Studies show that there are factors that influence nurse attitudes toward caring for people with mental illness. The results show that nurses who were ages 31 to 50, who had an advanced education, or who had more than 10 years of psychiatric nursing experience had the most positive attitudes toward people with mental illnesses. In addition, nurses working in the short-term units have more positive attitudes than those working in the long-term units (Tay, Pariyasami, Ravindran, Ali, & Rowsudden, 2004).

NURSING MANAGEMENT ISSUES IN FORENSIC CARE

Forensic mental health professionals who have been providing treatment of the mentally ill forensic patients have published research literature that documents evidence-based practice for forensic care. Several assessments and interventions are used predominately with forensic patients and are targeted at the specific legally relevant behaviors that are the basis for their involuntary treatment. The ultimate goals are rehabilitation and recovery.

Assessment

The nursing assessment should be completed according to accepted standards (see Chapter 5). The development of rapport and trust are important for a successful nursing assessment. Forensic patients may be uncomfortable discussing their crime for fear of rejection by the nursing staff and treatment team. They may also be reluctant to disclose personal information if they perceive themselves to be at risk for further prosecution if information about prior criminal activity is leaked to the district attorney's office. The nurse should reassure the patient that the focus of the assessment is mental health issues and behaviors, but not specific details of the crimes.

Risk Assessment

Risk assessment is an important determination to maintain the safety of the patient and others. Upon admission to a mental health treatment facility the staff performs a risk assessment. Patients' current level and past history of dangerousness are reviewed and a safety plan is developed. Some state mental health facilities perform a risk assessment screening to determine placement. The patient may be sent to a maximum secure mental health treatment facility based on this risk assessment. The data obtained in the risk assessment including the patient's known history, habits, legal status, and triggers are used to develop an individualized treatment plan.

Informed Consent

Informed consent is necessary prior to initiation of pharmacologic treatment of forensic patients. The nursing staff collaborates with the psychiatrist to educate patients about their medications and the need to take medication. The nurse also collaborates with the psychiatrist to obtain informed written or verbal consent from the patient to take medication. The informed consent is the legal responsibility of the physician, but the nurse often assists in obtaining the consent.

Forensic patients can refuse medication just as any other patient can. If patients refuse to take medication and then become a threat to themselves or others, treating psychiatrists may petition the court for enforced medication. Only after a court order is obtained is medication administered to someone who has not consented to it. If patients are not a threat to themselves or others, it is unlikely that the court will order medication administration. In these situations, the rights of the patient are respected but it is often at the expense of the patient receiving the best treatment available.

Documentation

Documentation is essential when caring for a patient with a mental illness in a forensic setting. Accurate and frequent recording of changes in mental condition, responses to treatment, and effectiveness of medication is useful information for the treatment team and the legal advocates. It is crucial that moods, behaviors, and overall mental health state are monitored and documented on a regular basis. Nursing interventions and the patient's response to the nursing care should always be documented. In addition, medical condition and the nursing care associated with these physical problems should be recorded.

The court report is a useful communication tool for mental health clinicians to provide technical information based on clinical assessment and current research to those governing the lives of the forensic person. Ideally, the report should reflect the careful balance of the rights of the individual, mental health needs, and public safety (Box 35.4).

BOX 35.4

Court Report Outline

1. Purpose
2. Methods of assessment (interview, testing, review of the files)
3. Confidentiality assurances
4. Human rights assurances
5. Current mental functioning with examples
6. Psychiatric history
7. Legal history
8. Medication history
9. Results of psychological testing
10. Detail significant history as it relates to mental status and psychological testing
11. Diagnosis and facts on which diagnosis is based
12. Other related diagnosis that may be relevant to the case
13. Give opinion of fitness or competence based on documentation in the report

Specific Interventions

Court Process Counseling

An understanding of the legal proceedings is essential for any person charged with crimes. **Court process counseling** educates mentally ill patients about the impending legal procedures and prepares them for courtroom appearances. This intervention is used for all forensic patients—those preparing for their fitness to stand trial hearing as well as those preparing for discharge. Factual information such as roles and functions of key courtroom personnel, potential pleas that might be offered in court, and the nature of the legal process are basic to this intervention. Fitness issues are discussed as appropriate.

Patients also have an opportunity to develop skills for interacting in a courtroom through mock trials and court process games. Groups and classes are often held for patients who are unfit to stand trial. These group sessions or class sessions teach the patient about fitness issues in order for the psychiatrist, forensic examiner, and the court to find them fit. These groups and classes usually test the patient's knowledge of the court by giving a written examination that the patient must pass prior to being found fit.

Physical Management of Aggression

Forensic patients frequently come from violent backgrounds and are normally physically aggressive. Confined to living with others who are also aggressive, these patients are easily provoked into verbal and physical aggression. Management of aggressive behavior is a priority and involves structuring the physical environment, de-escalation techniques, and pharmacological interventions.

Forensic mental health facilities focus on providing a safe and secure environment. Furniture and decorations are minimal and patient rooms are routinely inspected for any objects that can be used to cause injury to the patient or others. Patient movement and daily activities are carefully overseen and are very structured so that the staff knows the whereabouts of the patients and their activities at all times.

De-escalation techniques are commonly used in the forensic mental health setting. The primary goal of de-escalation is to resolve angry or violent conflicts in nonviolent ways (see Chapter 38). Most forensic mental health facilities use a nonviolent crisis intervention model that is based on the assumption that patients should not be further provoked if they are already in a state of agitation. These patients should be given space and time to calm down. They should be addressed in a calm, reasonable, and nonthreatening tone. For staff safety, agitated patients should be de-escalated by more than one staff member. Other de-escalation techniques include distraction, active listening, and sensory modulation and integration activities (Box 35.5). At all times, the patient should be involved in the decision-making process and their wishes and preferences for de-escalation techniques should be considered and honored if possible. For example, some patients may ask to talk to someone and others may want to be left alone. As a last resort, physical holds, seclusion, or restraints to protect the patient from harming themselves or others can be applied.

Antianxiety, mood stabilizers, or antipsychotic medication can be given to assist an agitated patient in calming down. Antipsychotic medications are used for patients with psychosis and mania. The disadvantage of antipsychotic medication is the risk of side effects such as acute muscular spasms and potentially irreversible tardive dyskinesia. Antianxiety and hypnotic medications such as lorezepam (Ativan) or diphenhydramine (Benadryl) are used for as-needed management of aggressive episodes that occur despite taking antipsychotic medication as prescribed. Other medications that have been found to be helpful in managing symptoms underlying aggressive behavior are the mood stabilizers (lithium, carbamazepine, valproic acid) and beta-blockers (propranolol, metoprolol).

BOX 35.5

Sensory Modulation and Integration Activities

Grounding physical activities
Holding
Weighted blankets
Arm massages
Aerobic exercise
Sour/fireball candies

Calming self-soothing activities
Hot shower/bath
Drumming
Decaf tea
Rocking in a rocking chair
Beanbag tapping
Yoga
Wrapping in a heavy quilt

Comfort rooms
The comfort room is a room that provides sanctuary from stress, and/or can be a place for persons to experience feelings within acceptable boundaries. The comfort room is set up to be physically comfortable and pleasing to the eye, including a recliner chair, walls with soft colors, murals, and colorful curtains.

Medication Compliance

Medication administration presents unique challenges for the nursing staff. Patients frequently do not believe or trust the staff to properly treat their mental illness. When patients do not trust the staff, they often refuse to take their medication as prescribed. Nursing staff should always be vigilant and observe patients carefully to ensure that they are taking their medications and not spitting, cheeking (hiding medication in their cheeks to avoid swallowing), hiding, or throwing it away. At the same time, the nurses need to work on developing a trusting therapeutic relationship with their patients. As nurses gain the trust of the patient, the individual often agrees to try the medication.

NURSING MANAGEMENT ISSUES IN A CORRECTIONAL SETTING

Correctional facilities are regulated by the judicial system, not by state departments of mental health. Nursing care in these facilities is held to the same standard of care as in any setting, but the circumstances are different. For example, medications are administered through a window or opening in the bars in the cell house and are usually crushed and dissolved in water prior to giving it to the patient. Refusal of medications is not an option. If an inmate refuses medication, the authorities take the necessary steps to enforce compliance.

The nursing care in the corrections setting is conducted in a call line system. Any inmate who becomes ill or has a medical complaint notifies the guard who in turn will contact the nurse who checks the inmate and administers first aid if indicated. Following the assessment, the nurse may place the inmate on the sick call line which is either medical or psychiatric. The inmate will then be seen by the nurse or physician during office hours. If indicated, medications will be ordered. Once seen, the inmate returns back to the cell house. If physically ill, the patient may be admitted to the health care unit for medical treatment until the illness is resolved. If psychiatric problems persist despite medication, the patient may be transferred to a psychiatric treatment facility within the correctional system.

PUBLIC SAFETY ON RELEASE

The issue of public safety is often raised regarding the care and discharge of patients with psychiatric disorders. The reality is that patients with psychiatric problems are more likely victims than perpetrators of criminal activity. For patients who are admitted to treatment facilities because they have committed a crime, the development of sound conditional release programs is one approach many states use. In **conditional release**, patients are discharged provided they are monitored on an ongoing basis by the court. The authority to release from hospitalization or to monitor and enforce mandatory outpatient treatment varies considerably across jurisdictions. The fate of the forensic patient may lie with a legal agent (court), a clinical agent (hospital staff), or a special administrative panel (clinical review board or psychiatric security review board).

Often social and political considerations influence judges and clinicians toward conservative placement and release decisions. Judges risk adverse publicity if they release a patient who again becomes violent in the community. Clinicians, on the other hand, may be fearful of malpractice litigation for wrongful imprisonment. In reality the treatment team's release decision is based on a variety of factors, including the patient's potential for future violence, the current political climate, and skillfulness of the attorney who portrays the patient as having no potential for violence.

FROM THE HOSPITAL TO THE COMMUNITY

Providing quality services to persons with mental illness who are involved with the legal system can be a long and complicated process. There are many opportunities for an individual to "fall in the cracks" and miss receiving services that are needed to live successfully in the community. Sometimes critical services are not available and sometimes service planners, family members, and the individuals do not know how to access available services. Some mental health agencies are unwilling to serve an "ex-offender." Patients discontinue treatment and services for a variety of reasons including medication side effects, substance abuse, long waiting lists, lack of services, and a lack of sufficient parole staff to monitor and encourage compliance.

When individuals do not receive the services they need, for whatever reason, their chances for repeat hospitalizations or legal difficulties are high.

In addition to mental health services, these patients need a wide range of other services, including medical and dental care, housing, food, and clothing. Financial and legal services along with support services such as self-help groups, and spiritual and recreational opportunities are also needed. Rehabilitation services are needed including education, training, and employment.

SUMMARY OF KEY POINTS

- There are special legal terms and considerations for individuals who have mental disorders and commit crimes. Those determined to be *unfit to stand trial* are mentally incompetent and unable to understand the proceedings against them or assist in their own defense. These patients are committed to a mental health facility for treatment until they achieve fitness. Those determined to be *not guilty by reason of insanity* are those who demonstrate that they had no understanding of their actions and no control over them when they committed the crime. These patients are committed to a mental health facility for treatment and then discharged after treatment.
- The patient found *guilty but mentally ill* applies to those who demonstrate that they knew the wrongfulness of their actions and had the ability to act otherwise. These patients enter the correctional system and receive treatment for their disorder but are returned after treatment to serve their sentences. For mentally disordered sex offenders, states usually have special statutes for hospitalization and discharge. Prisoners who develop mental illness while in prison are transferred to a mental hospital, treated, and returned to prison to complete their sentences.
- A major treatment issue in a forensic treatment facility is developing a trusting relationship and compliance with treatment.
- The role of the nurse in managing the forensic patient is to pharmacologically treat symptoms underlying aggression and at times utilize seclusion or restraints to manage physical aggression. The nurse needs to build a trusting therapeutic relationship with the patient to help the patient make informed choices about being compliant with their desired treatment plan. Another nursing intervention is to ensure that the teaching needs of the patient are met. These needs include medication education and court process education.
- Once the decision to release the forensic patient from the inpatient setting is made, often the commu-

nity providers have felt reluctant to accept recipients who have been involved with the criminal justice system. They express fears about the person's level of dangerousness, protection of staff and peers, and potential liability.

■ The goal is to coordinate mental health services and to provide the forensic patient with a wide range of services that will help them successfully live within his or her community.

CRITICAL THINKING CHALLENGES

1. Describe the differences between UST, NGRI, and GBMI.
2. If you were mentally ill, under what circumstances do you feel a forensic patient should no longer have the right to refuse medication? Keep in mind the patient's right for informed consent.
3. If you were responsible for a caseload at a community mental health center, would you be fearful of accepting a patient with a criminal background?

Sling Blade: 1996. Sling Blade is a drama set in rural Arkansas starring Billy Bob thornton who plays a man named Karl Childers who is released from a psychiatric hospital where he has lived since committing murder at age 12. He is a very simple man who thinks in concrete terms. He befriends a young boy and begins a friendship with the boys' mother. He then finally confronts the mother's abusive boyfriend. This film won many awards.

VIEWING POINTS: If Karl had been successfully rehabilitated, how would he have handled his rage? Would this film perpetuate the myth that people with mental illness are dangerous? Was the murder justified?

Inside/Outside Video: 2004. This video was developed by, and stars, consumers who have all reached recovery. The video envisions the patient on a journey to recovery and parallels𝑇heeo's primary focus is to give the consumers hope for the future, encouraging them to take responsibility for themselves and their actions and to try to seek recovery.

VIEWING POINTS: This video depicts the patient with a psychiatric illness as being able to recover and needing to be involved in their care in order to get well. It shows that there is hope for patients with a mental illness and that the patients who recovered were able to obtain jobs as a consumer specialist. The qualification needed in order to apply for a consumer specialist position is that you have to have been a patient in a psychiatric treatment facility.

REFERENCES

Beran, N. J., Tommey, B. G. (1979). Mentally ill offenders and the criminal justice system. *Issues in Forensic Services* (p. 1–23). New York: Proeger Publishers, Proeger Special Studios.

Goldstein, R. (1995). Paranoids in the legal system: The litigious paranoid and the paranoid criminal. *Psychiatric Clinics of North America, 18*(2), 303–315.

Schimmels, E. (2005). Rehabilitation of mentally ill offenders: Before and after the arrest. *Forensic Nurse,* Nov/Dec. Retrieved December 1, 2005 from www.forensicnursemag.com.

Tay, S. C., Pariyasami, S. D., Ravindran, K., Ali, M. I. A., Rowsudden, M. T. (2004) . Nurses' attitudes toward people with mental illnesses in a psychiatric hospital in Singapore. *Journal of Psychosocial Nursing, 42*(10), 41–47.

CHAPTER 36

Psychosocial Aspects of Medically Compromised Persons

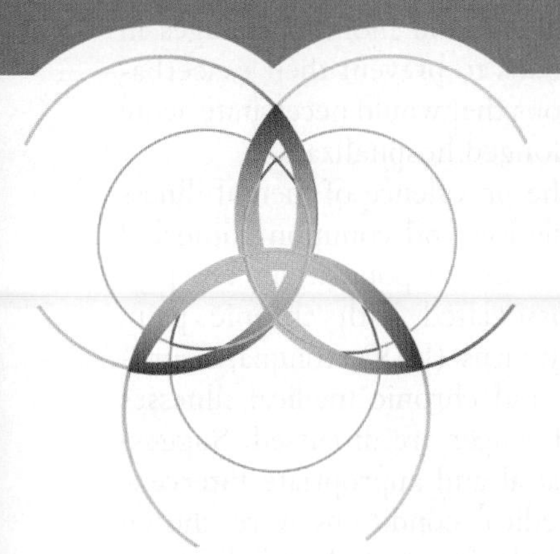

Gail L. Kongable

KEY CONCEPT

- chronic pain

LEARNING OBJECTIVES

After studying this chapter, you will be able to

- Identify medically ill populations at risk for secondary mental illness.
- Analyze the impact on patients and their families of mental illness associated with the medical illness.
- Discuss comorbid psychosocial and biological disorders seen in psychiatric settings and their treatments.
- Discuss neurobiological and psychological disturbances associated with specific medical illnesses and the medications used to treat them.
- Develop a plan of care for patients who are experiencing mental illness associated with medical illness.
- Discuss biopsychosocial interventions that promote patients' mental health in physical illness.

KEY TERMS

• acute pain • allodynia • endorphins • gate-control model • AIDS dementia complex • HIV-1-associated cognitive-motor complex • hyperalgia • hyperaesthesia • ischemic cascade • kindling • nociception • neurotransmitters • plasticity • prostaglandins • self-efficacy • substance P

Psychiatric illness often accompanies physical illness and is a significant health care problem in the medically ill population. People who have chronic medical illnesses have a nearly 41% higher rate of psychiatric disorders than people who are healthy. In addition, the chronically medically ill have a 28% higher lifetime prevalence of psychiatric disorders. Conversely, epidemiological studies indicate that up to 80% of psychiatric patients also have on average two physical diagnoses. These most commonly include diabetes mellitus, hypertension, cardiac disease, gastrointestinal disorders, chronic lung disease, and arthritis at rates higher than among the general population (Joffe, Brasche, & MacQueen, 2003; Stockton, Gonzales, Stern, & Epstein 2004). These comorbid conditions in chronically mentally ill patients have significant impact on functional impairment, often with additive effects that may or may not be related to psychopharmacological therapy (Evans et al., 2005).

Mood, bipolar, anxiety, and substance use disorders are the most prevalent psychiatric conditions of patients with chronic or terminal illnesses. Increasing clinical evidence suggests that the presence of these psychiatric disorders may be independent risk factors for increased morbidity and mortality, particularly in conditions such as chronic pain, acquired immunodeficiency syndrome (AIDS), acute trauma, stroke, and cancer. Finally, because most medically ill people are elderly, biological, psychological, and social changes may place them at even greater risk for mental illness and increased morbidity and mortality.

PSYCHOLOGICAL RESPONSES TO SPECIFIC PHYSIOLOGIC DISORDERS

Mental disorders associated with common medical illness have the same biologic changes as primary mental disorders. In fact, the neurochemical variations in catecholamine metabolism characteristic of primary depression, anxiety, and phobia may even cause some of the physical illnesses (Insel & Charney, 2003).

Unfortunately, mental illness is not commonly recognized and is usually under-treated in general medical settings. Psychiatric symptoms may be masked by physical symptoms. Additionally, some treatment regimens contribute to psychosocial dysfunction because many medications prescribed for chronic illness alter mood and thought processes. Generally, health care providers expect patients to exhibit depressed mood and anxiety as a normal response to illness. In fact, it is considered abnormal if a patient does not grieve over the loss of health or does not express discouragement or anxiety about treatment and the possibility of death.

When psychosocial dysfunction is not examined closely and is not treated, it can affect the course and outcome of associated medical illness. The presence of mental illness may weaken the motivation for self-care, impair symptom reporting, and delay the search for treatment. Symptoms of mental disorders may precede or occur during acute hospitalization and continue after discharge and apparent physical recovery. As a result, hospitalization may be prolonged and recovery delayed, or impaired, at increased emotional and financial cost to the patient and the family (Ciechanowski, Katon, Russo, & Hursch, 2003). In severe cases, mood disorders associated with medical illness predict morbidity and mortality (Burg, Benedetto, Rosenberg, & Soufer, 2003). Careful assessment to identify and evaluate symptoms of concomitant mental illness separately from those of medical illness is required, together with appropriate treatment, to achieve the patient's best psychological and medical outcome.

Another area of concern is the common comorbidity of physical disorders among people who require primary psychiatric care. Acute psychiatric settings, residential treatment settings, and psychiatric home health programs are reporting increasing numbers of patients with primary or secondary physical and medical problems (Stockton et al., 2004). Factors associated with increased hospital stays of psychiatric patients include the presence of physical disability and concomitant medical illness (Ciechanowski et al., 2003). Mental health care professionals must carefully evaluate and monitor changes in coexisting medical conditions to prevent their exacerbation or serious complications that would necessitate acute medical treatment or prolonged hospitalization.

This chapter reviews the prevalence of mental illness in the medically ill population and common comorbid medical disorders in the psychiatric population. The psychosocial disturbances associated with chronic pain, human immunodeficiency virus (HIV), trauma, neurological disorders, stroke, and chronic medical illnesses such as heart disease and cancer are discussed. Suggestions for diagnostic appraisal and appropriate intervention are given. These medical conditions were chosen because they are responsible for most hospitalizations and are frequently associated with psychiatric comorbidity. Psychiatric mental health liaison clinicians are consulted to see patients with these conditions in all phases of their illness, from acute hospitalization and treatment to rehabilitation and return to the community.

PSYCHOLOGICAL IMPACT OF PAIN

Physiologic pain is a protective response to noxious stimuli that serves as a warning of injury. Clinical pain related to inflammation and pathologic processes is characterized by low-threshold sensitization. Despite major advances in treatments that lessen its force, pain remains one of the most powerful and complex human experiences. Assessing and treating pain is difficult because the pain response is subjective and the degree of pain cannot be observed directly and may be difficult to localize. In addition, the person's discomfort may seem out of proportion to the observed conditions or influenced by disordered emotions, personality, or environmental conditioning. Severe or chronic pain may affect mentally healthy people in adverse ways. The prevalence and impact of pain have led to numerous approaches to therapy, including the use of antipsychotic drugs, antidepressants, antianxiety agents, and stimulants. Considerable evidence suggests that psychiatric medications and interventions can be effective in treating both acute and chronic pain.

The **gate-control model** of pain response is based on physiologic evidence that pain perception (**nociception**) involves pathways in the dorsal horn of the spinal cord that relay noxious stimuli to the brain. In addition, certain other nerve fibers function as an antagonistic "gate"

FAME AND FORTUNE

John Fitzgerald Kennedy (1917–1963):
President of the United States

Public Persona

As the very popular 35th President of the United States, John Kennedy promoted the civil rights movement in the United States, was instrumental in the space program, and successfully averted war with the Soviet Union over nuclear missiles placed in Cuba.

Personal Realities

On a day-to-day basis, however, Kennedy maintained mental health although he suffered with severe pain most of his adult life. Three fractured vertebrae caused by osteoporosis gave him so much pain that he could not put a sock or a shoe on his left foot without help. He also had persistent digestive problems and Addison's disease. He took several medications a day and he often received injections of procaine in his back in order to carry out his leadership duties.

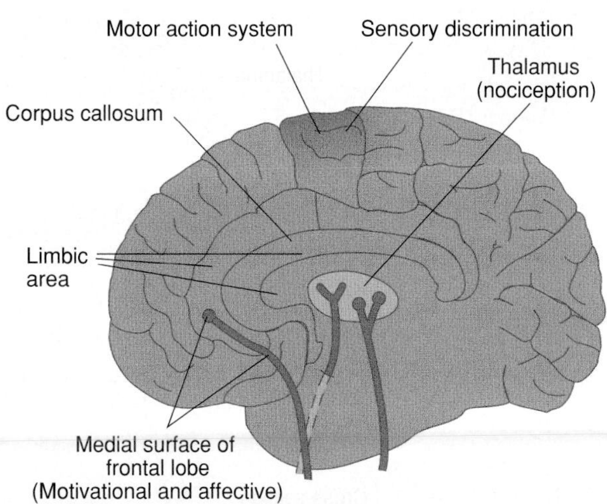

FIGURE 36.1. Pain stimuli activate regions of the brain that influence memory, emotion, and personality.

to augment or dampen the subjective experience of pain (Basbaum & Julius, 2006). The cognitive-behavioral model considers not only the patient's emotional and cognitive perception of pain but also the interaction of environmental influences, physical factors, and pain perception over time. From this perspective, patients' interpretation of pain, their coping and adaptation resources, and their emotive psychological processes interact with the experience of pain and can influence the physiologic activities that characterize pain (Kandel & Schwartz, 2000; Turk, 2004). Some pain theorists believe that the gate-control theory has been largely disproved (McCaffery & Pasero, 1999); others are working to refine the theory as more knowledge of pain becomes available (McMahon, Cafferty & Marchand, 2005).

Biologic Basis of the Pain Response

Pain is transmitted through specific neural pathways that carry information about touch and temperature (Figure 36.1). Painful stimuli also cause significant activation in areas of the brain responsible for memory, emotion, and personality (Tang et al., 2005) (Figure 36.2). Pain receptors (nociceptors) may be activated by mechanical, thermal, or chemical stimuli. When activated, **neurotransmitters** initiate, block, or modulate nerve signal transmission and ultimately control neural function under normal circumstances. Several specialized neurotransmitters within primary pain pathways are involved in pain transmission (Box 36.1).

When these neurotransmitters are released, they initiate local inflammatory reactions. In turn, cytokines are released that sensitize and stimulate central pain receptors. **Substance P** and **prostaglandins** are the most common nociceptive transmitters. They are released and transported along the central and peripheral pain synapses in the presence of noxious stimuli. **Endorphins**, neurotransmitters that exhibit opiate-like behavior, produce an inhibitory effect at opiate receptor sites and are probably responsible for pain tolerance. The release of endorphins is centrally mediated by serotonin (Kandel & Schwartz, 2000). Serotonin, histamine, and bradykinin sensitize and stimulate the pain receptors, causing the perception and experience of pain. The role of endorphins may go beyond pain modulation to include mood enhancement, behavior modification, and influence the development of tolerance or dependence on narcotics.

Acute and Chronic Pain

Acute pain is one of the most common symptoms of patients in emergency and acute care settings. It can result from a variety of physiologic abnormalities and trauma. It is characterized by a sudden, severe onset at the time of injury or illness and generally subsides as the injury heals. Postoperative incisional pain is an iatrogenic (treatment-induced) tissue injury most often seen in medical settings. Careful assessment and treatment of pain in these settings have a great impact on healing and recovery.

KEY CONCEPT Chronic pain, defined as pain on a daily basis or pain that is constant for more than 6 months, can be related to a variety of pathologies and takes the form of syndromes such as headache, temporomandibular pain disorders, back pain, and arthritis.

Chronic pain symptoms are associated with the clinical syndromes of neoplasia (cancer), thalamic stroke (central pain), diabetes mellitus (neuropathy), and reflex sympa-

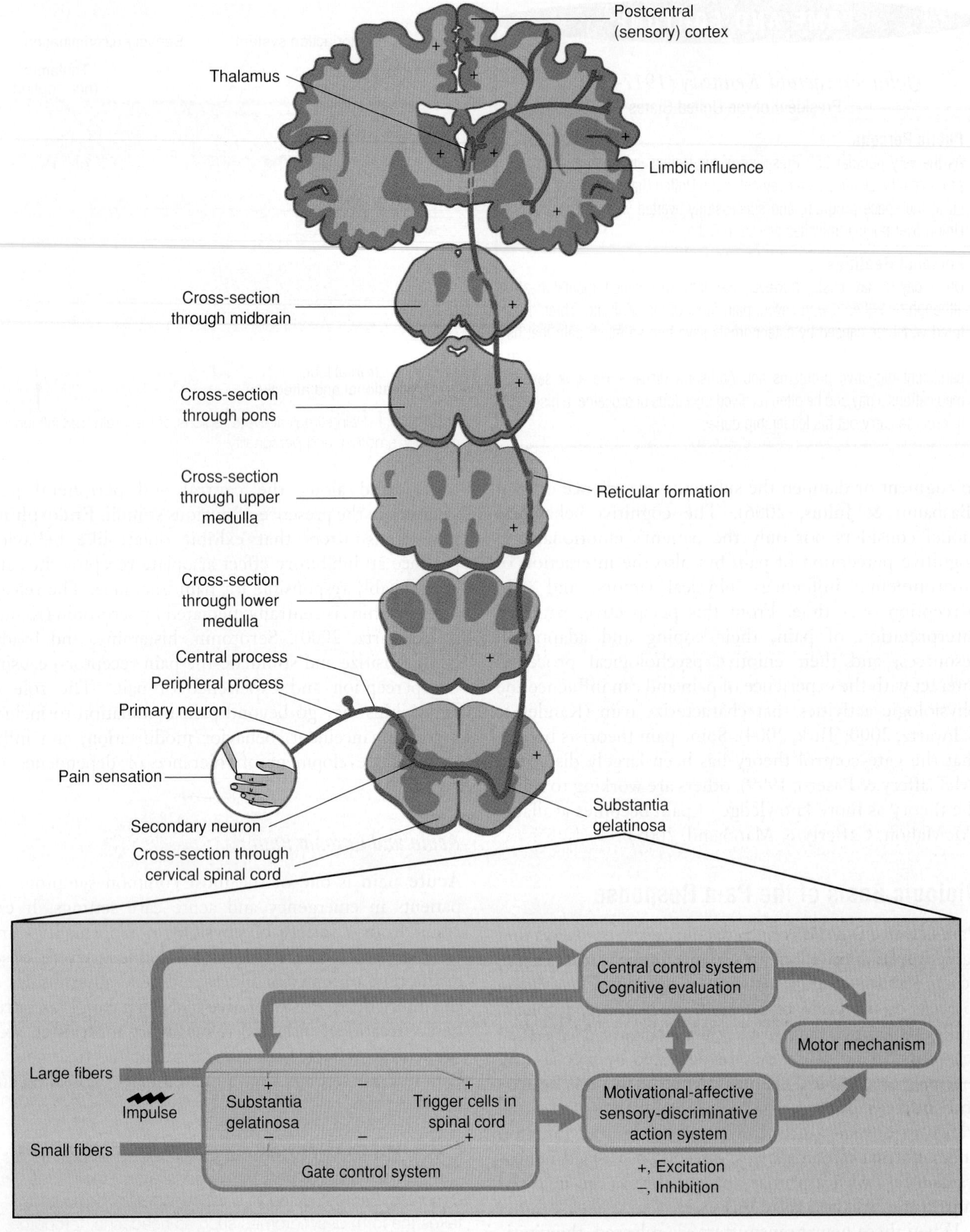

FIGURE 36.2. Ascending sensory pathways: anterior spinothalamic tract with a schematic diagram of the gate-control theory of pain mechanism.

BOX 36.1

Neurotransmitters Active in Pain Sensation and Induced Plasticity

C-Fiber Neuropeptides Released by Noxious Stimulation Peripherally
Substance P
Neurokinin A
Somatostatin
Prostaglandins
Calcitonin gene-related peptide (CGRP)
Galanin
Vasoactive intestinal polypeptide (VIP)
Cholecystokinin

Excitatory Amino Acids that have Widespread Activity in the CNS (Thalamus and Somatosensory Cortices)
L-glutamate
N-methyl-D-aspartate (NMDA)

Neurotransmitters Active as Pain Modulators
Endorphins
Enkephalin
Serotonin

thetic dystrophy (Box 36.2). Nervous tissue injury leads to neuropathic pain that may be described as burning, aching, pricking, or lancinating. This central or neuropathic pain is the underlying mechanism for most chronic pain and leads to **hyperalgia** (increased sensation of pain), **allodynia** (pain unrelated to noxious stimuli, lowered pain threshold), and **hyperaesthesia** (increased nociceptor sensitivity). Permanent change in central pain interpretation (**plasticity**) frequently results in abnormal physiologic, biochemical, cellular, and molecular responses that misinterpret nonpainful sensations as painful (Melzak, Coderre, Katz, & Vaccarino, 2001; Basbaum & Julius, 2006). This neural plasticity contributes to the development of errant firing and the pain syndromes of referred pain (pain felt in a body part other than where it was produced) and phantom pain (pain sensation in a missing [amputated] limb).

Psychological Aspects of the Pain Response

Pain is not only a sensation but also a perceptual phenomenon with an important affective component. When a patient's pain persists for an extended period, a range of psychosocial influences, such as the patient's mood, fears, expectancies, and coping efforts are engaged. External factors, such as financial and social resources, and the responses of significant others begin to influence the patient's perception of the pain. Affective and anxiety disorders are prevalent among people with chronic pain because of the respective neurochemical associations with serotonin and norepinephrine (Campbell, Clauw, & Keefe, 2003). They may be a symptom of or a defense against psychological stress caused by continuous nociceptive input. Severity and duration of chronic pain are directly proportional to severity of depression (Evans et

BOX 36.2

Pain Syndromes Seen in the Primary Care Setting

Migraine headache: a cerebrovasomotor disorder in which a focal reduction of cerebral blood flow initiates an ischemic headache. May be preceded by a visual aura and followed by nausea, vomiting, and incapacitating head pain.

Low back pain: pain arising from the vertebral column or surrounding muscles, tendons, ligaments, or fascia. Causes range from simple muscle strain to arthritis, fracture, or nerve compression from a ruptured disk.

Chronic benign orofacial pain: temporomandibular joint pain.

Rheumatoid arthritis: more than 100 different types of joint disease produce inflammation of the joints. Associated with varying degrees of pain and stiffness and eventual loss of use of the affected joints.

Reflex sympathetic dystrophy: causalgia. A painful burning syndrome that occurs after peripheral nerve injury. Associated with hyperesthesia, vasomotor disturbances, and dystrophic changes due to sympathetic hyperactivity.

Cancer pain: pain from malignant tumors that is caused by local infiltration or metastatic spread involving specific organs, bones, or peripheral or cranial nerves, or the spinal cord. Pain therapy is aimed at providing sufficient relief to allow maximum possible daily functioning and a relatively pain-free death.

Neuropathic pain
- *Polyneuropathy:* neuropathy involving multiple peripheral nerves
- *Diabetic neuropathy:* neuropathy due to diabetes mellitus; marked by diminished sensation secondary to vascular changes
- *Inflammatory neuropathy:* neuropathy related to the presence of chemical or microorganic pathogens
- *Traumatic neuropathy:* neuropathy caused by avulsion or compression
- *Plexopathy:* neuropathy involving a peripheral nerve plexus
- *Peripheral or central neuralgia:* abrupt, intense, paroxysmal pain due to intrinsic nerve injury or extrinsic nerve compression
- *Herpetic neuralgia:* pain associated with the dermatomal rash of acute herpes zoster
- *Radiculopathy:* pain radiating along a peripheral nerve tract, such as sciatica

Vasoocclusive pain: thrombotic crisis of sickle cell anemia in joints and peripheral muscles that is caused by ischemia

Myofascial pain: pain in palpable bands (trigger points) of muscle. Associated with stiffness, limitation of motion, and weakness.

al., 2005). Biopsychosocial stimuli and responses may cause the patient with chronic pain to become preoccupied with the pain and can contribute to depression. Also, the presence of persistent noxious sensations contributes to neurochemical and neurohormonal imbalances that lead to depressed mood and anxiety. Whether the psychological pain is primary or secondary may be difficult to determine because the neurovegetative symptoms of depression may resemble the patient's attempts to control the pain or the concomitant medical-physical conditions. Anorexia, sleep disturbance, and agitation or psychomotor retardation may be present. Also, affective disturbances, such as demoralization, sadness, loss of interest in life, feelings of worthlessness, self-reproach, excessive guilt, indecisiveness, and suicidal ideation, are all symptoms reported by patients with chronic pain (Evans et al., 2005). Substance use disorder may arise from the patient's search for relief through overuse of drugs that lessen the pain sensation. A formal psychiatric assessment is essential when these symptoms exist.

Assessment of the Patient with Chronic Pain

Appropriate diagnosis and treatment of pain as a primary presenting symptom must begin with a comprehensive history and physical examination. In talking with the nurse about the pain, a patient will not only describe its characteristics, location, and severity but may also provide information about possible psychosocial and behavioral factors that are influencing the pain experience. No direct relationship may be evident between the severity or extent of detectable disease and the intensity of the patient's pain. A number of assessment instruments have been developed to aid in evaluation, but a fundamental approach is necessary to determine the impact of pain on the patient's life. All systems must be examined in the patient to determine the degree to which biomedical, psychosocial, and behavioral factors interact to influence the nature, severity, and persistence of the patient's pain and disability. Box 36.3 presents a pain assessment tool.

Chronic pain occurs with a wide variety of medical illnesses. Proper diagnosis of the underlying condition determines primary treatment, which could eliminate or significantly reduce the need for analgesic drugs. Unsuspected medical conditions, such as alcoholism, autoimmune disease, or cancer, must be considered if pain develops in the absence of a known cause. Caregivers must know the mechanisms of action of analgesic drugs to administer them safely and monitor their effects. Patients' responses to individual drugs vary, and many agents at different doses may be tried before pain relief is achieved. Table 36.1 presents treatment approaches to pain. The use of physical and psychological modulation techniques as well as pharmacotherapy or physical therapy is more successful than the latter therapies alone. Combination treatment often affects mood and anxiety levels as well. Patients trained to use cognitive strategies such as biofeedback, a positive emotional state, relaxation, physical therapy or exercise, meditation, guided imagery, suggestion, hypnosis, placebos, and positive self-talk are able to tolerate higher levels of pain than patients without specific coping strategies. Most of these techniques involve redirecting the patient's attention away from the pain and

BOX 36.3

Assessing Patients Who Report Pain

A. What is the extent of the patient's disease or injury (physical impairment)?
B. What is the magnitude of the illness? That is, to what extent is the patient suffering, disabled, and unable to enjoy usual activities?
C. Does the person's behavior seem appropriate to the disease or injury, or is there any evidence of amplification of symptoms for any of a variety of psychological or social reasons or purposes?
D. How often and for how long does the patient perform specific behaviors, such as reclining, sitting, standing, and walking?
E. How often does the patient seek health care and take analgesic medication (frequency and quantity)?

The Multiaxial Assessment of Pain (MAP) (Rudy & Turk, 1991) includes evaluation of three axes: biomedical, psychosocial, and behavioral.

Pain Behavior Checklist

Pain behaviors have been characterized as interpersonal communications of pain, distress, or suffering. Pain behavior may be a more accurate indication of intensity and tolerance than verbal reports. Check the box of each behavior you observe or infer from the patient's comments.

- Facial grimacing, clenched teeth
- Holding or supporting of affected body area
- Questions such as, "Why did this happen to me?"
- Distorted gait, limping
- Frequent shifting of posture or position
- Requests to be excused from tasks or activities; avoidance of physical activity
- Taking of medication as often as possible
- Moving extremely slowly
- Sitting with rigid posture
- Moving in a guarded or protective fashion
- Moaning or sighing
- Using a cane, cervical collar, or other prosthetic device
- Requesting help in ambulation; frequent stopping while walking
- Lying down during the day
- Irritability

Table 36.1 Treatment Approaches to Pain

Principles of Pain Treatment	Second Step	Third Step	Fourth Step
• Establish the correct diagnosis. • Recognize that pain reduction, rather than complete pain control, is a reasonable goal. • Control other symptoms besides pain. This includes treating the symptoms that were present before treatment (such as depression and anxiety) and the adverse effects associated with the pain therapy. • Treat physical conditions that may Initiate or exacerbate the pain. **First Step** Analgesics for treatment of pain and: Nonsteroidal antiinflammatory drugs (NSAIDs) Acetaminophen Acetylsalicylic acid Ibuprofen Oral local anesthetics Flecainide Mexiletine Tocainide Topical agents Capsaicin EMLA Lidocaine gel Baclofen Neuroleptics Pimozide Corticosteroids Calcitonin Benzodiazepines Clonazepam Drugs for sympathetically maintained pain Nifedipine Phenoxybenzamine Prazosin Propranolol	Antidepressants, TENS, and psychosocial support, and/or: Tricyclic and tetracyclic antidepressants Amitriptyline Clomipramine Desipramine Doxepin Imipramine Maprotiline Nortriptyline Mirtazapine Selective and nonselective serotonin reuptake Inhibitors Buproprion Fluoxetine Fluvoxamine Nefazodone Olanzapine Paroxetine Sertraline Trazodone Venlafaxine Anticonvulsants Carbamazepine Neurontin Phenytoin Opioid analgesics Codeine Meperidine Morphine Monoamine oxidase inhibitors Isocarboxazid Phenelzine sulfate Tranylcypromine Herbal and alternative medicine SamE Ginseng Swedish massage Acupressure Acupuncture Zero balancing Reflexology Meditation Prayer *Note:* Treat the adverse effects of all the agents used.	Adrenergic agents, TENS, and psychosocial support, and/or: Clonidine Naloxone infusion, and/or: Other agents (mexiletine, diphenhydramine) *Note:* Add the third-step agents to partially helpful agents used in first step, or use alone and treat the adverse effects of all the agents used.	Psychiatric intervention Psychotherapy with pain patients: **Cognitive** • Explain the nature of the pain sensation. • Describe realistic expectations about the degree and course of pain. • Describe realistic expectations of treatment and side effects. • Use the placebo effect by supporting the treatment efficacy. • Relieve anxiety. **Behavioral** • Make the initial doses large rather than small, to effect some relief. • Reassure that medication will be available, not contingent on proof of need. • Reinforce healthy behavior/adaptation; do not reinforce obsession with pain. • Assure of regular evaluation not contingent on presence of pain. **Ablative Procedure for Selected Patients** *Neuroblockade* • Trigger point injection (TPI) • Epidural steroid injection (ESI) • Facet joint injection (FJI) • Nerve root blocks • Medial branch blocks • Peripheral nerve block • Sympathetic nerve block **Spinal Cord Stimulation** • Neurostimulator implants • TENS • Thalamic stimulation

TENS, transcutaneous electrical nerve stimulation
Note: If the patient has failed to experience response to all standard pharmacologic treatments, psychiatric evaluation for underlying problems (such as severe depression and risk for suicide) should be emphasized.

helping the patient learn strategies of **self-efficacy** (self-care effectiveness). Some of the biopsychosocial outcomes that can be measured to determine effectiveness of prescribed therapies include improvements in biologic, psychological, and sociocultural variables (Figure 36.3). The biologic basis for the effectiveness of these cognitive-behavioral strategies may be their ability to increase brain endorphin production (Basbaum & Julius, 2006).

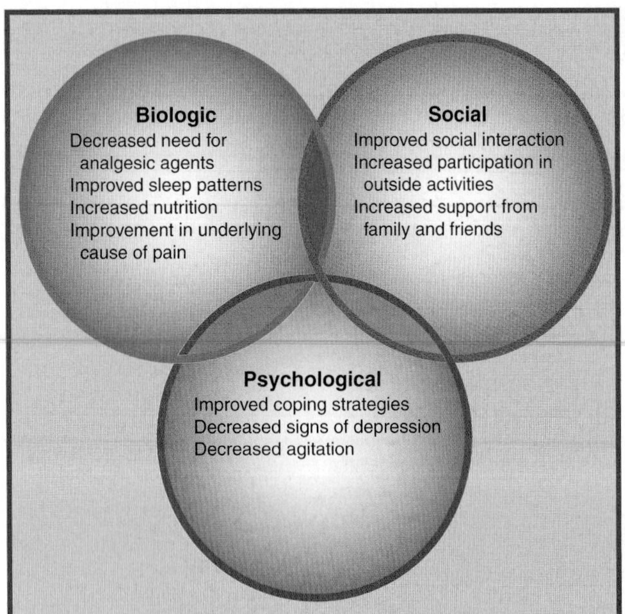

FIGURE 36.3. Biopsychosocial outcomes for patients with pain.

Many barriers to effective pain management exist (Box 36.4). Reluctance on the part of health professionals and the patient may contribute to persistent pain, which ultimately can adversely affect the patient's quality of life. Patients with chronic pain experience not only decreased functional capability but also diminished strength and endurance, nausea, poor appetite, and interrupted sleep. The psychological impact includes diminished leisure and enjoyment, anxiety and fear, depression, somatic preoccupation, and difficulty concentrating. Social impairment may exist in the form of diminished social and sexual relationships, altered appearance, and increased dependence on others. All these contribute to the suffering caused by the pain experience. Maladaptive coping by patients with chronic pain leads them to fear pain and to acquire a negative attitude about pain and how it affects their lives. These negative views can adversely influence biopsychological processes, thereby sustaining or even exacerbating the pain. Noncompliance by these patients with sequential prescription changes and combined treatments can be problematic as well. Strategies to assess compliance are regular self-report, assessment of behavioral change, biochemical assay, clinical improvement, and outcome-assessment. The nurse can enhance compliance by closely monitoring the therapeutic efficacy and untoward effects of the treatments being used, involving the patient and family in treatment planning, educating the patient and family about self-care, and instructing the patient in noninvasive approaches to pain control.

BOX 36.4

Barriers to Pain Management

Problems of Health Care Professionals

- Inadequate knowledge and experience with pain management
- Poor assessment of pain
- Concern about regulation of controlled substances
- Fear of patient tolerance and addiction
- Concern about side effects of analgesics

Problems of Patients

- Reluctance to report pain
- Concern about primary treatment of underlying disease
- Fear that pain means the disease is worse
- Concern about being a good patient and not a complainer
- Reluctance to take pain medications
- Fear of tolerance and addiction, fear of "addict" label
- Fear of unmanageable side effects

Problems of Health Care System

- Cost or inadequate reimbursement
- Restrictive regulation of controlled substances
- Problems with availability of treatment or access to it

PSYCHOPATHOLOGIC COMPLICATIONS OF AIDS

The medical syndrome of AIDS is characterized by multiple opportunistic infections and is associated with malignancy. People with AIDS are often overwhelmed by devastating disorders that cause profound fatigue, insomnia, anorexia, emaciation, pain, and disfigurement. The psychological impact of AIDS is considerably worsened by the social stigma associated with the infection and the special affinity of HIV for brain and central nervous system (CNS) tissue.

Biologic Basis of Cognitive and Motor Changes in AIDS

In about 60% of people with AIDS, neurologic complications occur that are directly attributable to infection of the brain. Important clinical manifestations include impaired cognitive and motor function. This aspect of the syndrome is referred to as the **HIV-1–associated cognitive-motor complex.** Neuronal injury and frank nerve cell loss probably contribute to the neurologic deficits (Manji & Miller, 2004). Evidence suggests that the presence of HIV stimulates brain cells to release neurotoxins and excitatory amino acids in excess. The resultant neurochemical changes and disrupted cell membrane integrity cause cell death similar to that which occurs with other types of brain injury. These neurochemical changes and eventual catecholamine depletion contribute to the cognitive, motor, and psychiatric manifestations of HIV infection (Cruess et al., 2003; Leserman, 2003). Comorbid neurologic infections such as encephalitis and meningitis can predispose the patient with AIDS to delirium.

Psychological Changes Associated with AIDS

The most common initial signs and symptoms of the **AIDS dementia complex** are changes in mentation and personality, followed by delirium, dementia, organic mood disorder, and organic delusional disorder. The onset of major depression and uncomplicated bereavement soon after diagnosis is common. The clinical symptoms reflect the areas of the brain invaded by HIV; however, physiologic conditions such as addiction to alcohol or drugs, brain damage, chronic illness, hypoxia related to pneumonia, infections, space-occupying brain lesions, and systemic reactions to medications may contribute to the progression of mental changes. Loss of normal cortical function may lead to abnormal social behavior, depression, psychosis, and anxiety. The psychological influences of stress and sleep and sensory deprivation can further contribute to the altered perception and mentation. Figure 36.4 shows the possible pathologic progression of HIV neuronal injury.

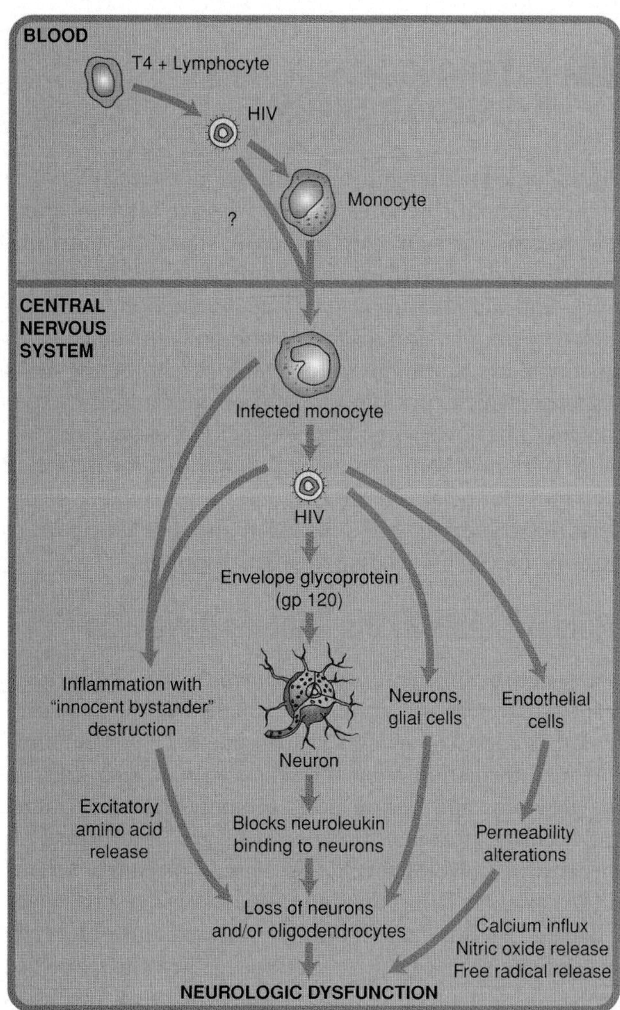

FIGURE 36.4. Possible pathologic progression of HIV neuronal injury.

Psychiatric disorders contribute to the course of AIDS in several ways. Mood disorder may be reflected in the patient who has an initial substance abuse disorder or an antisocial personality that predisposes him or her to a high-risk lifestyle that increases the risk for exposure to HIV. Depression and bipolar disorder are linked to biological changes in HIV/AIDS that might contribute to disease progression and mortality. Abnormalities in HPA axis and hypercortisolemia associated with physiological and psychological distress may alter immune response and diminish host defense in people with low CD4 counts (Leserman, 2003). The neuropathology associated with the presence of HIV then may also contribute to poor adherence to antiretroviral treatment, progression of the disease, and deterioration. AIDS-associated psychopathology is frequently unrecognized, misdiagnosed, and incorrectly treated. Diagnosis can be difficult when risk factors are not known or when cognitive or psychiatric symptoms precede the onset of other manifestations of HIV infection. Early CNS involvement is detected through neuropsychological testing and magnetic resonance imaging. The degree of cognitive dysfunction may not be a valid indication of the degree of organic involvement. Also, diagnostic findings on computed tomography scanning such as cerebral atrophy and prominent basal ganglia calcification may not correlate with the severity of the patient's dementia (Manji & Miller, 2004).

Assessment of the Patient with AIDS

Early recognition of psychiatric disorders associated with AIDS is important to enhance the understanding of the behavior of people with AIDS. Mental status changes and altered affect should be investigated through formal neurological and psychological testing to determine the extent of impairment. Successful coping and cognitive adaptation are often further hindered by the presence of psychiatric disorders associated with HIV (Box 36.5). These mental illnesses include mood disorders, adjustment disorders, anxiety disorders, substance use disorders, and personality disorders. Organic mood disorder may be characterized by symptoms of a major depressive or manic episode. The depressed mood, feelings of guilt, anhedonia, and hopelessness can be accompanied by insomnia or hypersomnia, psychomotor retardation, or agitation and suicidal ideation. Low self-esteem, feelings of worthlessness and hopelessness, and impaired thinking or concentration are other common findings. It is important to differentiate between major depression and complicated or uncomplicated grieving over the loss of health or of significant others to premature death due to HIV. When a patient receives the diagnosis of AIDS, he or she may withdraw into social

BOX 36.5

Psychiatric Disorders Associated With HIV Infection

Organic Mental Disorder
Dementia
- HIV dementia or AIDS–dementia complex
- Dementia associated with opportunistic infection
  - Fungal
    - Cryptococcoma
    - Cryptococcal meningitis
    - Candidal abscesses
  - Protozoal
    - Toxoplasmosis
  - Bacterial
    - *Mycobacterium avium–intracellulare*
  - Viral
    - Cytomegalovirus
    - Herpesvirus
    - Papovavirus progressive multifocal leukoencephalopathy
- Dementia associated with cancer
  - Primary cerebral lymphoma
  - Disseminated Kaposi's sarcoma

Delirium
Organic delusional disorder
Organic mood disorder
- Depression
- Mania
- Mixed

Affective disorders
- Major depression
- Dysthymic disorder

Adjustment disorders
- Adjustment disorder with depressed mood
- Adjustment disorder with anxious mood

Substance abuse disorder
Borderline personality disorder
Antisocial personality disorder
Bereavement
Anxiety disorders
- Obsessive-compulsive disorder
- Panic

isolation, unfamiliar and perhaps ineffective treatments, and the prospect of premature death.

Biopsychosocial Nursing Interventions

Interventions should focus on maintaining normal hydration, electrolyte balance, and nutrition, as well as a safe, comfortable environment. Antiviral agents, such as zidovudine, ribavirin, and phosphonoformate, and the HAART (highly active antiretroviral therapy) combinations cross the blood–brain barrier and achieve adequate anti-HIV concentrations in cerebrospinal fluid after systemic administration.

In addition, it is important to provide the patient and the patient's family, friends, and caregivers with emotional and educational support. Those close to the patient may especially need psychotherapy if the patient is young. Treatment of psychiatric disorders should include individual and family therapy, as well as psychotropic medications, in a manner similar to the treatment of primary psychiatric disorders. Selective serotonin reuptake inhibitors may be used in low doses for depressed mood. The administration of trazodone (Desyrel) or similar sedative for sleep support, may be appropriate in some cases.

Early diagnosis and treatment are imperative to maximize the patient's adherence to risk-reduction regimens and to prevent the transmission of infection. Treatment plans can often be tailored to meet the needs of the patient and family. The consultation-liaison psychiatric professional can recommend appropriate multidisciplinary interventions to meet the challenge of AIDS with compassion and dignity.

PSYCHOLOGICAL ILLNESS RELATED TO TRAUMA

Physiologic trauma activates the overall stress response of the autonomic nervous system. Massive catecholamine release causes certain cardiovascular, muscular, gastrointestinal, and respiratory symptoms that release energy stores and support survival. Tissue destruction, musculoskeletal pain, physical disability, and body image changes all contribute to the physiologic and psychological stress response, which continues long after the traumatic experience. The overwhelming behavioral responses are hypervigilance, fear, and anxiety; psychological sequelae may include social isolation, agitation, personality disorders, posttraumatic stress disorder, and depression or, in extreme cases, dissociative identity disorders.

Biologic Basis of the Trauma Response

The neurotransmitters responsible for behavioral responses to fear and anxiety are usually held in balance to maintain a level of arousal appropriate for environmental threat. Information from the sensory processing areas in the thalamus and cortex alerts the amygdala (the lateral and central nucleus). Events that are interpreted as threatening activate the hypothalamus–pituitary–adrenal (HPA) axis, initiating the generalized stress response (see Chapter 14). Adrenal steroids are released and trigger the physiologic reactions just described. When the perceived threat is sustained, complex neurochemical processes involving norepinephrine, gamma-aminobutyric acid (GABA), and serotonin are overwhelmed by the catecholamine release. For example, norepinephrine receptors adjust to the increased level of hyperstimulation. Then as the catecholamines are depleted, the norepinephrine receptors react to the relative catecholamine insufficiency. This depletion alters cognitive and affective function similar to the altered function that occurs in anxiety disorders. Persistent, severe distress leads to a general dysregulation of the HPA axis and inappropriate and prolonged secretion of high levels of catecholamines. The chronic stress disorder has been linked to increased susceptibility to diseases of immunosuppression, such as certain cancers, as well as infection, myocardial disease, and neurologic degenerative disorders (Radley et al., 2004).

Adaptation to trauma is related to such factors as the severity of the trauma, the person's maturity and age when the trauma occurs, available social support, and the person's ability to mobilize coping strategies (Heim et al., 2000). During adaptation to prolonged stress, the patient's cognitive thought processes and coping behaviors cause dopamine to be released in the prefrontal cortex of the brain. These dopaminergic systems are presumed to play a major role in physiologic and emotional coping responses, storage of the trauma experience into memory, and possibly the development of posttraumatic stress disorder (McAllister, Flashman, Sparling, & Saykin, 2004). Serotonin is also thought to influence adaptation and mobilize coping strategies.

Psychological Aspects of the Trauma Response

Individual behavior and perception are essential components of the stress reaction. Response to the challenge depends on prior experience, developmental history, and physical status. Individual differences in the extent of endocrine and autonomic activity occur during stress as well. Psychological sequelae of sustained stress and trauma may be manifested as flashbacks, intrusive recurring thoughts, panic or anxiety attacks, paranoia, inappropriate startle reactions, nightmares, or the extreme of posttraumatic stress disorder. Catecholamine depletion and activation of the dopamine pathways may contribute to deterioration in social and intellectual functioning after severe physical or emotional trauma. The patient may become so withdrawn and depressed that he or she stops participating in activities of daily living (ADLs). Toward the other extreme, the patient may become agitated and combative, perceiving any treatment as a continued threat.

Assessment of the Trauma Patient

Complete physical assessment after physical traumatic injury is imperative in life-threatening circumstances. Multiple trauma and head injury are the major causes of death and disability in young adults. Emergency care and intensive care providers are highly trained to recognize signs and symptoms of physiologic injury and to intervene to stabilize primary and secondary trauma in the general medical setting. Trauma scales and triage models have been developed to assist in immediate assessment and to measure neurologic and physical condition (Figure. 36.5) (Burkle, 1991). They have also been used to predict long-term outcome in patients in whom permanent cognitive and physical disability may limit recovery and challenge adaptive responses.

Psychological injury must be thoroughly evaluated through observation and interview to determine prevalent signs and symptoms of accompanying psychological disorders. This process includes evaluating the patient's adjustment and coping skills, personal way of dealing with the trauma, social circumstances, and environmental and life stressors. Assessment must be ongoing to help the patient deal with disfigurement, sudden disability, and changes in self-care. The evaluation should include assessment of the patient's perception of experienced stress, feelings related to the stress, dominant mood, cognitive functioning, defense and coping mechanisms, and available support systems. In addition, assessment of the risk for self-inflicted injury or suicide is critical.

Biopsychosocial Nursing Interventions

Psychiatric clinicians provide an important aspect of emergency care. Interventions that establish trust, reduce anxiety, promote adaptive coping, and cultivate a sense of control help the patient to begin recovery and maintain emotional health. Crisis intervention methods, stress management, cognitive behavioral therapies, psychotherapy, and psychotropic medications, alone or in combination, may be useful in achieving the best possible outcome.

When trauma causes the patient's death, the family must be informed of the death and allowed to grieve, to prevent the development of a pathologic or prolonged grief response. Traumatic death is sudden and unexpected, and the victim is often young. Surviving family members usually have a severe emotional reaction to the death. Dysfunctional family dynamics may become evident during this period. The psychiatric–mental health liaison nurse can use family intervention strategies to enhance or improve relationships while the family's motivation to do all that is possible is high.

PSYCHOLOGICAL ILLNESS RELATED TO CENTRAL NERVOUS SYSTEM DISORDERS

Neurological impairment is most often related to brain cell (neuron) destruction. The primary causes of neuronal damage are traumatic injury, ischemia, infarction (cere-

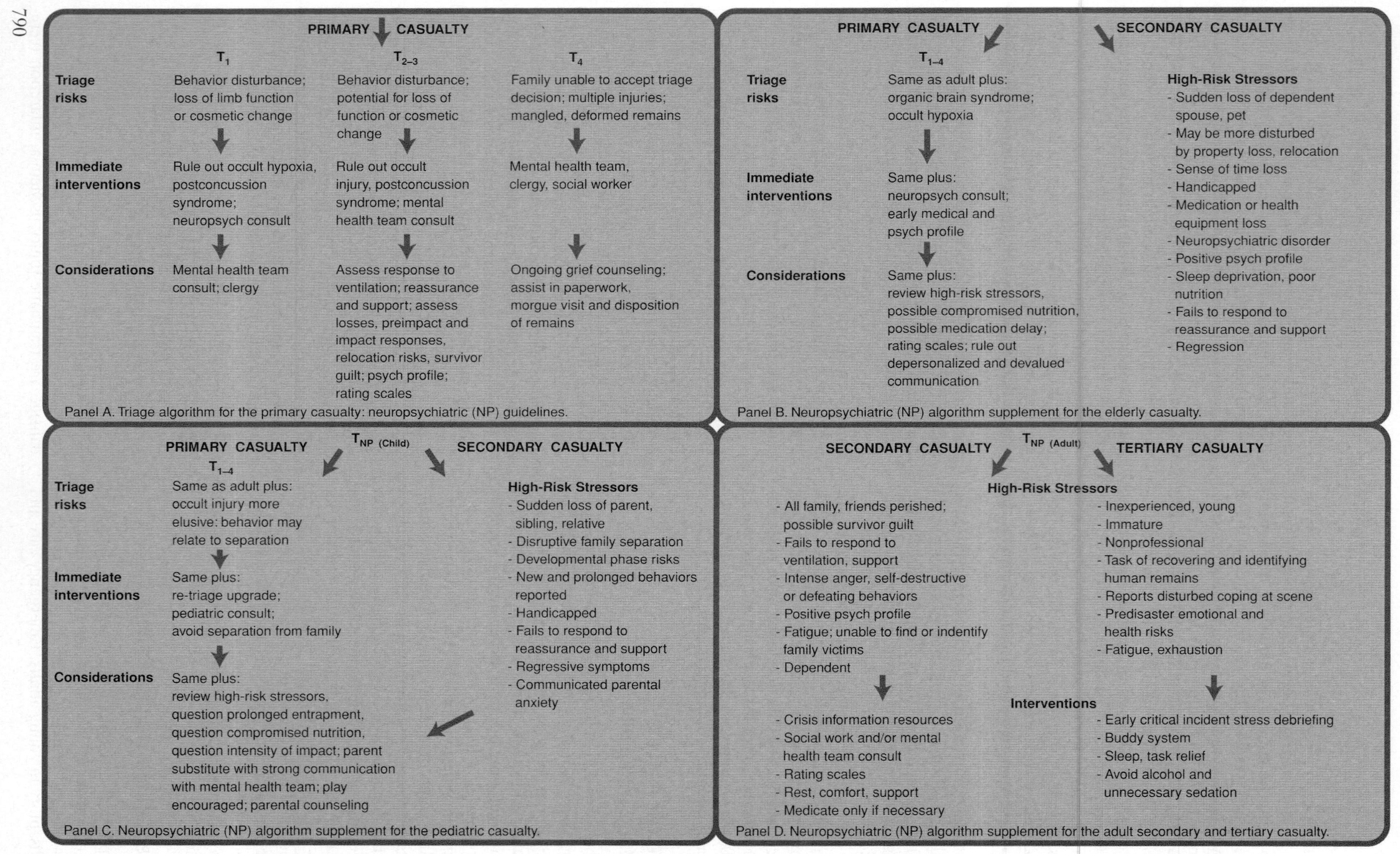

FIGURE 36.5. Triage algorithm for the primary casualty: neuropsychiatric guidelines. (Adapted from Burkle F. M., Jr. [1991]. Triage of disaster-related neuropsychiatric casualties. *Psychiatric Aspects of Emergency Medicine*, *9*[1], 87–104.)

brovascular accident), abnormal neuron growth (brain tumor), and metabolic poisoning associated with systemic disease. Brain cell loss may also be the result of degenerative processes, such as those that occur in Alzheimer's or Parkinson's disease. Psychological illness often is a complication of organic neurological disease and may be difficult to distinguish from the neuropathology itself. Therefore, appropriate intervention depends on skilled assessment to discriminate and detect mental status changes related to organic brain injury as well as disorders of mood and thought.

Biologic Basis of Neurological Impairment

All mechanisms of brain cell injury destroy brain cells directly or initiate a cascade of cell breakdown from ischemia. This **ischemic cascade** begins with hypoxia and is followed by paralysis of the ion exchange across the cell membrane, edema, calcium influx, free-radical production, and lipid peroxidation (Figure 36.6). The severity of brain injury is related to the degree and duration of ischemia. Complete ischemia results in brain infarction, commonly known as stroke. The resulting neurologic impairment is related to the size and location of the affected brain area (Figure 36.7). More eloquent areas of the brain, such as the internal capsule, are extremely sensitive to ischemia. They are typically injured first and contribute to more generalized impairment, such as memory loss or altered judgment. The primary psychological disorder experienced by people with brain injury is depression (Robinson, 2003). Depressive symptoms related to organic brain injury are generated by altered biochemical neurotransmitter systems. Hyperactivity and dysregulation of the HPA axis probably contribute to the elevated cortisol and catecholamine levels after cerebral insult. In addition, changes in the metabolism of biogenic amines after brain cell death and ischemia may mediate both mood disturbances and cognitive dysfunction in patients with stroke.

In cognitive brain function, dopamine is essential for normal neurotransmission of motor messages, motivation, and level of anxiety and mood; epinephrine establishes learning and memory; and serotonin regulates the level of alertness, the categorization of information, as well as the perception of well-being. These neurotransmitter pathways are temporarily interrupted or permanently disrupted during the acute injury. Secondary injury caused by swelling and compression may further compromise neurons in surrounding areas, causing marginal neurotransmitter function. In addition, circulating catecholamines can lead to oversecretion of dopamine or serotonin, which disrupts the necessary balance in production and uptake of the transmitters.

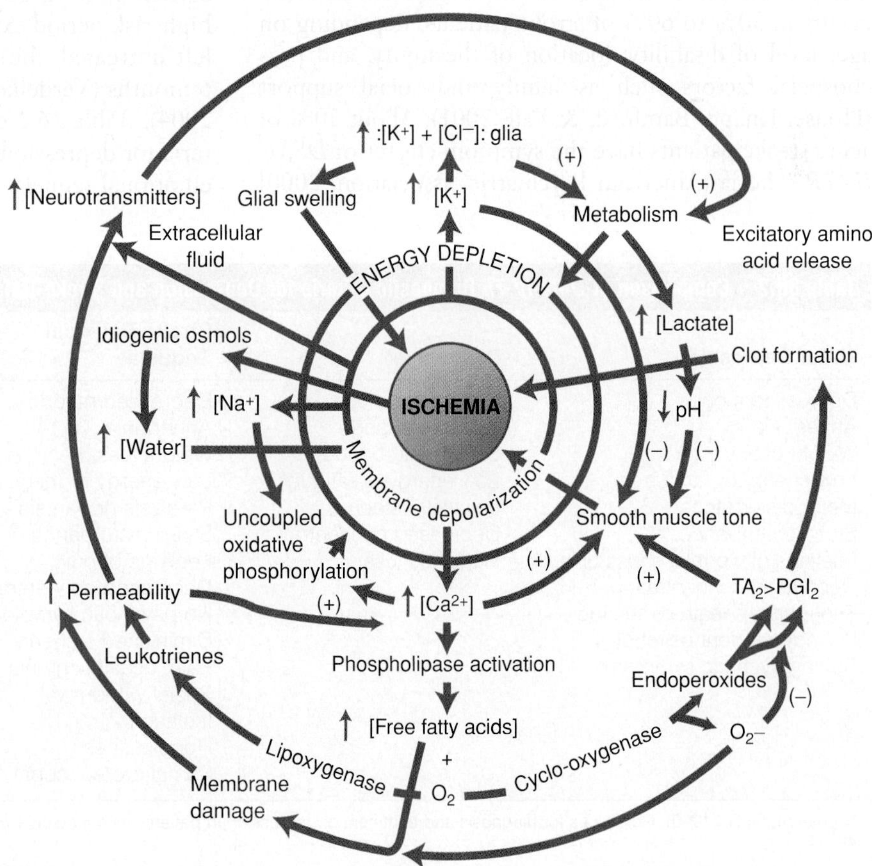

FIGURE 36.6. Ischemic cascade causes secondary brain injury and altered neurotransmitter function. (Based on Raichle, M.E. [1983]. The pathophysiology of brain ischemia. *Annals of Neurology*, 13[1], 2–10.)

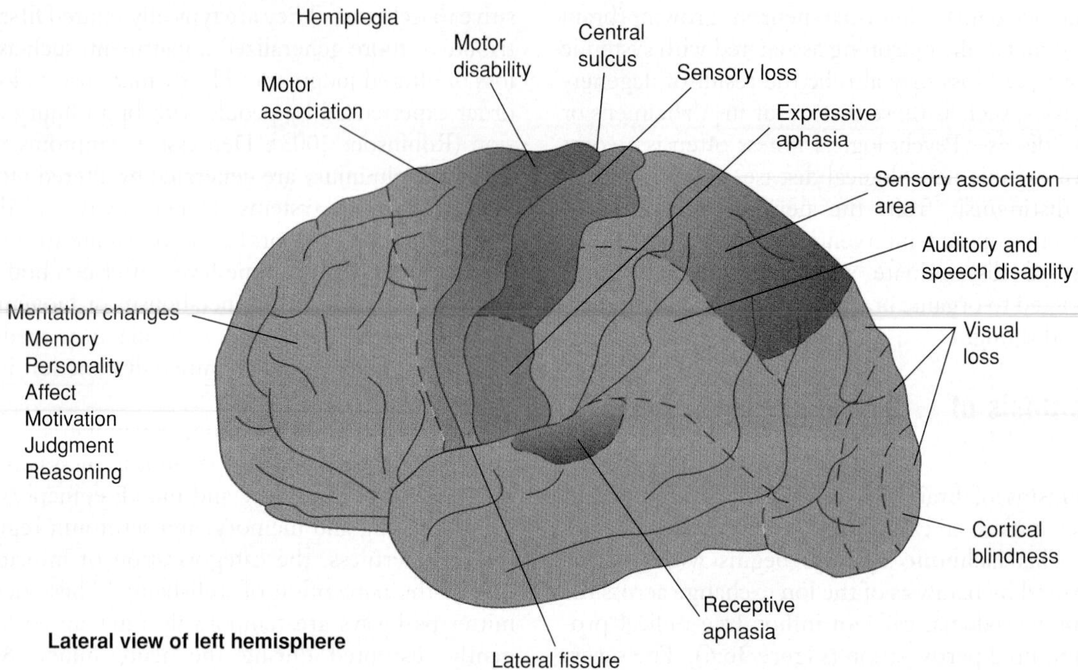

FIGURE 36.7. Functional cerebral anatomy and stroke.

Psychological Aspects of Neurological Impairment

Depressive disorder is a frequent complication of brain injury, particularly ischemic stroke. This mood disorder occurs in 30% to 60% of stroke patients, depending on age, level of disability, location of the injury, and psychosocial factors such as family and social support (House, Knapp, Bamford, & Vail, 2001). About 20% of acute stroke patients have the symptom cluster of *DSM-IV-TR* criteria (American Psychiatric Association, 2000) for major depression (see Chapter 20). Other symptoms, such as sleep disturbances, cognitive dysfunction, poor concentration, difficulty making decisions, somatic discomfort, poor appetite, social withdrawal, and fatigue or agitation, often accompany the mood disturbance. The high-risk period extends for 2 years after the stroke, and left untreated, the depression generally lasts for at least 6 months (Verdelko, Henon, Lebert, Pasquiere, & Leys, 2004). Table 36.2 compares *DSM-IV-TR* diagnostic criteria for depression and cerebrovascular accident–related emotional sequelae.

Table 36.2 Comparison of *DSM-IV-TR* Diagnostic Criteria for Depression and Stroke-Related Affective Sequelae

Major Depression	Dysthymia*	Stroke Residual Sequelae	Other Symptoms Associated With Depression
Depressed mood	Depressed mood	Depressed mood	Decreased sexual desire or sexual functioning
Anhedonia	Appetite change	Anhedonia	Loss of insight
Weight change	Sleep disturbance	Weight loss	Autonomic symptoms (e.g., sweating, tachycardia)
Low energy or fatigue	Low energy or fatigue	Low energy or fatigue	Somatic anxiety symptoms
Motor disturbance	Low self-esteem	Paralysis or paresis	Psychic anxiety symptoms
Sleep disturbance	Decreased concentration	Sleep disturbance	Somatic preoccupation (hypochondriasis)
Feelings of worthlessness or guilt	Hopelessness	Feelings of guilt	Pain, especially chronic pain
Decreased concentration		Decreased concentration	Diminished self-care
Thoughts of death or suicide		No psychotic symptoms	Social incapacitation
No independent psychosis		Diminished self-care	
Some psychotic symptoms		Pain, usually chronic	
		Social withdrawal	
		Isolation	
		Hopelessness	
		Somatic preoccupation	

*Cameron, O. G. (1990). Guidelines for diagnosis and treatment of depression in patients with medical illness. *Journal of Clinical Psychiatry, 51,* 7(Suppl.), 49–54.

Minor and moderate depression may go unrecognized and undiagnosed when patients with stroke describe somatic symptoms and demonstrate lack of motivation in ADLs. Depression is more likely to develop in stroke patients if they have altered speech or aphasia, severe hemiparesis, or both. Stroke patients, however, experience depression more frequently than other disabled and chronically ill patients, even though the level of functional disability is the same (Verdelko et al., 2004). This phenomenon is thought to be possibly related to the combination of permanent disability and altered neurotransmitter systems that persist after cerebral infarction.

Although the mechanism of neuronal injury is one of degeneration in Parkinson's disease and other neuromuscular diseases, the neurochemical changes in the brain are similar with respect to the loss of dopamine secretion and receptor sites in the internal capsule motor pathways. About 30% of patients with Parkinson's disease experience depression (Rojo, Aguilar, Garolera, Cubo, Navas, & Quintana, 2003). Although major depression may occur, the majority have less severe forms that contribute to impairment in daily functioning possibly as much as the underlying disease. Depression is the main factor negatively affecting quality of life and a source of distress for the patient and the family and caregivers. There is evidence suggesting that altered serotonergic function may be responsible, at least in part, for the depressive symptoms in Parkinson's disease and that altered noradrenergic function may underlie some of the associated anxiety symptoms (Zubenko et al., 2003). Recent clinical trials have demonstrated the SSRIs and SNRIs are more effective than traditional tricyclic antidepressants in reducing or relieving the depressive and anxiety symptoms in patients with neurological disease (Murai et al., 2001; Lyketsos et al., 2003). In addition, the serotonergic system is disrupted as the neuronal synapses are destroyed or injured. This generalized loss of dopaminergic activity and decreasing functional ability probably contribute to depressed mood in stroke patients as well.

Mental illness related to organic brain injury is consistently dependent on the degree of functional impairment, particularly loss of the ability to communicate and administer self-care. Depressed mood may become evident in the acute recovery phase or during rehabilitation. Depression often negatively affects survival and recovery. It impedes progress throughout the rehabilitation process and ultimately prevents an optimal outcome. Early evaluation assists in the detection of mental illness after brain injury (Robinson, 2003).

Assessment of the Neurological Patient

A thorough neurological examination is important in determining the location and degree of disability but even more critical in establishing the locus of retained function. Many scales exist that accurately assess neurological function and that are easy to administer and generally accepted as reliable tools to detect the degree and limitations of disability. Cognition and mentation can be more discretely measured by the Folstein Mini-Mental State Examination (Folstein, Folstein, & McHugh 1975), and functionability for self-care can be measured using the Barthel Index (Mahoney & Barthel, 1965). The evaluation of mood using the Center for Epidemiological Studies Depression Scale (CES-D) or the Beck Depression Inventory (Beck, Ward, Mendelson, Mock, & Erbaugh, 1961) provides important information for designing intervention strategies for the at-risk stroke patient. Findings of depressive symptoms indicate the need for a more definitive neuropsychological referral.

Biopsychosocial Interventions

Isolation, lack of companionship, bereavement, and poverty are associated with depressive symptoms in the general population and compound the relative risk of depression developing after brain damage. In addition, a prior history or family history of major depression increases the risk for depressed mood. Prevention strategies should be used as early as possible for patients known to have these risks. These strategies include the assessment and provision of social support resources while the patient is hospitalized and as an important component of discharge planning to rehabilitation services; the prescription of therapies to enhance competence in the performance of ADLs, with a focus on the use of retained function rather than on adaptation to disabilities only; formal psychosocial testing and psychopharmacologic treatment when appropriate (Robinson, 2003); and the education of the patient and family to increase their awareness of signs and symptoms of depressed mood, so that they will know when to seek medical attention and treatment to avert major depression, if possible. In addition, the presence of depressed mood and other symptoms of the depressive cluster indicate the need for cognitive, behavioral, biologic, and social interventions to support appropriate psychopharmacologic treatment.

PSYCHOLOGICAL ILLNESS RELATED TO ACUTE AND CHRONIC MEDICAL ILLNESS

Systemic medical illness is associated with a higher prevalence of concurrent psychiatric disorders. Disorders such as cancer, heart disease, endocrine abnormalities, and organ failure are often associated with more functional disability than most chronic medical illnesses and may be the basis of medically unexplained somatic symptoms. Among the psychiatric disorders, substance use disorder, anxiety, and depressive disorder occur most frequently in patients with chronic medical illnesses. Within the anxi-

Table 36.3 Prevalence of Psychiatric Disorders in Medically Ill Compared With Nonmedically Ill People

Prevalence of Psychiatric Disorders*	Medically Ill (%)	Nonmedically Ill (%)
Six-month prevalence	24.7	17.5
Substance abuse	8.5	
Anxiety	11.9	
Affective disorder	9.4	
Lifetime prevalence	42.4	33.0
Substance use	26.2	
Anxiety	18.2	
Phobias	12.1	
Panic disorder	1.5	
Obsessive-compulsive disorder	2.4	
Affective disorder	12.9	

*Prevalence rates are sex- and age-adjusted.
Adapted from National Institute of Mental Health Epidemiologic Catchment Area Program, Burkle, F. M., Jr. (1991). Triage of disaster-related neuropsychiatric casualties. *Psychiatric Aspects of Emergency Medicine, 9*(1), 87–104.

ety disorders, phobias are most common, with panic disorder and obsessive-compulsive disorder occurring less often (Harter, Conway, & Merikangas, 2003). Table 36.3 compares the prevalence rates of depressive and anxiety disorders in people who are medically ill with the rates in people who are not.

Biologic Aspects of Mental Illness Related to Medical Disease

The nervous, endocrine, and immune systems and their components are designed to communicate and interact through biochemical means. The cerebral cortex and limbic system initiate neuroendocrine HPA axis activity by thought processes in response to environmental stimuli. Various hormonal messengers travel between the hypothalamic, pituitary, and adrenal systems to initiate secondary peripheral responses. The immune system responds to signals from the HPA axis and returns messages as well. Its protective activities rely on neurochemicals to initiate the infection defense and stress response. At all levels, the circulating hormone levels serve as feedback messengers to inhibit HPA activity after sufficient response has occurred.

Dysregulation of the hypothalamic, pituitary, and adrenal systems at all levels leads to malfunction of the other systems. Abnormal nervous system firing in the hippocampus alerts the adrenal and immune systems unnecessarily, and vice versa. The principal neurochemical messengers in this regulation are thought to be norepinephrine, endorphins, cortisol, and dopamine. This trio of systems detects metabolic and cellular disease processes that eventually cause signs and symptoms of medical diseases, and activate body resources to stop these pathologic processes. Psychiatric conditions occur during the course of these medical illnesses and in some instances may contribute to the genesis of the physiologic disease.

A psychiatric disorder may be the first manifestation of a primary disease, such as depressive syndrome in Huntington's chorea, multiple sclerosis, Parkinson's disease, HIV, Cushing's disease, and systemic lupus erythematosus. Depressive symptoms are an intrinsic part of the primary pathophysiology of endocrine disorders, metabolic disturbances, malignancies, viral infections, inflammatory disorders, and cardiopulmonary conditions. Tables 36.4 and 36.5 list medical conditions associated with anxiety disorders and depression, respectively. Endocrine system pathologies involve abnormal HPA axis function, which affects neurotransmitter balance. Depression and anxiety are often present in patients with hyperthyroidism and hypothyroidism, Cushing's disease (hyperadrenalism), and Addison's disease (hypoadrenal-

Table 36.4 Medical Conditions Associated With Anxiety Disorders

Psychiatric Disorder	Medical Illness	Incidence (%)
Panic disorder	Parkinson's disease	20
	Primary biliary cirrhosis	10
	Chronic obstructive pulmonary diseases	24
	Cardiomyopathy	83
	Post-myocardial infarction	16
	Chronic pain	16
	Focal seizures	*
Social phobia	Parkinson's disease	17
Obsessive-compulsive disorder	Sydenham's chorea	13
Phobia	Multiple sclerosis	*
	Primary biliary cirrhosis	10
Generalized anxiety	Graves' disease	62

*Incidence not significant but reportable.

Table 36.5 Medical Illnesses Associated With Symptoms of Depression

Endocrinopathies	Hypothyroidism and hyperthyroidism
	Hypoparathyroidism and hyperparathyroidism
	Cushing's syndrome (steroid excess)
	Adrenal insufficiency (Addison's disease)
	Hyperaldosteronism
Malignancies	Abdominal carcinomas, especially pancreatic
	Brain tumors (temporal lobe)
	Breast cancer
	Gastrointestinal cancer
	Lung cancer
	Prostate cancer
	Metastases
Neurologic disorders	Ischemic stroke
	Subarachnoid hemorrhage
	Parkinson's disease
	Normal-pressure hydrocephalus
	Multiple sclerosis
	Closed head injury
	Epilepsy
Metabolic imbalance	Serum sodium and potassium reductions
	Vitamin B_{12}, niacin, vitamin C deficiencies; iron deficiency (anemias)
	Metal intoxication (thallium and mercury)
	Uremia
Viral/bacterial infection	Infectious hepatitis
	Encephalitis
	Tuberculosis
	AIDS
Hormonal imbalance	Premenstrual, premenopausal, postpartum periods
Cardiopulmonary	Acute myocardial infarction
	Post–cardiac arrest
	Post–coronary artery bypass graft
	Post–heart transplantation
	Cardiomyopathy
Inflammatory disorders	Rheumatoid arthritis

ism), complicating the clinical picture in up to 40% of cases (Gold, Licinio, Wong, & Chrousos, 1995). Although depression has been shown to be an independent risk factor for type 2 diabetes, the early onset of vascular disease, complications, and disability are associated with increased depressive symptoms (Ciechanowski et al., 2003).

Malignancies have also been associated with anxiety and depression. Depressive syndromes have been associated with cancer in up to 50% of cancer cases, and biologic relationships between the two disorders may exist such that the onset of depression may herald undetected carcinoma. Diagnoses range from major depression to adjustment disorder with depressed mood. Depression might also be a direct consequence of antineoplastic therapy (Brown, Levy, Rosberger, & Edgar, 2003) and consequently lead to poor adherence to cancer prevention behavior (e.g., smoking). Available evidence strongly suggests that depression in the patient with cancer responds to SSRIs and mirtazapine. Psychosocial interventions also have been shown to reduce depressive and anxiety symptoms, and result in longer survival (Fawzy, Canada, & Fawzy, 2003).

Systemic infections and generalized inflammatory disorders such as rheumatoid arthritis that acutely and chronically stress the immune system or that may be the result of immune dysfunction are associated with up to 50% of psychological disorders. In addition, renal, pancreatic, and hepatic transplant recipients, who are artificially immunosuppressed because of treatment with prophylactic anti-infectious agents, experience primary neuropsychiatric symptoms related to metabolic imbalances and neuropsychiatric side effects from treatment.

Diagnosing depression and anxiety in medically ill patients is not straightforward. Shared symptoms such as fatigue and weight loss can impede recognition in these patients. In addition to the disease process contributing to psychological complications, the drugs used to treat chronic disease may induce mental illness as well (see Table 36.6). The indications and pharmacologic activity of these medications often have biopsychosocial implications. In addition, medically ill elderly patients are particularly susceptible to medication effects at lower doses (Desai, 2003).

Cardiac disease deserves special attention because it has been associated with precipitated depressive syndromes in 20% to 50% of patients and anxiety disorders in up to 80%. The fact that more than 70% of patients who have an acute myocardial infarction remain depressed for up to a year after the event indicates that the mental illness may not be simply an adjustment disorder. The incidence of depression is similar in cardiac transplant recipients (54%) but is much lower in cardiac bypass surgery patients (6% to 15%) (Lesperance, Frasure-Smith, Talajic, & Bourassa, 2002). Risk of cardiac death in the 6 months after an acute MI is approximately four times greater in patients with depression compared with the non-depressed. Depressive and anxiety-related symptoms may in fact have an additive effect on patient function, well-being, and recovery when combined with medical illness. When a drug is suspected of causing mental changes, the recommended course of action is to withdraw the drug and find an effective alternative. When an adequate substitute is not available, the dosage should be decreased to an effective level at which symptoms resolve.

Psychological Aspects of Medical Illness

In all cases of medical illness, it is natural for patients to respond to the loss of health with hopelessness, particularly when the illness is demoralizing, life threatening,

Table 36.6 Medications Associated With Mental Illness in Medically Ill Patients

Analgesics and nonsteroidal anti-inflammatory drugs (NSAIDs)	Ibuprofen Indomethacin Opiates Pentazocine Phenacetin Phenylbutazone
Antihypertensives	Clonidine Hydralazine Methyldopa Propranolol Reserpine
Antimicrobials	Ampicillin (gram-negative agents) Clotrimazole Cycloserine Griseofulvin Metronidazole Nitrofurantoin Streptomycin Sulfamethoxazole (sulfonamides)
Neurologic agents	L-Dopa Levodopa
Antiparkinsonism drugs	Amantadine
Anticonvulsants	Carbamazepine Phenytoin
Antispasmodics	Baclofen Bromocriptine
Cardiac drugs	Digitalis Guanethidine Lidocaine Oxprenolol Procainamide
Psychotropic drugs	Benzodiazepines
Stimulants/sedatives	Amphetamines Barbiturates Chloral hydrate Chlorazepate Diethylpropion Ethanol Fenfluramine Haloperidol
Steroids and hormones	Adrenocorticotropic hormone Corticosteroids Estrogen Oral contraceptives Prednisone Progesterone Triamcinolone
Antineoplastic drugs	Bleomycin C-Asparaginase Trimethoprim Vincristine
Other miscellaneous drugs	Anticholinesterases Cimetidine Diuretics Metoclopramide

and without a clear prognosis. People who are chronically ill are distressed by loss of function and limitations on their daily activities. They are often forced to comply with treatments that add discomfort but no apparent benefit. Medical patients commonly experience weight loss, insomnia, and motor retardation, but perhaps not to the degree of "conspicuous" psychiatric illness. In addition, chronic life stress and mental illness may have set into motion a series of biologic processes ultimately resulting in the medical disorder, which may be further exacerbated by the stress of hospitalization. A vicious cycle of medical and mental disorders may arise.

Mental illness in medically ill people is potentially lethal because normal affects and cognitive functioning may be essential to recovery and compliance with the medical treatment plan. In addition, the use of excessive analgesics and reluctance to perform self-care and rehabilitative activities hinder recovery and expose the person to other potential complications. The detection and diagnosis of any secondary mental illnesses in patients with medical illnesses is critical. The physiologic and pharmacologic factors that contribute to the mental illness must be explored and ruled out before effective intervention can begin.

Assessment of the Patient with Medical Illness

Unfortunately, it may be very difficult for the clinician evaluating a medically ill patient, in whom psychiatric symptoms develop, to ascertain whether these symptoms are the result of direct psychobiologic changes brought about by the illness. People at obvious risk have a family or personal history of mental illness or were experiencing psychological problems before symptoms of the medical illness were present. The main challenge for the clinician is to determine which signs and symptoms are part of the medical illness and its treatment and which signify the presence of a psychological disorder. A complete health assessment and physical examination, including a psychological examination and a cognitive-affective assessment, will help determine the priority and severity of symptoms and interventions. In some instances, the primary diagnosis may be depression, although the symptoms may be similar to those of medical illness in the absence of diagnostic findings. Factors to be considered in diagnosing mental illness in medical patients are outlined in Box 36.6. Several important cognitive-affective symptoms best differentiate the effects of depression from those of medical illness. These include feelings of failure, low self-esteem, guilt feelings, loss of interest in people, feelings of being punished, suicidal ideation, dissatisfaction, difficulty with decisions, and crying (Evans et al., 2005). The severity of the vegetative symptoms generally increases with the severity of the depressive disorder as well as the severity of the medical illness. Decreased appetite, sleep disturbances, and loss of energy are not considered indicators of depression in the medically ill patient because these symptoms are common in medical illness as well.

BOX 36.6

Factors to Consider in Diagnosing Depression in Medical Patients

- One or more specific medical illnesses
- Defining criteria for one of the depressive syndromes
- Family psychiatric history
- Past psychiatric history of the patient
- Patient's response to treatment, if any, for any prior depressive episode
- Sex of the patient
- Patient's age at onset of depression
- Depression that preceded the medical illness
- Psychosocial precipitants before onset of depression
- Duration of depressive illness
- Biologic markers of depression
- Relative frequency in the population of diagnoses under consideration
- Diagnosis by commission, not omission

The Beck Depression Inventory and the CES-D are easy to administer and will provide some indication of whether a psychiatric liaison referral is needed.

Clinical Features of Special Significance

Two problems of special significance, psychosis and suicidal thoughts, are related in that patients with delusions or hallucinations tend to be at greater risk for suicide attempts or more likely to resist treatment (e.g., to refuse to eat or take medication) for their medical condition. It is important to distinguish between a mentally competent patient's right to refuse life-saving medical treatment and a depressed patient's desire to die. A clinical evaluation of the effect of depression on the patient's capacity to make competent decisions is imperative. If optimal medical and psychiatric treatments have been provided and the patient has been found competent enough to make decisions about further medical care, it may be appropriate to honor the patient's desire to die.

Patients with chronic medical illness and patients with primary mental illness may pose similar problems in psychiatric hospitals when their medical condition fails. The use of advance directives helps in addressing these problems.

Biopsychosocial Treatment Interventions

It is essential to provide optimal treatment of patients' medical illnesses without neglecting their mental distress. Most reports suggest that clinicians should be more aggressive in the pharmacologic treatment of mental illness in the medically ill. The basic rules for medicating patients include using the minimum dose initially, advancing the dose slowly, and performing frequent blood level monitoring. The doses required to achieve therapeutic blood levels may be lower or even half the usual therapeutic dose and take longer to titrate. It is important to understand the pharmacokinetics (absorption, distribution, metabolism, and elimination) of the treatment of choice, to prevent further systemic effects. SSRIs and SNRIs are used equally as the treatment for depression in the medically ill patient population. Because the side effects of psychopharmacologic agents can be especially troublesome in medically ill people, treatment must be changed or stopped if drug or illness interactions occur, or if treatment of the mental illness appears to be unsuccessful. SSRIs are increasingly popular in treating medically ill patients because their side-effect profile is more tolerable within a wider therapeutic range. Most patients respond to antidepressant therapy with a decrease in the severity of their vegetative symptoms in 4 to 8 days.

Both supportive individual psychotherapy and family therapy are helpful. Assisting the patient and family in understanding the nature and relationship of the medical and psychiatric diagnoses may strengthen the support system, alter the perception of caregiver burden, and identify appropriate coping strategies. Mutually agreed-upon goals and therapy actively involve the patient in progress toward recovery. At some point, the clinician may need to help the patient identify psychodynamic conflicts and maladaptive coping strategies that may be contributing to his or her distress. Cognitive intervention should address those areas of the patient's life that can be controlled, despite major lifestyle changes, to reinforce a feeling of competence. Also, it is important to convey the fact that although medical and mental illness are difficult to prevent, they are often treatable.

PHYSICAL ILLNESSES IN PERSONS WITH MENTAL DISORDERS

The relationship between stress and illness is becoming more apparent as studies increasingly disclose the effects of stress on the body (see Chapter 14). Chronic illness is viewed as a stressor and is associated with increased psychological distress; interventions can minimize that distress. Nurses are committed to preventing illness and promoting healthy living. It is essential, therefore, that they be aware of the physiologic and psychological impact of chronic stress, understand the coping process, and know appropriate alternative strategies for coping with illness. In addition, nurses can evaluate the effectiveness of strategies being used and revise care plans to improve outcomes for the patient.

Patients with primary mental illness in need of medical care are at particular risk when somatic complaints are viewed as part of the primary process. Undiagnosed pathophysiologic processes may progress to advanced stages while being attributed to somatization. A thorough medical history and physical examination with complementary laboratory evaluation are standard practice for these patients in all settings.

Ideally, a multidisciplinary team of care providers that includes a psychiatric liaison nurse should work closely together to deliver optimum treatment of complex medical and mental illness. All patients with chronic medical illnesses are at risk for psychological distress and should be approached with this understanding. Clinicians should include a general cognitive-affective status evaluation in their assessment of all medically ill patients and make appropriate psychiatric liaison consultation to offset the negative impact of mental illness on recovery.

A mental health assessment in the admission process helps in detecting stress, risks, and symptom relapse. This assessment provides the minimum information needed for each patient; neglect of even one area could compromise patient care. This information is useful in determining relevant nursing diagnoses and developing the plan of care.

Stress management training, systematic relaxation, supportive education, and stress monitoring should be built into the plan of care, regardless of the medical diagnosis. Assessment of anxiety and depression are ongoing, and crisis intervention with psychotherapy may be necessary to reduce the severity of mental distress. Physiologic stress factors, such as increased heart rate, blood pressure, and respiration, and signs of restlessness and sadness can be measured to determine the effectiveness of the intervention. Secondary mental illness can be approached using the same strategies that are effective for primary mental dysfunction. Interventions overlap across criteria, and all interventions provide some element of supportive therapy or social support.

Mental health can and should be monitored in patients who have physical illnesses. Certain kinds of pathologic processes place patients at greater risk for mental illness. These processes can be identified and interventions prescribed to prevent psychiatric disorders from developing or to minimize their severity. Cognitive and behavioral strategies have a place in the treatment regimen and offer the practitioner an opportunity to expand the boundaries of traditional patient-oriented practice in effective ways.

Alternatives to traditional medical intervention are increasingly employed as adjunct therapy in patients with pain related to cancer, neuropathy, or degenerative disorders. Natural and herbal therapies, therapeutic massage, zero balancing, thought-field therapy, imaging, prayer, and meditation have all been found to be useful in easing the mental and physical discomfort of the patient with medical illness. Also, these therapies are more satisfying to patients who otherwise must receive toxic medication as part of their conventional medical treatment.

SUMMARY OF KEY POINTS

- Psychiatric disorders are more common in people with systemic or chronic medical illnesses than in other people. Comorbid depression is common in certain medical diseases, such as endocrine and metabolic disturbances, viral infections, inflammatory disorders, and cardiopulmonary diseases. Specific anxiety disorders are associated with other medical conditions, such as Parkinson's disease, focal seizures, primary biliary cirrhosis, and chronic pain.
- Psychiatric illness that accompanies medical illness is seldom recognized and treated. Psychiatric symptoms may precede the onset of disease symptoms, and it may be difficult to distinguish between the symptoms of the two conditions.
- The biologic basis of mental illness associated with medical illness (e.g., catecholamine depletion, disorders in metabolism or production of neurotransmitters) is similar to that of primary psychiatric illness, and biopsychosocial treatment strategies are effective.
- Mental illness in medically ill people is potentially lethal because normal affective-cognitive function may be critical to recovery and compliance with the medical treatment plan. Therefore, it is imperative that mental health is included in the standard health assessment of all medically ill persons and that appropriate referrals be made.

CRITICAL THINKING CHALLENGE

1 You are caring for a stroke patient who refuses breakfast and a morning bath. Applying what you know about the neurological damage caused by stroke and the frequency of depression in stroke patients, develop a care plan addressing the patient's biopsychosocial needs.

2 As you care for an AIDS patient, you notice that his partner is pacing and hyperventilating. Using your knowledge of relationships, systems, and the interconnectedness of physical and psychological illness, how would you approach him?

3 Discuss the pain syndromes you may see in the primary care setting.

4 A patient is being seen for chronic pain. Discuss how you would go about assessing barriers to pain management with this patient.

5 You are a psychiatric–mental health liaison nurse and have been asked to prepare a program for the medical–surgical nursing staff on psychiatric aspects of medical illnesses. What topics would you include, and what would be your rationale for including each?

REFERENCES

American Psychiatric Association. (2000). *Diagnostic and statistical manual of mental disorders* (4th ed., text revision). Washington, DC: Author.

Basbaum A. I., & Julius, D. (2006). Pain control. *Scientific American, 294*(6), 60–67.

Beck, A. T., Ward, C. H., Mendelson, M., Mock, J., & Erbaugh, J. (1961). An inventory for measuring depression. *Archives of General Psychiatry, 4,* 561–656.

Brown, K. W., Levy, A. R., Rosberger, Z., & Edgar, L. (2003). Psychological distress and cancer survival: a followup 10 years after diagnosis. *Psychosomatic Medicine, 65,* 636–643.

Burg, M. M., Benedetto M. C., Rosenberg, R., & Soufer, R. (2003). Presurgical depression predicts medical morbidity 6 months after coronary artery bypass graft surgery. *Psychosomatic Medicine, 65,* 111–118.

Burkle, F. M., Jr. (1991). Triage of disaster-related neuro-psychiatric casualties. *Psychiatric Aspects of Emergency Medicine, 9*(l), 87–104.

Cameron, O. G. (1990). Guidelines for diagnosis and treatment of depression in patients with medical illness. *Journal of Clinical Pyschiatry, 7* (Suppl.), 49–54.

Campbell, L. C., Clauw, D. J., & Keefe, F. J. (2003). Persistent pain and depression: a biopsychosocial perspective. *Biological Psychiatry, 54,* 399–409.

Ciechanowski P. S., Katon W. J., Russo J. E., & Hirsch, I. B. (2003). The relationship of depressive symptoms to symptom reporting, self-care and glucose control in diabetes. *General Hospital Psychiatry, 25,* 246–252.

Cruess, D. G., Evans, D. L, Repetto, M. J., Gettes, D., Douglas, S. D., & Petitto, J. M. (2003). Prevalence, diagnosis and pharmacological treatment of mood disorders in HIV disease. *Biological Psychiatry, 54,* 307–316.

Desai, A. K. (2003). Use of psychopharmacologic agents in the elderly. *Clinics in Geriatric Medicine, 19,* 697–719.

Evans, D. L., Charney, D. S., Lewis, L., Golden, R. N., Gorman, J. M., Krishnan, K. R. R., et al. (2005). Mood disorders in the medically ill: scientific review and recommendations. *Journal of Biological Psychiatry, 58,* 175–189.

Fawzy, F. I., Canada, A. L., & Fawzy, N. W. (2003). Malignant melanoma: effects of a brief, structured psychiatric intervention on survival and recurrence at 10-year follow-up. *Archives of General Psychiatry, 60,* 100–103.

Folstein, M. F., Folstein, S. E., & McHugh, P. R. (1975). Mini-mental state: A practical method for grading the cognitive state of patients for the clinician. *Journal of Psychiatric Research, 12,* 189–198.

Gold, P. W., Licinio, J., Wong, M. L., & Chrousos, G. P. (1995). Corticotropin releasing hormone in the pathophysiology of melancholic and atypical depression and in the mechanism of action of antidepressant drugs. *Annals of the New York Academy of Sciences, 771,* 716–729.

Harter, M. C., Conway, K. P., & Merikangas, K. R. (2003). Associations between anxiety disorders and physical illness. *European Archives of Psychiatry and Clinical Neuroscience, 253*(6), 313–320.

House, A., Knapp, P., Bamford, J., & Vail, A. (2001). Mortality at 12 and 24 months after stroke may be associated with depressive symptoms at 1 month. *Stroke, 32,* 696–701.

Insel, T. R., & Charney, D. S. (2003). Research on major depression. *Journal of the American Medical Association, 289,* 3167–3168.

Joffe, R. T., Brasche, J. S., MacQueen, G. M. (2003). Psychiatric aspects of endocrine disorders in women. *Psychiatric Clinics of North America, 261*(3), 683–691.

Kandel, E. R., & Schwartz, J. H. (2000). *Principles of neural science* (3rd ed.). New York: Elsevier.

Leserman, J. (2003). HIV disease progression: Depression, stress and possible mechanisms. *Biological Psychiatry, 54,* 295–306.

Lesperance, F., Frasure-Smith, N., Talajic, M., & Bourassa, M. G. (2002). Five-year risk of cardiac mortality in relation to initial severity and one-year changes in depression symptoms after myocardial infarction. *Circulation, 105,* 1049–1053.

Lyketsos, C. G., delCampo, L., Steinberg, M., Miles, Q., Steele, C.D., Munro, C., et al. (2003). Treating depression in Alzheimer disease: Efficacy and safety of sertraline therapy, and the benefits of depression reduction. The DIADS. *Archives of General Psychiatry, 60,* 737–746.

Mahoney, F. T., & Barthel, D. W. (1965). Functional evaluation: Barthel index. *Maryland Medical Journal, 14,* 61–65.

Manji, H., & Miller, R. (2004). The neurology of HIV infection. *Journal of Neurology, Neurosurgery and Psychiatry, 75*(Suppl), 29–38.

McAllister, J. W., Flashman, L. A., Sparling, M. B., & Saykin, A. J. (2004). Working memory deficits after traumatic brain injury: catec-holeminergic mechanisms and prospects for treatment. *Brain Injury, 18*(4), 331–350.

McCaffery, M., & Pasero, C. (1999). *Pain clinical manual* (2nd ed.). St. Louis: Mosby.

McMahon, S. B., Cafferty, W. B., & Marchand, F. (2005). Immune and glial cell factors as pain mediators and modulators. *Experimental Neurology, 192*(2), 444–462.

Melzack, R., Coderre, T. J., Katz, J., & Vaccarino, A. L. (2001). Central neuroplasticity and pathological pain. *Annals of the New York Academy of Sciences, 993,* 157–174.

Murai T., Muller U., Werheid, K., Sorger, D., Reuter, M., Becker, T., et al. (2001). In vivo evidence for differential association of striatal dopamine and midbrain serotonin systems with neuropsychiatric symptoms in Parkinson's disease. *The Journal of Neuropsychiatry and Clinical Neurosciences, 13,* 222–228.

Radley, J. J., Sisti, H. M., Has, J., Rocker, A. B., McCall, T., Hef, P. R., et al. (2004). Chronic stress induces apical dendritic reorganization in pyramidal neurons of the medial prefrontal cortex. *Neuroscience, 125*(1), 1–6.

Raichle, M. E. (1983). The pathophysiology of brain ischemia. *Annals of Neurology, 13*(1), 2–10.

Robinson, R. G. (2003). Poststroke depression: Prevalence, diagnosis, treatment, and disease progression. *Biological Psychiatry, 54*(3), 376–387.

Rojo, A., Aguilar, M., Garolera, M. T., Cubo, E., Navas, I., & Quintana, S. (2003). Depression in Parkinson's disease: clinical correlates and outcomes. *Parkinsonism and Related Disorders, 10*(1), 23–28.

Rudy, T. E., & Turk, D. C. (1991). Psychological aspects of pain. *International Anesthesiology Clinics, 29*(1), 9–21.

Stockton, P., Gonzales, J. J., Stern, N. P., & Epstein, S. A. (2004). Treatment patterns and outcomes of depressed medically ill and non-medically ill patients in community psychiatric practice. *General Hospital Psychiatry, 26,* 2–8.

Tang, J., Ko, S., Ding, H. K., Qui, C. S., Caleje, A. A., & Zhuo, M. (2005). Pavlovian fear memory induced by activation in the anterior cingulate cortex. *Molecular Pain, 1*(1), 6.

Turk, D. C. (2004). Understanding pain sufferers: the role of cognitive successes. *Spine Journal, 4*(1), 1–7.

Verdelko, A., Henon, H., Lebert, F., Pasquiere, F., & Leys, D. (2004). Depressive symptoms after stroke and relationship with dementia: A three year follow-up study. *Neurology, 62*(6), 905–911.

Zubenko, G. S., Zubenko, W. N., McPherson, S., Spoor, E., Marin, D. B., Farlow, M. R., et al. (2003). A collaborative study of the emergence and clinical features of major depressive syndrome of Alzheimer's disease. *American Journal of Psychiatry, 160,* 857–866.

UNIT IX

Care Challenges in Psychiatric Nursing

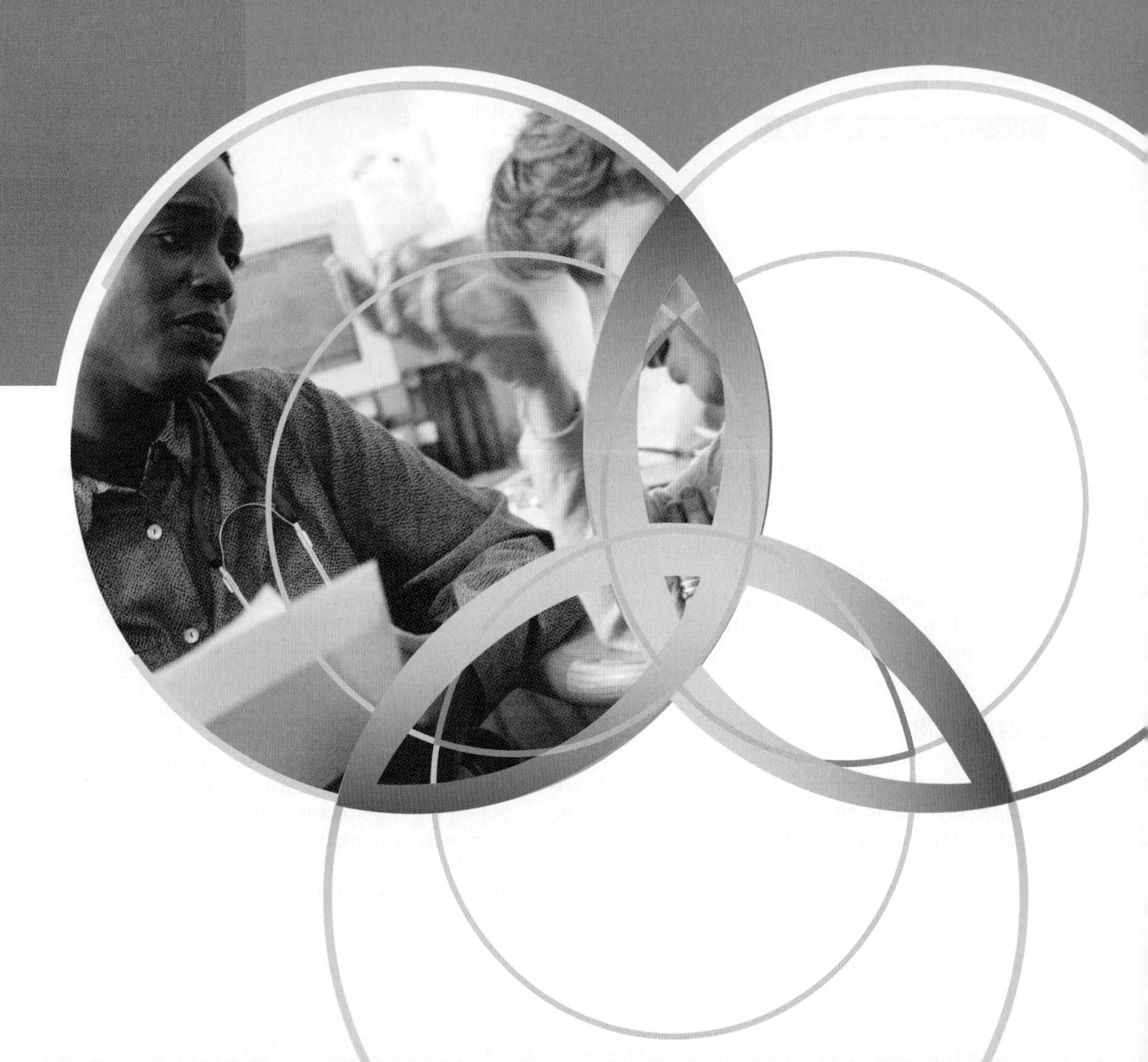

CHAPTER 37

Crisis, Grief, and Disaster Management

Lorraine D. Williams and Mary Ann Boyd

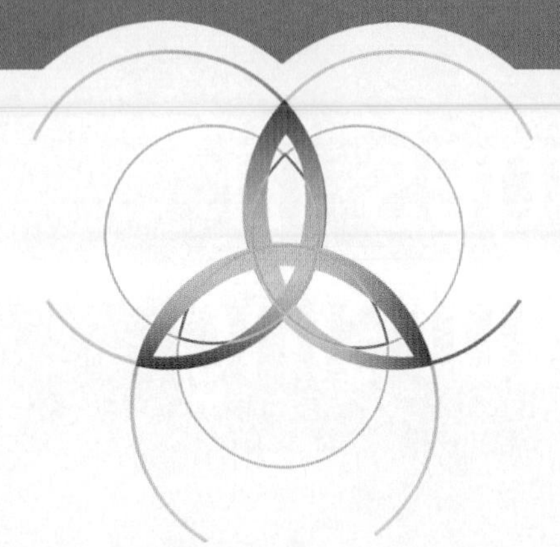

KEY CONCEPTS

- crisis
- grief
- disaster

LEARNING OBJECTIVES

After studying this chapter, you will be able to:

- Describe the types of crises including maturational, situational, and adventitious.
- Discuss grief and bereavement and the nursing process.
- Discuss nursing management for persons experiencing crises, grief, and disaster.
- Evaluate the effects of the crisis/disaster experience on lifestyle and survival.
- Explain the psychological impact of disaster on victims of catastrophic events.

KEY TERMS

• ABCs of psychological first aid • adventitious crisis • bereavement • dysfunctional grieving • maturational crisis • situational crisis • traumatic grief

This chapter focuses on broadening the scope and understanding of the responses of persons to crisis, loss, and disaster situations. Successfully surviving crises and disaster may make a difference between being mentally healthy or mentally ill. This chapter explores the concepts of crisis, grief, and disaster and describes how the nurse can use the nursing process to care for persons experiencing these events.

CRISIS

Adaptation and coping are a natural part of life (see Chapter 14). If children are protected from experiencing negative events and developing coping skills, they may be unable to cope and adapt to crisis situations in later life. Crisis occurs when there is a perceived challenge or threat that overwhelms the capacity of the individual to cope effectively with the event. A crisis disrupts the life of the individual experiencing the event.

KEY CONCEPT Crisis results from stressful events for which coping mechanisms fail to provide adequate adaptive skills to address the perceived challenge or threat. A crisis is a time-limited event that can trigger adaptive or nonadaptive biopsychosocial responses to maturational, situational, or interpersonal experiences.

In a crisis, the person's habits and coping patterns are suspended. Often, unexpected emotional (e.g., depression) and biologic (e.g., nausea, vomiting, diarrhea, headaches) responses occur. Although a person may become extremely anxious, depressed, or elated, feeling states do not determine whether a person is in a crisis. If functioning is severely impaired, a crisis is occurring (Yeager & Roberts, 2003).

A crisis is generally regarded as time limited, lasting no more than 4 to 6 weeks. At the end of that time, the person in crisis should have begun to come to grips with the event and to harness resources to cope with its long-term consequences. By definition, there is no such thing as a chronic crisis. People who live in constant turmoil are not in crisis but in chaos. A crisis can also represent a turning point in a person's life, with either positive or negative outcomes. It can be an opportunity for growth and change because new ways of coping are learned.

Either internal or external demands that are perceived as threats to a person's physical or emotional functioning can initiate a crisis. The precipitating event is not only stressful, but unusual or rare. Many life events can evoke a crisis, such as natural disasters (e.g., floods, tornadoes, earthquakes) and manmade disasters (e.g., wars, bombings, airplane crashes) as well as traumatic experiences (e.g., rape, sexual abuse, assault). In addition, interpersonal events (divorce, marriage, birth of a child) may create a crisis event in the life of any person.

A crisis is not the same as a psychiatric emergency that requires immediate intervention. A person in crisis may not need an immediate intervention and should not be viewed as having a mental disorder (Roberts, 2000). However, if the person is significantly distressed or social functioning impaired, a diagnosis of acute stress disorder should be considered (APA, 2000). The person with an acute stress disorder has dissociative symptoms and persistently re-experiences the event (APA) (Table 37.1).

Historical Perspectives of Crisis

The basis of our understanding of the biopsychosocial implications of a crisis began in the 1940s when Eric Lindemann (1944) studied bereavement reactions among the friends and relatives of the victims of the Coconut Grove nightclub fire in Boston in 1942. That fire, in which 493 people died, was the worst single building fire in the country's history at that time. Lindemann's goal was to develop prevention approaches at the community level that would maintain good health and prevent emotional disorganization. He described both grief and prolonged reactions as a result of loss of a significant person. From those results, he hypothesized that during the course of one's life, some situations, such as the birth of a child, marriage, and death, evoke adaptive mechanisms that lead either to mastery of a new situation (psychological growth) or impaired functioning.

In 1961, psychiatrist Gerald Caplan defined a crisis as occurring when a person faces a problem that cannot be solved by customary problem-solving methods. When the usual problem-solving methods no longer work, a person's life balance or equilibrium is upset. During the period of disequilibrium, there is a rise in inner tension and anxiety, followed by emotional upset and an inability to function. This conceptualization of phases of a crisis is used today (see Figure 37.1). According to Caplan, during a crisis, a person is open to learning new ways of coping to survive. The outcome of a crisis is governed by the kind of interaction that occurs between the person and available key social support systems.

Types of Crises

Recent research has focused on categorizing types of crisis events, understanding biopsychosocial responses to crisis, and developing intervention models that support people through crisis (Stone & Conley, 2004).

Table 37.1 Key Diagnostic Characteristics of Acute Stress Disorder DSM IV

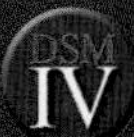

Diagnostic Criteria	Target Symptoms and Associated Findings
• Experienced, witnessed, or was confronted with an event or events that involved actual or threatened death or serious injury, or threat to the physical integrity of self or others • Intense fear, helplessness, or horror • Dissociative symptoms (at least three), including a subjective sense of numbing, detachment, or absence of emotional responsiveness, reduction in awareness of surroundings ("being in a daze"), derealization, depersonalization dissociative amnesia (inability to recall important aspects of trauma) • Traumatic event is persistently re-experienced—recurrent images, thoughts, dreams, flashback, illusions • Anxiety or increased arousal • Causes significant distress or impairment in social, occupational, or other important areas of functioning	• Disturbance lasts for at least 2 days and no more than 4 weeks; occurs within 4 weeks of the traumatic event • Disturbance is not due to direct physiologic effects of substance abuse or other medical conditions • Despair and hopelessness • Guilt (especially if patient survived a trauma and others did not) about not providing enough help to others • Neglects basic health and safety needs • Impulsive and risk-taking behavior • Increased risk for posttraumatic stress disorder ***Associated Physical Examination Findings*** • General medical conditions may occur as result of the trauma (e.g., head injury, burns)

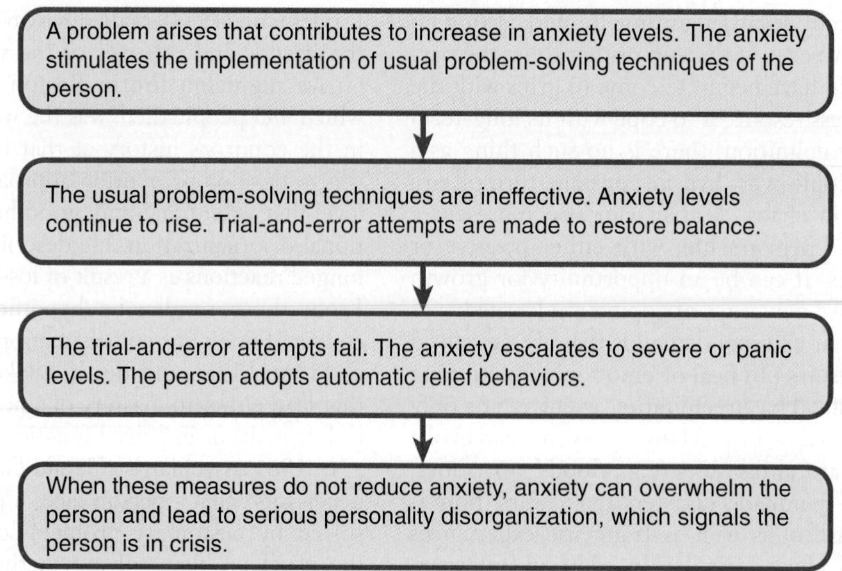

A problem arises that contributes to increase in anxiety levels. The anxiety stimulates the implementation of usual problem-solving techniques of the person.
The usual problem-solving techniques are ineffective. Anxiety levels continue to rise. Trial-and-error attempts are made to restore balance.
The trial-and-error attempts fail. The anxiety escalates to severe or panic levels. The person adopts automatic relief behaviors.
When these measures do not reduce anxiety, anxiety can overwhelm the person and lead to serious personality disorganization, which signals the person is in crisis.

FIGURE 37.1. Phases of crisis.

Maturational Crisis

While Lindemann and Caplan were creating their crisis model, Erik Erikson was formulating his ideas about crisis and development. He proposed that **maturational crises** are a normal part of growth and development, and that successfully resolving a crisis at one stage allows the child to move to the next. According to this model, the child develops positive characteristics after experiencing a crisis. If he or she develops less desirable traits, the crisis is not resolved. This concept of maturational crisis assumes that psychosocial development progresses by an easily identifiable, orderly process. However, the developmental models proposed by Gilligan (1994) and Miller (1994) do not fit into a stage model (see Chapter 6).

The concept of developmental crisis continues to be used today to describe unfavorable person–environment relationships that relate to maturational events, such as leaving home for the first time, completing school, or accepting the responsibility of adulthood. The accomplishment of developmental tasks throughout the life cycle will impact the interpretation of crisis events during the transition of an individual from one stage of life to another.

Situational Crisis

A **situational crisis** occurs whenever a specific stressful event threatens a person's biopsychosocial integrity and results in some degree of psychological disequilibrium. The event can be an internal one, such as a disease process or any number of external threats. A move to another city, a job promotion, or graduation from high school can initiate a crisis even though they are positive events. For example, graduation from high school marks the end of an established routine of going to school, participating in school activities, and doing homework assignments. When starting a new job after graduation, the former student must learn an entirely different routine and acquire new knowledge and skills. If a person enters a new situation without adequate coping skills, a crisis may develop that results in dissonance (inconsistency between attitude and behavior).

Adventitious Crisis

An **adventitious crisis** is initiated by unexpected, unusual events that can affect an individual or a multitude of people. In such situations, people face overwhelmingly hazardous events that may entail injury, trauma, destruction, or sacrifice. Such an event involves a physically aggressive and forced act by a person, a group, or an environment. National disasters (e.g., racial persecutions, kidnappings, riots, war); violent crimes (e.g., rape, murder, and assault and battery); and natural disasters (e.g., earthquakes, floods, forest fires, hurricanes) are examples of events that precipitate this type of crisis (Hazelwood & Burgess, 2001).

GRIEF AND BEREAVEMENT

One of the most common crisis-provoking events is the death of a loved one. Although death is a certainty, much is unknown about the process of death. Fear of the unknown contributes to the mystique of death for the person who is dying, as well as the loved one. The terms grief and bereavement are sometimes used interchangeably, but in this text they are differentiated. Normally, the death of a loved one produces feelings of grief. Any subsequent loss can also reactivate these feelings.

KEY CONCEPT Grief is an intense, emotional reaction to the loss of a loved one. The reaction is a biopsychosocial response that often includes spontaneous expression of pain, sadness, and desolation.

Phases of Bereavement

Bereavement, the process of mourning, begins immediately after the loss, but it can last months or years. Individual differences and cultural practices influence the grieving and the bereavement process. Although the following phases are discussed as if progression from one to another is linear, in reality, they may be concurrent and vary from the proposed phase sequence (Bonanno, 2004; see Box 37.1).

Shock and Disbelief

During the first phase, the person is in a state of shock and disbelief. This stage lasts from hours to weeks and is characterized by varying degrees of disbelief and denial of the loss. The length of time also will depend upon the type of crisis event. The person experiences tightness in the throat, choking, shortness of breath, a need to sigh, an empty feeling in the abdomen, and a lack of muscular power. The person has a sense of unreality, feels increased emotional distance from others, and is intensely preoccupied with the image of the deceased. In addition, the person may harbor exaggerated guilt feelings for minor negligence. Mourning rites, family, and friends facilitate the passage through this phase.

BOX 37.1

Stages of Bereavement

I. Shock: denial and disbelief
II. Acute mourning
   A. Intense feeling states: crying spells, guilt, shame, depression, anorexia, insomnia, irritability, emptiness, and fatigue
   B. Social withdrawal: preoccupation with health; inability to sustain usual work, family, and personal relationships
   C. Identification with the deceased: transient adoption of habits, mannerisms, and somatic symptoms of the deceased
III. Resolution: acceptance of loss, awareness of having grieved, return to well-being, and ability to recall the deceased without subjective pain

Reprinted from Zisook, S. (1987). Unresolved grief. In S. Zisook (Ed.), *Biopsychosocial aspects of bereavement* (p. 25). Washington, DC: American Psychiatric Press.

Acute Mourning

The acute mourning phase begins when the person becomes gradually aware of the loss. This phase, which may last several months, has three distinct periods:

1. *Intense feeling:* The person becomes disorganized and experiences waves of intense pain. An insatiable yearning for the deceased person occurs. The person cries, feels helpless, and possibly identifies with or idealizes the deceased.
2. *Social withdrawal:* In an attempt to avoid pain, the person avoids other people, including friends. The person feels irritable or angry, misses work, and emotionally distances self from others. The person spends time searching for evidence of failure in the relationship.
3. *Identification with the deceased:* The person's thought content and affect become consumed by the deceased. Mourners may adopt mannerisms, habits, and somatic symptoms of the deceased (Becker & Knudson, 2003).

Resolution

Gradually, the person experiences the return of feelings of well-being and the ability to continue with life. He or she reviews the relationship with the deceased and realizes the sorrow and sense of loss. The person recognizes that he or she has been grieving and now is ready to focus on the rest of the world. Finally, it is possible to re-experience pleasure and seek the companionship and love of others.

Variations in Grief and Bereavement

There is discussion in the literature about differences in the experience of grief and bereavement. Research presented by Arnold, Gemma, & Cushman (2005) described parental grieving as a sequential, organized response to loss and death that is bound by time that requires some kind of resolution for closure. They described parental grief as "non-linear, complex, and ongoing" (p. 253).

Traumatic grieving is a term that is used for a more difficult and prolonged grief. In traumatic grieving, external factors influence the reactions and potential long-term outcomes. The external circumstances of death include (1) suddenness and lack of anticipation, (2) violence, mutilation and destruction, (3) degree of preventability and/or randomness of the death, (4) multiple deaths (bereavement overload), and (5) mourner's personal encounter with death involving significant threat to personal survival, or a massive and shocking confrontation with the deaths (and/or mutilation) of others (Grief: what you should know, 2006).

Bereavement of family members for those who committed suicide seems to differ from other sudden deaths. Common experiences during the bereavement process include stigmatization, shame and guilt, and a sense of rejection. The bereaved may experience self-blame for contributing to their family member's death. Factors that influence bereavement after suicide include age of the deceased, quality of the relationship, the attitude of the bereaved to the loss, and cultural beliefs. These individuals benefit from psychological interventions (Hawton & Simkin, 2003).

There is evidence that men experience grief differently than women, who are more likely to confront and express negative emotion (Stinson, Lasker, Lohmann, & Toedter, 1992; Stroebe, Stroebe, & Schut, 2006). Suicide bereavement may be different because of the survivor's questions regarding the family member's suicide and the impact of the suicide on the family (Jordan, 2001) (see Chapter 17). More research is needed in this area.

The bereavement process is often applied to other situations in which a loss occurs, but not necessarily the death of a person, and has many of the same responses. The "empty nest syndrome" is an example of bereavement for children who have grown up and left home. This bereavement experience is less intense than that triggered by a loss through death, but the bereaved person has many of the same responses.

Dysfunctional Grieving

Grieving is a normal process of life. **Dysfunctional grieving** occurs when the grief response is either absent or exaggerated. However, it is difficult to exactly define abnormal grieving. The absence of a grief reaction to a loss of a significant person is considered abnormal. If a person does not grieve in response to a significant loss, he or she may eventually have an adverse biopsychosocial reaction that may lead to mental health problems (Becker & Knudson, 2003).

Dysfunctional grieving occurs if a person fails to move from one bereavement phase to another (Table 37.2). When a person becomes stuck in one phase, he or she experiences exaggerated grief feelings associated with that phase. For example, depressive symptoms in a person who remains in the acute mourning phase become a full-blown depressive episode. In dysfunctional grieving, the bereaved becomes a chronic mourner fixed on the deceased and events surrounding the person's death. Dysfunctional grieving often leads to depression.

NURSING MANAGEMENT: HUMAN RESPONSE TO CRISIS

The goal for people experiencing a crisis is to return to the precrisis level of functioning. The role of the nurse is to provide a framework of support systems that guide the patient through the crisis and facilitate the development and use of positive coping skills. The nurse must be acutely aware that a person in crisis may be at high risk for suicide or homicide. To determine the level of effectiveness of coping capabilities of the person, the nurse should complete a careful assessment for suicidal or homicidal risk. If a person is at high risk for either, the nurse should consider the possible need for the person to be referred for admission to the hospital. When assessing the coping mechanisms and ability of the client to use those mechanisms for adaptation, the nurse should assess for unusual behaviors and determine the level of involvement of the person with the crisis. In addition, assess for evidence of self-mutilation activities that may indicate the use of self-preservation measures to avoid suicide. It is critical to assess the client's perception of the problem and the availability of support mechanisms (emotional and financial) for use by the person (Litz, Gray, Bryant, & Adler, 2002).

Table 37.2 Syndromes Associated With Nonresolution of Grief

Phase	Resolution	Nonresolution
I. Shock denial	Acceptance	Psychotic denial
II. Acute mourning		
A. Intense feeling states	Equanimity	Depression
B. Withdrawal	Reinvolvement	Hypochondriasis
C. Identification	Individuation	Grief-related facsimile illness
III. Resolution	Work, love, play	Chronic mourning

Reprinted from Zisook, S. (1987). Unresolved grief. In S. Zisook (Ed.), *Biopsychosocial aspects of bereavement* (p. 25). Washington, DC: American Psychiatric Press.

• NCLEXNOTE

During a crisis, the behaviors and verbalizations of a person may provide data that are indicative of a mental illness. Nursing care should be prioritized according to severity of responses. Once the crisis is resolved, assess whether the abnormal thoughts or feelings disappear.

During an adventitious crisis (e.g., flood, hurricane, forest fire), that affects the well-being of many people, the interventions of the nurse will be a part of the community's efforts to respond to the event. On the other hand, when a personal crisis occurs, the person in crisis may have only the nurse to respond to his or her needs. After the assessment, the nurse must decide whether to provide the care needed or to refer the person to a mental health specialist. The decision tree in Box 37.2 offers guidance in making that decision.

Biologic Domain

Biologic Assessment

Biologic assessment focuses on areas that usually undergo initial changes. Eliciting information about changes in health practices provide important data that the nurse can use to determine the severity of the disruption in functioning. Biologic functioning is important because a crisis can be physically exhausting. Disturbances in sleep and eating patterns and the reappearance of physical or psychiatric symptoms are common. Changes in body function may include tachycardia, tachypnea, profuse perspiration, nausea, vomiting, dilated pupils, and extreme shakiness. Some victims may exhibit loss of control and have total disregard for their personal safety. The victims are at high risk for injury, which may include infection, trauma, and head injuries (France, 2002). If the victim's sleep patterns are disturbed or nutrition is inadequate, the victim will not have the physical resources to deal with the crisis.

Nursing Diagnoses for the Biologic Domain

Biologic responses can be very severe during crises. All the body systems can be affected. Possible Nursing Diagnoses may include Risk for Body Temperature Imbalance, Diarrhea, Impaired Urinary Elimination, and Stress Urinary Incontinence. In addition, the person may report a variety of somatic complaints. Implement appropriate nursing interventions to address the nursing diagnosis of assessed needs of the victim and make appropriate referrals (Carpenito-Moyet, 2006).

Interventions for the Biologic Domain

Any negative physiological responses should be treated immediately. Triage the victims according to the level of care needed. If the crisis involves a life-threatening physical injury, those types of injuries should be treated immediately. Throughout the triage process, the victims should be reassured that the caregiver is concerned and committed to providing quality nursing care. *Be careful not to give unrealistic or false reassurances of positive outcomes over which you have no control.* Other interventions focusing on the biologic domain will be those implemented for nursing diagnoses developed from assessment findings. Make referrals as appropriate (Davidhizar & Shearer, 2005). Ideally, a mental health specialist would be an integral part of the triage team. Pharmacologic interventions may be needed to help maintain a high level of psychophysical functioning.

• NCLEXNOTE

Individual responses to a crisis can be best understood by assessing the usual responses of the victim to stressful events.

The response to the crisis will also depend on the meaning of the event to the victim. The use of therapeutic communication principles is a priority when caring for a person who has experienced a crisis/disaster.

BOX 37.2

Decision Tree for Determining Referral

Situation: A 35-year-old woman is being seen in a clinic because of minor burns she received during a house fire. Her home was completely destroyed. She is tearful and withdrawn, and she complains of a great deal of pain from her minor burns. Biopsychosocial assessment is completed.

Patient has psychological distress but believes that her social support is adequate. She would like to talk to a nurse when she returns for her follow-up visit. → Provide counseling and support for the patient during her visit. Make an appointment for her return visit to the clinic for follow-up.

Patient is severely distressed. She has no social support. She does not know how she will survive. → Refer the patient to a mental health specialist. The patient will need crisis intervention strategies provided by a mental health specialist.

Medication cannot resolve a crisis, but the judicious use of psychopharmacologic agents can help reduce its emotional intensity. For example, Mrs. Brown has just learned that both of her parents have perished in an airplane crash. When she arrives at the emergency department to identify their bodies, she is shaking, sobbing, and unable to answer questions. The emergency physician orders lorazepam (Ativan) (see Box 37.3). The phases of treatment include initiation of treatment, assessment of stabilization from the treatment, and timeframe for maintenance of treatment (Frykberg, 2002).

Initiation

Because Mrs. Brown is overcome by grief and severe anxiety from seeing her parents' bodies, 2 mg of lorazepam is administered intramuscularly as ordered by the doctor. The nurse monitors the patient for onset of action and any side effects. If Mrs. Brown does not have some relief within 20 to 30 minutes, another injection can be given as ordered by the doctor.

Stabilization

During the next half-hour, Mrs. Brown regains some of her composure. She is no longer shaking, and her crying is occasional. She is reluctant to identify her parents but can do so when accompanied by the nurse. Once the paperwork is completed, Mrs. Brown is sent home with a prescription for lorazepam, 2 to 4 mg every 12 hours.

Maintenance

Mrs. Brown takes the medication during the next week as she plans and attends her parents' funeral and manages the affairs surrounding their deaths. The medication keeps her anxiety at a manageable level, enabling her to do the tasks required of her.

BOX 37.3

Drug Profile: Lorazepam (Ativan)

DRUG CLASS: Benzodiazepine; antianxiety/sedative hypnotic agent

RECEPTOR AFFINITY: Acts mainly at the subcortical levels of the central nervous system (CNS), leaving the cortex relatively unaffected. Main sites of action may be the limbic system and reticular formation. It potentiates the effects of α-aminobutyric acid, an inhibitory neurotransmitter. Exact mechanism of action is unknown.

INDICATIONS: Management of anxiety disorders or for short-term relief of symptoms of anxiety or anxiety associated with depression (oral forms). Also used as preanesthetic medication in adults to produce sedation, relieve anxiety, and decrease recall of events related to surgery (parenteral form). Unlabeled parenteral uses for management of acute alcohol withdrawal.

ROUTE AND DOSAGE: Available in 0.5-, 1-, and 2-mg tablets; 2 mg/mL concentrated oral solution and 2 mg/mL and 4 mg/mL solutions for injection.

Adult Dosage: Usually 2–6 mg/d orally, with a range of 1–10 mg/d in divided doses, with largest dose given at night. 0.05 mg/kg IM up to a maximum of 4 mg administered at least 2 h before surgery. Initially 2 mg total or 0.044 mg/kg IV (whichever is smaller). Doses as high as 0.05 mg/kg up to a total of 4 mg may be given 15–20 min before the procedure to those benefiting by a greater lack of recall.

Geriatric: Dosage not to exceed adult IV dose. Orally, 1–2 mg/d in divided doses initially, adjusted as needed and tolerated.

Children: Drug should not be used in children younger than 12 years.

HALF-LIFE (PEAK EFFECT): 10–20 h (1–6 h [oral]; 60–90 min [IM]; 10–15 min [IV]).

SELECT ADVERSE REACTIONS: Transient mild drowsiness, sedation, depression, lethargy, apathy, fatigue, light-headedness, disorientation, anger, hostility, restlessness, confusion, crying, headache, mild paradoxical excitatory reactions during first 2 weeks of treatment, constipation, dry mouth, diarrhea, nausea, bradycardia, hypotension, cardiovascular collapse, urinary retention, drug dependence with withdrawal symptoms.

WARNING: Contraindicated in psychoses, acute narrow angle glaucoma, shock, acute alcoholic intoxication with depression of vital signs, and during pregnancy, labor and delivery, and while breast-feeding. Use cautiously in patients with impaired liver or kidney function or those who are debilitated. When given with theophylline, there is a decreased effect of lorazepam. When using the drug IV, it must be diluted immediately prior to use and administered by direct injection slowly or infused at a maximum rate of 2 mg/min. When giving narcotic analgesics, reduce its dose by at least half in patients who have received lorazepam.

SPECIAL PATIENT/FAMILY EDUCATION:

- Take the drug exactly as prescribed; do not stop taking the drug abruptly.
- Avoid alcohol and other CNS depressants.
- Avoid driving or other activities that require alertness.
- Notify prescriber before taking any other prescription or over-the-counter drug.
- Change your position slowly and sit at the edge of the bed for a few minutes before arising.
- Report to the prescriber any severe dizziness, weakness, drowsiness that persists, any rash or skin lesions, palpitations, edema of the extremities, visual changes, or difficulty urinating.

Medication Cessation

Two weeks after the death of her parents, Mrs. Brown is no longer taking lorazepam. She is grieving normally, has periods of teariness and sadness about her loss, but can cope. She visits with friends, reminisces with family members, and reads inspirational poems. All of these activities help her navigate the changes in her life brought about by her parents' sudden death.

This example demonstrates how a medication can be used to assist a person through a crisis. Once that crisis is past, the person can use personal coping mechanisms to adapt.

Psychological Domain

Psychological Assessment

Psychological assessment focuses on the victim's emotions and coping strengths. In the beginning of the crisis, the victim may report the feeling of numbness and shock. Responses to psychological distress should be differentiated from symptoms of psychiatric illnesses of the victim. Later, as the reality of the crisis sinks in, the victim will be able to recognize and describe the felt emotions. The nurse should expect those emotions to be intense and will need to provide some support during their expression by that victim. At the beginning of a crisis, assess the victim for behaviors that indicate a depressed state, the presence of confusion, uncontrolled weeping or screaming, disorientation, or aggression. The victim may be suffering from loss of feelings of well-being and safety. In addition, panic responses, anxiety, and fear may be present (Hall, Norwood, Ursano, & Fullerton, 2003). The ability to cope by problem-solving may be disrupted. By assessing the victim's ability to solve problems, the nurse can evaluate whether the victim can cognitively cope with the crisis situation and determine the kind and amount of support needed. The survivor of a disaster may experience traumatic bereavement because of feelings of guilt for survival of the crisis.

Nursing Diagnoses for the Psychological Domain

Many nursing diagnoses generated from assessment of the psychological may be appropriate for the person experiencing crisis. The nursing diagnoses may include Grieving, Post-Trauma Syndrome, Confusion, Ineffective Coping, Risk for Violence (self-directed or directed toward others), Impaired Communication, Interrupted Family Processes, Anxiety, Powerlessness, and many other diagnoses. The nurse should make sure that the diagnoses are based on the victim's appraisal of the situation. In addition, any diagnosis should be determined from the assessment data that has been clustered and prioritized to address identified needs (Carpenito-Moyet, 2006).

Interventions for the Psychological Domain

Safety interventions to protect the person in crisis from harm should include preventing the person from committing suicide or homicide, arranging for food and shelter (if needed), and mobilizing social support. Once the person's safety needs are met, the nurse can address the psychosocial aspects of the crisis. Prepare the victims for recovery. Guidelines for crisis intervention and examples are presented in Table 37.3. Victims should be encouraged to report any depression, anxiety, or interpersonal difficulties during the recovery period. There may be a need for support groups to be established to help victims and their families deal with the psychological effects of the phenomenon (McCloskey & Bulechek, 2000).

Counseling reinforces healthy coping behaviors and interaction patterns. Counseling, which focuses on identifying the victim's emotions and positive coping strategies for the corresponding nursing diagnosis, helps the victim to integrate the effects of the crisis into a real life experience. Responses to crisis differ with individuals. Some victims may present with behaviors that indicate transient disruptions in their ability to cope. Others may be totally devastated (Bonanno, 2004). At times, telephone counseling may provide the victim with enough help that face-to-face counseling is not necessary. If counseling strategies do not work, other stress reduction and coping enhancement interventions can be used (see Chapter 14). For anyone who cannot cope with a crisis, the nurse should refer that victim to a mental health specialist for short-term therapy.

Social Domain

Social Assessment

Assessment of the impact of the crisis on the victim's social functioning is essential because a crisis usually severely disrupts social proficiencies. The nurse should assess the severity of the crisis to determine the capability of the individual or the community to respond in a supportive way. Assist the victims to maintain a calm demeanor, obtain and distribute information about the crisis and the victims of the crisis. Initiate attempts to reunite victims and their families. Shelter, food, and other resources may not be available. In a crisis, the first priority is to meet the basic human needs of the victims.

Table 37.3 Guidelines for Crisis Intervention

Approach	Rationale	Example
Assist the person in confronting reality.	During the crisis experience, the person may use denial as a coping mechanism. Denial is ineffective in resolving the crisis. Emotional support will help the person face reality.	Accompany the husband to view the body of his deceased wife.
Encourage the expression of feelings (within limits).	Identification and expression of feelings about the crisis events help the person understand the significance of the crisis.	Encourage a woman who survived a house fire but lost her home to explore the meaning of the lost home.
Encourage the person to focus on one implication at a time.	Focusing on all the implications at once can be too overwhelming.	A woman left her husband because of abuse. At first, focus only on living arrangements and safety. At another time, discuss the other implications of the separation.
Avoid giving false reassurances, such as "It will be all right."	Giving false reassurances blocks communication. It may not be all right.	Patient: "My doctor told me that I have a terminal illness." Nurse: "What does that mean to you?"
Clarify fantasies with facts.	Accurate information is needed to problem solve.	A young mother believes that her comatose child will regain consciousness, although the medical evidence contradicts it. Gently clarify the meaning of the medical evidence.
Link the person and family with community resources, as needed.	Strengthening the person's social network so that social support can be obtained reduces the effect of the crisis.	Provide information about a meeting of a support group such as that of the American Cancer Society.

Adapted from Lazarus, R. (1991). *Emotion and adaptation* (p. 122). New York: Oxford University Press.

Nursing Diagnoses for the Social Domain

Nursing diagnoses appropriate for the social domain include Impaired Adjustment, Impaired Social Interaction, and Impaired Interrupted Family Processes. Other diagnoses may be Ineffective Role Performance and Relocation Stress Syndrome. Any diagnosis generated by the nurse will be dependent on the assessment findings related to the needs of the victims (Carpenito-Moyet, 2006).

Interventions for the Social Domain

The nursing interventions for the social domain include the individual, the family, and the community. A crisis often disrupts a victim's social network leading to changes in available social support. Development of a new social support network may help the victim cope more effectively with the crisis. Supporting the development of new support contacts within the context of available social networks can be done by contacting available local and state agencies for assistance as well as specific private support groups and religious groups (McCloskey & Bulechek, 2000).

Telephone Hot Lines

Public and private funding and the efforts of trained volunteers permit most communities to provide crisis services to the public. For example, telephone hot lines for problems ranging from child abuse to suicide are a part of health delivery systems of most communities. Crisis services permit immediate access to the mental health system for people who are experiencing an emergency (such as threatened suicide) or for those who need help with stress or a crisis.

Residential Crisis Services

Many communities provide, as part of the health care network, residential crisis services for people who need short-term housing. The specific residential crisis services available within a community reflect those problems that it judges as particularly important. For example, some communities provide shelter for teenage runaways; others offer shelter for abused spouses. Still others provide shelter for people who would otherwise require acute psychiatric hospitalization. These settings provide residents with a place to stay in a supportive, homelike atmosphere. The people who use these services are linked to other community services such as financial aid.

Evaluation and Outcomes

Outcomes, developed in cooperation with the person experiencing the crisis, will guide the evaluation. When assessment data are clustered and prioritized to determine the nursing diagnosis and the outcomes and interventions are developed and implemented in cooperation with the victim, the victim should come through the crisis well, with improved health, well-being, and social function. If complications occur, the nurse should make appropriate alterations in the entire nursing process or make appropriate referrals.

DISASTER AND TERRORISM

A disaster is a sudden ecological or man-made phenomenon that is of sufficient magnitude to require external help to address the psychosocial needs as well as the physical needs of the victims. Acts of terrorism present situations that mimic disasters and can be categorized as a type of disaster.

KEY CONCEPT Disaster is a sudden overwhelming catastrophic event that causes great damage and destruction that may involve mass casualties and human suffering that requires assistance from all available resources.

Although crises and disasters are usually viewed as negative experiences, the outcomes can be positive. Some survivors of disasters draw on resources that they never realized they had and grow from those experiences (Walter & Berkovitz, 2005). However, the survivors of disasters may present with severe psychological problems that begin with expressed feelings of fear, anger, and distress that elevate to severe anxiety at the panic level with deterioration to more severe mental illnesses (Norris, Friedman, Watson, Byrne, Diaz, & Kaniasty, 2002). Unresolved crisis and/or disastrous events can lead to disorganized thinking and responses that are inappropriate and traumatic for the person experiencing the situation (Flynn & Norwood, 2004). In addition, the victims may experience the development of acute stress disorder (that has a strong emphasis on dissociative symptoms), and posttraumatic stress disorder (PTSD) (Harvey & Pauwels, 2000).

Historical Perspectives of Disasters in the United States

Throughout history, disasters have been portrayed from a fatalistic perspective that humans have little control over catastrophic events. Some cultures contend that natural disasters are an act of God. Other cultures express their belief that natural disaster events can be attributed to gods dwelling within such places as volcanoes, with eruptions being an expression of the gods' anger (van Griensven, et al., 2006). Although often caused by nature, disasters can have human origins. Wars and civil disturbances that destroy homelands and displace people are included among the causes of disasters. Other causes can be a building collapse, blizzard, drought, earthquake, epidemic, explosion, famine, fire, flood, hazardous material or transportation incident (such as a chemical spill), hurricane, nuclear incident, terrorist attack, tornado, or volcano eruptions. Often, it is the unpredictability of such disasters that causes fear, confusion, and stress that can have lasting effects on the health of affected communities and their sense of well-being (Norwood, Ursano, & Fullerton, 2001).

In recent history, we have experienced several attacks of violence and terrorism that are unprecedented in North America. The bombing of the federal office building in Oklahoma City on April 19, 1995; the shooting massacre of Columbine High School students on April 20, 1999; the destruction of the World Trade Center in New York and the attack on the Pentagon in Washington, DC, on September 11, 2001; and later, the dispersal of anthrax spores in the United States mail shattered North Americans' sense of safety and security (Miller, 2002; North et al., 2002).

Since September 11, 2001, the emergency response planning of federal, state, and local agencies has focused on possible terrorist attacks with chemical, biological, radiological, nuclear, or high-yield explosive weapons. Before September 11, government agencies and public health leaders had not incorporated mental health into their overall response plans to bioterrorism. In the aftermath of the mass destruction of human life and property in 2001, government and health care leaders are recognizing the need for monumental mental health efforts to be implemented during episodes of terrorism and disaster. The psychological and behavioral consequences of a terrorist attack are now included in most disaster plans (Hall, Norwood, Ursano, & Fullerton, 2003).

The hurricane Katrina disaster 2005 highlighted the importance of government preparedness for natural disasters as well as terrorism. The lack of government response and breakdown in communication resulted in thousands of hurricane victims being displaced and injured. Consequences of Hurricane Katrina are being felt months and years after the event (www.trynova.org/crisis/katrina/reactions-coping.html).

Phases Of Disaster

Natural and man-made disaster can be conceptualized in three phases:

1. *Pre-warning of the disaster.* This phase entails preparing victims for possible evacuation of the environment, mobilization of resources, and review of community disaster plans.
2. *Disaster event occurs.* Here the rescuers provide resources, assistance, and support as needed to pre-

serve the biopsychosocial functioning and survival of the victims.

3. *Recuperative effort*. The focus here is to implement strategies for healing the sick and injured, preventing complications of health problems, repairing damages, and reconstructing the community (Flynn & Norwood, 2004).

NURSING MANAGEMENT: HUMAN RESPONSE TO DISASTER/TERRORISM

Psychiatric nurses encounter three different types of disaster victims. The first category is the victims who may or may not survive. If they survive, the victims often suffer severe physical injuries. The more serious the physical injury, the more likely the victim will experience a mental health problem such as PTSD, depression, anxiety, or other mental health problems (North, McCutcheon, Spitznagel, & Smith, 2002; Pfefferbaum et al., 2001). Victims and families will need ongoing health care to prevent complications related to both physical and mental health.

The second category of victims includes the professional rescuers. These are persons who are less likely to suffer physical injury but who often suffer psychological stress. The professional rescuers, such as policemen, firefighters, nurses, and so on, have more effective coping skills than do volunteer rescuers who are not prepared for the emotional impact of a disaster (North et al., 2002). However, many professional responders have reported experiencing PTSD for many months following the traumatic event in which they were involved (Puig & Glynn, 2003).

The third category includes everyone else involved in the disaster. Psychological effects may be experienced worldwide by millions of people as they experience terrorism or disaster vicariously or as direct victims of the terrorism/disaster event (Hall et al., 2003). After an act of terrorism, most people will experience some psychological stress, including an altered sense of safety, hypervigilance, sadness, anger, fear, decreased concentration, and difficulty sleeping. Others may alter their behavior by traveling less, staying at home, avoiding public events, keeping children out of school, or increasing smoking and alcohol use. In a nationwide interview of 560 adults after September 11, 2001, 90% reported at least one stress symptom and 44% had several symptoms of stress (Schuster et al., 2001). In New York state, almost half a million people reported symptoms that would meet the criteria for acute PTSD (see Chapter 34). In Manhattan, the estimated prevalence of acute PTSD was 11.2%, increasing to 20% in people living close to the World Trade Center (Galea et al., 2002; Schlenger et al., 2002).

The interventions developed by the nurse in collaboration with the victim should address the outcomes that are individualized for each diagnosis. Victims experiencing head injuries or psychic trauma after a disaster may have to be hospitalized. During a disaster, a victim with a mental illness may experience regression to his or her pretreatment condition. If community mental health facilities are available, they should be directed to seek assistance from mental health care professionals. The victims should receive follow-up care for the disaster response after they are discharged (McCloskey & Bulechek, 2000).

Biologic Domain

Biologic Assessment

The nurse should assess physical reactions that may involve many changes in body functions, such as tachycardia, tachypnea, profuse perspiration, nausea, vomiting, dilated pupils, and extreme shakiness. Virtually any organ may be involved. Some victims may exhibit panic reactions and loss of control and have a total disregard for their personal safety. The victims may be suicidal or homicidal and are at high risk for injuries that may include infection, trauma, and head injuries (France, 2002).

Nursing Diagnoses for the Biologic Domain

Because the responses are so varied, almost any nursing diagnosis can be generated from the assessment data. Ineffective Thermoregulation, Ineffective Breathing Patterns, Insomnia and Risk for Self-harm are examples of possible nursing diagnoses. Utilize assessment data that have been clustered and prioritized to determine the nursing diagnosis (Carpenito-Moyet, 2006).

Interventions for the Biologic Domain

Any physiological problems or injuries should be treated quickly. During the emergency response, individuals will be triaged to the appropriate level of care. Victims who are primarily distressed and may have somatic symptoms will be treated after those suffering from exposure with critical injuries. All patients need to be reassured of the caring and commitment of the nurse to their safety, comfort, and well-being throughout the triage process. Ideally, a mental health specialist is an integral member of the triage team. Many of the same interventions used for persons experiencing stress or crisis will be used for these victims.

Psychological Domain

Psychological Assessment

Therapeutic communication is key to understanding the extent of the psychological responses to a disaster and to establishing a bridge of trust that communicates respect, commitment, and acceptance. By developing rapport with the victim or victims, the nurse communicates reassurance and support (Flynn & Norwood, 2004).

The nurse should assess the victim for behaviors that indicate a depressed state, presence of confusion, uncontrolled weeping or screaming, disorientation, or aggressive behavior. Ideally, the nurse should assess the coping strategies the victim uses to normally manage stressful situations. The victims may suffer from loss of feelings of well-being and various psychological problems, including panic responses, anxiety, and fear (Hall et al., 2003). In addition, the victims may demonstrate behaviors indicative of acute stress disorder (ASD) and PTSD. The survivors of the disaster may experience traumatic bereavement because of their feelings of guilt that they survived the disaster (Norwood, Ursano, & Fullerton, 2001; Ozer, Best, Lipsey, and Weiss, 2003). Responses to psychological distress need to be differentiated from any psychiatric illness that the person may be experiencing. A response to a disaster may leave the person feeling overwhelmed, incapacitated, and disoriented.

Nursing Diagnoses for the Psychological Domain

Assessment data may support any number of nursing diagnoses (Anxiety, Powerlessness, Fear, Fatigue, Spiritual Distress, and Low Self-esteem). The challenge of generating nursing diagnoses is to make sure that the diagnoses are based on the victim's appraisal of the situation (Carpenito-Moyet, 2006).

Interventions for the Psychological Domain

The **ABCs of psychological first aid** include focusing on A (arousal), B (behavior), and C (cognition). When arousal is present, the intervention goal is to decrease excitement by providing safety, comfort, and consolation. When abnormal or irrational behavior is present, survivors should be assisted to function more effectively in the disaster and when cognitive disorientation occurs, reality testing and clear information should be provided. In the initial phases, the nurse should assist the victim in focusing on the reality of problems that are immediate, with specific goals that are consistent with available resources as well as the culture and lifestyle of the victim.

After the initial interventions, the nurse should support the development of resilience, coping, and recovery while providing technical assistance, training, and consultation. During the treatment process, it may become necessary to administer an antianxiety medication or sedative, especially in the early phases of recovery (Centers for Disease Control, 2005; Dochterman & Bulechek, 2004). The goals of care include helping the victims prioritize and match available resources with their needs, and preventing further complications, monitoring the environment, disseminating information, and implementing disease control strategies (Centers for Disease Control, 2005; Noji, 2000).

Debriefing (the reconstruction of the traumatic events by the victim) may be helpful for some. Long a common practice, debriefing was believed to be necessary in order for the person to develop a healthy perspective of the event and ultimately prevent PTSD. However, research does not support debriefing as a useful treatment for the prevention of PTSD after traumatic incidents. Compulsory debriefing is not recommended (Rose, Bisson, Churchill, & Wessely, 2006). If the victim has symptoms of PTSD, referral to a mental health clinic for additional evaluation and treatment is important (see Chapter 35). The nurse should prepare the victim for recovery by teaching about the effects of stress and helping the victim identify personal strengths and coping skills. Positive coping skills should be supported. The victims should be encouraged to report any depression, anxiety, or interpersonal difficulty during the recovery period. After most disasters, support groups are established that help victims and their families deal with the psychological effects of the disaster (Dochterman & Bulechek, 2004).

• NCLEXNOTE

NCLEXNOTE Individual responses to a disaster can be best understood by examining the victim's usual response to stressful events. A response to a disaster will also depend on the meaning of the event to the person having the experience and any previous encounters with that type of experience. Therapeutic communication is a priority in caring for a person who has experienced a disaster.

Women exhibit higher levels of distress than men after a disaster, especially older women (Norris et al., 2002). Assess the ages of the female victims, their capability to participate in problem-solving activities related to the devastation left by the disaster, and their level of self-confidence/self-esteem that would allow each to participate as a team member or a team leader in addressing the needs of others. This includes encouraging the victims to do necessary chores and participate in decision making, and to take advantage of the opportunity to serve as a leader or team member, as dictated by their abilities.

Educating the public and emphasizing the natural recovery process is important. There are information gaps and rumors that add to the anxiety and stress of the situation. By giving information and direction, it will help the public and victims to use the coping skills they already possess. Initially, the event may leave individuals and families in a stage of ambiguity with frantic disorganized behavior. In addition, individuals and family members are concerned about their own physical and psychological responses to the disastrous event. Children are especially vulnerable to disasters and respond according to their age and family experiences (Davidhizar & Shearer, 2005; Hoven, Duarte, & Mandell, 2003). Traumatized children and adolescents are high risk victims of a wide range of behavioral, psychological, and neurological problems after experiencing various traumatic events (Caffo, Forresi, & Lievers, 2005; Davidhizar & Shearer, 2005).

When the nurse explains anticipated reactions and behaviors, this helps the victims gain control and improve coping. For example, after a major disaster, there may be excessive worry, preoccupation with the event, and changes in eating and sleeping patterns. With time, counseling, and group work, these symptoms will lessen. Active coping strategies can be presented in multiple media forums, such as television and radio (Hall et al., 2003). After the initial shock, victims react by trying to do something to resolve the situation. When victims begin working to remedy the disaster situation, their physical responses become less exaggerated and they are more able to work with less tension and fear.

Social Domain

Social Assessment

The nurse should assess the kind and severity of a natural or man-made disaster or terrorist act to determine the capability of individuals and communities to respond in a supportive way. The nurse should maintain a calm demeanor, obtain and distribute information about the disaster and the victims, and reunite victims and their families. In addition, there is a need to monitor the news media's impact on the mental health of the victims of the crisis. Sometimes, the persistence of the news media diminishes the ability of the survivors to achieve closure to the crisis (Duggar, 2001; Majer et al. 2002). Constant rehearsal of the disaster in the newspapers and on television can increase and prolong the severity or initiate feelings of anxiety and depression.

In a disaster, the victims may experience economic distress because of job loss and loss of other resources. This may ultimately lead to psychological distress. In addition, acts of aggression and other mental health problems may emerge (Dooley, Prause, & Ham-Rowbottom, 2000; Bonanno, 2004). Again, shelter, money, and food may not be available. The absence of basic human needs such as food, a place to live, or immediate transportation quickly becomes a priority that may precipitate acts of violence.

Nursing Diagnoses for the Social Domain

Nursing diagnoses appropriate for the social domain include Impaired Adjustment, Impaired Social Interaction, and Interrupted Family Processes. Ineffective Role Performance and Relocation Stress Syndrome are also diagnoses that could be generated during a disaster. Other nursing diagnoses may be generated from the assessment findings of the nurse related to the needs of the victims (Carpenito-Moyet, 2006).

Interventions for the Social Domain

The nursing interventions for the social domain include the individual, family, and community. The individual should learn about the community resources that can be made available. Family support systems may need to be re-established. The health care community should actively reach out to the media and keep the press engaged. Direct attention to stories that inform and help the public respond should be encouraged. There are federal agencies that assist victims of disasters. This assistance is available for individual, families, and communities. One of those agencies is the Federal Emergency Management Agency (FEMA). When a disaster occurs, FEMA sends a team of specialists who review the devastation of disaster. They provide counseling and mental health services, and arrange for many of the victims to access other services needed for survival including training programs. In addition, the Substance Abuse and Mental Health Services Administration (SAMHSA) of the Department of Health and Human Services are available to assist both victims of and responders to the disaster. When a disaster disrupts the victim's social network, other resources must be made available for social support. The social support system provides an environment in which the victims experience respect and caring from the caregivers, the opportunity to ventilate and examine personal feelings regarding the tragedy, as well as the opportunity to begin the healing and recovery process (Everly, 2000). Supporting the development of more contacts within the social network can be done by organizing support groups within the area of the disaster that address grief and loss, trauma, psychoeducational needs, and substance abuse. In addition, the nurse may refer the victims to nearby support groups or religious groups that are appropriate to meet their needs (Herman, Kaplan, & LeMelle, 2002).

Evaluation and Treatment Outcomes

To determine the effectiveness of nursing interventions, the nurse should evaluate the outcomes based on the success of resolution of the disaster. The outcomes will depend on the specific disaster and its meaning (appraisal) to the survivors. For example, are the survivors in a safe place? Are the victims involved able to cope with the disaster? Were the appropriate supports given so that the victims could draw upon their own strengths?

SUMMARY OF KEY POINTS

- A crisis is a severely stressful situation that causes exaggerated stress responses. Use the nursing process to address the identified needs of a victim experiencing a crisis or disaster event. With both events, provide close scrutiny to safety issues.
    - Grief is an intense emotional response to loss, and bereavement is the process of mourning. There are variations in grief responses that are influenced by the characteristics of the individual and the situation of loss. Dysfunctional grieving occurs when grief is absent or exaggerated.
    - Bereavement can be conceptualized in phases, shock, acute mourning, and resolution, and may last months or years.
- Disaster is a sudden, overwhelming catastrophic event that causes great damage, destruction, mass casualties, and human suffering that require assistance from all available resources.

CRITICAL THINKING CHALLENGES

1 Compare nursing interventions used for crises with those used for disasters. What are the similarities? What are the differences?

2 After the death of his mother, a 24-year-old single man with schizophrenia moves into an apartment. He continues to take his medication but feels sad about his mother's death. He is not adjusting well to living alone and tells his nurse that he no longer wants to go to work. In tears, he admits that he is lonely and can no longer cope with the apartment. The nurse generates the following nursing diagnosis: Ineffective Coping related to inadequate support system. Develop a plan of care for this young man.

3 Discuss the relationship of *crisis, disaster*, and a *psychiatric emergency*.

4 Discuss the role of medication when used in crises.

5 List the phases of bereavement that can be considered a crisis, and discuss the difference between normal and dysfunctional grief.

6 There is a threat of anthrax in your community. A patient appears in the emergency room convinced that his mail is contaminated. How would you proceed with assessing this patient?

Schindler's List: 1993. The film presents the true story of Oskar Schindler, a member of the Nazi party, womanizer, and war profiteer, who saved the lives of more than 1,000 Jews during the Holocaust. The movie shows how during long periods of political turmoil and terror, life can become somewhat normalized. Yet, fear underlies people's daily lives. Crises erupt at different times during the very long period of chronic stress.

VIEWING POINTS: Differentiate the periods of chronic stress from crisis in this film. Observe the reactions of different characters under stress. Is the behavior different from what you would expect? Observe your own feelings throughout the movie. Did you experience stress?

REFERENCES

American Psychiatric Association (APA). (2000). *Diagnostic and statistical manual of mental disorders* (4th ed., text revision). Washington, DC: Author.

Arnold, J., Gemma, P. B., Cushman, L. F. (2005). Exploring parental grief: Combining quantitative and qualitative measures. *Archives of Psychiatric Nursing, 19*(6), 245–255.

Becker, S. H., & Knudson, R. M. (2003). Visions of the dead: Imagination and mourning. *Death Studies, 27*(8), 691–716.

Bonanno, G. A., (2004). Loss, trauma, and human resilience: How can we underestimate the human capacity to thrive after extremely aversive events? *American Psychologist, 59*(1), 20–28.

Caffo, E., Forresi, B., & Lievers, L. S. (2005). Impact, psychological sequelae and management of trauma affecting children and adolescents. *Current Opinion in Psychiatry, 18*(4), 422–428.

Caplan, G. (1961). *An approach to community mental health*. New York: Grune & Stratton.

Carpenito-Moyet, L. (2006). *Nursing diagnosis: Application to clinical practice* (11th ed.). Philadelphia: Lippincott Williams & Wilkins.

Centers for Disease Control (2005). Disaster mental health for states: Key principles, issues, and questions. *Department of Health and Human Services, August 30*, 1–4.

Davidhizar, R., & Shearer, R. (2005). Helping children cope with public disasters. *American Journal of Nursing, 102*(3), 26–33.

Dochterman, J., & Bulechek, G. (2004). *Nursing interventions classification* (NIC) (4th ed.). St. Louis: Mosby.

Dooley, D., Prause, J., & Ham-Rowbottom, K. A. (2000). Underemployment and depression: Longitudinal relationships. *Journal of Health and Social Behavior, 41*(4), 421–436.

Duggar, D. (2001). Crisis intervention in public schools: Building a collection for parents and professionals. *References and Cheer Service Quarterly, 40*(4), 328–336.

Everly, G. S. (2000). Crisis management briefings (CMB): Large group crisis intervention in response to terrorism, disasters, and violence. *International Journal of Emergency Mental Health*, 2(1), 53–57.

Flynn, B. W., & Norwood, A. E. (2004). Defining normal psychological reactions to disaster. *Psychiatric Annals, 34*, 597–603.

France, K. (2002). *Crisis intervention: A handbook of immediate person-to-person help*. Springfield, IL: Charles C. Thomas.

Frykberg, E. R. (2002). Medical management of disasters and manmade casualties from terrorist bombings: How can we cope? *Journal of Trauma, 53*, 201–212.

Galea, S., Ahern, J., Resnick, H., Kilpatrick, D., Bucuvalas, M., Gold, J., & Vlahov, D. (2002). Psychological sequelae of the September 11 terrorist attacks in New York City. *New England Journal of Medicine, 346*(13), 982–987.

Gilligan, C. (1994). Joining the resistance: Psychology, politics, girls and women. In M. Berger (Ed.), *Women beyond Freud: New concepts of feminine psychology* (pp. 99–145). New York: Brunner/Mazel.

Grief: what you should know. Late Life Depression Evaluation and Treatment, University of Pittsburgh Medical Center. (2006). Retrieved on July 23, 2006, from www.wpic.pitt.edu/research/depr/ hrief.htm

Hall, M. J., Norwood, A. E., Ursano, R. J., & Fullerton, C. S. (2003). The psychological impacts of bioterrorism. *Biosecurity & Bioterrorism, 1*(2), 139–144.

Harvey, J. J., & Pauwels, B. G. (2000). Post traumatic stress theory: Research and application, Brunner/Mazel: Levittown, PA.

Hawton, K., & Simkin, S. (2003). Helping people bereaved by suicide? (Editorial). *British Medication Journal, 327*, 177–178.

Hazelwood, R.R., & Burgess, A. W. (2001). Practical aspects of rape: A multidisciplinary approach. 3rd ed. Boca Raton, FL: CRC Press.

Herman, R., Kaplan, M., & LeMelle, S. (2002). Psychoeducational debriefings after the September 11 disaster. *Psychiatric Services, 53*(4), 479–80.

Hoven, C. W., Duarte, C. S., & Mandell, D. J. (2003). Children's mental health after diagnostics: the impact of the World Trade Center attack. *Current Psychiatry Reports, 5*(2), 101–107.

Jordan, J. R. (2001). Is suicide bereavement different? A reassessment of the literature. *Suicide and Life-Threatening Behavior, 31*(1), 91–102.

Lazarus, R. (1991). *Emotion and adaptation* (p. 122). New York: Oxford University Press.

Lindemann, E. (1944). Symptomatology and management of acute grief. *American Journal of Psychiatry, 101*, 141–148.

Litz, B. T., Gray, M. J., Bryant, R. A., & Adler, A. B. (2002). Early intervention for trauma: Current status and future directions. *Clinical Psychology: Science and Practice, 9*, 112–134.

Majer, J. M., Jason, L. A., Ferrarie, J. R., Venable, L. B., & Olson, B. D. (2002). Social support and self-efficacy for abstinence: Is peer identification an issue? *Journal of Substance Abuse Treatment, 23*(3), 209–215.

Miller, J. (1994). Women's psychological development connections, disconnections, and violations. In M. Berger, *Women Beyond Freud: new concepts of feminine psychology* (79–97). New York: Brunner/Mazel.

Miller, J. (2002). Affirming flames: Debriefing survivors of the World Trade Center attack. *Brief Treatment and Crisis Intervention, 21*, 85–94.

Noji, E. K. (2000). The public health consequences of disasters: A review. *Prehospital and Disaster Medicine, 15*(1), 32–53.

Norris, F. H., Friedman, M. J., Watson, P. J., Byrne, C. M., Diaz, E., & Kaniasty, K. (2002). 60,000 disaster victims speak: Part I. An empirical review of the empirical literature, 1981–2001. *Psychiatry, 65*(3), 207–239.

North, C. S., McCutcheon, V., Spitznagel, E. L., & Smith, E. M. (2002). Three-year follow-up of survivors of a mass shooting episode. *Journal of Urban Health, 79* (3), 383–391.

North, C. S., Tivis, L., McMillen, J. C., Pfefferbaum, B., Spitznagel, E. L., Cox, J., et al. (2002). Psychiatric disorders in rescue workers after the Oklahoma City bombing. *American Journal of Psychiatry, 159*(5), 857–859.

Norwood, A. E., Ursano, R. J., & Fullerton, C. S. (2001). *Disaster psychiatry: Principles and practice*. American Psychiatric Association. Retrieved on May 23, 2003 from www.psych.org/pract_of_psych/principles_and_practice3201.cfm.

Ozer, E. J., Best, S. R., Lipsey, T. L., & Weiss, D. S. (2003). Predictors of posttraumatic stress disorder and symptoms in adults: A meta analysis. *Psychological Bulletin, 129*, 52–71.

Pfefferbaum, B., North, C. S., Flynn, B. W., Ursano, R. J., McCoy, G., DeMartino, R., et al. (2001). The emotional impact of injury following an international terrorist incident. *Public Health Review, 29*(2–4), 271–280.

Puig, M. E., & Glynn, J. B. (2003). Disaster responders: A cross cultural approach to recovery and relief work. *Journal of Social Service Research, 30*(2), 55–66.

Roberts, A. R. (2000). *Crisis intervention handbook: Assessment, treatment, and research* (2nd ed.). Oxford & New York: Oxford University Press.

Rose, S., Bisson, J., Churchill, R., & Wessely, S. (2006). Psychological debriefing for preventing post traumatic stress disorders. EMB Review: Cochrane Database of Systematic Reviews. Retrieved July 23, 2006, from http://gateway.ut.ovid.com/gw2/ovidweb.cgi.

Schlenger, W. E., Caddell, J. M., Ebert, L., Jordan, B. K., Rourke, K. M., Wilson, D., et al. (2002). Psychological reactions to terrorist attacks: Findings from the national study of Americans' reactions to September 11. *Journal of the American Medical Association, 288*(5), 581–588.

Schuster, M. A., Stein, B. D., Jaycox, L., Collins, R. L., Marshall, G. N., Elliott, M. N., et al. (2001). A national survey of stress reactions after September 11, 2001, terrorist attacks. *New England Journal of Medicine, 345*(20), 1507–1512.

Stinson, KM., Lasker, J.N., Lohmann, J., & Toedter, L.J. (1992). Parent's grief following pregnancy loss: A comparison of mothers and fathers. *Family Relations, 41*(2), 218–223.

Stroebe, M., Stroebe, W., & Schut, D. (2006). Bereavement research: methodological issues and ethical concerns, *Palliative Medicine, 17*, 235–240.

Stone, D. A., & Conley, J. A. (2004). A partnership between Roberts' crisis intervention model and the multicultural competencies. *Brief Treatment and Crisis Intervention, 4*(4), 367–375.

van Griensven, F., Chakkraband, S., Thienkrua, W., Pengjuntr, W., Cardozo, B. L., Tantipiwatanaskul, P., et al. (2006). Mental health problems among adults in Tsunami-affected areas in Southern Thailand. *JAMA, 296*(5), 527–548.

Walter, H. J., & Berkovitz, I. H. (2005). Practice parameter for psychiatric consultation to schools. *Journal of the American Academy of Child & Adolescent Psychiatry 44*(10), 1068–1083.

Yeager, K. R., & Roberts, A. R. (2003). Differentiating among stress, acute stress disorder, crisis episodes, trauma, and PTSD: Paradigm and treatment goals. *Brief Treatment and Crisis Intervention*, 3:1.

Zisook, S. (1987). Unresolved grief. In S. Zisook (Ed.), *Biopsychosocial aspects of bereavement* (pp. 21–34). Washington, D.C.: American Psychiatric Press.

CHAPTER 38

Management of Anger, Aggression, and Violence

Sandra P. Thomas

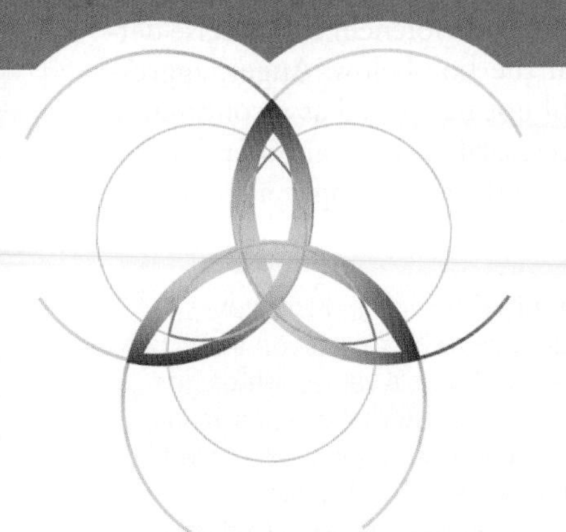

KEY CONCEPTS

- anger
- aggression
- violence
- assertiveness

LEARNING OBJECTIVES

After studying this chapter, you will be able to:

- Explore healthy and unhealthy styles of anger management.
- Discuss principles of anger management as a psychoeducational intervention.
- Discuss the biopsychosocial factors that influence aggressive and violent behaviors.
- Discuss biopsychosocial theories used to explain anger, aggression, and violence.
- Identify behaviors or actions that escalate and de-escalate violent behavior.
- Recognize the risk for "nurse abuse" (attacks on nurses).
- Generate options for responding to the expression of anger and violent behaviors in clinical nursing practice.
- Apply the nursing process to the management of anger, aggression, and violence in patients.

KEY TERMS

- anger management • catharsis • emotional circuit

It has been said that we are living in an age of anger (Knafo, 2004). Dysfunctional anger and potentially lethal violent behavior are increasingly evident in contemporary Western society.

Temper tantrums of athletes, episodes of road rage, and school shootings often dominate the evening news. Bullying incidents in schools occur every $7^1/_2$ minutes (Paquette, 2001). Fear of bullying by their classmates causes more than 160,000 American children to skip school every day (Orecklin, 2000). A Yale University study showed that nearly one quarter of American workers feel chronic anger because of heavy workloads and feelings of betrayal by their employers (cited in Malmgren, 2000). Vengeful attacks in the workplace have occurred often enough that the term "going postal" has entered common parlance.

Assaults by patients toward the staff of hospitals and nursing homes are also on the increase (Poster & Drew, 2006). More than 70% of psychiatric-mental health nurses report that they have been assaulted (Poster & Drew, 2006). It is a myth that patients who have psychiatric problems are more violent than other patients, but astute clinicians know which patients *might* become aggressive, given a combination of known risk factors with specific environmental conditions. One of the goals of this chapter is to outline those risk factors and describe preventive interventions. It is clear that all nurses must develop expertise in prevention and management of aggression.

A second aim of this chapter is to dispel confusion between anger as a normal, healthy response to violation of one's integrity and maladaptive anger that is detrimental to one's mental and physical health. Maladaptive anger is linked to psychiatric conditions, such as depression (Koh, Kim, & Park, 2002), as well as a plethora of medical conditions. For example, *excessive outwardly directed anger* is linked to coronary heart disease (Kubzansky & Kawachi, 2000), reduced left ventricular ejection fraction (Ironson et al., 1992), myocardial infarction (Mittleman et al., 1995), and restenosis after angioplasty (Goodman, Quigley, Moran, Meilman, & Sherman, 1996). *Suppressed anger* is related to arthritis, breast and colorectal cancer, and hypertension (Everson, Goldberg, Kaplan, Julkunen, & Salonen, 1998; Thomas et al., 2000). Furthermore, suppressed anger was a predictor of early mortality for both men and women in a large 17-year study (Harburg, Julius, Kaciroti, Gleiberman, & Schork, 2003). In contrast to these dysfunctional anger management styles, research shows that anger discussed with other people in a constructive way has a beneficial effect on blood pressure (Davidson, MacGregor, Stuhr, Dixon, & Maclean, 2000; Thomas, 1997a), as well as statistically significant associations with better general health, a higher sense of self-efficacy, less depression, and lower likelihood of obesity (Thomas, 1997b). Thus, effective anger management is important in maintenance of holistic health. Additionally, skillful anger control is a vital aspect of "emotional intelligence," which is essential to social and occupational success (Mayer, 1999). People with poor anger control have more conflict at work, change jobs more frequently, take more unwise risks, and have more accidents than people with adaptive anger behavior (Deffenbacher, Filetti, Richards, Lynch, & Oetting, 2003; Lench, 2004). Nurses are well positioned to teach health-promoting anger management classes in diverse practice settings, such as outpatient clinics, schools, and corporate sites. Classes for children and adolescents can be of great benefit, because young people are forming the anger habits that will continue into adulthood. Two examples of teaching programs on anger management are provided by Thomas (2001) and Frey and Weller (2000).

WHAT ANGER IS AND IS NOT

Language pertaining to anger is imprecise and confusing. Some of the words used interchangeably with anger include annoyance, frustration, temper, resentment, hostility, hatred, and rage. To avoid perpetuating the confusion, three key concepts were selected for use in this chapter (anger, aggression, and violence) and precise definitions are presented in the box below. Anger, aggression, and violence should not be viewed as a continuum, because one does not necessarily lead to another. That is a myth. In fact, cultural myths about anger abound (see Table 38.1).

KEY CONCEPTS **Anger** is "a strong, uncomfortable emotional response to a provocation that is unwanted and incongruent with one's values, beliefs, or rights" (Thomas, 1998). Anger is an internal affective state and may not be expressed in overt behavior. If expressed, anger behavior can be constructive or destructive.

Aggression involves overt behavior intended to hurt, belittle, take revenge, or achieve domination and control. Aggression can be verbal (sarcasm, insults, threats) or physical (property damage, slapping, hitting). Mentally healthy people stop themselves from aggression by realizing the negative consequences to themselves and/or their relationships.

Violence involves the use of strong force or weapons to inflict bodily harm to another person, and in some cases, to kill. **Violence** connotes greater intensity and destruction than aggression (Liu, 2004). It can be predatory (purposefully planned and nonemotional) or emotionally reactive (enacted in response to irrational fear of attack) (Meloy, 1992).

It is one of the six emotions with identifiable facial features across the diverse cultures of the world (Ekman, 1993). Mayne and Ambrose (1999, p. 354) assert that people across the globe "will largely agree about the possible causes of anger, and what an angry individual would like to do, though culture is perhaps the most important

Table 38.1 Cultural Myths About Anger

Myth	Truth
Anger is a knee-jerk reaction to external events.	Humans can choose to slow down their reactions and to think and behave differently in response to events.
Anger can be uncontrollable, resulting in crimes of passion such as "involuntary manslaughter."	In societies that believe anger can be controlled, there are far fewer violent crimes than in America. Compare statistics of Japan and the United States.
Anger behavior in adulthood is determined by temperament and childhood experiences.	While temperament and early experiences are important, emotional development continues throughout life. Adults can acquire knowledge and skills to handle emotions more effectively.
Men are angrier than women.	Women experience anger as frequently as men, but societal constraints may inhibit their expression of it.
People have to behave aggressively to get what they want.	Making an assertive request is more likely to lead to the desired outcome.

determinant of what an angry individual actually *does.*" Thus, in Japan, a wife might indicate anger to her husband by creating a disorderly flower arrangement. Such a subtle nonverbal cue is unlikely to be understood (or even noticed) by a husband from another culture.

In nonclinical samples, anger is usually a temporary state of emotional arousal, not an enduring negative attitude. Anger offers a signal to those experiencing it that something is wrong in themselves, others, or their relationships with others (Lerner, 1997). It is commonly provoked by an interpersonal offense such as unjust or disrespectful treatment (a spouse lying, a coworker taking advantage) (Thomas, 2006). The meaning of angry episodes must be understood within a relational context. For example, anger is intermingled with considerable hurt when loved ones violate the implicit relational contract ("If he loved me, how could he lie about that? How can I trust him again?") The violation that produces angry emotion is more substantive than minor irritations such as slow grocery lines or inefficient sales clerks. Therefore, most people feel an urge to take an action of some kind. If anger is expressed assertively to an intimate partner or coworker, beneficial outcomes are possible. In Averill's classic study (1983) of everyday anger, 76% of those who were on the receiving end of someone else's anger reported that they recognized their own faults as a result of the anger incident. Contrary to popular misconception, the relationship with the angry person was strengthened, not weakened. Thomas (2001) contends that the expression of honest anger may actually prevent aggression and help to resolve a situation. Suppression of anger, prolonged rumination about the grievance, and malevolent fantasies of revenge do not resolve a problem and may result in negative consequences at a later time.

Experience of Anger

The physiology of anger experience is powerful, involving the cerebral cortex, sympathetic nervous system, adrenal medulla (which secretes adrenaline and noradrenaline), the adrenal cortex (which secretes cortisol), the cardiovascular system, and even the immune system. When you are angry, your heart pounds, your blood pressure rises, you breathe faster, your muscles tense, and you clench your jaw or fists as you experience an impulse to do something with this physical energy. Some individuals experience anger arousal as pleasurable, while others find its strong physical manifestations scary and unpleasant. People who were taught that anger is a sin may immediately try to ban it from awareness and deny its existence. However, suppression actually results in greater, more prolonged, physiological arousal. A better option is finding a way to safely release the physical energy, either through vigorous physical activity (e.g., jogging) or through a calming activity (e.g., deep breathing). Later, at an opportune time, calmly discussing the incident with the provocateur permits clarification of misunderstandings and resolution of grievances. Box 38.1 invites the reader to explore variations in anger experience.

BOX 38.1

*Self-Awareness Exercise: **Personal Experience of Anger***

People's reactions differ when they experience anger. Some people report a sense of power, control, and calmness different from their usual experience; others report feeling shaky, tearful, and on the verge of collapse. Still others describe physical sensations of nausea and dizziness.

Think about the last time that you felt angry. List the body sensations and other emotions that you experienced. Now ask a friend, colleague, or family member to do the same. Compare lists. What are the similarities and differences between you? How will awareness of these differences help you in your clinical practice?

Expression of Anger

The physiological arousal of anger is similar in all people, but ways of expressing anger differ. The most common modes, or styles, of anger expression are listed in Table 38.2.

In Western culture, control of anger was the dominant stance from Greco-Roman times to the 20th century. Anger was viewed as sinful, dangerous, and destructive—an irrational emotion to be contained, controlled, and denied. This pejorative view contributed to the development of a powerful taboo against feeling and expressing anger. People who have accepted this persistent taboo may have difficulty even knowing when they are angry (Lerner, 1997). During the early 20th century, based on the animal research of ethologists such as Lorenz and Freud's conceptualization of "strangulated affect," some mental health care providers advocated the use of **catharsis.** Rather than containing anger, people were urged to "vent it," lest there be a dangerous "slush fund" of unexpressed anger building up in the body (Rubin, 1970). The legacy of the ill-advised "ventilationist movement" is still with us, visible in rude, uncivil behavior in the nation's classrooms, offices, roadways, and other public places, as well as in countless homes where loud arguments are a daily occurrence.

There is interest in developing communication techniques that promote the expression of anger in nondestructive ways (Davidson et al., 2000; Thomas, 1997b). However, most people lack skill in handling anger constructively. Few people had healthy role models to observe while growing up. Therefore, education in anger

Table 38.2 Styles of Anger Expression

Style	Characteristic Behaviors	Gender Socialization Issues
Anger suppression	Feeling anxious when anger is aroused Acting as though nothing happened Withdrawing from people when angry Conveying anger nonverbally by body language Sulking, pouting, or ruminating	In North America, girls are often discouraged from openly expressing anger, lest they hurt someone's feelings. Females are more likely than males to engage in passive-aggressive tactics, to ruminate about unresolved conflict, and to have somatic anger symptoms, such as headaches
Unhealthy outward anger expression	Flying off the handle Expressing anger in an attacking or blaming way Yelling, saying nasty things Calling the other person names or using profanity Using fists rather than words to express angry feelings	In North America, boys are encouraged to be aggressive and competitive, to express their anger in "manly" ways. Throughout life, males are more likely to express anger physically than females are.
Constructive anger discussion	Discussing the anger with a friend or family member, even if the provocateur cannot be confronted at the time Approaching the person with whom one is angry and discussing the concern directly Using "I" language to describe feelings and request changes in another's behavior	Most research shows that females, more so than males, prefer to talk through anger episodes and restore relationship harmony. Both men and women may benefit from assertiveness training, problem-solving skills training, and conflict resolution workshops.

management can be valuable, both for psychological growth and improved interpersonal relations.

Assessment of Anger

Both outwardly directed anger (particularly the hostile, attacking forms) and inwardly directed anger (i.e., anger that is stifled despite strong arousal) produce adverse consequences, indicating a need for anger management (AM) intervention. Complicating matters, however, most people's anger styles cannot be neatly categorized as "anger-in" or "anger-out," because they behave differently in different environments (for example, yelling at secretaries in the office, stifling anger at spouse). Therefore, it is necessary to conduct a careful assessment of a patient's behavior pattern across various situations. The manner of anger expression is not the only important aspect of assessment. The nurse must also assess the difficulty in regulating the frequency and intensity of anger, the extent to which it is creating problems in social, occupational, or intimate relationships, and the presence or absence of self-soothing techniques (Carrere, Mittman, Woodin, Tabares, & Yoshimoto, 2005). Given the current climate of evidence-based practice, it may be advantageous to administer a questionnaire that has been extensively used with thousands of people, permitting comparison of your client to established norms. The Spielberger State-Trait Anger Expression Inventory (STAXI) is one such tool (Spielberger, 1999). This instrument is particularly useful because it measures the general propensity to be angry (trait anger), as well as current feelings (state anger) and several styles of anger expression.

Accurate client assessment and appropriate nursing intervention would be facilitated by the kind of precise diagnostic nomenclature for anger disorders that is available in the *Diagnostic and Statistical Manual of Mental Disorders* (4th ed., text revision) (*DSM-IV-TR*) for other conditions. At present, only one anger-related disorder appears in the *DSM-IV-TR*: Intermittent Explosive Disorder (see box 38.2). Once thought to be rare, Intermittent Explosive Disorder (IED) is receiving heightened attention because it is reported to affect 16 million Americans (Kessler et al., 2006). The disorder usually appears during the teen years, and persists over the life course. A national study indicates that the average number of lifetime anger attacks per person is large (43 per person). Because the disorder involves inadequate production or functioning of serotonin, IED is commonly treated with selective serotonin reuptake inhibitors

BOX 38.2

Diagnostic Characteristics of Intermittent Explosive Disorder (DSM-IV-TR 312.34)

- A history of several episodes of failure to control aggressive impulses resulting in serious assault or property destruction
- The degree of aggression during these episodes is grossly out of proportion to any precipitating stressors
- The aggressive episodes cannot be accounted for by another mental disorder (e.g., personality disorder), a medical condition (e.g., Alzheimer's), or effects of a drug

BOX 38.3

Proposed Nomenclature for Anger Disorders

- Adjustment disorder with angry mood: A diagnosis suitable for a patient who has no evidence of personality disorder or other pathology, but has experienced an identifiable psychosocial stressor within the past 3 months (e.g., a painful divorce following the affair of a spouse)
- Situational anger disorder without aggression: A diagnosis for a client whose situational anger is intense for 6 months or more (e.g., having to deal daily with a critical or sexist supervisor)
- Situational anger disorder with aggression: A diagnosis for a client whose situational anger has progressed to aggressive behaviors such as obscene language or property damage
- General anger disorder: A diagnosis for a client with pervasive, chronic anger for a year or longer, and inability to control its eruption despite costly consequences (e.g., frequently losing job because of angry outbursts toward coworkers).
- General anger disorder with aggression: Same as general anger disorder, with addition of habitual aggressive acts (e.g., frequent confrontation with others resulting in physical assault or destruction of property)

Adapted from Eckhardt & Deffenbacher, 1995.

(SSRIs). However, behavior therapy should also be included. Only 28.8% of patients with IED ever receive treatment for their anger (Kessler, 2006), although the IED population is just as responsive to treatment as non-IED populations are (Galovski, 2001).

Scholars (Eckhardt & Deffenbacher, 1995) have proposed that five additional anger disorders be included in the *DSM-IV-TR* (see Box 38.3). These diagnoses could be applied when anger is the primary affective disruption, obviating the need to give an angry patient a label such as borderline personality disorder, a diagnosis too hastily applied to an angry woman. An individual with situational anger (e.g., because of spousal infidelity) does not need the same type of intervention as a person with more global, chronic anger. Clinicians are encouraged to participate in the ongoing process of validating the diagnoses and testing the efficacy of various anger treatments.

Culture and Gender Considerations in Anger Assessment

Even when diagnostic classifications are further refined and validated, patients can never be neatly categorized because gender, culture, and ethnic differences in the experience and expression of anger also must be taken into consideration before planning interventions.

Cultural differences in anger behavior can emanate from the historical trajectories, religions, languages, and customs of a group of people (Thomas, 2006). The same event can provoke different emotional responses in culturally different persons (e.g., a random act by a stranger could be perceived as insulting by one individual but dismissed with a laugh by someone from another culture). The nurse must explore what the client learned about anger, and its display, in his or her culture and family of origin (the primary bearer of that culture).

Gender role socialization influences beliefs about the appropriateness of "owning" angry emotionality and revealing it to others. Western cultures generally promote more aggressive behavior in males and more conciliatory behavior in females (see Table 38.2). However, these generalizations may not apply to marginalized individuals, such as ethnic minorities (Thomas, 2006). For example, black mothers prepare their daughters to mobilize anger in order to cope with the harsh realities of racist treatment (Greene, 1990). The nurse should also be aware that some clients from Eastern cultures disapprove of anger for both genders, particularly those cultures emphasizing connectedness rather than individualism (e.g., Japanese). A more extensive discussion of culture and gender factors can be found in Thomas (2006).

Anger Management Intervention

Anger management (AM) is a psychoeducational intervention for persons whose behavior is dysfunctional in some way (i.e., interfering with success in work or relationships) but *not violent.* In recent years, there has been an increase in court-mandated AM for persons whose behavior is violent, as opposed to angry. When these individuals do not greatly benefit, a conclusion may be drawn that AM is ineffective. However, AM courses cannot be expected to modify violent behavior (interventions designed for aggressive and violent individuals are presented later in the chapter).

The desired outcomes of any AM intervention are to teach people to: (1) effectively modulate the physiological arousal of anger; (2) alter any irrational thoughts fueling the anger; and (3) modify maladaptive anger behaviors (e.g., blaming, attacking, or suppressing) that prevent problem-solving in daily living. Group work is valuable to AM clients, because they need to practice new behaviors in an interpersonal context that offers feedback and support. The leader of an AM group functions as a teacher and coach, not a therapist. Therefore, potential participants should be screened and referred to individual counseling or psychotherapy if their anger is deep-seated and chronic. Exclusion criteria are paranoia, organic disorders, and severe personality disorders (Thomas, 2001). Candidates for AM must have some insight that their behavior is problematic and some desire to enlarge their behavioral repertoire.

AM includes both didactic and experiential components. Ideally, participants commit to attendance for a series of weekly meetings, ranging from 4 to 10 weeks. Between the group meetings, participants are given homework assignments such as keeping an anger diary and applying the lessons of the class in their homes and work sites. It may be useful to conduct gender-specific or race-specific groups (Thomas, 2001). Effectiveness of AM has been demonstrated in studies of college students, angry drivers, angry veterans, and parents who have difficulty controlling anger toward their children (Deffenbacher, Oetting, & Di Giuseppe, 2002). When patients are screened properly, differentiating between anger and violence, even prisoners have benefited from AM (see Box 38. 4).

AGGRESSION AND VIOLENCE

Aggression and violence are serious societal problems commanding the attention of the criminal justice system as well as the mental health care system. During periods when people are a danger to others, they are separated from the larger society and confined in prisons or locked psychiatric units. Because nurses frequently practice in these settings, management of aggressive and violent behavior is an essential skill. Violence *can* be understood; it is not senseless and random (Paquette, 2001). The violent individual may feel trapped, frightened, or desperate, perhaps at the end of his rope. The nurse would do well to remember that many violent individuals have experienced childhood abandonment, physical brutality, and/or sexual abuse. Confinement that replicates earlier experiences of degrading treatment may provoke aggressive response, while humane care may kindle hope of recovery and rehabilitation. The response of the nurse may be critical in determining whether aggression escalates or diminishes. Aggressive or violent behavior does not occur in a vacuum. Both the patient and the context must be considered. Therefore, a multidimensional framework (Fig. 38.1) is essential for understanding and responding to these behaviors (Morrison & Love, 2003).

BOX 38.4

Anger Management Success

Ireland, J. (2004). Anger management therapy with young male offenders: An evaluation of treatment outcome. Aggressive Behavior, 30, 174–185.

QUESTION: Is a brief group-based anger management intervention effective with young male offenders?

METHOD: A quasi-experimental pre- and posttest, non-equivalent group was used in this study. Eighty-seven prisoners were assigned to experimental (n = 50) and control (n = 37) groups. The two groups were similar in terms of age, offense, and levels of anger. The cognitive-behavior intervention consisted of 12 1-hour sessions that included triggers to anger, consequence of anger, and the importance of behavior, thoughts, and feelings. Daily homework and group participation were required. All members of the experimental group attended all sessions. Changes in managing were determined by staff observations and self-report angry behaviors.

RESULTS: The number of angry incidents significantly decreased in the anger management group compared with the control group. The number of self-reported angry behaviors, thoughts, and feelings also decreased in the group that participated in the intervention. These changes were maintained for 8 weeks following completion of the group work.

IMPLICATIONS FOR NURSING: Anger management classes can be effective in helping patients learn to understand and modify the experience of anger. Cognitive-behavior anger management could be a standard intervention in psychiatric mental health settings. Patients should be informed of the success of anger management groups.

MODELS OF ANGER, AGGRESSION, AND VIOLENCE

This section discusses some of the main theoretical explanations for anger, aggression, and violence. A single model or theory cannot fully explain anger, aggression, and violence; instead, the nurse must choose the most useful models for explaining a particular patient's experience and for planning interventions.

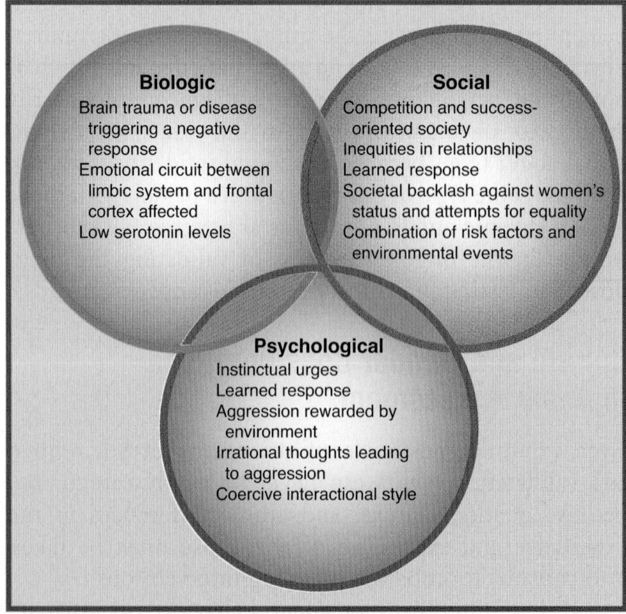

FIGURE 38.1. Biopsychosocial etiologies for patients with aggression.

Biologic Theories

From a biologic viewpoint, a tendency to have more frequent angry episodes may partially originate from developmental deficits, anoxia, malnutrition, toxins, tumors, neurodegenerative diseases, or trauma affecting the brain. Patients with a history of damage to the cerebral cortex are more likely to exhibit increased impulsivity, decreased inhibition, and decreased judgment than are those who have not experienced such damage. The interaction of neurocognitive impairment and social history of abuse or family violence increases the risk for violent behavior (Scarpa & Raine, 1997). An aggression-related gene (monoamine oxidase A), which affects norepinephrine, serotonin, and dopamine, may play a significant role in the violence enacted by abused children, especially boys (Caspi et al., 2002; Meyer-Lindenberg & Weinberg, 2006). Sex hormones also play a role in some aggressive behavior. Violent male offenders have higher testosterone than controls, and female offenders are more likely to commit crimes during the low progesterone phase of the menstrual cycle (Liu, 2004). The odds of violent behavior also increase when separate risk factors, such as schizophrenia, substance abuse, and not taking prescribed medications, coexist in the same person. Before reading additional research evidence, try the anger exercise in Box 38.5. What does daily experience suggest about biologically based aspects of the experience and expression of anger?

Cognitive Neuroassociation Model

The cognitive neuroassociation model is one explanation for the interplay of biologic and other internal influences (Berkowitz, 1989; Miller, Pedersen, Earleywine, & Pollock, 2003). Initially, an adverse event (such as pain from tripping over a skateboard) triggers a primitive negative response. Peripheral receptors communicate this response to the spinal cord through the spinothalamic tract to the hypothalamus. The hypothalamus, which synthesizes input from the nervous system, is part of the limbic system. The limbic system mediates primitive emotion and basic drives to produce behaviors for survival, such as the fight-or-flight response (Harper-Jaques & Reimer, 1992).

At first, cognitive appraisal is not involved in these rudimentary feelings of fear or anger, other than identifying the stimulus as aversive; however, higher order cognitive processing quickly begins to take over. The brain associates the current experience of physiologic sensations with memories, ideas, and previously experienced expressive-motor reactions. It then interprets and differentiates the experience. Depending on prior experience and associations, the response may be intensified or suppressed. It is this latter part of the process that is most amenable to modification through psychotherapy.

BOX 38.5

Self-Awareness Exercise: Intensity of Anger

Imagine this scene:

You are coming home late at night. You've been at the library studying for midterm examinations and are tired. As you come up the front walk, you trip over a skateboard, probably left by one of the neighborhood children. Before you know it, you are sprawled across the front step.

What emotions threaten to overwhelm you at that moment? What contributes to the intensity of the anger that you feel?

- The pain where you scraped your leg across the cement?
- Your general state of tiredness?
- The fact that you skipped dinner?
- The five cups of coffee you had today?
- The careless children who left a toy in your way?

If the same thing had happened when you were well rested and feeling good, would the feeling and the intensity be the same?

• NCLEXNOTE

In caring for a potentially aggressive patient, the nurse should recognize that biochemical imbalance contributes to the person's inability to control aggression.

Neurostructural Model and the Emotional Circuit

The brain structures most frequently associated with aggressive behavior are the limbic system and the cerebral cortex, particularly the frontal and temporal lobes. Harper-Jaques and Reimer (1992) proposed the phrase **emotional circuit** to describe the interrelationship between the emotional processes of the limbic system and the neurocognitive processes of the frontal lobe and other parts of the cortex. They hypothesize that the functioning of this system determines the meaning a person gives to a particular situation. Thus, meaning is influenced by physiologic capability to perceive incoming messages, prioritize among competing stimuli, and interpret these messages in relation to stored ideas, beliefs, and memories.

Neurochemical Model and Low Serotonin Syndrome

In recent decades, knowledge has exploded about the complex role of neurotransmitters in human behavior. Serotonin is a major neurotransmitter involved in mood, sleep, and appetite. Low serotonin levels are associated not only with depression, but also with irritability, increased pain sensitivity, impulsiveness, and aggression (Kavoussi, Armstead, & Coccaro, 1997). Serotonin is sensitive to fluctuations in dietary intake of its precursor, tryptophan, which is found in high-carbohydrate foods. Once it crosses the blood–brain barrier, tryptophan is synthesized into serotonin within the 5-hydroxytryptophan (5-HTP) neurons by interaction with the enzyme tryptophan hydroxylase. Normally, the amount of tryptophan available in the plasma is below saturation (i.e., below the amount that could be used if available). Tryptophan intake and the availability of binding sites on the plasma proteins affect synthesis of serotonin. Thus, assessing overall dietary intake is relevant, particularly of good tryptophan sources, such as wheat, flour, corn, milk, and eggs. Preliminary research evidence suggests that tryptophan depletion may increase anger levels in individuals already prone to aggressive behavior (Schmeck et al., 2002).

People with a history of aggressive behavior have been found to have a lower-than-average level of serotonin. Studies of humans with known aggressive tendencies, such as violent offenders, have repeatedly shown lower-than-average concentrations of 5-hydroxyindoleacetic acid (5-HIAA), the major metabolite for serotonin (Kavoussi et al., 1997) and prefrontal cortex dysfunction (Best, Williams, & Coccaro, 2002). Similarly, the plasma concentration of tryptophan is lower in people with alcoholism who have a history of aggressive behavior than in people with alcoholism and no such history. Criminals whose acts of violence were committed impulsively have lower levels of 5-HIAA than do criminals whose acts of violence were premeditated. Hyperarousal, such as may occur through being constantly vigilant against possible attack (e.g., in guerrilla warfare), also may contribute to aggressive behavior.

This evidence for a biologic component to aggressive behavior does not mean that only biologic means of treatment can be effective. Feedback between human behavior and biochemistry is continuous; verbal suggestions can affect biochemistry, just as biochemistry affects behavior (Pardo, Pardo, & Raichle, 1993). Environmental and learned behaviors influence the type and degree of aggression expressed, even by those for whom there is a biologic component (Kavoussi et al., 1997).

Psychological Theories

Several psychological explanations exist for aggressive and violent behaviors. This section discusses psychoanalytic, behavioral, and cognitive theories, as well as treatment approaches consistent with these theories. Treatment may be lengthy for individuals with severe psychopathology.

Psychoanalytic Theories

Psychoanalytic theorists view emotions as instinctual drives. They view suppression of these drives as unhealthy and possible contributors to the development of psychosomatic or psychological disorders. Freud struggled to understand the nature and expression of human aggressive behavior. In his early works, he linked aggression with libidinal factors; however, this association did not explain destructive actions during wars and armed conflict. In his later writings, Freud identified aggression as a separate instinct, like the sexual instinct. Because the language of hydraulics is evident in Freud's use of terms such as cathexis (filling) and catharsis (release), some psychoanalysts recommended the use of cathartic approaches to release patients' pent-up anger (Tavris, 1989). Following this theoretical formulation, nurses in the mid-20th century often employed interventions that directed the patient to "let it out" by pounding a pillow or ripping up telephone books (Thomas, 1990). However, recent studies have not supported the theory that catharsis reduces aggression. In fact, it can cause aggression to escalate by amplifying signals in the internal neural feedback loop (Mayne & Ambrose, 1999).

Contemporary psychoanalysts do not adhere to any single explanatory model of aggression, often focusing on patients' tendencies to reenact old childhood conflicts or their defensive attempts to deny vulnerability (Feindler & Byers, 2006). In working with angry patients, they focus on issues such as improved control over outbursts, heightened empathy for others, and repair of deficits in the personality structure. During analytic therapy, patients gradually achieve greater insight into unconscious processes (Feindler & Byers, 2006). Thus, they become aware of the reasons they developed maladaptive anger behaviors.

Behavioral Theories

As behavioral theories came into prominence, anger was viewed as a learned response to a stimulus, rather than an instinctual drive. In the 1930s, the frustration-aggression hypothesis was advanced, in which a person may experience anger and act violently in response to interference with or blocking of a goal. Laboratory experiments and the reality of everyday experience have proved the limitations of this theory (Thomas, 1990). Not all situations in which one's goal is blocked lead to anger or violence.

Another behavioral theory is social learning theory. In his research, Bandura (1973) drew attention to the role of learning and rewards in the expression of anger and violence. He studied interactions between mothers and children. The children learned that anger and aggressive behavior helped them get what they wanted from their mothers. Children's observation of aggressive behavior between family members and in their communities fosters a context for learning aggressive behavior. It may also lead to an assumption that aggressive behavior is appropriate. According to this view, people learn to be aggressive by participating in an aggressive environment.

Angry outbursts are strengthened by reinforcement contingencies such as compliance of others.

Behavioral treatment of anger could involve avoidance of provoking stimuli, self-monitoring regarding cues of anger arousal, stimulus control, response disruption, and guided practice of more effective anger behaviors. Relaxation training is often introduced early in the treatment because it strengthens the therapeutic alliance and convinces clients that they can indeed learn to calm themselves when angry (Deffenbacher, 2006). When the body relaxes, there is less physical impetus to act impulsively in a way that one will later regret.

Cognitive Theories

Cognitive theorists are interested in how people transform internal and external stimuli into useful information. They emphasize understanding how a person takes new information and fits it into an already developed schema. Beck (1976) proposed that cognitive schema such as judgments, self-esteem, and expectations influence angry responses. In a situation perceived as intentional, dangerous, and unprovoked, the recipient's reaction will be intensified. The person's reaction will be further intensified if he or she views the offender as undesirable. In Beck's therapeutic approach, Socratic questioning is used to challenge distorted cognitions. A meta-analysis of 50 studies found that the average recipient of Beck's cognitive therapy for anger scored better on outcome measures than 76% of untreated control subjects (Beck & Fernandez, 1998). Participants in the 50 studies included abusive spouses and parents, aggressive children, adolescents in residential treatment, college students, and prison inmates.

Rational-emotive theory, another type of cognitive theory, considers cognition, affect, and behavior to be interrelated psychological processes (Ellis, 1977). This theory regards anger as an inappropriate negative emotion because it stems from irrational beliefs. Emphasized in rational-emotive therapy are common irrational beliefs that fuel anger, such as one-track thinking ("they are doing that deliberately to get to me"), catastrophizing ("I'm never going to get over this awful insult"), and overgeneralization ("All of these doctors are idiots"). Patients may think that the world should be just and fair, that they should get whatever they want, and that other people should act the way they want them to. Notice that the word "should" appears as a significant element of these irrational thoughts. Change is directed at altering irrational beliefs by identifying and working to change them and their associated inappropriate anger behaviors. Patients are guided to moderate their unrealistic expectations of other people and to practice new behaviors in role-playing situations and (if possible) in real-world homework assignments. A limitation of the rational-emotive approach is that anger is always considered as a negative emotion. Some practitioners of this approach advocate complete elimination of angry emotion, failing to consider the benefits of defending one's boundaries and rights in situations of genuine injustice. Another limitation of all the cognitive approaches is that cognitive processing is compromised in many psychological disorders (Rubinsztein, Sahakian, & Dolan, 2002; Sergi & Green, 2003).

To date, cognitive and cognitive-behavioral therapies have the most extensive empirical evidence of efficacy for anger-related disorders (Deffenbacher, 2006), but much of the research has been conducted with nonclinical samples, such as college students who voluntarily seek treatment. Not all individuals with dysfunctional anger recognize that they have a problem or willingly enter treatment. Persons who wish to place blame outside the self ("she *made* me so angry!" "He was asking for it!") may resist examining their irrational thoughts and the consequences of their actions.

Sociocultural Theories

Western society is characterized by a competitive, success-oriented ideology that values the individual and individual accomplishments over collaboration and a sense of community. Self-esteem, particularly for men, may be based on social and economic status and influence over others and the environment (Jenkins, 1990). The pursuit of status produces inequities in relationships, whereby one person is superior and the other is subordinate. A hazard inherent in the pursuit of status is the view that the "entitled person" has the right to use whatever means necessary to obtain status (Jenkins, 1990). These means may include force or disregarding the rights and needs of others. The entitled person may also begin to consider other people responsible for his or her thoughts, feelings, or actions.

Men have used a belief in entitlement to justify such actions as threatening, hurting, or murdering women. In 2001, the United Nations (UN) Commission on Human Rights issued a resolution on the elimination of violence against women. This resolution implored the governments of UN member nations to develop policies and provide funding for violence prevention and treatment programs. However, violence against women remains a worldwide problem of staggering magnitude (one in three females will experience abusive treatment during her lifetime). In the developed world, women now have greater access to education, increased economic independence, and opportunities to control the frequency and number of pregnancies. These changes have led some to suggest that the continuing prevalence of violence toward women (Tjaden & Thoennes, 2000) is a backlash against their increased efforts toward achieving equality.

A disturbing new phenomenon in North America is the rise in aggressive and violent behavior in girls and women. For several decades, arrests of girls for assault and weapons charges have been increasing at rates exceeding those for boys (Poe-Yamagata & Butts, 1996; Thomas, 2003). Are females choosing to fight back, rather than be victims of violence? That is one theoretical explanation, and research by Jack (1999) provides some support for this. However, other theories are plausible. Some girls may be emulating aggressive role models, such as female boxers and wrestlers, or the physical fighting they are observing in their own homes and neighborhoods. Large percentages of girls in a national study admitted hitting another person within the past year because they were angry (64% of middle school girls, 61% of high school girls) (Thomas & Smith, 2004).

Babcock, Miller, and Siard (2003) identified two groups of violent adult women: those who were only abusive toward intimate partners, and those who were generally violent. The generally violent women had more frequently witnessed their mothers engaging in aggression toward their fathers, had assaulted a wider variety of individuals (e.g., family, friends, strangers, coworkers), and were more likely to admit using violence as a means to control others. Both groups of women reported high rates of childhood maltreatment as well as abuse by adult intimate partners.

Interactional Theory

Morrison (1998) challenges research and theories suggesting that aggression and violence are biologically or psychologically based. She asserts that these views lead to excusing the person's behavior. She proposes that violence among people in psychiatric settings is the same as violence in other settings. Therefore, the patient's behavior should be considered a social problem and responded to on that basis. This challenge is grounded in several studies that examined the interactional style of the aggressive and violent individual. People with interactional styles that were argumentative or coercive were more likely to engage in aggressive or violent interchanges. Such people are often described as having a "chip on their shoulders." Morrison argues that the antecedent variables (i.e., history of violence, psychiatric diagnosis, length of hospitalization) and the mediating variable of interactional style are the primary reasons for the behavior.

NURSING MANAGEMENT: HUMAN RESPONSE TO ANGER AND AGGRESSION

The paramount aim of psychiatric nurses, particularly those staffing inpatient facilities, is *prevention* of patient violence. Noting the lack of theoretical understanding of violence prevention, Johnson and Delaney (2006) recently conducted a study that resulted in a theory of keeping the unit safe. The researchers interviewed both staff and patients as well as observing behavior on inpatient psychiatric units for 400 hours. Keeping the unit safe involved a proactive approach to reducing risk and enhancing predictability of aggressive behavior. Dimensions of keeping the unit safe included maintenance of a structured and respectful therapeutic milieu, careful timing of admissions and discharges, expert use of space and personnel, and a conviction that staff needed to understand the *meaning* of patients' behaviors.

Aggression and violence often arise from one party's belief that his or her view of a situation is the only correct one. The first party considers other views wrong and in need of changing. A second party's refusal to give in to the view of the first may lead to violence (Capra, 2002). Box 38.6 illustrates such a scenario in the clinical setting. Low self-esteem that may be further eroded during hospitalization or treatment may influence a patient to use force to meet his or her needs or to experience some sense of empowerment. Many people who have chronic mental health problems "fight" the experience and refuse to accept medical treatment. When admitted to the hospital, they may experience turmoil from both the illness and the anger at the additional loss of control associated with hospitalization. Patients may use aggression and violence to force change or to regain or maintain control. Rewards from violence include attention from nursing staff and status and prestige among the patient group (Harris & Morrison, 1995). For example, the patient who behaves

BOX 38.6

Clinical Vignette: Paul's Anger

Paul, a new patient on the unit, appears to be experiencing auditory hallucinations. The nurse approaches Paul, careful not to invade his personal space, and begins to walk with him. In an attempt to assess his current mental status, the nurse points out that he seems restless and asks if the voices have returned. Paul responds, "They are telling me this place isn't safe. The angel in the corner is signaling to me. She wants me to leave!" Paul starts to walk toward the door. The nurse understands that what the patient is seeing and hearing are hallucinations. The nurse attempts to increase Paul's feeling of safety by identifying his perceptions as hallucinations and reassuring him of his safety. "No, I won't stay and you can't make me." Paul pushes the nurse aside and runs to the door.

What Do You Think?

If you were the nurse in this situation, what would be your next response? How would you acknowledge Paul's concerns and encourage him to stay?

violently is observed more frequently and has more opportunities to discuss concerns with nurses.

Nurses' perceptions and beliefs about themselves as individuals and professionals will influence their responses to aggressive behaviors. For example, the nurse who considers any expression of anger or aggression inappropriate will approach an agitated patient differently from a nurse who considers agitated behavior to be meaningful. Varying beliefs about appropriate ways to express anger become apparent when a patient and a nurse enter into a therapeutic relationship. Understandably, nurses often shrink from patient anger when their own family backgrounds have been characterized by out-of-control anger and/or abuse. The incidence of childhood abuse is high within the nursing profession (Rew & Christian, 1993).

The nurse's ability to maintain personal control is challenged when faced with angry, provoking patients. Some patients who are experiencing emotional problems have an uncanny ability to verbally target a nurse's vulnerable characteristics. It is a usual response to become defensive when one feels vulnerable. However, when nurses lose control of their own responses, the potential for punitive interventions or the use of threats or sarcasm is greater. Furthermore, threatening the patient (e.g., "You are going to get an injection if you don't calm down") will only worsen a volatile situation.

Studies show that nurses often withdraw from angry patients (Smith & Hart, 1994). Disconnecting from the patient occurs when nurses feel threatened and appraise the anger as a personal attack on their competence or integrity. Nurses studied by Smith and Hart tried to hide their own anger because "good nurses" do not get angry at patients. Only one study participant reported talking to a patient afterward about the anger episode, and this conversation occurred after the patient apologized. Coldness and distancing on the part of staff were acutely painful to psychiatric patients interviewed by Carlsson and colleagues (2006) (see Box 38.7). What patients want are steady, dependable, confident caregivers who will remain connected with them when they are angry.

Predictors of Violence

To develop a means of predicting aggressive and violent behaviors, some researchers have examined demographics, patient characteristics, and unit climate. Others have attempted to determine the relationship between medical diagnosis and violence. A third area of inquiry has been the role of the patient's history in predicting violence.

Several research reports suggest that particular characteristics are predictive of violent behaviors. Suspiciousness, impulsivity, agitation, and unwillingness to follow unit rules were among the predictors identified in Johnson's (2004) systematic review of the literature about violence on inpatient psychiatric units. Other predictors were involuntary hospitalization in a locked unit, past history of violence, crowding and density during times of high patient census, and anger-producing staff actions (such as limit-setting). Age, gender, and race of patients were *not* good predictors. Research findings regarding number of staff have been mixed,

BOX 38.7

What do Patients Want from Caregivers?

Carlsson, G., Dahlberg, K., Ekebergh, M., & Dahlberg, H. (2006). Patients longing for authentic personal care: A phenomenological study of violent encounters in psychiatric settings. Issues in Mental Health Nursing, 27(3), 287–305.

QUESTION: How does the patient experience violent encounters?

METHODS: This qualitative study is approached from the reflective lifeworld approach. This methodology focuses on the patient experiences of their violent encounters. Seven men and two women, ages 20–38, agreed to an interview based on the reflective model. The interviews were transcribed verbatim and the text was analyzed for meaning that was recorded and then transcribed. The goal of the analysis was to describe the essential structure of the phenomenon and its meaning.

RESULTS: The researchers found that patients wanted steady, dependable, confident caregivers who remained connected with them when they were angry. When caregivers were cold and distant, patients felt a sense of despair and their aggression increased:

- "My most lasting memory from these moments is the encounter with an expressionless, blank face with expressionless, cold eyes staring back at me" (p. 295)
- "I don't think they [the staff] really care whether I'm dead or alive…nobody is trying to help me to live, to stay alive" (p. 299)

In contrast, when caregivers displayed authentic sensitivity to their suffering, patients' aggression was diffused:

- "I could see in his face then that he liked me, he was not scared…He was sort of calm and had loving eyes, it was very disarming" (p. 293)
- "You could tell that there is some warmth and authenticity. You can tell that she is serious, that she cares about you… it is authentic, not ingratiating just so that I will behave" (P. 299)

IMPLICATIONS FOR NURSING: This study helps nurses understand the needs of patients who are violent. Being authentic and sensitive are valued nursing attributes. Demonstration of these attributes can help reduce patients' risk for aggressive behavior.

although some researchers continue to assert that inadequate staffing must be acknowledged as a contributing factor in units with high incidence of assault (Kindy, Petersen, & Parkhurst, 2005).

Specific diagnoses are not consistently predictive of violence, although some reports suggest that patients who have reduced impulse control (i.e., diagnoses such as schizophrenia, bipolar disorder, organic brain syndrome, brain injury, or attention-deficit hyperactivity disorder) are at increased risk for violent episodes (Tasman, 1997). One 7-year study in a forensic mental health unit found that paranoid schizophrenic patients committed the most violent acts, often compelled to act by internal psychotic phenomena (Green and Robinson, 2005). A British study found that young men with dual diagnoses (psychiatric illness and substance misuse) were most likely to be violent (Royal College of Psychiatrists, 1998). Impaired communication, disorientation, and depression have been found to be consistently associated with aggressive behavior among nursing home residents with dementia (Talerico, Evans, & Strumpf, 2002). Temporal lobe epilepsy has also been discussed as a possible predictor of violence (Harper-Jaques & Reimer, 1992; Mesulam, 2000), although this remains a matter of controversy (Citrome & Volavka, 1999). Aggressive behavior that occurs in the interictal period (i.e., between seizures) could be related to the intense frustration that people who have epilepsy often experience. Certain antiepileptic drugs, particularly barbiturates, may contribute to irritability and aggressive behavior. However, mood-stabilizing medications such as carbamazepine (Tegretol) and divalproex sodium (Depakote) have reduced aggressive behavior. The nurse should include any history of seizures, current medications, and compliance with pharmacotherapy in patient assessments.

The patient's history is probably the most important predictor of potential for violence. Important markers include previous episodes of rage and violent behavior, escalating irritability, intruding angry thoughts, and fear of losing control. The Nurses' Observational Scale for In-patient Evaluation (NOSIE) has been used to rate patients. Swett and Mills (1997) reported that a high score on the irritability factor of the NOSIE may be useful to clinicians in predicting which patients may be assaultive. The nurse should be mindful, however, that not all violence is enacted in anger. Some violent individuals are acting on frightening paranoid delusions rather than the heat of angry emotion. Others commit predatory violence (Meloy, 1992) that is deliberately planned for a time when a disliked staff member is on duty and the unit is short-staffed. Staff on duty during afternoons and evenings may be more vulnerable to assault (Green & Robinson, 2005).

Analysis and Outcome Identification

The nurse analyzes all assessment data across the biologic, psychological, and social domains to understand the dangers that the patient's behavior poses for self or others. The most common nursing diagnoses for patients experiencing intense anger and aggression are Risk for Self-Directed Violence and Risk for Other-Directed Violence (North American Nursing Diagnosis Association [NANDA], 2003). Outcomes focus on aggression control.

Planning and Implementing Interventions

This section emphasizes the development of a partnership between the nurse and patient, who work together to find solutions to prevent the recurrence of explosive episodes and to de-escalate volatile situations. However, sometimes the patient's condition (e.g., advanced dementia) or the situation will prevent the development of a partnership. In such instances, the nurse must take charge. The nurse who intervenes from within the context of the therapeutic relationship must be cognizant of the fit of a particular intervention. Blanket interventions not only may fail but could even be counterproductive (Davey, Day, & Howells, 2005). Interventions that are appropriate in early phases of escalation differ from those used when the patient's agitation is greater. The patient's affective, behavioral, and cognitive response to the intervention provides information about its effects and guides the nurse's next response (Wright & Leahey, 2000) (Fig. 38.2). The following assumptions are important to consider in planning interventions with this patient population (Harper-Jaques & Masters, 1994):

- The nurse and patient collaborate to find solutions and alternatives to aggressive and violent outbursts.
- While anger is a normal emotion, aggression and violence are not. Other people should never be threatened or harmed.
- In most instances, the person who behaves aggressively or violently can assume responsibility for the behavior.
- The nurse views the patient from the perspective of acknowledging that the patient has solved problems before and is only temporarily in need of help.
- The nurse understands that norms for behavior are created within the context of a particular environment and are influenced by the patient's history and culture.

Nurses who work with potentially violent patients must also keep in mind that they can take actions to minimize personal risk:

- Using nonthreatening body language
- Respecting the patient's personal space and boundaries
- Positioning themselves so that they have immediate access to the door of the room in case they need to leave the room
- Choosing to leave the door open to an office while talking to a patient
- Knowing where colleagues are and making sure those colleagues know where they are
- Removing or not wearing clothing or accessories that could be used to harm them, such as scarves, necklaces, or dangling earrings

The nurse who works with potentially aggressive patients does so with respect and concern. The goal is to work with patients to find solutions. The nurse approaches these patients calmly, empathizing with the patient's perspective and avoiding a power struggle (Johnson & Hauser, 2001). In dealing with aggression, as in other aspects of nursing practice, the nurse will find that at times the best intervention is silence. It is easy to equate intervention with activity, the sense that "I must do something." But quiet calmness on the nurse's part may be enough to help a patient regain control of his or her behavior.

When a violent outburst appears imminent or occurs, immediate intervention is required and should be directed by a designated leader (Box 38.8). Preassigning a crisis intervention leader at the change of shift or during a staff meeting can reduce confusion and time-consuming delays during a crisis. The crisis leader assumes responsibility for requesting additional staff, assigning staff duties, and designing and directing interventions (Brasic & Fogelman, 1999; Carpenito, 2003). The unit environment can be modified by closing off parts of the space and regulating the flow of people into and out of various spaces (Johnson & Delaney, 2006). For example, a smoking room could be locked for a period of time.

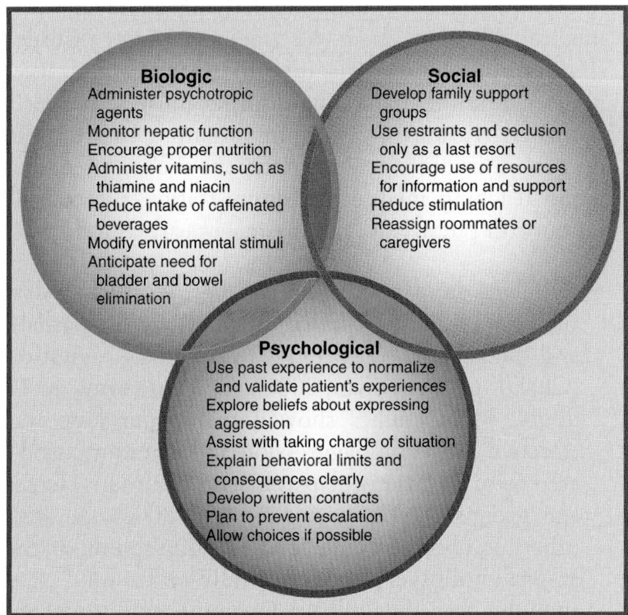

FIGURE 38.2. Biopsychosocial interventions for patients with aggression.

BOX 38.8

Guidelines for Crisis Intervention

1. Call for assistance (e.g., other nurses, security staff).
2. Brief all staff; plan intervention.
3. Assign staff to limbs should physical restraint or movement of the patient become necessary.
4. Remove other patients from the area. Also, remove any items that may impede the staff's movement.
5. Crisis intervention leader talks to the patient firmly and calmly. Other staff are present.
6. Leader gives patient choices (e.g., go to room to calm down, talk with someone, lose privileges, take medication).
7. If patient continues to argue, leader tells the patient that staff will escort him or her to his or her room. If the patient refuses to walk, staff carry patient to the room.

Trying to clarify what has upset the patient is important, although not all patients are capable of articulating what provoked them, and some analyses will have to take place after a crisis has been diffused. The nurse can use therapeutic communication techniques to prevent a crisis or diffuse a critical situation (see Box 38.9). During daily interactions with patients, nurses intervene in many creative and useful ways. The intervention alone does not serve as the solution; it is the process or art of offering the intervention within the context of the nurse–patient relationship that is more likely to be successful. No intervention will be successful with all patients all the time. However, it is not the nurse's or patient's fault when an intervention is ineffective. The intervention simply did not fit the situation at that particular time.

Biologic Domain

Biologic Assessment

The nurse may encounter patients whose aggressive tendencies have been exacerbated by a biochemical imbalance. However, nurses must recognize that biologic alterations are neither necessary nor sufficient to account for most aggressive behaviors. In taking the patient's history, the nurse listens for evidence of industrial exposure to toxic chemicals, missed doses of medications, alcohol intoxication, and withdrawal, or premenstrual dysphoric disorder. Similarly, a history of even minor structural changes resulting in trauma, hem-

BOX 38.9

***Therapeutic Dialogue:* The Potentially Aggressive Patient**

Paul is a 23-year-old patient in the high observation area of an inpatient unit. He is pacing back and forth. He is pounding one fist into his other hand. In the last 24 hours Paul has been more cooperative and less agitated. The behavior the nurse observes now is more like the behavior that Paul displayed 2 days ago. Yesterday the psychiatrist told Paul that he would be granted more freedom in the unit if his behavior improved. The psychiatrist has just seen Paul and refused to change the restrictions on Paul's activities.

Ineffective Approach

Nurse: Paul, I can understand this is frustrating for you.

Paul: How can you understand? Have you ever been held like a prisoner?

Nurse: I do understand, Paul. Now you must calm down or more privileges will be removed.

Paul: [voice gets louder] But I was told that calm behavior would mean more privileges. Now you are telling me calm behavior only gets me what I have got! Can't you talk to the doctor for me?

Nurse: No, Paul, I can't talk to the doctor. [Paul appears more frustrated and agitated as the conversation continues]

Effective Approach

Nurse: Paul, you look upset (observation). What happened in your conversation with the psychiatrist? (seeking information)

Paul: Yesterday he said calmer behavior would mean more freedom in the unit. I have tried to be calmer and not to swear. You said you noticed the difference. But today he says "no" to more freedom.

Nurse: Some people might feel cheated if this happened to them. (Validation). Is that how you feel?

Paul: Yeah, I feel real cheated. Nothing I do makes a difference. That's the way it is here and that's the way it is when I am out of the hospital.

Nurse: Sounds like experiences like this leave you feeling pretty powerless. (Validation).

Paul: I don't have any power, anywhere. Sometimes when I have no power I get mean. At least then people pay attention to me.

Nurse: In this situation with your doctor, what would help you feel that you had some power? (Inviting patient partnership).

Paul: Well if he would listen to me; if he would read my chart.

Nurse: I am a bit confused by the psychiatrist's decision. I won't make promises that your privileges will change but would it be okay with you if I talk with him?

Paul: That would make me feel like someone is on my side.

Critical Thinking Challenge

- In the first scenario, how did the nurse escalate the situation?
- Compare the first scenario with the second. How are they different?

orrhage, or tumor may contribute to lowering a patient's anger threshold, and thus requires investigation.

Aggressive episodes that are mainly biologic in origin share certain characteristics (Corrigan, Yudofsky, & Silver, 1993):

- The patient has a history or evidence of central nervous system (CNS) lesion or dysfunction.
- Onset of the episode is sudden and relatively unprovoked.
- The outburst is less controlled than those associated with external influences.
- The episode has a clear beginning and ending.
- The patient expresses remorse after the episode.

Sensory Impairment

Sensory impairment and difficulties in communicating have been reported as one precipitant of agitation in older adults (Allen, 1999). The most common impairments are hearing loss and reduced visual acuity. A common component of nursing assessment documents is visual and hearing impairments. If a patient cannot provide information about his or her hearing and vision, the nurse should ask a family member or friend. If there are impairments, the nurse should ensure that hearing aids are working for patients who use them and assess patients for access to glasses or contact lenses.

Interventions for the Biologic Domain

Administering and Monitoring Medications

Several classes of drugs are used in the management of aggressive behavior. Because anger and aggression can be symptomatic of many underlying psychiatric or medical disorders, from posttraumatic stress disorder (PTSD) and bipolar disorder to toxicities and head injuries, first the underlying disorder must be properly evaluated (Edwards, 2006). Important points for the nurse to consider in making decisions about patient and family teaching, medication administration, and consultation with physicians and pharmacists are as follows:

- Evidence supports the use of *atypical antipsychotics*, such as clozapine (Clozaril), risperidone (Risperdal), and olanzapine (Zyprexa), in reducing agitation (Chakos & Lieberman, 2001). A recent review of 19 double-blind studies showed that risperidone was effective in treating aggression and agitation associated with a variety of psychiatric disorders, across age groups (DeDeyn & Buitelaar, 2006). As with other psychotropic medications, the action of the atypical antipsychotics is not fully understood. It is thought that they block dopamine and serotonin receptors. Extrapyramidal side effects are few, which makes these drugs easier to tolerate than the typical antipsychotics (see the drug profile on risperidone [Risperdal] in Chapter 18 for more information).

- *Selective serotonin reuptake inhibitors* (SSRIs) (e.g., fluoxetine [Prozac], paroxetine [Paxil]) are increasingly being used for their antiaggressive effects, as well as for their antidepressant effects. Because their onset of action is gradual, SSRIs are not used when immediate control of dysfunctional anger is desired. However, their effects on aggressive behavior usually occur before their effects on depression.
- *Anxiolytic medications* exert a calming effect by increasing brain levels of gamma-aminobutyric acid (GABA). Therefore, drugs such as alprazolam (Xanax) or lorazepam (Ativan) may be employed to quickly calm an angry patient (Edwards, 2006).
- *β-adrenergic receptor blockers*, such as propranolol (Inderal), may be used for their effect in decreasing the peripheral manifestations of rage that are associated with excitement of the sympathetic nervous system (Silver et al., 2000).
- *Lithium carbonate* has been effective in treating explosive aggression and aggressive behavior associated with head injury.
  - *Divalproex sodium* (Depakote), *carbamazepine* (Tegretol), and *oxcarbazepine* (Trileptal) have been shown to reduce aggressive behavior.
  - Psychotropic drugs often interact with antiepileptic and antispasmodic agents, altering pharmacokinetics. For example, chlorpromazine may increase the risk for seizures in patients taking antiepileptic drugs (Fahs, Potiron, Senon, & Perivier, 1999).
  - The liver metabolizes most psychotropic drugs (except lithium). The nurse should be alert to possible hepatic dysfunction in patients with a history of alcohol or drug abuse.

Managing Nutrition

Patients with longstanding poor dietary habits (e.g., indigent patients, patients with alcoholism) often have deficiencies of thiamine and niacin. Prolonged use of alcohol can block as much as 70% of thiamine uptake. Increased irritability, disorientation, and paranoia may result. Encouraging patients to eat more whole grains, nuts, fruits, vegetables, organ meats, and milk, instead of "junk" foods, is important. The nurse may need to help patients with obtaining the resources needed to buy and prepare healthier food choices.

Caffeine is a potent stimulant (Lorist & Tops, 2003). Some inpatient psychiatric units have restricted patients' accessibility to coffee and other caffeinated beverages as a means to reduce aggressive behavior. Results have been mixed.

Anticipating Needs

The nurse can anticipate many biologic needs of patients. In assuming responsibility for patients with cognitive impairment, the nurse needs to know when the patient last voided and the pattern of bowel movements. Regular toileting routines are not just interventions to prevent incontinence. Similarly, the anticipation of basic needs such as thirst and hunger is important, especially when working with adults or children who cannot readily express their needs. Other discomforts can arise from such conditions as ingrown toenails and adverse medication reactions.

The urge to void can be a powerful stimulus to agitated behavior. For example, a 75-year-old woman was pacing around a psychogeriatric unit, crying for her mother. Various people spoke kindly to her, trying to explain that her mother was not there. Donna, a graduate student, was studying the wandering behaviors of patients with Alzheimer's disease on the unit. Hypothesizing that there is purpose behind these actions, she walked alongside the woman. After talking a bit with her about the patient's mother, Donna asked the patient what she would like to do if her mother were there. Gradually the patient confided that she needed her mother to help her find the bathroom. Donna then offered to help the woman, walking her to the bathroom. After voiding copiously, the patient seemed greatly relieved and settled down.

Psychological Domain

Psychological Assessment

The nurse working with patients to prevent and manage aggression should observe them for disturbances in thought processing. This is especially important for newly admitted patients, who should be under closer surveillance while careful assessment takes place. Patients may have disordered thoughts for various reasons, including psychiatric diagnoses such as major depressive episode, bipolar disorder, delusional disorders, PTSD, schizophrenia, and depersonalization. The nurse should also look for a current or past history of substance abuse because patients who abuse drugs, alcohol, or solvents may also exhibit disordered thought processing. Intoxication can trigger erratic thought processes and unpredicted violence. Some form of thought disorder may remain after a person is detoxified, becoming a permanent feature of the person's way of processing ideas. In addition, the nurse must look for acute and chronic medical conditions, such as brain tumor, encephalitis, electrolyte imbalance, and hepatic failure, which may also alter thought-processing (Citrome & Volavka, 1999). The thought processes of greatest interest to the nurse in assessing a patient's potential for aggression and violence are perception and delusion.

Perception

Perception is awareness of events and sensations and the ability to make distinctions between them. Patients with disordered perceptions may misinterpret objects or events. Such misperception is called an *illusion*. For example, a patient may assume that a person walking toward him or her is going to strike out and thus take action to defend against this illusionary foe. The nurse can explore a patient's perception by asking such questions as, "I noticed you were looking very cautious as I approached you. I wonder what you are thinking?"

Delusions

Patients may maintain false or unreasonable beliefs, known as delusions. The nurse may not notice any abnormalities in the patient's behavior or appearance until the patient begins to discuss the delusional ideas. Discussion of the delusions may precipitate aggressive or violent behavior. To explore these false beliefs, the nurse could, with the patient's consent, ask questions respectfully. The nurse should match the pacing of such questions to the patient's responses. Attempts to dissuade the patient from his or her beliefs are usually ineffective.

Interventions for the Psychological Domain

Psychological interventions help patients gain control over their expression of anger and aggressive behavior, thereby reducing the need for chemical or mechanical restraints. De-escalating potential aggression is always preferable to challenging or provoking a patient. Anger control assistance, as set forth by the *Nursing Interventions Classification* (*NIC*) (Dochterman & Bulechek, 2004), is useful and can prevent deterioration of a patient's control of behavior (Box 38.10). For example, nurses at a psychiatric center in New York state (Visalli, McNasser, Johnstone, & Lazzaro, 1997) developed an anger management assessment tool and a handout for use by patients. In a 1-year follow-up study, they reported a reduction in the use of seclusion and restraint and an increase in the successful use of alternative interventions to respond to aggression.

Affective Interventions

Affective interventions are designed to reduce intense emotions that may hinder the patient from finding alternatives to the use of aggression or violence (Wright & Leahey, 2000). They include validating, listening to the patient's illness experience, and exploring beliefs.

Validating. Patients who experience intense anger and rage can feel isolated and anxious. The nurse can acknowledge these intense feelings by reflecting "This

BOX 38.10

Anger Control Assistance

Definition: Facilitation of the expression of anger adaptively and nonviolently

Activities

- Establish basic trust and rapport with patient.
- Use a calm, reassuring approach.
- Determine appropriate behavior expectations for expression of anger, given patient's level of cognitive and physical functioning.
- Limit patient's access to frustrating situations until he or she can express anger adaptively.
- Encourage patient to seek assistance of nursing staff or responsible others during periods of increasing tension.
- Monitor patient's potential for inappropriate aggression and intervene before its expression.
- Prevent physical harm (e.g., apply restraint, remove potential weapons) if patient directs anger at self or others.
- Provide reassurance to patient that nursing staff will intervene to prevent him or her from losing control.
- Use external controls (e.g., physical or manual restraint, time-outs, seclusion) as needed to calm a patient who is expressing anger destructively.
- Provide feedback on behavior to help patient identify anger.
- Assist patient in identifying the source of anger.
- Identify the function that anger, frustration, and rage serve for the patient.
- Identify consequences of inappropriate expressions of anger.
- Assist patient in planning strategies to prevent the inappropriate expression of anger.
- Identify with patient the benefits of expressing anger adaptively and nonviolently.
- Establish expectation that patient can control his or her behavior.
- Instruct patient on use of calming measures (e.g., time-outs, deep breaths).
- Assist patient to develop appropriate methods of expressing anger to others (e.g., assertiveness, use of statements).
- Provide role models who express anger appropriately.
- Support patient in implementing anger-control strategies and appropriately expressing anger.
- Provide reinforcement for appropriate expression of anger.

Adapted from McCloskey, J., & Bulechek, G. (2000): *Nursing interventions classification (NIC)* (3rd ed.). St. Louis: Mosby.

must be scary for you." Empathic responding can reduce emotional arousal because the patient feels understood and supported (Jarry & Paivio, 2006). By drawing on past experience with other patients, the nurse can also reassure the patient that others have felt the same way.

Listening to the Patient's Illness Experience. Patients and their family members are routinely requested to provide details about past medical treatments, medications, hospitalizations, and therapies. What is often overlooked is the subjective experience of the health problem (Thomas & Pollio, 2002). Many patients with persistent mental illness have had frightening medication reactions and unpleasant side effects of treatments (such as memory loss due to electroconvulsive therapy). Understandably, they may harbor distrust of mental health clinicians. Disappointment with "playing little games with staff" or "attending classes" has been expressed by hospitalized psychiatric patients who longed for a deeper connection with nursing staff and more intensive insight-oriented therapies (Thomas, Shattell, & Martin, 2002). Inviting patients and families to talk about their previous experiences with the health care system may highlight both their concerns and resources.

Exploring Beliefs. Exploring the patient's beliefs about the expression of angry feelings can be useful. Obviously, this type of discussion is not undertaken when the patient is too agitated to think clearly.

Cognitive Interventions

Cognitive interventions provide new ideas, opinions, information, or education about a particular problem. The nurse offers a cognitive intervention with the goal of inviting the patient to consider other possibilities (Wright & Leahey, 2000). Examples include giving commendations, offering information, providing education, and using thought stopping and contracting.

• NCLEXNOTE

NCLEXNOTE

The best time to teach the patient techniques for managing anger and aggression is when the patient is not experiencing the provoking event. Cognitive therapy approaches are useful and can be prioritized according to responses.

Giving Commendations. Often, in clinical settings, the focus becomes "problem saturated" (White, 1988/89) and what the patient does well is overlooked. A commendation focuses on the patient's behavior pattern over time and highlights his or her strengths and resources (Limacher & Wright, 2003). For example, commending a patient's decision to request medication or to remove herself from an overstimulating environment highlights the woman's ability to assume responsibility for thoughts and feelings that have previously precipitated aggressive behavior.

Offering Information. Nurses can offer information or arrange opportunities for patients to receive information from other professionals. Patients may sometimes become agitated and threaten to harm the nurse because they do not know what is expected of them or they do not remember why they need to be in treatment. The nurse can tell them about unit expectations or the reasons for hospitalization.

In the inpatient setting, the nurse must make behavioral limits and consequences clear. Many units prohibit patients from entering other patients' rooms and from borrowing personal items (Johnson & Delaney, 2006). Consequences for rule violations should be explained on admission and applied consistently thereafter. When possible, the nurse should match consequences for rule infractions to the patient's interests and desires. For example, Jane was slamming doors and banging dishes in the kitchen of the group home. The nurse approached her to discuss other means of expressing her anger. During the conversation, the nurse reminded Jane that further disruptive behavior would mean that Jane would not participate in a shopping trip planned that day. The trip was important to Jane, so she chose to discuss her concern with the nurse.

Providing Education. Inpatient hospitalization offers opportunities for education of patients and families about a variety of topics. Nurses can seize "teachable moments" to convey important principles of anger management. For example, after an outburst of loud cursing by John, who mistakenly thought another patient (Jim) had stolen his cigarettes, the nurse helped him consider what he could have done differently in the situation. John was more amenable to learning about calming techniques and problem-solving strategies at this time because his behavior had resulted in adverse consequences (estrangement from Jim, disruption of the dayroom during a popular bingo game, and cancellation of his weekend pass). This incident could also be used for teaching in a subsequent group meeting of inpatients. Many units have daily meetings that permit processing of such conflicts. Jim could be invited to express his feelings about being falsely accused of stealing. Other patients may reveal how distressed they were when John was cursing loudly, providing John useful peer feedback about his outburst. Together, group members could generate ideas for more appropriate behavior.

Thought Stopping. In thought stopping, the nurse asks the patient to identify thoughts that heighten feelings of anger and invites the patient to "turn the thoughts off" by focusing on other thoughts or activities. Ideas of other activities include talking to someone, reading, baking, or thinking about a future event.

Contracting. A contract is a written document that the nurse and patient develop. The document clearly states acceptable and unacceptable behaviors, consequences and rewards, and the role of both the patient and nurse in preventing and managing aggressive behavior (Morrison, 1998).

Behavioral Interventions

Behavioral interventions are designed to assist the patient to behave differently (Wright & Leahey, 2000). Examples of such interventions include assigning behavioral tasks, using bibliotherapy, interrupting patterns, and providing choices.

Assigning Behavioral Tasks. Sometimes, the nurse may assign a behavioral task as a way to help the patient maintain or regain control over aggressive behaviors. Behavioral tasks might include writing down a list of grievances that the patient will discuss with the nurse or observing how other people take charge of anger and aggression. For example, the nurse may ask the patient to observe patients or staff on the unit, people at a shopping mall, or particular movies or television shows to evaluate how other people in real or fictitious situations handle anger. Because many patients say they never learned to discuss angry feelings at home (Lanza, Kayne, Pattison, Hicks, & Islam, 1996), staff can model assertive anger statements ("I feel angry because ______ and here is what I would like to be different") and oversee the practice of new behaviors with staff or other patients in role-playing scenarios.

> **KEY CONCEPTS Assertiveness** is a set of behaviors and a communication style that is open, honest, direct, and confident. Assertiveness enables the expression of emotions, including anger, in a manner that assumes responsibility. It allows placement of boundaries and prevents acceptance of inappropriate aggression from others.

Using Bibliotherapy. In bibliotherapy, the nurse may ask the patient to read a particular pamphlet or article on anger management. The nurse and patient then discuss what the patient read to decide which, if any, of the ideas the patient can use when angry.

Interrupting Patterns. Although patients are not usually aware of it, escalation of feelings, thoughts, and behavior from calmness to violence usually follows a particular pattern. Disruption of the pattern can sometimes be a useful means for preventing escalation and can help the patient regain composure. Nurses can suggest several strategies to interrupt patterns:

- Counting to 10
- Using a relaxation or breathing technique (see chapter 13)
- Removing oneself from interactions or stimuli that may contribute to increased distress (voluntarily taking "time-out")
- Doing something different (e.g., reading, listening to quiet music, watching television)

Providing Choices. When possible, the nurse should provide the patient with choices, particularly patients who have little control over their situation because of their condition. Offering concrete choices is better than offering open-ended options (Johnson & Hauser, 2001). For example, the patient who is experiencing a manic episode and is confined to her room may have few options in her daily schedule. However, she may be allowed to make choices about food, personal hygiene, and which pajamas to wear.

Social Domain

Social Assessment

The nurse should evaluate factors related to the social domain that may be contributing to aggression or violence in a patient. Are crisis conditions in the patient's home, family, or community leading to aggression or violent episodes? Are financial or legal troubles placing increased stress on the patient? Is the patient experiencing conflict with other patients on the unit, or with certain staff? People re-enact in new relationships the same behaviors that created problems in old ones. Thus, behavior in a mental health facility provides important clues to a patient's habitual responses to authority figures, opposite-sex peers, and same-sex peers. Assessment data provide direction for interventions such as reassigning roommates or caregivers.

If assessment reveals stressful actions by family members, such as evicting the patient from the home, attention must be devoted to mobilizing resources for support and alternative housing.

Interventions for the Social Domain

Reducing Stimulation

People differ as to the level of stimulation that they need or prefer (Kolanowski, Hurwitz, Taylor, Evans, & Strumpf, 1994). Normally, they adjust their environments accordingly: Some people like their music loud, whereas others want it soft; some people seek out the thrill of high-risk sports, whereas others prefer to be spectators. Within the context of a brain disorder or an unusually restrictive environment, such adjustments may not be within the patient's control. The patient with a brain injury, progressive dementia, or distorted vision may be experiencing intense and highly confusing stimulation, even though the environment, from the nurse or family's perspective, seems calm and orderly.

For people whose perceptions or thoughts are disordered from brain damage, degeneration, or other thought-processing difficulties, modification of the environment may be one of the main interventions. Likewise, introducing more structure into a chaotic environment can help decrease the risk for aggressive behavior (Citrome & Volavka, 1999). The nurse can make stimuli meaningful or can simplify and interpret the environment in many practical ways, such as by identifying people or equipment that may be unfamiliar, providing cues as to what is expected (e.g., posting signs with directions, putting toothbrush and toothpaste by the sink), and removing or silencing unnecessary stimuli (e.g., turning off paging systems). A good place to start is with the NIC environmental management interventions (Box 38.11). Considering the environment from the patient's viewpoint is essential. For instance, if the surroundings are unfamiliar, the patient will need to process more information. Lack of a recognizable pattern or structure further taxes the patient's capacity to encode information. Appropriate interventions include clarifying the meaning and purpose of people and objects in the environment, enhancing the patient's sense of control and the predictability of the environment, and reducing other stimuli as much as possible (Stolley, Gerdner, & Buckwalter, 1999).

Using Seclusion and Restraint

Seclusion and restraint are used when patients need to be separated from other patients on the unit. However, as noted in Chapter 10, these are controversial interventions to be used judiciously and only when other interventions have failed to control the patient's behavior. Reasons traditionally cited for using them are to protect the patient from injury to self or others, to help the patient re-establish behavioral control, and to minimize disruption of unit treatment regimens. Only recently has there been recognition that these interventions cause considerable psychological damage, in some cases replicating childhood traumas. Seclusion may be extremely painful to a patient who has already experienced abandonment and rejection (Holmes, Kennedy, & Perron, 2004). Restraint may re-create trauma comparable to a rape ("They held me down, they pulled my drawers down") (Benson et al., 2003). Gerolamo (2006) strongly argues that restraint use in acute psychiatric settings should be considered an *adverse outcome*. The controversy over these interventions and their potential to be applied punitively provided impetus for issuance of federal guidelines for their use. American institutions that receive Medicare or Medicaid reimbursement must adhere to guidelines issued by the Center for Medicare and Medicaid Services. Restraint-related injuries and deaths have prompted many facilities to ban their use entirely and train staff in alternative techniques.

BOX 38.11

Environmental Management: Violence Prevention

Definition: Monitoring and manipulating the physical environment to decrease the potential of violent behavior directed toward self, others, or environment

Activities

- Remove potential weapons (e.g., sharps, ropelike objects) from the environment.
- Search environment routinely to maintain it as hazard free.
- Search patient and belongings for weapons or potential weapons during inpatient admission procedures as appropriate.
- Monitor the safety of items that visitors bring to the environment.
- Instruct visitors and other caregivers about relevant patient safety issues.
- Limit patient use of potential weapons (e.g., sharps, ropelike objects).
- Monitor patient during use of potential weapons (e.g., razors).
- Place patient with potential for self-harm with a roommate to decrease isolation and opportunity to act on self-harm thoughts, as appropriate.
- Assign single room to patient with potential for violence toward others.
- Place patient in a bedroom located near a nursing station.
- Limit access to windows, unless locked and shatterproof, as appropriate.
- Lock utility and storage rooms.
- Provide paper dishes and plastic utensils at meals.
- Place patient in the least restrictive environment that still allows for the necessary level of observation.
- Provide ongoing surveillance of all patient access areas to maintain patient safety and therapeutically intervene, as needed.
- Remove other individuals from the vicinity of a violent or potentially violent patient.
- Maintain a designated safe area (e.g., seclusion room) for patient to be placed when violent.
- Provide plastic, rather than metal, clothes hangers, as appropriate.

Adapted from Dochterman, J., & Bulechek, G. (2000). *Nursing interventions classification (NIC)* (4th ed.). St. Louis: Mosby.

Interactional Processes

The skills the nurse uses in interactions with the patient may invite escalation or de-escalation of a tense situation (Morrison, 1998). When the nurse uses communication skills to draw out the patient's experience, together the nurse and patient coevolve an alternative view of the problem. Some nursing writers (Leahey & Harper-Jaques, 1996; Vosburgh & Simpson, 1993; Wright & Leahey, 2000) have highlighted the importance of attending to notions of reciprocity and circularity when providing nursing care. For example, the nurse explores the meaning of the expression of aggressive behaviors with the patient and the patient's beliefs about the ability to control aggressive impulses. Or the nurse and patient could discuss the effects of the nurse's behaviors on the patient and the effects of the patient's behaviors on the nurse. Such an approach facilitates the development of an accepting and equal nurse–patient relationship. The patient is a partner invited to assume responsibility for inappropriate actions. This approach is in contrast to a hierarchical nurse–patient relationship that emphasizes the nurse's role in controlling the patient's behaviors and defining changes the patient must make. In a collaborative approach, the nurse values the patient's experience and acknowledges his or her strengths. The nurse asks the patient to use those strengths to either maintain or resume control of behavior.

Responding to Assault on Nurses

Because nurses have extended contact with patients during highly stressful circumstances, there is always the risk that they may be the recipients of patient aggression. Nurses are the targets of patient violence more often than any other health care professional (Arnetz, Arnetz, & Soderman, 1998). Assaults tend to occur in situations in which the patient perceives the nurse's actions as restricting, controlling, or aggressive (e.g., the use of physical restraints) (Morrison, 1998). The reported rates of assaults on nurses vary greatly. The incidence is higher in general hospitals and psychiatric facilities, but nurses who work in ambulatory care settings or community clinics are not immune to assault. Variations in statistics result from differences in definitions of violence, reporting practices, and data collection and analysis, as well as underreporting. Nurses seldom prosecute their attackers.

Assaults on nurses by patients can have both immediate and long-term consequences, as shown in Lanza's research (1992) (see Table 38.3). Reported assaults range from verbal threats and minor altercations to severe injuries, rape, and murder. Any assault can produce severe sequelae for the victim. Because of their role as caregivers, nurses may suppress the normal range of feelings after an assault, believing that it is wrong to experience strong feelings of anger and fear in this situation. This belief may relate to the conflict nurses experience in having to care for patients who have hurt them. The conflict between one's professional role as caregiver and one's own needs as an assault victim has been explored in a support group for nurses and nursing assistants who had been assaulted (Lanza, Demaio, & Benedict, 2005). The support group met twice per week for 6 weeks, allowing expression of anger, blame, and anxiety, and concluding with development of personal plans for working with potentially assaultive patients.

Unfortunately, patient aggression directed toward nurses is often minimized or tolerated by nurses as "part of the job" (Poster & Drew, 2006). Aggression by patients

Table 38.3 Nurses' Respones to Assault

Response Type	Personal	Professional
Affective	• Irritability • Depression • Anger • Anxiety • Apathy	• Erosion of feelings of competence, leading to increased anxiety and fear • Feelings of guilt or self-blame • Fear of potentially violent patients
Cognitive	• Suppressed or intrusive thoughts of assault	• Reduced confidence in judgment • Consideration of job change
Behavioral	• Social withdrawal	• Possible hesitation in responding to other violent situations • Possible over-controlling • Possible hesitation to report future assaults • Possible withdrawal from colleagues • Questioning of capabilities by coworkers
Physiologic	• Disturbed sleep • Headaches • Stomach aches • Tension	• Increased absenteeism from somatic complaints

must be addressed more vigorously because it can threaten the other patients, other health care professionals, family members, and visitors, as well as the nursing staff. Steps can be taken to reduce the incidence of patient assault. Nurses must be provided with training programs in the prevention and management of aggressive behavior. These programs, like courses on cardiopulmonary resuscitation (CPR), impart both knowledge and skills. Like CPR training, the courses need to be made available to nurses regularly so that they have opportunities to reinforce and update what they have learned. Nurses who have participated in preventive training programs as students or as professionals become more confident in coping with patient aggression (Needham et al., 2005). Those with no training are at greater risk (Brasic & Fogelman, 1999). Less experienced staff with poor communication skills are at higher risk for assault (Wright, Dixon, & Tompkins, 2003). Morrison and Love (2003) caution that many commercially marketed training programs fail to consider the predatory aspect of some patients' violence and fail to cite nursing research. The quality of training programs must be systematically evaluated.

Evaluation and Treatment Outcomes

Treatment outcomes can be considered at both individual and aggregate levels. The desired outcome at the individual level is for the patient to regain or maintain control over aggressive or potentially aggressive thoughts, feelings, and actions. *Aggression Control* is the term used in the *Nursing Outcomes Classification* (*NOC*) (Moorhead, Johnson, & Maas, 2003). The nurse may observe that the patient shows decreased psychomotor activity (e.g., less pacing), has a more relaxed posture, speaks more directly about feelings of anger and personal needs, requires less sedating medication, shows increased tolerance for frustration and the ability to consider alternatives, and makes effective use of other coping strategies. Evidence of a reduction in risk factors may include decreased noise and confusion in the immediate environment, calmness on the part of nursing staff and others, and a climate of safety, clear expectations, and mutual acceptance and respect. In units, day hospitals, or group home settings, indicators of positive treatment outcomes would be a reduction in the number and severity of assaults on staff and other patients, fewer incident reports, and increased staff competency in de-escalating potentially violent situations.

Research and Policy Initiatives

Additional understanding of the phenomena of anger, aggression, and violence as they occur in the clinical setting is needed. Research studies that have illuminated this problem from a nursing perspective need to be continued and expanded. The links among biology, neurology, and psychology must be further elucidated. In addition, further explorations of the reciprocal influence of patient interactional style and treatment setting culture will assist in the development and management of humane treatment settings. Finally, and perhaps most importantly, nurses must research the effectiveness of particular anger and aggression management interventions (see Box 38.12). Although much of this chapter

BOX 38.12

Research for Best Practice: How Nurses and Patients Experience Patients' Aggression

Duxbury, J., & Whittington, R. (2005). Causes and management of patient aggression and violence: Staff and patient perspectives. Journal of Advanced Nursing, 50, 469–478.

QUESTION: (1) How do the views of patients and staff about the causes of aggression on 3 mental health wards compare? (2) What are patients' perspectives on existing aggression management approaches?

METHODS: A survey was conducted, using the Management of Aggression and Violence Scale (MAVAS), with follow-up audiotaped interviews of a subsample; 80 nurses and 82 patients (with diagnoses ranging from depression to schizophrenia) participated in the study.

MAVAS responses were analyzed using descriptive statistics, and a *t* test was used to compare staff and patients. Content analysis was employed with the interview data.

FINDINGS: Disagreements between patients and nurses were found on more than half of the MAVAS items. Patients were more likely to attribute their aggression to factors such as staff failure to listen and to the negative and restrictive atmosphere of the wards. Patients wanted alternatives to sedation and seclusion, such as negotiation.

Nurses were more likely to attribute patient aggression to psychopathology, consistent with the biomedical perspective that Duxbury (2002) found in an earlier study. Unlike the patients, nurses wanted seclusion to continue. Both staff and patients expressed dissatisfaction with the current status of aggression management.

IMPLICATIONS FOR NURSING: Despite the study limitations (convenience sample from 3 British inpatient units and use of a new survey tool), the study provides impetus for psychiatric nurses' self-assessment of their aggression management behaviors and thoughtful consideration of negative aspects of the inpatient environments in which they practice. This research study is suitable for conceptual utilization, that is, expanding ways of thinking about nursing practice.

focused on individuals who need to *down*-regulate anger, the reader must remember that anger suppressors have a need to *up*-regulate their anger and express it more assertively (Mayne & Ambrose, 1999). Treatments should be tailored accordingly, and patients' progress documented by administering questionnaires such as the STAXI both before and after the treatments. A practitioner's guide to comparative treatments of anger-related disorders was recently published (Feindler, 2006). However, authors in this edited volume caution that research is sparse regarding the efficacy of some treatments, especially for culturally diverse clients whose heritage is quite different from the Euro-American heritage of most mental health clinicians in the United States. Thomas (2006) points out the inadequacy of most training programs in preparing mental health professionals for work with culturally diverse clients. It is unknown what adaptations may be needed to deliver appropriate anger treatments to these individuals. Only by accruing sufficient empirical evidence can we obtain definitive guidance for clinical practice with angry and aggressive individuals.

There is a moral imperative for nurses to be involved in combating violence in the larger community. Lessening violence in the workplace and the home demands involvement of all mental health professionals. Nurses can share their expertise with parents, children, teachers, and community agencies. For example, Jones and Selder (1996) conducted groups for children at a community "safe house" to teach them how to cope with violence in their neighborhood. Compelling scientific evidence is now available to show that violence portrayed in the media is harmful to children. As a result, television networks have limited violent programming during hours when children are generally watching programs. However, this gain is offset by the growing availability of violent websites and videogames. Videogames actively involve players in violence and reward them for it (Winerman, 2006). Nurses can add their voices to those of activists who object to the content of these games and to offensive media offerings. As concerned citizens, nurses can advocate for changes in public policy such as those recommended by the World Health Organization in its "World Report on Violence and Health" (2002). Finally, nurses can support legislation to make assault on nurses a felony, like assault on lifeguards, bus drivers, jurors, umpires, and emergency medical technicians. The American Academy of Nursing Expert Panel on Violence (Love & Morrison, 2003) and other nursing organizations support such legislation, but few states have passed it. The epidemic of violence cannot be curtailed unless all of us become involved.

SUMMARY OF KEY POINTS

- Anger, aggression, and violence should not be viewed as a continuum. The anger of ordinary people seldom progresses to aggression or violence.
- Anger management is a useful psychoeducational intervention that is effective with a wide variety of nonviolent individuals. However, AM is not designed to modify violent behavior.
- Biopsychosocial theories used to explain anger, aggression, and violence include the following types:
  - —Neurobiologic, including the cognitive neuroassociation model, neurostructural model (the emotional circuit), and neurochemical model (low serotonin syndrome)
  - —Psychological, including psychoanalytic theories, behavioral theories, and cognitive theories
  - —Sociocultural theories
  - —Interactional theory
- Biologic factors to assess in patients who display aggressive and violent behaviors include exposure to toxic chemicals, use of medications, substance abuse, premenstrual dysphoric disorder, trauma, hemorrhage, and tumor.
- Biologic intervention choices include administering medications, anticipating needs, and managing nutrition.
- Psychological factors to assess in patients who display aggressive and violent behaviors include thought processing (e.g., perception, delusion) and sensory impairment.
- Psychological intervention choices can be affective (e.g., validating, listening, exploring beliefs), cognitive (e.g., giving commendations, offering information, providing education, using thought stopping or contracting), or behavioral (e.g., assigning tasks, using bibliotherapy, interrupting patterns, providing choices).
- Social intervention choices include reducing stimulation and using seclusion or restraints.
- Patient aggression and violence are serious concerns for nurses in all areas of clinical practice. Training in and policies and procedures for the prevention and management of aggressive episodes should be available in all work settings.

CRITICAL THINKING CHALLENGES

1 Mary Jane, a 24-year-old single woman, has just been admitted to an inpatient psychiatry unit. She was transferred to the unit from the emergency room, where she was treated for a drug overdose. She is sullen when she is introduced to her roommate and

refuses to answer the questions the nurse has that are part of the admission procedure. The nurse tells Mary Jane that he will come back later to see how she is. A few minutes later, Mary Jane approaches the nursing station and asks in a demanding tone to talk with someone and complains that she has been completely ignored since she came into the unit. What frameworks can the nurse use to understand Mary Jane's behavior? At this point in time, what data does he have to develop a plan of care? What interventions might the nurse choose to use to help Mary Jane behave in a manner that is consistent with the norms of this inpatient unit?

2 Discuss the influence of gender and cultural norms on the expression of anger. When a nurse is caring for a patient from a culture that the nurse is not familiar with, what could the nurse ask to ensure that her/his expectations of the patient's behavior are consistent with the gender and cultural norms of the patient?

3 Under what circumstances should people who are aggressive or violent be held accountable for their behavior? Are there any exceptions?

4 When a nurse minimizes verbally abusive behavior by a patient, family member, or health care colleague, what implicit message does she or he send?

The Insider: 1999. Russell Crowe plays a tobacco industry insider with scientific evidence that cigarettes are made to increase their addictive qualities. Al Pacino plays a news program producer who tries to get the story. Throughout the movie, many attempts are made to suppress the story.

VIEWING POINT: What is the goal of the people who use aggression and violence in this film?

Girl Interrupted: 2000. This movie tells the story of a young woman who is committed to a mental hospital after a suicide attempt.

VIEWING POINTS: In what way do the behaviors of the staff encourage aggression and violence? How do nurses intervene to help the patients regain or maintain control of aggressive behaviors?

REFERENCES

Allen, L. A. (1999). Treating agitation without drugs. *American Journal of Nursing, 99*(4), 36–42.

Arnetz, J. E., Arnetz, B. B., & Soderman, E. (1998). Violence toward health care workers. *American Association of Occupational Health Nurses Journal, 46*(3), 107–114.

Averill, J. R. (1983). Studies on anger and aggression: Implications for theories of emotion. *American Psychologist, 38*, 1145–1160.

Babcock, J. C., Miller, S. A., & Siard, C. (2003). Toward a typology of abusive women: Differences between partner-only and generally violent women in the use of violence. *Psychology of Women Quarterly, 27*, 153–161.

Bandura, A. (1973). *Aggression: A social learning analysis*. New York: Prentice-Hall.

Beck, A. T. (1976). *Cognitive therapy and emotional disorders*. New York: International Universities Press.

Beck, R., & Fernandez, E. (1998). Cognitive-behavioral therapy in the treatment of anger: A meta-analysis. *Cognitive Therapy and Research, 22*, 63–74.

Benson, A., Secker, I., Balfe, E., Lipsedge, M., Robinson, S., & Walker, J. (2003). Discourse of blame: Accounting for aggression and violence on an acute mental health inpatient unit. *Social Science and Medicine, 57*, 917–926.

Berkowitz, L. (1989). Frustration-aggression hypothesis: Examination and reformulation. *Psychological Bulletin, 106*(1), 59–73.

Best, M., Williams, J. M., & Coccaro, E. F. (2002). Evidence for a dysfunctional prefrontal circuit in patients with an impulsive aggressive disorder. *Proceedings of the National Academy of Sciences, 99*(12), 8448–8453.

Brasic, J. R., & Fogelman, D. (1999). Clinician safety. *Psychiatric Clinics of North America, 22*(4), 923–940.

Capra, F. (2002). *The hidden connections: Integrating the biological, cognitive and social dimensions of life into a science of sustainability*. New York: Doubleday.

Carlsson, G., Dahlberg, K., Ekeburgh, M., & Dahlberg, H. (2006). Patients longing for authentic personal care: A phenomenological study of violent encounters in psychiatric settings. *Issues in Mental Health Nursing, 27*, 287–305.

Carpenito, L. J. (2006). *Nursing diagnosis: Application to practice* (10th ed.). Philadelphia: Lippincott Williams & Wilkins.

Carrere, S., Mittmann, A., Woodin, E., Tabares, A., & Yoshimoto, D. (2005). Anger dysregulation, depressive symptoms, and health in married women and men. *Nursing Research, 54*, 184–192.

Caspi, A., McClay, J., Moffitt, T., Mill, J., Martin, J., Craig, I., Taylor, A., & Poulton, R. (2002). Role of genotype in the cycle of violence in maltreated children. *Science, 297*, 851–853.

Chakos, M., & Lieberman, J. A. (2001). Effects of clozapine, olanzapine, risperidone, and haloperidol on hostility among patients with schizophrenia. *Psychiatric Services, 52*(11), 1510–1514.

Citrome, L., & Volavka, J. (1999). Violent patients in the emergency setting. *Psychiatric Clinics of North America, 22*(4), 789–801.

Corrigan, P. W., Yudofsky, S. C., & Silver, J. M. (1993). Pharmacological and behavioral treatment for aggressive psychiatric in-patients. *Hospital and Community Psychiatry, 44*(3), 125–133.

Davey, L., Day, A., & Howells, K. (2005). Anger, over-control and serious violent offending. *Aggression and Violent Behavior, 10*, 624–635.

Davidson, K., MacGregor, M., Stuhr, J., Dixon, K., & Maclean, D. (2000). Constructive anger verbal behavior predicts blood pressure in a population-based sample. *Health Psychology, 19*, 55–64.

DeDeyn, P. P., & Buitelaar, J. (2006). Risperidone in the management of agitation and aggression associated with psychiatric disorders. *European Psychiatry, 21*, 21–28.

Deffenbacher, J. L. (2006). Evidence for effective treatment of anger-related disorders. In E. L. Feindler (Ed.), *Anger-related disorders: A practitioner's guide to comparative treatments* (pp. 43–69). New York: Springer.

Deffenbacher, J. L., Filetti, L. B., Richards, T. L., Lynch, R. S., & Oetting, E. R. (2003). Characteristics of two groups of angry drivers. *Journal of Counseling Psychology, 50*, 123–132.

Deffenbacher, J. L., Oetting, E. R., & Di Giuseppe, R. A. (2002). Principles of empirically supported interventions applied to anger management. *The Counseling Psychologist, 30*, 262–280.

Di Giuseppe, R. A. (1999). End piece: Reflections on the treatment of anger. *Journal of Clinical Psychology in Session: Psychotherapy in Practice, 55*, 365–379.

Dochterman, J., & Bulechek, G. (2004). *Nursing interventions classification (NIC)* (3rd ed.). St. Louis: Mosby.

Duxbury, J. (2002). An evaluation of staff and patient views of and strategies employed to manage inpatient aggression and violence on one mental health unit: A pluralistic design. *Journal of Psychiatric & Mental Health Nursing, 9*(3), 325–327.

Duxbury, J., & Whittington, R. (2005). Causes and management of patient aggression and violence: Staff and patient perspectives. *Journal of Advanced Nursing, 50*, 469–478.

Eckhardt, C., & Deffenbacher, J. L. (1995). Diagnosis of anger disorders. In H. Kassinove (Ed.), *Anger disorders: Definition, diagnosis, and treatment* (pp. 27–47). Washington, DC: Taylor and Francis.

Edwards, H. (2006). Psychopharmacological considerations in anger management. In E. L. Feindler (Ed.), *Anger-related disorders: A practitioner's guide to comparative treatments* (pp. 189–202). New York: Springer.

Ekman, P. (1993). Facial expression and emotion. *American Psychologist 48*, 384–392.

Ellis, A. (1977). *Anger: How to live with and without it*. Secaucus, NJ: Citadel Press.

Everson, S. A., Goldberg, D. E., Kaplan, G. A., Julkunen, J., & Salonen, J. (1998). Anger expression and incident hypertension. *Psychosomatic Medicine, 60*, 730–735.

Fahs, H., Potiron, G., Senon, J. L., & Perivier, E. (1999). Anticonvulsants in agitation and behavior disorders in demented subjects. *Encephale, 25*(2), 169–174.

Feindler, E.L. (2006). *Anger-related disorders: A practitioner's guide to comparative treatments*. New York: Springer.

Feindler, E. L., & Byers, A. (2006). Multiple perspectives on the conceptualization and treatment of anger-related disorders. In E. L. Feindler (Ed.), *Anger-related disorders: A practitioner's guide to comparative treatments* (pp. 303–320). New York: Springer.

Frey, R. E. C., & Weller, J. (2000). Rehab rounds: Behavioral management of aggression through teaching interpersonal skills. *Psychiatric Services, 51*, 607–609.

Galovski, T. (2001). Pre- and post-treatment psychophysiological reactivity of individuals diagnosed with IED: A controlled comparison. Paper presented at the Society of Behavioral Medicine, Seattle. March 21–24, 2007.

Gerolamo, A. M. (2006). The conceptualization of physical restraint as a nursing-sensitive adverse outcome in acute care psychiatric treatment settings. *Archives of Psychiatric Nursing, 20*, 175–185.

Goodman, M., Quigley, J., Moran, G., Meilman, H., & Sherman, M. (1996). Hostility predicts restenosis after percutaneous transluminal coronary angioplasty. *Mayo Clinic Proceedings, 71*, 729–734.

Green, B. (1990). What has gone before: The legacy of racism and sexism in the lives of black mothers and daughters. *Women and Therapy, 9*(1–3), 207–230.

Green, B., & Robinson, L. (2005). Reducing violence in a forensic mental health unit: A 7-year study. *Mental Health Practice, 9*(4), 40–44.

Harburg, J., Julius, M., Kaciroti, N., Gleiberman, L., & Schork, M. (2003). Expressive/suppressive anger-coping responses, gender, and types of mortality: A 17-year follow-up (Tecumseh, Michigan, 1971–1988). *Psychosomatic Medicine, 65*, 588–597.

Harper-Jaques, S., & Masters, A. (1994). Powerful words: The use of letters with sexual abuse survivors. *Journal of Psychosocial Nursing and Mental Health Services, 32*(8), 11–16.

Harper-Jaques, S., & Reimer, M. (1992). Aggressive behavior and the brain: A different perspective for the mental health nurse. *Archives of Psychiatric Nursing, 6*(5), 312–320.

Harris, D., & Morrison, E. F. (1995). Managing violence without coercion. *Archives of Psychiatric Nursing, 9*(4), 203–210.

Holmes, D., Kennedy, S., & Perron, A. (2004). The mentally ill and social exclusion: A critical examination of the use of seclusion from the patient's perspective. *Issues in Mental Health Nursing, 25*, 559–578.

Ireland, J. (2004). Anger management therapy with young male offenders: An evaluation of treatment outcome. *Aggressive Behavior, 30*, 174–185.

Ironson, G., Taylor, C. B., Boltwood, M., Bartzokis, T., Dennis, C., Chesney, M., et al. (1992). Effects of anger on left ventricular ejection fraction in coronary artery disease. *American Journal of Cardiology, 70*, 281–285.

Jack, D.C. (1999). *Behind the mask: Destruction and creativity in women's aggression*. Cambridge, MA: Harvard University Press.

Jarry, J., & Paivio, S. (2006). Emotion-focused therapy for anger. In E. L. Feindler (Ed.), *Anger-related disorders: A practitioner's guide to comparative treatments* (pp. 203–229). New York: Springer.

Jenkins, A. (1990). *Invitations to responsibility*. Adelaide, NSW, Australia: Dulwich Centre Publications.

Johnson, M. E. (2004). Violence on inpatient psychiatric units: State of the science. *Journal of the American Psychiatric Nurses Association, 10*(3), 113–121.

Johnson, M. E., & Hauser, P. M. (2001). The practices of expert psychiatric nurses: Accompanying the patient to a calmer personal space. *Issues in Mental Health Nursing, 22*, 651–668.

Johnson, M. E., & Delaney, K. R. (2006). Keeping the unit safe: A grounded theory study. *Journal of the American Psychiatric Nurses Association, 12*(1), 13–21.

Jones, F. C., & Selder, F. (1996). Psychoeducational groups to promote effective coping in school-age children living in violent communities. *Issues in Mental Health Nursing, 17*, 559–571.

Kavoussi, R., Armstead, P., & Coccaro, E. (1997). The neurobiology of aggression. *Psychiatric Clinics of North America, 20*(2), 395–403.

Kessler, R., Coccaro, E., Fava, M., Jaeger, S., Jin, R., & Walters, E. (2006). The prevalence and correlates of DSM-IV intermittent explosive disorder in the National Comorbidity Survey replication. *Archives of General Psychiatry, 63*, 669–678.

Kindy, D., Petersen, S., & Parkhurst, D. (2005). Perilous work: Nurses' experiences in psychiatric units with high risks of assault. *Archives of Psychiatric Nursing, 19*, 169–175.

Knafo, D. (2004). Introduction. In D. Knafo (Ed)., *Living with terror, working with trauma: A clinician's handbook* (pp. 1–15). Lanham, MD: Aronson.

Koh, K. B., Kim, C. H., & Park, J. K. (2002). Predominance of anger in depressive disorders compared with anxiety disorders and somatoform disorders. *Journal of Clinical Psychiatry, 6*, 486–492.

Kolanowski, A., Hurwitz, S., Taylor, L. A., Evans, L., & Strumpf, N. (1994). Contextual factors associated with disturbing behavior of institutionalized elders. *Nursing Research, 43*(2), 73–79.

Kubzansky, L. D., & Kawachi, I. (2000). Going to the heart of the matter: Do negative emotions cause coronary heart disease? *Journal of Psychosomatic Research, 48*, 323–337.

Lanza, M. L. (1992). Nurses as patient assault victims: An update, synthesis, and recommendations. *Archives of Psychiatric Nursing, 6*(3), 163–171.

Lanza, M. L., Demaio, J., & Benedict, M. A. (2005). Patient assault support group: Achieving educational objectives. *Issues in Mental Health Nursing, 26*, 643–660.

Lanza, M. L., Kayne, H. L., Pattison, I., Hicks, C., & Islam, S. (1996). The relationship of behavioral clues to assaultive behavior. *Clinical Nursing Research, 5*, 6–27.

Leahey, M., & Harper-Jaques, S. (1996). Family–nurse relationship: Core assumptions and clinical implications. *Journal of Family Nursing, 2*(2), 133–151.

Lench, H. (2004). Anger management: Diagnostic differences and treatment implications. *Journal of Social and Clinical Psychology, 23*, 512–531.

Lerner, H. (1997). *The dance of anger: A woman's guide to changing the patterns of intimate relationships*. New York: Harper & Row.

Limacher, L. H., & Wright, L. M. (2003). Commendations: Listening to the silent side of a family intervention. *Journal of Family Nursing, 9*(2), 130–150.

Liu, J. (2004). Concept analysis: Aggression. *Issues in Mental Health Nursing, 25*, 693–714.

Lorist, M. M., & Tops, M. (2003). Caffeine, fatigue, and cognition. *Brain and Cognition, 53*(1), 82–94.

Love, C. C., & Morrison, E. (2003). American Academy of Nursing Expert Panel on Violence Policy Recommendations on Workplace Violence. *Issues in Mental Health Nursing, 24*, 599–604.

Malmgren, J. (2000, March 20). Controlled burn. *Knoxville News-Sentinel*, B1.

Mayer, J. D. (1999). Emotional intelligence: Popular or scientific psychology? *American Psychological Association Monitor, 30*(8), 20.

Mayne, T. J., & Ambrose, T. K. (1999). Research review on anger in psychotherapy. *Journal of Clinical Psychology/In Session: Psychotherapy in Practice, 55*, 353–363.

Meyer-Lindenberg, A., & Weinberger, D. (2006, March 20). Aggression-related gene weakens brain's impulse control circuits. *Proceedings of the National Academy of Sciences*. Retrieved March 20, 2006, from www.nimh.nih.gov.

Meloy, J. R. (1992). *Violent attachments*. Northvale, NJ: Aronson.

Mesulam, M. (2000). *Principles of behavioral and cognitive neurology* (2nd ed.). Oxford: Oxford University Press.

Miller, N., Pedersen, W. C., Earleywine, M., & Pollock, V. E. (2003). Artificial theoretical model of triggered displaced aggression. *Personality Social Psychology Review, 7*(1), 57–97.

Mittleman, M., Maclure, M., Sherwood, J., Mulry, R., Tofler, G., Jacobs, S., et al. (1995). Triggering of acute myocardial infarction onset by episodes of anger. *Circulation, 92,* 720–725.

Moorhead, S., Johnson, M., & Maas, M. (2003). *Nursing Outcomes Classification* (3rd ed.). Philadelphia: Elsevier.

Morrison, E. F. (1998). The culture of caregiving and aggression in psychiatric settings. *Archives of Psychiatric Nursing, 12*(1), 21–31.

Morrison, E. F., & Love, C. C. (2003). An evaluation of four programs for the management of aggression in psychiatric settings. *Archives of Psychiatric Nursing, 17*(4), 146–155.

Needham, I., Abderhalden, C., Zeller, A., Dassen, T., Haug, H-J., Fischer, J., & Halfens, R. (2005). The effect of a training course on nursing students' attitudes toward, perceptions of, and confidence in managing patient aggression. *Journal of Nursing Education, 44,* 415–420.

North American Nursing Diagnosis Association (NANDA). (2003). *Nursing diagnoses: Definitions and classification 2003–2004*. Philadelphia: Author.

Orecklin, M. (2000, August 21). Beware of the in crowd. *Time,* 69.

Paquette, M. (2001, April). Prevention of violence in children and adolescents. Paper presented at the International Society of Psychiatric–Mental Health Nurses, Phoenix, AZ. April 25–28, 2001.

Pardo, J. V., Pardo, P. J., & Raichle, M. E. (1993). Neural correlates of self-induced dysphoria. *American Journal of Psychiatry, 150*(5), 713–719.

Poe-Yamagata, E., & Butts, J.A. (1996). Female offenders in the juvenile justice system: Statistics summary. Pittsburgh, PA: National Center for Juvenile Justice.

Poster, L., & Drew, B. (2006, July-August). Presidents' message. *American Psychiatric Nurses Association News, 18*(4), 2–3.

Rew, L., & Christian, B. (1993). Self-efficacy, coping, and well-being among nursing students sexually abused in childhood. *Journal of Pediatric Nursing, 8,* 392–399.

Royal College of Psychiatrists. (1998). Management of imminent violence: Occasional paper. OP 41. London, UK: Author.

Rubin, T. I. (1970). *The angry book*. New York: Collier.

Rubinstein, E. R., Sahakian, B. J., & Dolan, R. J. (2002). The neural basis of mood congruent processing biases in depression. *Archives of General Psychiatry, 59*(7), 597–604.

Scarpa, A., & Raine, A. (1997). Psychophysiology of anger and violent behavior. *Psychiatric Clinics of North America, 20*(2), 375–394.

Schmeck, K., Sadigorsky, S., Englert, E., Demisch, L., Dierks, T., Barta, S., & Poustka, F. (2002). Mood changes following acute tryptophan depletion in healthy adults. *Psychopathology, 35*(4), 234–240.

Sergi, M. J., & Green, M. F. (2003). Social perception and early visual processing in schizophrenia. *Schizophrenia Research, 59*(2–3), 233–241.

Silver, J. M., Yudofsky, S. C., Slater, J. A., Gold, R. K., Stryer, B. L., Williams, D. T., et al. (2000). Propranolol treatment of chronically hospitalized aggressive patients. *Journal of Neuropsychiatry & Clinical Neuroscience, 12*(3), 413.

Smith, M. E., & Hart, G. (1994). Nurses' response to patients' anger: From disconnecting to connecting. *Journal of Advanced Nursing, 20,* 643–651.

Spielberger, C. D. (1999). Manual for the State Trait Anger Expression Inventory-2. Odessa, FL: Psychological Assessment Resources.

Stolley, J. M., Gerdner, L. A., & Buckwalter, K. C. (1999). Dementia management. In G. M. Bulechek & J. C. McCloskey (Eds.), *Nursing interventions: Effective nursing treatments* (3rd ed., pp. 533–548). Philadelphia: WB Saunders.

Swett, C., & Mills, T. (1997). Use of NOSIE to predict assaults among acute psychiatric patients. Nurses' Observation Scale for Inpatient Evaluation. *Psychiatric Services, 48*(9), 1177–1180.

Tjaden, P., & Thoennes, N. (2000). *Findings from national violence against women survey*. Washington, DC: U.S. Department of Justice.

Talerico, K. A., Evans, L. K., & Strumpf, N. E. (2002). Mental health correlates of aggression in nursing home residents with dementia. *Gerontologist, 42*(2), 169–177.

Tasman, A. (1997). *Psychiatry*. Philadelphia: WB Saunders.

Tavris, C. (1989). *Anger: The misunderstood emotion*. New York: Simon & Schuster.

Thomas, S. P. (1990). Theoretical and empirical perspectives on anger. *Issues in Mental Health Nursing, 11,* 203–216.

Thomas, S. P. (1997a). Women's anger: Relationship of suppression to blood pressure. *Nursing Research, 46,* 324–330.

Thomas, S. P. (1997b). Angry? Let's talk about it! *Applied Nursing Research, 10*(2), 80–85.

Thomas, S. P. (1998). Assessing and intervening with anger disorders. *Nursing Clinics of North America, 33*(1), 121–133.

Thomas, S. P., Groer, G., Davis, M., Droppleman, P., Mozingo, J., & Pierce, M. (2000). Anger and cancer: An analysis of the linkages. *Cancer Nursing, 23,* 344–349.

Thomas, S. P. (2001). Teaching healthy anger management. *Perspectives in Psychiatric Care, 37*(2), 41–48.

Thomas, S. P. (2003). Women's anger, aggression, and violence. *Health Care for Women International, 26,* 504–522.

Thomas, S. P. (2006). Cultural and gender considerations in the assessment and treatment of anger-related disorders. In E. L. Feindler (Ed.), *Anger-related disorders: A practitioner's guide to comparative treatments* (pp. 71–95). New York: Springer.

Thomas, S. P., & Pollio, H. R. (2002). *Listening to patients*. New York: Springer.

Thomas, S. P., Shattell, M., & Martin, T. (2002). What's therapeutic about the therapeutic milieu? *Archives of Psychiatric Nursing, 16*(3), 99–107.

Thomas, S. P., & Smith, H. (2004). School connectedness, anger behaviors, and relationships of violent and nonviolent American youth. *Perspectives in Psychiatric Care, 40*(4), 135–148.

United Nations High Commission on Human Rights. (2001). Human rights resolution 2001.49. *Elimination of violence against women*. Available at www.unhchr.ch.

Visalli, H., McNasser, G., Johnstone, L., & Lazzaro, C. A. (1997). Reducing high-risk interventions for managing aggression in psychiatric settings. *Journal of Nursing Care Quality, 11*(3), 54–61.

Vosburgh, D., & Simpson, P. (1993). Linking family theory and practice: A family nursing program. *Image—The Journal of Nursing Scholarship, 25*(3), 231–235.

White, M. (1988/89, Summer). The externalizing of the problem and the re-authoring of lives and relationships. *Dulwich Centre Newsletter,* 3–21.

Winerman, L. (2006, June). Psychologists testify at Senate video-game hearing. *Monitor on Psychology, 37*(6), 11.

World Health Organization. (2002). *World report on violence and health*. Geneva, Switzerland: Author.

Wright, L. M., & Leahey, M. (2000). *Nurses and families: A guide to family assessment and intervention* (3rd ed.). Philadelphia: FA Davis.

Wright, N. M. J., Dixon, A. J., & Tompkins, C. N. E. (2003). Managing violence in primary care: An evidence-based approach. *British Journal of General Practice, 53,* 557–562.

CHAPTER 39

Caring for Abused Persons

Mary R. Boyd and Stephanie Burgess

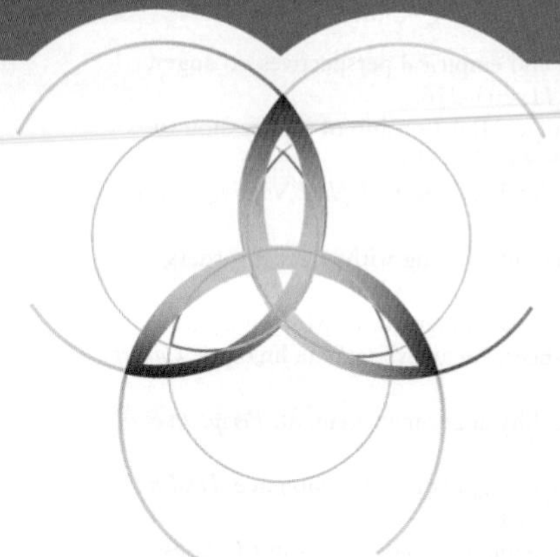

KEY CONCEPTS

- empowerment
- self-esteem

LEARNING OBJECTIVES

After studying this chapter, you will be able to:

- Describe woman, child, and elder abuse.
- Describe biopsychosocial theories of abuse.
- Discuss theories explaining why some men become abusive and why some women remain in violent relationships.
- Describe biopsychosocial consequences of abuse.
- Describe the diagnostic criteria for posttraumatic stress disorder (PTSD).
- Discuss the three major symptom categories found in PTSD and their associated etiologic factors.
- Describe the diagnostic criteria for dissociative identity disorder (DID).
- Integrate biopsychosocial theories into the analysis of human responses to survivors of abuse.
- Formulate nursing care plans for survivors of abuse.

KEY TERMS

• acute stress disorder (ASD) • alexithymia • behavioral sensitization • complex posttraumatic stress disorder (PTSD) • cycle of violence • dissociation • dissociative identity disorder (DID) • emotional abuse • extinction • factitious disorder by proxy (Münchausen syndrome by proxy) • fear conditioning • intergenerational transmission • neglect • physical abuse • posttraumatic stress disorder (PTSD) • sexual abuse • traumatic bonding

Violence manifested in the abuse of women, children, and elders is a national health problem that causes significant impairment in survivors. Abuse of any type permanently changes the survivor's construction of reality and the meaning of his or her life. It wounds deeply, endangering core beliefs about self, others, and the world. It can damage or destroy the survivor's self-esteem.

Nurses encounter survivors of abuse in all health care settings. For this reason, nurses must be knowledgeable about abuse. They must possess knowledge of abuse risk factors, indicators, causes, assessment techniques, and effective nursing interventions. Unfortunately, few nurses ask about abuse because doing so is often uncomfortable. It requires nurses to acknowledge evil in human nature and their own vulnerability to that evil. Protection and recovery from abuse requires survivors to remember and discuss terrible events. However, secrecy and silence protect perpetrators and seriously endanger survivors. Nurses communicate a powerfully disturbing message with their silence: that the most traumatic event of a patient's life is too upsetting for others to hear. If nurses do not empower survivors to tell their stories, the abuse experiences will continue to haunt patients, often manifesting as symptoms of mental disorders.

This chapter focuses on the nursing process with women, children, and elders who are survivors of abuse. It provides basic nursing information required to address the multiple, complex problems of these patients.

KEY CONCEPT Self-esteem is how one feels about oneself. Its components are self-acceptance, self-worth, self-love, and self-nurturing.

TYPES OF ABUSE

Most abuse that women, children, and the elderly experience is intimate violence; that is, the perpetrator is a loved and trusted partner or family member. As a result, the world and home are no longer safe, people seem dangerous, and life may become a tortured existence of warding off ever-present threats. Empowerment is a foreign concept to those who are being abused.

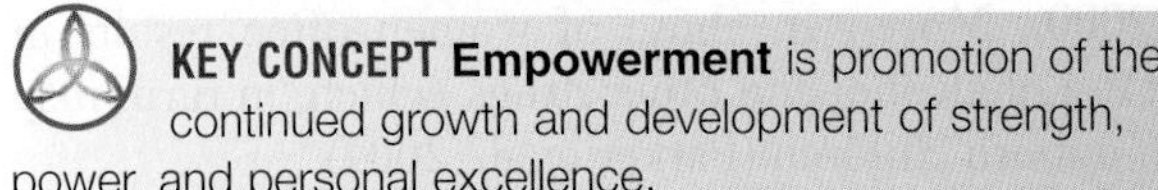

KEY CONCEPT Empowerment is promotion of the continued growth and development of strength, power, and personal excellence.

Woman Abuse

Woman abuse, domestic violence, spouse abuse, partner abuse, wife abuse, and battered wives are all terms used interchangeably to denote violence directed toward women. However, some of these terms do not specifically refer to the abuse of a woman by an intimate partner. For example, the term *domestic violence* may be used in cases in which one person directs abuse against an entire family. The terms *spouse abuse* and *partner abuse* could indicate that women abuse their male partners with the same frequency and similar consequences as when men direct violence against women (Ryan & King, 1998), which is simply not true. Among violent crimes against a spouse, 86% of the offenders are men (U.S. Department of Justice [DOJ], 2005). When women use force against their male partners, they often do so in self-defense, and the injuries women receive are typically more severe than those they inflict (Swann, Ganbone, Fields, Sullivan, Snow 2005). For these reasons, *woman abuse* has been chosen as the most appropriate term to use in this chapter in designating violence, including rape, directed toward a woman by an intimate partner.

Woman abuse is a significant health problem that crosses all ethnic, racial, and socioeconomic lines (Basile, 2002; Boris, Heller, Sheperd, & Zeanah, 2002; Centers for Disease Control & Prevention, 2003a; Coker, Smith, McKeown, & King, 2000; Dienemann, Boyle, Baker, Resnick, Wiederhorn, & Campbell, 2000; Vest, Catlin, Chen, & Brownson, 2002). Approximately four million women are abused by a partner each year (Brady & Dansky, 2002). These figures may be low, because underreporting or barriers to getting help contribute to low estimates (Kershner & Anderson 2002; Lapidus, Cooke, & Gelven, 2002). Many women are afraid or reluctant to identify their abusers. In some cases, they fear retaliation against themselves or their children. In other cases, they continue to hold strong feelings for their partners, despite the abuse. In other scenarios, health care providers are reluctant to inquire about abuse.

Evidence suggests that younger, single, divorced, and separated women may actually be at greater risk for abuse than are married women (Burgess & Tavakoli, 2005; Fishwick, Campbell, & Taylor, 2004). Moreover, this group is at particularly high risk for severe violence. Danger assessments show that abusive ex-partners often exhibit obsessive threatening behavior after their relationships end and pose significant dangers to women. Forty-three percent of women seen in emergency departments (EDs) attributed their abuse to a past partner. These findings emphasize that ending a relationship often does not end violence (Fishwick et al., 2004). This information is important for health care providers, who frequently pressure women to end abusive relationships. Rates of woman abuse vary among women of different racial backgrounds. Asian/Pacific Islander women report the lowest rates of intimate partner violence, and African American and Native American/Alaska Native women report the highest rates (Centers for Disease Control and Prevention [CDC], 2000b). However, differences among minority groups decrease when other sociodemographic and relationship variables are controlled. Other women at higher risk of abuse include lower income women; less educated women; and women in relationships with income, educational, or occupational status disparities (Burgess & Tavakoli, & CDC, 2003b).

The perpetuation of violence begins early in dating relationships (Burgess & Tavakoli, 2005; James, West, Deters, & Armijio, 2000). The prevalence of dating violence is unknown because, as with other forms of violence, it usually takes place in private and is not always reported or disclosed. A few studies provide some data on the extent of the problem. One study found that of 1,870 cases of domestic assaults, 51.5% were classified as boyfriend or girlfriend violence. About 20% to 50% of men and women in college-aged dating relationships have admitted physically abusing a dating partner. These figures do not include date rape. One study found that behaviors that would qualify as date rape or sexual assault occurred at a rate of 15.4% or 38 per 1,000 women (Barnett, Miller-Perrin, & Perrin, 1997). More recent sources suggest that prevalence of dating violence ranges from 9% to 46% of adolescent females (Burgess & Tavakoli, 2005; King & Ryan, 2004; Roberts & Klein, 2003), with gender differences in predictors of adolescent dating violence (Forshee, Linder, & MacDougall, 2001). For example, females perpetrate more violence than males towards partners even when controlling for self-defense, but males perpetrate more sexual dating violence than females. One study conducted in an ethnically and economically diverse urban community found that dating violence affected 45.5% of participating girls and boys (Watson, Cascardi, Avery-Leaf, & O'Leary, 2001).

To understand woman abuse, one must understand the dynamics of violent intimate relationships. Woman abuse is not just physical or sexual abuse. Rather, it is a chronic syndrome characterized by emotional abuse, degradation, restrictions on freedom, destruction of property, threatened or actual child abuse, threats against one's family, stalking, and isolation from family and friends (Mechanic, Weaver, & Resick, 2000; Morewitz, 2001). Violence of this nature has at its core a pattern of coercive control and domination over all aspects of a woman's life (Flitcraft, 1995, 1997). Threats of violence against the woman and her loved ones are among the tactics that the batterer uses to enforce the woman's submission and secrecy (King & Ryan, 2004). Many battered women report that physical violence is much less damaging than the accompanying emotional abuse. Relentless emotional and psychological violence destroys and isolates women (Boyd & Mackey, 2000a). The varieties of abuse used to exert power and control over women are represented in Figure 39.1.

Battering

Battering is the single greatest cause of serious injury to women. Estimates of injury related to battering seen in EDs range from 14% to 50% (Campbell, Torres, McKenna, Sheridan, & Landenburger, 2004). Woman abuse contributes to a high rate of completed and attempted suicides in women; 40% to 81% of women reporting suicide attempts have experienced abuse by an intimate partner (Thompson, Kaslow, & Kingree, 2002; Thompson et al., 1999). Moreover, many women who experience abuse experience PTSD (Lang, Kennedy, & Stein, 2002; Norris, Foster, & Weisshaar, 2002; Stein & Kennedy, 2001). Individuals with PTSD are 15 times more likely to attempt suicide than are individuals in the general population (Thompson et al., 1999).

Battered women are also in danger of being murdered by their abusers, especially when they take deliberate action to leave an abusive relationship (Paulozzi, Saltzman, Thompson, & Holmgreen, 2001). In 1996, 75% of 1,800 homicides perpetrated by intimate partners had female victims (Sisley, Jacobs, Poole, Campbell, & Esposito, 1999). Indeed, the realistic fear of being killed is one factor that keeps many women from leaving abusive partners, even after years of severe abuse. A recent study found that 44% of women murdered by their intimate partner had visited an ED within 2 years of the homicide (Crandall et al., 2004). Of those women, 93% had at least one injury visit. Those results suggest that health care professionals need to be more vigilant in screening for violence and lethality in EDs.

Battering also poses a significant danger for pregnant women and adolescents. Estimates of the prevalence of battering during pregnancy and the postpartum period vary from 4% (Harrykissoon, Rickert, & Wiemann, 2002; Sisley et al., 1999) to as high as 22% (Parker, Bullock, Bohn, & Curry, 2004). Differences in prevalence rates may be attributed to differences in definitions of abuse used by study authors. Abuse during pregnancy is a significant risk factor for several fetal and maternal complications, including low birth weight, low maternal weight gain, infections, and anemia (Anderson, Marshak, & Hebbeler, 2002; Clark, Martin, Petersen, Cloutier, Covington, Buescher, & Beck-Warden, 2000; Cloutier, Martin, Moracco, Garro, Clark, & Brody, 2002; Durant, Colley, Saltzman, & Johnson, 2000; Weiss, Lawrence, & Tiller, 2002; Wiemann, Agurcia, Berenson, Volk, & Rickert, 2000). Moreover, abuse of women often results in their use of alcohol and other drugs, which, in turn, may harm unborn children (Parker et al., 2004).

Rape and Sexual Assault

Rape and sexual assault are common in the United States; however, prevalence rates are difficult to determine because of underreporting. Between 1998 and 2002, fewer than 4 out of 10 sex offenses (rape or sexual assault) were reported to law enforcement (DOJ, 2005). A sexual assault occurs once every 6.4 minutes (Petter & Whitehill, 1998). Expressed in another way, one in every three to four Caucasian women and one in every four African American women will be raped in their lifetime (Starling, 1998). In a study of sexual assault among college women, 69.8% of women reported at least one victimization experience by the fourth year of college (Humphrey & White, 2000). In a national study of violence against women, 18% of women reported that they had been raped (Abbey, Zawacki, Buck, Clinton, & McAuslan, 2003). Sexual assault includes any form of nonconsenting sexual activity, ranging from fondling to penetration. Most sexual assaults are underreported for the same reason that domestic violence is underreported—women are embarrassed and ashamed and fear being blamed for the assault. These reactions to sexual assault persist, even though rape is a felony (Abbey et al.).

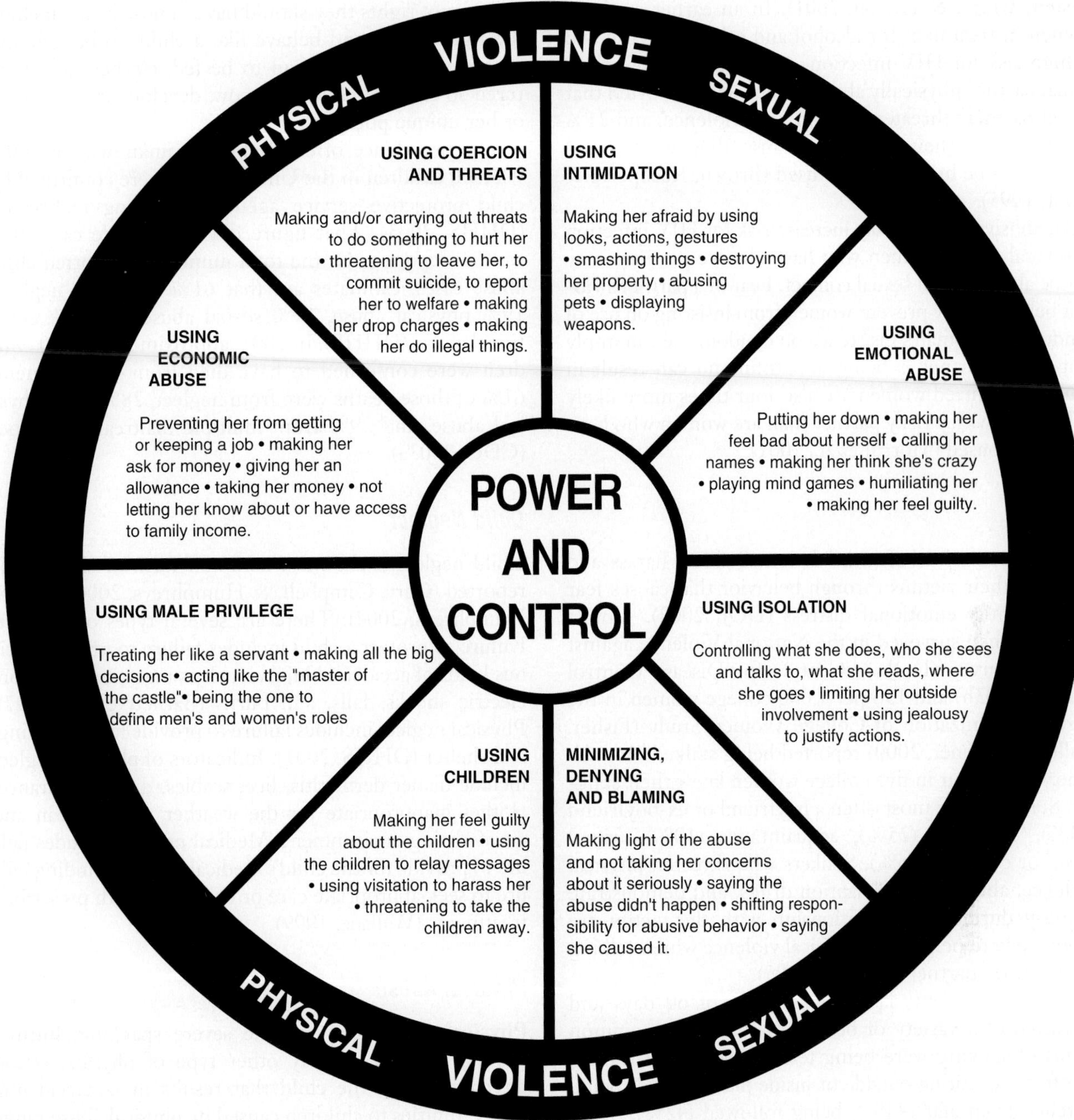

FIGURE 39.1. Power and control wheel (courtesy of Domestic Abuse Intervention Project, 202 East Superior Street, Duluth, MN).

Rapists can be classified into three categories: the power rapist, the anger rapist, and the sadistic rapist (Petter & Whitehill, 1998). Power rapists account for 55% of sexual assaults. They often attack people their own age and use intimidation and minimal physical force to control their victims. Their assaults are generally premeditated. Anger rapists account for 40% of sexual assaults. These rapists tend to target either very young or elderly victims. They may use extreme force and restraint that results in physical injury to the victim. Sadistic rapists account for 5% of sexual assaults; however, they are the most dangerous. Their crimes are premeditated, and they often torture and kill their victims. Sadistic rapists derive erotic gratification from their victim's suffering (Petter & Whitehill).

Coerced Sex and Increased Risk for Human Immunodeficiency Virus

Woman abuse is also a risk factor for human immunodeficiency virus (HIV) infection among women. Among women who test positive for HIV, the lifetime prevalence of adult coerced sexual activity perpetrated by a male partner has been estimated to be 74% or higher (Morrill,

Kasten, Urato, & Larson, 2001). In an earlier study of women in treatment for alcohol and other drug use and at high risk for HIV infection, 42% reported that their sexual partner physically abused them, 45% reported that sexual partners threatened them with violence, and 21% reported that they had sex because they were afraid they would be hurt if they refused (Brown, Recupero, & Stout, 1995).

An abusive partner may increase risk for HIV infection in several ways. Women who have abusive partners may not be able to avoid sexual contact. Fear of a partner's violent behavior may prevent women from insisting on use of condoms. A woman's insistence on condom use can imply that either partner is being unfaithful and can result in abuse. Victimized women are also four times more likely to have sex with a risky partner than are women who have not been abused (Morrill et al., 2001).

Stalking

Stalking is a crime of intimidation. Stalkers harass and terrorize their victims through behavior that causes fear or substantial emotional distress (DOJ, 2002). Almost 5% of women surveyed in the National Violence against Women Survey (DOJ & Centers for Disease Control [CDC], 2003b) and 156 per 1,000 college women in the Sexual Victimization of College Women Study (Fisher, Cullen, & Turner, 2000) reported being stalked. As with other abuse, four in five college women knew their stalkers. Stalkers were most often a boyfriend or ex-boyfriend (43%), classmate (25%), acquaintance (10%), friend (6%), or coworker (6%). Stalkers who threaten physical violence, abuse nonprescription drugs, and demonstrate jealousy during their relationship with the victim are more likely to perpetuate physical violence while stalking their former partner (Roberts, 2005).

Stalking incidents lasted an average of 60 days and consisted of a variety of behaviors. The most common forms of stalking were being telephoned (78%), having an offender waiting outside or inside places (48%), being watched from afar (44%), being followed (42%), being sent letters (31%), and being sent electronic mail messages (25%) (NIJ & BJS, 2000). Stalking occurred two to six times a week and caused victims extreme psychological stress (Fisher, Cullen, & Turner, 2000). Every state has a stalking law, but laws and their enforcement vary in each state. In most states, stalking is a Class A or first-degree misdemeanor, except under certain circumstances, which include stalking in violation of a protective order, with a weapon, and repeat offenses (NIJ & BJS).

Child Abuse

Child abuse can take several forms, and the definition of each type varies by state. All forms of child abuse rob children of rights they should have. Those rights include the rights to be and behave like a child; to be safe and protected from harm; and to be fed, clothed, and nurtured so that the child can grow, develop, and fulfill his or her unique potential.

The prevalence of child abuse is unknown. In 2003, 906,000 children in the United States were confirmed by child protective service agencies as being maltreated (DHHS, 2003). That figure did not include cases that were unreported. Of the total number of reported child abuse cases, estimates are that 61% represent neglect, 19% physical abuse, 10% sexual abuse, and 5% emotional abuse (DHHS). In 2003, approximately 1,500 children were confirmed to have died from maltreatment: 61% of those deaths were from neglect, 28% from physical abuse, and 29% from multiple maltreatment types (CDC, 2003a).

Child Neglect

Child neglect is the most common form of child abuse reported (Gary, Campbell, & Humphreys, 2004; Gary & Humphreys, 2004). There are several types of **neglect.** Failure to protect a child includes failure to prevent various kinds of accidental injury, such as ingestion of poison, electric shocks, falls, and burns (Barnett et al., 1997). Physical neglect includes failure to provide food, clothing, and shelter (DHHS, 2001). Indicators of physical neglect include diaper dermatitis, lice, scabies, dirty appearance, clothes inappropriate for the weather, and unclean and unsafe living environment. Medical neglect includes failure to provide for the child's medical needs, including failure to seek appropriate care or to comply with prescribed treatments (Wallace, 1999).

Physical Abuse

Physical abuse may include severe spanking, hitting, kicking, shoving, or any other type of physical action directed toward the child that results in nonaccidental injury. Injuries to children caused by physical abuse range from mild to severe and life-threatening. Types of injuries include skin and soft tissue injuries; internal injuries; dislocations and fractures; tooth loss; burns; abrasions or bruises made by fists or belts; hair loss from pulling the hair; wounds from guns, knives, razors, or other sharp objects; retinal hemorrhage; and conjunctival hemorrhage (Gary et al., 2004; Gary & Humphreys, 2004; DHHS, 2001; Wallace, 1999). Often, clothing hides these injuries, and practitioners must look for other signs of abuse, such as fear, aggressive or withdrawn behavior, poor social relations, learning problems, delinquent behavior, and wearing clothing that is meant to cover injuries but is inappropriate for the weather. In addition, when treating a child with such injuries, professionals should suspect abuse when explanations are implausible and inconsistent with injuries, involved parties give different versions of the incident, or treatment seeking is delayed (Wallace, 1999).

Sexual Abuse

Behaviors that constitute child **sexual abuse** range from mild, covert behaviors to overt sexual acts. Examples of sexual abuse include exhibitionism, voyeurism, touching the child's sexual organs, and oral, anal, and vaginal sex (Gary et al., 2004; Gary & Humphreys, 2004; DHHS, 2003; Urbancic, 2004; Wallace, 1999). There are three categories of sexual abuse: incest, sexual abuse perpetrated by a nonfamily member, and pedophilia. Incest is defined as any form of sexual activity between a child younger than age 18 years and an immediate family member (parent, stepparent, sibling), extended family member (grandparent, uncle, aunt, cousin), or surrogate parent (DHHS). Extrafamilial child sexual abuse is any form of sexual contact between a nonfamily member and a child younger than age 18 years. Pedophilia describes those who have a sexual fixation on young children that usually translates into sexual acts with the victims (Wallace). The following conditions qualify as pedophilia:

- For at least 6 months, the person has recurrent intense sexual urges and sexually arousing fantasies involving sexual activity with a prepubescent child.
- The person has acted on or is extremely distressed by these urges.
- The person is at least 16 years old and at least 5 years older than the child (Wallace, 1999).

Research shows that about 8% to 10% of child sexual abuse offenders are strangers, 47% are family members, and 40% are acquaintances. The high-risk years for child sexual abuse range between ages 4 and 9 years (Wallace, 1999).

Several factors may mediate the effects of child sexual abuse. In general, younger children with a history of emotional difficulties may be more traumatized than will be older and more stable children. Repeated abuse for long periods with more violence and bodily penetration results in greater traumatization. Sexual abuse by someone that the child knows and trusts causes more severe trauma. The child abused by a family member experiences a devastating breach of trust, loss of a safe home, and threats to fundamental survival requirements (Boyd & Mackey, 2000a). Finally, negative reactions by significant others, health care professionals, or others may exacerbate the effects of trauma (Wallace, 1999).

Emotional Abuse

Emotional abuse includes acts or omissions that psychologically damage the child (Gary et al., 2004). The emotionally abused child does not have visible injuries to alert others. Nevertheless, emotional abuse severely affects a child's self-esteem and often leaves permanent emotional scars. Survivors of abuse frequently report that emotional abuse is worse than physical abuse (Wallace, 1999).

There are several types of emotional abuse. *Rejecting* involves refusing to acknowledge the child's worth and the legitimacy of his or her needs. The child receives the message that he or she is no good and is unwanted. *Isolating* involves cutting the child off from normal social experiences, preventing the child from forming friendships, and hindering the development of social skills. *Terrorizing* involves creating a climate of fear and making the child believe that the world is a capricious and hostile place. *Ignoring* means being psychologically unavailable to the child and, therefore, starving him or her emotionally. Normal self-development depends on emotional connection to others. *Corrupting* involves mis-socializing the child to engage in destructive and antisocial behaviors and reinforcing deviance. This type of abuse makes the child unfit for normal social experience and sets him or her up for additional rejection (Barnett et al., 1997; Wallace, 1999).

Factitious Disorder by Proxy: Münchausen Syndrome by Proxy

Factitious disorder by proxy is another form of child abuse (see Chapter 23). This disorder includes "the intentional production or feigning of physical or psychological signs or symptoms in another person who is under the individual's care for the purpose of indirectly assuming the sick role" (American Psychiatric Association [APA], 2000, p. 781). The signs of this disorder include repeated hospitalizations and medical evaluations of the child without definitive diagnosis; symptoms or medical signs that are inappropriate or inconsistent; symptoms that disappear when the child is away from the parent; a parent who encourages medical tests for the child; parental uneasiness as the child recovers; and a parent who is less concerned with the child's health than with spending time with caregivers (Bartsch, Risse, Schutz, Weigand, & Weiler, 2003). One source estimates that approximately 10% of children who are victims of factitious disorder by proxy will die at the hands of their parents (Wallace, 1999).

Secondary Abuse: Children of Battered Women

At least 1.5 million children are exposed to their mothers' abuse by an intimate partner (Kernic et al., 2003). Children of battered women are often overlooked as abuse victims unless they demonstrate evidence of physical or sexual abuse themselves (Rhea, Chafey, Dohner, &

Terragno, 1996). However, these children often demonstrate numerous problems. One study found that children exposed to maternal interpersonal violence without concomitant child abuse were 40% more likely to demonstrate behavioral problems than normative children, and children who experienced both maternal interpersonal violence and concomitant child abuse were over twice as likely to demonstrate behavioral problems as normative children (Kernic et al.). Externalizing behavior problems (aggressive/delinquent behaviors) were particularly common in children exposed to their mother's violent victimization. Many children of these abused children also develop depression and PTSD (Berman, Hardesty, & Humphreys, 2004). Children may witness their mother being choked, threatened with a weapon, or threatened with death (Berman et al.; Boyd & Mackey, 2000a; Campbell & Lewandowski, 1997). These children fear for both their own and their mother's safety (Boyd & Mackey, 2000a). In addition, children who grow up in violent families experience living with secrecy, relocations as the mother leaves home to seek safety, economic hardship, maternal depression that may reduce her ability to nurture, and frightening interactions with the police and court systems (Berman et al., Boyd & Mackey; Campbell & Lewandowski, 1997). Moreover, many children who witness violence begin to accept it as a normal part of relationships and a way to deal with problems (Sisley et al., 1999).

Victimization by Family Courts

Women and children often sustain further victimization by family courts after they leave the abuser (Slote et al., 2005). In many instances, battered women are expected to abide by custody and visitation orders that require them and their children to maintain long-term, unprotected contact with their batterers. If women fail to comply, they risk being held in contempt of court or even losing custody of their children to the batterers. Custody and visitation can provide a context for batterers to continue to control and victimize women and their children. Research shows that fathers who seek custody obtain either primary or joint physical custody 70% to 90% of the time (Slote et al., 2005). Some abusive men have even been granted unsupervised visitation with children, including overnight visits.

Abusive men may also use the courts as a tool for ongoing harassment, retaliation, and intimidation (Slote et al., 2005). Tactics include multiple harassing, baseless, or retaliatory motions in court that force a woman to go back to court endlessly with devastating economic consequences. Abusive men also use the courts to avoid paying child support. In addition, battered women relate that judges and probation officers often treat them with condescension, scorn, and disrespect, and do not consider them to be credible and dismiss their allocations of partner or child abuse (Slote et al.).

Elder Abuse

Elder abuse is increasingly recognized as a serious problem in the United States and other countries. As the population continues to age, it is likely that the problem will worsen. As with other types of abuse, the prevalence of elder abuse is unknown; however, one report estimated 1.5 million cases of elder abuse each year in the United States (Wallace, 1999). The most recent statistics on elder abuse in the United States found that approximately 1.2% or approximately 12 per 1,000 individuals older than 60 years are abused annually (National Center on Elder Abuse, 1998).

Types of elder abuse and their estimated prevalence rates are as follows: neglect (58.5%), physical abuse (15.7%), financial or material mistreatment (12.3%), emotional abuse (7.3%), and sexual abuse (0.04%) (Comijs et al., 1998; Wallace, 1999). Neglect and physical, sexual, and emotional abuse are similar to that described for women and children. Financial or material mistreatment may include improper or illegal acts to obtain and use an elderly person's resources for personal benefit (Wallace).

Risk factors for elder abuse include older age, impairment in activities of daily living (ADLs), cognitive disability or other mental illness, dependency on the caregiver, isolation, stressful events, and a history of intergenerational conflict between the elder and the caregiver (Sengstock, Ulrich, & Barrett, 2004).

Teen Partner Abuse

Partner abuse of teen girls is recognized as an emerging health problem in the United States (Coker et al., 2000). Studies suggest an incidence rate of 21% to 60% in all teen girls (Burgess & Tavakoli, 2005; Forshee et al., 2001; James, West, Deters, & Armijio, 2000; Rickert, Vaughan, & Wiemann, 2003; Roberts & Klein, 2003) and 10% to 22% in pregnant teen girls (Harrykissoon, et al., 2002; Wiemann et al., 2000). Likewise, other studies report that annually 6% of teen girls are murdered by partners and 8% are sexually assaulted by partners (Perrin, Dindial, Eaton, Harrison, Matthews, & Henry, 2000; Rhynard, Krebs, & Glover, 1997; Wood, Maforah, & Jewkes, 1998). Problems reported with teen partner abuse include depression (Ackard & Neumark-Sztainer, 2002; Boris et al., 2002; Burgess & Tavakoli, 2005; Roberts & Klein, 2003), hopelessness (Bolland, McCallum, Lian, Bailey, & Rowan, 2002), peer violence/harassment (Smith & Thomas, 2000; Wiemann et al., 2000), and substance abuse (Abbey, Zawacki, & Buck, 2001; Rickert et al., 2003; Roberts & Klein).

THEORIES OF ABUSE

Many theories have attempted to explain violence between intimate partners and in the family. The theories reviewed here have been categorized as biologic, psychological, and social. In all likelihood, family violence is truly a biopsychosocial phenomenon that no one of these theories can fully explain (Figure 39.2). A separate section presents additional theories that are more specific to the phenomenon of woman abuse.

Biologic Theories

Neurologic Problems

Aggressive behavior may be associated with several neurologic conditions, including traumatic brain injury, seizure disorder, and dementia (see Chapter 32). Neurodevelopmental factors and traumatic brain injury can produce seizure disorders, attentional dysfunction, or focal neurobehavioral syndromes, all of which are associated with aggressive behavior. The most common association between seizures and aggressive behavior occurs during the postictal period (the period immediately after the seizure), during which the individual may be confused and react aggressively.

Damage to the orbitofrontal cortex often causes impulsive, labile, irritable, and socially inappropriate behavior. Individuals with such damage often respond aggressively to trivial stimuli. In addition, damage to the neocortex, limbic system, and hypothalamus may result in aggressive behavior. These systems have hierarchic control over one another. Damage to higher centers may disinhibit aggression from lower centers. Aggressive behavior also may be related to disruptions in neurotransmitter systems. Disruption in serotonin, dopamine, and gamma-aminobutyric acid (GABA) systems has been linked with several psychiatric disorders, including depression, schizophrenia, impulsive behavior, suicide, and aggression (Rosenbaum, Geffner, & Benjamin, 1997).

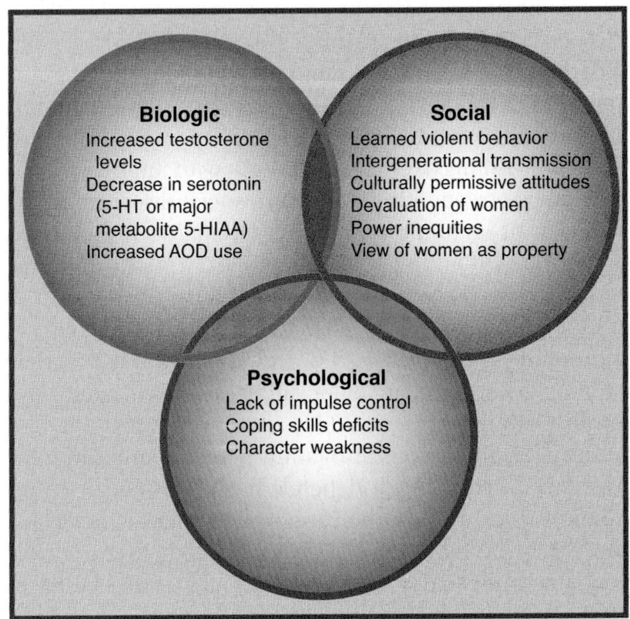

FIGURE 39.2. Biopsychosocial etiologies for violent behavior.

Links With Substance Abuse

The use of alcohol and other drugs (AOD) is commonly associated with violent incidents. Alcohol has been found to be present in approximately one half to two thirds of sexual assaults (Ulman, 2003). Of the 32.1 million nonfatal violent crimes that took place within families between 1998 and 2002, 30% of victims said the offender had been drinking or using drugs (DOJ, 2005). However, AOD use alone is rarely sufficient to account for violence. Other factors, such as low family income, stress, and abuse in the family of origin, are often more important (Collins & Messerschmidt, 1993; Wallace, 1999). The relationship of AOD to violence may result from three factors: (1) AOD-induced cognitive impairment, (2) the user's expectations that AOD increases the tendency toward aggression, and (3) socioculturally grounded beliefs that people are unaccountable for their behavior while intoxicated (Abbey et al., 2003).

Studies have demonstrated that drinking alcohol may change perceptions about accountability for behavior (Abbey et al., 2003). The belief that intoxicated behavior will be judged less harshly may encourage and provide an excuse for those who abuse substances to engage in normally unacceptable behavior. Research shows that people attempt to justify their criminal behavior by blaming alcohol after the fact (Abbey et al., 2003). However, the rules about AOD and accountability appear to be applied differently to men and women. One early study that examined the effects of intoxication on attributions of blame in a rape incident found that both men and women judged the rapist as less responsible if intoxicated, whereas they held the victim more responsible if intoxicated (Richardson & Campbell, 1982).

Psychosocial Theories

Psychopathology Theory

Psychopathology theory seeks to understand violence by examining characteristics of individual men and women (Wallace, 1999). Theorists from this perspective focus on personality traits, internal defense systems, and mental disorders. An outdated theory that was particularly damaging labeled women masochistic, paranoid, or depressed (Bograd, 1999). One underlying assumption of this labeling was that some women enjoy abuse and deliberately provoke attacks because they need to suffer.

Research on batterers has shown that there is not a common profile or a typical batterer. Studies have found evidence of personality disorders including antisocial, borderline, narcissistic, and dependent. Others have found mood disorders such as depression and anxiety (see Guille, 2004, for an integrated review). Although research has not consistently found one common mental disorder or set of characteristics in violent individuals, a recently identified typology of men who batter shows promise (Emery & Laumann-Billings, 1998). Type I batterers are violent in many situations, have many victims, and display antisocial characteristics. Type II batterers abuse only their family, commit less severe violence, are generally less aggressive, and demonstrate remorse. These men tend to be dependent, jealous, and unlikely to have personality or other disorders. Type III batterers display dysphoric-borderline or schizoid characteristics, such as emotional volatility, depression, feelings of inadequacy, and social isolation (Emery & Laumann-Billings, 1998). Type III batterers also tend to be violent only within their families.

Social Learning Theory

Violent families create an atmosphere of tension, fear, intimidation, and tremendous confusion about intimate relationships (Boyd & Mackey, 2000a). Children in violent homes often learn violent behavior as an approved and legitimate way to solve problems, especially within intimate relationships. Social learning theory posits that men who witness violence in their homes often perpetuate violent behavior in their families as adults (Dewey, 2004; Emery & Laumann-Billings, 1998; Wallace, 1999). Moreover, women who grow up in violent homes learn to accept violence and expect it in their own adult relationships (Boyd & Mackey, 2000a). These concepts are often referred to as the **intergenerational transmission** of violence.

Findings of extreme violence in the parental homes of battered individuals and individuals who grew up witnessing violence are common and support the intergenerational transmission of violence theory (Dewey, 2004). However, not all those who batter or are abused come from violent homes. Estimates are that approximately 40% of those who experienced abuse or witnessed abuse in childhood will consequently abuse their wives or children (Dutton, 1998).

Social Theories

Covering the many sociologic theories of violence is beyond the scope of this chapter. Sociologic theories posit that abuse occurs because of cultural norms that permit and even glamorize violent behavior (Dewey, 2004). The permissive attitude toward violence in the United States is reflected in violence in the media, choice of heroes, spiraling rates of violent crimes, and lack of or inadequate response by the criminal justice system. For instance, some continue to view O. J. Simpson as a hero, and he was never arrested or prosecuted for battering his wife.

Violence as normal behavior appears widespread among young people (Rickert et al., 2003; Rickert, Wiemann, Harrykissoon, Berenson, & Kolb, 2002). In another study, as many as 70% of a group of female college students listed at least one form of violence as acceptable in dating relationships. Even more disturbing is that 80% of these women mentioned situations in which physical force between partners was tolerable. Slapping was cited most often (49%), whereas punching was seen as acceptable by 21% of these women (Girshick, 1993). In addition, as many as 34% of women marry someone who abused them in a dating relationship (Barnett et al., 1997).

Family violence is also related to qualities of the community in which the family is embedded. Poverty, absence of family services, social isolation, lack of cohesion in the community, and stress contribute to family violence (Dewey, 2004). The relationship of poverty, social isolation, and child abuse has been well established (Emery & Laumann-Billings, 1998). Families with annual incomes of less that $15,000 are approximately 22 times more likely to abuse or neglect a child, compared with families whose income is $30,000 or more (Gary et al., 2004). However, not all poor families abuse their children. One difference between poor families who do and do not abuse their children lies in the degree of social cohesion and mutual caring found in their communities (Emery & Laumann-Billings). Neighborhoods with high levels of child abuse frequently have severe social disorganization and lack of community identity. In addition, they have higher rates of juvenile delinquency, drug trafficking, and violent crime (Emery & Laumann-Billings).

One of the most accepted theories of elder abuse is the family stress theory. The theory hypothesizes that providing care for an elder induces stress within the family. Family stress includes economic hardship, loss of sleep, and intrusions into family activities and routines. Moreover, caring for a dependent elder takes an enormous physical toll on the caregiver. If there is no relief, the caregiver may become overwhelmed, lose control, and abuse the elder (Sengstock et al., 2004; Wallace, 1999). Other characteristics of caregivers that may predispose them to abuse elderly parents include alcohol or drug abuse, dementia, restricted outside activities, unrealistic expectations, and a blaming, hypercritical personality.

Theoretic Dynamics Specific to Woman Abuse

Feminist Theories

Feminist theory focuses on issues of gender, inequality, power and privilege, patriarchy, and the subordination of women as explanations for woman abuse (Landenburger, Campbell, & Rodriguez, 2004). According to the feminist perspective, woman abuse results from a patriarchal society that perpetuates attitudes that support violence against women (Lloyd & Emery, 2000; Wallace, 1999). Three major characteristics of such a patriarchal society are the devaluation of women, power inequities, and the view of women as property (Barnett et al., 1997; Wallace, 1999).

Feminists charge that patriarchal society is the product of a predominately white, male-dominated majority that believes that women are inherently inferior to men. Such societies value women primarily for their reproductive capacity and potential to please men (Sampselle et al., 1992; Wallace, 1999).

Feminists also point to a power inequity in society as a contributing factor to woman abuse. Women have made many advances in recent years; however, men continue to control most institutions (Lloyd & Emery, 2000). Women continue to earn less than men for paid work and are less likely to advance to positions of authority and power (Nolen-Hoeksema, 2002; Sampselle et al., 1992). Moreover, marriage often victimizes women in ways other than through violence. Although men now contribute to household work, most women who hold jobs outside the home continue to perform most household and child care tasks (Lloyd & Emery). This power inequity is reflected in higher depression rates among married women than among married men (Nolen-Hoeksema, 2002). In cases of divorce, most women become single parents with a standard of living significantly lower than that of their former spouse (Wallace, 1999).

Until the early 1900s, women legally were the property of men in the United States (Sampselle et al., 1992). Ownership of women continues in many parts of the world and continues to influence attitudes toward women. The entertainment and advertising industries perpetuate the image of women as property by depicting them as objects and often portraying the dismembering of women's bodies (Kilbourne, 1987, 1999). The focus on women's body parts in advertising dehumanizes women, and that dehumanization is often the first step in making women acceptable targets of violence. Moreover, the explicit portrayal in the media of women in various states of undress and in seductive postures suggests that they are vulnerable and openly welcome sexual advances. Frequently, the message is, "Buy the product and get the woman" (Kilbourne, 1987).

Theory of Borderline Personality Organization and Violence

In a 1998 publication, Donald Dutton discussed the relationship of borderline personality organization (BPO) to the type of batterer who is chronically and intermittently abusive but abusive only within his family (see Chapter 22). Dutton's work combines aspects from social learning theory, reinforcement principles from learning theory, and evidence that early trauma can alter personality through changes that occur biologically or through learning. He bases his theory on his own research and that of others, such as Bandura (social learning theory) (1977) and van der Kolk (1997) (traumatic stress and its consequences).

Dutton (1998) describes three characteristics or cycles of BPO that shift with time and seem to coincide with the cycle of violence first proposed by Walker in 1979 and described later in this chapter. These characteristics can apply to men or women with BPO; however, because this discussion focuses on men's aggression toward their female partners, it addresses the individual with BPO as male. Phase I of the male borderline personality, or "cyclic personality," consists of an internal buildup of tensions, in which the man feels depressed and irritable but does not know how to verbalize his inner dysphoria. In fact, he may not even be able to recognize or label the painful feelings, a condition called **alexithymia** (Dutton). The inability to recognize or express painful feelings and ask for what he needs traps the man in a downward spiral of bad feelings, compounded by an inability to maintain his own self-integrity. He is dependent on his partner for his sense of self. Therefore, the loss of the partner carries the risk that he will lose himself. According to Dutton, the reason that men with BPO become so abusive in their intimate relationships, but not in other relationships, is linked to their extreme dependency on their partners for sense of self and their inability to tolerate aloneness. This type of dependency is often called a "masked or hostile dependency." To maintain this relationship, the man with BPO must control his partner; therefore, his controlling behavior masks his dependency. The man with BPO expects his partner to do the impossible. When she fails, he erupts in extreme anger because his sense of self is threatened. He converts dysphoria into abuse through (1) the belief that the partner should be able to soothe the bad feelings, and (2) conversion of feelings of terror into rage. His use of projection, a defense mechanism, leads him to believe that it is her fault. The explosive combination of ego needs, an inability to communicate them, chronic irritability, jealousy, and projective blaming combine to ensure a violent relationship (Dutton).

As this phase continues, the man with BPO becomes verbally abusive, and the partner withdraws. The man wants closeness, not withdrawal, but he does not have the skills to ask for it. In addition to increasing anger, the man with BPO becomes increasingly demanding. At this stage, the dichotomous thinking or splitting characteristic of BPO is evident, and the man sees the partner as "all bad"—unfaithful, unloving, and malevolent. The unexpressed rage builds until the man with BPO erupts with violence. The violence drives the partner further away, increasing the man's feelings of abandonment. As a result, the abusive man promises anything to get the partner back. (This phase coincides with Walker's contrition phase in the cycle of violence.) The opposite side of splitting is now in evidence, as the man describes his partner as "all good"—"a madonna" (Dutton, 1998, p. 96). This example of splitting is sometimes referred to as "madonna/whore."

It is hypothesized that the abuser's BPO results from early physical abuse. Researchers suggest that early physical abuse causes long-term problems in modulating emotion and aggression and may lead to chronic anger (Dutton, 1998). The difficulty in modulating emotion often manifests first in affective numbing and constriction or in alexithymia. Hyperarousal follows emotional numbing, a process that culminates in violence (Dutton). These symptoms are manifestations of PTSD, described later in this chapter. Abusive men also score higher than do control subjects on other measures of trauma, such as depression, anxiety, sleep disturbances, and dissociation (Dutton). However, the form that the violence takes appears to be learned. That is, boys tend to identify with the aggressor and act out, whereas girls often identify with the victim and turn to self-destructive acts, such as substance abuse and self-mutilation (Dutton).

One other aspect of this cycle appears to ensure its continuation—that of positive reinforcement. The type of violence perpetrated by men with BPO has been labeled "deindividuated violence;" that is, the violence is responsive only to internal cues from the perpetrator and unresponsive to cues from the victim (Dutton, 1998). The violence feeds on itself because it is rewarding; it reduces the perpetrator's aversive arousal and tension. As a result, batterers often continue the assault until they are exhausted. Expressing rage through violent acts is the only way they know to reduce their tension or aversive arousal, and it becomes addictive (Dutton).

The cycle described by Dutton helps explain the descriptions of violent men provided by more than 200 women with whom he has worked. The following are examples of their descriptions of violent partners: "He's like Jekyll and Hyde"; "He's completely different sometimes"; and "His friends never see the other side of him; they think he's just a nice guy, just one of the boys" (Dutton, 1998, p. 53).

Theories of Why Women Stay in Violent Relationships

A more appropriate question than "Why do women stay in violent relationships?" is to ask "How does she ever manage to leave given all the strikes against her?" (Anderson & Saunders, 2003). There are many reasons women stay in violent relationships. One of the strongest reasons is economic (Wallace, 1999). Despite years of progress, women still earn less than men for equal work. Many women lack the education or skills that would allow them to earn an adequate living outside the home. For these women, leaving their abusive partners means that they and their children would be homeless and without any source of support for even basic necessities. Furthermore, many shelters for battered women have long waiting lists and provide only temporary housing. The socialization of women to assume major responsibility for marriages and childrearing is often another barrier to leaving abusive relationships. Society teaches women that their proper place is at home and their primary responsibility is caring for their husbands and children (Chodorow, 1974; Gilligan, 1982; Wallace, 1999). Many women believe that making their marriage a success is their responsibility. Therefore, when they are abused, they assume that it is their fault and that their duty is to remain and try harder for their children's sakes (Boyd & Mackey, 2000a; Lloyd & Emery, 2000). Moreover, many women who were abused in childhood or witnessed abuse of their mothers think that abuse is part of a normal relationship (Boyd & Mackey).

Women also face political and legal obstacles in leaving abusive partners. Although the legal response to wife battering is improving, police response remains inadequate in many areas of the United States (Boyd & Mackey, 2000a). If a man is arrested for assault and no action is taken to prevent future violence, he may be released shortly and retaliate against his partner. Fear for their lives and the lives of their children and other relatives often keeps women from attempting to leave abusive relationships (Anderson & Saunders, 2003; Boyd and Mackey, 2000a).

Even more difficult to understand is why some women stay in violent dating relationships. About 30% to 50% of dating couples continue their relationships despite violence (Barnett et al., 1997). One factor is that dating violence often does not occur until the relationship has been sustained for a long time. By then, many women feel that they have invested too much in the relationship to end it. Research has shown that the length of the relationship and the commitment level are positively correlated with physical and sexual abuse. Moreover, about 30% of those who stay in violent dating relationships interpret the violence as an act of love (Barnett et al.). Another explanation is that abused women stay because they believe they can change their partners and save their relationships.

Survivors may go though a process consisting of several phases in leaving an abusive relationship (Anderson & Saunders, 2003). Women may leave and return several times as they are learning new coping skills. The phases may involve cognitive and emotional "leaving" before actually leaving the relationship. The phases may include (1) enduring and managing the violence while disconnecting from self and others; (2) acknowledging the abuse, reframing it, and counteracting it; and (3) disengaging and focusing on her own needs (Anderson & Saunders).

Cycle of Violence

Many cases of woman abuse reflect a recognized **cycle of violence** (Wallace, 1999). The cycle consists of three recurring phases that often increase in frequency and severity (Walker, 1979, 2000). The cycle is fully described in Figure 39.3.

Traumatic Bonding

The formation of strong emotional bonds under conditions of intermittent maltreatment has been reported in several studies with human and animal subjects. For example, people taken hostage may show positive regard for their captors. Abused children often show strong attachment to their abusing parents. Cult members show strong loyalty to malevolent cult leaders (Dutton, 1995). Therefore, the relationship between battered women and their partners may be just one example of **traumatic bonding**—the development of strong emotional ties between two people, one of whom intermittently abuses the other. Traumatic bonding suggests that

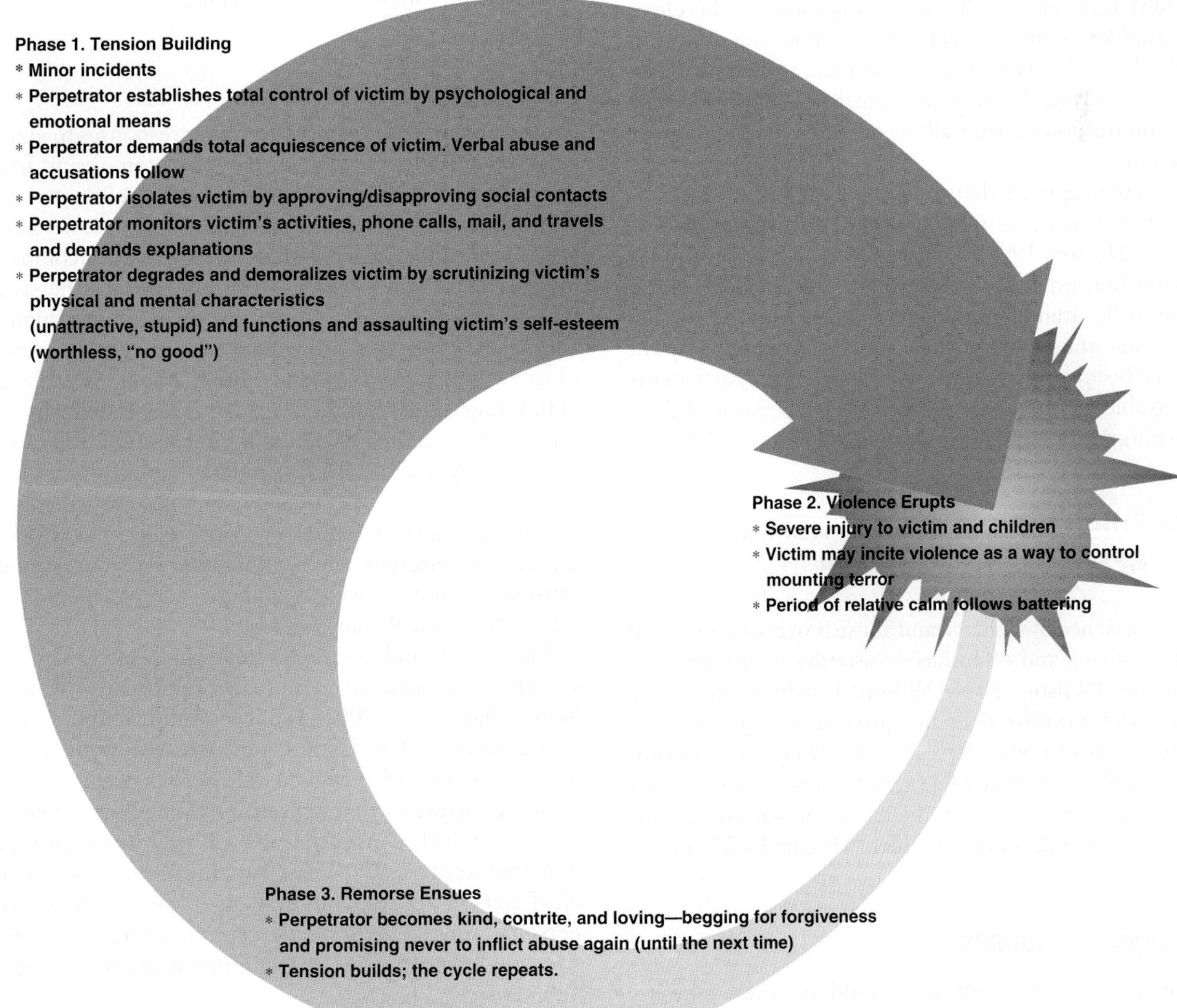

Phase 1. Tension Building
* Minor incidents
* Perpetrator establishes total control of victim by psychological and emotional means
* Perpetrator demands total acquiescence of victim. Verbal abuse and accusations follow
* Perpetrator isolates victim by approving/disapproving social contacts
* Perpetrator monitors victim's activities, phone calls, mail, and travels and demands explanations
* Perpetrator degrades and demoralizes victim by scrutinizing victim's physical and mental characteristics (unattractive, stupid) and functions and assaulting victim's self-esteem (worthless, "no good")
Phase 2. Violence Erupts
* Severe injury to victim and children
* Victim may incite violence as a way to control mounting terror
* Period of relative calm follows battering
Phase 3. Remorse Ensues
* Perpetrator becomes kind, contrite, and loving—begging for forgiveness and promising never to inflict abuse again (until the next time)
* Tension builds; the cycle repeats.

FIGURE 39.3. The cycle of violence.

a power imbalance and intermittent abuse help to form extremely strong emotional attachments. Traumatic bonding theory (Dutton & Painter, 1993) explains why the cycle of violence is so powerful in entrapping a woman in a violent relationship.

The woman in a power imbalance perceives herself to be in a powerless position in relation to her partner, whom she perceives as extremely powerful. As the power imbalance intensifies, she feels increasingly worthless, less capable of fending for herself and, therefore, more in need of her partner. This cycle of dependency and lowered self-esteem is continually repeated, eventually creating a strong affective bond to the partner (Dutton, 1995).

Intermittent reinforcement or punishment is one of the strongest learning paradigms in behavioral theory, especially in maintaining a particular behavior (Dutton, 1995). An example that is often used to illustrate this concept is the gambler who persistently puts coins in a slot machine. Despite substantial losses, the gambler persists because the next time just might be the big payoff. Therefore, the gambler is not rewarded every time, but intermittently. To apply this to battered women, women may stay because this time the man may actually mean what he says and stop the abuse. After all, he has been kind and loving intermittently.

Research suggests that traumatic bonding is especially important when a woman attempts to leave her abusive partner (Dutton, 1995). When a woman leaves an abusive relationship, especially after a battering incident, she is emotionally drained and vulnerable. As time passes, her fear of her abuser diminishes, and needs supplied by the partner become evident. At this time, she is particularly susceptible to the abuser's attempts to persuade her to return to the relationship (Dutton & Painter, 1993).

SURVIVORS OF ABUSE: HUMAN RESPONSES TO TRAUMA

The experience of violence and abuse is overwhelming for most survivors and often has devastating long-term consequences (Wilson, 2001; Wilson, Friedman, & Lindy, 2001). Victimization does not produce a single uniform syndrome or response. Research on the effects of victimization reflects considerable consistency in the biopsychosocial responses to overwhelming trauma, whether the victim is a child, adult, or elder (Hendricks-Matthews, 1993).

Biologic Responses

Victims of violence experience mild to severe physical consequences. Mild injuries may include bruises and abrasions of the head, neck, face, trunk, and extremities (Hathaway, Mucci, Silverman, Brooks, Mathews, & Pavlos (2000). Severe injuries include multiple traumas, major fractures, major lacerations, and internal injuries, including chest and abdominal injuries and subdural hematomas (Campbell et al., 2004). Loss of vision and hearing can result from blows to the head. Physical or sexual violence may result in head injuries that can produce changes in cognition, affect, motivation, and behavior. Victims of sexual abuse may have vaginal and perineal trauma that is sufficient to require surgical repair (Barnett et al., 1997). Anorectal injuries may also be present, including disruption of anal sphincters, retained foreign bodies, and mucosal lacerations. The following section covers the most common responses to violence and abuse:

- Depression (the dysregulated stress response theory of depression)
- Acute stress disorder (ASD)
- Posttraumatic stress disorder (PTSD)
- Dissociative identity disorder (DID)

Depression

Depression, one of the most common responses to abuse, is a biologically based disorder that can result from the effects of chronic stress on neurotransmitter and neuroendocrine systems. The body's response to stress is a complex, integrated system of reactions, encompassing body and mind. Threat or stress engages the stress system, which consists of the hypothalamus–pituitary–adrenal (HPA) axis and the sympathetic nervous system (Thase, Jindal, & Howland, 2002; Wong & Yehuda, 2002). Engagement of the HPA axis is associated with the release of corticotropin-releasing hormone (CRH) from the pituitary gland. CRH stimulates the pituitary gland to secrete adrenocorticotropic hormone (corticotropin), which stimulates the adrenal cortex to secrete cortisol. Stress also engages the sympathetic nervous system, causing the locus ceruleus and the adrenal medulla to release norepinephrine.

The CRH and locus ceruleus and norepinephrine systems participate in a mutually reinforcing feedback loop (Thase et al., 2002; Wong & Yehuda, 2002). That is, increases in CRH stimulate increased firing of the locus ceruleus and increased release of norepinephrine. Similarly, stressors that activate norepinephrine neurons increase CRH concentrations in the locus ceruleus (Charney et al., 1993). These systems prepare the threatened person to respond to danger by enhancing the person's arousal, attention, perception, energy, and emotion and by suppressing the immune response (Wong & Yehuda).

The stress response is meant to be of limited duration (Thase et al., 2002). However, when resistance or escape is impossible, the human stress system becomes overwhelmed and disorganized (Herman, 1997). Exposure to severe stressors early in life has been shown to compromise the regulation of HPA activity for a lifetime (Thase et al.). Most types of abuse are extreme forms of chronic stress. A protracted or dysregulated stress response has been associated with the development of major depression, especially the melancholic type (Chrousos & Gold, 1992; Henry, 1992). Melancholic features include dysphoric hyperarousal that is reflected in agitation, early morning awakening, anorexia, anxiety, excessive guilt, and hypervigilance (APA, 2000). Survivors of abuse report many of these symptoms.

Acute Stress Disorder and Posttraumatic Stress Disorder

The experience of trauma exerts tremendous physical and psychological stress on survivors. The cluster of signs and symptoms that frequently occur after major trauma is now labeled **acute stress disorder** (ASD) and **posttraumatic stress disorder** (PTSD). Dysregulation of the HPA axis may be the basis for the link between trauma and these disorders (Olff, Langeland, & Gersons, 2005). Originally, the diagnosis of PTSD was given only to men who demonstrated symptoms after combat experiences. In such cases, PTSD has been given several names, including *shell shock* after World War I, *traumatic neurosis* after World War II, and PTSD after the Vietnam War (Hollander & Simeon, 2003). However, subsequent research has demonstrated that symptoms of ASD and PTSD occur not only after war but also after many types of severe trauma, including physical abuse, sexual abuse, and rape.

ASD was a new disorder included in the *Diagnostic and Statistical Manual of Mental Disorders*, (4th ed., text revision) (*DSM-IV-TR*) (APA, 2000). It is diagnosed when a barrage of stress-related symptoms occurs within 1 month of a traumatic event and persists for at least 2 days, causing significant distress. If symptoms persist beyond 1 month, the diagnosis changes to PTSD. Research has indicated that symptoms of ASD predict the development of PTSD (Raphael & Matthew, 2002). The diagnostic criteria for ASD are similar to those for PTSD.

Because ASD is a new diagnostic category in *DSM-IV*, its prevalence is unknown. Community-based studies show a lifetime prevalence for PTSD of 1% to 14% (APA, 2000). Researchers studying at-risk people, including survivors of abuse, have found prevalence rates ranging from 3% to 64% (APA; Epstein, Saunders, Kilpatrick, & Resnick, 1998). A comprehensive review of research on the epidemiology of PTSD suggests several gender differences (Norris et al., 2002). Men are more exposed to traumatic events than are women. However, women are approximately twice as likely as men to experience PTSD, and the median time from onset to remission for women is 4 years, compared with 1 year for men. Several factors may contribute to these differences. One factor is that men and women experience different types of traumatic events. More men report exposure to events such as fire/disaster, life-threatening accidents, physical assault, combat, being threatened with a weapon, and being held captive. More women report child abuse, sexual molestation, and sexual assault. Sexual violence is associated with a high risk for the development of PTSD. Another factor is differing reactions to traumatic events. To meet criteria for a diagnosis of PTSD, the traumatized individual must experience terror, horror, or helplessness in response to the trauma (Criterion A2 in *DSM-IV-TR*, APA, 2000, p. 467). More women than men meet this criterion, suggesting that women may be more distressed than men by traumatic events. However, neither types of events nor perceptions of threat fully account for the difference in prevalence rates of PTSD in men and women (Norris et al.).

Other factors that may contribute to higher prevalence of PTSD in women include higher rates of anxiety and depressive disorders and traumatic events before the age of 15 years (Breslau et al., 1997; Orsillo, Raja, & Hammond, 2002). In one study of childhood exposure to trauma, a greater percentage of women (27%) than men (8%) reported rape, assault, or ongoing physical or sexual abuse. More men (28%) than women (11%) with childhood trauma reported serious accidents or injury. Exposure to accidents or injury in childhood did not lead to PTSD in respondents of either gender, whereas rape and abuse resulted in a high rate of early PTSD in women (63%), but no cases in men (Breslau et al.).

PTSD may develop any time after the trauma. The delay may be as short as 1 week or as long as 30 years (Hollander & Simeon, 2003). Symptoms may fluctuate in intensity with time and usually are worse during periods of stress. Some 30% of patients with PTSD recover completely, 40% continue to have mild symptoms, 20% continue to have moderate symptoms, and 10% remain unchanged or become worse (Sadock & Sadock, 2004).

Young children and the elderly have special difficulty with traumatic events. Young children may not have developed adequate coping mechanisms to deal with severe stressors, and older people are likely to have rigid coping mechanisms, making successful coping with the trauma more difficult (Hollander & Simeon, 2003).

Women with PTSD frequently have comorbid anxiety, depressive disorders, or both, and the association between childhood abuse, PTSD, and substance abuse is also becoming well established (Boyd, 2000, 2003; Boyd & Mackey, 2000b; Brady & Dansky, 2002; Stewart,

Ouimette, & Brown, 2002). The neurobiology of ASD and PTSD involves the stress response previously described. In addition, stress is manifested in three broad symptom categories associated with ASD and PTSD: hyperarousal, intrusion, and avoidance and numbing (APA, 2000; Rothschild, 1998).

Hyperarousal

After a traumatic experience, the stress system seems to go on permanent alert, as if the danger might return at any time (Hollander & Simeon, 2003; Rasmusson & Friedman, 2002; Wong & Yehuda, 2002). In this state of physiologic hyperarousal, the traumatized person is hypervigilant for signs of danger, startles easily, reacts irritably to small annoyances, and sleeps poorly. These symptoms are characteristic of increased noradrenergic function, particularly in the locus ceruleus and limbic system (hypothalamus, hippocampus, and amygdala), and of increased dopamine activity, particularly in the prefrontal cortical dopamine system (Rasmusson & Friedman; Wong & Yehuda). Dopamine hyperactivity is associated with the hypervigilance seen in PTSD. Many people with PTSD do not return to their normal baseline level of alertness. Instead, they seem to have a new baseline of elevated arousal, as if their "thermostat" had been reset (Bremner, Southwick, & Charney, 1999).

Behavioral sensitization may be one mechanism underlying the hyperarousal seen in PTSD. This phenomenon, sometimes referred to as *kindling*, occurs after exposure to severe, uncontrollable stressors. The sensitized person reacts with a magnified stress response to later, milder stressors (Bremner et al., 1999; Charney et al., 1993; Krystal et al., 1989). Research shows that a single or repeated exposure to a severe stressor potentiates the capacity of a subsequent stressor to increase synaptic levels of norepinephrine and dopamine in the forebrain (Charney et al., 1993). This finding would account for the fact that some survivors with PTSD experience intense fear, anxiety, and panic in response to minor stimuli. One example of behavioral sensitization is that PTSD after combat exposure is more likely to develop in veterans who are survivors of childhood abuse than in those who have not experienced prior trauma (Southwick, Bremner, Krystal, & Charney, 1994).

The state of hyperarousal causes other problems for survivors. The loss of neuromodulation leads to loss of affect regulation, so that the survivor is irritable and overreacts to others (van der Kolk & Fisler, 1993). This type of behavior may cause others to avoid the survivor. The continual arousal may desensitize the survivor to real threat and decrease the probability that she will respond to perceived danger (Messman-Moore & Long, 2003). This development may cause the person to miss clues of danger and place himself or herself in situations that can lead to revictimization.

Intrusion

Long after abuse has stopped, survivors relive it as though it were continually recurring. Flashbacks and nightmares, which the survivor experiences with terrifying immediacy, are vivid and often include fragments of traumatic events exactly as they happened (Bremner et al., 1999). Moreover, a wide variety of stimuli that may have been associated with the trauma can elicit flashbacks and dreams. Consequently, survivors avoid such stimuli (Bremner et al.).

Three related but somewhat different explanations may account for the vivid, disturbing flashbacks and dreams that individuals with PTSD have: disturbances of memory, classic conditioning (fear conditioning), and extinction.

Memory function is altered in PTSD. Memory deficits include short-term memory and potentiation of recall of traumatic experiences and dissociative flashbacks. Human beings are bombarded constantly by sensory stimuli yet attend to and remember only a fraction of it (Bremner et al., 1999; Southwick et al., 1994). People seem to remember best those events that have emotional effects and occur when they are alert, aroused, and responsive to their internal and external environment.

During stress, there is a massive release of neurotransmitters, particularly norepinephrine, epinephrine, and opioid peptides. This flood of "stress hormones" may lead to structural changes in the brain that potentiate long-term memory. In most situations, this type of memory has survival value: remembering events that occur during danger may protect oneself during similar future situations. However, in PTSD the memories occur when the individual is not in danger. Research supporting this hypothesis demonstrated that if norepinephrine is administered to animals immediately after training, long-term memory is enhanced. Epinephrine and endogenous opioids may influence memory consolidation (transforming short-term memory to long-term memory) by affecting norepinephrine (Bremner et al., 1999; Hollander & Simeon, 2003; Southwick et al., 1994).

The hippocampus and amygdala are involved in memory consolidation. The hippocampus is involved in object memory and placement of memory traces in space and time (Bremner et al., 1999; Cohen, Perel, DeBellis, Friedman, & Putnam, 2002). High levels of stress have been shown to damage the hippocampus and decrease its volume, producing memory deficits such as amnesia and deficits in autobiographical memory (memory of one's life story) (Bremner et al., 1999). The amygdala integrates sensory information for storage in and retrieval from memory. The amygdala also attaches emotional significance to sensory information and transmits this information to all the other systems involved in the stress response. Overreactivity of the amygdala might explain the recurrent and intrusive traumatic memories and the excessive fear associated with traumatic reminders characteristic of PTSD (Cohen et al.). Moreover, electrical stimulation of the amygdala and hippocampal area has been associated with dream-like and memory-like hallucinations that are similar to flashbacks reported by patients with PTSD (Bremner et al., 1999).

Classic conditioning, or **fear conditioning**, occurs when a neutral stimulus (the conditioned stimulus [CS]) is paired with an aversive unconditioned stimulus (US) that elicits an unconditioned fear response (UR). After repeated pairing, the CS alone will elicit the fear response, which is now the conditioned response (CR). For example, certain sights, sounds, or smells that occurred in close proximity to the traumatic event may elicit a fear response in the future. The result of this process is that an individual becomes fearful and anxious in response to a wide variety of stimuli (Bremner et al., 1999; Southwick et al., 1994); therefore, a wide variety of stimuli can elicit symptoms of PTSD.

The amygdala and hippocampus also appear to be important players in fear conditioning (Bremner et al., 1999; Southwick et al., 1994). Other important brain sites include the thalamus, locus ceruleus, and sensory cortex. Interaction between the cortex and the amygdala may be necessary for specific stimuli to elicit traumatic memories (Bremner et al.; Charney et al., 1993).

Several neurochemical systems are involved in regulating fear conditioning, including norepinephrine, dopamine (DA), opiate, and corticotropin-releasing systems. In addition, N-methyl-D-aspartate (NMDA), one of the major excitatory neurotransmitters in the brain, appears necessary for this type of learning to occur. NMDA antagonists applied to the amygdala prevent the development of fear-conditioned responses (Bremner et al., 1999; Charney et al., 1993).

Extinction is the loss of a learned conditioned emotional response after repeated presentations of the conditioned fear stimulus without a contiguous traumatic event. In other words, the individual no longer responds with fear to the conditioned response. For example, many children are afraid of the dark; however, after many uneventful nights, children gradually lose their fear. Failure of the neuronal mechanisms involved in extinction also may explain the continued ability of conditioned stimuli to elicit traumatic memories and flashbacks in PTSD (Bremner et al., 1999; Charney et al., 1993). Recent research on brain dysfunction associated with PTSD resulting from childhood abuse of women has shown that damage to the medial prefrontal cortex interferes with extinguishing fear responses. In addition, individuals with damage to the medial prefrontal cortex show emotional dysfunction and an inability to relate in social situations that require correct interpretation of the emotional expressions of others. These findings suggest that dysfunction of this area of the brain may play a role in pathologic emotions that follow exposure to extreme stressors, such as childhood sexual abuse (Bremner et al., 1999).

Avoidance and Numbing (Dissociative Symptoms)

Survivors try to avoid people or situations that might provoke memories of the trauma. This restriction in their activities may interfere with normal functioning. Survivors also report anhedonia (loss of ability to sense pleasure), and may report that they feel as if parts of themselves have died. These disturbing symptoms may lead them to engage in acts of self-mutilation to feel alive or ultimately to suicide (van der Kolk & Fisler, 1993).

A person who is completely powerless may go into a state of surrender. In that state, the person escapes the situation by altering his or her state of consciousness, that is, by dissociating (Herman, 1997). **Dissociation** is defined as a disruption in the normally occurring linkages between subjective awareness, feelings, thoughts, behavior, and memories (APA, 2000; Briere & Elliott, 1994).

Dissociation is a complex psychophysiologic process that produces alterations in sense of self, accessibility of memory and knowledge, and integration of behavior (Putnam, 1994; Rothschild, 1998). In simpler words, a person who dissociates is making themselves "disappear." That is, the person has the feeling of leaving their body and observing what happens to them from a distance. During trauma, dissociation enables a person to observe the event while experiencing no pain, or only limited pain, and to protect themselves from awareness of the full impact of the traumatic event (van der Kolk, 1996). Examples of dissociation include (1) derealization and depersonalization (the experience of self or the environment as strange or unreal); (2) periods of disengagement from the immediate environment during stress, such as "spacing out"; (3) alterations in bodily perceptions; (4) emotional numbing; (5) out-of-body experiences; and (6) amnesia for abuse-related memories (Briere & Elliott, 1994; Rothschild). Fear activates the endogenous opioid system, producing stress-induced analgesia (SIA) (Bremner et al., 1999; van der Kolk). SIA may be associated with avoidance and numbing. The purpose of SIA is to protect against pain in dangerous situations so that the individual (animal or human) can defend itself (fight) or escape the situation (flight). In severely stressed animals, opiate withdrawal symptoms can be produced by removing the stressor or by injecting naloxone, an opiate antagonist. In people with PTSD, SIA can become conditioned to stimuli resembling the original trauma. Research with humans showed that as long as 20 years after the original trauma, people with PTSD developed SIA equivalent to 8 mg of morphine in response to such stimuli. Excessive opioid and norepinephrine secretion can interfere with memory. Freezing or numbing responses may prevent animals from remembering situations of overwhelming stress.

Trauma-related dissociative reactions after prolonged exposure to severe, uncontrollable stress may be analogous to this effect in animals (van der Kolk).

Dissociative Identity Disorder

Dissociation exists on a continuum, with most people experiencing short, situation-specific episodes, such as daydreaming (Putnam, 1994). Among survivors of abuse, dissociative symptoms may be part of the symptom picture of ASD and PTSD, or they may be the predominant symptom. In such cases, the disorder is **dissociative identity disorder** (DID) (formerly multiple personality disorder) (Hollander & Simeon, 2003; Rothschild, 1998). The hallmarks of DID are two or more distinct identities with unique personality characteristics and an inability to recall important information about self or events that is too extensive to be explained by ordinary forgetfulness (APA, 2000). Other memory disturbances linked with dissociation include intermittent and disruptive intrusions of traumatic memories into awareness and difficulties in determining whether a given memory reflects an actual event or information acquired through another source (Putnam). The diagnostic criteria for DID are found in Table 39.1.Three most common symptoms of DID are amnesia, conversion symptoms, and voices (Dell, 2006).

The overall prevalence of DID is unknown (Hollander & Simeon, 2003). Estimates are that 1% of the American population may be affected and as many as 5% to 20% of people in psychiatric hospitals (National Women's Health Information Center [NWHIC], 2003). The cause of DID is unknown. However, the patient history invariably involves a traumatic event in childhood. Four types of causative factors have been identified: a traumatic event, a psychological or genetic vulnerability to develop the disorder, formative environmental factors, and the absence of external support (Sadock & Sadock, 2004). Examples of psychological vulnerability include being suggestible or easily hypnotized. Formative environmental events may include a lack of role models who demonstrate healthy problem solving or practices to relieve anxiety or stress. Many who experience DID lack supportive others, such as parents, siblings, other relatives, and supportive people outside the family (e.g., teachers) (Sadock & Sadock).

Complex Trauma

In her book *Trauma and Recovery*, Judith Herman proposed a new diagnosis: "**complex post-traumatic stress disorder**" (1997, p. 119). Her proposal was based on experience that none of the diagnostic categories in the APA's *Diagnostic and Statistical Manual* (3rd ed., rev., APA, 1987) were appropriate for survivors of extreme, prolonged trauma, especially interpersonal trauma (i.e., severe, prolonged child abuse), including the diagnosis of PTSD. She noted that survivors of prolonged, repeated trauma experience characteristic personality changes, including problems of relatedness, identity, and vulnerability to repeated harm, inflicted by others or self. Complex PTSD was considered for inclusion in the fourth edition of the *DSM* as "disorders of extreme stress not otherwise specified (DESNOS)" (van der Kolk, 1996, p. 203). DESNOS was eventually incorporated into the *DSM-IV* under the "Associated Features and Disorders" section. The symptoms include impaired affect modulation (difficulty modulating anger or sexual behaviors; self-destructive and suicidal behavior); impulsive/risk-taking behavior; alterations in attention and consciousness (amnesia, dissociation); somatization; chronic characterological changes, including alterations in rela-

Table 39.1  **Key Diagnostic Characteristics for Dissociative Identity Disorder** 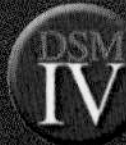

Diagnostic Criteria	Target Symptoms and Associated Findings
• Presence of two or more distinct personality states or identities • At least two identities or personality states recurrently take control of the person's behavior • Inability to recall important information that is too extensive to be explained by ordinary forgetfulness • Not due to direct physiologic effects of substances or general medical condition • In children, symptoms not attributable to imaginary playmates or other fantasy play	• Posttraumatic symptoms (nightmares, flashbacks, startle responses) • Posttraumatic stress disorder • Self-mutilation • Suicidal behavior • Aggressive behavior • Repetitive relationships characterized by physical and sexual abuse **Associated Physical Examination Findings** • Scars from self-inflicted injuries or physical abuse • Migraine and other types of headaches, irritable bowel syndrome and asthma **Associated Laboratory Findings** • Physiologic functioning may vary across personality states • High scores on measures of hypnotizability and dissociative capacity

tions with others (inability to trust or maintain relationships, tendency to be revictimized or to victimize others); and alterations in systems of meaning (despair, hopelessness, loss of previously sustaining beliefs) (APA, 2000; van der Kolk).

These symptoms are similar to those of borderline personality disorder (BPD). Many people with BPD were severely abused in childhood. Splitting self and others into *all-good* or *all-bad* may result from a developmental arrest: a fragmentation of self, based on modes of organizing experiences that were common in earlier developmental stages. Self-mutilation, often labeled as masochism or manipulative behavior, may be a way of regulating psychological and biological equilibrium when ordinary means of self-regulation have been disturbed by trauma. Psychotic episodes in patients with BPD are similar to flashbacks, intrusive recollections of traumatic memories that were stored on a somatosensory level (van der Kolk, 1996).

PTSD, as presently conceptualized, does not adequately capture the nature of violence against women (Mechanic, 2004). The first criterion for PTSD in the *DSM-IV-TR* states that "the person experienc*ed*, witness*ed*, or was confront*ed* with an event or events that involv*ed* actual or threatened death or serious injury, or threat to the physical integrity of self or others" (italics added). In other words, the danger is no longer present. According to diagnostic criteria, PTSD is an appropriate diagnosis when individuals display symptoms of traumatic stress when they are no longer in danger, that is, their reaction is now pathological. However, we know that harassment, stalking, and other types of threats continue even when women leave a violent relationship. In that light, symptoms such as hyperarousal are not pathological; they are survival-based fear reactions to real danger (Mechanic). Pathologizing appropriate reactions to real danger further victimizes women. Moreover, treatment aimed to reduce fear in the face of real danger is not appropriate.

Substance Abuse and Dependence

Childhood abuse, PTSD, and substance abuse are known to be associated. Investigators have reported that as many as 84% of female inpatient substance abusers had a history of sexual or physical assault (Brady & Dansky, 2002; Stewart et al., 2002). High rates of abuse have also been found in samples of outpatient, rural women (Boyd, 2000, 2003).

Survivors who experience PTSD, depression, and other forms of dysphoric hyperarousal or emotional distress often abuse substances, including alcohol and other sedative drugs, that lessen stress and reduce hyperarousal and distress by inhibiting noradrenergic activity (Brady & Dansky, 2002; Stewart et al., 2002). Sexually abused adolescents and adults may use alcohol and other drugs as alternatives to psychological dissociation (Roesler & Dafler, 1993). Increasing numbers of women reportedly abuse cocaine to wipe out dysphoric feelings caused by abuse. These women report that the intense high of cocaine totally obliterates painful feelings, if only for a short time (Boyd, 2000). Substance abuse in a person with PTSD is particularly problematic. The comorbidity worsens the symptoms and courses of both disorders, increases suicidality, and makes treatment more difficult (Boyd; Hana & Grant, 1997).

Psychological Responses

Low Self-esteem

The consequences of abuse are devastating, and the term "low self-esteem" seems inadequate. Women who are abused as children often experience "alienation from self and others" (Boyd & Mackey, 2000a). Alienation from self includes painful feelings that go to the "core of a woman being"—experiencing self as fundamentally flawed and having no purpose in life. Alienation from others, especially significant others, is associated with painful feelings of loneliness, depression, anger, shame, guilt, and feeling hurt, unloved, and unwanted (Boyd & Mackey, 2000a). Women who experience alienation from self and others often turn to substance abuse to cope with their intense pain (Boyd & Mackey, 2000b).

Low self-esteem or alienation may be attributable to the direct effects of physical or sexual abuse or to the accompanying psychological abuse. One technique that perpetrators use to control and disempower women is to erode their sense of self-worth with a constant barrage of criticism. Perpetrators frequently tell women that they are stupid, ugly, inadequate wives and mothers, inadequate sexually, and incompetent. Other contributing factors include a sense of being different from other people, the need to maintain secrecy, lack of trust, and self-blame (Boyd & Mackey, 2000a).

Low self-esteem may be one factor contributing to a battered woman's reluctance to disclose her abuse. Because of low self-esteem, battered women, even many who are successful outside the home, underestimate their ability to do anything about the abuse (Boyd & Mackey, 2000a).

Guilt and Shame

A history of abuse is often associated with excessive guilt and shame. These feelings stem from survivors' mistaken beliefs that they are somehow to blame for their abuse (Boyd & Mackey, 2000a; Campbell et al., 2004; Long & Smyth, 1998). Feelings of humiliation and shame may prevent women from seeking medical care and reporting abuse to authorities. The experience of being battered is so degrading and humiliating that women are often afraid to disclose it. Many women fear that they will not be taken seriously or will be blamed for inciting the abuse or for staying with their abusers (Boyd & Mackey; Campbell et al.; Long & Smyth).

Anger

Chronic irritability, unexpected or uncontrollable feelings of anger, and difficulties with the expression of anger are frequent experiences for survivors of abuse (Campbell et al., 2004). They may express anger toward the perpetrator, fate, those who have been spared suffering, or someone whom the victim believes could have prevented the abuse (Barnett et al., 1997).

Feelings of anger may signal that a person is an incest survivor. However, some incest survivors have difficulty expressing anger and mask it with compliance and perfectionism (Campbell et al., 2004; Hendricks-Matthews, 1993).

Social And Interpersonal Responses

Problems With Intimacy

The abused child experiences intrusion, abandonment, devaluation, or pain in the relationship with the abuser, instead of the closeness and nurturing that are normal for intimate relationships, such as those between parent and child (Briere & Elliott, 1994; Long & Smyth, 1998; Urbancic, 2004). As a result, many survivors have difficulty trusting and forming intimate relationships.

Sexual problems are common among survivors of abuse. Among the most common and chronic problems are fear of intimate sexual relationships, feelings of repulsion toward sex, lack of enjoyment of sex, dysfunctions of desire and arousal, and failure to achieve orgasm. Some survivors engage in compulsive promiscuity and prostitution, reflecting their internalization of the message that the only thing that they are good for is sex (Hendricks-Matthews, 1993; Long & Smyth, 1998; Urbancic, 2004).

Revictimization

Many women who have been sexually abused as children are revictimized on multiple occasions later in life. Among women with a history of sexual assault, rates of revictimization range from 15% to 79% (Arata, 2002; Breitenbecher, 2001; Messman-Moore & Long, 2003). Numerous factors have been related to revictimization, including PTSD symptoms, dissociation, alexithymia, use of alcohol and other drugs, boundary issues, and sexual behavior (Breitenbecher, 2001; Messman-Moore & Long, 2003). Proneness to revictimization may result from a general vulnerability in dangerous situations that may be associated with dissociation. Dissociation makes women unaware of their environment and also may make them look confused or distracted. Thus, women in a dissociative state may be easy targets (Cloitre, Scarvalone, & Difede, 1997; Messman-Moore & Long,).

Alexithymia may also add to a woman's risk for revictimization. Difficulty in labeling and communicating feelings may make it difficult for a woman to set limits on sexual advances. Moreover, these women may not be able to read accurately the emotional cues of others, which diminishes their ability to respond effectively in interpersonally dangerous situations (Cloitre et al., 1997).

Women with abuse histories frequently have difficulty with boundaries. During childhood abuse, they experienced boundary violations as normal and connected with their expectations of intimate relationships. Confusion over boundaries may result in confusion about appropriate behavior in adult intimate relationships (Cloitre et al., 1997; Messman-Moore & Long, 2003).

The sexual behavior pattern of survivors may place them at risk for revictimization. One effect of sexual victimization is that the child's sexuality is shaped by "traumatic sexualization." Traumatic sexualization occurs when a child is rewarded for sexual behavior with affection, attention, privileges, and gifts. As a result, the child may learn that her self-worth is tied to her sexuality, and she may use sexual behavior to manipulate others (Breitenbecher, 2001; Messman-Moore & Long, 2003).

Other Consequences of Child Abuse

Other acute responses to child abuse may include lower academic performance, behavioral problems, higher incidences of depression, more dissociative symptoms, and a propensity toward sexual acting-out behaviors (Noll, 2005). Other consequences include early coital initiation, teen pregnancy, obesity, and poor physiological health (Noll). Consequences that may persist into adulthood include dysregulation of the HPA axis and stress sensitivity, PTSD, and pathological dissociation (Noll).

NURSING MANAGEMENT: HUMAN RESPONSE TO ABUSE

Nurses encounter survivors of abuse in many health care settings. The percentage of ED visits that are attributed to domestic violence ranges from 4% to 18% (Campbell et al., 2004); however, reports have been as high as 80% (McGrath et al., 1997). Approximately 50% of female patients admitted to psychiatric facilities are victims of either child or adult abuse (Seeman, 2002). Other settings in which the nurse encounters battered women include primary care settings, obstetrics-gynecology settings, pediatric units, well-child clinics, geriatric units, and nursing homes.

The pediatric ED provides a unique opportunity to identify and respond to child survivors, as well as battered mothers (Campbell et al., 2004). As many as 59% of mothers of child abuse victims are battered women, and child abuse occurs disproportionately in homes with woman abuse (Wright, Wright, & Isaac, 1997). Identifying battered mothers may be the most important means of identifying child abuse. Conversely, when a nurse suspects child abuse, he or she cannot ignore the possibility that the mother is also a victim. Identifying children who are traumatized by witnessing the battering of their mothers also is essential. However, despite the opportunity the pediatric ED affords, disturbingly few battered women are identified there. Health care providers in pediatric EDs have reported several obstacles to identification, including lack of training, time constraints, powerlessness, lack of comfort, lack of control over the victim's circumstances, and fear of offending the patient (Wright et al.). Nurses may encounter elder abuse in virtually any setting. Examples include EDs, medical–surgical units, psychiatric units, and homes during home care visits. In addition, nurses may encounter elder abuse in nursing homes. Events such as unnecessary chemical (medications) or physical restraints used to control an elder's behavior may be abusive and should be investigated.

Although some aspects of care are specific to adult, child, or elderly survivors of abuse, many elements are common in the nursing management of all survivors, regardless of age or setting. The goals of all nursing interventions in cases of abuse are to stop the violence and ensure the survivor's safety (Walton-Moss & Campbell, 2002). Victimization removes all power and control from a woman, child, or elder. Therefore, as appropriate for age and ability, all nursing interventions should empower survivors to act on their own behalf and must be done in a collaborative partnership. To that end, nurses must be willing to offer support and information and not impose their own values on survivors by encouraging them to leave abusive relationships. Strong psychological and economic bonds tie many women to their perpetrators. Moreover, adult survivors who are capable of making decisions are the experts on their situations. They are the best judges of when leaving the relationship is appropriate (Walker, 1994).

However, removing children and elders from their families or caregivers often is necessary to ensure immediate safety. If the home of an abused or neglected child or elder cannot be made safe, the nurse must support other professionals involved in placing the child or elder in a foster or nursing home (Gary & Humphreys, 2004; Sengstock et al., 2004). However, intervening in cases of elder abuse is not a clear-cut issue. Nurses must allow elders whose decision making is not impaired (*competence* is a legal term) an appropriate degree of autonomy in deciding how to manage the problem, even if they choose to remain in the abusive situation (Allan, 1998). Forcing an elder to do something against his or her wishes is itself a form of victimization.

Intervention strategies for elders depend on whether the elder accepts or refuses assistance and whether he or she can make decisions. If the elder refuses treatment, the nurse must remain nonjudgmental and provide information about available services and emergency numbers. The nurse must contact the adult protective services department (APS) if mandated to do so in his or her state. If the elder appears incapable of making decisions, the nurse should contact APS and assist in making arrangements for guardianship, foster care, nursing home placement, or court proceedings as needed (Sengstock et al., 2004).

Biologic Domain

Biologic Assessment

Research indicates that health care providers often fail to respond therapeutically to survivors of abuse. In many instances, they neglect to identify abuse as the cause of traumatic injuries or mental health problems (Campbell et al., 2004). Even more damaging, many health care professionals treat abuse survivors derogatorily, blaming them for the abuse or for staying in abusive situations. Unfortunately, nursing staff may revictimize survivors with BPD. Often these women have been severely traumatized, and their behavior is difficult and disruptive. In some cases, caregivers react negatively, labeling this behavior attention seeking and manipulative. When nurses react to the patient in a negative, punitive manner, they retraumatize these women. It is not uncommon to see this behavior punished by staff avoidance, time in seclusion rooms, and overmedication. BPD symptoms should be interpreted as ineffective coping strategies, developed in response to severe trauma, rather than as deliberate attempts to manipulate staff (Hattendorf & Tollerud, 1997).

To improve providers' responses, the American Nurses Association (ANA) recommends instruction for all nurses and health care providers in the skills necessary to prevent violence and manage the treatment of survivors. Moreover, the ANA recommends that nurses assess all women for abuse in every setting. That recommendation should be expanded to include people of all age groups. Nurses should assess everyone for violence—both women and men, no matter what age or presenting problem. An awareness of violence and a high index of suspicion are the most important elements in assessing the problem (Campbell et al., 2004).

If suspected abuse is never assessed, it will never be uncovered.

Establishing a trusting nurse–patient relationship is one of the most important steps in assessing any type of abuse. Survivors are unlikely to disclose sensitive information unless they perceive the nurse to be trustworthy and nonjudgmental. Important considerations in establishing open communication are ensuring confidentiality and providing a quiet, private place in which to conduct assessment. The law mandates that nurses report child and elder abuse to the authorities, and nurses must make that responsibility clear before beginning the assessment. Child abuse is usually reported to the department of social services (DSS), and elder abuse is reported to APS. In states in which reporting woman abuse is mandatory, the nurse must also inform women of that responsibility before assessment. Mandatory reporting is controversial because it may act as a barrier to disclosure, especially in cases in which the woman fears that the abuser will retaliate (Sheridan, 2004).

Lethality Assessment First

The most important assessment and the one to be done first is a lethality assessment (Walker, 1994). The nurse must ascertain whether the survivor is in danger for his or her life, either from homicide or suicide and, if children are in the home, whether they are in danger (Campbell et al., 2004). The nurse should take immediate steps to ensure the survivor's safety. Those steps may include reporting to police, DSS, or APS. In the case of suspected child abuse assessed in a health care agency, an interdisciplinary team consisting of physicians, psychologists, nurses, and social workers usually makes this decision. In other settings, the nurse may be the person to make that decision. Nurses do not have to obtain proof of abuse, only a reasonable suspicion. The Danger Assessment Screen developed by Jacquelyn Campbell and colleagues is a useful tool for assessing the risk that either the adult survivor or perpetrator will commit homicide (Box 39.1).

Most survivors do not report abuse to health care workers without being asked specifically about it. Only 13% of women seen in the ED after a battering incident either told or were asked by staff about abuse (Sisley et al., 1999). Survivors may be reluctant to report abuse because of shame and fear of retaliation, especially if the victim depends on the abuser as caregiver. In addition, children may be afraid that they will not be believed. Asking specific abuse screening questions has been shown to increase the detection of abuse substantially (from 3% to 15%) (Sisley et al., 1999). For that reason, nurses must develop a repertoire of age-appropriate, culturally sensitive abuse-related questions (Burgess & Tavakoli, 2005).

BOX 39.1

Danger Assessment

Several risk factors have been associated with homicides (murders) of both batterers and battered women in research that has been conducted after the killings have taken place. We cannot predict what will happen in your case, but we would like you to be aware of the danger of homicide in situations of severe battering and to see how many of the risk factors apply to your situation. (The "he" in the questions refers to your husband, partner, ex-husband, ex-partner, or whoever is currently physically hurting you.)

1. Has the physical violence increased in frequency during the past year?
2. Has the physical violence increased in severity during the past year, or has a weapon or threat with weapon been used?
3. Does he ever try to choke you?
4. Is there a gun in the house?
5. Has he ever forced you into sex when you did not wish to do so?
6. Does he use drugs? By drugs, I mean "uppers" or amphetamines, speed, angel dust, cocaine, "crack," street drugs, heroin, or mixtures.
7. Does he threaten to kill you, or do you believe he is capable of killing you?
8. Is he drunk every day or almost every day? (In terms of quantity of alcohol.)
9. Does he control most or all of your daily activities? For instance, does he tell you whom you can be friends with, how much money you can take with you shopping, or when you can take the car? (If he tries, but you do not let him, check here—.)
10. Has he ever beaten you while you were pregnant? (If never pregnant by him, check here—.)
11. Is he violently and constantly jealous of you? (For instance, does he say, "If I can't have you, no one can.")
12. Have you ever threatened or tried to commit suicide?
13. Has he ever threatened or tried to commit suicide?
14. Is he violent toward the children?
15. Is he violent outside the home?

TOTAL YES ANSWERS:—.

THANK YOU. PLEASE TALK TO YOUR NURSE, ADVOCATE, OR COUNSELOR ABOUT WHAT THE DANGER ASSESSMENT MEANS IN TERMS OF YOUR SITUATION.

Adapted from Campbell, J., & Humphreys, J. (Eds.). (1993). *Nursing care of survivors of family violence* (p. 259). St. Louis: Mosby.

BOX 39.2

Abuse Assessment Screen

1. Have you ever been emotionally or physically abused by your partner or someone important to you?
   YES ________
   NO ________
2. Within the past year, have you been hit, slapped, kicked or otherwise physically hurt by someone?
   YES ________
   NO ________
   If YES, by whom: ________________
   Number of times: ________
   Mark the area of injury on body map.
3. Within the past year, has anyone forced you to have sexual activities?
   If YES, who: ________________
   Number of times: ________
4. Are you afraid of your partner or anyone you listed above?
   YES ________
   NO ________

Appropriate questions to ask in assessing abuse in women are found in the Abuse Assessment Screen (Box 39.2) and in the Burgess-Partner Abuse Scale for Teens (Box 39.3). Other questions that might be useful in eliciting disclosure are: "When there are fights at home, have you ever been hurt or afraid?" "It looks like someone has hurt you. Tell me about it." "Some women have described problems like yours and have told me that their partner has hurt them. Is that happening to you?" (Campbell et al., 2004). When survivors are disclosing abuse, they need privacy and time to tell their story. They need to know that the nurse is listening, believes them, and is concerned for their safety and well-being (Long & Smyth, 1998).

Most survivors are not offended when health care providers ask about abuse directly, as long as they conduct the interview nonjudgmentally. Survivors may perceive failure to ask about abuse as evidence of lack of concern, adding to feelings of entrapment and helplessness. The high prevalence of abuse and the reluctance of survivors to volunteer information about it mandates routine screening of every patient for abuse by explicit questioning. Perhaps even more important, the nurse must complete such screening in privacy, away from the woman's partner, the child's parents or legal guardians, or the elderly person's relative or companion (Campbell et al., 2004; Sisley et al., 1999). If a partner, parent, other relative, or companion accompanies the patient to the health care facility, protocols should be in place to separate the patient from these individuals until assessment is completed. One approach is to ask the other person to wait in the reception area, explaining that assessments are always done in private.

After assessment is completed in a health care agency, the nurse should offer the adult survivor use of the telephone. The agency appointment may be the only time that the survivor can make calls in private to family, who might offer support, or to the police, lawyers, or shelters. Scheduling future appointments may provide the survivor with a legitimate reason to leave the perpetrator temporarily and continue to explore her options.

History and Physical Examination

All survivors who report or for whom the nurse suspects abuse should receive a complete history and physical examination. Throughout, the nurse must remain nonjudgmental and communicate openly and honestly (Campbell et al., 2004; Long & Smyth, 1998). It is not the nurse's responsibility to judge any situation, whether that is a woman's decision to remain in an abusive relationship, the abusive actions of children's parents, or abuse perpetrated by caregivers of the elderly. Therefore, nurses must continually monitor their own feelings toward the abuser and survivor, especially in cases of child abuse. Working with child survivors often causes distress and feelings of anger and inadequacy. Seeking supervision may prevent negative feelings from influencing the nurse–patient relationship in a nontherapeutic manner and perhaps retraumatizing the survivor (Long & Smyth).

The history should include past and present medical history, ADLs, and social and financial support. The nurse should obtain a detailed history of how injuries occurred. As with any history, the nurse begins with the complaint that brought the patient to the health care facility. The nurse assesses whether the explanation for the injuries or symptoms is plausible, given their nature. Discrepancies between the history and physical examination findings may suggest abuse or neglect. The nurse moves from safe to more sensitive topics, such as the nature of the injuries. Walker (1994) suggests using what she calls the "four-incident technique" to elicit a complete abuse history. The nurse asks the survivor to describe four battering incidents: the first incident that she remembers, the most recent incident, the worst incident, and a typical incident. This series of questions is designed to elicit a complete picture of the cycle of violence and its progression. If the child is too young or an elder is too impaired to give a history, the nurse should interview one or both parents of the child or the caregiver of the elder. If the survivor is a child or dependent elder who cannot describe what happened or make decisions about personal safety and care, the health care team may take steps to place the survivor in protective custody and defer additional assessment to the appropriate agency (DSS or APS). The physical examination should include a neurologic examination,

BOX 39.3

Burgess-Partner Abuse Scale for Teens

Directions: During the past 12 months, you and one of your partners may have had a fight. Below is a list of things one of your partners may have done to you. Please circle the number of how often this partner did these things to you. This is not a test and there are no right or wrong answers. Remember, having a partner (s) does not mean you are having sex with the partner (s).

If you have not had a partner in the past 12 months, do not fill this form out.

	Never	Once	A few times	More than a few times	Routinely or a lot
1. My partner doesn't let me go out with my friends	0	1	2	3	4
2. My partner tells me what to wear	0	1	2	3	4
3. My partner says if I don't have sex with him/her then I don't love him/her	0	1	2	3	4
4. My partner says he/she will hurt me if I talk to another guy/girl	0	1	2	3	4
5. My partner calls me bad names like bitch	0	1	2	3	4
6. My partner says he/she will hurt me with a weapon	0	1	2	3	4
7. My partner forces me to have sex	0	1	2	3	4
8. My partner tells me I am stupid or dumb	0	1	2	3	4
9. My partner follows me when I do things with my friends or family	0	1	2	3	4
10. My partner hits or kicks something when he/she gets mad at me	0	1	2	3	4
11. My partner kicks me	0	1	2	3	4
12. My partner says he/she can have sex with other people even though he/she said I can't	0	1	2	3	4
13. My partner gives me sex infections	0	1	2	3	4
14. My partner hurts me using a weapon	0	1	2	3	4
15. My partner forces me to use drugs even though I don't want to	0	1	2	3	4
16. My partner beats me up so bad	0.	1	2	3	4
17. My partner says he/she will hurt my family if I don't do what he/she says	0	1	2	3	4
18. My partner tells me what school activities I can and can't do	0	1	2	3	4
19. My partner tells me what friends I can hang out with	0	1	2	3	4
20. My partner chokes me if he/she gets mad at me	0	1	2	3	4
21. My partner yells at me if he/she doesn't know where I am	0	1	2	3	4
22. My partner says we can't break up even though I want to	0	1	2	3	4

How many partners have you had in the past 12 months?_________

 Burgess, S., & Tavakoli, A. (2005). Psychometric assessment of the Burgess-Partner Abuse Scale for Teens (B-PAST). *Aquichan*, 5, 96–107.

radiographs to identify any old or new fractures, and examination for sexual abuse. Nurses, assessing the elderly, need to be familiar with normal aging and signs and symptoms of common illnesses in the elderly to distinguish those conditions from abuse (Allan, 1998). Similarly, nurses need to know healthy child development to detect deviations that abuse or neglect may cause. For children, assessing developmental milestones, school history, and relationships with siblings and friends is important (Walker). Any discrepancies between history and physical examination and implausible explanations for injuries and other symptoms should alert the nurse to the possibility of abuse. Box 39.4 lists indicators of actual or potential abuse that need to be thoroughly assessed for all survivors. The nurse should thoroughly document all findings. Injuries should be photographed if possible, but this can be done only with written permission from an adult survivor or one of the child's parents. If the survivor will not permit photographing, the nurse should document the injuries on a body map. Survivors may need assurance that their medical records will not be released to anyone without written permission and that documentation of injuries will be important if legal action is taken. If the survivor does not admit abuse, the nurse cannot note abuse in the record. However, the

BOX 39.4

History and Physical Findings Suggestive of Abuse

Presenting Problem
- Vague information about cause of problem
- Delay between occurrence of injury and seeking of treatment
- Inappropriate reactions of significant other or family
- Denial or minimizing of seriousness of injury
- Discrepancy between history and physical examination findings

Family History
- Past family violence
- Physical punishment of children
- Children who are fearful of parent(s)
- Father and/or mother who demands unquestioning obedience
- Alcohol or drug abuse
- Violence outside the home
- Unemployment or underemployment
- Financial difficulties or poverty
- Use of elder's finances for other family members
- Finances rigidly controlled by one member

Health and Psychiatric History
- Fractures at various stages of healing
- Spontaneous abortions
- Injuries during pregnancy
- Multiple visits to the emergency department
- Elimination disturbances (e.g., constipation, diarrhea)
- Multiple somatic complaints
- Eating disorders
- Substance abuse
- Depression
- Posttraumatic stress disorder
- Self-mutilation
- Suicide attempts
- Feelings of helplessness or hopelessness
- Low self-esteem
- Chronic fatigue
- Apathy
- Sleep disturbances (e.g., hypersomnia, hyposomnia)
- Psychiatric hospitalizations

Personal and Social History
- Feelings of powerlessness
- Feelings of being trapped
- Lack of trust
- Traditional values about home, partner, and children's behavior
- Major decisions in family controlled by one person
- Few social supports (isolated from family, friends)
- Little activity outside the home
- Unwanted or unplanned pregnancy
- Dependency on caregivers
- Extreme jealousy by partner
- Difficulties at school or work
- Short attention span
- Running away
- Promiscuity
- Child who has knowledge of sexual matters beyond that appropriate for age
- Sexualized play with self, peers, dolls, toys
- Masturbation
- Excessive fears and clinging in children
- Verbal aggression
- Themes of violence in artwork and school work
- Distorted body image
- History of chronic physical or psychological disability
- Inability to perform activities of daily living
- Delayed language development

Physical Examination Findings

General Appearance
- Fearful, anxious, hyperactive, hypoactive
- Watching partner, parent, or caregiver for approval of answers to questions
- Poor grooming or inappropriate dress
- Malnourishment
- Signs of stress or fatigue
- Flinching when approached or touched
- Inappropriate or anxious nonverbal behavior
- Wearing clothing inappropriate to the season or occasion to cover body parts

Vital Statistics
- Elevated pulse or blood pressure
- Other signs of autonomic arousal (exaggerated startle response, excessive sweating)
- Underweight or overweight

Skin
- Bruises, welts, edema, or scars
- Burns (cigarette, immersion, friction from ropes, pattern like electric iron or stove)
- Subdural hematoma
- Missing hair
- Poor skin integrity: dehydration, decubitus ulcers, untreated wounds, urine burns or excoriation

Eyes
- Orbital swelling
- Conjunctival hemorrhage
- Retinal hemorrhage
- Black eyes
- No glasses to accommodate poor eyesight

Ears
- Hearing loss
- No prosthetic device to accommodate poor hearing

Mouth
- Bruising
- Lacerations
- Missing or broken teeth
- Untreated dental problems

Abdomen
- Abdominal injuries during pregnancy
- Intra-abdominal injuries

Genitourinary System or Rectum
- Bruising, lacerations, bleeding, edema, tenderness
- Untreated infections

(Continued on following page)

BOX 39.4

History and Physical Findings Suggestive of Abuse (continued)

Musculoskeletal System
- Fractures or old fractures in various stages of healing
- Dislocations
- Limited range of motion in extremities
- Contractures

Neurologic System
- Difficulty with speech or swallowing
- Hyperactive reflexes
- Developmental delays
- Areas of numbness
- Tremors

Mental Status
- Anxiety, fear
- Depression
- Suicidal ideation
- Difficulty concentrating
- Memory loss

Medications
- Medications not indicated by physical condition
- Overdose of drugs or medications (prescribed or over the counter)
- Medications not taken as prescribed

Communication Patterns/Relations
- Verbal hostility, arguments
- Negative nonverbal communication, lack of visible affection
- One person answers questions and looks to other person for approval
- Extreme dependency of family members

nurse can document that the description of injuries is inconsistent with the injury pattern.

Biologic indicators, such as elevated pulse and blood pressure, sleep and appetite disturbances, exaggerated startle responses, flashbacks, and nightmares, may suggest PTSD or depression. Signs and symptoms of dissociation include memory difficulties, a feeling of unreality about oneself or events, a feeling that a familiar place is strange and unfamiliar, auditory or visual hallucinations, and evidence of having done things without remembering them (Carlson & Putnam, 1993). If any of these signs or symptoms is present, the survivor requires a thorough diagnostic workup for PTSD and DID.

• NCLEXNOTE

In caring for persons with DID, the nurse should intervene with the personality that is present.

The nurse should assess every adult or adolescent who discloses victimization for substance abuse. The Michigan Alcoholism Screening Test (MAST) (Selzer, 1971) and the Drug Abuse Screening Test (DAST) (Skinner, 1982) are two screening instruments for use in any health assessment. An adolescent version of the MAST is available. If the results of these tests or the answers to any alcohol-related or drug-related questions are positive, the nurse should evaluate the survivor further for an alcohol or drug disorder.

Nursing Diagnoses for the Biologic Domain

Selected nursing diagnoses focusing on the human responses that nurses manage in the biologic domain may include Post-Trauma Syndrome, Delayed Growth and Development, Impaired Memory, and Rape-Trauma Syndrome.

Interventions for the Biologic Domain

Restoring health is a primary concern for survivors of abuse. When injuries are severe and surgery is required, the survivor may require hospital admittance.

Treating Physical Symptoms

Treatment of trauma symptoms may include cleaning and dressing burns or other wounds and assisting with casting of broken bones (see Box 39.5 for more information). Malnourished and dehydrated children and elders may require nursing interventions such as intravenous therapy or nutritional supplements that alleviate the alteration in nutrition and fluid and electrolyte balance.

• NCLEXNOTE

Women who are experiencing abusive relationships need their basic needs met (safety, housing, food, child care) before their psychological traumas can be addressed.

Promoting Healthy Daily Activity

Teaching sleep hygiene (practices conducive to healthy sleep patterns) and promoting exercise, leisure time, and nutrition will help battered survivors regain a healthy physical state and learn self-care. Taking care of themselves may be difficult for survivors who have spent years trying to separate themselves from their bodies (dissociate) to survive years of abuse (Walker, 1994). Techniques such as going to bed and arising at

BOX 39.5

Special Concerns for Victims of Sexual Assault

Assessment Focus

The history and physical examination of the survivor of sexual assault differ significantly from other assessment routines because the evidence obtained may be used in prosecuting the perpetrator (Sheridan, 2004). Therefore, the purpose is twofold:

- To assess the patient for injuries
- To collect evidence for forensic evaluation and proceedings.

Usually, someone with special training, such as a nurse practitioner who has taken special courses, examines a rape or sexual assault victim. Generalist nurses may be involved in treating the injuries that result from the assault, including genital trauma, such as vaginal and anal lacerations, and extragenital trauma, such as injury to the mouth, throat, wrists, arms, breasts, and thighs (Sheridan, 2004).

Key Interventions

Nursing intervention to prevent short- or long-term psychopathology after sexual assault is crucial. Psychological trauma following rape and sexual assault includes immediate anxiety and distress and the development of PTSD, depression, panic, and substance abuse (McNutt, Carlson, & Rose, 2002; Resnick et al., 1999).

Key interventions include:

- Early treatment because initial levels of distress are strongly related to later levels of PTSD, panic, and anxiety (Resnick et al., 1999).
- Supportive, caring, and nonjudgmental nursing interventions during the forensic rape examination are also crucial. This examination often increases survivors' immediate distress because they must recount the assault in detail and submit to an invasive pelvic or anal examination.
- Anxiety-reducing education, counseling, and emotional support, particularly in regard to unwanted pregnancies and sexually transmitted diseases, including HIV. All survivors should be tested for these possibilities. Treatment may include terminating a pregnancy; administering medications to treat gonorrhea, chlamydia, trichomoniasis, and syphilis; and administering medications that may decrease the likelihood of contracting HIV infection.
- Interventions that are helpful for survivors of domestic violence; these also apply to survivors of sexual assault.

consistent times, avoiding naps and caffeine, and scheduling periods for relaxation just before retiring may be useful in promoting sleep. Aerobic exercise is a useful technique for relieving anxiety and depression and promoting sleep.

Administering and Monitoring Medications

Survivors with a comorbid mood or anxiety disorder including PTSD may require pharmacologic interventions. Although only nurses with advanced preparation and prescriptive authority may prescribe medications, all nurses must be familiar with medications used to treat mood and anxiety disorders and the side effects of these drugs. Medications may be contraindicated for young and elderly survivors.

The autonomic nervous system is involved in many of the symptoms of depression and PTSD. Therefore, the use of agents that decrease its activity, such as the benzodiazepines, beta-blockers, and antidepressants, can help treat these symptoms (Friedman, 2001; Sutherland & Davidson, 1999). Tricyclics and other antidepressants are effective in treating depression and some symptoms of PTSD, such as nightmares, sleep disorders, and startle reactions. They are less effective in treating other PTSD symptoms, such as numbing (Friedman; Sutherland & Davidson). The benzodiazepines are useful in treating anxiety and sleep disturbances in PTSD, but because they can cause dependence, they are contraindicated in women who also have a substance abuse disorder.

Approved for treating PTSD, the selective serotonin reuptake inhibitor (SSRI) sertraline (Zoloft) has improved PTSD symptoms in women but not in men (Henney, 2000) (see Chapters 20 and 21 for information on monitoring medications and their side effects).

Managing Care of Patients with Comorbid Substance Abuse

Survivors who have a comorbid substance abuse disorder need referral to a treatment center for alcohol and drug disorders. The treatment center should have programs that address the special needs of survivors. Alcohol-dependent and drug-dependent survivors frequently stop treatment and return to alcohol and drug abuse if their abuse-related problems are not addressed appropriately (Boyd, 2000; Ouimette, Moos, & Brown, 2003).

Survivors, especially those with substance abuse problems, are at high risk for HIV infection and AIDS. If women do not know their HIV status, they should be encouraged to get tested. Those with positive test results should receive counseling and begin taking appropriate medication. Those without HIV need to be taught about the high-risk behaviors for HIV infection and how to protect themselves from contracting HIV infection.

Psychological Domain

Psychological Assessment

A mental status evaluation should be part of every health assessment. Symptoms such as anhedonia, difficulties concentrating, feelings of worthlessness or guilt, and thoughts of death or suicide suggest depression or PTSD. A thorough assessment of suicidal intent is crucial.

Nursing Diagnoses for the Psychological Domain

Selected nursing diagnoses focusing on the human responses that nurses manage in the psychological domain may include Ineffective Coping, Hopelessness, Chronic Low Self-Esteem, Anxiety, Risk for Self-Directed Violence, and Risk for Other-Directed Violence.

Interventions for the Psychological Domain

Assisting With Psychotherapy or Counseling

Psychotherapy may include individual, group, family, or marital therapy. Only psychiatric nurse specialists at the master's or doctoral levels who have had training in these therapeutic methods may conduct psychotherapy. In addition, the nurse therapist should have training in conducting therapy specifically with survivors of abuse. That training should include management of PTSD, DID, depression, and substance abuse. The goal of therapy is to integrate the patient's traumatic memories with the remainder of the patient's personal history and identity, manage painful affect, and restructure the meaning of the traumatic experiences (Wilson, 2001). The ultimate goal is for the survivor to integrate the trauma in memory as a past event that no longer has the power to terrorize.

Family or marital therapy may be unwise unless the perpetrator of abuse has obtained therapy for himself or herself and demonstrated change. Otherwise, survivors are placed in a very difficult situation. If they disclose abuse in family or marital therapy, perpetrators may retaliate with violence, but if they do not disclose the abuse, the crucial issue will not be addressed (Landenburger et al., 2004).

Several issues must be addressed for all survivors in psychotherapy or counseling (Campbell et al., 2004). All nurses can implement these interventions, using skills appropriate to their educational level and training. Nurses must address the guilt, shame, and stigmatization that survivors experience. They can approach these issues in several ways. Assisting survivors to verbalize their experience in an accepting, nonjudgmental atmosphere is a first step. Nurses must challenge directly attributions of self-blame for the abuse and feelings of being dirty and different. Helping survivors to identify their strengths and validating thoughts and feelings may help to increase self-esteem.

Working with Children

Children may need to learn a "violence vocabulary" that allows them to talk about their abuse and assign responsibility for abusive behavior. Children also need to learn that violence is not okay, and it is not their fault (Berman et al., 2004). Allowing children to discuss their abuse in the safety of a supportive, caring relationship may alleviate anxiety and fear (Berman et al.).

Re-enacting the abuse through play is another technique that may be helpful in assisting children to express and work through their anxiety and fear. Play therapy uses dolls, human or animal figures, or puppets to work through anxiety or fears (Hill, 2003). Other techniques used with children to reduce fear include reading stories about recovery from abusive experiences (literal or metaphoric), using art or music to express feelings, and psychodrama. In addition, teaching strategies to manage fear and anxiety, such as relaxation techniques, coping skills, and imagery, may give the child an added sense of mastering his or her fear (Barnett et al., 1997).

Managing Anger

Anger and rage are part of the healing process for survivors (Walker, 1994). Expression of intense anger is uncomfortable for many nurses. However, they should expect anger expression and develop comfortable ways to respond. Moreover, an important nursing intervention is teaching and modeling anger expression appropriately. Inappropriate expressions of anger might drive supportive people away. Anger management techniques include appropriately recognizing and labeling anger and expressing it assertively, rather than aggressively or passive-aggressively. Assertive ways of expressing anger include owning the feeling by using "I feel" statements and avoiding blaming others. Teaching anger management and conflict resolution may be especially important for children who have seen nothing but violence to resolve problems (Lowenthal, 2001).

Teaching Skills and Clarifying Identity 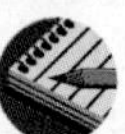

Other nursing interventions include teaching self-protection skills, healthy relationship skills, and healthy sexuality. Again, this teaching may be especially important for children who have no role models for healthy relationships. Children also need to know what constitutes controlling and abusive behavior and how to get help for abuse.

Children who have been sexually abused may become confused about their sexuality. They may regard sex as dirty and as something that can be used against other people. Discussions about healthy sexuality and feelings about sex may help these children regain a healthy perspective on sex-related matters (Peled, Jaffe, & Edleson, 1995).

Group therapy with survivors offers a powerful method to counter self-denigrating beliefs and to confront issues of secrecy and stigmatization (Urbancic, 2004). Moreover, one of the therapeutic factors in group therapy, universality or the discovery that others have had similar experiences, may be a tremendous relief, especially to child survivors.

Providing Education

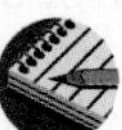

Education is a key nursing intervention for survivors. As appropriate to age or condition, survivors must understand the cycle of violence and the danger of homicide that increases as violence escalates or the survivor attempts to leave the relationship. Survivors also need information about resources, such as shelters for battered women, legal services, government benefits, and support networks (Walker, 1994). Before giving the survivor any written material, the nurse must discuss the possibility that if the perpetrator were to find the information in the survivor's possession, he or she might use it as an excuse for battering.

Survivors also need education appropriate for age and cognitive ability about the symptoms of anxiety, depression, dissociation, and PTSD. They must understand that these symptoms are common in anyone who has sustained significant stressors and are not signs of being "crazy" or weak. If survivors require medication for these symptoms, they must know how to monitor symptoms so that the effectiveness of pharmacologic management can be determined (see Box 39.6). One of the most important teaching goals is to help survivors develop a safety plan (Walker, 1994). The first step in developing such a plan is helping the survivor recognize the signs of danger. Changes in tone of voice, drinking and drug use, and increased criticism may indicate that the perpetrator is losing control. Detecting early warning signs helps survivors to escape before battering begins (Campbell et al., 2004; Urbancic, 2004; Walker, 2000).

The next step is to devise an escape route (Walker, 1994, 2000). This involves mapping the house and identifying where the battering usually occurs and what exits are available. The survivor needs to have a bag packed and hidden, but readily accessible, that has what is needed to get away. Important things to pack are clothes, a set of car and house keys, bank account numbers, birth certificate, insurance policies and numbers, marriage license, valuable jewelry, important telephone numbers, and money (Walker, 2000). The survivor must carefully hide the bag so that the perpetrator cannot find it and use it as an excuse for assault. If children are involved, the adult survivor should make arrangements to get them out safely. That might include arranging a signal to indicate when it is safe for them to leave the house and to meet at a prearranged place (Walker, 2000). A safety plan for a child or dependent elder might include safe places to hide and important telephone numbers, including 911 and those of the police and fire departments and other family members and friends.

BOX 39.6

Psychoeducation Checklist: Abuse

When caring for the patient who has been abused, be sure to address the following topics in the teaching plan:

- Cycle of violence
- Access to shelters
- Legal services
- Government benefits
- Support network
- Symptoms of anxiety, dissociation, and posttraumatic stress disorder
- Safety or escape plan
- Relaxation
- Adequate nutrition and exercise
- Sleep hygiene
- HIV testing/counseling

Finding Strength and Hope

Providing hope and a sense of control is important for survivors of trauma (Campbell et al., 2004). Nurses can help survivors find hope and view themselves as survivors by assisting them to identify specific strengths and aspects of their lives that are under their control. This type of intervention may empower women to find options to remaining in an abusive relationship.

Using Behavioral Interventions

Treatment for depression, anxiety, and PTSD symptoms can be divided into two categories: exposure therapy and anxiety management training (Rothbaum & Foa, 1996). Only professionals trained in exposure therapy techniques can use them; however, nurses need to be familiar with this approach. The goal of exposure therapy, which includes flooding and systematic desensitization, is to promote the processing of the traumatic memory by exposing the survivor to the traumatic event through memories or some cue that reactivates trauma memories. Through repeated exposure, the event loses its ability to cause intense anxiety (Coffey, Dansky, & Brady, 2003).

Coping with Anxiety

Anxiety management is a crucial intervention for all survivors. There is a high comorbidity among trauma, PTSD, and anxiety disorders (Orsillo et al., 2002). During treatment, survivors will experience situations and memories that provoke intense anxiety and must know how to soothe themselves when they experience painful feelings. Moreover, most survivors struggle with control issues, especially involving their bodies. Anxiety management skills offer one way to maintain some control over their bodies (Lundberg-Love, 1997).

Anxiety management training may include progressive relaxation, deep breathing, imagery techniques, and cognitive restructuring. Progressive relaxation entails systematically tensing and then relaxing the major muscle groups. Visualization consists of imagining a scene that is especially relaxing (e.g., spending a day at the beach), while practicing relaxation and deep breathing. Any interventions that reduce dysphoric symptoms can help survivors feel more in control of their situation.

Anxiety disorders, including PTSD, and depression are associated with cognitive distortions that cognitive therapy techniques can challenge (Zust, 2000). Self-defeating thoughts in anxiety disorders involve perceptions of threat and danger, and those in depression involve negative self-perceptions (Blackburn & Davidson, 1990). Nurses can teach survivors how to identify and challenge these self-defeating thought patterns. Cognitive therapy techniques may be especially useful in helping survivors to stop blaming themselves for their abuse.

Nurses must become accustomed to measuring gains in small steps when working with survivors. Making any changes in significant relationships has serious consequences and can be done only when the adult survivor is ready. It is easy for nurses to become angry or discouraged, and they must be careful not to communicate these feelings to survivors (Campbell et al., 2004; Urbancic, 2004). Discussing such feelings with other staff provides a way of dealing with them appropriately. In such discussions with supervisors or other staff, the nurse must protect the patient's confidentiality by discussing feelings around issues, not particular patients. The nurse should frame the discussion in such a way that individual patients cannot be identified.

Social Domain

Social Assessment

An evaluation of social networks and daily activities may provide additional clues of psychological abuse and controlling behavior (Burgess & Tavakoli, 2005; Gary & Humphreys, 2004; Wallace, 1999). When a nurse assesses social isolation, evaluating the reasons behind it is crucial. Many perpetrators isolate their family from all social contacts, including other relatives. Some survivors isolate themselves because they are ashamed of the abuse or fear nonsupportive responses. An evaluation of social support is important for other reasons. Having supportive family or friends is crucial in short-term planning for developing a safety plan and is also important to long-term recovery (Coker, Smith, Thompson, McKeown, Bethea, & Davis, 2002). A survivor cannot leave an abusive situation if she has nowhere to go. Supportive family and friends may be willing to provide shelter and safety.

Nurses can assess restrictions on freedom that may suggest abuse and control by asking such questions as: "Are you free to go where you want?" "Is staying home your choice?" and "Is there anything that you would like to do that you cannot?"

The degree of dependency on the relationship is another important variable to assess. Women who have young children and are economically dependent on the perpetrator may feel that they cannot leave the abusive relationship. Those who are emotionally dependent on the perpetrator may experience an intense grief reaction that further complicates their leaving (Campbell et al., 2004; Wallace, 1999). Elders and children are often dependent on the abuser and cannot leave the abusive situation without alternatives.

Nursing Diagnoses for the Social Domain

Selected nursing diagnoses focusing on the human responses that nurses manage in the social domain may include Hopelessness, Powerlessness, and Ineffective Role Performance.

Interventions for the Social Domain

Working with Abusive Families

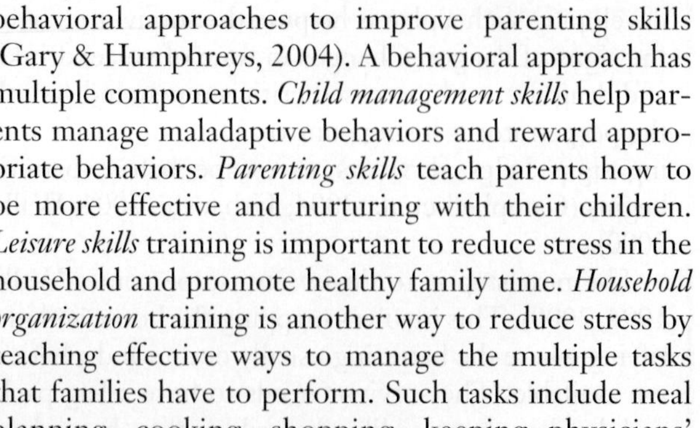

Family interventions in cases of child abuse focus on behavioral approaches to improve parenting skills (Gary & Humphreys, 2004). A behavioral approach has multiple components. *Child management skills* help parents manage maladaptive behaviors and reward appropriate behaviors. *Parenting skills* teach parents how to be more effective and nurturing with their children. *Leisure skills* training is important to reduce stress in the household and promote healthy family time. *Household organization* training is another way to reduce stress by teaching effective ways to manage the multiple tasks that families have to perform. Such tasks include meal planning, cooking, shopping, keeping physicians' appointments, and planning family activities (Gary & Humphreys).

Anger control and stress management skills are important parts of behavioral programs for families. Anger control programs teach parents to identify events that increase anger and stress and to replace anger-producing thoughts with more appropriate ones. Parents learn self-control skills to reduce the expression of uncontrolled anger. Stress-reduction techniques include relaxation techniques and methods for coping with stressful interactions with their children (Lowenthal, 2001). These skills may be especially important in families in which elder abuse is occurring. Both caregivers and abused elders may need to learn assertive ways to express their anger and healthy ways to manage their stress. Helping caregivers find ways to get some relief from their caregiving burdens may be crucial in reducing abuse that comes from exhaustion in trying to manage multiple roles. Examples might be to identify agencies that offer respite care or agencies that offer day care for elders and support groups in which caregivers can share experiences and gain support from others dealing with similar issues.

Working in the Community

Nurses may be involved in interventions to reduce violence at the community level. Many abusive parents and battered women are socially isolated. Assistance in developing support networks may help reduce stress and, therefore, reduce abuse. Community contacts vary for each survivor but might include crisis hot lines, support groups, and education classes (Gary & Humphreys, 2004).

Nurses may also make home visits to abusive parents. Home visits provide support to families and provide them with knowledge about child development and management (Barnett et al., 1997). Abuse of any kind is a volatile situation, and nurses may place themselves or the survivor in danger if they make home visits. Nurses should carefully assess this possibility before proceeding. If necessary, the nurse and adult survivor may need to arrange a safe place to meet.

Evaluation and Treatment Outcomes

Evaluation and outcome criteria depend on the setting for interventions. For instance, if the nurse encounters a survivor in the ED, successful outcomes might be that injuries are appropriately managed and the patient's immediate safety is ensured. For long-term care, outcome criteria and evaluation might center on ending abusive relationships. Examples of other outcome criteria that would indicate successful nursing intervention are recognizing that one is not to blame for the violence, demonstrating knowledge of strengths and coping skills, and re-establishing social networks.

Evaluation of nursing care for abused children depends on attaining goals mutually set with the parents. An end to all violence is the optimal outcome criterion; however, attainment of smaller goals indicates progress toward that end. Outcomes such as increased problem-solving and communication skills within the family, increased self-esteem in both children and parents, and increased use of nonphysical forms of discipline may all indicate progress toward the total elimination of child abuse.

Follow-up efforts are important in evaluating the outcomes of elder abuse. The optimal outcome is to end all abuse and keep the elderly person in his or her own living environment, if appropriate. Although the abuse may have been resolved temporarily, it may flare up again. Ongoing support for the caregiver and assistance with caregiving tasks may be necessary if the elder is to remain at home. Nursing home or assisted living may be the most desirable option if the burden is too great for the family and the likelihood of ongoing abuse or neglect is high.

Another important outcome of nursing intervention with survivors is appropriate treatment of any disorder resulting from abuse (e.g., ASD, PTSD and other anxiety disorders, DID, major depression, substance abuse). Follow-up nursing assessments should monitor symptom reduction or exacerbation, adherence to any medication regimen, and side effects of medication. The ultimate outcome is to end violence and enable the survivor to return to a more productive, safe, and nurturing life without being continually haunted by memories of the abuse.

Treatment for the Batterer

Participants in programs that treat batterers are usually there because the court has mandated the treatment. Programs are often outpatient groups that meet weekly for an extended period of time, often 36 to 48 weeks. Some programs advocate longer programs, believing that chronic offenders require from 1 to 5 years of treatment to change abusive behavior.

Groups often use cognitive-behavioral techniques and/or a psychoeducational, skill building approach (Healey, Smith, & O'Sullivan, 1998). This approach offers the batterer tools that help him see that his violent acts are not uncontrollable outbursts but rather foreseeable behavior patterns that he can learn to interrupt. Cognitive-behavioral interventions target three elements: (1) what the batterer thinks about just before a battering incident; (2) the batterer's physical and emotional response to these thoughts; and (3) what the batterer does that progresses to violence (yelling, throwing things). The group teaches members to recognize and interrupt negative feelings about their partners and to reduce physiological arousal through relaxation techniques.

Psychoeducational topics are often similar to those covered by the Duluth Curriculum, which is a model program. Topics may include nonviolence; nonthreatening behavior; respect; support and trust; honesty and accountability; sexual respect; and partnership, negotiation, and fairness. Other programs also offer more in-depth counseling, arguing that psychoeducational approaches do not address the true problem (Healey et al., 1998). If the problem were simply a deficit in skills, the batterer would be dysfunctional in work or relationships outside the family. Batterers need resocialization that convinces them that they do not have the right to abuse their partners. Other programs add a moral aspect by taking a value-laden approach against violence and confronting the batterer's behavior as unacceptable and illegal.

Accountability for violent acts is an important early goal in treating batterers (Healey et al., 1998). Most batterers deny responsibility for their actions and refuse to look at battering as a choice. Therefore, it is important that batterers become accountable for their actions. Interventions aim at getting the batterer to acknowledge his violence across the full range of abusive acts that he has committed, for example, verbal abuse, intimidation, controlling behavior, and sexual abuse. Batterers may use several tactics to avoid accountability, and all must be addressed. Those tactics include denying the abuse ever happened ("I never touched her"); minimizing the abuse by downplaying the violent acts or underestimating its effects ("It was just a slap" or "she bruises easily"); and blaming the abuse on the victim ("she pushed me too far"), alcohol or other drugs ("I was high"), or other life circumstances ("I had too many pressures at work").

Some states require that batterer programs contact partners (Healey et al., 1998). Because batterers typically minimize or deny their violent behavior, it is often necessary to interview the survivor to gain a complete picture of the batterer's behavior. A trained victim advocate usually contacts partners. There are other reasons for contacting partners. This may be the first contact the partner has had with professionals, and she may benefit by telling her story. Many partners do not know that services are available to them, and this is an opportunity to tell her what is available. In addition, advocates often explain the batterer program and emphasize that it takes a long time and requires the batterer to take responsibility for his violent behavior. Partners need to hear that many batterers are not willing to change their behavior. Another important point that partners need to know and discuss with professionals is that batterers often use entry into treatment as a justification for pressuring partners to remain in the relationship, but that this behavior is a good indicator that abuse will continue.

There are four points in treating batterers when it is essential to contact the partner for safety reasons. Those points are (1) when the batterer begins attending the program; (2) if and when he is terminated from treatment for noncompliance; (3) when he has completed treatment; and (4) if he is an imminent threat to the partner's safety (Healey et al., 1998).

Batterer intervention must be culturally competent (Healey et al., 1998). Many factors can affect violence against women, including socioeconomic status, racial or ethnic identity, country of origin, and sexual orientation, and those differences must be addressed. Another factor that must be addressed is alcohol and other drug use. Intervention programs may require batterers to undergo substance abuse treatment concurrently, and batterers are required to remain sober and submit to random drug testing.

Treatment programs alone are not sufficient to stop many batterers (Healey et al., 1998). To be effective, programs must operate within a comprehensive intervention effort that includes criminal justice support. The criminal justice response includes arrest, incarceration, adjudication, and probation supervision that includes issuing a warrant if the batterer does not attend the batterer program or supervision. The combination of criminal justice response and batterer treatment may convey a more powerful message to the batterer about the seriousness of his actions than a batterer program alone. Unfortunately, many offenders never show up for batterer intervention, and arrests for violation of probation may be rare because of overload and staffing shortages. Inaction by the criminal justice system is serious; it sends the message that there is little concern for violence against women and that batterers can get away with it. Several approaches to batterer intervention are controversial (Healey et al., 1998).

Anger management attributes battering to out-of-control anger and teaches anger management techniques. There are several arguments against this approach. It does not address the real issue—batterers' desire to control their partners. Batterers are able to control their behavior in other difficult situations but choose anger and intimidation to control their partners. Anger management may merely teach batterers nonviolent methods to exert control. Couples counseling may endanger the survivor. Women will not be free to disclose, and any disclosures may give the batterer reason to retaliate. Self-help groups modeled on Alcoholics Anonymous are inappropriate for initial intervention for several reasons. Without trained facilitators who will confront denial and excuses, batterers may never accept accountability for their violence. On the other hand, an untrained facilitator may use an excessively confrontational approach that is abusive and models antagonistic behavior.

How effective is batterer treatment? Results from an extended follow-up of court-ordered batterer intervention programs show that many men continue to be assaultive during and/or on completion of treatment. Based on partners' reports, 32% had reassaulted their partners by 15 months after treatment; 38% had done so by 30 months, and 42% had done so at 48 months. Twenty-five percent of the men repeatedly reassaulted their partners through 48 months of follow-up. However, the results did show that reassaults de-escalated somewhat with time (Gondolf, 2001).

SUMMARY OF KEY POINTS

- The abuse of women, teens, children, and elders is a national health problem that requires awareness and sensitivity from nurses.
- The abuse of women may be physical, emotional and psychological, or social.
- Child abuse may be neglectful, physical, sexual, or emotional. Other forms of child abuse include Münchausen syndrome by proxy and witnessing abuse of their mothers or significant caregivers.
- Elder abuse may be physical, emotional, neglectful, or financial.
- Among the many theories that have been proposed to explain abuse are psychopathology, social learning, sociologic, feminist, neurobiologic, borderline personality disorder, and substance abuse.
- A well-documented cycle of violence consists of three phases of increasing frequency and severity.
- Child abuse leaves many scars that can lead to such problems in adulthood as depression, anxiety, self-destructive behavior, poor self-esteem, and lack of trust.
- Responses to abuse include depression, acute stress disorder (ASD), posttraumatic stress disorder (PTSD), and dissociative identity disorder (DID).
- Nurses need to be familiar with signs and symptoms of abuse and to be vigilant when assessing patients.
- Nurses can help victims of abuse to view themselves as survivors.

CRITICAL THINKING CHALLENGES

1 Abuse is a pervasive problem, and anyone can be a victim (women, men, children, elders, gays, lesbians). Why do so few nursing units and nurses make it routine to ask questions about abuse?
2 Abuse is not just a "women's issue." The prevalence of abuse might decrease if men make it a "men's issue" as well. What is preventing this from happening?
3 What are your thoughts and feelings about women who are victims of abuse in which both partners (victim and perpetrator) abuse alcohol and other drugs?
4 What are your thoughts and feelings about women who will not leave an abusive relationship?
5 What are some reasons that women remain in abusive relationships?
6 Why do some women become involved in more than one abusive relationship?
7 How do you handle your feelings toward abusive parents or relatives who abuse elders?
8 What are the issues in mandatory reporting of violence toward women, particularly violence?

Sleeping With the Enemy: 1990. Julia Roberts plays a woman who escapes her abusive husband and moves to a small town to start over. Her peace is shattered when her husband finds her and discovers she is involved with another man. The movie ends with a fatal confrontation.

VIEWING POINTS: What are the effects of the husband's behavior on the woman in this film? What evidence can you find in this film of the "theory of borderline personality organization" and "traumatic bonding"?

Once Were Warriors: 1994. A mother of five re-evaluates her 18-year marriage to her alcoholic, hot-tempered husband when his bar-room violence tragically encroaches into their home life. Produced and filmed in New Zealand, this film also presents how urbanization has undermined the culture and strength of the indigenous Maori people.

VIEWING POINTS: What evidence can you find in this film that may reflect intergenerational transmission of violence? In what ways do you think that culture can influence attitudes toward abuse (both positive and negative)? What are positive and negative cultural influences in this film?

Sybil: 1976. Sally Field plays Sybil, a woman who experiences DID after suffering horrible abuse during childhood. Help from a psychiatrist (Joanne Woodward) uncovers the memories that have led to the splitting of Sybil's personality. The movie contains harrowing scenes of the abuse Sybil experienced.

VIEWING POINTS: What signs of DID does Sybil show in the film? How does the psychiatrist work with Sybil's different personalities in this film?

REFERENCES

Abbey, A., Zawacki, T., & Buck, P. (2001). Alcohol and sexual assault. *Alcohol Research and Health, 25*, 43–51.

Abbey, A., Zawacki, T., Buck, P. O., Clinton, A. M., & McAuslan, P. (2003). Sexual assault and alcohol consumption: What do we know about their relationship and what types of research are still needed? *Aggression and Violent Behavior, 277*, 1–33.

Ackard, D., & Neumark-Sztainer, D. (2002). Date violence and date rape among adolescents with disordered eating behaviors and psychological health. *Child Abuse & Neglect, 26*(5), 455–473.

Allan, M. A. (1998). Elder abuse: A challenge for home care nurses. *Home Health Care Nurse, 16*(2), 103–110.

American Psychiatric Association (APA). (2000). *Diagnostic and statistical manual of mental disorders* (4th ed., text revision). Washington, DC: Author.

Anderson, B., Marshak, H., & Hebbeler, D. (2002). Identifying intimate partner violence at entry to prenatal care clustering routine clinical information. *Journal of Midwifery Women's Health, 47*(5), 353–359.

Anderson, D. K., & Saunders, D. G. (2003). Leaving an abusive partner: An empirical review of predictors, the process of leaving, and psychological well-being. *Trauma, Violence, & Abuse, 4(2)*, 163–191.

Arata, C. M. (2002). Child sexual abuse and sexual revictimization. *Clinical Psychological: Science and Practice, 9*, 135–164.

Basile, K. (2002). Prevalence of wife rape and other intimate partner asexual coercion in a nationally representative sample. *Violence and Victims, 17*(5), 511–524.

Bandura, A. (1977). *Social Learning Theory*. New York: General Learning Press.

Barnett, O. W., Miller-Perrin, C. L., & Perrin, R. D. (1997). *Family violence across the life span: An introduction*. Thousand Oaks, CA: Sage.

Bartsch, C., Risse, M., Schutz, H., Weigand, N., & Weiler, G. (2003). Munchausen syndrome by proxy (MSBP): An extreme form of child abuse with a special forensic challenge. *Forensic Science International, 137*(2–3), 147–151.

Berman, H., Hardesty, J., & Humphreys, J. C. (2004). Children of abused women. In J. C. Campbell & J. C. Humphreys (Eds.), *Family violence and nursing practice* (pp. 160–185). Philadelphia: Lippincott Williams & Wilkins.

Blackburn, I., & Davidson, K. (1990). *Cognitive therapy for depression and anxiety*. Boston: Blackwell Scientific Publications.

Bograd, M. (1999). Strengthening domestic violence theories: Intersections of race, class, sexual orientation, and gender. *Journal of Marital and Family Therapy, 25*(3), 275–289.

Bolland, J., McCallum, D., Lian, B., Bailey, C., & Rowan, P. (2002). Hopelessness and violence among inner-city youths. *Journal of Maternal Child* Health, *5*, 237–244.

Boris, N., Heller, S., Sheperd, T., & Zeanah, C. (2002). Partner violence among homeless young adults: Measurement issues and associations. *Journal of Adolescent Health, 30*(5), 355–363.

Boyd, M. R. (2000). Predicting substance abuse and comorbidity in rural women. *Archives of Psychiatric Nursing, 14*(2), 64–72.

Boyd, M. R. (2003). Vulnerability to alcohol and other drug disorders in rural women. *Archives of Psychiatric Nursing, 17*(1), 33–41.

Boyd, M. R., & Mackey, M. (2000a). Alienation from self and others: The psychosocial problem of rural alcoholic women. *Archives of Psychiatric Nursing, 14*(3), 134–141.

Boyd, M. R., & Mackey, M. (2000b). Running away to nowhere: Rural women's experience of becoming alcohol dependent. *Archives of Psychiatric Nursing, 14*(3), 142–149.

Brady, K. T., & Dansky, B. S. (2002). Effects of victimization and posttraumatic stress disorder on substance use disorders in women. In F. L. Hall, T. S. Williams, J. A. Panetta, & J. M. Herrera (Eds,), *Psychiatric illnesses in women* (pp. 449–466). Washington, DC: American Psychiatric Publishing.

Breitenbecher, K. H. (2001). Sexual victimization among women: A review of the literature focusing on empirical investigations. *Aggression and Violent Behavior, 6*, 415–432.

Bremner, J. D., Southwick, S. M., & Charney, D. S. (1999). The neurobiology of posttraumatic stress disorder: An integration of animal and human research. In P. A. Saigh & J. D. Bremner (Eds.), *Posttraumatic stress disorder: A comprehensive text*. Boston: Allyn and Bacon.

Breslau, N., Davis, G. C., Andreski, P., Peterson, E. L., & Schultz, L. R. (1997). Sex differences in posttraumatic stress disorder. *Archives of General Psychiatry, 54*(11), 1044–1048.

Briere, J. N., & Elliott, D. M. (1994). Immediate and long-term impacts of child sexual abuse. *The Future of Children, 4*(2), 54–69.

Brown, P. J., Recupero, P. R., & Stout, R. (1995). PTSD substance abuse comorbidity and treatment utilization. *Addictive Behaviors, 20*, 251–254.

Burgess, S., & Tavokoli, A. (2005). Psychometric Assessment of the Burgess-Partner Abuse Scale for Teens (B-PAST). *Aquichan, 5*, 96–107.

Campbell, J. C., Torres, S., McKenna, L. S., Sheridan, D. J., & Landenburger, K. (2004). Nursing care of survivors of intimate partner violence. In J. C. Campbell & J. C. Humphreys (Eds.), *Family violence and nursing practice* (pp. 307–360). Philadelphia: Lippincott Williams & Wilkins.

Carlson, E. B., & Putnam, F. W. (1993). An update on the Dissociative Experiences Scale. *Dissociation, 6*(1), 16–27.

Centers For Disease Control, National Center for Injury Prevention and Control. (2003a). Child maltreatment: Fact sheet. Retrieved November 22, 2006, from http://www.cdc.gov/ncipc/factsheets/cmfacts.htm.

Centers for Disease Control & Prevention. (2003b). National Center for Injury Prevention and Control: *Intimate Partner Violence Fact Sheet*. Atlanta, Georgia: Author.

Charney, D. S., Deutch, A. Y., Krystal, J. H., Southwick, S. M., & Davis, M. (1993). Psychobiologic mechanisms of posttraumatic stress disorder. *Archives of General Psychiatry, 50*(4), 294–305.

Clark, K., Martin, S., Petersen, R., Cloutier, S., Covington, D., Buescher, P., & Beck-Warden, M. (2000). Who gets screened during pregnancy for partner violence? *Archives of Family Medicine, 9*(10), 1093–1099.

Cloutier, S., Martin, S., Moracco, K., Garro, J., Clark, K., & Brody, S. (2002). Physically abused pregnant women's perceptions about the quality of their relationships with their male partners. *Women's Health, 35*(2–3), 149–163.

Chodorow, N. (1974). Family structure and feminine personality. In M. R. Rosaldo & L. Lamphere (Eds.), *Woman, culture, and society* (pp. 43–66). Stanford: Stanford University Press.

Chrousos, G. P., & Gold, P. W. (1992). The concepts of stress and stress system disorders. *Journal of the American Medical Association, 267*(9), 1244–1252.

Cloitre, M., Scarvalone, P., & Difede, J. (1997). Posttraumatic stress disorder, self- and interpersonal dysfunction among sexually retraumatized women. *Journal of Traumatic Stress, 10*(3), 437–452.

Coffey, S. F., Dansky, B. S., & Brady, K. T. (2003). Exposure-based, trauma-focused therapy for comorbid posttraumatic stress disorder-substance use disorder. In P. Ouimette & P. J. Brown (Eds.), *Trauma and substance abuse: Causes, consequences, and treatment of comorbid disorders* (pp. 127–146). Washington, DC: American Psychiatric Association.

Cohen, J. A., Perel, J. M., DeBellis, M. D., Friedman, M. J., & Putnam, F. W. (2002). Treating traumatized children: Clinical implications of the psychobiology of posttraumatic stress disorder. *Trauma, Violence, & Abuse, 3*(2), 91–108.

Coker, A., Smith, P., McKeown, R., & King, M. (2000). Frequency and correlates of intimate partner violence by type: Physical, sexual, and psychological battering. *American Journal of Public Health, 90*(4), 553–559.

Coker, A., Smith, P., Thompson, M., McKeown, R., Bethea, L., & Davis, S. (2002). Social support protects against the negative effects of partner violence on mental health. *Journal of Women's Health & Gender Based-Medicine, 11*(5), 465–476.

Collins, J. J., & Messerschmidt, P. M. (1993). Epidemiology of alcohol-related violence. *Alcohol Health and Research World, 17*(2), 93–100.

Comijs, H. C., Pot, A. M., Smit, J. H., Bouter, L. M., & Jonker, C. (1998). Elder abuse in the community: Prevalence and consequences. *Journal of the American Geriatrics Society, 46*(7), 885–888.

Crandall, C. S., Jost, P. F., Broidy, L. M., Doday, C., Sklar, D. P. (2004). Previous emergency department use among homicide victims and offenders: A case-control study. *Annals of Emergency Medicine, 44*(6), 646–655.

Dell, P. F. (2006). A new model of dissociative identity disorder. *Psychiatric Clinics of North America, 29*, 1–26.

Dewey, J. (2004). Theories of aggression and family violence. In J. C. Campbell & J. C. Humphreys (Eds.), *Family violence and nursing practice* (pp. 3–28). Philadelphia: Lippincott Williams & Wilkins.

Dienemann, J., Boyle, E., Baker, D., Resnick, W., Wiederhorn, N., & Campbell, J. (2000). Intimate partner abuse among women diagnosed with depression. *Issues in Mental Health Nursing, 21*(5), 499–513.

Durant, T., Colley, G., Saltzman, L., & Johnson, C. (2000). Opportunities for intervention: Discussing physical abuse during prenatal care visits. *American Journal of Preventive Medicine, 19*(4), 238–244.

Dutton, D. G. (1995). *The domestic assault of women*. Vancouver, British Columbia, Canada: UBC Press.

Dutton, D. G. (1998). *The abusive personality*. New York: Guilford.

Dutton, D. G., & Painter, S. (1993). Emotional attachments in abusive relationships: A test of traumatic bonding theory. *Violence and Victims, 8*(2), 105–120.

Emery, R. E., & Laumann-Billings, L. (1998). An overview of the nature, causes, and consequences of abusive family relationships: Toward differentiating maltreatment and violence. *American Psychologist, 53*(2), 121–135.

Epstein, J. N., Saunders, B. E., Kilpatrick, D. G., & Resnick, H. S. (1998). PTSD as a mediator between childhood rape and alcohol use in adult women. *Child Abuse & Neglect, 22*(3), 223–234.

Fisher, B., Cullen, F., & Turner, M. G. (2000). The sexual victimization of college women. U.S. Department of Justice. National Institute of Justice Statistics Research Report. NCJ182369.

Fishwick, N. J., Campbell, J. C., & Taylor, J. Y. (2004). Theories of intimate partner violence. In J. C. Campbell & J. C. Humphreys (Eds.), *Family violence and nursing practice* (pp. 29–57). Philadelphia: Lippincott Williams & Wilkins.

Flitcraft, A. (1997). Learning from the paradoxes of domestic violence. *Journal of the American Medical Association, 277*(17), 1400–1401.

Flitcraft, A. H. (1995). Clinical violence intervention: Lessons from battered women. *Journal of Health Care for the Poor and Underserved, 6*(2), 187–197.

Forshee, V., Linder, G., & MacDougall, J. (2001). Gender differences in the longitudinal predictors of adolescent dating violence. *Preventive Medicine, 32*, 128–141.

Friedman, M. J. (2001). Allostatic versus empirical perspective in pharmacotherapy for PTSD. In J. P. Wilson, M. J. Friedman, & J. Lindy (Eds.), *Treating psychological trauma and PTSD* (pp. 94–124). New York: Guilford.

Gary, F. A., Campbell, D. W., & Humphreys, J. (2004). Theories of child abuse. In J. C. Campbell & J. C. Humphreys (Eds.), *Family violence and nursing practice* (pp. 58–73). Philadelphia: Lippincott Williams & Wilkins.

Gary, F. A., & Humphreys, J. C. (2004). Nursing care of abused children. In J. C. Campbell & J. C. Humphreys (Eds.), *Family violence and nursing practice* (pp. 252–287). Philadelphia: Lippincott Williams & Wilkins.

Gilligan, C. (1982). In a different voice: Psychological theory and women's development. Cambridge, MA: Harvard University Press.

Girshick, L. B. (1993). *Teen dating violence. Violence update*. Thousand Oaks, CA: Sage.

Gondolf, E. W. (2001). *An extended follow-up of batterers and their partners*. Atlanta: Centers for Disease Control and Prevention. Available at www.iup.edu/maati/publications/CDCFinalReport.shtm

Guille, L. (2004). Men who batter and their children: An integrated review. *Aggression and Violent Behaviour, 9*(2) 129–163.

Hana, E. Z., & Grant, B. F. (1997). Gender differences in *DSM-IV* alcohol use disorders and major depression as distributed in the general population: Clinical implications. *Comprehensive Psychiatry, 38*(4), 202–212.

Harrykissoon, S., Rickert, V., & Wiemann, C. (2002). Prevalence and patterns of intimate partner violence among adolescent mothers during the postpartum period. *Archives of Pediatric Adolescent Medicine, 156*(4), 325–330.

Hathaway, J., Mucci, L., Silverman, J., Brooks, D., Mathews, R., & Pavlos, C. (2000). Health status and health care use of Massachusetts women reporting partner abuse. *American Journal of Preventive Medicine, 19*(4), 302–307.

Hattendorf, J., & Tollerud, T. R. (1997). Domestic violence: Counseling strategies that minimize the impact of secondary victimization. *Perspectives in Psychiatric Care, 33*(1), 14–23.

Healey, K., Smith, C., & O'Sullivan, C. (1998). *Batterer intervention: Program approaches and criminal justice strategies*. Washington, DC: U.S. Department of Justice, National Institute of Justice. Available at http://www.ojp.usdoj.gov.

Hendricks-Matthews, M. K. (1993). Survivors of abuse: Health care issues. *Primary Care, 20*(2), 391–406.

Henney, J. E. (2000). Sertraline approved for posttraumatic stress disorder. *Journal of the American Medical Association, 283*(5), 596.

Henry, J. P. (1992). Biological basis of the stress response. *Integrative Physiological and Behavioral Science, 1*, 66–83.

Herman, J. (1997). *Trauma and recovery: The aftermath of violence—from domestic abuse to political terror*. New York: Basic Books.

Hill, A. (2003). Issues facing brothers of sexually abused children: Implications for professional practice. *Child & Family Social Work, 8*(4), 281–291.

Hollander, R., & Simeon, D. (2003). Anxiety disorders. In R. E. Hales & S. C. Yudofsky, (Eds.). American Psychiatric Publishing *Textbook of clinical psychiatry* (4th ed, pp. 543–630). Washington, DC: American Psychiatric Publishing, Inc.

Humphrey, J. A., & White, J. W. (2000). Women's vulnerability to sexual assault from adolescence to young adulthood. *Journal of Adolescent Health, 27*, 419–424.

James, W., West, C., Deters, K., & Armijio, E. (2000). Youth dating violence. *Adolescence, 35*(319), 455–465.

Kernic, M. A., Wolf, M. E., Holt, V. L., McKnight, B., Huebner, C. E., & Rivara, F. P. (2003). Behavioral problems among children whose mothers are abused by an intimate partner. *Child Abuse & Neglect 27*, 1231–1246.

Kershner, M., & Anderson, J. (2002). Barriers to disclose abuse among rural women. *Minnesota Medicine, 85*(3), 32–27.

Kilbourne, J. (1987). *Still killing us softly*. Cambridge, MA: Cambridge Documentary Films.

Kilbourne, J. (1999). *Can't buy my love: How advertising changes the way we think and feel*. New York: Simon & Schuster.

King, M. C., & Ryan, J. M. (2004). Nursing care and adolescent dating violence. In J. C. Campbell & J. C. Humphreys (Eds.), *Family violence and nursing practice* (pp. 288–306). Philadelphia: Lippincott Williams & Wilkins.

Krystal, J. H., Kosten, T. R., Southwick, S., et al. (1989). Neurobiological aspects of PTSD: Review of clinical and preclinical studies. *Behavior Therapy, 20*, 177–198.

Landenburger, K., Campbell, D. W., & Rodriguez, R. (2004). Nursing care of families using violence. In J. C. Campbell & J. C. Humphreys (Eds.), *Family violence and nursing practice* (pp. 220–251). Philadelphia: Lippincott Williams & Wilkins.

Lang, A., Kennedy, C., & Stein, M. (2002). Anxiety sensitivity and PTSD among female victims of intimate partner violence. *Depression and Anxiety, 16*(2), 77–83.

Lapidus, G., Cooke, M., & Gelven, E. (2002). A statewide survey of domestic violence screening behaviors among pediatricians and family physicians. *Archives of Pediatric Medicine, 156*, 332–336.

Lloyd, S. A., & Emery, B. C. (2000). The context and dynamics of intimate aggression against women. *Journal of Social and Personal Relationships, 17*(4–5), 503–521.

Long, A., & Smyth, A. (1998). The role of mental health nursing in the prevention of child sexual abuse and the therapeutic care of survivors. *Journal of Psychiatric and Mental Health Nursing, 5*, 129–136.

Lowenthal, B. (2001). Teaching resilience to maltreated children. *Reclaiming Children and Youth, 3*, 169–173.

Lundberg-Love, P. K. (1997). Current treatment strategies of adult incest survivors and their partners. In R. Geffner, S. B. Sorenson, & P. K. Lundberg-Love (Eds.), *Violence and sexual abuse at home: Current issues in spousal battering and child maltreatment* (pp. 293–311). New York: Haworth Maltreatment & Trauma Press.

McGrath, M. E., Bettacchi, A., Duffy, S. J., Peipert, J. F., Becker, B. M., & St. Angelo, L. (1997). Violence against women: Provider barriers to intervention in emergency departments. *Academic Emergency Medicine, 4*, 297–300.

McNutt, I., Carlson, B., & Rose, I. (2002). Partner violence intervention in the busy primary care environment. *American Journal of Preventive Medicine, 22*, 84–91.

Mechanic, M. B. (2004). Beyond PTSD: Mental health consequences of violence against women: A response to Briere and Jordan. *Journal of Interpersonal Violence, 19*(11), 1283–1289.

Mechanic, M., Weaver, T., & Resick, P. (2000). Intimate partner violence and stalking behavior: Exploration of patterns and correlates in a sample of acutely battered women. *Violence and Victims, 15*(1), 55–72.

Messman-Moore, T. L., & Long, P. J. (2003). The role of childhood sexual abuse sequelae in the sexual revictimization of women: An empirical review and theoretical reformulation. *Clinical Psychology Review, 23*, 537–571.

Morewitz, S. J. (2001). Domestic violence and stalking during pregnancy. *Journal of Obstetrics and Gynecology, 97*(4 Supplement), 53.

Morrill, A. C., Kasten, L., Urato, M., & Larson, M. J. (2001). Abuse, addiction, and depression as pathways to sexual risk in women and men with a history of substance abuse. *Journal of Substance Abuse, 13*, 169–184.

National Center on Elder Abuse. (1998). *National elder abuse incidence study: Final report*. Washington, DC: Author.

National Women's Health Information Center. (2003). Women with disabilities: dissociative disorders. Available at http://www.4woman.gov/wwd.cfm?page=45

Nolen-Hoeksema, S. (2002). Gender differences in depression. In I. H. Gotlib & C. L. Hammen (Eds.), *Handbook of depression* (pp.492–509). New York: Guilford.

Noll, J.G. (2005). Does childhood sexual abuse set in motion a cycle of violence against women? What we know and what we need to learn. *Journal of Interpersonal Violence, 20,* 455–462.

Norris, F. H., Foster, J. D., & Weisshaar, D. L. (2002). The epidemiology of sex differences in PTSD across developmental, social, and research contexts. In R. Kimmerling, P. Ouimette, & J. Wolfe (Eds.), *Gender and PTSD* (pp. 3–42). New York: Guilford.

Olff, M., Langeland, W., & Gersons, B. P. R. (2005). The psychobiology of PTSD: Coping with trauma. *Psychoneuroendocrinology, 30,* 974–982.

Orsillo, S. M., Raja, S., & Hammond, C. (2002). Gender issues in PTSD with comorbid mental health disorders. In R. Kimerling, P. Ouimette, & J. Wolfe (Eds.), *Gender and PTSD* (pp. 207–231). New York: Guilford.

Ouimette, P., Moos, R. H., & Brown, P. J. (2003). Substance use disorder–posttraumatic stress disorder comorbidity: A survey of treatments and proposed practice guidelines. In P. Ouimette & P. J. Brown (Eds.), *Trauma and substance abuse: Causes, consequences, and treatment of comorbid disorders* (pp. 91–110). Washington, DC: American Psychiatric Association.

Parker, B., Bullock, L., Bohn, D., & Curry, M. A. (2004). In J. C. Campbell & J. C. Humphreys (Eds.), *Family violence and nursing practice* (pp. 77–96). Philadelphia: Lippincott Williams & Wilkins.

Paulozzi, L., Saltzman, L., Thompson, M., & Holmgreen, P. (2001). Surveillance for homicide among intimate partner: United States 1981–1998. *Centers for Disease Surveillance Summaries 2001, 50*(SS-3), 1–16.

Peled, E., Jaffe, P. G., & Edleson, J. L. (1995). *Ending the cycle of violence.* Thousand Oaks, CA: Sage.

Perrin, K., Dindial, K., Eaton, D., Harrison, V., Matthews, T., & Henry, T. (2000). Responses of seventh grade students to "Do you have a partner with whom you would like to have a baby?" *Psychology Reports. 86*: 109–118.

Petter, M., & Whitehill, D. L. (1998). Management of female sexual assault. *American Family Physician, 58*(4), 920–929.

Putnam, F. W. (1994). Dissociative disorders in children and adolescents. In S. J. Lynn & J. W. Rhue (Eds.), *Dissociation: Clinical and theoretical perspectives* (pp. 175–189). New York: Guilford.

Raphael, B., & Matthew, M. (2002). Acute posttraumatic interventions. In F. Lewis-Hall, T. S. Williams, J. A. Panetta, & J. M. Herrera (Eds.), *Psychiatric illnesses in women* (pp. 139–158). Washington, DC: American Psychiatric Press.

Rasmusson, A. M., & Friedman, M. J. (2002). Gender issues in the neurobiology of PTSD. In R. Kimerling, P. Ouimette, & J. Wolfe (Eds.), *Gender and PTSD* (pp. 43–75). New York: Guilford.

Resnick, H., Acierno, R., Holmes, M., Kilpatrick, D. G., & Jager, N. (1999). Prevention of post-rape psychopathology: Preliminary findings of a controlled acute rate treatment study. *Journal of Anxiety Disorders, 13*(4), 359–370.

Rhea, M. H., Chafey, K. H., Dohner, V. A., & Terragno, R. (1996). The silent victims of domestic violence—Who will speak? *Journal of Child and Adolescent Psychiatric Nursing, 9*(3), 7–15.

Rhynard, J., Krebs, M., & Glover, J. (1997). Sexual assault in dating relationships. *Journal of School Health*, 67: 89–95.

Richardson, D., & Campbell, J. L. (1982). Alcohol and rape: The effect of alcohol on attributions of blame for rape. *Personality and Social Psychology Bulletin, 8*(3), 468–476.

Rickert, V., Vaughan, R., & Wiemann, C. (2003). Violence against young women: Implications for clinicians. *Contemporary OB/GYN, 48*(2), 30–45.

Rickert, V., Wiemann, C., Harrykissoon, S., Berenson, A., & Kolb, E. (2002). The relationship among demographics, reproductive characteristics, and intimate partner violence. *American Journal of Obstetric Gynecology, 187*(4), 1002–1007.

Roberts, T., & Klein, J. (2003). Intimate partner abuse and high-risk behavior adolescents. *Archives of Pediatric & Adolescent Medicine, 157*(4), 375–380.

Roberts, K. A. (2005). Women's experience of violence during stalking by former romantic partners. *Violence against Women, 11*(1), 89–114.

Roesler, T. A., & Dafler, C. A. (1993). Chemical dissociation in adults sexually victimized as children: Alcohol and drug use in adult survivors. *Journal of Substance Abuse Treatment, 10,* 537–543.

Rosenbaum, A., Geffner, R., & Benjamin, S. (1977). A biopsychosocial model for understanding relationship aggression. In R.Geffner, S. B. Sorenson, & R. K. Lundburg-Love (Eds.), *Violence and sexual abuse at home* (pp. 57–80). New York: Haworth Maltreatment & Trauma Press.

Rothbaum, B. O., & Foa, E. B. (1996). Cognitive-behavioral therapy for posttraumatic stress disorder. In B. A. van der Kolk, A. C. McFarlane, & L. Weisaeth (Eds.), *Traumatic stress: The effects of overwhelming experience on mind, body, and society* (pp. 491–509). New York: Guilford.

Rothschild, B. (1998). Post-traumatic stress disorder: Identification and diagnosis. *Swiss Journal of Social Work.* Available at http://www.healing-arts.org

Ryan, J., & King, M. C. (1998). Scanning for violence: Educational strategies for helping abused women. *AWHONN Lifelines, 2*(3), 36–41.

Sadock, B.J., & Sadock, V.A. (2004). *Kaplan & Sadock's Comprehensive Textbook of Psychiatry* (8th ed.). New York: Lippincott, Williams, & Wilkins.

Sampselle, C. M., Bernhard, L., Kerr, R. B., et al. (1992). Violence against women: The scope and significance of the problem. In C.M. Sampselle (Ed.), *Violence against women: Nursing research, education, and practice issues* (pp. 3–16). New York: Hemisphere.

Seeman, M. V. (2002). Single-sex psychiatric services to protect women. *Medscape General Medicine*, 4(3) [formerly published in *Medscape Women's Health eJournal* 7(4), 2002. Available at http://www.medscape.com/viewarticle/440095].

Selzer, M. L. (1971). The Michigan Alcoholism Screening Test: The quest for a new diagnostic instrument. *American Journal of Psychiatry, 127,* 89–94.

Sengstock, M. C., Ulrich, Y. C., & Barrett, S. A. (2004). Abuse and neglect of the elderly. In J. C. Campbell & J. C. Humphreys (Eds.), *Family violence and nursing practice* (pp. 97–149). Philadelphia: Lippincott Williams & Wilkins.

Sheridan, D. (2004). Legal and forensic nursing responses to family violence. In J. C. Campbell & J. C. Humphreys (Eds.), *Family violence and nursing practice* (pp. 386–406). Philadelphia: Lippincott Williams & Wilkins.

Sisley, A., Jacobs, L. M., Poole, G., Campbell, S., & Esposito, T. (1999). Violence in America: A public health crisis—domestic violence. *The Journal of Trauma 46*(6), 1105–1112.

Skinner, H. A. (1982). The drug abuse screening test. *Addictive Behavior,* 7, 363–371.

Slote, K. Y., Cuthbert, C., Mesh, C. J., Driggers, M. G., Bancroft, L., & Silverman, J.G. (2005). Battered mothers speak out. *Violence against Women, 11(11),* 1367–1395.

Smith, H. & Thomas, S. (2000). Violent and nonviolent girls: Contrasting perceptions of anger experiences, school, and relationships. *Issues in Mental Health Nursing*, 21, 547–575.

Southwick, S. M., Bremner, D., Krystal, J. H., & Charney, D. S. (1994). Psychobiologic research in post-traumatic stress disorder. *Psychiatric Clinics of North America, 17*(2), 251–264.

Starling, K. (1998). Black women and rape: The shocking secret no one talks about. *Ebony, 54*(1), 140–144.

Stein, M. & Kennedy, C. (2001). Major depressive and post-traumatic stress disorder comorbidity in female victims of intimate partner violence. *Journal of Affective Disorders, 66*(2–3), 133–138.

Stewart, S. H., Ouimette, P., & Brown, P. J. (2002). Gender and the comorbidity of PTSD with substance use disorders. In R. Kimerling, P. Ouimette, & J. Wolfe (Eds.), *Gender and PTSD* (pp. 232–270). New York: Guilford.

Sutherland, S. M., & Davidson, J. T. (1999). Pharmacological treatment of posttraumatic stress disorder. In P. A. Saigh & J. D. Bremner (Eds.), *Posttraumatic stress disorder: A comprehensive text* (pp. 327–353). Boston: Allyn & Bacon.

Swan, S. C., Gambone, L. J., Fields, A. M., Sullivan, T. P., & Snow, D. L. (2005). Women who use violence in intimate relationships: The role of anger, victimization, and symptoms of posttraumatic stress and depression. *Violence and Victims, 20*(3), 267–284.

Swan, S. C. (2001). Women's use of violence in intimate relationships: Myths and facts. Paper presented at the Effects of Domestic Violence in Children: A Fathers Role Conference, Southern Connecticut State University, New Haven, Connecticut.

Thase, M. E., Jindal, R., & Howland, R. H. (2002). Biological aspects of depression. In I. H. Gotlib & C. L. Hammen (Eds.), *Handbook of depression* (pp. 192–218). New York: Guilford.

Thompson, M., Kaslow, N., & Kingree, J. (2002). Risk factors for suicide attempts among African-American women who experience recent intimate partner violence. *Violence and Victims, 17*(3), 283–295.

Thompson, M. P., Kaslow, N. J., Kingree, J. B., Puett, R., Thompson, N. J., & Meadows, L. (1999). Partner abuse and posttraumatic stress disorder as risk factors for suicide attempts in a sample of low-income, inner-city women. *Journal of Traumatic Stress, 12*(1), 59–71.

Ulman, S. E. (2003). A critical review of field studies on the link of alcohol and adult sexual assault in women. *Aggression and Violent Behavior, 8*, 471–486.

U. S. Department of Health and Human Services (U.S. DHHS). (2001).

United States Department of Justice. (2005). Family violence statistics. Washington, DC: Author.

United States Department of Justice. (2002). Strengthening antistalking statutes. Available at http://www.ojp.usdoj.gov/ovc/publications/bulletins/legalseries/bulletin1/ncj189192.pdf.

United States Department of Justice (U.S. DOJ) & Centers for Disease Control and Prevention (CDC). (2000). *Extent, nature, and consequences of intimate partner violence: Findings from the National Violence against Women Survey*. Available at http://www.usdoj.gov/ nij/pubs-sum/181867.htm.

United States Department of Health and Human Services, Administration for Children & Families (2003). Child Maltreatment 2003. Retrieved November, 2006, from http://www.acf.hhs.gov/programs/cb/pubs/cm03/chapterthree.htm#types.

Urbancic, J. C. (2004). Sexual abuse in families. In J. C. Campbell & J. C. Humphreys (Eds.), *Family violence and nursing practice* (pp. 186–219). Philadelphia: Lippincott Williams & Wilkins.

Van der Kolk, B. A. (1996). The complexity of adaptation to trauma self-regulation, stimulus discrimination, and characterological development. In B. A. van der Kolk, A. C. McFarlane, & L. Weisaeth (Eds.), *Traumatic stress: The effects of overwhelming experience on mind, body, and society*. New York: Guilford.

Van der Kolk, B. A., & Fisler, R. E. (1993). The biologic basis of posttraumatic stress. *Primary Care, 20*(2), 417–432.

Van der Kolk, B. A., McFarlane, A. C., & Weisaeth, L. (Eds.). (1996). *Traumatic stress: The effects of overwhelming experience on mind, body, and society*. New York: Guilford.

Vest, J., Catlin, T., Chen, J., Brownson, R. (2002). Multi-state analysis of factors associated with intimate partner violence. *American Journal of Preventive Medicine, 22*(3), 156–164.

Walker, L. (1979). *The battered woman*. New York: Harper & Row.

Walker, L. E. (2000). *The battered woman syndrome*. New York: Springer Publishing Company.

Walker, L. (1994). The abused woman: A survivor therapy approach [Film]. Available from Psychotherapy.net, 4625 California street, San Francisco, CA 94118.

Wallace, H. (1999). *Family violence: Legal, medical, and social perspectives* (2nd ed.). Boston: Allyn & Bacon.

Walton-Moss, B., & Campbell, J. (2002). Intimate partner violence: Implications for nursing. *Online Journal Issues in Nursing*, 7 (1), 6.

Watson, J. M., Cascardi, M., Avery-Leaf, S., & O'Leary, K. D. (2001). High school students' responses to dating aggression. *Violence and Victims, 16*, 339–348.

Weiss, H., Lawrence, B., & Tiller, T. (2002). Pregnancy associated assault hospitalizations. *Journal of Obstetrics and Gynecology, 100*(4), 773–780.

Wiemann, C., Agurcia, C., Berenson, A., Volk., R., & Rickert, V. (2000). Pregnant adolescents: Experiences and behaviors associated with physical assault by an intimate partner. *Maternal & Child Health, 4*(2), 93–101.

Wilson, J. P. (2001). An overview of clinical considerations and principles in the treatment of PTSD. In J. P. Wilson, M. J. Friedman, & J. Lindy (Eds.), *Treating psychological trauma and PTSD* (pp. 59–93). New York: Guilford.

Wilson, J. P., Friedman, M. J., & Lindy, J. D. (2001). A holistic, organismic approach to healing trauma and PTSD. In J. P. Wilson, M. J. Friedman, & J. Lindy (Eds.), *Treating psychological trauma and PTSD* (pp. 28–56). New York: Guilford.

Wong, C. M., & Yehuda, R. (2002). Sex differences in posttraumatic stress disorder. In F. Lewis-Hall, T. S. Williams, J. A. Panetta, & J. M. Herrera (Eds.), *Psychiatric illnesses in women* (pp. 57–96). Washington, DC: American Psychiatric Press.

Wood, K., Maforah, F., & Jewkes, R. (1998). He forced me to have sex: Putting violence on adolescent sexual health agendas. *Social Science Medicine, 47*, 233–242.

Wright, R. J., Wright, R. O., & Isaac, N. E. (1997). Response to battered mothers in the pediatric emergency department: A call for an interdisciplinary approach to family violence. *Pediatrics, 99*(2), 186–192.

Zust, B. L. (2000). Effect of cognitive therapy on depression in rural battered women. *Archives of Psychiatric Nursing, 14*(2), 51–63.

APPENDIX A

DSM-IV-TR Classification: Axes I and II Categories and Codes

DISORDERS USUALLY FIRST DIAGNOSED IN INFANCY, CHILDHOOD, OR ADOLESCENCE

Mental Retardation

Note: These are coded on Axis II.

317 Mild Mental Retardation
318.0 Moderate Mental Retardation
318.1 Severe Mental Retardation
318.2 Profound Mental Retardation
319 Mental Retardation, Severity Unspecified

Learning Disorders

315.00 Reading Disorders
315.1 Mathematics Disorders
315.2 Disorder of Written Expression
315.9 Learning Disorder NOS

Motor Skills Disorder

315.4 Developmental Coordination Disorder

Communication Disorders

315.31 Expressive Language Disorder
315.31 Mixed Receptive-Expressive Language Disorder
315.39 Phonological Disorder
307.0 Stuttering
307.9 Communication Disorder NOS

Pervasive Developmental Disorders

299.00 Autistic Disorder
299.80 Rett's Disorder
299.10 Childhood Disintegrative Disorder
299.80 Asperger's Disorder
299.80 Pervasive Developmental Disorder NOS

Attention-Deficit and Disruptive Behavior Disorders

314.xx Attention-Deficit/Hyperactivity Disorder
.01 Combined Type
.00 Predominantly Inattentive Type
.01 Predominantly Hyperactive-Impulsive Type
314.9 Attention-Deficit/Hyperactivity Disorder NOS
312.8 Conduct Disorder
Specify type: Childhood-Onset/Adolescent-Onset
313.81 Oppositional Defiant Disorder
312.9 Disruptive Behavior Disorder NOS

Feeding and Eating Disorders of Infancy or Early Childhood

307.52 Pica
307.53 Rumination Disorder
307.59 Feeding Disorder of Infancy or Early Childhood

Tic Disorders

307.23 Tourette's Disorder
307.22 Chronic Motor or Vocal Tic Disorder

NOS = not otherwise specified.
An x appearing in a diagnostic code indicates that a specific code number is required.
An ellipsis (. . .) is used in the names of certain disorders to indicate that the name of a specific mental disorder or general medical condition should be inserted when recording the name (e.g., 293 Delirium Due to Hypothyroidism).
*Indicate the General Medical Condition.
**Refer to Substance-Related Disorders for substance-specific codes.
***Indicate the Axis I or Axis II Disorder.
American Psychiatric Association. (2000). *Diagnostic and statistical manual of mental disorders.* (4th ed., Text revision). Washington, DC: Author.

307.21 Transient Tic Disorder
Specify if: Single Episode/Recurrent
307.20 Tic Disorder NOS

Elimination Disorders

—.- Encopresis
787.6 With Constipation and Overflow Incontinence
307.7 Without Constipation and Overflow Incontinence
307.6 Enuresis (Not Due to a General Medical Condition)
Specify type: Nocturnal Only/Diurnal Only/Nocturnal and Diurnal

Other Disorders of Infancy, Childhood, or Adolescence

309.21 Separation and Anxiety Disorder
Specify if: Early Onset
313.23 Selective Mutism
313.89 Reactive Attachment Disorder of Infancy or Early Childhood
Specify type: Inhibited/Disinhibited
307.3 Stereotypic Movement Disorder
Specify if: With Self-Injurious Behavior
313.9 Disorder of Infancy, Childhood, or Adolescence NOS

DELIRIUM, DEMENTIA, AND AMNESTIC AND OTHER COGNITIVE DISORDERS

Delirium

293.0 Delirium Due to. . .*
—.- Substance Intoxication Delirium**
—.- Substance Withdrawal Delirium**
—.- Delirium Due to Multiple Etiologies (code each of the specific etiologies)
780.09 Delirium NOS

Dementia

294.xx Dementia of the Alzheimer's Type, With Early Onset
.10 Without Behavioral Disturbance
.11 With Behavioral Disturbance
294.xx Dementia of the Alzheimer's Type, With Late Onset
.10 Without Behavioral Disturbance
.11 With Behavioral Disturbance
294.xx Vascular Dementia
.40 Uncomplicated
.41 With Delirium
.42 With Delusions
.43 With Depressed Mood
Specify if: With Behavioral Disturbance
294.1x Dementia Due to HIV Disease
294.1x Dementia Due to Head Trauma
294.1x Dementia Due to Parkinson's Disease
294.1x Dementia Due to Huntington's Disease
294.10 Dementia Due to Pick's Disease
290.10 Dementia Due to Creutzfeldt-Jakob Disease
294.1 Dementia Due to . . . [Indicate the General Medical Condition not listed above]
—.- Substance-Induced Persisting Dementia**
—.- Dementia Due to Multiple Etiologies (code each of the specific etiologies)
294.8 Dementia NOS

Amnestic Disorders

294.0 Amnestic Disorder Due to . . .*
Specify if: Transient/Chronic
—.- Substance-Induced Persisting Amnestic Disorder**
294.8 Amnestic Disorder NOS

Other Cognitive Disorders

294.9 Cognitive Disorder NOS

MENTAL DISORDERS DUE TO A GENERAL MEDICAL CONDITION NOT ELSEWHERE CLASSIFIED

293.89 Catatonic Disorder Due to . . .*
310.0 Personality Change Due to . . .*
Specify type: Labile/Disinhibited/Aggressive/Apathetic/Paranoid/Other/Combined/Unspecified
293.9 Mental Disorder NOS Due to . . .*

SUBSTANCE-RELATED DISORDERS

The following specifiers may be applied to Substance Dependence:

With Physiological Dependence/Without Physiological Dependence
Early Full Remission/Early Partial Remission
Sustained Full Remission/Sustained Partial Remission
On Agonist Therapy/In a Controlled Environment

The following specifiers apply to Substance-Induced Disorders as noted:

With Onset During Intoxication/[W] With Onset During Withdrawal

Alcohol-Related Disorders

Alcohol Use Disorders

303.90 Alcohol Dependence
305.00 Alcohol Abuse

Alcohol-Induced Disorders

303.00 Alcohol Intoxications
291.8 Alcohol Withdrawal
Specify if: With Perceptual Disturbances
291.0 Alcohol Intoxication Delirium
291.0 Alcohol Withdrawal Delirium
291.2 Alcohol-Induced Persisting Dementia
291.1 Alcohol-Induced Persisting Amnestic Disorder
291.x Alcohol-Induced Psychotic Disorder
.5 With Delusions[I,W]
.3 With Hallucinations[I,W]
291.8 Alcohol-Induced Mood Disorder[I,W]
291.8 Alcohol-Induced Anxiety Disorder[I,W]
291.8 Alcohol-Induced Sexual Dysfunction[I]
291. Alcohol-Induced Sleep Disorder[I,W]
291.9 Alcohol-Related Disorder NOS

Amphetamine (or Amphetamine-Like)-Related Disorders

Amphetamine Use Disorders

304.40 Amphetamine Dependence*
305.70 Amphetamine Abuse

Amphetamine-Induced Disorders

292.89 Amphetamine Intoxication
Specify if: With Perceptual Disturbances
292.0 Amphetamine Withdrawal
292.81 Amphetamine Intoxication Delirium
292.xx Amphetamine-Induced Psychotic Disorder
.11 With Delusions[I]
.12 With Hallucinations[I]
292.84 Amphetamine-Induced Mood Disorder[I,W]
292.89 Amphetamine-Induced Anxiety Disorder[I]
292.89 Amphetamine-Induced Sexual Dysfunction[I]
292.89 Amphetamine-Induced Sleep Disorder[I,W]
292.9 Amphetamine-Related Disorder NOS

Caffeine-Related Disorders

Caffeine-Induced Disorders

305.90 Caffeine Intoxication
292.89 Caffeine-Induced Anxiety Disorder[I]
292.89 Caffeine-Induced Sleep Disorder[I]
292.9 Caffeine-Related Disorder NOS

Cannabis-Related Disorders

Cannabis Use Disorders

304.30 Cannabis Dependence*
305.20 Cannabis Abuse

Cannabis-Induced Disorders

292.89 Cannabis Intoxication
Specify if: With Perceptual Disturbances
292.81 Cannabis Intoxication Delirium
292.xx Cannabis-Induced Psychotic Disorder
.11 With Delusions[I]
.12 With Hallucinations[I]
292.89 Cannabis-Induced Anxiety Disorder
292.9 Cannabis-Related Disorder NOS

Cocaine-Related Disorders

Cocaine Use Disorders

304.20 Cocaine Dependence*
305.60 Cocaine Abuse

Cocaine-Induced Disorders

292.89 Cocaine Intoxication
Specify if: With Perceptual Disturbances
292.0 Cocaine Withdrawal
292.81 Cocaine Intoxication Delirium
292.xx Cocaine-Induced Psychotic Disorder
.11 With Delusions[I]
.12 With Hallucinations[I]
292.84 Cocaine-Induced Mood Disorder[I,W]
292.89 Cocaine-Induced Anxiety Disorder[I,W]
292.89 Cocaine-Induced Sexual Dysfunction[I]
292.89 Cocaine-Induced Sleep Disorder[I,W]
292.9 Cocaine-Related Disorder NOS

Hallucinogen-Related Disorders

Hallucinogen-Use Disorders

304.50 Hallucinogen Dependence*
305.30 Hallucinogen Abuse

Hallucinogen-Induced Disorders

292.89 Hallucinogen Intoxication
292.89 Hallucinogen Persisting Perception Disorder (Flashbacks)
292.81 Hallucinogen Intoxication Delirium
292.xx Hallucinogen-Induced Psychotic Disorder
.11 With Delusions[I]
.12 With Hallucinations[I]
292.84 Hallucinogen-Induced Mood Disorder[I]
292.89 Hallucinogen-Induced Anxiety Disorder[I]
292.9 Hallucinogen-Related Disorder NOS

Inhalant-Related Disorders

Inhalant Use Disorders

304.60 Inhalant Dependence*
305.90 Inhalant Abuse

Inhalant-Induced Disorders

292.89 Inhalant Intoxication
292.81 Inhalant Intoxication Delirium
292.82 Inhalant-Induced Persisting Dementia
292.xx Inhalant-Induced Psychotic Disorder
.11 With Delusions[I]
.12 With Hallucinations*
292.84 Inhalant-Induced Mood Disorder[I]
292.89 Inhalant-Induced Anxiety Disorder[I]
292.9 Inhalant-Related Disorder NOS

Nicotine-Related Disorders

Nicotine Use Disorder

305.10 Nicotine Dependence*

Nicotine-Induced Disorder

292.0 Nicotine Withdrawal
292.9 Nicotine-Related Disorder NOS

Opioid-Related Disorders

Opioid Use Disorders

304.00 Opioid Dependence*
305.50 Opioid Abuse

Opioid-Induced Disorders

292.89 Opioid Intoxication
Specify if: With Perceptual Disturbances
292.0 Opioid Withdrawal
292.81 Opioid Intoxication Delirium
292.xx Opioid-Induced Psychotic Disorders
.11 With Delusions[I]
.12 With Hallucinations[I]
292.84 Opioid-Induced Mood Disorder[I]
292.89 Opioid-Induced Sexual Dysfunction[I]
292.89 Opioid-Induced Sleep Disorder[I,W]
292.9 Opioid-Related Disorder NOS

Phencyclidine (or Phencyclidine-Like)-Related Disorders

Phencyclidine Use Disorders

304.90 Phencyclidine Dependence*
305.90 Phencyclidine Abuse

Phencyclidine-Induced Disorders

292.89 Phencyclidine Intoxication
Specify if: With Perceptual Disturbances
292.81 Phencyclidine Intoxication Delirium
292.xx Phencyclidine-Induced Psychotic Disorders
.11 With Delusions[I]
.12 With Hallucinations[I]
292.84 Phencyclidine-Induced Mood Disorder[I]
292.89 Phencyclidine-Induced Anxiety Disorder[I]
292.9 Phencyclidine-Related Disorder NOS

Sedative-Hypnotic- or Anxiolytic-Related Disorders

Sedative-Hypnotic- or Anxiolytic Use Disorders

304.10 Sedative, Hypnotic, or Anxiolytic Dependence*
305.40 Sedative, Hypnotic, or Anxiolytic Abuse

Sedative, Hypnotic, or Anxiolytic-Induced Disorders

292.89 Sedative, Hypnotic, or Anxiolytic Intoxication
292.0 Sedative, Hypnotic, or Anxiolytic Withdrawal
Specify if: With Perceptual Disturbances
292.81 Sedative, Hypnotic, or Anxiolytic Intoxication Delirium
292.81 Sedative, Hypnotic, or Anxiolytic Withdrawal Delirium
292.82 Sedative-, Hypnotic-, or Anxiolytic-Induced Persisting Delirium
292.83 Sedative-, Hypnotic-, or Anxiolytic-Induced Persisting Amnestic Disorder
292.xx Sedative-, Hypnotic-, or Anxiolytic-Induced Psychotic Disorder
.11 With Delusions[I,W]
.12 With Hallucinations[I,W]
292.84 Sedative-, Hypnotic-, or Anxiolytic-Induced Mood Disorder[I,W]
292.89 Sedative-, Hypnotic-, or Anxiolytic-Induced Anxiety Disorder[W]
292.89 Sedative-, Hypnotic-, or Anxiolytic-Induced Sexual Dysfunction[I]
292.89 Sedative-, Hypnotic-, or Anxiolytic-Induced Sleep Disorder[I,W]
292.9 Sedative-, Hypnotic-, or Anxiolytic-Induced Disorder NOS

Polysubstance-Related Disorder

304.80 Polysubstance Dependence*

Other (or Unknown) Substance-Related Disorders

Other (or Unknown) Substance Use Disorders

304.90 Other (or Unknown) Substance Dependence*
305.90 Other (or Unknown) Substance Abuse

Other (or Unknown) Substance-Induced Disorders

292.89 Other (or Unknown) Substance Intoxication
Specify if: With Perceptual Disturbances
292.0 Other (or Unknown) Substance Withdrawal
Specify if: With Perceptual Disturbances
292.81 Other (or Unknown) Substance-Induced Delirium
292.82 Other (or Unknown) Substance-Induced Persisting Dementia
292.83 Other (or Unknown) Substance-Induced Persisting Amnestic Disorder
292.xx Other (or Unknown) Substance-Induced Psychotic Disorder
.11 With Delusions[I,W]
.12 With Hallucinations[I,W]
292.84 Other (or Unknown) Substance-Induced Mood Disorder[I,W]
292.89 Other (or Unknown) Substance-Induced Anxiety Disorder[I,W]
292.89 Other (or Unknown) Substance-Induced Sexual Dysfunction[I]
292.89 Other (or Unknown) Substance-Induced Sleep Disorder[I,W]
292.9 Other (or Unknown) Substance-Induced Disorder NOS

SCHIZOPHRENIA AND OTHER PSYCHOTIC DISORDERS

295.xx Schizophrenia

The following Classification of Longitudinal Course applies to all subtypes of Schizophrenia:

Episodic With Interepisode Residual Symptoms
(*Specify if:* With Prominent Negative Symptoms)/
Episodic With No Interepisode Residual Symptoms/Continuous
(*Specify if:* With Prominent Negative Symptoms)
Single Episode in Partial Remission
(*Specify if:* With Prominent Negative Symptoms)
Single Episode in Full Remission
Other or Unspecified Pattern
.30 Paranoid Type
.10 Disorganized Type
.20 Catatonic Type
.90 Undifferentiated Type
.60 Residual Type
295.40 Schizophreniform Disorder
Specify if: Without Good Prognostic Features/With Good Prognostic Features
295.70 Schizoaffective Disorder
Specify type: Bipolar/Depressive
297.1 Delusional Disorder
Specify type: Erotomanic/Grandiose/Jealous/Persecutory Somatic/Mixed/Unspecified
298.8 Brief Psychotic Disorder
Specify if: With Marked Stressor(s) Without Marked Stressor(s) With Postpartum Onset
297.3 Shared Psychotic Disorder
293.xx Psychotic Disorder Due to . . .*
.81 With Delusions
.82 With Hallucinations
—.- Substance-Induced Psychotic Disorder (refer to Substance-Related Disorders for substance-specific codes)
Specify if: With Onset During Intoxication/With Onset During Withdrawal
298.9 Psychotic Disorder NOS

MOOD DISORDERS

Code current state of Major Depressive Disorder or Bipolar I Disorder in fifth digit
1 = Mild
2 = Moderate
3 = Severe Without Psychotic Features
4 = Severe With Psychotic Features
Specify: Mood-Congruent Psychotic Features/Mood-Incongruent Psychotic Features
5 = In Partial Remission
6 = In Full Remission
0 = Unspecified

The following specifiers apply (for current or most recent episode) to Mood Disorders as noted:

[a]Severity/Psychotic/Remission Specifiers/[b]Chronic/[c]With Catatonic Features/[d]With Melancholic Features/[e]With Atypical Features/[f]With Postpartum Onset

The following specifiers apply to Mood Disorders as noted:

[g]With or Without Full Interepisode Recovery/With Seasonal Pattern/[i]With Rapid Cycling

Depressive Disorders

296.xx Major Depressive Disorder,
.2x Single Episode[a,b,c,d,e,f]
.3x Recurrent[a,b,c,d,e,f,g,h]
300.4 Dysthymic Disorder

Specify if: Early Onset/Late Onset
Specify if: With Atypical Features
311 Depressive Disorder NOS

Bipolar Disorders

296.xx Bipolar I Disorder,
.0x Single Manic Episode[a,c,f]
Specify if: Mixed
.40 Most Recent Episode Hypomanic[a,h,j]
.4x Most Recent Episode Manic[a,c,f,g,h,i]
.6x Most Recent Episode Mixed[a,c,f,g,h,i]
.5x Most Recent Episode Depressed[a,b,c,d,e,f,g,h,i]
.7 Most Recent Episode Unspecified[g,h,i]
296.89 Bipolar II Disorder[a,b,c,d,e,f,g,h,i]
Specify (current or most recent episode): Hypomanic/Depressed
301.13 Cyclothymic Disorder
296.80 Bipolar Disorder NOS
293.83 Mood Disorder Due to . . .*
Specify type: With Depressive Features/ With Major Depressive-Like Episode/ With Manic Features/With Mixed Features
—.- Substance-Induced Mood Disorder**
Specify type: With Depressive Features/ With Manic Features/With Mixed Features
Specify if: With Onset During Intoxication/ With Onset During Withdrawal
296.90 Mood Disorder NOS

ANXIETY DISORDERS

300.01 Panic Disorder Without Agoraphobia
300.21 Panic Disorder With Agoraphobia
300.22 Agoraphobia Without History of Panic Disorder
300.29 Specific Phobia
Specify type: Animal Type/Natural Environment Type/Blood-Injection-Injury Type/Situational Type/Other Type
300.23 Social Phobia
Specify if: Generalized
300.3 Obsessive-Compulsive Disorder
Specify if: With Poor Insight
309.81 Posttraumatic Stress Disorder
Specify if: Acute/Chronic
Specify if: With Delayed Onset
308.3 Acute Stress Disorder
300.02 Generalized Anxiety Disorder
293.80 Anxiety Disorder Due to. . .*
Specify if: With Generalized Anxiety/With Panic Attacks/With Obsessive Compulsive Symptoms. . .*
293.84 Substance-Induced Anxiety Disorder
Specify if: With Generalized Anxiety/With Panic Attacks/With Obsessive-Compulsive Symptoms/With Phobic Symptoms
Specify if: With Onset During Intoxication/ With Onset During Withdrawal
300.00 Anxiety Disorder NOS

SOMATOFORM DISORDERS

300.81 Somatization Disorder
300.82 Undifferentiated Somatoform Disorder
300.11 Conversion Disorder
Specify type: With Motor Symptom or Deficit/With Sensory Symptom or Deficit/With Seizures or Convulsions/ With Mixed Presentation
307.xx Pain Disorder
.80 Associated With Psychological Factors
.89 Associated with Both Psychological Factors and a General Medical Condition
Specify if: Acute/Chronic
300.7 Hypochondriasis
Specify if: With Poor Insight
300.7 Body Dysmorphic Disorder
300.82 Somatoform Disorder NOS

FACTITIOUS DISORDERS

300.xx Factitious Disorder
.16 With Predominantly Psychological Signs and Symptoms
.19 With Predominantly Physical Signs and Symptoms
.19 With Combined Psychological and Physical Signs and Symptoms
300.19 Factitious Disorder NOS

DISSOCIATIVE DISORDERS

300.12 Dissociative Amnesia
300.13 Dissociative Fugue
300.14 Dissociative Identity Disorder
300.6 Depersonalized Disorder
300.15 Dissociative Disorder NOS

SEXUAL AND GENDER IDENTITY DISORDERS

Sexual Dysfunctions

The following specifiers apply to all primary Sexual Dysfunctions:
Lifelong Type/Acquired

Type Generalized Type/Situational Type
Due to Psychological Factors. Due to Combined Factors

Sexual Desire Disorders

302.71 Hypoactive Sexual Desire Disorder
302.79 Sexual Aversion Disorder

Sexual Arousal Disorders

302.72 Female Sexual Arousal Disorder
302.72 Male Erectile Disorder

Orgasmic Disorders

302.73 Female Orgasmic Disorder
302.74 Male Orgasmic Disorder
302.75 Premature Ejaculation

Sexual Pain Disorders

302.76 Dyspareunia (Not Due to a General Medical Condition)
306.51 Vaginismus (Not Due to a General Medical Condition)

Sexual Dysfunction Due to a General Medical Condition

625.8 Female Hypoactive Sexual Desire Disorder Due to . . .*
608.89 Male Hypoactive Sexual Desire Disorder Due to . . .*
607.84 Male Erectile Disorder Due to . . .*
625.0 Female Dyspareunia Due to . . .*
608.89 Male Dyspareunia Due to . . .*
625.8 Other Female Sexual Dysfunction Due to . . .*
608.89 Other Male Sexual Dysfunction Due to . . .*
—.- Substance-Induced Sexual Dysfunction**
Specify if: With Impaired Desire/With Impaired Arousal/With Impaired Orgasm/With Sexual Pain
Specify if: With Onset During Intoxication
302.70 Sexual Dysfunction NOS

Paraphilias

302.4 Exhibitionism
302.81 Fetishism
302.89 Frotteurism
302.2 Pedophilia
Specify if: Sexually Attracted to Males/Sexually Attracted to Females/Sexually Attracted to Both
Specify if: Limited to Incest
Specify type: Exclusive Type/Nonexclusive Type
302.83 Sexual Masochism
302.84 Sexual Sadism
302.3 Transvestic Fetishism
Specify if: With Gender Dysphoria
302.82 Voyeurism
302.9 Paraphilia NOS

Gender Identity Disorders

302.xx Gender Identity Disorder
.6 in Children
.85 in Adolescents or Adults
Specify if: Sexually Attracted to Males/Sexually Attracted to Females/Sexually Attracted to Both/Sexually Attracted to Neither
302.6 Gender Identity Disorder NOS
302.9 Sexual Disorder NOS

EATING DISORDERS

307.1 Anorexia Nervosa
Specify type: Restricting, Binge-Eating/Purging
307.51 Bulimia Nervosa
Specify type: Purging/Nonpurging
307.50 Eating Disorder NOS

SLEEP DISORDERS

Primary Sleep Disorders

Dyssomnias

307.42 Primary Insomnia
307.44 Primary Hypersomnia
Specify if: Recurrent
347 Narcolepsy
380.59 Breathing-Related Sleep Disorder
307.45 Circadian Rhythm Sleep Disorder
Specify type: Delayed Sleep Phase/Jet Lag/Shift Work/Unspecified
307.47 Dyssomnia NOS

Parasomnias

307.47 Nightmare Disorder
307.46 Sleep Terror Disorder
307.46 Sleepwalking Disorder
307.47 Parasomnia NOS

Sleep Disorders Related to Another Mental Disorder

307.42 Insomnia Related to . . . ***
307.44 Hypersomnia Related to . . . ***

Other Sleep Disorders

780.xx Sleep Disorder Due to . . . *
.52 Insomnia Type
.54 Hyposomnia Type
.59 Parasomnia Type
.59 Mixed Type
—.- Substance-Induced Sleep Disorder (refer to Substance-Related Disorders for substance-specific codes)
Specify type: Insomnia/Hypersomnia/Parasomnia/Mixed
Specify if: With Onset during Intoxication/With Onset During Withdrawal

IMPULSE-CONTROL DISORDERS NOT ELSEWHERE CLASSIFIED

312.34 Intermittent Explosive Disorder
312.32 Kleptomania
312.33 Pyromania
312.31 Pathological Gambling
312.39 Trichotillomania
312.30 Impulse-Control Disorder NOS

ADJUSTMENT DISORDERS

309.xx Adjustment Disorder
.0 With Depressed Mood
.24 With Anxiety
.28 With Mixed Anxiety and Depressed Mood
.3 With Disturbance of Conduct
.4 With Mixed Disturbance of Emotions and Conduct
.9 Unspecified
Specify if: Acute/Chronic

PERSONALITY DISORDERS

Note: These are coded on Axis II

301.0 Paranoid Personality Disorder
301.20 Schizoid Personality Disorder
301.22 Schizotypal Personality Disorder
301.7 Antisocial Personality Disorder
301.83 Borderline Personality Disorder
301.50 Histrionic Personality Disorder
301.81 Narcissistic Personality Disorder
301.82 Avoidant Personality Disorder
301.6 Dependent Personality Disorder
301.4 Obsessive-Compulsive Personality Disorder
301.9 Personality Disorder NOS

OTHER CONDITIONS THAT MAY BE A FOCUS OF CLINICAL ATTENTION

Psychological Factors Affecting Medical Condition

316. . . [Specified Psychological Factor] Affecting . . .*
Choose name based on nature of factors:
Mental Disorder Affecting Medical Condition
Psychological Symptoms Affecting Medical Condition
Personality Traits or Coping Style Affecting Medical Condition
Maladaptive Health Behaviors Affecting Medical Condition
Stress-Related Physiological Response Affecting Medical Condition
Other or Unspecified Psychological Factors Affecting Medical Condition

Medication-Induced Movement Disorders

332.1 Neuroleptic-Induced Parkinsonism
333.92 Neuroleptic Malignant Syndrome
333.7 Neuroleptic-Induced Acute Dystonia
333.99 Neuroleptic-Induced Acute Akathisia
333.82 Neuroleptic-Induced Tardive Dyskinesia
333.1 Medication-Induced Postural Tumor
333.90 Medication-Induced Movement Disorder NOS

Other Medical-Induced Disorder

995.2 Adverse Effects of Medication NOS

Relational Problems

V61.9 Relational Problem Related to a Mental Disorder or General Medical Condition
V61.1 Partner Relational Problem
V61.20 Parent-Child Relational Problem
V61.8 Sibling Relational Problem
V62.81 Relational Problem NOS

Problems Related to Abuse or Neglect

(code 995.5 if focus of attention is on victim)
V61.21 Physical Abuse of Child
V61.21 Sexual Abuse of Child
V61.21 Neglect of Child

V61.12 Physical Abuse of Adult
V61.1 Sexual Abuse of Adult
V62.83 Person Other Than Partner

Additional Conditions That May be Focus of Clinical Attention

V15.81 Noncompliance With Treatment
V65.2 Malingering
V71.01 Adult Antisocial Behavior
V71.02 Child or Adolescent Antisocial Behavior
V62.89 Borderline Intellectual Functioning
Note: This is code on Axis II.
780.9 Age-Related Cognitive Decline
V62.82 Bereavement
V62.3 Academic Problem
V62.2 Occupational Problem
313.82 Identity Problem
V62.89 Religious or Spiritual Problem
V62.4 Acculturation Problem
V62.89 Phase of Life Problem

ADDITIONAL CODES

300.9 Unspecified Mental Disorder (nonpsychotic)
V71.09 No Diagnosis or Condition on Axis I
799.9 Diagnosis or Condition Deferred on Axis I
V71.09 No Diagnosis on Axis II
799.9 Diagnosis Deferred on Axis II

APPENDIX B

Brief Psychiatric Rating Scale

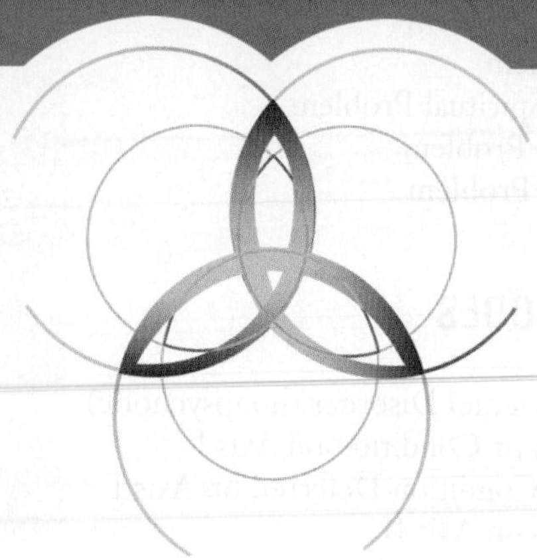

DIRECTIONS: Place an X in the appropriate box to represent level of severity of each symptom.

	Not Present	Very Mild	Mild	Moderate	Mod. Severe	Severe	Extremely Severe
SOMATIC CONCERN—preoccupation with physical health, fear of physical illness, hypochondriasis.	☐	☐	☐	☐	☐	☐	☐
ANXIETY—worry, fear, overconcern for present or future, uneasiness.	☐	☐	☐	☐	☐	☐	☐
EMOTIONAL WITHDRAWAL—lack of spontaneous interaction, isolation deficiency in relating to others.	☐	☐	☐	☐	☐	☐	☐
CONCEPTUAL DISORGANIZATION—thought processes confused, disconnected, disorganized, disrupted.	☐	☐	☐	☐	☐	☐	☐
GUILT FEELINGS—self-blame, shame, remorse for past behavior.	☐	☐	☐	☐	☐	☐	☐
TENSION—physical and motor manifestations of nervousness, over-activation.	☐	☐	☐	☐	☐	☐	☐
MANNERISMS AND POSTURING—peculiar, bizarre unnatural motor behavior (not including tic).	☐	☐	☐	☐	☐	☐	☐
GRANDIOSITY—exaggerated self-opinion, arrogance, conviction of unusual power or abilities.	☐	☐	☐	☐	☐	☐	☐
DEPRESSIVE MOOD—sorrow, sadness, despondency, pessimism.	☐	☐	☐	☐	☐	☐	☐
HOSTILITY—animosity, contempt, belligerence, disdain for others.	☐	☐	☐	☐	☐	☐	☐
SUSPICIOUSNESS—mistrust, belief others harbor malicious or discriminatory intent.	☐	☐	☐	☐	☐	☐	☐
HALLUCINATORY BEHAVIOR—perceptions without normal external stimulus correspondence.	☐	☐	☐	☐	☐	☐	☐
MOTOR RETARDATION—slowed weakened movements or speech, reduced body tone.	☐	☐	☐	☐	☐	☐	☐
UNCOOPERATIVENESS—resistance, guardedness, rejection of authority.	☐	☐	☐	☐	☐	☐	☐
UNUSUAL THOUGHT CONTENT—unusual, odd, strange, bizarre thought content.	☐	☐	☐	☐	☐	☐	☐
BLUNTED AFFECT—reduced emotional tone, reduction in formal intensity of feelings, flatness.	☐	☐	☐	☐	☐	☐	☐
EXCITEMENT—heightened emotional tone, agitation, increased reactivity.	☐	☐	☐	☐	☐	☐	☐
DISORIENTATION—confusion or lack of proper association for person, place, or time.	☐	☐	☐	☐	☐	☐	☐
Global Assessment Scale (Range 1–100)	☐	☐	☐	☐	☐	☐	☐

Reprinted with permission from Overall J. E. (1988). The Brief Psychiatric Rating Scale (BPRS): Recent developments in ascertainment and scaling. *Psychopharmacology Bulletin*, 24, 97–99.

APPENDIX C

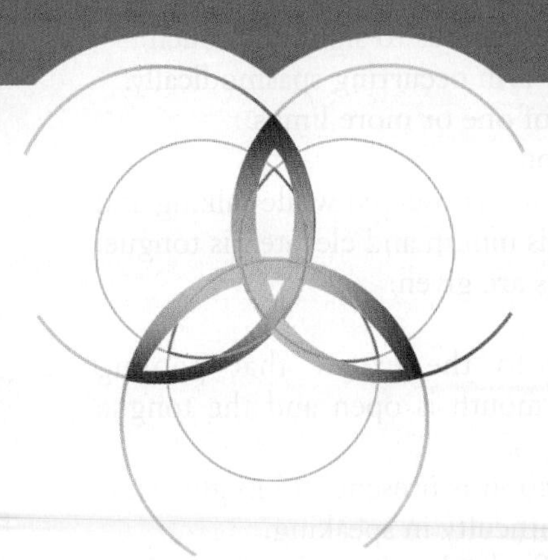

Simpson-Angus Rating Scale

1. GAIT: The patient is examined as he walks into the examining room; his gait, the swing of his arms, his general posture, all form the basis for an overall score for this item. This is rated as follows:
   0 Normal
   1 Diminution in swing while the patient is walking.
   2 Marked diminution in swing with obvious rigidity in the arm.
   3 Stiff gait with arms held rigidly before the abdomen.
   4 Stooped shuffling gait with propulsion and retropulsion.
2. ARM DROPPING: The patient and the examiner both raise their arms to shoulder height and let them fall to their sides. In a normal subject, a stout slap is heard as the arms hit the sides. In the patient with extreme Parkinson's syndrome, the arms fall very slowly.
   0 Normal, free fall with loud slap and rebound.
   1 Fall slowed slightly with less audible contact and little rebound.
   2 Fall slowed, no rebound.
   3 Marked slowing, no slap at all.
   4 Arms fall as though against resistance; as though through glue.
3. SHOULDER SHAKING: The subject's arms are bent at a right angle at the elbow and are taken one at a time by the examiner who grasps one hand and also clasps the other around the patient's elbow. The subject's upper arm is pushed to and fro, and the humerus is externally rotated. The degree of resistance from normal to extreme rigidity is scored as follows:
   0 Normal
   1 Slight stiffness and resistance.
   2 Moderate stiffness and resistance.
   3 Marked rigidity with difficulty in passive movement.
   4 Extreme stiffness and rigidity with almost a frozen shoulder.
4. ELBOW RIGIDITY: The elbow joints are separately bent at right angles and passively extended and flexed, with the subject's biceps observed and simultaneously palpated. The resistance to this procedure is rated. (The presence of cogwheel rigidity is noted separately.) Scoring is from 0 to 4, as in the Shoulder Shaking test.
   0 Normal
   1 Slight stiffness and resistance.
   2 Moderate stiffness and resistance.
   3 Marked rigidity with difficulty in passive movement.
   4 Extreme stiffness and rigidity with almost a frozen shoulder.
5. FIXATION OF POSITION OR WRIST RIGIDITY: The wrist is held in one hand and the fingers held by the examiner's other hand, with the wrist moved to extension flexion and both ulnar and radial deviation. The resistance to this procedure is rated as in Items 3 and 4.
   0 Normal
   1 Slight stiffness and resistance.
   2 Moderate stiffness and resistance.
   3 Marked rigidity with difficulty in passive movement.
   4 Extreme stiffness and rigidity with almost a frozen shoulder.
6. LEG PENDULOUSNESS: The patient sits on a table with his legs hanging down and swinging free. The ankle is grasped by the examiner and raised until the knee is partially extended. It is then allowed to fall. The resistance to falling and the lack of swinging form the basis for the score on this item.
   0 The legs swing freely.
   1 Slight diminution in the swing of the legs.
   2 Moderate resistance to swing.
   3 Marked resistance and damping of swing.
   4 Complete absence of swing.
7. HEAD DROPPING: The patient lies on a well-padded examining table and his head is raised by the

examiner's hand. The hand is then withdrawn, and the head allowed to drop. In the normal subject, the head will fall upon the table. The movement is delayed in extrapyramidal system disorder, and in extreme parkinsonism, it is absent. The neck muscles are rigid, and the head does not reach the examining table. Scoring is as follows:

0 The head falls completely, with a good thump as it hits the table.
1 Slight slowing in fall, mainly noted by lack of slap as head meets the table.
2 Moderate slowing in the fall, quite noticeable to the eye.
3 Head falls stiffly and slowly.
4 Head does not reach examining table.

8. GLABELLA TAP: Subject is told to open his eyes wide and not to blink. The glabella region is tapped at a steady, rapid speed. The number of times patient blinks in succession is noted:
   0 0 to 5 blinks
   1 6 to 10 blinks
   2 11 to 15 blinks
   3 16 to 20 blinks
   4 21 or more blinks
9. TREMOR: Patient is observed walking into examining room and then is re-examined for this item:
   0 Normal
   1 Mild finger tremor, obvious to sight and touch.
   2 Tremor of hand or arm occurring spasmodically.
   3 Persistent tremor of one or more limbs.
   4 Whole body tremor.
10. SALIVATION: Patient is observed while talking and then asked to open his mouth and elevate his tongue. The following ratings are given:
   0 Normal
   1 Excess salivation to the extent that pooling takes place if the mouth is open and the tongue raised.
   2 When excess salivation is present and might occasionally result in difficulty in speaking.
   3 Speaking with difficulty because of excess salivation.
   4 Frank drooling.

Scoring: Each item is rated on a 5-point scale, with 0 meaning the complete absence of the condition, and 4 meaning the presence of the condition in extreme form. The score is obtained by adding the items and dividing by 10.

APPENDIX D

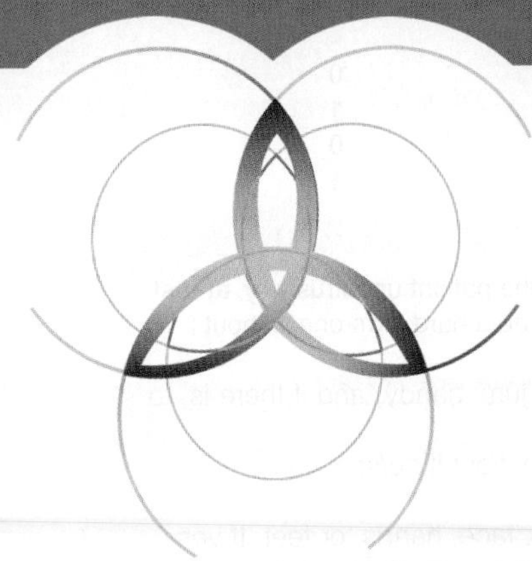

Abnormal Involuntary Movement Scale (AIMS)

		None	Minimal	Mild	Moderate	Severe
Facial and Oral Movements vvbb	1: Muscles of Facial Expression e.g., movements of forehead, eyebrows, periorbital area, cheeks; include frowning, blinking, smiling, grimacing	0	1	2	3	4
	2: Lips and Perioral Area e.g., puckering, pouting, smacking	0	1	2	3	4
	3: Jaw e.g., biting, clenching, chewing, mouth opening, lateral movement	0	1	2	3	4
	4: Tongue Rate only increase in movement both in and out of mouth, NOT inability to sustain movement	0	1	2	3	4
Extremity Movements	5: Upper (arms, wrists, hands, fingers) Include choreic movements (i.e., rapid, objectively purposeless, irregular, spontaneous), athetoid movements (i.e., slow, irregular, complex, serpentine). Do NOT include tremor (i.e., repetitive, regular, rhythmic).	0	1	2	3	4
	6: Lower (legs, knees, ankles, toes) e.g., lateral knee movement, foot tapping, heel dropping, foot squirming, inversion and eversion of foot	0	1	2	3	4
Trunk Movements	7: Neck, shoulders, hips e.g., rocking, twisting, squirming, pelvic gyrations	0	1	2	3	4
	8: Severity of abnormal movements	0	1	2	3	4
Global Judgment	9: Incapacitation due to abnormal movements	0	1	2	3	4
	10: Patient's awareness of abnormal movements Rate only patient's report	No awareness			0	
		Aware, no distress			1	
		Aware, mild distress			2	
		Aware, moderate distress			3	
		Aware, severe distress			4	

		None	Minimal	Mild	Moderate	Severe
Global Judgment						
	11: Current problems with teeth and/or dentures		No		0	
			Yes		1	
	12: Does patient usually wear dentures?		No		0	
			Yes		1	

Examination Procedures for AIMS

Either before or after completing the Examination Procedure, observe the patient unobtrusively, at rest (e.g., in waiting room). The chair to be used in this examination should be a hard, firm one without arms.

1: Ask patient whether there is anything in his/her mouth (e.g., gum, candy) and if there is, to remove it.
2: Ask patient about the *current* condition of his/her teeth. Ask patient if he/she wears dentures. Do teeth or dentures bother patient *now*?
3: Ask patient whether he/she notices any movements in mouth, face, hands, or feet. If yes, ask to describe and to what extent they *currently* bother patient or interfere with his/her activities.
4: Have patient sit in chair with hands on knees, legs slightly apart, and feet flat on floor. (Look at entire body for movements while in this position.)
5: Ask patient to sit with hands hanging unsupported. If male, between legs, if female and wearing a dress, hanging over knees. (Observe hands and other body areas.)
6: Ask patient to open mouth. (Observe tongue at rest within mouth.) Do this twice.
7: Ask patient to protrude tongue. (Observe tongue at rest within mouth.) Do this twice.
*8: Ask patient to tap thumb, with each finger, as rapidly as possible for 10–15 seconds; separately with right hand, then with left hand. (Observe facial and leg movements.)
9: Flex and extend patient's left and right arms (one at a time). (Note any rigidity and rate on NOTES.)
10: Ask patient to stand up. (Observe in profile. Observe all body areas again, hips included.)
*11: Ask patient to extend both arms outstretched in front with palms down. (Observe trunk, legs, and mouth.)
*12: Have patient walk a few paces, turn, and walk back to chair. (Observe hand and gait.) Do this twice.

---

*Activated movements

Reprinted from Guy, W. (1976). ECDEU: Assessment manual for psychopharmacology (DHEW Publ No 76–338). Washington, DC: Department of Health, Education, and Welfare, Psychopharmacology Research Branch.

APPENDIX E

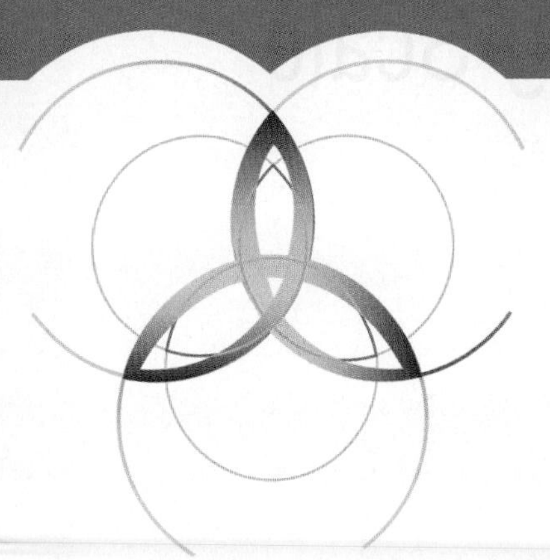

Abnormal Involuntary Movement Scale (AIMS)

PREREQUISITES.—The three prerequisites are as follows. Exceptions may occur.

1. A history of at least 3 months' total cumulative neuroleptic exposure. Include amoxapine and metoclopramide in all categories below as well.
2. **SCORING/INTENSITY LEVEL.** The presence of a **TOTAL SCORE OF FIVE (5) OR ABOVE.** Also be alert for any change from baseline or scores below five which have at least a "moderate" (3) or "severe" (4) movement on any item or at least two "mild" (2) movements on two items located in different body areas.
3. Other conditions are not responsible for the abnormal involuntary movements.

DIAGNOSES.—The diagnosis is based upon the current exam and its relation to the last exam. The diagnosis can shift depending upon: (a) whether movements are present or not, (b) whether movements are present for 3 months or more (6 months if on a semiannual assessment schedule), and (c) whether neuroleptic dosage changes occur and effect movements.

- **NO TD.**—Movements **are not** present on this exam **or** movements are present, but some other condition is responsible for them. The last diagnosis must be NO TD, PROBABLE TD, or WITHDRAWAL TD.
- **PROBABLE TD.**—Movements **are** present on this exam. This is the first time they are present or they have never been present for 3 months or more. The last diagnosis must be NO TD or PROBABLE TD.
- **PERSISTENT TD.**—Movements are present on this exam **and** they have been present for 3 months or more with this exam or at some point in the past. The last diagnosis can be any except NO TD.
- **MASKED TD.**—Movements **are not** present on this exam **but** this is due to a neuroleptic dosage increase or reinstitution after a prior exam when movements were present. Also use this conclusion if movements are not present due to the addition of a non-neuroleptic medication to treat TD. The last diagnosis must be PROBABLE TD, PERSISTENT TD, WITHDRAWAL TD, or MASKED TD.
- **REMITTED TD.**—Movements **are not** present on this exam **but** PERSISTENT TD has been diagnosed and neuroleptic dosage increase or reinstitution has occurred. The last diagnosis must be PERSISTENT TD or REMITTED TD. If movements re-emerge, the diagnosis shifts back to PERSISTENT TD.
- **WITHDRAWAL TD.**—Movements **are not seen while** receiving neuroleptics or at the last dosage level **but are seen within** 8 weeks following a neuroleptic reduction or discontinuation. The last diagnosis must be NO TD or WITHDRAWAL TD. If movements continue for 3 months or more after the neuroleptic dosage reduction or discontinuation, the diagnosis shifts to PERSISTENT TD. If movements do not continue for 3 months or more after the reduction or discontinuation, the diagnosis shifts to NO TD.

INSTRUCTIONS

1. The rater completes the Assessment according to the standardized exam procedure. If the rater also completes Evaluation items 1–4, he/she must also sign the preparer box. The form is given to the physician. Alternatively, the physician may perform the assessment.
2. The physician completes the Evaluation section. The physician is responsible for the entire Evaluation section and its accuracy.
3. IT IS RECOMMENDED THAT THE PHYSICIAN EXAMINE ANY INDIVIDUAL WHO MEETS THE THREE PREREQUISITES OR WHO HAS MOVEMENTS NOT EXPLAINED BY OTHER FACTORS. NEUROLOGICAL ASSESSMENTS OR DIFFERENTIAL DIAGNOSTIC TESTS WHICH MAY BE NECESSARY SHOULD BE OBTAINED.
4. File form according to policy or procedure.

OTHER CONDITIONS (partial list)

1. Age
2. Blind
3. Cerebral Palsy
4. Contact Lenses
5. Dentures/No Teeth
6. Down Syndrome
7. Drug Intoxication (specify)
8. Encephalitis
9. Extrapyramidal Side-Effects (specify)
10. Fahr's Syndrome
11. Heavy Meta Intoxication (specify)
12. Huntington's Chorea
13. Hyperthyroidism
14. Hypoglycemia
15. Hypoparathyroidism
16. Idiopathic Torsion Dystonia
17. Meige Syndrome
18. Parkinson's Disease
19. Stereotypies
20. Sydenham's Chorea
21. Tourette's Syndrome
22. Wilson's Disease
23. Other (specify)

Sprague, R. L., & Kalachnik, J. E. (1991). Reliability, validity, and a total score cutoff for the Dyskinesia Identification System, Condensed User Scale (DISCUS) with mentally ill and mentally retarded populations. *Psychopharmacology Bulletin, 27*(1), 51–58.

APPENDIX F

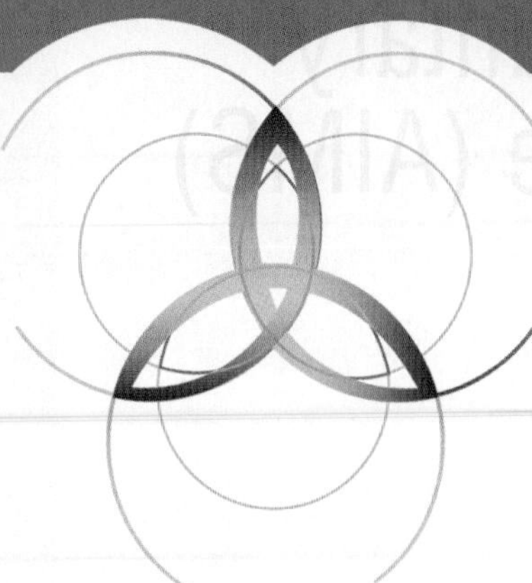

Hamilton Rating Scale for Depression

Clinic No.________ Date________ Rating No.________ Code Number________
Sex________ Age________ Patient's Name________________________________
Patient's Address____ Tel________________

Item	Range	Score
1. Depressed mood	0–4	
2. Guilt	0–4	
3. Suicide	0–4	
4. Insomnia initial	0–2	
5. Insomnia middle	0–2	
6. Insomnia delayed	0–2	
7. Work and interest	0–4	
8. Retardation	0–4	
9. Agitation	0–4	
10. Anxiety (psychic)	0–4	
11. Anxiety (somatic)	0–4	
12. Somatic gastrointestinal	0–2	
13. Somatic general	0–2	
14. Genital	0–2	
15. Hypochondriasis	0–2	
16. Insight	0–4	
17. Loss of weight	0–2	
	Total Score	
Diurnal variation (M.A.E.)	0–2	
Depersonalization	0–4	
Paranoid symptoms	0–4	
Obsessional symptoms	0–4	

The scale is designed to measure the severity of illness of patients already diagnosed as suffering from depressive illness. It is obviously not a diagnostic instrument because that requires much more information (e.g., previous history, family history, precipitating factors).

As far as possible, the scale should be used in the manner of a clinical interview. The first time the interview should be conducted in a relaxed, free, and easy manner, giving the patients time to unburden themselves and giving them the opportunity to speak of their problems and ask whatever questions they wish. It may then be necessary to obtain further information by asking them questions. At subsequent assessments, the interview can be briefer and more to the point.

An observer rating scale is not a checklist in which each item is strictly defined. The raters must have sufficient clinical experience and judgment to be able to interpret the patients' statements and reticences about some symptoms, and to compare them with other patients. They should use all sources of information (e.g., from relatives and nurses).

The scale consists of 17 items, the scores on which are summed to give a total score. There are four other items, one of which (diurnal variation) is excluded on the grounds that it is not an additional burden on the patient. The last three are excluded from the total score because they occur infrequently, although information on them may be useful for other purposes.

The method of assessment is simple. For some symptoms it is difficult to elicit such information as will permit of full quantification. If present, score 2; if absent, score 0; and if doubtful or trivial, score 1. For those symptoms where more detailed information can be obtained, the score of 2 is expanded into 2 for mild, 3 for moderate, and 4 for severe. In case of difficulty, the raters should use their judgment as clinicians.

Hamilton, M. (1960). A rating scale for depression. *Journal of Neurology, Neurosurgery and Psychiatry, 23,* 56.

APPENDIX G

CAGE Questionnaire

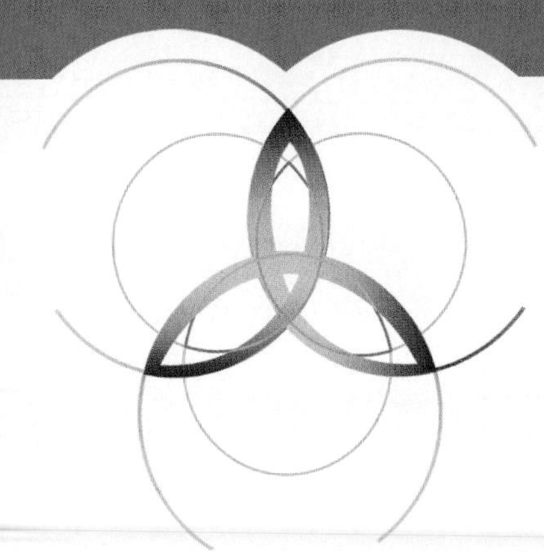

The CAGE is a very brief questionnaire for detection of alcoholism. Item responses on the CAGE are scored 0 for *no* and 1 for *yes*, with a higher score an indication of alcohol problems. A total score of 2 or more is considered clinically significant and requires a more focused and detailed assessment. The following are the four questions that comprise the CAGE questionnaire.

Have you ever felt you should *Cut down* on your drinking?	Yes	No
Have people *Annoyed* you by criticizing your drinking?	Yes	No
Have you ever felt bad or *Guilty* about your drinking?	Yes	No
Have you ever had a drink first thing in the morning to steady your nerves to get rid of a hangover? (*Eyeopener*)	Yes	No

Ewing, J. A. (1984). Detecting alcoholism. *Journal of the American Medical Association. 252,* 1905–1907.

Additional readings:

Burge, S., & Schneider, F. (1999). Alcohol-related problems: Recognition and intervention. *American Family Physician,* American Academy of Family Physicians Home Page (www.aafp.org. 1/15/99).

Davis, M. (2000). Alcohol and drug addiction. *Medical Library* (www.medical-library.org. 9/30/00).

Wesson, D. (1995). *Detoxification from alcohol and other drugs.* Rockville, MD: Substance Abuse and Mental Health Services Administration, Center for Substance Abuse Treatment, Treatment Improvement Protocol #19.

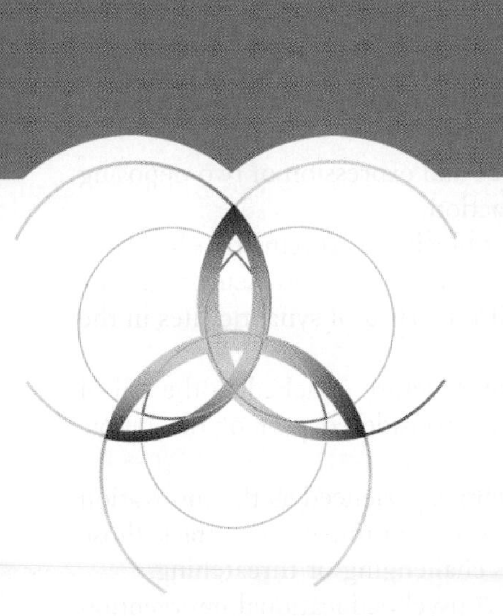

Glossary

23-hour observation a short-term treatment that serves the patient in immediate but short-term crisis. This type of care admits individuals to an inpatient setting for as long as 23 hours, during which time services are provided at a less-than-acute care level.

ABCDE An acronym for the basic framework of Rational Emotive Cognitive Therapy.

ABCs of psychological first aid Focusing on A (arousal), B (behavior), and C (cognition).

absorption Movement of drug from the site of administration into plasma.

abuse Use of alcohol or drugs for the purpose of intoxication or, in the case of prescription drugs, for purposes beyond the intended use.

accommodation Adjustment in cognitive organization that results from the demands of reality (Piaget).

accreditation Process by which a mental health agency is judged by established standards to be providing acceptable quality of care.

acculturation Act or process of assuming the beliefs, values, and practices of another, usually dominant culture.

acetylcholine (ACh) An important neurotransmitter associated with cognitive functioning; disruption of cholinergic mechanisms damages memory in animals and humans.

acetylcholinesterase (AChE) Key enzyme that inactivates the neurotransmitter acetylcholine. AChE is found in high concentrations in the brain and is one of two cholinesterase enzymes capable of breaking down ACh.

acetylcholinesterase inhibitors (AChEI) Mainstay of pharmacologic treatment of dementia; these drugs inhibit AChE, resulting in an enhancement of cholinergic activity.

activating event The "A" in the RECT framework that represents the external or internal stimulus; not necessarily an actual event; may be an emotion, or thought/expectation that is interpreted according to a set of beliefs.

active listening Focusing on what the patient is saying in order to interpret and respond to the message in an objective manner, while using techniques such as open-ended statements, reflection, and questions that elicit additional responses from the patient.

acute pain a sudden onset of pain at the time of injury or illness that generally subsides as the injury heals.

acute stress disorder (ASD) A mental disorder characterized by persistent, distressing stress-related symptoms that last between 2 days and 1 month and that occur within 1 month after a traumatic experience.

addiction Severe psychological and behavioral dependence on drugs or alcohol.

adherence An individual's ability to follow directions for self-administration of medications and other biologic therapies; compliance.

advanced practice psychiatric–mental health nurse A licensed registered nurse who is educationally prepared at the master's level and is nationally certified as a specialist by the American Nurses Credentialing Center (AANC).

advance care directives Treatment directives (living wills) and appointment directives (power of attorney or health proxies) that apply only if the individual is unable to make his or her own decisions because the patient is incapacitated or, in the opinion of two physicians, is otherwise unable to make decisions for himself or herself.

adventitious crisis A crisis initiated by unexpected, unusual events that can affect an individual or a multitude of people.

adverse reactions Unwanted medication effects that may have serious physiologic consequences.

affect An expression of mood manifest in a pattern of observable behaviors.

affective flattening or blunting Flat or blunted emotion.

affective instability Rapid and extreme shifts in mood, erratic emotional responses to situations, and intense sensitivity to criticism or perceived slights; one of the core characteristics of borderline personality disorder.

affective lability Abrupt, dramatic, unprovoked changes in the types of emotions expressed.

afferent Toward the central nervous system or a particular structure.

affinity Degree of attraction or strength of the bond between a drug and its receptor.

aggression Behaviors or attitudes that reflect rage, hostility, and the potential for physical or verbal destructiveness; usually occurs if the person believes someone is going to do him or her harm.

agitation Inability to sit still or attend to others, accompanied by heightened emotions and tension.

agnosia Failure to recognize or identify objects despite intact sensory function, or a disturbance in executive functioning (ability to think abstractly, plan, initiate, sequence, monitor, and stop complex behavior).

agonists Chemicals producing the same biologic action as the neurotransmitter.

agoraphobia Anxiety about being in places from which escape might be difficult or embarrassing, or about being in places in which help may not be readily available if a panic attack should occur.

agranulocytosis Dangerously low level of circulating neutrophils.

AIDS dementia complex Changes in mentation and personality, followed by delirium, dementia, organic mood disorder, and organic delusional disorder in persons with AIDS.

akathisia An extrapyramidal side effect from phenothiazine, which includes restlessness that is easily mistaken for anxiety or increased psychotic symptoms.

Alcoholics Anonymous The first 12-step, self-help program; a worldwide fellowship of people with alcoholism who provide support, individually and at meetings, to others who seek help.

alcohol-induced persisting amnestic disorder Cognitive impairment deficits related to substance abuse.

alcohol tolerance A phenomenon producing a more rapid metabolism of alcohol and a decreased response to its sedating, motor, and anxiolytic effects.

alcohol withdrawal syndrome A syndrome that occurs after the reduction of alcohol consumption, or when abstaining from alcohol after prolonged use, causing changes in vital signs, diaphoresis, and other adverse gastrointestinal and central nervous system side effects.

alexithymia Inability to experience and communicate feelings consciously.

algorithms Systematic decision trees that depict the flow of decisions and outcomes.

allodynia Lowered pain threshold.

allostasis Regulatory systems that have a wide range of functioning (e.g., blood pressure, heart rate) and achieve stability through adaptation or change.

alogia Brief, empty verbal responses; often referred to as *poverty of speech*.

ambivalence Presence and expression of two opposing forces, leading to inaction.

amino acids Building blocks of proteins that have different roles. Amino acids function as neurotransmitters in as many as 60% to 70% of synaptic sites in the brain.

amygdala A bulb-like structure attached to the tail of the caudate and often considered part of the limbic system.

anger An affective state experienced as the motivation to act in ways that warn, intimidate, or attack those who are perceived as challenging or threatening.

anger management A psychoeducational intervention for persons whose behavior is dysfunctional in some way (i.e., interfering with success in work or relationships) but *not violent*.

anhedonia Inability to gain pleasure from activities.

animism A child's belief that inanimate objects are alive.

anorexia nervosa A life-threatening eating disorder characterized by refusal to maintain body weight appropriate for age, intense fear of gaining weight or becoming fat, a severely distorted body image, and refusal to acknowledge the seriousness of weight loss.

antagonists Chemicals blocking the biologic response at a given receptor site.

anticholinergic crisis A potentially life-threatening medical emergency that occurs as a result of overdose or sensitivity to drugs with anticholinergic properties.

antimotivational syndrome Attributed to long-term marijuana use, a syndrome marked by apathy, diminished interest in activities and goals, poor job performance, and reduced short-term memory.

anxiety Energy that arises when expectations that are present are not met (Peplau).

anxiogenic Anxiety provoking.

anxiolytics Drugs that reverse or diminish anxiety.

apathy Reactions to stimuli that are decreased, along with a diminished interest and desire.

aphasia Alterations in language ability.

apraxia Impaired ability to execute motor activities despite intact motor functioning.

arachnoid layer A thin, delicate sheet of collagenous tissue under the meningeal layer that follows the contours of the brain but does not dip down inside them.

area restriction Limitation of patient mobility to a specified area for purposes of safety or behavior management.

ascertainment bias a bias that occurs when the method of identifying cases creates a sample that differs from the population it purports to represent.

assault The threat of unlawful force to inflict bodily injury upon another. The threat must be imminent and cause reasonable apprehension in the individual.

assertive community treatment Direct and individualized treatment and services provided by a selectively chosen interdisciplinary team that follows on a patient's progress during reintegration into the community.

assessment Deliberate and systematic collection of biopsychosocial information or data to determine current and past health and functional status and to evaluate present and past coping patterns.

association areas Areas of the cortex in which neighboring nerve fibers are related to the same sensory modality.

assortative mating Tendency for individuals to select mates who are similar in genetically linked traits such as intelligence and personality styles.

atropine flush Flushing of the face, neck, and upper arms due to a reflex blood vessel dilation that results from increased body temperature.

attachment Emotional bond between the infant and parental figure.

attachment disorganization A consequence of extreme insecurity that results from feared or actual separation from the attached figure. Infants appear to be unable to maintain the strategic adjustments in attachment behavior.

attention A complex mental process that involves concentrating on one activity to the exclusion of others, as well as sustaining interest over time.

atypical antipsychotics Newer antipsychotics that are equally or more effective than conventional antipsychotics, but have fewer side effects.

augmentation A strategy of adding another medication to enhance effectiveness.

autism A form of thinking or a style of relating that focuses subjectively on "me" to the exclusion of "not me."

autistic thinking Thinking restricted to the literal and immediate so that the individual has private rules of logic and reasoning that make no sense to others.

automatic thinking Thinking that influences the person's actions or other thought; it is often subject to errors or tangible distortions of reality that contradict objective appraisals.

autonomic nervous system Part of the nervous system that regulates involuntary vital functions including cardiac muscle, smooth muscles, and glands. It is composed of the sympathetic and parasympathetic systems.

autonomy Concept that each person has the fundamental right of self-determination.

avolition Inability to complete projects, assignments, or work.

axes A term used to describe domains of information. In a psychiatric diagnosis, there are five domains: Axis I, clinical domain that is the focus of treatment; Axis II, personality disorders or mental retardation; Axis III, general medical condition; Axis IV, psychosocial stress; and Axis V, level of functioning.

basal ganglia One set of structures in each hemisphere; areas of gray matter containing many cell bodies or nuclei.

basic level of practice According to the *Scope and Standards of Psychiatric–Mental Health Nursing*, this level includes two groups of nurses. The first group includes registered nurses who practice in psychiatric settings; the second includes those who have a baccalaureate degree in nursing and have worked in the field for 2 years.

behavior modification A specific therapy technique that can be applied to individuals, groups, or systems. The aim of behavior modification is to reinforce desired behaviors and extinguish undesired ones.

behavior therapy Interventions that reinforce or promote desirable behaviors or alter undesirable ones.

behavioral sensitization A phenomenon by which a person has a magnified stress response to milder stressors after one or more exposures to a severe, uncontrollable stressor.

behaviorism A paradigm shift in understanding human behavior that was initiated by Watson, who theorized that human behavior is developed through a stimulus–response process rather than through unconscious drives or instincts.

belief system Beliefs underlying thoughts and emotions.

beneficence The health care provider uses knowledge of science and incorporates the art of caring to develop an environment in which individuals achieve maximum health care potential.

bereavement A period of profound grieving following a loss.

beta-amyloid plaques Dense, mostly insoluble deposits of protein and cellular material outside and around neurons; pathology of Alzheimer's disease.

bibliotherapy The use of books and other reading materials to help individuals cope with various life stressors.

binge eating Episodes of uncontrollable, ravenous eating of large amounts of food within discrete periods of time, usually followed by feelings of guilt that result in purging.

binge eating disorder A newly identified eating disorder in its infancy relative to research; individuals binge in the same way as those with bulimia nervosa but do not purge or compensate for binges through other behaviors.

bioavailability Amount of a drug that reaches the systemic circulation for targeted treatment.

biogenic amines Small molecules manufactured in the neuron that contain an amine group. These include dopamine, norepinephrine, and epinephrine (all synthesized from the amino acid tyrosine), serotonin (from tryptophan), and histamine (from histidine).

biologic domain Part of the biopsychosocial model that explains the biologic knowledge of mental health, including pathogenesis and treatment of mental illness.

biologic markers Physical indicators of disturbances within the central nervous system that differentiate one disease state from another.

biologic view A theoretic view or argument of the early 1900s that mental illness has a biologic cause and can be treated with physical interventions.

biopsychosocial model An organizational model consisting of three separate but interdependent domains: biologic, psychological, and social. Each domain has an independent knowledge and treatment focus but can interact and be mutually interdependent with the other dimensions.

biosexual identity Anatomic and physiologic state of being male or female that results from genetic and hormonal influences.

biotransformation Metabolism of a drug or substance.

bipolar A mood disorder characterized by manic or hypomanic and depressive episodes; manic-depressive disorder.

bipolar type A subtype of schizophrenic disorder in which the patient exhibits manic symptoms alone or with a mix of manic and depressive symptoms.

board-and-care homes Facilities that provide 24-hour supervision and assistance with medications, meals, and some self-care skills, but in which individualized attention to self-care skills and other activities of daily living is generally not available.

body dysmorphic disorder Disorder in which there is a preoccupation with an imagined or slight defect in appearance, such as a large nose, thinning hair, or small genitals.

body image How each individual perceives his or her own body, separate from how the world or society views him or her.

body image disturbance Extreme discrepancy between one's perception of one's own body image and others' perceptions of one.

boundaries Limits in which a person may act or refrain from acting within a designated time or place.

boxed warning Serious adverse effects that can occur with the use of a specific medication found in the package insert.

bradykinesia An extrapyramidal condition characterized by a slowness of voluntary movement and speech.

brain stem Area of the brain containing the midbrain, pons, and medulla, which continues beneath the thalamus.

breach of confidentiality Release of patient information without the patient's consent in the absence of legal compulsion or authorization to release information.

brief intervention A negotiated conversation between professional and patient designed to reduce alcohol and drug use; any short-term intervention.

Broca's area A section of the left frontal lobe of the brain thought to be responsible for the articulation of speech.

bulimia nervosa An eating disorder in which the individual engages in recurrent episodes of binge eating and compensatory behavior to avoid weight gain through purging methods such as self-induced vomiting, or use of laxatives, diuretics, enemas, or emetics, or through nonpurging methods such as fasting or excessive exercise.

butyrylcholinesterase (BuChE) A nonspecific cholinesterase found in the brain and especially in the glial cells.

carrier protein A membrane protein that transports a specific molecule across the cell membrane.

case finding Identifying people who are at risk for suicide to initiate proper treatment. Identification of depression and risk factors associated with suicide.

case management Problem solving and coordinating services for the patient to ensure continuity of services and overcome system rigidity, fragmentation of services, misuse of facilities, and inaccessibility.

cataplexy Bilateral loss of muscle tone triggered by a strong emotion such as laughter. This muscle atonia can range from subtle (drooping eyelids) to dramatic (buckling knees). Eye and respiratory muscles are not affected. Cataplexy usually lasts only seconds. Individuals are fully conscious, oriented, and alert during the episode. Prolonged episodes of cataplexy may lead to sleep episodes.

catastrophic reactions Overreactions or extreme anxiety reactions to everyday situations.

catatonic excitement Hyperactivity characterized by purposeless activity and abnormal movements like grimacing and posturing.

catharsis A Freudian concept meaning release of feelings.

central sulcus Posterior boundary of the frontal lobe that separates it from the parietal lobe.

cerebellum Part of the brain that is responsible for controlling movement and postural adjustments; it receives information from all parts of the body.

cerebrospinal fluid Cushioning fluid that circulates around the brain beneath the arachnoid layer in the subarachnoid space; it is colorless and contains sodium chloride and other salts.

chemical restraints Use of medication to control patients or manage behavior.

child abuse and neglect Child abuse is any action (or lack of) which endangers or impairs a child's physical, psychological, or emotional health and development. Child abuse occurs in different ways. All forms of child abuse and neglect are detrimental to the child; both physical and sexual abuse are crimes.

choroid plexus A collection of cells within the ventricles that produces cerebrospinal fluid.

chronic syndromes Symptom patterns that last for long periods of time.

chronobiology Study and measure of time structures or biologic rhythms.

chronopharmacotherapy Resetting the biologic clock by using short-acting hypnotics to induce sleep.

chronotherapy Manipulation of the sleep schedule by progressively delaying bedtime until an acceptable bedtime is attained.

circadian rhythm (cycle) From the Latin *circa* and *dies*, meaning "about a day"; refers to a biologic system that fluctuates or oscillates in a pattern that repeats itself in about a day.

circumstantiality Extremely detailed and lengthy discourse about a topic.

clang association Repetition of word phrases that are similar in sound but in no other way, for example, "right, light, sight, might."

classical conditioning A learning situation in which an unconditioned stimulus initially produces an unconditioned response; over time, a conditioned response is elicited for a specific stimulus (Pavlov).

clearance Total amount of blood, serum, or plasma from which a drug is completely removed per unit of time.

clinical reasoning Using critical thinking and reflection to address patient problems and interventions.

closed group A group in which all the members begin at one time. New members are not admitted after the first meeting.

clubhouse model Psychosocial rehabilitation approach with the goal of integrating individuals with mental illness back into the community; these houses are run entirely by the patients or "clubhouse members."

codependence A maladaptive coping pattern in family members or others closely related to a substance abuser that results from prolonged exposure to the behaviors of the alcohol- or drug-dependent person; characterized by boundary distortions, poor relationship and friendship skills, compulsive and obsessive behaviors, inappropriate anger, sexual maladjustment, and resistance to change.

cognition A high level of intellectual processing in which perceptions and information are acquired, used, or manipulated.

cognitive appraisal The process of examining the demands, constraints, and resources of the environment and of negotiating them with personal goals and beliefs.

cognitive distortions Automatic thoughts generated by organizing distorted information and/or inaccurate interpretation of a situation.

cognitive interventions or cognitive therapy Interventions or psychotherapy that reinforce and promote desirable cognitive functioning or alter undesirable cognitive functioning.

cognitive reserve The brain's ability to operate effectively even when there is disruption in functioning.

cognitive triad Thoughts about oneself, the world, and the future.

cognitive schema Patterns of thoughts that determine how a person interprets events. Each person's cognitive schema screen, code, and evaluate incoming stimuli.

commitment to treatment statement Patient verbally or in writing agrees to seek treatment.

communication blocks Interruptions in the content flow of communication that can be identified in process recordings as such changes in topic that either the nurse or patient makes.

communication disorders Disorders that involve speech or language impairments.

communication triad A technique used to provide a specific syntax and order for patients to identify and express their feelings and seek relief. The "sentence" consists of three parts: (1) an "I" statement to identify the prevailing feeling, (2) a nonjudgmental statement of the emotional trigger, and (3) a statement of what the person would like differently or what would restore comfort to the situation.

comorbidity (comorbid) Disease that coexists with the primary disease.

competence The degree to which the patient is able to understand and appreciate the information given during the consent process; the patient's cognitive ability to process information at a specific time; the patient's ability to gather and interpret information and make reasonable judgments based on that information to participate fully as a partner in treatment.

complex posttraumatic stress disorder (PTSD) A new and proposed diagnosis: for survivors of extreme, prolonged trauma, especially interpersonal trauma (i.e., severe, prolonged child abuse), including the diagnosis of PTSD.

compliance The individual's ability to follow directions for self-administration of medications and other biologic therapies; adherence.

compliments Affirmations of the patient.

concordant Mutually affected.

concrete thinking Lack of abstraction in thinking, in which people are unable to understand punch lines, metaphors, and analogies.

conditional release Discharge of patients whose psychiatric symptoms have been stabilized and are no longer considered a danger to the community. Similar to parole for inmates released from a correctional facility.

confabulation Telling a plausible, but imagined scenario that fills in memory gaps.

confidentiality An ethical duty of nondisclosure; the patient has the right to disclose personal information without fear of it being revealed to others.

conflict resolution A specific type of counseling in which the nurse helps the patient resolve a disagreement or dispute.

confrontation Presenting evidence of inconsistencies in thoughts, feelings, and actions.

confused speech and thinking Symptoms of schizophrenia that render the patient unable to respond accurately to the ordinary signs and sounds of daily living.

connections Mutually responsive and enhancing relationships.

conservation The child's awareness that a quantity remains the same despite its shape.

constraints Limitations that are both personal (internalized cultural values and beliefs) and environmental (finite resources such as money and time).

containment The process of providing safety and security; involves the patient's access to food and shelter.

content themes Repetition of concerns or feelings that occur within the therapeutic relationship. Themes may emerge as symbolic representations of fears.

continuum of care Providing care in an integrated system of settings, services (physical, psychological, and social), and care levels appropriate to the individual's specific needs in a continuous manner over time, with channels of communication among the service providers.

conventional antipsychotics Medications used to treat psychotic disorders that are primarily dopamine antagonists; also referred to as typical antipsychotics.

coordination of care Integration of the various components of the continuum of care, including the pre-entry, entry, pre-exit, and exit phases.

coping Thinking and acting in ways to manage specific external and internal demands and conflicts that are taxing or exceeding one's resources.

corpus callosum Functional link between the two hemispheres of the brain, made up of a thick band of fibers.

cortex Outer surface of the mature brain.

cortical dementia A type of dementia that is characterized by amnesia, aphasia, apraxia, and agnosia.

counseling (counseling interventions) Specific time-limited interactions between a nurse and a patient, family, or group experiencing intermediate or ongoing difficulties related to their health or well-being.

countertransference The nurse's reactions to a patient that are based on the nurse's unconscious needs, conflicts, problems, and views of the world. It can significantly interfere with the nurse–patient relationship.

court process counseling An approach that educates mentally ill patients about the impending legal procedures and prepares them for courtroom appearances.

craving The urge or desire to engage in a behavior such as drinking.

crisis A severely stressful experience for which coping mechanisms fail to provide any adaptation, whether the experience is positive or negative.

crisis intervention A specialized short-term (usually no longer than 6 hours) goal-directed therapy designed to assist patients in an immediate manner, after which they are usually transferred to an inpatient unit or to an intensive outpatient setting.

critical pathways An interdisciplinary plan of care for patients with a common problem represented by flow charts that usually specifies expected length of stay.

critical thinking An analytic and complex process that involves observing behaviors and responses; making purposeful, objective judgments; and constantly re-evaluating.

cue Stimuli that lead to behavior.

cue elimination Emotional and environmental cues are identified and alternative responses are suggested, tried, and reinforced. When a cue or stimulus leads to a dysfunctional or unhealthy response, the response can be eliminated, or an alternate, healthier response to the cue can be substituted, tried, and then reinforced.

cultural-bound syndrome A recurrent, locality-specific pattern of aberrant behavior and troubling experience that is limited to specific societies or culture areas.

cultural brokering Act of bridging, linking, or mediating between groups or individuals of different cultural systems for the purpose of reducing conflict or producing change.

cultural competence A process (developed through cultural awareness, acquisition of cultural knowledge, development of cultural skills, and engagement in numerous cultural encounters) in which the nurse continually strives to achieve the ability to work effectively within the cultural context of an individual or community from a diverse cultural or ethnic background.

culture Any group of people who identify or associate with each other on the basis of some common purpose, need, or similarity of background; the set of learned, socially transmitted beliefs and behaviors that arise from interpersonal transactions among members of the cultural group.

culture of poverty A term that describes the norms and behaviors of people living in poverty.

cycle of violence A three-phase pattern of tension, abuse, and kindness in which the abuser engages first in abuse and then in seemingly sincere expressions of love, contrition, and remorse.

cyclothymic disorder Periods of hypomanic episodes and depressive episodes that do not meet full criteria for a major depressive episode.

cytochrome P-450 (CYP450) a set of microsomal enzymes (usually hepatic) referred to as CYP1, CYP2, and CYP3.

day treatment A bridge between institutional and community care for severely mentally ill and substance-abusing people. Participation in structured day treatment programs provides emotional and practical support and strengthens ties to community services and potentially to family and friends.

de-escalation An interactive process of calming and redirecting a patient who has an immediate potential for violence directed at others or self.

defense levels Division of defense mechanisms that includes high adaptive, mental inhibitions (compromise formation), minor image-distorting, disavowal, major image-distorting, action level, and defense dysregulation.

defense mechanisms Coping styles; the automatic psychological process protecting the individual against anxiety and creating awareness of internal or external dangers or stressors.

defining characteristics Clues given by the signs and symptoms that join together in the nurse's mind to form a cluster that leads to a specific nursing diagnosis.

deinstitutionalization Release of patients with severe and persistent mental illness from state mental hospitals to community settings.

delirium Characterized by a disturbance in consciousness and a change in cognition that develops over a short period of time.

delirium tremens An acute withdrawal syndrome that occurs often in alcoholics after 10 or more years of heavy drinking and is characterized by tachycardia, sweating, hypertension, irregular tremor, delusions, vivid hallucinations, and wild, agitated behavior.

delusion Erroneous belief that usually involves a misinterpretation of perception of experience. These beliefs are false, fixed, and fall outside of the patient's social, cultural, or religious background.

delusional disorder A disorder in which there is the presence of nonbizarre delusions; includes several subtypes: ergotomania, grandiose, jealous, somatic, mixed, and specified.

demands External pulls (crowding, crime, noise, pollution) imposed by the physical environment, and internal pulls (behavior and role expectations) imposed by the social environment.

dementia From the Latin de (from or out of) and *mens* (mind); several cognitive deficits (one of which is impaired memory) that are due to the direct physiologic effects of a general medical condition, the persisting effects of a substance, or multiple biologic etiologies.

denial The patient's inability to accept loss of control over substance use or the severity of the consequences associated with substance abuse.

dependence The state of being psychologically or physiologically dependent on a drug after a prolonged period of use.

depersonalization A nonspecific experience in which the individual loses a sense of personal identity and feels strange or unreal.

depressive episode In a major depressive episode, either a depressed mood or a loss of interest or pleasure in nearly all activities must be present for at least 2 weeks. Four of seven additional symptoms must be present: disruption in sleep, appetite (or weight), concentration, energy; psychomotor agitation or retardation; excessive guilt or feelings of worthlessness; suicidal ideation.

depressive type A subtype of schizophrenia disorder in which the patient displays only symptoms of a major depressive episode during the illness.

desensitization A rapid decrease in drug effects that may develop within a few minutes or over a period of days, months, years, or lifetime of exposure to a drug.

desynchronized Two or more circadian rhythms reaching their peaks at different times.

detoxification Process of safely and effectively withdrawing a person from an addictive substance, usually under medical supervision.

developmental delay The impairment of normal growth and development that may not be reversible.

Dialectical Behavior Therapy (DBT) An important biosocial approach to treatment that combines numerous cognitive and behavior therapy strategies. It requires patients to understand their disorder by actively participating in formulating treatment goals by collecting data about their own behavior, identifying treatment targets in individual therapy, and working with the therapists in changing these target behaviors.

diathesis A constitutional predisposition to a disorder.

dichotomous thinking Tendency to view things as absolute, either black or white, good or bad, with no perception of compromise.

differentiation of self An individual's resolution of attachment to his or her family's emotional chaos. It involves an intrapsychic separation of thinking from feelings and an interpersonal freeing of oneself from the chaos.

direct leadership behavior The leader controls the interaction of the group by giving directions and information and allowing little discussion.

disconnections Lack of mutually responsive and enhancing relationships.

discrimination The differential treatment of others because they are members of a particular group.

disinhibition A concept borrowed from physics and biology and based on the idea of a dynamic, self-regulatory model of equilibrium in which equilibrium is defined (Piaget) as compensation for external disturbance; a mechanism for providing the self-regulation by which intelligence adapts to internal and external changes.

disordered water balance A state of chronic fluid imbalance, vacillating between normal and hyponatremic, that commonly occurs in psychiatric patients with chronic illnesses.

dissociation A disruption in the normally occurring linkages among subjective awareness, feelings, thoughts, behavior, and memories.

dissociative identity disorder (DID) A mental disorder characterized by the existence of two or more distinct identities with unique personality characteristics and the inability to recall important information about oneself or events.

distraction Consciously changing behaviors to take the focus off the physical sensations or unwanted thoughts, feelings, or behaviors.

distribution The amount of a drug that may be found in various tissues at the site of the drug action for which it is intended.

disturbances of executive functioning Problems in the ability to think abstractly, plan, initiate, sequence, monitor, and stop complex behavior.

diurnal weight gain Weight gain that occurs throughout a day that is caused by fluid and food intake that is regulated by the circadian rhythm.

domestic abuse Violence, including rape, directed toward a person by an intimate partner.

dopamine An excitatory neurotransmitter found in distinct regions of the CNS involved in cognition, motor, and neuroendocrine function.

dosing Administration of medication over time so that therapeutic levels may be achieved or maintained without reaching toxic levels.

drug–drug interaction Reaction of two or more drugs with each other; may cause unexpected side effects.

drug overdose A dose of a drug that causes an acute reaction such as agitation, delirium, coma, or death.

DSM-IV-TR Abbreviation for the *Diagnostic and Statistical Manual of Mental Disorders*, 4th edition, text revision.

dura mater The tough layer of collagen fibers that forms a loose sac around the central nervous system (in Latin, "hard mother") and contains three layers: meningeal, arachnoid, and pia mater.

dyad A group of only two people who are usually related, such as a married couple, siblings, or parent and child.

dysfunctional consequences The result of the interaction between A (activating event) and B (belief system) that follows from absolute, rigid, irrational beliefs.

dysfunctional family A family whose interactions, decisions, or behaviors interfere with the positive development of the family and its individual members.

dysfunctional grieving Absent or exaggerated grief response.

dyslexia Significantly lower score for mental age on standardized test in reading that is not due to low intelligence or inadequate schooling.

dysphagia Difficulty swallowing.

dysphoric (mood) Depressed, disquieted, and/or restless.

dyssomnia A disorder of initiating or maintaining sleep or of excessive sleepiness.

dysthymic disorder A milder but more chronic form of major depressive disorder.

dystonia An impairment in muscle tone that is generally the first extrapyramidal symptom to occur, usually within a few days of initiating an antipsychotic. Dystonia is characterized by involuntary muscle spasms, especially of the head and neck muscles.

early intervention programs Community outreach efforts designed to work with infants and preschool-aged children and their caretakers to foster healthy physical, psychological, social, and intellectual development.

echolalia Parrot-like repetition of another's words; inappropriate choice of topics.

echopraxia Involuntary imitation of another person's movements and gestures; regressed behavior that is child-like or immature.

efferent Away from the central nervous system or other particular structure.

efficacy Ability of a drug to produce a response as a result of the receptor or receptors being occupied.

egocentrism Tendency to view the world as revolving around oneself.

emotion Psychophysiologic reaction that defines a person's mood and can be categorized as negative (anger, fright, anxiety, guilt, shame, sadness, envy, jealousy, and disgust), positive (happiness, pride, relief, and love), or somewhat ambiguous, or borderline (hope, compassion, empathy, sympathy, and contentment).

emotional abuse In reference to adults: degrading, threatening, stalking, or otherwise using psychological violence; in reference to children: rejecting, isolating, terrorizing, ignoring, or corrupting.

emotional circuit The interrelationship between the emotional processes of the limbic system and the neurocognitive processes of the frontal lobe and other parts of the cortex.

emotional cutoff If a member cannot differentiate from his or her family, that member may flee from the family, either by moving away or avoiding personal subjects of conversation. A brief visit from parents can render these individuals helpless.

emotional dysregulation Inability to control emotion in social interactions.

emotional regulation A biosocial interaction between the innate emotional vulnerability of the individual and the ability to modulate that emotion in social interactions.

emotional vulnerability Sensitivity and reactivity to environmental stress.

emotion-focused coping A type of coping that changes the meaning of the situation.

empathic linkage Ability to feel in oneself the feelings being expressed by another person or persons.

empathy A voluntary, nonprimordial experiencing of the situation of another within some form of interaction or relationship.

empty nest Home of parents whose children have grown up and moved out.

encopresis Soiling clothing with feces or depositing feces in inappropriate places.

endorphins Neurotransmitters that have opiate-like behavior and produce an inhibitory effect at opiate receptor sites; probably responsible for pain tolerance.

engagement Establishing a treatment relationship and enhancing motivation to make behavior changes and a commitment to treatment.

enuresis Involuntary excretion of urine after the age at which a child should have attained bladder control.

enzymes Any of numerous proteins produced in living cells that accelerate or catalyze the metabolic processes of an organism.

epidemiology The study of patterns of disease distribution in time and space that focuses on the health status of population groups or aggregates, rather than on individuals, and involves quantitative analysis of the occurrence of illnesses in population groups; basic science of public health.

episode A period of a minimal duration of 2 weeks during which an individual experiences symptoms that meet the diagnostic criteria for that disorder.

epithalamus Area above and medial to the thalamus and adjacent to the roof of the third ventricle.

equilibration Compensation for external disturbances; a mechanism for providing the self-regulation by which intelligence adapts to external and internal changes (Piaget).

erectile dysfunction Inability of a male to achieve or maintain an erection sufficient for completion of sexual activity.

erotomania Delusional belief that the person is loved intensely by the loved object, who is usually married and of a higher socioeconomic status, making him or her unattainable.

ethnic (ethnicity) People representing common traits, customs, thinking, and judgment.

ethnopsychopharmacology The study of cultural variations and differences that influence the effectiveness of pharmacotherapies used in mental health; includes genetics and psychosocial factors.

euphoric (mood) An elated mood.

euthymic (mood) A normal mood.

exception questions Questions used to help the patient identify times when whatever is bothering them is not present, or is present with less intensity, based on the underlying assumption that during these times the patient is usually doing something to make things better.

excretion Elimination of the products of metabolism from living organisms.

expansive (mood) A mood characterized by inappropriate lack of restraint in expressing one's feelings and frequently overvaluing one's own importance. Expansive qualities include an unceasing and indiscriminate enthusiasm for interpersonal, sexual, or occupational interactions.

exposure therapy The treatment of choice for agoraphobia that puts the patient into contact with the feared situations until the stimuli no longer produce anxiety.

expressed emotion Family members' responses that include one or more of the following dynamics: critical comments, hostility, or emotional over-involvement.

extended family Several nuclear families who may or may not live together and function as one group.

external advocacy system Organizations that operate outside mental health agencies and serve as advocates for the treatment and rights of mental health patients.

externalizing disorders Disorders that are characterized by acting-out behavior.

extinction Elimination of a classically conditioned response by the repeated presentation of the conditioned stimulus without the unconditioned stimulus, or elimination of an operantly conditioned response by no longer presenting the reward after the response.

extrapyramidal motor system Collection of neuronal pathways that provides significant input in involuntary motor movements.

extrapyramidal side effects See extrapyramidal syndromes.

extrapyramidal syndromes (EPS) Acute abnormal movements developing early in the course of treatment with antipsychotic agents.

factitious disorder A type of psychiatric disorder characterized by somatization, in which the person intentionally causes an illness for the purpose of becoming a patient.

factitious disorder by proxy (Münchausen syndrome by proxy) The intentional production or feigning of physical or psychological signs or symptoms in another person who is under the individual's care for the purpose of indirectly assuming the sick role.

family development A broad term that refers to all the processes connected with the growth of a family, including changes associated with work, geographic location, migration, acculturation, and serious illness.

family dynamics The patterned interpersonal and social interactions that occur within the family structure over the life of a family.

family life cycle A process of expansion, contraction, and realignment of relationship systems to support the entry, exit, and development of family members.

family preservation Efforts made by professionals to preserve the family unit by preventing the removal of children from their homes through parental support and education and through work to facilitate a secure attachment between the child and parent.

family projection process The family projects its conflicts onto the child or spouse, and this member becomes the center of family conflicts.

family structure According to Minuchin, the organized pattern within which family members interact.

fear conditioning A type of classic conditioning in which a previously neutral stimulus (conditioned stimulus) elicits a fear response (conditioned response) after it has been paired with an aversive stimulus (unconditioned stimulus) that produces fear (unconditioned response).

fetal alcohol syndrome A syndrome that occurs in infants whose mothers ingested alcohol during pregnancy; includes symptoms such as permanent brain damage, often resulting in mental retardation.

fidelity Faithfulness to obligations and duties.

first-pass effect Metabolism of part of oral drugs after being absorbed from the gastrointestinal tract and carried through the portal circulation to the liver. Only part of the drug dose reaches systemic circulation.

fissures The grooves of the cerebrum.

fitness to stand trial Ability to consult with a lawyer with a reasonable degree of rational understanding of the facts of the alleged crime and of the legal proceedings.

flight of ideas Repeated and rapid changes in the topic of conversation, generally with just one sentence or phrase.

flooding A type of therapy for agoraphobia in which highly anxiety-provoking stimuli are presented to the patient in vivo or with imagery, with no relaxation until the anxiety dissipates.

forensic examiner A mental health specialist, usually a psychiatrist or psychologist, who is certified as a forensic examiner and assigned by the judge to assess and testify to the patient's competency and responsibility for the crime, including the mental state at the time of an offense.

formal group roles The designated leader and members of a group.

formal operations The ability to use abstract reasoning to conceptualize and solve problems.

formal support system Large organizations that provide care to individuals, such as hospitals and nursing homes.

frontal, occipital, parietal, temporal lobes Lobes of the brain located on the lateral surface of each hemisphere.

functional activities Activities of daily living necessary for self-care (i.e., bathing, toileting, dressing, and transferring).

functional consequences The results of the interaction between A (activating event) and B (belief system) that follow from flexible, rational beliefs.

functional status Extent to which a person has the ability to carry out independent personal care, home management, and social functions in everyday life that has meaning and purpose.

GABA Gamma-aminobutyric acid, the primary inhibitory neurotransmitter for the CNS. The pathways of GABA exist almost exclusively in the CNS, with the largest GABA concentrations in the hypothalamus, hippocampus, basal ganglia, spinal cord, and cerebellum.

gate-control model Pain response based on the theory that pain perception involves pathways in the dorsal horn of the spinal column that relay noxious stimuli to the brain and that certain other nerve fibers function as an antagonistic "gate" to augment or dampen the subjective experience of pain.

gender identity A sense of self as being male or female.

gender role How one functions and behaves as a male or a female in relation to others in society, also referred to as *sex role identity.*

generic caring A phrase coined by Leininger to mean the foundational prototype included in local home remedies and folklore.

genogram A multigenerational schematic diagram that lists family members and their relationships.

genome A complete set of chromosomes derived from one parent.

genotype Genetic make-up of the individual with reference to a specific trait or traits.

gentrification The refurbishing of homes and buildings in rundown neighborhoods and the subsequent raising of rents.

gerotranscendence A concept of Erikson; continued growth in dimensions such as spirituality and inner strength.

glia (white matter) A fatty or lipid substance with a white appearance that surrounds the pathways of the cell body axons.

global risk factors Risk factors such as poverty, prejudice, and inadequate living situations that are associated with the risk for a mental disorder.

glutamate The most widely distributed excitatory neurotransmitter; the main transmitter in the associational areas of the cortex.

gray matter The cortex, with its gray-brown color because of the capillary blood vessels.

group Two or more people who are in an interdependent relationship with one another.
group cohesion Forces that act on the members to stay in a group.
group dynamics Interactions within groups.
group process The culmination of the session-to-session interactions of the members that move the group toward its goals.
groupthink The tendency of many groups to avoid conflict and adopt a normative pattern of thinking that is often consistent with the group leader's ideas.
guided imagery The purposeful use of imagination to achieve relaxation or direct attention away from undesirable sensations.
Guilty But Mentally Ill (GBMI) Persons with a mental illness who demonstrate they knew the wrongfulness of their actions and had the ability to act otherwise.
gyri Bumps and convolutions in the brain.
half-life The time required for plasma concentrations of a drug to be reduced by 50%.
hallucinations Perceptual experiences that occur in the absence of actual external sensory stimuli and may be auditory, visual, tactile, gustatory, or olfactory.
hallucinogen A class of drug that produces euphoria or dysphoria, altered body image, distorted or sharpened visual and auditory perception, confusion, uncoordination, and impaired judgment and memory.
harm reduction A community health intervention designed to reduce the harm of substance use to the individual, the family, and society that has replaced a moral or criminal approach to drug use and addiction.
hippocampus Subcortical gray matter embedded within each temporal lobe that may be involved in determining the best way to store information or memory; "time-dating" memory.
histamine A Neurotransmitter that originates predominantly in the hypothalamus and projects to all major structures in the cerebrum, brain stem, and spinal cord. Its functions are not well known.
HIV-1–associated cognitive-motor complex Neurologic complications that occur with HIV-1 that are directly attributable to infection of the brain and include impaired cognitive and motor function.
homeless A description of a person who lives for a sustained period of time on the street, in a public shelter, or in other temporary living quarters.
homelessness State of being without a consistent dwelling place.
home visits Delivery of nursing care in a patient's living environment.
homeostasis A balanced state achieved by the physiologic and psychological mechanism's response to the environment.
Housing First A mental health approach that places people who are homeless, usually also experiencing severe mental illness, substance abuse, or release from prison, into affordable housing.
hyperactivity Excessive motor activity, movement, and/or utterances that may be either purposeless or aimless.
hyperalgia Increased nociceptor sensitivity.
hyperaesthesia Increased sensation of pain.
hyperkinetic delirium A type of delirium in which the patient demonstrates behaviors most commonly recognized as delirium, including psychomotor hyperactivity, marked excitability, and a tendency toward hallucinations.
hypersexuality Inappropriate and socially unacceptable sexual behavior. The patient begins talking and behaving in ways that are uncharacteristic of the patient's behavior.
hypersomnia Oversleeping.
hypervigilance Sustained attention to external stimuli as if expecting something important or frightening to happen.
hypervocalization Screams, curses, moans, groans, and verbal repetitiveness that are common in the later stages of cognitively impaired elders, often occurring during a hospitalization or nursing home placement.
hypnagogic hallucinations Intense dream-like images that occur when an individual is falling asleep and usually involve the immediate environment.
hypofrontality Reduced cerebral blood flow and glucose metabolism in the prefrontal cortex.
hypokinetic delirium A type of delirium in which the patient is lethargic, somnolent, and apathetic and exhibits reduced psychomotor activity.
hypomanic episode Mildly dysphoric mood that meets the same criteria as for a manic episode except that it lasts at least 4 days rather than 1 week and that no marked impairment in social or occupational functioning is present.
hyponatremia Decreased sodium concentration in the blood.
hyposthenuria Secretion of urine with a low specific gravity.
hypothalamus Immediately ventral and slightly anterior to the thalamus, forming the floor and part of the walls of the third ventricle.
hypothalamic–pituitary–adrenal (HPA) axis Neurotransmitters responsible for behavioral responses to fear and anxiety that are usually held in balance until information from the sensory processing areas in the thalamus and cortex alerts the amygdala. If events are interpreted as threatening, this axis is activated, initiating the stress response.
identity An integration of a person's social and occupational roles and affiliations, self-attributed personality traits, attitudes about gender roles, beliefs about sexu-

ality and intimacy, long-term goals, political ideology, and religious beliefs.

identity diffusion Occurs when parts of a person's identity are absent or poorly developed; a lack of consistent sense of identity.

illusions Disorganized perceptions that create an oversensitivity to colors, shapes, and background activities, which occur when the person misperceives or exaggerates stimuli in the external environment.

impaired consciousness Less environmental awareness and loss of the ability to focus, sustain, and shift attention. Associated cognitive changes include problems in memory, orientation, and language.

implosive therapy An imaginal technique useful in treating agoraphobia in which the therapist identifies individual phobic stimuli for the patient and then presents highly anxiety-provoking imagery in a dramatic fashion.

impulsiveness A sudden, irresistible urge or desire resulting from a particular feeling that can lead to an action.

impulsivity Acting without considering the consequences of the act or alternative actions.

incidence A rate that includes only new cases that have occurred within a clearly defined time period.

incompetent A person is legally determined not to be able to understand and appreciate the information given during the consent process.

indirect leader Leader who primarily reflects the group members' discussion and offers little guidance or information to the group.

individual roles Group roles that either enhance or detract from the group's functioning but have nothing to do with either the group task or maintenance.

individual treatment plan A plan of care that identifies the patient's problems, outcomes, interventions, the individuals assigned to implement interventions, and evaluation criteria.

inducer Drugs or substances that stimulate liver cells to produce larger amounts of enzymes that results in acceleration of the metabolism of another drug or substance.

informal caregivers Unpaid individuals who provide care.

informal group roles Positions in the group with rights and duties directed toward other group members. These positions are not formally sanctioned.

informal support systems Family members, friends, and neighbors who can provide care and support to the individual.

informed consent The right to determine what shall be done with one's own body and mind. To provide informed consent, the patient must be given adequate information on which to base decisions about care. The patient ultimately decides the course of treatment.

inhalants Organic solvents, also known as volatile substances, that are central nervous system depressants and when inhaled cause euphoria, sedation, emotional lability, and impaired judgment.

inhibited grieving a pattern of repetitive, significant trauma and loss, together with an inability to fully experience and personally integrate or resolve these events.

inhibitor Drugs or substances that delay or decrease the activity of the metabolism enzymes that results in a decrease in the rate of another drug or substance.

in-home mental health care The provision of skilled mental health nursing care under the direction of a psychiatrist or physician for individuals in their residences.

initial outcomes Those outcomes written after the patient interview and assessment.

insight The ability of the individual to be aware of his or her own thoughts and feelings and to compare them with the thoughts and feelings of others.

insomnia (initial) Difficulty falling asleep.

instrumental activities Activities that facilitate or enhance the performance of activities of daily living (e.g., shopping, using the telephone, transportation). These aspects are critical to consider for any older adult living alone.

integrated treatment Treatment for both mental illness and substance use disorders is combined in a single session or interaction or series of interactions.

intensive case management An approach targeted for adults with serious mental illnesses or children with serious emotional disturbances. Managers of such cases have fewer caseloads and higher levels of professional training than do traditional case managers.

intensive residential services Intensively staffed residential care and mental health that may include medical, nursing, psychosocial, vocational, recreational, or other support services.

intensive outpatient program Program focused on continued stabilization and prevention of relapse in vulnerable individuals who have returned to job or school, usually with sessions running 3 days per week and lasting 3 to 4 hours per day.

interdisciplinary approach Interventions from different disciplines integrated into the delivery of patient care.

interdisciplinary treatment plan A plan of care that identifies the patient's problems, outcomes, interventions, and members of different disciplines assigned to implement interventions, and evaluation criteria.

intergenerational transmission Social learning theory concept that explains the process of violence being transmitted from one generation to the next. Men who witness violence in their homes often perpetuate violent behavior in their families as adults.

internal rights protection system Patient protective mechanisms developed by the United States mental health care system's organizations to help combat any violation of mental health patients' rights, including investigating any incidents of abuse or neglect.

internalizing disorders Anxiety disorders and depression in which the symptoms tend to be within the individual.

interoceptive conditioning Pairing a somatic discomfort, such as dizziness or palpitations, with an impending panic attack.

interpersonal relations Characteristic interaction patterns that occur between human beings that are the basis of emotional and social connections.

intrinsic activity The ability of a drug to produce a biologic response when it becomes attached to its receptor.

introspective The self-examination of personal beliefs, attitudes, and motivations.

invalidating environment A highly personal social situation that negates the individual's emotional responses and communication.

involuntary commitment The confined hospitalization of a person without his or her consent, but with a court order (because the person has been judged to be a danger to self or others).

ischemic cascade Cell breakdown resulting from brain cell injury.

judgment The ability to reach a logical decision about a situation and to choose a course after looking at and analyzing various possibilities.

justice Duty to treat all fairly, distributing the risks and benefits equally.

kindling Repetitive stimulation of certain tracts may facilitate conduction of impulses in the future and lead to enhancement of intense behaviors after even mild stimulation.

kleptomania A disorder in which the patient is unable to resist the urge to steal and independently steals items that he or she could easily afford. These items are not particularly useful or wanted. The underlying issue is the act of stealing.

Korsakoff's psychosis An amnestic syndrome in which there is a profound deficit in the ability to form new memories; associated with a variable deficit in recall of old memories despite a clear sensorium.

labile (lability of mood) Rapid alternations of mood, usually between euphoria and irritability.

larks A term referring to people who are more alert and perform best in the early morning.

lateral (sylvian) fissure Separates the inferior aspects of the frontal and parietal lobes from the temporal lobe.

lateral ventricles The horn-shaped first and second ventricles that are the largest of the brain's ventricles.

learning disorder A discrepancy between actual achievement and expected achievement that is based on a person's age and intellectual ability.

least restrictive environment The patient has the right to treatment in an environment that restricts the exercise of free will to the least extent; an individual cannot be restricted to an institution when he or she can be successfully treated in the community.

life events Major times or events such as marriage, divorce, and bereavement.

life review A therapeutic intervention using recall and memory to conduct a critical analysis of one's life.

limbic system (limbic lobe) Structures including the septum and the fornix, as well as the amygdala, hippocampus, cingulate, parahippocampal gyrus, epithalamus, portions of the basal ganglia, paraolfactory area, and the anterior nucleus of the thalamus.

locus ceruleus A tiny cluster of neurons that fans out and innervates almost every part of the brain, including most of the cortex, the thalamus and hypothalamus, cerebellum, and the spinal cord.

longitudinal fissure The longest and deepest groove of the cerebrum that separates the right and left hemispheres.

loose associations Absence of the normal connectedness of thoughts and ideas; sudden shifts without apparent relationship to preceding topic.

luminotherapy Light therapy used to manipulate the circadian system.

maintenance function A term used to describe the informal role of group members that encourages the group to stay together.

malingering To produce illness symptoms intentionally with an obvious self-serving goal such as being classified as disabled or avoiding work.

managed care organizations Large health care organizations whose goals are to increase access to care and to provide the most appropriate level of services in the least restrictive setting, which includes more outpatient and alternative treatment programs, while trying to avoid costly inpatient hospitalizations; in the long term, allowing patients better access to quality services while using health care dollars wisely.

manic episode A distinct period during which there is an abnormally and persistently elevated, expansive, or irritable mood.

marginalization Relegation to a lower social standing or to the outskirts of society.

maturation Healthy development of the brain and nervous system during childhood and adolescence.

maturational crisis Developmental crisis.

medical battery Intentional and unauthorized (without informed consent) treatment that is harmful or offensive.

memory One aspect of cognitive function; an information storage system composed of short-term memory (retention of information over a brief period of time) and long-term memory (retention of an unlimited amount of information over an indefinite period of time); the ability to recall or reproduce what has been learned or experienced.

meningeal layer The inner layer of dura mater that becomes continuous with the spinal dura mater and sends extensions into the brain for support and protection of the different lobes or structures.

mental disorder A disorder that is associated with the presence of psychological distress; impairment in psychological, social, or occupational functioning; or a significantly increased risk for death, pain, disability, or an important loss of freedom.

mental health problem A term used when signs and symptoms of mental illnesses occur but do not meet specified criteria for a disorder.

mental illness A term used to mean all diagnosable mental disorders.

mental retardation Significantly below-average intelligence accompanied by impaired adaptive functioning.

mental status examination An organized systematic approach to assessment of an individual's current psychiatric condition.

mesocortical Medial aspects of the cortex.

metabolism Biotransformation, or the process by which a drug is altered.

metabolites Substance necessary for or taking part in a particular metabolic process.

methadone maintenance The treatment of opiate addiction with a daily, stabilized dose of methadone.

metonymic speech Use of words with similar meanings interchangeably.

middle insomnia Waking up during the night and having difficulty returning to sleep.

middle-old A term used to describe adults ages 75–84 years.

mild cognitive impairment (MCI) A transitional state between normal cognition and AD.

milieu therapy An approach using the total environment to provide a therapeutic community; a therapeutic environment.

miracle questions Patients are asked to use their imagination in crafting their response to very specific questions.

misidentification Delusions in which the person believes that a familiar person is replaced by an imposter.

mixed episode Irritability or excitement and depression occurring at the same time.

mixed variant delirium Behavior that fluctuates between the hyperactive and hypoactive states.

modeling Pervasive imitation; one person trying to be like another person.

mood A pervasive and sustained emotion that colors a person's perception of the world.

mood disorder A clinically significant behavioral or psychological syndrome or pattern that occurs in an individual whereby the primary alteration is evident in mood rather than in thought or perception.

moral treatment An approach to curing mental illness, popular in the 1800s, which was built on the principles of kindness, compassion, and a pleasant environment.

motivational interventions One to several sessions delivered within a few weeks or less where the patient is motivated to become involved in treatment.

motivational interviewing Interviewing that helps the patient clarify personal goals and increases commitment to recovery; often used in treating people with substance abuse.

multiaxial diagnostic system A diagnostic structure that includes more than one domain of information, such as the psychiatric diagnoses of the *DSM-IV-TR.*

multidisciplinary approach Several disciplines providing services to a patient at one time.

multigenerational transmission process The transmission of emotional processes from one generation to the next.

multiple sleep latency test (MSLT) A standardized procedure that measures the amount of time a person takes to fall asleep during a 20-minute period.

music therapy The controlled use of music to promote physiologic or psychological well-being.

myoclonus Twitching or clonic spasms of a muscle group.

myoglobinuria The presence of myohemoglobin in the urine due to sustained muscular rigidity and necrosis.

neglect Failure to protect from injury or to provide for the physical, psychological, and medical needs of a child or dependent elder.

negligence A breach of duty of reasonable care for a patient for whom the nurse is responsible that results in personal injuries. A clinician who does get consent, but does not disclose the nature of the procedure and the risks involved, is subject to a negligence claim.

neologisms Words that are made up that have no common meaning and are not recognized.

neurofibrillary tangles Fibrous proteins, or *tau proteins,* that are chemically altered and twisted together and spread throughout the brain, interfering with nerve functioning in cholinergic neurons. It is hypothesized that formation of these neurofibrillary tangles are related to the apolipoprotein E_4 (apoE_4).

neurohormones Hormones produced by cells within the nervous system, such as antidiuretic hormone (ADH).

neuroleptic malignant syndrome A syndrome caused by neuroleptic medications that are dopamine receptor blockers. The classic signs and symptoms include hyperthermia, lead-pipe rigidity, changes in mental status, and autonomic nervous system changes.

neuromodulators Chemical messengers that make the target cell membrane or postsynaptic membrane more or less susceptible to the effects of the primary neurotransmitter.

neuron Nerve cells responsible for receiving, organizing, and transmitting information. Each neuron has a cell body, or soma, which holds the nucleus containing most of the cell's genetic information.

neuropeptide Y A recently discovered 36-amino-acid peptide that is a potent stimulator of feeding behavior especially selective for foods heavy in carbohydrates.

neuropeptides Short chains of amino acids that exist in the central nervous system and have a number of important roles, including as neurotransmitters, neuromodulators, or neurohormones.

neurotransmitters Small molecules that directly and indirectly control the opening or closing of ion channels.

NIC taxonomy Standardized classification of interventions that nurses perform.

night terrors Childhood disorder in which a child awakes screaming with fright.

nociception Pain perception.

nociceptive Pertaining to a neural receptor for painful stimuli.

nonbizarre delusions Beliefs that are characterized by adherence to possible situations that could appear in real life and are plausible in the context of the person's ethnic and cultural background.

nonmaleficence The duty to cause no harm, both individually and for all.

non-REM (NREM) sleep A sleep cycle state of non-rapid eye movement.

nontherapeutic relationships A nontrusting relationship between the nurse and patient. Both feel very frustrated and keep varying their approach with each other in an attempt to establish a meaningful relationship.

nonverbal communication The gestures, expressions, and body language used in communications between the nurse and the patient.

norepinephrine An excitatory neurochemical that plays a major role in generating and maintaining mood states. Heavily concentrated in the terminal sites of sympathetic nerves, it can be released quickly to ready the individual for a fight-or-flight response to threats in the environment.

normalization Teaching families what are normal behaviors and expected responses.

no-suicide contract Written or verbal agreement between the health care professional and the patient that the patient will not engage in suicidal behavior for a specific period of time.

Not Guilty by Reason of Insanity (NGRI) Persons who demonstrate they had no understanding of their actions and no control over them when they committed the crime.

nuclear family Two or more people related by blood, marriage, or adoption.

nuclear family emotional process Patterns of emotional functioning in a family within single generations.

nurse–patient relationship A time-limited interpersonal process with definable phases during which the patient is able to consider alternative behaviors, try new health care strategies, and discuss complex health problems.

nursing diagnosis A clinical judgment about the individual, family, or community response to actual or potential health problems and life processes. It provides the basis for the selection of interventions and outcomes.

nursing intervention Nursing activities that promote and foster health, assess dysfunction, assist patients to regain or improve their coping abilities, or prevent further disabilities.

negative symptoms A lessening or loss of normal functions, such as restriction or flattening in the range of intensity of emotion; reduced fluency and productivity of thought and speech; withdrawal and inability to initiate and persist in goal-directed activity; and inability to experience pleasure.

nursing process The basis of clinical decision making and nursing actions.

object permanence The awareness that an object or person exists when not physically seen; behavior that results in a person attaining or retaining proximity to some other differentiated and preferred individual.

object relations The psychological attachment to another person or object.

observation Ongoing assessment of the patient's mental and health status to identify and subvert any potential problems.

obsessive-compulsive disorder (OCD) A disorder characterized by intrusive thoughts that are difficult to dislodge (obsessions) and ritualized behaviors that the person feels driven to perform (compulsions).

oculogyric crisis A medication side effect resulting from an imbalance of dopamine and acetylcholine, in which the muscles that control eye movements tense and pull the eyeball so that the patient is looking toward the ceiling; may be followed by torticollis or retrocollis.

off-label Use of medication for a condition that is not approved by the FDA.

old-old A term used to describe adults ages 85 years and older.

oligomers Fragments of beta-amyloid peptides (ADDLs) that clump together.

ongoing assessments Shorter and more focused assessments made to monitor the progress and outcomes of the interventions implemented.

open communication Willingness to share personal information about relevant topics.

open group A group in which new members can join at any time.

operant behavior A type of learning that is a consequence of a particular behavioral response, not a specific stimulus.

opiate Any substance that binds to an opiate receptor in the brain to produce an agonist action.

orientation phase The first phase of the nurse–patient relationship in which the nurse and the patient get to know each other. During this phase, the patient develops a sense of trust.

outcome indicators Representation or description of patient status, behaviors, or perceptions evaluated during a patient's assessment.

outcomes A patient's response to care received; the end result of the process of nursing.

outpatient detoxification A specialized form of partial hospitalization for patients requiring medical supervision during withdrawal from alcohol or other addictive substances, with or without use of a 23-hour bed during the initial withdrawal phase, including a requirement of attending a program 5 or 6 days per week for a period of 1 to 2 weeks.

owls A term used to describe people who are more alert and perform better during the late evening hours.

Oxford House A self-help, communal-living setting created to foster recovery in persons who abuse alcohol and substances.

oxidative stress A condition of increased oxidant production in cells characterized by the release of free radicals and resulting in cellular degeneration.

package insert The approved FDA product labeling that includes approved indications for the medication, side effects, adverse effects, contraindications, and other important information.

panic A normal but extreme overwhelming form of anxiety often experienced when an individual is placed in a real or perceived life-threatening situation.

panic attacks Discrete periods of intense fear or discomfort that are accompanied by significant somatic or cognitive symptoms.

panic control treatment Systematic structured exposure to panic-invoking sensations such as dizziness, hyperventilation, tightness in chest, and sweating.

panicogenic Substances that produce panic attacks.

paranoia Suspiciousness and guardedness that is unrealistic and often accompanied by grandiosity.

paranoid schizophrenia One of the types of schizophrenia characterized by prominent delusions or auditory hallucinations; cognitive functioning is relatively uninvolved; delusions are usually persecutory.

parasomnia Disorders of abnormal physiologic or behavioral events that occur in relationship to sleep, specific sleep stages, or during transition from sleep to wakefulness.

parasuicide or parasuicidal behavior Deliberate self-injury with an intent to harm oneself.

parietal-occipital sulcus Separates the occipital lobe from the parietal lobe.

partial agonist A drug that has the ability to block a receptor if it is overstimulated and to stimulate a receptor if it is understimulated.

partial hospitalization A type of outpatient program that provides services to patients who spend only part of a 24-hour period in the facility but that does not provide overnight care; usually, the programs run 5 days per week for about 6 hours per day.

passive listening A nontherapeutic mode of interaction that involves sitting quietly and allowing the patient to talk without focusing on guiding the thought process; includes body language that communicates boredom, indifference, or hostility.

paternalism The belief that knowledge and education authorizes professionals to make decisions for the good of the patient.

peak marriage age An age when the person is most likely to have a successful marriage.

peer assistance programs Programs developed by state nurses' associations to assist nurses in securing evaluation, treatment, monitoring, and ongoing support.

perceptions The awareness reached as a result of sensory inputs of real stimuli that are usually altered.

persecutory delusions Delusions in which the person believes that he or she is being conspired against, cheated, spied on, followed, poisoned, drugged, maliciously maligned, harassed, or obstructed in the pursuit of long-term goals.

personal identity Knowing "who I am" formed through the numerous biologic, psychological, and social challenges and demands faced throughout the stages of life.

personality A complex pattern of psychological characteristics, largely outside a person's awareness, that are not easily altered.

personality disorder An enduring pattern of inner experience and behavior that deviates markedly from the expectations of the individual's culture; is pervasive and inflexible; has an onset in adolescence or early adulthood; is stable over time; and leads to distress or impairment.

person–environment relationship The interaction between the individual and the environment that changes throughout the stress experience.

pet therapy The therapeutic use of animals as pets to promote physical, psychological, or social well-being.

pharmacodynamics The study of the biologic actions of drugs on living tissue and the human body in general.

pharmacogenomics Blends pharmacology with genetic knowledge; understanding and determining an individual's specific CYP450 makeup, then individualizing medications to match the person's CYP450 profile.

pharmacokinetics The study of how the human body processes a drug, including absorption, distribution, metabolism, and elimination.

phenomena of concern Human responses to actual or potential health problems.

phenotype Observable characteristics or expressions of a specific trait.

phobia Persistent, unrealistic fears of situations, objects, or activities that often lead to avoidance behaviors.

phonologic processing Thought to be the cause of reading disability; a process that involves the discrimination and interpretation of speech sounds. Reading disability is believed to be caused by some disturbance in the development of the left hemisphere.

phototherapy Also known as *light therapy;* involves exposing the patient to an artificial light source during winter months to relieve seasonal depression.

physical abuse Using physical force or a weapon against a person to do bodily injury.

physical restraints The application of wrist, leg, and body straps made of leather or cloth for the purpose of controlling or managing behavior.

pia mater The third layer of the central nervous system; in Latin, "soft mother."

pineal body Located in the epithalamus; contains secretory cells that emit the neurohormone melatonin (as well as other substances), which has been associated with sleep and emotional disorders and modulation of immune function.

plasticity Capability to change or adapt in form or physiology.

point prevalence Basic measure that refers to the proportion of individuals in a population who have a particular disorder at a specified point in time.

polydipsia Excessive thirst that can be chronic in patients with severe mental illness.

polypharmacy Use of several different medications at one time.

polysomnography A special procedure that involves the recording of the electroencephalogram throughout the night. This procedure is usually conducted in a sleep laboratory.

polyuria Excessive excretion of urine.

population genetics The study of inheritance.

positive self-talk Countering fearful or negative thoughts by using preplanned and rehearsed positive coping statements.

positive symptoms An excess or distortion of normal functions, including delusions and hallucinations.

posttraumatic stress disorder A mental disorder characterized by persistent, distressing symptoms lasting longer than 1 month after exposure to an extreme traumatic stressor.

potency The dose of drug required to produce a specific effect.

prejudice A hostile attitude toward others who belong to a particular group that is considered by some to have objectionable characteristics.

pressured speech Speech that is rapid and difficult to interrupt; the amount of speech produced is greater than that considered normal.

prevalence The total number of people who have a particular disorder within a given population at a specific time.

prevention Interventions used before the initial onset of a disorder that become distinct from the treatment.

priapism A rare condition of prolonged and painful erection, usually without sexual desire; often the result of neurologic or vascular impairment.

privacy That part of an individual's personal life that is not governed by society's laws and governmental intrusion.

probation A sentence of conditional or revocable release under the supervision of a probation officer for a specified time.

problem-focused coping A type of coping that actually changes the person–environment relationship.

process recording A verbatim transcript of a verbal interaction usually organized according to the nurse–patient interaction. It often includes analysis of the interaction.

prodromal An early symptom indicating the development of a disease or syndrome.

professional caring Cognitively learned, practiced, and transmitted knowledge learned formally and informally through various schools of professional nursing education (Leininger).

projective identification A psychoanalytic term used to describe behavior of people with borderline personality disorder when they falsely attribute to others their own unacceptable feelings, impulses, or thoughts.

prostaglandins One of the most common nociceptive transmitters.

protective factors Characteristics that reduce the probability that a person will develop a mental health disorder or problem or decrease the severity of existing problems.

protein binding Drugs from a compound with plasma proteins (mainly albumin) that act as carriers. Drugs are inactive when bound to protein.

pseudodementia Memory difficulties in older adults with major depression (may be mistaken for early signs of dementia).

pseudologia fantastica Stories that are not entirely improbable and often contain a matrix of truth and falsehood.

pseudoparkinsonism Sometimes referred to as *drug-induced parkinsonism;* presents identically as Parkinson's disease without the same destruction of dopaminergic cells.

psychiatric pluralism An integration of human biologic functions with the environment that was advocated by Meyer.

psychiatric rehabilitation programs Programs that are focused on reintegrating people with psychiatric disabilities back into the community through work, educational, and social avenues while also addressing their medical and residential needs.

psychoanalytic movement Freud's radical approach to psychiatric mental health care, which involved using a new technique called *psychoanalysis* based on unconscious motivations for behavior or drives.

psychodrama A group role-playing technique used to encourage expression of emotion and exploration of problems.

psychoeducation An educational approach used to enhance knowledge and shape behavior.

psychoeducational programs A form of mental health intervention in which basic coping skills for dealing with various stressors are taught.

psychoneuroimmunology The study of relationships among the immune system, nervous system, and endocrine system and our behaviors, thoughts, and feelings.

psychopath A term often used by the general public to refer to persons with an antisocial personality disorder.

psychopathy Refers to individuals who behave impulsively and are interpersonally irresponsible, act hastily and spontaneously, are shortsighted, and fail to plan ahead or consider alternatives; equated with antisocial personality disorder.

psychopharmacology Subspecialty of pharmacology that includes medications used to affect the brain and behaviors related to psychiatric disorders.

psychosis A state in which the individual is experiencing hallucinations, delusions, or disorganized thoughts, speech, or behavior.

psychosocial domain Part of the biopsychosocial model that explains the importance of the internal psychological processes of thoughts, feelings, and behavior (interpersonal dynamics) in influencing one's emotion, cognition, and behavior.

psychosocial theory A theoretic argument or view from the early 1900s that mental disorders result from environmental and social deprivation.

psychosomatic Conditions in which a psychological state contributes to the development of a physical illness.

purging A compensatory behavior to rid oneself of food already eaten by means of self-induced vomiting or the use of laxatives, enemas, or diuretics.

pyromania Irresistible impulses to start fires.

quadrants of care A conceptual framework that classifies patients according to symptom severity, not diagnosis.

rapid cycling In bipolar disorder, the occurrence of four or more mood episodes that meet criteria for manic, mixed, hypomanic, or depressive episode during the previous 12 months.

rapport A series of interrelated thoughts and feelings that describe purposeful interactions between individuals; including empathy, compassion, sympathy, a nonjudgmental attitude, and respect for others.

rate A proportion of the cases in the population when compared to the total population. It is expressed as a fraction in which the numerator is the number of cases, and the denominator is the total number in the population, including the cases and noncases.

reaction time The lapse of time between stimulus and response.

reappraisal Appraisal after coping based on feedback about the outcomes.

receptor Site to which a neurotransmitter substance can specifically adhere to produce a change in the cell membrane, serving a physiologic regulatory function.

recovery A period of full remission for a minimum of 8 weeks.

referential thinking Belief that neutral stimuli have special meaning to the individual, such as a television commentator speaking directly to the individual.

referral Act of recommending another provider or service.

reflection Continual self-evaluation through observing, monitoring, and judging nursing behaviors with the goal of providing ideal interventions.

regressed behavior Behaving in a manner of a less mature life stage; childlike and immature.

reintegration A term used to describe the process of returning to the community through work, educational, and social avenues.

relapse Recurrence or marked increase in severity of the symptoms of the disease, especially following a period of apparent improvement or stability; the recurrence of alcohol- or drug-dependent behavior in an individual who has previously achieved and maintained abstinence for a significant time beyond the period of detoxification.

relapse prevention An approach that focuses on preventing recurrence of symptoms.

related factors Those factors (biologic, maturational, social, and treatment-related) that influence a health status change.

relationship questions Questions used to amplify and reinforce positive responses to the other questions.

relaxation A mental health intervention that promotes comfort, reduces anxiety, alleviates stress, reduces pain, and prevents aggressive behavior.

relaxation training A variety of procedures to reduce somatic arousal, such as progressive muscle relaxation, autogenic training, and biofeedback.

religiosity A psychiatric symptom characterized by excessive or affected piety.

religiousness The participation in a community of people who gather around common ways of worshiping.

REM sleep A sleep cycle state of rapid eye movement.

reminiscence Thinking about or relating past experiences.

reminiscence therapy The process of looking back on specific times or events in one's life.

remission A restoration of baseline psychological functioning.

remotivation therapy The encouragement of interest and enthusiasm about events in one's life or the world.

residential services A place for people to reside during a 24-hour period or any portion of the day, on an ongoing basis.

residential treatment facility A facility that requires special accreditation and specialized licensing from the state that generally treats patients for 6 months or longer.

resilience Ability to recover readily from illness, depression, adversity, or the like.

resolution The last phase of the nurse–patient relationship in which the patient learns to manage the problems and the relationship is terminated.

resolution phase The termination phase of the nurse–patient relationship that lasts from the time the problems are resolved to the close of the relationship.

restraint The use of any manual, physical, or mechanical device or material, which when attached to the patient's body (usually to the arms and legs) restricts the patient's movements.

retrocollis The neck muscles pull the head back.

revised outcomes Those outcomes written after each evaluation.

reward-seeking behavior A behavior that is initiated to gain a pleasurable outcome, such as feeling good, being rewarded, or gaining recognition or attention.

risk factors Characteristics that do not cause the disorder or problem and are not symptoms of the illness, but rather are factors that have been shown to influence the likelihood of developing a disorder.

role An individual's social position and function within an environment.

ruminations Repetitive thoughts that are forced into a patient's consciousness even when unwanted; when a person goes over and over the same ideas endlessly; part of an obsessive style of thinking.

Safe Havens A form of supportive housing that serves hard-to-reach people with severe mental illness.

safety Care that supports protection against harm.

sandwich generation A generation of people who give care to their children and their parents at the same time.

satiety Internal signals that indicate one has had enough to eat.

scaling questions Questions that quantify exceptions noted in intensity, and in tracking change over time.

schema A cognitive structure that screens, codes, and evaluates the incoming stimuli through which the individual interprets events.

schizoaffective disorder An interrupted period of illness during which at some point there is a major depressive, manic, or mixed episode, along with two of the following symptoms of schizophrenia: delusions, hallucinations, disorganized speech, disorganized or catatonic behavior, or negative symptoms (affective flattening, alogia, or avolition).

school phobia Anxiety in which the child refuses to attend school in order to stay at home and with the primary attachment figure. School phobia is a common presenting complaint in child psychiatric clinics and may be part of separation anxiety, general anxiety, social phobia, obsessive-compulsive disorder, depression, or conduct disorder.

seclusion Solitary confinement in a full protective environment for the purpose of safety or behavior management.

section 8 housing Federally subsidized housing units that are supervised or operated by the state or city; tenants are responsible for paying one third of the monthly income toward rent.

sedative-hypnotics Medications that induce sleep and reduce anxiety.

segregation Separation of a cultural group from the majority through legally sanctioned societal practices.

selectivity The ability of a drug to be specific for a particular receptor, interacting only with specific receptors in the areas of the body where the receptors occur and therefore not affecting tissues and organs where these receptors do not occur.

self-awareness Being cognizant of one's own beliefs, thought motivations, biases, physical and emotional limitations, and the impact one may have on others.

self-concept The sum of beliefs about oneself, which develops over time.

self-determinism The right to choose one's own health-related behaviors, which at times differ from those recommended by health professionals.

self-disclosure The act of revealing personal information about oneself.

self-efficacy Self-effectiveness.

self-esteem Attitude about oneself.

self-identity Formed through the integration of social and occupational roles and affiliations, self-attributed personality traits, attitudes about gender roles, beliefs about sexuality and intimacy, long-term goals, political ideology, and religious beliefs. Without an adequately formed identity, goal-directed behavior is impaired and interpersonal relationships are disrupted.

self-medicate Using medication, usually over-the-counter or substances without professional prescription or supervision, to alleviate an illness or condition.

self-monitoring Observing and recording one's own information, usually behavior, thoughts, or feelings.

self-system An important concept in Peplau's model. Drawing from Sullivan, Peplau defined the self as an "anti-anxiety system" and a product of socialization.

separation-individuation A process during which the child develops a sense of self, a permanent sense of significant others (object constancy), and an integration of both bad and good as a component of the self-concept.

serotonin Centrally mediates the release of endorphin. Along with histamine and bradykinin, serotonin stimulates the pain receptors to generate experienced pain. Serotonin is involved in inhibiting gastric secretion, stimulating smooth muscle, and serving as a central neurotransmitter.

serotonin syndrome A toxic side effect that occurs as a result of the newer serotonergic drugs; this syndrome is thought to be caused by hyperstimulation of the 5-HT receptor in the brain stem and spinal cord.

severe and persistent mental illness Mental disorders that are long term and have recurring periods of exacerbation and remission.

sex role identity Outward expression of gender.

sexual abuse Sexual misconduct toward another person.

sexual desire Ability, interest, or willingness to receive, or a motivational state to seek, sexual stimulation.

sexual orientation (sexual preference) An individual's feelings of sexual attraction and erotic potential.

sexuality Basic dimension of every individual's personality, undergoing periods of growth and development, and influenced by biologic and psychosocial factors.

Shelter Plus Care Program A continuum of care program that allows for various housing choices and a range of supportive services funded by other sources.

sibling position The relative social status of the children in the family.

side effects Unwanted or untoward effects of medications.

simple relaxation techniques Interventions that encourage and elicit relaxation to decrease undesirable signs and symptoms.

situational crisis A crisis that occurs whenever a specific stressful event threatens a person's biopsychosocial integrity and results in some degree of psychological disequilibrium.

skills groups An integral part of DBT; skills are taught in group settings in which patients practice emotional regulation, interpersonal effectiveness, distress tolerance, core mindfulness, and self-management skills.

sleep architecture A predictable pattern during a night's sleep that includes the timing, amount, and distribution of REM and NREM stages.

sleep debt Interruption of basic restoration following recurrent long-term sleep deprivation.

sleep diary A written account of the sleep experience.

sleep disorders Ongoing disruptions of normal waking and sleeping patterns that lead to excessive daytime sleepiness, inappropriate naps, chronic fatigue, and the inability to perform safely or properly at work, school, or home.

sleep efficiency Expressed as a percentage of time in bed spent asleep.

sleep latency Amount of time it takes for an individual to fall asleep.

sleep paralysis Being unable to move or speak when falling asleep or waking.

sleep restriction Deliberately spending less time in bed and avoiding napping.

sleepiness The urge to fall asleep.

slow-wave sleep Deepest state of sleep.

social change The structural and cultural evolution of society, which is dependent on a complex interaction between economic and productivity factors as well as among political, religious, philosophical, and scientific ideas.

social distance Degree to which the values of a formal organization and its primary group members differ.

social domain Part of the biopsychosocial model that accounts for the influence of social forces encompassing family, community, and cultural settings.

social functioning Performance of daily activities within the context of interpersonal relations and family and community roles.

social network Linkages among a defined set of people, among whom there are personal contacts.

social skills training A psychoeducational approach that involves instruction, feedback, support, and practice with learning behaviors that helps people interact more effectively with peers, and also children with adults.

social support Positive and harmonious interpersonal interactions that occur within social relationships.

sociopath A term often used by the general public to refer to persons with an antisocial personality disorder.

solubility Ability of a drug to dissolve.

somatization The manifestation of psychological distress as physical symptoms.

somatization disorder A polysymptomatic disorder that begins before age 30 years, extends over a period of years, and is characterized by a combination of pain, gastrointestinal, sexual, and psychoneurologic symptoms.

somatoform disorders Chronic relapsing conditions characterized by multiple physical symptoms of unknown origin that develop during times of emotional distress and include somatization disorder, undifferentiated somatoform disorder, conversion disorder, pain disorder, hypochondriasis, and body dysmorphic disorder.

somnambulism Sleep walking.

speech The motor aspects of speaking.

spinal cord A long, cylindrical collection of neural fibers continuous with the brain stem, housed within the vertebral column.

spirituality Beliefs and values related to hope and meaning in life.

spiritual support Assisting patients to feel balance and connection within their relationships; involves listening to expressions of loneliness, using empathy, and providing patients with desired spiritual articles.

stabilization Short-term care, lasting 7 to 14 days, with a primary focus on control of precipitating symptoms with medications, behavioral interventions, and coordination with other agencies for appropriate aftercare.

stage-wise treatment Treatment that moves the patient towards recovery through commonly recognized stages of treatment: engagement, persuasion or motivation, active treatment, and relapse prevention.

standards of care Standards that are organized around the nursing process and include assessment, diagnosis, outcome identification, planning, and implementation.

standards Authoritative statements established by professional organizations that describe the responsibilities for which nurses are accountable but that are not legally binding unless they are incorporated into a legal document, such as a nurse practice act or state board rules and regulations.

steady state Absorption equals excretion and the therapeutic level plateaus.

stereotypic behavior Repetitive, driven, nonfunctional, and potentially self-injurious behavior, such as head banging, rocking, and hand flapping, seen in autistic disorder, with an extraordinary insistence on sameness.

stereotyping Expecting individuals to behave in a manner that conforms to a negative perception of the cultural group to which they belong.

stereotypy Repetitive, purposeless movements that are idiosyncratic to the individual and to some degree outside of the individual's control.

stigmatization A process of assigning negative characteristics and identity to a person or group and causing that person or group to feel unaccepted, devalued, ostracized, and isolated from the larger society.

stilted language Overly and inappropriately artificial formal language.

stimulus control A technique used when the bedroom environment no longer provides cues for sleep but has become the cue for wakefulness. Patients are instructed to avoid behaviors in the bedroom incompatible with sleep.

stranger anxiety Fear when approached by a person unknown to oneself.

stress (stressors) A pressure or force that puts strain on the system; can be either positive or negative but most often is used to mean a negative mental or physical tension or strain.

stress response Physiological, behavioral and cognitive reaction to an appraised threatening person–environment event.

structured interaction Purposeful interaction that allows patients to interact with others in a way that is useful to them.

subcortical dementia Dementia that is caused by dysfunction or deterioration of deep gray or white matter structures inside the brain and brain stem.

subcortical Structures inside the hemispheres and beneath the cortex.

substance P The most common nociceptive transmitter that is released and transported along the central and peripheral pain synapses in the presence of noxious stimuli.

substance-related disorders Disorders related to taking a drug of abuse, including alcohol, amphetamines, cannabis (marijuana), cocaine, hallucinogens, inhalants, nicotine, opioids, phencyclidine, sedatives-hypnotics, anxiolytics, caffeine, or other unknown substances.

substrate The drug or compound that is identified as a target of an enzyme.

subsystems A systems term used by family theorists to describe subgroups of family members who join together for various activities.

suicidal ideation Thinking about and planning one's own death without actually engaging in self-harm.

suicidality All suicide-related behaviors and thoughts of completing or attempting suicide and suicide ideation.

suicide The act of killing oneself voluntarily.

suicide attempt A nonfatal, self-inflicted destructive act with explicit or implicit intent to die.

suicide contagion One person commits suicide and several more follow.

supportive housing Permanently subsidized housing with attendant social services.

surveillance The ongoing collection and analysis of information about patients and their environments for use in promoting and maintaining patient safety.

symbolism The use of a word or a phrase to represent an object, event, or feeling.

synapse The region across which nerve impulses are transmitted through the action of a neurotransmitter.

synaptic cleft A junction between one nerve and another; the space where the electrical intracellular signal becomes a chemical extracellular signal.

synchronized Two or more circadian rhythms reaching their peak at the same time.

systematic desensitization A method used to desensitize patients to anxiety-provoking situations by exposing the patient to a hierarchy of feared situations. Patient is taught to use muscle relaxation as levels of anxiety increase through multisituational exposure.

tangentiality When the topic of conversation changes to an entirely different topic that is within a logical progression but causes a permanent detour from the original focus.

tardive dyskinesia A late-appearing extrapyramidal side effect of antipsychotic medication that includes abnormal involuntary movements of the mouth, tongue, and jaw such as lip smacking, sucking, puckering, tongue protrusion, the bon-bon sign, athetoid (worm-like) movements of the tongue, and chewing.

target risk factors Specific biopsychosocial stressors, such as genetic predisposition and traumatic situations, which are associated with mental disorders.

target symptoms Specific symptoms for which psychiatric medications are prescribed, such as hallucinations, delusions, paranoia, agitation, assaultive behavior, bizarre ideation, social withdrawal, disorientation, catatonia, blunted affect, thought blocking, insomnia, and anorexia.

task function The group role that focuses on the task of the group.

temperament A person's characteristic intensity, rhythmicity, adaptability, energy expenditure, and mood.

terminal insomnia Waking up too early and being unable to return to sleep.

thalamus Thought to play a role in controlling electrical activity in the cortex; provides the relay mechanism for information to and from the cerebrum.

themes Concerns or feelings expressed symbolically by the patient.

therapeutic communication The ongoing process of interaction in which meaning emerges; may be verbal or nonverbal.

therapeutic foster care The placement of patients in residences of families specially trained to handle individuals with mental illnesses.

therapeutic index A ratio of the maximum nontoxic dose to the minimum effective dose.

thought stopping A practice in which a person identifies negative feelings and thoughts that exist together, says "stop," and then engages in a distracting activity.

thymoleptic Mood stabilizing.

token economy The application of behavior modification techniques to multiple behaviors. In a token economy, patients are rewarded with tokens for selected desired behaviors.

tolerance A gradual decrease in the action of a drug at a given dose or concentration in the blood.

torticollis The neck muscles pull the head to the side.

toxicity The point at which concentrations of a drug in the bloodstream become harmful or poisonous to the body.

transaction Transfer of value between two or more individuals.

transcranial magnetic stimulation Noninvasive, painless method to stimulate the cerebral cortex, which activates inhibitory and excitatory neurons.

transfer The formal shifting of responsibility for the care of an individual from one clinician to another or from one care unit to another.

transference The unconscious assignment to others of feelings and attitudes that were originally associated with important figures such as parents or siblings.

transitional object A symbolic attachment figure, such as a blanket or a stuffed animal, that a child may cling to when a parent is not available.

transitional housing Temporary housing such as a halfway house, short-stay residence or group home, or a room at a hotel designated for people who are homeless and looking for permanent housing.

transition times A term used to describe times of addition, subtraction, or change in status of family members.

traumatic bonding A strong emotional attachment between an abused person and his or her abuser, formed as a result of the cycle of violence.

traumatic grief A difficult and prolonged grief.

triad A group consisting of three people.

triangles A three-person system and the smallest stable unit in human relations.

trichotillomania Chronic, self-destructive hair pulling that results in noticeable hair loss, usually in the crown, occipital, or parietal areas, though sometimes of the eyebrows and eyelashes.

twelve-step programs Anonymous self-help groups such as Alcoholics Anonymous that use 12 steps to recovery as part of their program.

twenty-three–hour beds A specialized type of short-term treatment that is a relatively new trend for inpatient treatment (previously referred to as *observation units*); admits individuals to an inpatient setting, then discharges them before 24 hours.

Unfit to Stand Trial (UST) Persons who are determined to be mentally incompetent and are unable to understand the proceedings against them or assist in their own defense.

unipolar A term used to describe one abnormal mood state, usually depression.

untoward effects Unwanted side effects.

uptake receptors See carrier proteins.

use The drinking of alcohol or the swallowing, smoking, sniffing, or injecting of a mind-altering substance.

validation An interactive process that affirms the patient's beliefs, no matter how bizarre.

ventricles The four cavities of the brain.

veracity The duty to tell the truth.

verbal communication The use of the spoken word, including its underlying emotion, context, and connotation.

verbigeration Purposeless repetition of words or phrases.

violence (violent behavior) A physical act of force intended to cause harm to a person or an object and to convey the message that the perpetrator's, and not the victim's, point of view is correct.

voluntary admission (voluntary commitment) The legal status of a patient who has consented to being admitted to the hospital for treatment, during which time he or she maintains all civil rights and is free to leave at any time, even if it is against medical advice.

water intoxication A severe state of fluid overload; this disorder develops when large amounts of water are ingested and serum sodium levels rapidly fall to a level below 120 mEq/L. The specific etiology of this disorder is unknown.

waxy flexibility Posture held in an odd or unusual fixed position for extended periods of time.

Wernicke's area An area in the left superior temporal gyrus of the brain thought to be responsible for comprehension of speech.

Wernicke's syndrome An alcohol-induced amnestic disorder caused by a thiamine-deficient diet and characterized by diplopia, hyperactivity, and delirium.

withdrawal The adverse physical and psychological symptoms that occur when a person ceases to use a substance.

win-win A situation in which the parties involved are satisfied with the outcomes.

word salad A string of words that are not connected in any way.

working phase The second phase of the nurse–patient relationship, in which patients can examine specific problems and learn new ways of approaching them.

xerostomia Dry mouth.

young-old A term used to describe adults ages 65–74 years.

zeitgebers Specific events that function as time givers or synchronizers and that result in the setting of biologic rhythms.

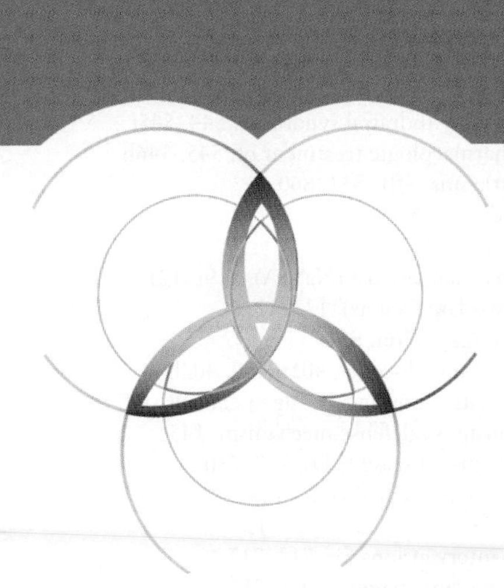

Index

Note: Page numbers followed by "b" indicate boxed materials; page numbers followed by "f" indicate figures; page numbers followed by "t" indicate tables.

A

B

C

D

G

H

N

O

Q

X

Y

Z

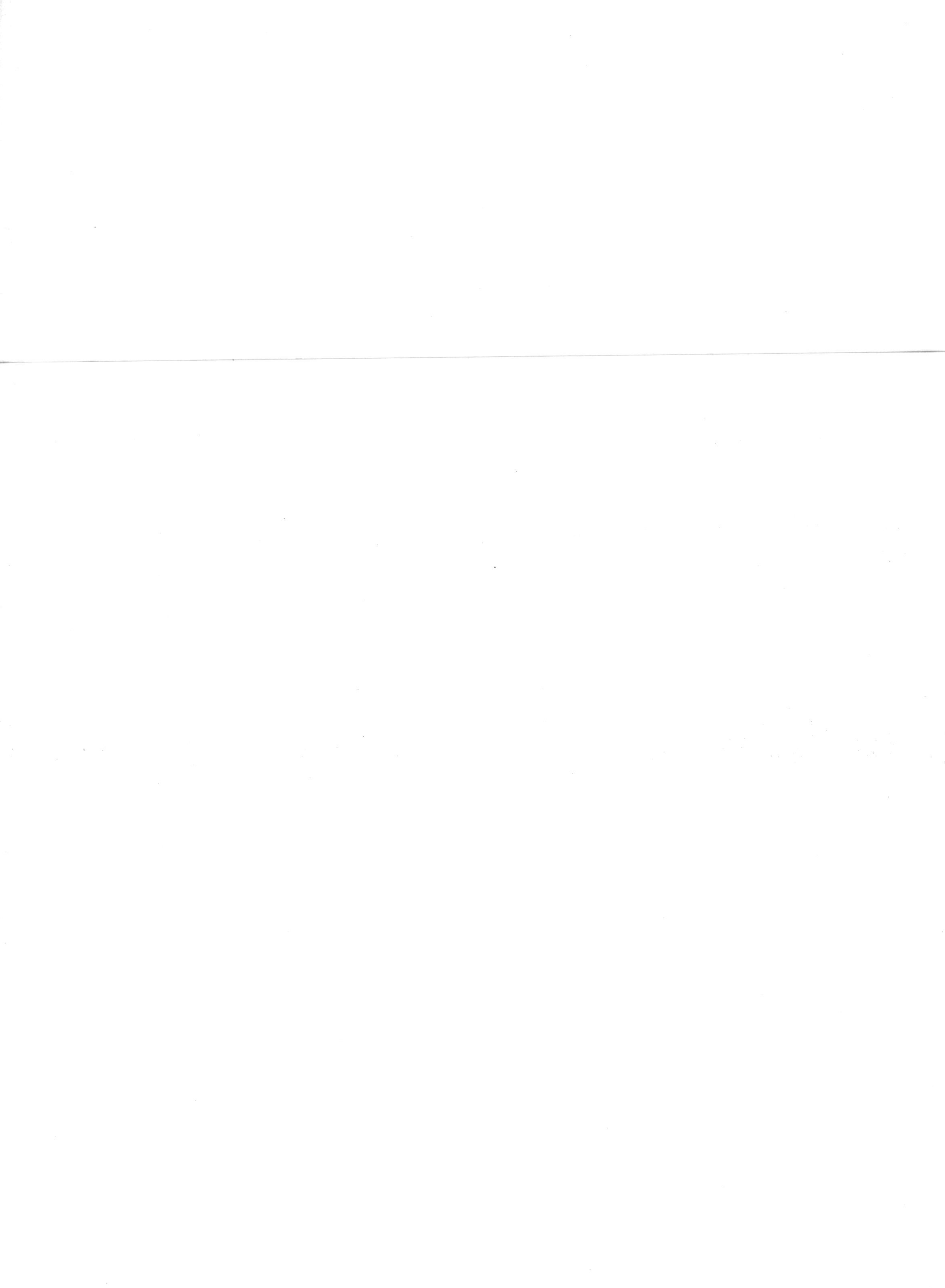